Lecture Notes in Medical Informatics 45

Editors:
O. Rienhoff, Marburg
D. A. B. Lindberg, Washington

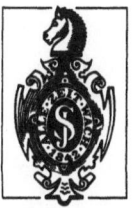

Lecture Notes in Medical Informatics

45

Edited by
D. A. B. Lindberg and
P. L. Reichertz

K.-P. Adlassnig   G. Grabner
S. Bengtsson R. Hansen (Eds.)

Medical Informatics Europe 1991

Proceedings, Vienna, Austria, August 19-22, 1991

Springer-Verlag

Berlin Heidelberg New York
London Paris Tokyo
Hong Kong Barcelona
Budapest

Editors

Klaus-Peter Adlassnig
Georg Grabner
Department of Medical Computer Sciences, University of Vienna
Währinger Gürtel 18-20, 1090 Wien, Austria

Stellan Bengtsson
Department of Clinical Microbiology, Akademiska Hospital
P. O. Box 552, 751 85 Uppsala, Sweden

Rolf Hansen
National Institute of Public Health
Geitmyrsveien 75, 0462 Oslo, Norway

Programme Committee

S. Bengtsson, Sweden (Chairman)	W. Dorda, Austria	R. O'Moore, Ireland
J. Bryant, United Kingdom	G. Gell, Austria	A. Reichert, Israel
R. Hansen, Norway (Vice-Chairman)	H. Grabner, Austria	O. Rienhoff, Germany
	P. Grösser, Austria	F. H. Roger, EFMI WG 1
K.-P. Adlassnig, Austria	B. Haidl, Austria	J. R. Scherrer, Switzerland
B. Barber, EFMI WG 2	J. Hofdijk, The Netherlands	E. Schuster, Austria
M. Barbosa, Portugal	E. Karjalainen, Finland	A. Serio, Italia
J. Bou, Spain	P. Le Beux, France	K. Staehr Johansen, WHO
C. Cobelli, IFAC	P. McNair, Denmark	M. Tallberg, EFMI WG 5
G. de Moor, Belgium	A. Naszlady, Hungary	L. Thayer, Council of Europe
G. Deželić, Yugoslavia	J. M. Noothoven van Goor, EC	

Executive Committee

S. Bengtsson, Sweden
J. Bryant, United Kingdom
R. Hansen, Norway
G. Grabner, Austria
K.-P. Adlassnig, Austria

Organizing Committee

G. Grabner (Chairman)
K.-P. Adlassnig (Secretary General)
W. Dorda
G. Gell
H. Grabner
P. Grösser
Ch. Hay
A. Marksteiner
E. Schuster

ISBN-13: 978-3-540-54392-3   e-ISBN-13: 978-3-642-93503-9
DOI: 10.1007/978-3-642-93503-9

© Springer-Verlag Berlin Heidelberg 1991

2127/3140-543210 - Printed on acid-free paper

INTRODUCTION

This volume contains the proceedings of the *Tenth International Congress on Medical Informatics*, MIE 91, that will be held in Vienna, Austria, August 19–22, 1991.

The MIE 91 Congress was organized by the *European Federation for Medical Informatics* (EFMI) in cooperation with the *Austrian Computer Society* (OCG) and the *Austrian Society for Biomedical Engineering* (OGBMT). It follows the previous congresses in Cambridge (1978), Berlin (1979), Toulouse (1981), Dublin (1982), Brussels (1984), Helsinki (1985), Rome (1987), Oslo (1988), and the Congress 1990 in Glasgow.

The proceedings contain 199 contributions to the MIE 91 Congress. They cover all presentations which are part of the scientific programme of MIE 91, among them 157 paper presentations with an average of five pages, 28 poster presentations again with an average of five pages, and 14 abstracts of demonstrations with an average of one page. The papers included were selected by an International Programme Committee out of over 300 submissions after careful review by at least two international reviewers (for whose estimable efforts we are especially thankful). The recommendations of the reviewers were incorporated in the final texts. Some papers were reworked by a professional translator to obtain a high quality of presentation. Several submissions could not be considered for presentation at MIE 91 because of shortage of congress time and limitations in the number of pages of the proceedings.

The scientific topics present in the proceedings volume at hand range from information and communication systems, knowledge-based systems, signal and image processing, health care, biometry and biomathematics, research and epidemiology, classification and coding, and nursing, up to computer-assisted education, medical curricula, and even robotics in medicine. They are interdisciplinary in nature and may therefore be of interest to a variety of professionals: medical informatics and health information scientists, medical computing specialists, public health and hospital administrators, physicians, nurses, other allied health personnel, and consultants in the various health fields.

There are several prominent themes that are the main topic of a paper, poster, or demonstration or occur again and again within various contexts:

First, a highly prevalent topic is medical information and communication systems: hospital, medical, clinical, ward, nursing, health, and executive information systems, hospital and data communication networks and PACS, drug information systems (database, interaction, monitoring), and related issues such as standardization of information exchange. The proceedings' Subject Index, for example, contains a total of 40 cross-references to the above-mentioned keywords. Although industry has already offered several types of information systems for hospitals, clinical wards, departments, laboratories, and physicians' offices, their application is at least partially not advanced enough and therefore not to the contentment of the medical user, so research seems still highly necessary.

Second, a "hot" topic is knowledge-based systems with 62 cross-references in the Subject Index. This topic is not only discussed in several Medical Expert Systems' sessions but is also part of sessions such as biosignal and image processing, computer-assisted instruction, and information systems and decision support. Some areas of knowledge-based systems are discussed in detail. This concerns, for example, knowledge representation, knowledge acquisition and learning, knowledge models, and evaluation issues. Several contributions report on clinical applications of knowledge-based systems and thus demonstrate their achieved practical usefulness.

Moreover, some recent topics of great research interest were part of the MIE 91 Congress and reports are included in the proceedings: fuzzy set theory, fractals, neural networks, parallel computation, and bioinformatics. These presentations provide an indication of some future developments and may act as a starting point for those becoming more interested.

The MIE 91 Congress gathered participants from all over the world, although mainly Europeans. This is reflected by the authors of the proceedings' contributions; altogether, over 550 researchers have reported their results in this volume. By considering only the first author of each paper, 27 different countries can be counted that contributed to this volume.

The great variety of scientific topics and countries that will be present should guarantee both an interesting international MIE 91 Congress in Vienna in August and a fruitful study of the proceedings by those interested in Medical Informatics.

K.-P. Adlassnig, G. Grabner, S. Bengtsson, and R. Hansen (Eds.)
June 1991

Contents

PAPER PRESENTATIONS

DEPARTMENTAL INFORMATION SYSTEMS

EXPERT SYSTEMS

EXPERT SYSTEMS—KNOWLEDGE REPRESENTATION

EXPERT SYSTEMS—KNOWLEDGE ACQUISITION AND LEARNING

EXPERT SYSTEMS—EVALUATION

CURRICULA AND COMPUTER-ASSISTED EDUCATION

RESEARCH AND EPIDEMIOLOGY

HEALTH CARE SYSTEMS AND SERVICES

CLASSIFICATION AND CODING

QUALITY ASSURANCE AND INFORMATION TECHNOLOGY

NURSING

HEALTH SERVICES ADMINISTRATION

STANDARDIZATION

POSTER PRESENTATIONS

INFORMATION SYSTEMS AND HEALTH CARE

DEMONSTRATIONS

PAPER PRESENTATIONS

PAPER PRESENTATIONS

KEYNOTE ADDRESSES

KNOWLEDGE-BASED SYSTEMS IN MEDICINE

Edward H. Shortliffe
Section on Medical Informatics, Stanford University
300 Pasteur Drive, Stanford, CA 94305-5479, USA

Introduction

In early 1990, Miller and Maserie described their belief that early approaches to computer-based decision support in medicine had been flawed in their adoption of the "Greek oracle" model of consultation [1]—computer programs to which a physician would turn for advice, answering patient-related questions but otherwise deferring to the dialog style and recommendations of the machine. The authors correctly observed that this model, adopted by many knowledge-based systems during the first decade of medical artificial-intelligence (AI) research [2], failed to capitalize on the special observational skills of physicians and failed to allow the user adequately to control the interaction, selecting the ways in which the program's knowledge could most effectively be brought to bear in the consideration of a particular case. Their redesign of Internist-1's interactive model in the development of the QMR system reflected their belief that the "Greek oracle" model should be laid to rest and replaced by a much more interactive and user-controlled approach to decision support.

I fully agree with Miller and Maserie's assessment of the early approaches to computer-based consultation, but I think that the reasons for the limited success and adoption of knowledge-based tools in medicine run much deeper than the issue of their interactive style and philosophy. In this paper I will briefly summarize some of my concerns and suggest solutions that may help define an agenda for efforts during the decade ahead.

The Evolution of Medical AI Research

The first decade of AI in Medicine (AIM) research was, appropriately, largely focused on basic-research issues in the development of knowledge-based decision-support systems. Although all the work in the field was motivated by pressing real-world problems drawn from biomedicine, the research issues were largely fundamental topics such as knowledge representation, knowledge acquisition, causal reasoning, problem-solving methods, temporal reasoning, and models for managing uncertainty. All these topics remain pressing concerns in AIM research, but great strides have been made in each of these areas since the early 1970s when the field began. Ironically, many of the lessons from medical AI research during that era have subsequently been adopted by the general computer-science community, have appeared in operational systems implemented in other segments of society, and have begun to show their commercial value and effectiveness [3]. The medical world is still struggling to deliver such tools, however, and it is not uncommon to hear disparaging remarks about the "failure of medical AI" and the undelivered promises that were early touted for the field.

There is little doubt that AI was oversold in the early 1980s, in large part by the media which, in their eagerness to predict the next great technological breakthroughs emerging from the computer field, failed to understand or to convey the inherent complexities in developing and delivering knowledge-based systems. As one who has worked in the field of medical AI since the early 1970s, I have done a great deal of soul-searching about why the field has encountered the difficulties that it has and why we still do not see a medical AI industry and routine use of decision support by clinicians and other health workers. Although I believe that challenging research issues certainly remain, and there continues to be great promise for a beneficial impact of AIM on health-care delivery and its cost-effectiveness, I have become convinced that the limited use of medical AI in health care today has little to do with the quality of the products themselves; resistance to system use has occurred despite the inherent merit of the methods that have been developed. As I will argue below, many of the problems are, instead, a reflection of the disarray of our health-care system and, more importantly, its failure to build the local, regional, national, and international infrastructure for biomedical computing and communications which will be required before computer-based decision support tools can become routine elements in the clinical setting.

AIM In Perspective

If the 1970s were the era of basic medical AI research, the 1980s were the period of adolescence during which the field learned that its promise and effectiveness are tightly linked to other developments in computing hardware and software. I believe that it is no longer wise to view AIM as a discipline separate from other areas of medical informatics; AIM is rather best viewed as a set of methods that must be merged with other key technologies in computer science when building systems and doing research in this field. If we are driven by pragmatic goals to benefit the health-care community, AI provides one set of techniques, but we must be selective in choosing them and must understand how they complement or compare with the other options that may exist. The interdisciplinary nature of medical informatics requires a willingness to be eclectic and to avoid "religious" dedication to any single technique or set of approaches. Our group at Stanford, for example, has in the last decade explicitly attempted to broaden its perspective and expertise beyond medical AI to embrace the wide range of pertinent topics in medical informatics that may be crucial to the effective delivery of decision-support tools: database methods, human-computer interaction, classical statistics, computer graphics, distributed systems, and information retrieval (to name just a few examples). As recent work at the intersection of (for example) AI and decision analysis, AI and Bayesian statistics, AI and databases, and AI and graphical interfaces have shown, it is in the synergies between AI methods and other techniques that the greatest hope for effective systems may lie.

We must resist the temptation to blame practitioners themselves for their failure to embrace the decision-support systems that we have offered to them. In the late 1970s, when I was attending my first scientific meeting in Japan, I was encouraged to hear of an advisory system there that was in routine use by all physicians in a prenatal-care obstetrical clinic in Tokyo. I thought I had finally discovered a system that had been successfully implemented and accepted for routine use and was eager to see it in action. Then I learned the secret of this particular system: it had been developed by the clinic chief and he required all physicians in the clinic to use it if they wanted to keep working for him. Many used it grudgingly, apparently, but they felt they had no choice.

I mention this anecdote for two reasons in addition to its entertainment value. First, it suggests a contrast between the medical world and those environments in which knowledge-based systems had their greatest success during the past decade: Fielded systems have tended to be introduced in settings where employees are told by supervisors that use of the system is part of their job. In most medical settings it has been difficult to produce systems that have sufficiently clear value, cost-effectiveness, and time-saving characteristics that practitioners themselves have been drawn to use the system on its merits alone. Furthermore, there are still limited numbers of settings in which physicians work in a managerial structure where someone else can force them to use a tool unless they want to do so. Most physicians would resist such pressure, and it is not clear that external requirements for system use would be wise unless the value of the system can be clearly documented—often a challenge for the system developers.

The second lesson of the Japanese anecdote, however, is the importance of high-level support for medical computing applications in clinical settings. I am not arguing for blind adherence to computational innovations, but I do believe that we must accept the impossibility of viewing the introduction of decision-support tools as a grass roots activity that emerges from the research lab, appears as an isolated entity in a clinic or on a hospital ward, and then grows by some kind of mass effect to encompass an entire medical community. It is naiveté about this point which has characterized our efforts to introduce computer-based decision-support systems in the past. Instead, the greatest hope for effective systems will be realized when the infrastructure for introducing computational tools in medicine has been put in place by visionary leaders who understand the importance of networking, integration, shared access to patient data bases, and the use of standards for data exchange, communications, and knowledge sharing.

The reason for emphasizing the need to facilitate integration of computational tools relates to a point that R. Greenes and I have made about physicians as "horizontal" rather than "vertical" users of information technology [4]. I believe that the greatest barrier to routine use of decision support by clinicians has been inertia; systems have been designed for single problems that arise infrequently and have generally not been integrated into the routine data-management environment of the user. Physicians will be attracted to computers when they are useful for essentially every patient that he or she sees and when the metaphor for system use is consistent across the varied applications that are offered (see, for example, the futuristic scenario that I presented in [5]). The recent emphasis on developing integrated workstations for physicians is clearly in response to this realization; many groups are seeking to develop single environments which offer, using consistent conventions for human-computer interaction, everything from medical-record review and order entry to bibliographic retrieval and use of expert systems. Our limited success with dissemination of knowledge-based systems in medicine is, in my opinion, due more to this failure of integration than it is to any other basic problem with the AI technologies that have been developed.

Moving To The Future

In the United States the need for integration of information technologies has received increasing recognition in recent years. It accounts, in large part, for the emergence of Integrated Academic Information Management Systems (IAIMS) as a concept for support by the National Library of Medicine [6]. IAIMS proponents have argued that individual academic medical centers must have a coordinated plan for networking and shared information access if patient-care, administrative, and information-retrieval innovations are to be integrated effectively in support of practitioners and their decision-making tasks.

Once the basic infrastructure is in place, it is much easier for individual systems to be added to the environment, drawing on patient databases as needed and adhering to interface standards that will allow the programs' seamless integration into the routine data-management activities of the institution's workers. Viewed in this context, for example, QMR should not only cast off the "Greek oracle" model of consultation but should also exist as one element in an integrated environment from which it can gather pertinent patient information and be instantaneously available to the physician when he or she is reviewing a patient's record and realizes that diagnostic support would be useful. If standards for such integration do not exist, however, QMR will continue to exist as a stand-alone resource that requires special effort and redundant entry of patient-specific data.

If individual institutions need to have visionary leaders who define an information-management environment for their health workers, the same can be said of regional and national health planning activities. In the United States there has been no single organization with the responsibility, or the credibility, to take on the task of defining connectivity standards, data exchange standards, and the similar requirements for integration that will be necessary before individual institutions can link to one another, share patient data appropriately, pool data for research purposes, and provide direct feedback in the form of guidelines for care or other decision-support functions. In the past two years a committee of the Institute of Medicine of the National Academy of Sciences has been considering the future of the computer-based patient record and has recently released its recommendations on the subject [7]. Among its suggestions is a call for a Computer-Based Patient Record Institute (CPRI) that would serve as the national center for coordinating and planning the infrastructure necessary for developing integrated patient records. The report of the committee is scheduled for publication in August 1991 and it will provide in some detail the rationale for a CPRI and its functions.

Conclusions

In summary, twenty years of research on knowledge-based systems in medicine, plus a failure to introduce such tools widely in medicine despite the significant progress in developing the underlying methodologies, has taught us that AIM is not a field that can be set off to the side, separate from the rest of medical informatics or the world of health planning and policy making. Effective decision-support systems will be dependent upon the development of integrated environments for communication and computing that allow integration of knowledge-based tools with other patient data-management and information-retrieval applications. This kind of infrastructure will be created only by visionary leaders who realize that the practice of medicine is inherently an information-management task and that biomedicine must make the same kind of coordinated commitment to information technologies as have other segments of our society in which the importance of information management is well understood. We can draw from these observations a set of items that sit squarely on the agenda for the medical informatics community in the decade ahead:

- The enhancement of training opportunities so that a large cadre of professionals who are broadly educated regarding the interdisciplinary nature of medical informatics is available to assume leadership roles in both research and in information technology management.

- The need to develop national and international biomedical networking infrastructures that use existing and future technologies for communication, data exchange, and information retrieval.

- The need for credible international standards for communications, data, and knowledge exchange that will allow both commercial and academic developers of medical information systems to know what to do in order to assure the integration of their products with other developing systems.

- The creation of leadership organizations, closely tied to the medical informatics community but with a broad mandate, from both the public and private sectors, for representing biomedicine's interests in negotiations regarding networking and other standards development for the information technologies.

References

[1] Miller, R.A. and Maserie, F.E. "The Demise of the 'Greek Oracle' Model for Medical Diagnostic Systems." Meth. Info. Med. (1990) 29:1-2.

[2] Clancey, W.J. and Shortliffe, E.H. (eds). Readings in Medical Artificial Intelligence: The First Decade. Reading, MA: Addison-Wesley, 1984.

[3] Feigenbaum, E.A., McCorduck, P., and Nii, H.P. The Rise of the Expert Company: How Visionary Companies are Using Artificial Intelligence to Achieve Higher Productivity and Products. New York: Times Books, 1988.

[4] Greenes, R.A. and Shortliffe, E.H. "Medical Informatics: An Emerging Academic Discipline and Institutional Priority." JAMA (1990) 263:1114-1120.

[5] Shortliffe, E.H., Perreault, L.E., Wiederhold, G., and Fagan, L.M. (eds). Chapter 1 in Medical Informatics: Computer Applications in Health Care. Reading, MA: Addison-Wesley, 1990.

[6] Matheson, N.W. and Cooper, J.A.D. "Academic Information in the Academic Health Sciences Center: Roles for the Library in Information Management." J. Med. Educ. (1982) 57:1-93.

[7] Institute of Medicine. Report of the Committee to Improve the Patient Record. Washington, D.C.: National Academy Press, 1991.

PERSPECTIVES OF COMPUTER ASSISTED MEDICAL IMAGING

Karl-Heinz Höhne
Institute of Mathematics and Computer Science in Medicine
University of Hamburg, Martinistraße 52, D-2000 Hamburg 20

1. Introduction

Over decades after the discovery of the X-rays by Wilhelm Konrad Röntgen medical imaging techniques did not change: X-rays were cast through the patient and the shadows caused by the anatomical structures were recorded on photographic film. Beside the fact that the shadows of different objects are overlaid, the low contrast for soft tissue requires highly trained and experienced radiologists to read those images. With the advent of modern computers, imaging techniques could be developed, that deliver cross-sectional images, such as Computer Tomography (CT) and Magnetic Resonance Imaging (MRI) as shown in fig. 1. They do not have the problem of overlays, but they still show only a limited two-dimensional aspect of the anatomy, which is three-dimensional in nature.

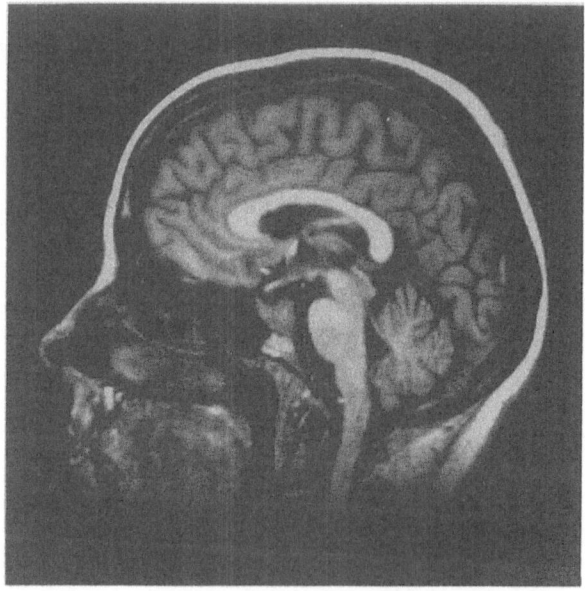

Fig. 1   Magnetic resonance image of a brain.

In principle there is no reason to image the human body just this way, it is more or less a consequence of the technical development. If we were asked nowadays to design an imaging system without the knowledge about X-ray projection and cross-sectional techniques, we would certainly aim at a technique that shows the human body as we know it from our experience or the anatomy textbook. Here we find perspective views as they were already drawn by Leonardo da Vinci 400 years ago (fig. 2).

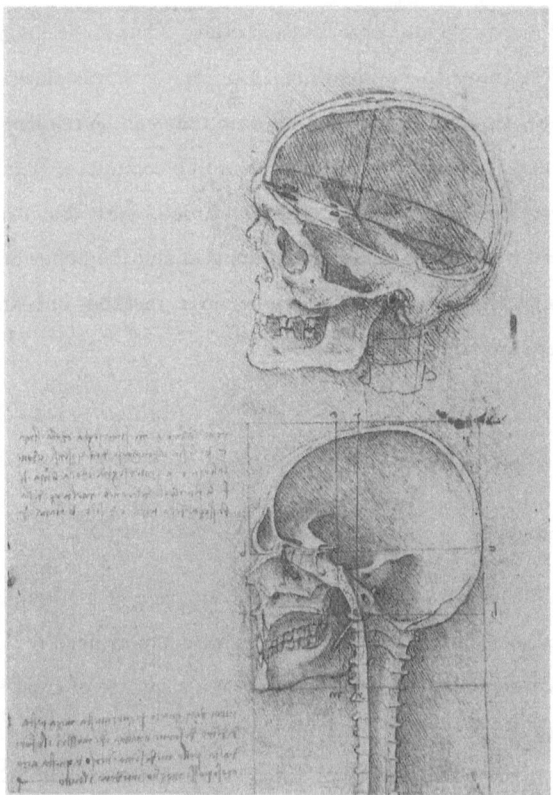

Fig. 2 Leonardos famous anatomical drawings of a skull.

It turns out that using methods of image processing and computer graphics we are on the way to make clinical imaging as realistic as in anatomy textbooks. Actually we also see many new applications which we could not think of before. This article reviews applications presently under investigation and their perspectives for the future.

2. Method

A variety of methods have been described by several authors [1-10]. We describe here just their general principle, while details can be found in the respective literature. Basically all methods start with a spatial sequence of tomograms (represented as image matrices of up to 512x512 picture elements), which include the organ to be imaged. This sequence of images can be considered as an image volume. One of the main problems of 3D visualization comes from the fact that unlike in 2D imaging objects in the volume may obscure each other. Thus for the display of real anatomy the outlines of the objects have to be identified in order to be visualized or removed [10-14]. Once we know the outlines through a segmentation step they can be rendered by simulating light reflection. For this purpose the surface inclination has to be computed, which is again not trivial for tomographic imagery. Fig. 3 shows as an example those objects that can easily be identified in a 3D volume recorded by computer tomography, the skin and the bone surface. Methods of 3D display have advanced such that in a variety of applications, methods of realistic 3D imaging can be applied usefully. These are now shortly reviewed.

3. Fields of Application

3.1 Diagnostic Radiology

At first glance one would expect radiology to be the main field of 3D imaging. This has turned out not to be the case because of two reasons. On one hand experienced radiologists are very well capable of a "mental reconstruction" of a 3D scene from a sequence of cross-sectional images. On the other hand due to segmentation problems not all desired objects can be displayed in 3D. Thus diagnostic radiology does not profit too much today. In some cases the 3D image may help in finding an optimum orientation of the cross-sectional images as shown in fig. 4 where different cuts are shown in the context of the body and the liver.

3.2 Surgical Planning

The situation is different in all fields where therapeutical decisions have to be made by non-radiologists on the basis of images . Here the realistic presentation of the operation site prior to surgery can be of decisive importance [15-17]. This surgery planning becomes more and more standard in craniofacial surgery, e. g. of congenital malformations. The problem of pre- and postoperative 3D visualization of bony anatomy can be considered to be solved. However, it would help the surgeons even more if they could rehearse their operation prior to the real surgery. Although this is by far more difficult to accomplish such applications are under development.

While planning time may be long for congenital malformations, in traumatology no long delays are affordable. Nonetheless, with the increasing speed of modern computers also here these techniques are being introduced. Especially in pelvic surgery, where the morphology is difficult to assess, 3D imaging is considered as a great help as shown in fig. 5. The fractures can even be visualized from views that are not possible even under surgery.

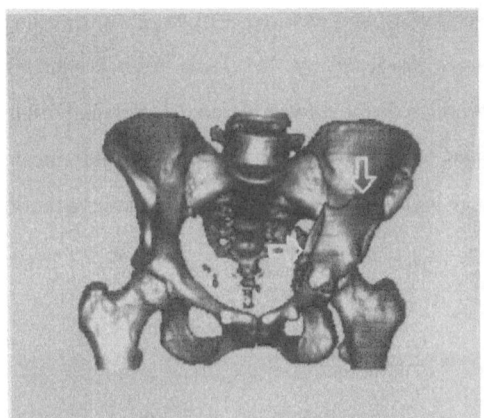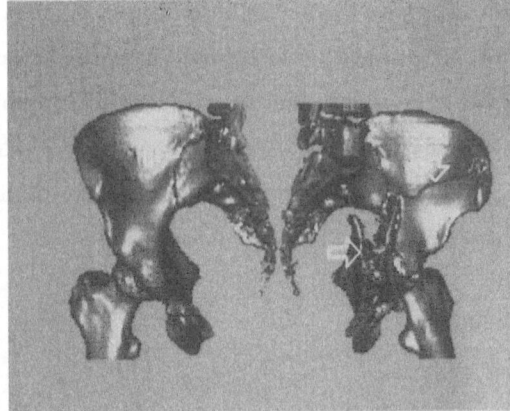

Fig. 5   Pelvis (from CT) with a severe fracture; a) frontal view, b): frontal view, cut at the central sagittal plane.

An application that becomes more and more attractive with the increasing resolution and specifity of MRI is neurosurgery planning. Here the proper choice of the access path to a lesion is of extreme importance. 3D visualization of brain tissue and blood vessels before a surgical intervention allows to know the access path with minimal risk in advance. Fig. 6 shows the kind of image that can be used for this purpose.

3.3 Radiotherapy Planning

One other potential application that is reducing the risk of a therapeutical intervention, is radiotherapy planning. Here the objective is to focus the radiation to the target volume while avoiding radiation for healthy organs. In present practice this is done in a rather crude fashion only of 2D cross-sections. The 3D visualization of target volume, organs at risk and the simulated radiation dose will allow the rehearsal of the treatment procedure without risk for the patient (fig. 7). Preliminary results show promising results.

3.4 Medical Education

An application that was not thought of in the beginning, but will be standard in the near future is education especially in anatomy. Once an image volume of the human body is labelled, e. g. with anatomical and functional descriptions, programs can be written that allow preparation and surgical training at the computer screen. We have developed the first version of a true 3D brain atlas, that allows the exploration of the human brain by sectioning and cutting. Unlike in multimedia atlasses where stored images are called, the images are produced by the viewer from a volume model. Thus e. g.the function and anatomical membership of any volume element can be inquired by the student (fig. 8). The other way round the student can browse through the list of anatomical constituents and can get them labelled on the 3D image he has chosen. Various teaching programs can be built upon this basic data structure.

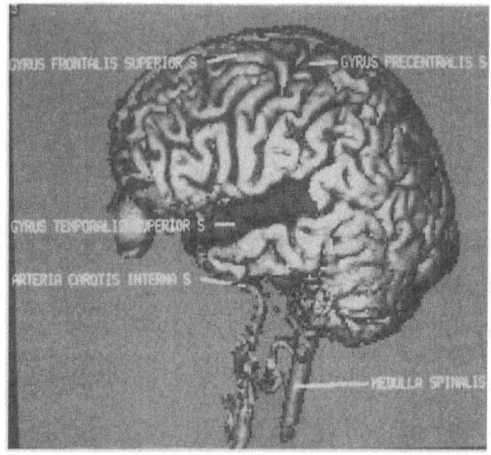

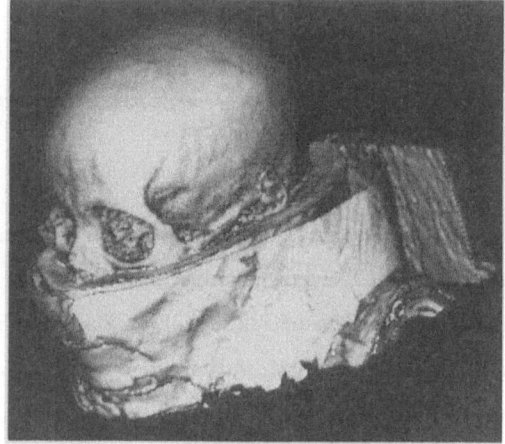

Fig. 8   Learning anatomy using a brain
volume model (from MR).

Fig. 9   Skull of a 2600 year old mummy
(from CT).

3.5 Physical Anthropology

Although the described techniques of 3D visualization have been developed for clinical medicine it has turned out that they can be applied to other non-medical problems such as material testing or physical anthropology. Physical anthropologists are e. g. interested in the non-destructive examination of old egyptian mummies. Using computer tomography the bony structures can be reconstructed and measured with high accuracy (fig.9).

4. Current Problems

Despite the beauty of the shown images there are still a lot of problems to be solved. One could expect that computer capacity is one of the problems. In fact, it is at present, but it will certainly disappear when the cost-performance ratio develops as fast as in the past. The main problem to be solved is still that of segmentating the image volume into 3D regions, that represent the objects such as the different tissue types, bone, lesions. This process that is rather easy for a human viewer has turned out extremely difficult to formalize e. g. in a knowledge based system. An alternative that makes use of the viewers knowledge is interactive segmentation. Here the viewer controls segmentation parameters such as intensity threshold and assesses the result by visual inspection. This is similar to the enhancement of objects in a 2D image by using the brightness and contrast control. Still a general solution of the segmentation problem is not visible.

The second major problem is that of the man-machine interface. The number of ways a 3D object can be visualized is virtually infinite. A user-interface that allows this spectrum of possibilities cannot be simple. Thus nowadays the production of the images even in routine applications is in the hands of specialists. A break-through will certainly be achieved when we have computer power such, that the visualization system can react instantaneously to our requests thus giving the impression of manipulating the object itself.

5. The Future

Although the vast majority of radiological examinations is at present still based on the classical X-ray techniques, many research projects aiming at the realistic visualization of the human body are going on. In applications dealing with patient treatment such as surgery planning they have already become operational in clinical practice, at least for complicated cases. Here the usefulness of previewing and even rehearsing surgery is obvious. While at present practical applications suffer from long computing times (up to some minutes/picture) the next generations of computers will probably solve this problem automatically. For many applications the main bottleneck is the user interface. There is no doubt that the described techniques will have a decisive impact on medical education especially in anatomy and surgery very soon. In general it can be expected for the future that the information content of medical images will no longer be extracted by reading static images. Instead we will explore anatomy and function at the computer screen like an anatomist or a surgeon who in addition has "radiological" eyes.

Acknowledgement

The example images of this paper have been produced using methods developed at our institute. My special thanks go to M. Bomans, B. Pflesser, A. Pommert, M. Riemer, T. Schiemann, and U. Tiede. The anatomical atlas is a result of the excellent cooperation with Prof. Dr. W. Lierse (Dept. of Neuroanatomy). I am grateful to Dr. Schmidt (Dept. of Radiotherapy), and Dr. Wening (Dept. of Traumatology) for their cooperation. The MRI data sets from which the 3D reconstructions have been made were kindly provided by Siemens, Erlangen. We also thank the Werner-Otto-Stiftung, Hamburg, which has supported this work in part.

References

[1] Herman GT, Liu HK. Three-dimensional Display of Human Organs from Computed Tomograms. Comput. Graph. Image Process. 1979; 9,1

[2] Vannier MW, Marsh JC, Warren JD. Three-Dimensional Computer Graphics for Craniofacial Surgical Planning and Evaluation. Comput. Graph. 1983; 17,263

[3] Höhne KH, Riemer M, Tiede U. Viewing Operations for 3D-Tomographic Gray Level Data, In: Lemke HU et al. (eds), Computer Assisted Radiology (Proc. CAR '87), Springer, Berlin 1987; 599-609

[4] Höhne KH, DeLaPaz RL, Bernstein R, Taylor RC. Combined Surface Display and Reformatting for the 3D-Analysis of Tomographic Data. Investigative Radiology 1987; 22: 658-664

[5] Höhne KH. 3D-Bildverarbeitung und Computer-Graphik in der Medizin. Informatik-Spektrum 1987; 10: 192-204

[6] Levoy M. Display of surface from volume data. IEEE Computer Graphics and Applications 1988; 8: 29-37

[7] Drebin RA, Carpenter L, Hanrahan P. Volume Rendering. Computer Graphics Proc. SIGGRAPH 1988; 22,3: 65-74

[8] Tiede U, Hoehne KH, Bomans M, Pommert A, Riemer M, Wiebecke G. Surface Rendering, Investigation of Medical 3D-Rendering Algorithms. Computer Graphics and Applications 1990; 10,2: 41-53

[9] Hoehne KH, Bomans M, Pommert A, Riemer M, Schiers C, Tiede U, Wiebecke G. 3D-Visualization of Tomographic Volume Data Using the Generalized Voxel Model. The Visual Computer 1990; 6,1: 28-36

[10] Höhne KH, Fuchs H, Pizer SM (eds). 3D Imaging in Medicine, NATO ASI Series, F 60, Springer Berlin 1990

[11] Bomans M, Höhne KH, Tiede U, Riemer M. 3-D Segmentation of MR Images of the Head for 3-D Display. IEEE Transactions on Medical Imaging 1990; 9,2:177-183

[12] Cline HE, Lorensen WE, Kikinis R, Jolesz F. Threedimensional Segmentation of MR Images of the Head Using Probability and Connectivity. J Comput Assist Tomogr 1990; 14: 1038-1045

[13] Pizer SM, Gauch JM, Cullip TJ, Fredericksen RE. Toward Interactive Object Definition in 3D Scalar Images. In: Höhne KH, Fuchs H, Pizer SM (eds). 3D Imaging in Medicine, NATO ASI Series, F 60, Springer Berlin 1990; 45-62

[14] Höhne KH, Hanson WA. Interactive 3D-Segmentation of MRI and CT Volumes Using Morphological Filters, to be published.

[15] Witte G, Höltje W-H, Tiede U, Riemer M. Die dreidimensionale Darstellung Computertomographischer Untersuchungen Craniofacialer Mißbildungen. Forschr. Röntgenstr. 1986; 144,4: 400-405

[16] Zonneveld FW, Lobregt S, van der Meulen JCH, Vaandrager JM. Three-Dimensional Imaging in Craniofacial Surgery. World Journal of Surgery 1989; 13: 328-342

[17] Fishman EK, Ney DR, Magid D. Three-Dimensional Imaging: Clinical Applications in Orthopedics. In: Höhne KH, Fuchs H, Pizer SM (eds). 3D Imaging in Medicine, NATO ASI Series, F 60, Springer Berlin 1990; 425-440

[18] Schlegel W. Computer Assisted Radiation Therapy Planning. In: Höhne KH, Fuchs H, Pizer SM (eds). 3D Imaging in Medicine, NATO ASI Series, F 60, Springer Berlin 1990; 399-410

[19] Schmidt R, Schiemann T, Höhne KH, Hübener KH. 3-D Treatment Planning for Fast Neutrons. In: Proc. *Advanced Radiation Therapy (ART) 91*, Munich 1991, in press

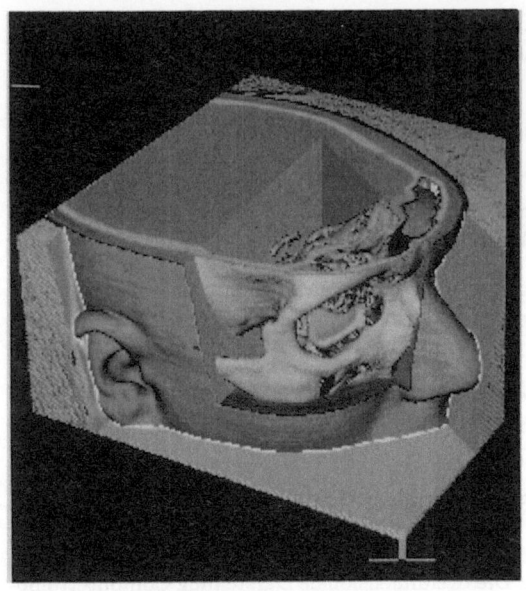

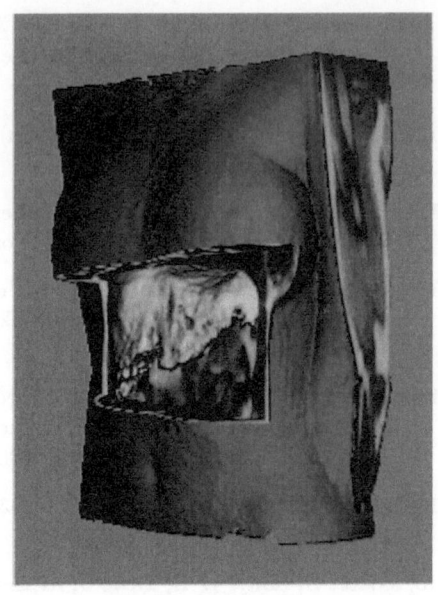

Fig. 3 Objects that can easily be identified from a CT volume: skin and bone surface.

Fig. 4 3D image of the liver within its anatomical surroundings (from MRI).

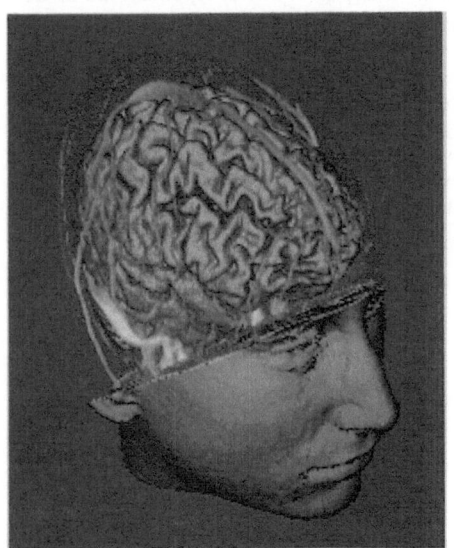

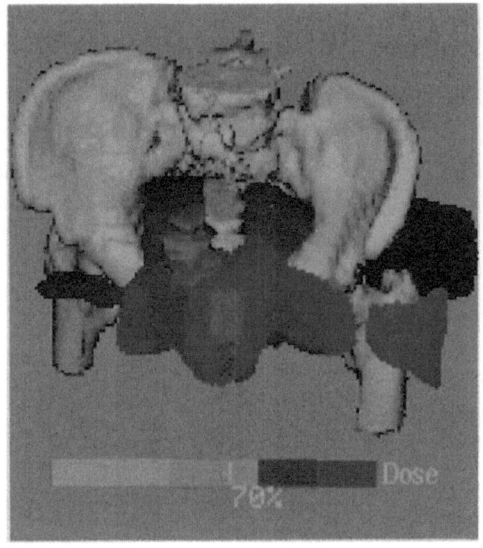

Fig. 6 3D image of the brain and the extra-cerebral blood vessels (from MRI).

Fig. 7 Planning the radiation treatment of a prostate. Organs at risk: rectum (orange) and bladder (green). The blue object is the 70% dose volume (from CT).

MEDICAL LANGUAGES: USE, DEFINITION AND PROCESSING IN WARD INFORMATION SYSTEMS (WIS)

J.-R. SCHERRER
Hospital Information Center
Cantonal University Hospital of Geneva
CH-1211 Geneva 4

It is quite commonplace to observe nowadays how medical records are reduced to a huge mass of poorly structured information, that is to say a mixture of texts, images and numbers. Within medical institutions, particularly hospitals, the situation becomes worse when there is the least attempt to retrieve specific, relevant information, let us say, first patient-to-patient and then by medical entities or on an institutional statistical basis. It is not always a surprise why the bibliographical research is so paramount, since it is generally accepted that the easiest accessible relevant information is from medical literature thanks to powerful tools like MEDLINE, Excerpta Medica or Pergamon. Regarding MEDLINE, the facility in terms of user-friendliness, is going to be enforced by the availability of the new UMLS developments [1]. Before entering into more detail the medical reference model of behaviour should be highlighted here [Fig. 1] in the following way: The daily medical decision-making is relying upon updated "standards of medical behaviour" at a time when it is uniformly shared within the medical practicing community. Quite a few of these standards are collected physician-to-physician in a personal "cook-book". However, to be and to remain pertinent such "cook-book" information has to fit the present stage of how to apply knowledge, in the form of literature, to a given problem. The "cook-book" has a necessary extension, that is the local expertise in the same field based upon the support of local statistics related to similar patients [2]. C. Safran et al. [3] have given emphasis to the fact that clinical and administrative data are routinely stored on all patients as a regular part of the hospital information system (HIS) process. Booleian seaching expressions can easily be built taking into account features of the following kind: Age (i.e. the user specifies a value "larger, lower or equal to" or "being between" such and such value) the more-or-less detailed diagnostic medical expressions, selected laboratory tests issued by different laboratories, x-ray findings, etc. The system is properly called "ClinQuery" and is well suited for selecting patients according to a profile of patients set by the user himself, in order to compare his/her patients both with those similar to the literature and with those similar to his/her own institution, getting a critical insight into clinical investigation patterns, effectiveness and appropriateness of treatment than of prognosis based upon follow-up assessments.

Now, back to Figure 1, we really deal with the two pillars of bibliographical research and of "ClinQuery" or equivalents supporting the bridge of standards of medical behaviour this is in order to allow the vehicle of "decision making" to cross the gap of uncertainly as safely as possible. Regarding the once attractive perspective of automated medical diagnosis, it would be tempting to consider Mazone's claims here in order to accurately prepare human diagnosticians since, according to political clamour, human physician diagnosis is fraught with error [4]! Going along with R.A. Miller's thoughts about the medical diagnostic process we discard first the Mazone's approach [4], that is defined as "a mapping from patient data (normal and abnormal history, physical examination, and laboratory data) to a nosology of disease states", in order to feel more comfortable with the Random House Collegiate Dictionary [5] as R.A. Miller said that defines diagnosis as "the process of determining by examination the nature and circumstances of a diseased condition", it elicits a portion of the patient's life story, it is not merely another case of some disease [6]. It becomes a text. It is also meaningful in this respect to quote R.A. Miller again about "The demise of the Greek Oracle Model for medical diagnostic systems" and to acknowledge that the authors of the former INTERNIST - I, who have called QMR (Quick Medical Reference) the successor to INTERNIST - 1, left aside the Greek Oracle metaphor for diagnostic reasoning [7]. Now since QMR offers easy to use tools for building up patient profiles in terms of positive, as well as negative, findings to be abstracted from the patient history, physical examination and laboratory studies, it would be i.e. more attractive again to start from the free medical text of the reports rather than from a kind of an awkward menu selection. [8]. Besides, it is worth stressing here that the Figure 1 could even better be illustrated by the creation of a link from QMR to the NLM's "Grateful Med" bibiographical retrieval program back to 1988 already [9] to trigger the appropriate medical references to seek and to retrieve abstracts or even full papers downloaded and printed locally.

Besides this, patient histories and charts are supposed to be available from the ClinQuery or equivalent tools that should belong to any HIS by design already. However, most of the time only a combination of medical diagnosis, Rx-diagnosis, laboratory tests etc. associated with demographic and financial patient information, are accessible. It is not too common that the access mode is interactive with a user-friendly interface! Furthermore, it appears that the detailed clinical information is either missing or embedded within the discharge summaries, letters to the practitioners, radiology or consultant reports. A.H. Pratt already in 1973 [10] expressed his view regarding the importance of natural language processing for a more extensive use of medical information:
"It is emphasized that the data that the medical profession reduces or aggregates by logical inference and deduction to provide for the care of a patient or to communicate a medical concept to a student or colleague or to describe a research opportunity are in the large majority nonnumeric in form and are formulated almost exclusively within the constructs of natural language [...]. The data are language data [...]. The larger goal in information retrieval must be the recognition and evaluation of the input language data by some measure of information - information that can be used in turn

to form higher levels of information and information patterns essential to man's capability of analysis and decision-making. It is difficult to see how this larger goal can be achieved without extensive linguistic augmentation of the computing design and execution of such information retrieval projects".

It used to be said that whilst humans work better with "natural languages", computers are more efficient with coded data. Amongst the objectives of the joint conference IMIA-WHO, in Geneva in 1988, about the use of computerised natural medical language processing [11] it was stressed that health professionals and medical institutions could benefit most from the availability and use of natural language encoding tools. However, it was requested as being the major concern of the conference to make an assessment of the role, the state-of-the-art and the future trends of natural language processing feasibility and use in medicine at acceptable costs.

OVERVIEW OF THE NATURAL MEDICAL LANGUAGE PROCESSING (NMLP) STATE-OF-THE-ART

Let us look first to a short history of NMLP that is reaching as far back as the history of machine translation as given by M. King [11]: It begins in 1949 when "Warren Weaver, then Director of the Natural Science Division of the Rockefeller Foundation, circulated a memorandum called "Translation" to some 200 influential people in the USA." Very rapidly a substantial funding for research in this new area was constituted. Back in those years we have to remember that both computer science and computational linguistics were in their infancy. The quality of the translations produced was not too good and a US National Committee in a 1966 report of conclusions (ALPAC) emphasised that the efforts should be devoted to fundamental research within the same field.

After this first lesson, the research on natural-language processing (NLP) has been motivated mostly by its potential use for communicating with software systems as it has been pointed out by C.R. Perrault and B.J. Grosz in an exhaustive review of about 113 references related to natural language interfaces (NLI) issued in 1986 [12]. It is seen that NLI have been developed to extract information from database management systems to control or simulate robots, to interact with graphic systems, to specify simulation problems or to communicate with systems embodying expertise like, for instance, in our field the UMLS project [1]. This quoted review paper is even declaratively focussing onto the use of NLI to DBMS, that is to say on interpreting queries, although some other efforts have been invested on the use of natural language (NL) to update DBMS like Davidson, Kaplen 1983 [13] or, moreover, to feed a relational DBMS, N. Sager [14, 15]. However, despite the apparent opposition between the two approaches: NLI uses for query languages (QL) and NLI uses for feeding and updating a DBMS, from the mere standpoint of NMLS and having clearly Figure 1 in front of us, we have to agree that we are interested by both approaches. Nevertheless, if more emphasis is given here to the process of feeding in and of updating a DBMS it is because the last SCAMC 1990 was partly dedicated to that side of QL (with ULMS, Alert Systems), and that there is already an increasing broad literature about these subjects [16]. However, it is worthwhile briefly to highlight the reasons for NLI attractiveness from the side of QL. Indeed, in this respect there is quite a symmetry between the two approaches (feeding in and updating of DBMS on one side and queries to the DBMS on the other). In both approaches:

. There is a given immediate controlled medical vocabulary for
   describing the contents of the DBMS.
. The access means to information are independent of DBMS
   structure and encoding modes.
. It is easy to use by every medical professional without
   special training or without need to enter into the esoteric
   folk-lore of too many different systems.

Now, to see where we stand and where we go, let us resume the overview of the NLP history. From 1960 to 1970, two main approaches were explored that did not seek meaning as a goal. One of them was dealing with the transformational grammars, the other one was using keywords or also "patterns", in order to extract directly one part of the information from a sentence. The latter approach has been famously illustrated by J. Weizenbaum with ELIZA in 1966 [17].

However, recovering after the shock of the ALPAC report the researchers restarted in a new era with T. Winograd setting a new cornerstone that is the SHRDLU programme [18], allowing a robot to "understand" complex orders in rudimentary English. From this research onwards new ways have been opened-up: representation of the meaning of the text being kept independent of the superficial structure of the language. The process is characterised by the set up of a necessary intermediate stage or "intermediate representation language" (IRL). Here only two programmes are necessary along with the translation process: A parser that is going from the NL text of one language to IRL and then a generator that is going from IRL to the other language, Warren [19].

The system architecture in NLI [12] reflect choices of what information is to be applied and, therefore, what interpretation problems to attempt. Every system has at least to build one internal representation of a query expressed in QL:

. One approach is based on the addition of a purely syntactic
   representation following i.e. a three stage process: a parser,
   a semantic interpretation, a query interpreter.
. Semantic grammar systems also produce a single intermediate
   representation.
. Systems that produce a separate representation of the meaning
   of the query in terms of the concepts of the domain of the DB.

"Intermediate-representation language" (IRL) refer to the
languages in which these representations are expressed (they
also may be called "logical forms" or "meaning representation
language".

It is worthwhile to highlight then that phrase-structure grammars have provided the
basis for the syntactic components of NLI. Most of these grammars are context-
free(CF)! However, the major arguments, supporting the concept that NL's are not
context-free in a weak way, are recent like in Shieber (1985) [20] for the Swiss-German
language. Those approaches involve constructions not treated by grammars in existing
NLI's. "Definite clause grammars" as elaborated by Pereira and Warren [19] try to
simplify the syntactic analysers that hence become quite close to the "Augmented
Transition Networks" (ATN) parsers. This is the first major extension of CF grammars
based upon a two-step generalisation of the "Finite-State Automaton" of Hopcroft and
Ullman in 1979 (FSA). The language that may be recognised by FSAs are "Type 3
Languages". The "recursive transition networks" (RTN) generalise FSA's. These RTN's
recognise precisely the class of CF languages. In the early top-down ATN parsers, the
grammar and the lexicon were encoded as LISP structures and then interpreted by the
parser. However, these top-down parsers suffered from quite a few problems namely
the backtracking problem that I will not develop here.

If we turn now to semantic interpretation, we have to deal with the process of
translating syntactic analyse into IRL like Schank and others have done [20], that is to
say an attempt towards semantic parsing without the support of a fully syntactic
component. The semantic representation of the text in a rigourous formal model
becomes necessary. The use of well-defined graph operation in natural language
processing has become prominent particularly when J.F. Sowa [21] introduced his so-
called "Conceptual Graph Model" as a promising unifying model.

Sowa developed the formalism of conceptual schemes based on the "First Order Logic"
(FOL) that is to say on sound theoretical grounds. The well defined representation of
concepts and relations makes easy the incremental growth of the conceptual graphs
without being worried too much about the complexity of knowledge. Our Geneva Group
[22] has stressed that knowledge-base queries are easily formulated using FOL and a
knowledge-matching algorithm can be designed with the help of a pure, formal basis.
According to Rassinoux et al. [23] the overall process of knowledge representation
acquired from discharge summaries may be divided into two major phases: (1) proximity
processing of sentences, (2) assembling components according to knowledge frames,
transforming them automatically into conceptual schemes. Then two other phases should
take place: database representations of conceptual schemes and the matching of queries
with the graphs. The proximity processing has been detailed in [23]. A detailed
example from digestive surgery is given in [22]. In all sentences the system is

discovering concepts and relations itself. The type of the sentence is determined by the presence of a dominent concept, the so-called "vehicle concept" that has its knowledge frame. As it will be seen from the detailed example of [22] the whole approach is now feasible. However, considerable work is still necessary to complete the knowledge frames, the lexicon and the refinement of the sentence processing.

Now it is time to pay attention to the results obtained from the fifteen year Linguistic String Project (LSP) from Naomi Sager [14] that is soundly based upon the design and use of a chained English grammar that was easy to adapt to French. Besides this, it should be remembered here that the LSP has one of the most extensive, fully written grammars today as needed by most of the NLP's anyway and has been applied to medical texts since its early years. Very briefly, the structure is the following:

. One parser able to handle one Backus-Nauer Form (BNF)
    grammar with backtracking, dealing when necessary with several
    interpretations related to ambiguous sentences.
. Several grammars written in BNF, handling the same sentence one
    after the other with its semantic content.

It follows that after multiple transformations the syntactic tree of the sentence becomes standardised on a unified basis that is to say: Verb + subject + object. This standardised structure is then the target of formatting operations to such an extent that all the information belonging to the tree may be mapped in a predefined general table. The type-formats are progressively established on a kind of apprenticeship basis of several texts dealing with the same subjects. The trouble is, however, that the formatting has to be predefined in terms of semantic categories before any registration of new elements. Nevertheless, such an approach has revealed not only its usefulness but its demonstrative richness when being used with digestive surgery discharge letters. Examples will be shown regarding associations of symptoms and signs, reasoning, clinical investigation with lab tests and images and finally with one major diagnostic more or less combined with associated diagnostics. In the present state-of-the-art, the system is usable and is able to feed on SQL DB automatically (INGRES in our case).

CONCLUSIONS

The richness of patient to patient collected information on a text basis, if dealing with discharge letters and consultant reports, is unquestionably far richer than any other encoding methodology. For meeting the stage of quasi scientific critique, without being concerned with the detailed data, there is nothing really relevant that can be done. The condition to enter into the detailed data gathering implies representing the contents of discharge letters as a final critical appraisal of what the patient has been about.
At the end of the present paper, it is possible to obtain evidence that the approach is not only feasible but obviously fruitful and not as costly as we at first thought. It should in future, therefore, be enforced.

As an extension of the medical office automation effort, that is to say, all discharge
letters or consultant reports are written on micro-computers and might be collected
within some archiving device, it would be frustrating not to be able to extract
automatically from this material all detailed, relevant information and to have it stored
in a SQL DB to which you may address your queries in a way that is close to the
UMLS or NLI facilities.

REFERENCES

[1]   D.A.B. Lindberg, B.L. Humphreys: "The UMLS Knowledge Sources :
       Tools for Building Better User Interfaces" In: Proceedings of
       the 14th Annual Symposium in Medical Care, R.A. Miller (Ed.),
       New York : IEEE Comp. Soc. Press 1990 : 121-125.

[2]   F.R. Borst, J.-C. Chevrolet, P.-F. Unger, J.-R. Scherrer: "How
       to Promote High Level Medical Standards of Care in a Teaching
       Hospital"; In: Medical Informatics Europe '88, R. Hansen, B.G.
       Solheim, R.R. O'Moore, F.H. Roger (Eds.) : Springer-Verlag,
       Berlin 1988 : pp.133-136.

[3]   C. Safran, D. Porter, J. Lightfoot, C.D. Rury, L.H. Underhill,
       H.L. Bleich, W.V. Slack: "ClinQuery: A System for Online
       Searching of Data in a Teaching Hospital" : Ann. Int. Med.
       1989 : 113 (9): 751-756.

[4]   J.G. Mazone: "Diagnosis without Doctors" : Journal of Medicine
       and Philosophy : 1990.

[5]   S.B. Flexma, J.Stein, (Editors): 1988 "The Random House College
       Dictionary" : Revised Edition, Random House, Inc. New York :
       pp.366.

[6]   R.A. Miller: "Why The Standard View is Standard : People, Not
       Machines, Understand Patients' Problems" : 1991 (to be
       published).

[7]   R.A. Miller and F.E. Masarie Jr.: "The Demise of the Greek
       Oracle Model for Medical Diagnostic Systems" : Meth.
       Inform. Med. 29 (1990) : 1-2.

[8]   "QMR User Manual-Version 1.0 for the DOS Operating System" :
       University of Pittsburgh, Camdat Corp. 1990 : pp.161-171.

[9]   R.A. Miller, F.E. Masarie,Jr.: "Quick Medical Reference (QMR)-
       An Evolving, Microcomputer-based Diagnostic Decision-Support
       Program For General Internal Medicine" In: Proceedings of the
       13th Annual Symposium in Medical Care. New York: IEEE Comp.
       Soc. Press 1989: 947-8.

[10]   A.W. Pratt: "Medicine, Computers and Linguistics", Adv. Biomed.
       Eng. Academic Press, New York, 1973 : 3-97-140.

[11]   M. King: "Are There Any Lessons to be Learned from Machine

Translation?" In: Computerised Natural Medical Language Processing for Knowledge Representations: J.-R. Scherrer, R.A. Côté, S.H. Mandil (Eds.): Elsevier Science Publishers, B.V. (North-Holland): IMIA (1989) : pp.73-82.

[12] C.R. Perrault, B.J. Grosz: "Natural-Language Interfaces" : Ann. Rev. Comp. Sc., 1986, 1:47-82.

[13] J. Davidson, S.J. Kaplen: "Natural Language Access to Databases Interpreting update requests" : Am. J. Comp. Linguist. 9(2):57-68.

[14] N. Sager, C. Friedman, M.S. Lyman: "Medical Language Processing: Computer Management of Narrative Data" : Addison-Wesley, Reading 1987.

[15] N. Sager, M. Lyman, L.J. Tick, F. Borst, Ngo Thanh Nhan, C. Revillard, Yu Su, J.-R. Scherrer: "Adapting & Medical Language Processor From English to French" In: MEDINFO 89 Proceedings, B. Barber, D. Cao, D. Qin, G. Wagner (Eds.), North-Holland, Amsterdam 1989: pp. 795-799.

[16] Fourteenth Annual Symposium on Computer Applications In Medical Care, American Medical Informatics Association, IEEE Comp. Sor Press, Washington 1990: R.A. Miller (Ed.); Sections 4A-4B; pp. 121-179.

[17] J. Weizenbaum: "ELIZA", Communication of the ACM, (1966) 9:36.

[18] T. Winograd: "Understanding Natural Languages", New York Academic Press (1972).

[19] D.H.D. Warren, F.C.N. Pereira: "An Efficient Easily Adaptable System for Interpreting Natural Language Queries" Am. J. Comput. Linguist. 8(3-4):110-22.

[20] S.M. Shieber: "Evidence Against the Context-Freeness of Natural Language" Linguist. Philos. 8:333-43.

[21] J.F. Sowa: "Conceptual Structures : Information Processing in Mind and Machine" : Addison-Wesley Pub. Co., New York 1984.

[22] A.M. Morel, R.H. Baud, J.-R. Scherrer: "Proximity Processing of Medical Text" In: Medical Informatics Europe 90, R.O'Moore, S. Bengtsson, J.R. Bryant, J.S. Bryden (Eds.), Springer-Verlag Heidelberg 1990 pp.625 - 620.

[23] R.H. Baud, A.-M. Rassinoux, J.-R. Scherrer: "Knowledge Representation of Discharge Summaries" : AIME (Artificial Intelligence in Medicine, Europe - accepted for presentation) 1991.

The Clinical Methodology

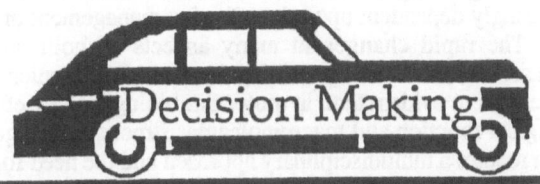

Decision Making

Standards of Medical Behaviour

Biblio-
graphic
search

MEDLINE

Similar
cases

CLIN-
QUERY

FIGURE   1

Informatics in Molecular Biology

Howard Bilofsky

European Molecular Biology Laboratory
Meyerhofstrasse 1, D-6900 Heidelberg, Germany

Abstract. There is growing recognition that advances in basic biological research and biotechnology are increasingly dependent upon the effective management of information using computer technology. The rapid changes in many aspects of both the science and the technology have led to a serious problem of providing for the bioinformatics needs of European scientists. This is nowhere more evident than in molecular biology where efforts to understand the relationship of biological function and macromolecular structure have generated relatively large databases and often require a multidisciplinary approach and the need for information from new and diverse sources. Recent initiatives to map and sequence a number of genomes will lead to considerable new biological understanding, but will only exacerbate these problems.

Meeting this challenge will require new approaches to organising and funding bioinformatics resources in Europe. Long-term infrastructural support is required to ensure that stable multidisciplinary expertise is focused on bioinformatics and is widely available. The European Molecular Biology Laboratory (EMBL) is home to the EMBL Data Library, a key component of the international sequence database community, which is on the front-line facing these challenges. A European Bioinformatics Institute (EBI) is planned which will address the expected growth in our own database management and distribution activities, provide consulting and training, encourage the development of new designs, tools and interfaces for relevant databases and computational resources, enhance the professional and cooperative nature of the bioinformatics community and represent European interests as a leader in the international arena.

Keywords: molecular biology, bioinformatics, European infrastructure.

Progress in basic and applied biological research is increasingly dependent on bibliographic and factual databases and on computing tools for organising, analysing and modelling data. More and more bioscientists find themselves in front of keyboards and computer screens, capturing data, doing statistics, graphing and examining results, searching out information, communicating with colleagues, writing grants and papers, and managing their projects. Yet the traditional view of computer related activities being the domain of the programmer, the theoretician or the instrumentation engineer but not the laboratory scientist is changing only slowly in biology and seldom is this viewed as a fundamental dependence [1]. The richness of biological knowledge is at the heart of this dependence. Bioinformatics becomes a critical policy issue in the context of rapid change and growth in the information and broad industrial importance of biotechnology [2].

Molecular biology is a relatively new and interdisciplinary science which uses and contributes to knowledge in a wide range of other sciences beyond biology. These include the clinical, chemical, physical and mathematical. Of course, in each of these other fields there are to various degrees already well-established informatics activities which can be important to a molecular biologist and makes it difficult to narrow the scope of our interest. So, for example, data acquisition and image analysis may be an essential computational need for one scientist and computer simulations for structure prediction may be for another. The term bioinformatics is often used to encompass all applications of computer and information technologies to the management and understanding of biological and biotechnology information [3,4,5].

One view of the rich biological information spectrum and the relationship between various types of information is provided by Figure 1 which is based on a simple natural hierarchy of cells, genes and proteins. There are databases and associated software tools available to European biologists from a variety of European and US sources in all these areas, though there is great variety in the quantity of information and how well organised the maintenance and distribution is for each [6]. Biological sequences and associated information are just part of the spectrum of information required by molecular biologists and biotechnologists, but represent perhaps the most rapidly changing area of bioinformatics and provide a useful perspective from which to examine informatics needs.

The EMBL Data Library [7,8] has been providing molecular biology information services internationally since being established in 1980. The two major databases at the Data Library are the Nucleotide Sequence Database with over 50 million bases and the Swiss-Prot protein sequence with over 6 million amino acids. Both are the result of extensive international collaborations; the former with GenBank in the US and DDBJ in Japan and the latter with the University of Geneva. Figure 2 shows that they are doubling almost every two years. The well-engineered application of advanced hardware and software technology has long been needed to keep pace with this growth [9]. The increasing diversity of data and the widening scope of users' needs present a newer challenge. This can be seen in Figure 3, where we have shown just those databases available in EMBL. The arrows indicate existing cross-links which allow experienced scientists to combine information from each database. However, for many scientists only the most facile user interface will do; one which is transparent to these

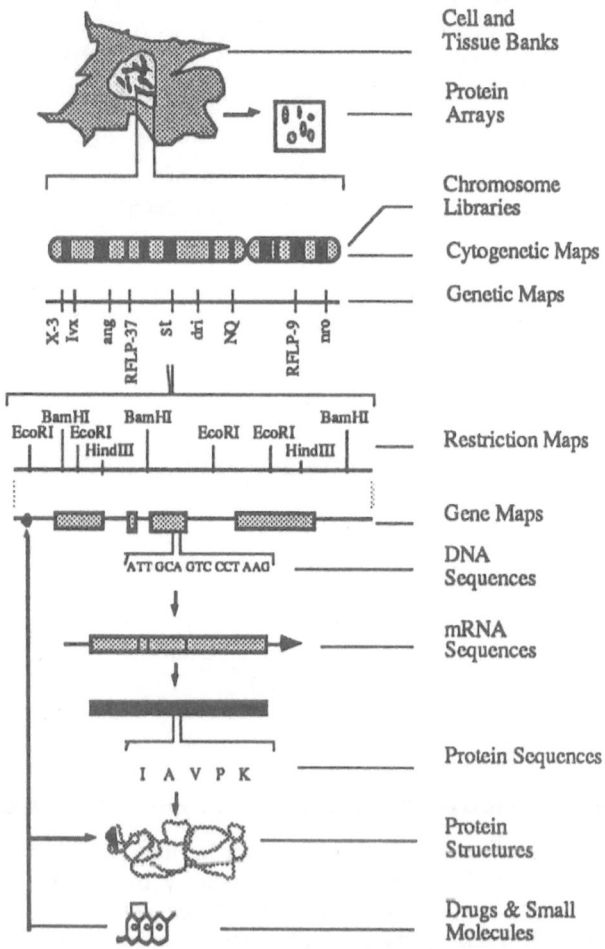

Figure 1. The spectrum of biological knowledge (with permission.)

links and permits easy access to all relevant databases and provides extensive knowledge of the underlying science and technology. This is a key problem for bioinformatics. There is no one right solution to this problem; progress requires diverse experiments which result from collaborations between scientists (both data generators and users) and technologists.

Encouraging these collaboration, and providing access to the fundamental data, the necessary tools and underlying technology is a critical mission. One not easily accomplished within the framework of existing organisational options. There are a number of problems with the infrastructure of biologically-oriented computer and information resources in Europe. Present activities are generally funded by short term grants and contracts from competitive research budgets. There is too little coordination and cooperation on broad European initiatives aimed at encouraging the use of new bioinformatics technologies. Thus the resources presently available tend to be underfunded and narrowly focussed, resulting in short-lived, incomplete and relatively costly projects. A third problem is the difficulty in establishing new facilities. Finally, Europe needs resources comparable in scope to those in the US and Japan in order to participate as equals in international bioinformatics initiatives. If left unsolved, these problems will rapidly become a significant hindrance to European science and technology. A solution is therefore urgently needed.

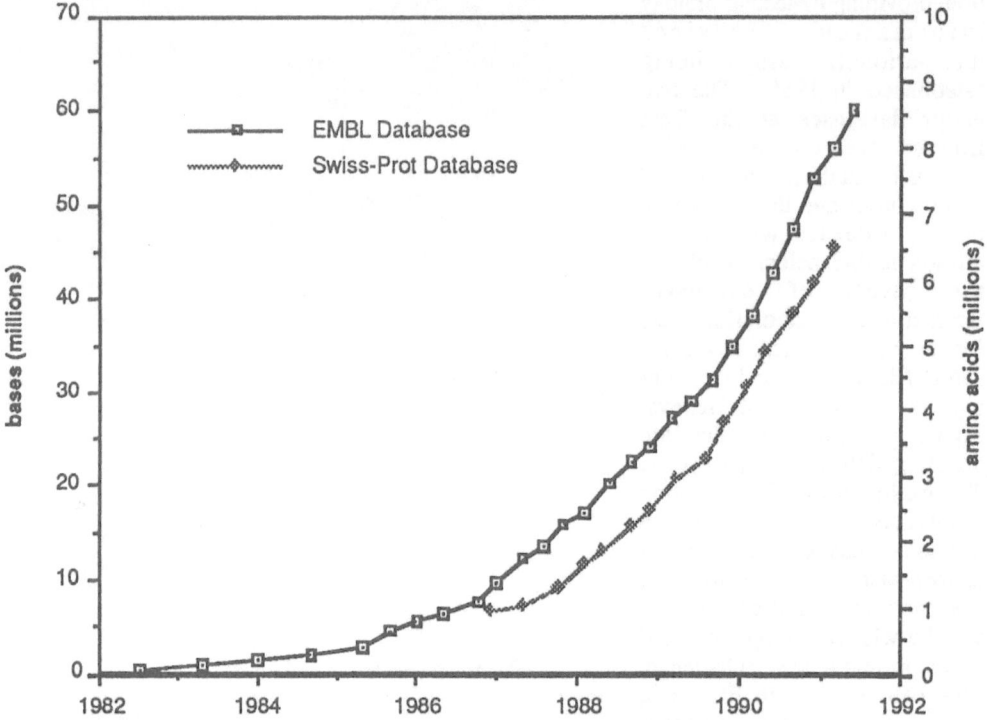

Figure 2. EMBL nucleotide sequence and Swiss-Prot protein database growth.

The non-profit European Bioinformatics Institute (EBI) is designed to serve the entire European bioscience and biotechnology community by encouraging the development and wide availability of comprehensive computer and information resources (products, services and expertise). These resources will be aimed at a user community with varying levels of computer expertise. It will particularly focus on the unmet needs of those who are trying to create value-added database-related products and provide end-user services. It will support a program of research and development and that will help it and its user community to understand and quickly apply new technologies to essential scientific problems. The EBI will continue the present EMBL Data Library activities of collecting, organising and making available the nucleotide sequence database and related information and services. Coping with the anticipated increases in the volume, demand and complexity of the data, particularly in view of the many large-scale genome sequencing projects [10,11,12] now being initiated, will require exploration of new data structures and distributed database designs and interfaces that will benefit from collaborations with independent database, knowledge engineering and network experts.

Fostering an environment which encourages diverse cooperative new initiatives and integrates them into a new pan-European bioinformatics infrastructure will ensure that European bioscientists have unhindered access to the tools and opportunities they need to continue to make outstanding contributions to science, health and the economy.

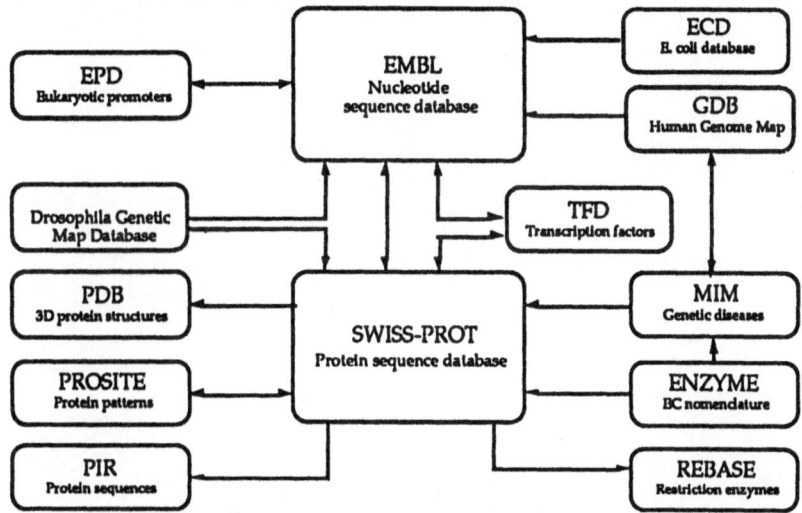

Figure 3. Databases and cross-links.

Acknowledgements. I would like to thank my colleagues at the EMBL who have been essential in the formulation and articulation of these ideas and in the effort to create the EBI, in particular Graham Cameron, Patricia Kahn and Lennart Philipson. I would also like to thank Dan Masys of the U.S. NLM for permission to base Figure 1 on one of his figures.

References.
[1] Gilbert, W., Towards a paradigm shift in biology. *Nature,* 349: 99; 1991.
[2] Bioinformatics in Europe 2. Strategy for a European biotechnology information infrastructure. *European Chemical Industry Federation*; 1990.
[3] FAST - Research Activities, *CEC*, EUR-7102; 1980.
[4] Cantley, M.F., Bio-informatics in Europe, Foundations and Visions. *Swiss Biotech*, 4: 7-14; 1984.
[5] Berendsen, H.J.C., A Bio-Informatics Workstation, Report for the *European Economic Community* under the "IT for BT" Initiative; June, 1986.
[6] Doolittle, R.F., ed., "Molecular Evolution: Computer Analysis of Protein and Nucleic Acid Sequences" *Methods Enzymol.*, **183**; 1990.
[7] Kahn, P. and Cameron, G., EMBL Data Library, *Methods Enzymol.*, **183**: 23-31; 1990.
[8] Stoehr, P.J., and Cameron, G., The EMBL Data Library, *Nucl. Acids Res.* (in press); 1991.
[9] Bilofsky, H., Advanced technology for sequence data banks. "Biotechnology Information '86", R. Wakeford ed., IRL Press, 31-34; 1987.
[10] Report on Genome Research 1991. *The European Science Foundation*; 1991.
[11] Research on the Human Genome in Europe and its Relationship to Activities Elsewhere in the World. *Academia Europaea*; 1991.
[12] Pearson, M.L., and Söll, D., The Human Genome Project: a paradigm for information management in the life sciences, *FASEB J.*, 5: 35-39; 1991.

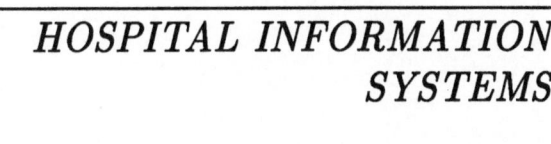

*HOSPITAL INFORMATION
SYSTEMS*

WAMIS—HEURISTIC APPROACHES
TO A MEDICAL INFORMATION NETWORK

Alois Marksteiner

Department of Medical Computer Sciences
(Director: Univ.Prof. Dr. G. Grabner)
University of Vienna, Garnisongasse 13, A - 1090 Vienna, Austria

Abstract

WAMIS is a Medical Information System that has been applied successfully at the Vienna General Hospital (University of Vienna Medical School) for many years. The centralized architecture of WAMIS used in former years was more and more developed to a solution that integrates independent systems into the central computer system. The argument is that this approach will probably be a successful solution of software and hardware architectures used in hospitals in the near future.

1. Introduction

For more than two decades, computers have been used to assist people working in the field of medical health care. And the amount of tasks than can be assisted by computers is increasing continuously. In Vienna, a general-purpose computer was purchased for the university hospital in 1966, and a small team of young scientists was hired to operate it. The members of this team were looking forward to solving a lot of problems by "computerizing" all the patient's data contained in the patient's medical records. Very soon, however, they got acquainted with one of the most important problems in hospital: acquisition and storage of these data. For only if the data are stored in the computer in a suitable manner, they can be retrieved by programs to gain information for scientific as well as for managerial purposes. Therefore in the course of some 15 years, a Hospital Information System—the "Wiener Allgemeines Medizinisches Informations-System" or WAMIS—was developed [1].

2. Hospital information system

2.1. Goals

Health care is done by a network of fairly independent units. A hospital consists of a huge number of such units: inpatient and outpatient wards, laboratories, X-ray department, kitchen, pharmacy, laundry, etc. Each of these units performs its duties fairly independently from all the others, although it accepts orders from, and exchanges information with, other units. When analyzing the different worksteps within these units, high redundancies are to be found. Each unit registers incoming orders and outgoing results. Since in a hospital all activities are connected with patients, the patient data such as name, age, sex, etc. are transcribed from one form to another and from one index book to another several times. It is really amazing what a complex organization has to be run through just in order to obtain the results of one simple blood or urine test.

All this work of registering and indexing the patient's personal and medical data is mainly done to be able to retrieve it in case of readmission. Another reason is the wish to prove the efficiency of a department as well as the necessity of planning and ordering new supplies.

To reduce the amount of work that goes into patient registration and data acquisition is one of the most important goals of computer assistance in health care. In general there are different ways towards a satisfactory solution:

- centralized systems;
- a network of independent systems;
- the integration of independent computer systems into a centralized EDP (electronic data processing) system.

However, each of these solutions has its advantages and disadvantages.

2.2. Centralized solution

Its main advantage is that there is only one type of hardware and software. The staff operating the system can become highly familiar with it because they only have to deal with one type.

The disadvantages of a centralized system, however, are just as evident. It is much more difficult and time-consuming to change programs and applications which are used by many users. New applications must be tested thoroughly in order to prevent them from destroying or interfering with existing ones. If the workload increases, the response time of the system goes down significantly and is often insufficient for a lot of urgent tasks. Upgrading of the system ("increasing the core memory as a solution to nearly every performance problem") can be expensive and is even impossible in some cases if the limits of the system are reached.

2.3. Network solution

The idea behind this is to use very specialized hardware and software for each different task. This solution seems to offer nothing but advantages, as long as the different systems are successfully linked together. A lot of hardware and software manufacturers offer special packages for different types of health care units. There are packages for patient administration, various types of laboratory tasks, for the X-ray department, the pharmacy, for diet planning, etc. These systems are sold under the motto of "turn on key system", i.e. with the manufacturers' implicit promise that upon the turn of a key the system will work and perform every task that the customer wants and needs. The problems in interconnecting these systems to a Medical Information Network are often ignored. Actually, however, it proves quite difficult to interconnect different systems, a task which can often only be solved by an EDP crew that is familiar with both the different software packages and the hospital problems. If this experience is lacking, people will often copy data from one computer system to another via keyboard, instead of a network of computer systems exchanging information among each other themselves. In this case, the cheap registration forms and index books are merely replaced by expensive computer equipment—data exchange is done via alphanumeric keyboards instead of paper and pencil. In other words, paper is replaced by electronics, but the workload remains nearly the same.

2.4. Integration of independent systems into a central computer system

This path was taken in Vienna. (It would be incorrect to say "this solution was chosen in Vienna" since it was an evolutionary development.)

A large variety of different computers and software products, either bought from EDP suppliers or developed by our staff, are now in operation in the Vienna University Hospital. What all these systems have in common is that they generate medical data which pertain to individual patients but are of general interest. Data exchange between the different systems is only achieved via the central database stored in the mainframe.

Compared with the modern slogan of "data exchange between everybody and every system in the network" this seems a serious restriction.

Figure 1 explains the benefits of this restriction, however. If there are n different systems that want to communicate with each other, a general communication routine has to handle z different conditions, where $z >> n$ for $n > 3$ and $z = \sum_{i=1}^{n-1} n_i$.

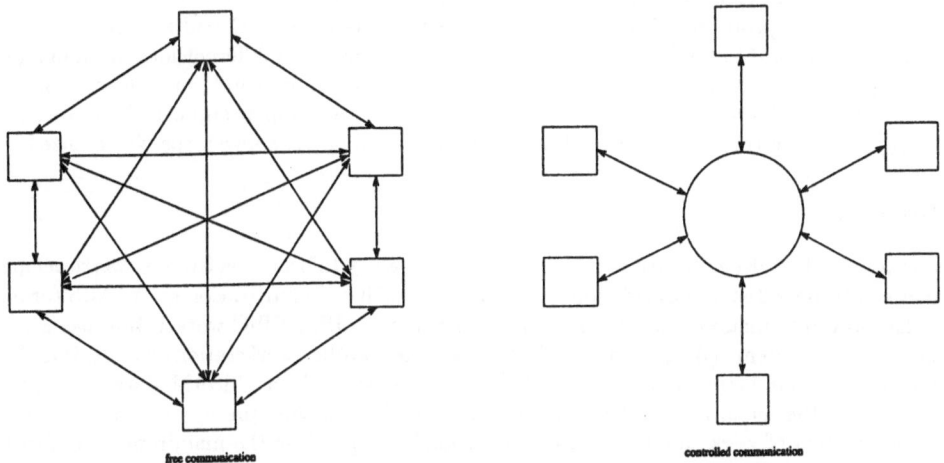

free communication   controlled communication

Figure 1: Pathes of communication between 6 different partners (local systems).

If data exchange is done via mainframe, only n different conditions have to be taken into account, where the conditions are:

- different computer systems;
- different network technologies.

Protocols allowing the interconnection of different computer worlds are already available, but to solve all problems of direct data exchange between different types of computers run with different software and having their data stored in different types of files or databases is still far beyond the capabilities of commercially available software. Great efforts are made by the various manufacturers in this fields but to establish a real "program to program" communication between applications which are run on different systems still requires the skills of experienced EDP personnel and is very time-consuming and costly. The sensitivity of the stored data imply even more particular problems of privacy and integrity.

The linking of external systems to WAMIS must be achieved by IBM methods because the mainframe is an IBM. IBM's philosophy of communication between different computer systems and devices is SNA (System Network Architecture). Therefore all external systems and devices have to emulate SNA, which can be done either by software or by the hardware. Serial devices are linked up by means of the IBM software NTO (Network Terminal Options) run on a controller unit or by data converters (e.g., IBM 3708) which convert the ASCII data stream from the serial device according to IBM specifications.

Access to the IBM mainframe from external computer systems is handled by the IBM program APPC (Advanced Program to Program Communication). External computer systems can access the mainframe if they have either installed a communication program according to the rules of APPC or a "gateway" handling communication with the IBM mainframe. APPC communication software is not commercially available for every type of local computer system. In a lot of cases, individual communication between the local systems and the mainframe was therefore established by simple teletype protocols. The local systems are connected via NTO and behave like ASCII terminals with regard to the host. The ASCII data string from each different local system starts a special program in the mainframe which processes the incoming data and sends the appropriate response. The requirements for these different programs are very similar and can therefore easily be changed. During the course of evolution of WAMIS, each of the above steps was realized.

3. Examples

Based upon the knowledge gained over the years, a Laboratory Information System was developed [2] that can be operated as a stand-alone workstation as well as in integration to WAMIS (or any other Hospital Information System). The system runs on an IBM RISC workstation using AIX as its operating system. (AIX is an IBM UNIX; porting to other workstations should therefore be possible without larger modification.) All data are stored in a C-ISAM database. Data exchange with the mainframe is done by APPC. Even if the mainframe is not available, there is no interruption of work as all data that are normally supplied by the mainframe can also be presented by the CRT displays.

During evaluation and release of the results, however, a connection with the mainframe is desirable. WAMIS contains a lot of information (drugs administered, diagnosis) which is of importance to the lab physician who is responsible for the quality of the tests. Results outside the normal range become often plausible when seen in the light of a patient's diagnosis or of his or her medication.

There are also other laboratory systems that are connected to WAMIS, either by means of individual communication routines or by means of APPC. As an example, a small system in a research laboratory shall be mentioned here. This hepatitis research laboratory performs a lot of immunoassays. The laboratory organization is assisted by a small computer system (WILAS) to which the analyzer and the WAMIS system are connected. During registration of the requested tests and during release of the results, the system is connected with the mainframe. The local computer system behaves like an ASCII terminal to the mainframe. The results are sent from the WILAS system to the WAMIS database, where the data are stored for use by entitled WAMIS participants.

The expert system HEPAXPERT-II [3] was developed at our Institute. This system can be run either on the mainframe or on a PC. It uses the results of the immunoassays from the hepatitis research lab as an input, producing an interpretation of the tests in the form of neat printouts and graphic presentation.

Since WILAS is run on an S-9000 IBM lab computer that has been withdrawn from sale for several years, the programming of a direct communication routine between the S-9000 and the PC system would not only be difficult but of no general use. Therefore the PC system uses the APPC communication routine to access the data in the mainframe. This example illustrates in an excellent manner the power of the "centralized" network.

4. Conclusions

Medical Information Networks will be developed to a high degree of complexity in the near future. To wait for a commercially available network software that allows every participant of the network to communicate with all the others, even though they might use different hardware or software looks like a hopeless prospect. The pragmatic way of a mixture between centralization and networking is one of the possible solutions. The Medical Information System WAMIS has direct access to medical data of more than 1.15 million patients. Every entitled participant of WAMIS can use these data for inquiries according to the security and privacy rules established in WAMIS for different types of data. The response time is amazingly short. It would have been absolutely impossible to manually key in this large amount of data. Only by using the different local computer systems as input sources for WAMIS, this big medical database could be built up. Figure 2 shows parts of the WAMIS structure. This large medical network was not planned in advance but developed in an evolutionary manner according to the hardware and software possibilities that could be afforded by the various departments and according to the manpower of the small EDP group of the Institute of Medical Computer Sciences.

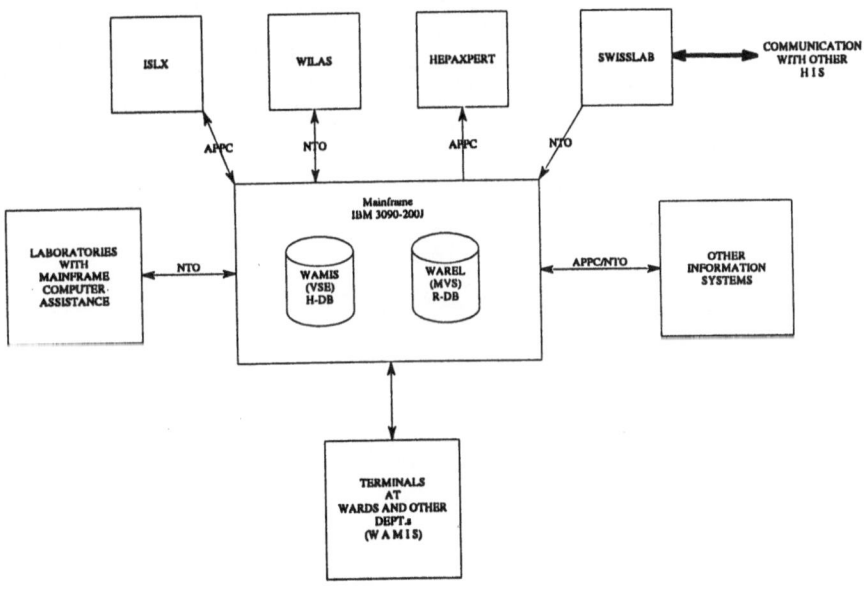

Figure 2: Part of the WAMIS Information Network.

References

[1] G. Grabner (Ed.). (1985) WAMIS: Wiener Allgemeines Medizinisches Informations-System. Springer-Verlag, Berlin/Heidelberg/New York/Tokyo.

[2] G. Hoffmann, A. Marksteiner. (1991) ISLX, a UNIX-Based Laboratory Information System for Stand-Alone Use and for Integration into Hospital Information Systems on IBM Mainframes (in press).

[3] K.-P. Adlassnig, W. Horak. (1990) Routinely-Used, Automated Interpretive Analysis of Hepatitis A and B Serology Findings by a Medical Expert System. In *Proc. MIE'90*, Springer-Verlag, Berlin, 313–318.

"THE VIENNA HOSPITAL INFORMATION SYSTEM"

EDP-ASSISTED MANAGEMENT OF THE CITY OF VIENNA

OSR Dipl.Ing. Heinz Sack
EDP Department Municipal Administration of the City of Vienna (Austria)
A-1082 Wien, Rathausstraße 1

1 *ABSTRACT.* Conceived in 1982 the Hospital Information System ("Krankenhausinformation-ssystem", KIS) constitutes a system for the support of all administrative and clinical functions in hospitals. Through modularization it provides a flexible answer to the protean nature of the organisational workload, allowing the combination of basic functions to meet the requirements of the individual users (customization) while at the same time ensuring maximum compatibility between and within existing and prospective hardware configurations.

2 *KEYWORDS.* Administrative and clinical functions management, patient-oriented database, modularization, customization, commonly interpretable data, defined standard interfaces.

3 *INTRODUCTION.* The 18 hospitals and 8 nursing homes run by the City of Vienna have a total of some 12,000 acute-care beds and another 8,000 geriatric-care beds. EDP was introduced to the hospital environment in 1975, and by 1980 some 400 terminals and approximately 200 printers were operating. The machines handled all administrative activities of hospital management besides running jobs in the central supply field (dietary department, stores, pharmacy, etc.). Since 1982 work has been under way to develop a comprehensive Hospital Information System (KIS) to extend EDP to all the medical areas as well. The system is based on the Patient Administration Package conceived in 1975 and expands EDP support to encompass clinical, medical and medical-technical functions. What makes the system so unique is that the design and development of all KIS components reflect the notion of the hospital being a uniform whole. Thus, the EDP system provides important support for the functioning of the hospital in its entirety, dealing less with specific, i.e. local processes. At present (July 1990), a staff of 150 and 50 in the EDP Department and hospitals respectively work with and on the system, using a total of 1,000 terminals.

4 HOSPITAL INFORMATION SYSTEM.

4.1 *SOFTWARE.* When EDP began to conquer the hospital environment, it was clear that while it was not desirable to have a multitude of individual systems, integration into a single overall system would be impossible. Also, the repeated demand was heard that a common patient-oriented database should be established and double entries avoided. Medical research also attached growing importance to having access to commonly interpretable information within the whole of the hospital network. It soon became evident that existing database storage systems were not powerful enough to meet the requirements of the task and store, process and integrate data for extended periods of time, ensure flexible screen handling and show enough flexibility to allow the optimum utilization of a variety of hardware configurations. To develop a system that would answer these needs, we broke down hospital operations into basic routines and tried to identify similarities. Then we matched these physical routines against EDP functions, defining what we call "AGF (Allgemeiner Geschäftsfall) Modules" for generalized routine work processes.

The system takes into account the fact that the majority of processes going on in a hospital can be reduced to three distinct phases: "the requesting of a service", "the processing of a request" and "the presenting of the results." The Hospital Information System (KIS) aims at coordinating these three phases, which may run off at different times, in different places and at different organizational levels. Thus, any department may request a service, and any department can have the final result of this service presented. KIS is equipped with a special transport mechanism which transmits requests to the service-rendering department and returns the results to the requesting department. Other tasks such as patient identification and archiving of data are integrated into this three-component structure of the system. The Hospital Information System (KIS) has been developed for seven-days-a-week round-the-clock operation. Data backup and data protection are an integral part of the system and of the on-going operation so that no downtimes occur. Since the tasks to be carried out in a hospital are extremely diversified and comprehensive, it was not undertaken to develop specific programmes for individual areas such as pharmacy, kitchen, X-ray, clinics, etc.; instead, an overall system was designed that would accommodate all partial functions. Specific needs of individual users can be met through customization.

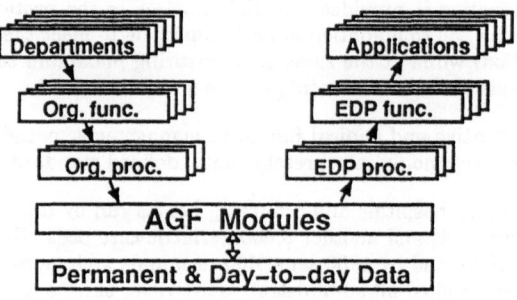

Figure 1. Modularization of administrative processes

For functions that cannot be run on KIS or to communicate with systems outside the actual hospital environment (e.g. social security), appropriate interfaces have been built in. They are standard interfaces with constant characteristics for the next years to come and allow the transmission of data between KIS and other systems such as the SAS (Statistical Analysis System), which is of considerable importance in the research field.

4.2 *FUNCTIONS OF KIS.* Customization forms one of the tenets of the KIS philosophy and implementation. But in order to be able to meet specific requirements with such an overall system, we needed great flexibility in the basic building blocks, of our system. Therefore, we initiated a long process of painstaking analysis of organisational structures to define the "AGF".

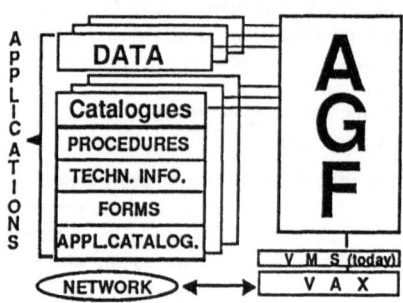

Figure 2. Basic elements to create higher functions

Having determined these, we set out to combine these (approximately 100) basic elements to create functions of different complexity and "interconnectedness". In this way, for instance, we are able to make data generated or entered at any location within the system electronically interpretable at any other location within the system.

4.2.1 *Patient Identification and Administration.*

KIS features patient identification and patient administration functions. Patient identification allows access to medical records of present and previous hospital stays. Thus, it is also possible to have access to a patient's previous case history and include relevant parts in his/her present history. The identification process is not limited to one hospital so that data from another hospital to which a given patient was at one time admitted can also be retrieved. Patient administration handles all information necessary for carrying out such patient management-related activities as billing, etc.

4.2.2 *Diagnosis and Therapy.*

4.2.2.1 *Controlling examinations and treatment at the service-requesting departments.*

The instructions a physician gives with regard to a particular patient are entered directly via a terminal at the service-requesting department (i.e. out-patient facility and ward). They may concern both medical services as well as kitchen, pharmacy and central supply services. The instructions are transmitted electronically to the appropriate service departments, such as laboratory, ECG and X-ray departments, etc.

All instructions are stored in the patient database to retrieve them for follow-up or report-writing (e.g. writing physicians' letters, case histories). The system allows the display of requests for a given patient according to the status of the request, e.g. "available", "not completed", "under way", "completed", "deleted", "confirmed", etc. Typical inquiries would be "What lab services for a given department are still available, unfinished, under way or have been completed?" or "What time, on a particular day, does the X-ray department have dates available for a CT scan?"

4.2.2.2 *Controlling examinations and treatment at the service-rendering departments (laboratory, X-ray, ECG, e.g.).*

The fact that the requested department has access to the requester's information allows it to plan services ranging from the utilization of therapy rooms or X-ray equipment to the reservation of operating rooms. This helps to avoid clashes in reservations. In this way, an overview of dates available and dates booked is possible at any time.

To further assist in organizing work at the service-rendering departments, work-lists, e.g. of certain workstations in the laboratory, are printed. Like the requesters, the service-rendering departments have inquiry functions, i.e. the X-ray department, lab, etc. have at their disposal patient-oriented and/or service-oriented retrieval. Typical inquiries would be "For how many out-patients/in-patients has a CT scan been requested today?" or "Which X-ray requests are unfinished, under way, completed, etc. at a given workstation?" Both the requesting and the requested department are thus enabled by the system to perform patient scheduling.

4.2.2.3 *Report-writing.*

KIS also supports the documentation of medical results.

An X-ray, for instance, is examined by the physician immediately after it has been taken. His diagnosis is then recorded on tape, typed (verbal report), subsequently checked by the physician in question and signed electronically. At a laboratory the situation is different because here reports consist mainly of readings from automatic analyzing devices that are taken over automatically.

All reports, regardless of where they originate, are sent electronically to the out-patient departments and wards where they are printed out and entered into the patient's individual file. An essential function in this context is the putting together of partial results to form an overall report. A typical task would consist in establishing a chronology of all the lab results of a given patient, from the day of his/her admission onwards.

4.3 ADMINISTRATION. The system is capable of supporting all major administrative processes, such as personnel management, billing of patients, management of fixed assets, inventory and consumption goods, cost accounting and statistics, financial management and accounting, management of central supply, management of the dietary department and pharmacy, etc.

4.4 SYSTEM-SIDE FUNCTIONS.

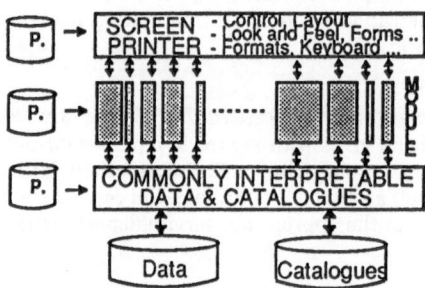

Figure 3. A "cross-section" through KIS: internal variability as determined by external parameters

The above-described administrative functions would be incomplete, however, if they were not complemented by highly flexible keyboard and screen handling, comprehensive catalogue management, and multi-tier help functions. Since there is such a large number of different users and, hence, generators of data, it is vitally important that the users are given a large scope within which they can use, define and select scroll areas and fixed-position fields on the screen. Thus, it is the incoming data that govern the layout on the screen. Closely linked with this is the system's capability of hardware- and context-dependent keyboard utilization. Context sensitivity is also a principal characteristic of the system's help function, which is available at any stage during the work process. The function provides information not only on the on-going work process, but also on the significance of any processing step in terms of the overall system and its applications.

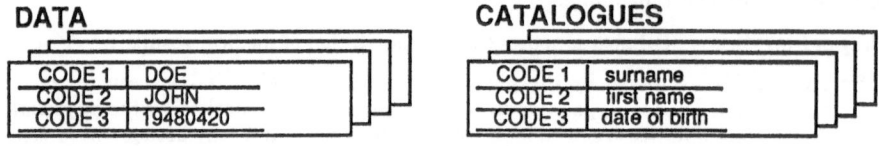

Figure 4. A simplified schematic representation of data/catalogue interaction in KIS

A pivotal feature of the system is the catalogues, which constitute the contact area between the permanent data, which must be available at all times and to all users in a commonly interpretable form, and the constant flow of changing day-to-day data, which are generated in large quantities by a diverse hospital environment. Catalogues are tables of codes and meanings assigned to them and form the key to the standardized interpretability of data.

4.5 *HARDWARE.* KIS' capability of being tailored to very specific individual requirements also extends to the hardware level. Although by essence an overall system, KIS is flexible enough to permit hardware configurations ranging from single-user stations to multi-user networks which may be expanded as the need arises.

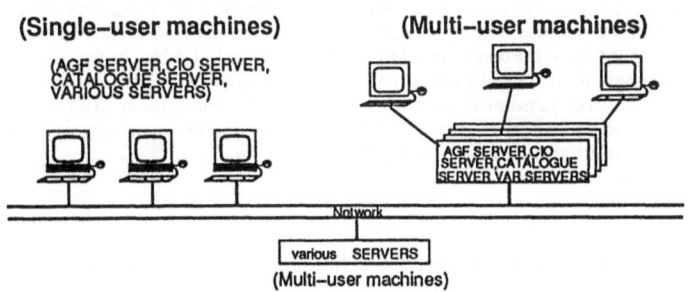

Figure 5. Hardware configurations and individual user needs

5 *CONCLUSION AND OUTLOOK.* KIS is an information system that covers all clinical and administrative aspects of hospital operation. Although uniform in design, it is highly variable so that it is readily customized to meet special requirements.

Full implementation of KIS in the City's hospital network will take some 5 - 8 more years. By that time more than 4,000 terminals will be installed in all of Vienna's hospitals; at the City's biggest hospital alone (Allgemeines Krankenhaus Wien), there will be some 1,000 EDP workstations.

REFERENCES

1. City of Vienna ed., KIS
    Krankenhausinformationssystem der Stadt Wien, Documentation of EDP Department, 1988

2. City of Vienna ed., Eine Übersicht über Konzepte,
    Ziele und Anwendungen des Krankenhausinformationssystems der ADV, Documentation of EDP Department, 1990

3. City of Vienna ed., AGF Module (Laufzeitsystem), Documentation of EDP Department, 1989

4. Sack, H., The AGF Style Guide—An Approach to Programming and Design, Documentation of EDP Department, 1988

5. City of Vienna ed., AGF Standards, Documentation of EDP Department, 1990

THE INFORMATION SYSTEM OF THE FREIBURG
UNIVERSITY HOSPITAL

R.KLAR, A.ZAISS, U.TIMMERMANN, U.SCHRADER
Abteilung für Medizinische Informatik, Universitätsklinikum Freiburg, Stefan-Meier-Str.27,
D-7800 Freiburg

Abstract

The Freiburg University Hospital (2 000 beds, 530 000 outpatient visits per year) has developed the second generation of its computerized information system. Mainframe computers with 560 terminals (display terminals, printers, PCs, card imprinters) and an ISDN based PBX System, especially for transmission of findings, are used centrally. Decentrally organized department systems were bought or developed for the Radiology, Hygiene, Central Laboratory, Pathology etc. and connected with the central systems. Most of the department systems are based on mini computers but there are also PC-LAN e.g. for the Tumor Center, Surgery and Neurophysiology. We designed a new relational patient data base with some deviations from the normal forms and a special error tolerant patient identification. The non patient oriented administrative applications are mainly based on commercially available SAP software. The most sophisticated subsystem is the PACS which stores and transmits radiological pictures.

Introduction

The Albert-Ludwig-University Freiburg operates one of the largest German hospitals (2 000 beds, 530 000 outpatient visits per year, 5 000 employers) and installed in 1983 a first generation of a hospital information system (HIS) which mainly supported administrative procedures. In 1986 the clinical computer center and the new founded department of Medical Informatics started the development of the second generation of the HIS with more emphasis on physician and nursing support, a better integration of the information flow, a not only case- but also patientoriented record keeping and less effort for software maintenance. The experiences and analyses of own and other HIS e.g. (1),(2) were taken into consideration and so we designed a mainly centrally organized HIS with some decentralized aspects.

The central patient data base and patient administration system

Our old central patient data base was only case oriented, used a technically obsolete (ISAM files) hierarchical DB model and required high efforts of maintenance. After a detailed analysis of commercial HIS and HIS of other Universities we decided to develope a new patient administration system by ourself with the help of a fourth generation language (NATURAL II) using a relational oriented data base management system (ADABAS) and a modern data dictionary (PREDICT). The main principle of the new design was the patient orientation and the long term medical record (3).

With our new patient identification optionally we can search for a patient via an identification number (free of semantics) or an arbitrary combination of family name, prename, name of birth and date of birth. This algorithm standardizes in an error tolerant manner the search name with regard on spelling, uses a German phonetic code and handles names consisting of several word independently of the word sequences. This patient identification must operate more than 30 000 online transactions per day and that is why a high performance is essential. We achieved this by a controlled violation of the normalization rules for a relational data base using multiple fields and an iterative search with retain sets in our large data base with more than 30 0000 patient records. In this way the response time could be reduced by the factor four in contrast to pure normal form (3).

Data Processing Systems at the University Hospital Freiburg

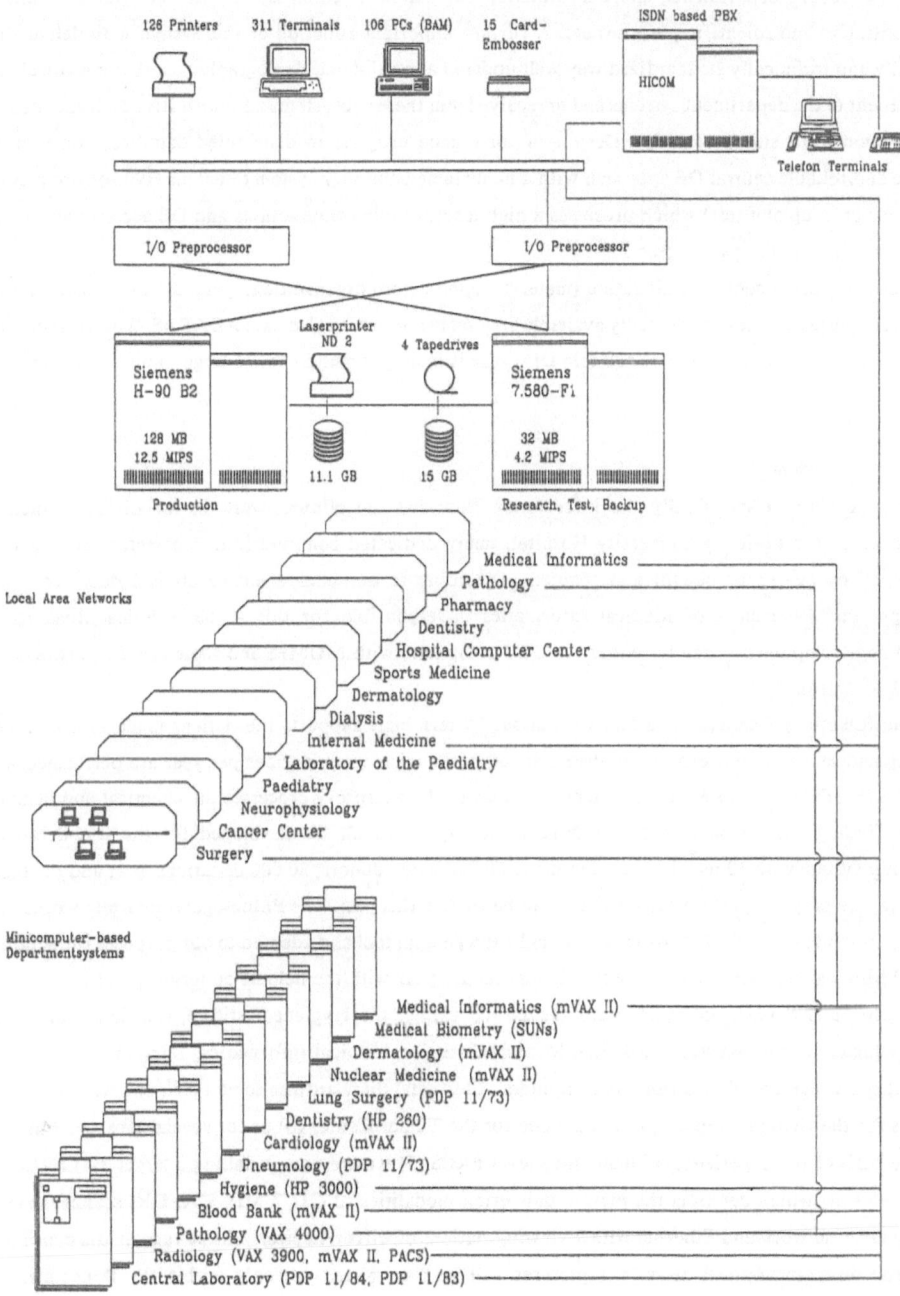

Figure 1

Stand 03.91
us clinic

This new patient administration system includes in- and outpatient admission, patient management, reimbursement, bookkeeping etc. as well as more medically procedures like basic documentation, support of patient record departments, short information for patient's readmission, case retrieval for clinical, administrative and scientific purposes etc. A further important function of this system is to deliver in a logically and technically standardized way well updated and validated demographic and basic medical data of a patient to the department systems and to receive from these subsystems administrative data and medical information to be stored centrally. Despite of some good progress in distributed data bases we prefer a simple and reliable central DB approach with a mainframe computer system (Siemens H90 for production, 7.580 for back up and test) which processes a high load of online transactions and DB accesses and works as a server for the subsystems (see Fig.1).

The patient independent administration (material supply, store organization, general ledger, bookkeeping etc.) is supported by the commercially available SAP software, which also uses ADABAS. With this software tool our hospital with a budget of 500 mio DM/year is managed similar like a large industrial business.

Department Systems

In order to support specifically the information flow and the clinical work in the different medical specialties of the Freiburg University Hospital, many dedicated computerized department system were developed by our us or bought and adapted. According to our comprehensive clinical data processing concept- the department of Medical Informatics is responsible for this - the technical diversity of department computers is mainly reduced to DEC computers with MUMPS and some few LAN (MS-DOS, Novell Netware).

For the **Radiology Department** a RIS with about 75 terminals supports the patient management, report writing and scientific retrieval, more than 100 000 radiological examinations per year are performed with this RIS (RADOS, Philips Medical Systems). The **Central Laboratory** processes the chemical and hematological findings with a modified LABOSYS (Philips), see Fig.2. We developed for the **Blood Bank** a computer system with 12 terminals to administer 50 000 blood donors, 20 000 donations/year and the blood findings; the program part for the receivers will be written this year. The **Pathological Institute** works with the department system PATSY which was bought as a general tool and adapted to our purposes for handling 36 000 histological, cytological and autoptic reports per year with the help of 50 terminals (4).

There are other department systems for the Dental Clinic, the Hygiene Institute, Cardiological Clinic, Pneumological Clinic, Nuclear Medicine, Medical Statistics, Medical Informatics, Lung Surgery, Neurophysiology, which are all based an minicomputers. Additional there are also some LAN, one with more than 24 PCs for the General Surgery (5), a small one for the Tumor Center (6) or for special labs, see Fig. 1.

On the basis of the experience with an entry level PACS (7) we are now installing a larger PACS (Comm View, Philips) which connects the picture delivering modalities (2 CT, 2 MR, DA, DR, scanner) via an optical fiber network and Ethernet with 7 viewing stations of different sizes. The storage media consists of magnetic disks and optical disks. The pictures will be transmitted not only within the Department of Diagnostic Radiology but also into the Surgical Clinic.

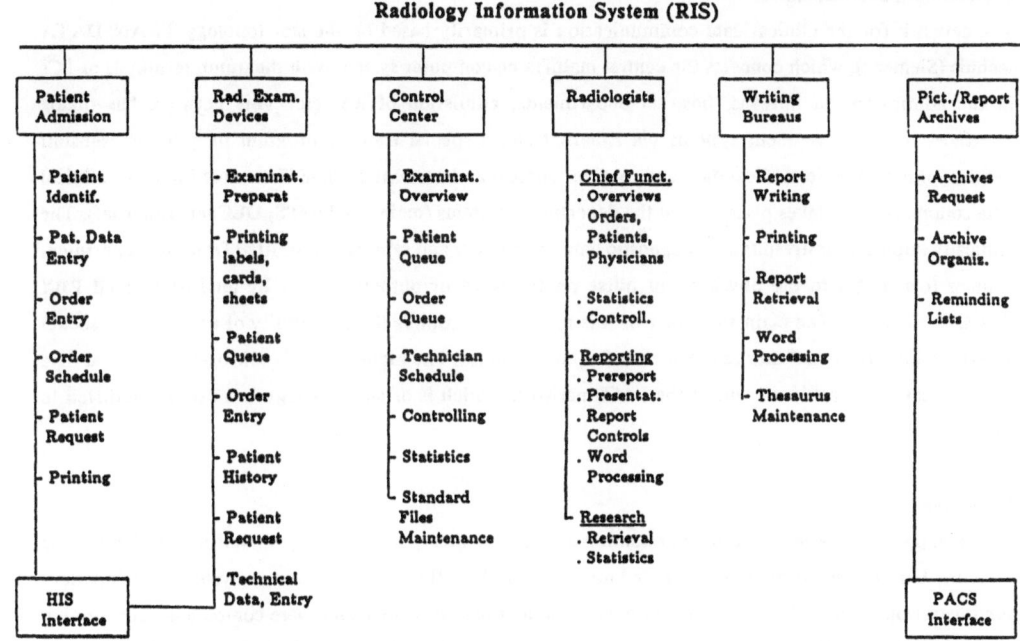

Fig. 2: Main Junctions of the Radiology Information System at Freiburg University Hospital

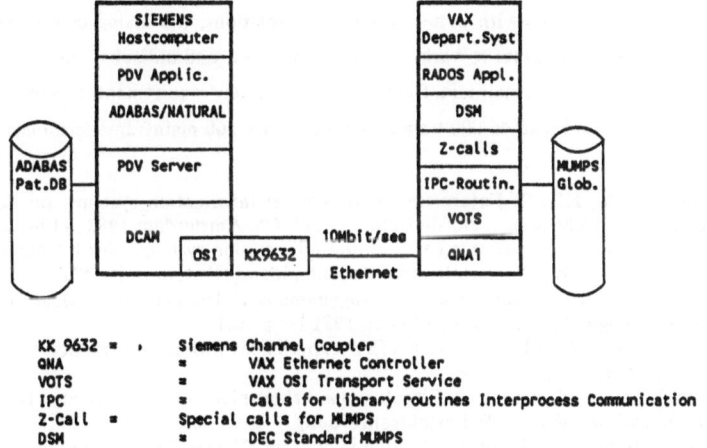

KK 9632 = ,	Siemens Channel Coupler	
QNA	=	VAX Ethernet Controller
VOTS	=	VAX OSI Transport Service
IPC	=	Calls for library routines Interprocess Communication
Z-Call =	Special calls for MUMPS	
DSM	=	DEC Standard MUMPS

Fig. 3: Dialog interface between the central host computer with the large patient datebase and the MUMPS based departement systems, here the Radiology Information System RADOS as example

Clinical data communication

The network for the clinical data communication is primarily based on the star topology TRANSDATA technic (Siemens), which connects the central mainframe computer system with the dumb terminals or PCs in the administration bureaus, hospital departments, admission offices etc. This network has dialog interfaces to the department systems via Ethernet and a special transfer program in order to transmit demographic and basic medical data and receives clinical and accounting data. The most intensive clinical data communication takes place within the department systems (mainly MUMPS, DECnet, Ethernet). The clinically important testresults and diagnostic data are reliably and rapidly transmitted from the department systems (e.g. Labs) to the physician or nurse on the ward or outpatient unit by an ISDN based PBX (HICOM, Siemens). The main advantage of this ISDN application is the availability of any telefone socket as terminal interface and thus reduced costs for laying cables. The highest speed (40Mb/s) for clinical data communications is achieved within the PACS network, which is of star topology but can be modified to form a FDDI ring.

Discussion

On the experiences with an old patient administration system we developed by ourself a new HIS for the Freiburg University Hospital. The first components of this HIS consist of central systems for inpatient administration, medical basic dokumentation and patient record archive and these components are running routinely since Jan. 1991. The other parts especially for outpatients have been installed in a pilot policlinic in April 91 and the other outpatient departments will follow within this year. Overall these central components of our HIS required a development effort of 9 person years, yield to high user's acceptance with dialog response time of less than one second and provide further improvements: The software engineering with hardware independent tools like ADABAS/NATURAL or SAP offers the opportunity of portability to open systems with better cost/benefit relations, the dialog connection to the department systems of our HIS proved that it works effectively for new and old subsystems, and the whole centrally organized HIS is now easy to maintain, flexible to adapt to new requirements and offers a high performance to process reliably more than 46 000 transactions/day with 560 mainframe terminals.

References

(1)   Ehlers,C.Th., Klar,R: Future trends in hospital information systems. In: Fokkens,O. et al.(eds): MEDINFO-83 Seminars. North-Holland Publ. Co. Amsterdam 1983, 112-116

(2)   Bakker, A.R. et al.: Towards new hospital information systems. North Holland, Amsterdam 1988

(3)   Zaiss,A., Klar,R.: Fehlertolerante Patientenidendifikation mit ADABAS, Performanz durch Verletzung der Normalform. In: Guggenmoos-Holzmann (ed.): Quantitative Methoden der Epidemiologie. Springer Verlag Berlin 1991 (in print)

(4)   Zaiss,A., Schäfer,H.E., Klar,R.: PATSY-experiences with an information system for pathology (see these proceedings)

(5)   Salm,R. et al.:Planung und Einsatz von Arbeitsplatz Computern zur Unterstützung der OP-Organisation und OP-Berichtschreibung. In: Selbmann, Dietz (eds.) Medizinische Informationsverarbeitung und Epidemiologie im Dienste der Gesundheit. Springer Verlag Berlin 1988, 348-35

(6)   Kaufmehl,K., Klar,R., Simonis: Auswertung eines klinischen Krebsregisters und vergleichende Interpretation der Ergebnisse. In: Giani, Repges (eds.): Biometrie und Informatik. Springer Verlag Berlin 1990, 26-29

(7)   Timmermann,U. et al.: Erste Erfahrungen mit einem PACS-Entry-Level System in der Universitätsklinik Freiburg. In: Giani, Repges (eds): Biometrie und Informatik. Springer Verlag Berlin 1990, 261-265

OVERVIEW OF AN ARCHITECTURAL APPROACH TO THE DEVELOPMENT OF THE A.Z. - V.U.B. DISTRIBUTED CLINICAL INFORMATION SYSTEM

R. Van de Velde
Department of medical informatics
University Hospital of Brussels - A.Z.-V.U.B.

ABSTRACT

The greatest challenge facing hospitals today is finding an harmony between the quality of patient care and the need for reduction of healthcare costs. As for the next decade we can be certain of two issues:hospital's reliance on computerized information will increase and like medical technology the ongoing change of hospital information systems. The current healthcare system is in a state of transition. This transition is primarily concerned with the transition from analog to digital information from a paper patient medical record to an electronic patient medical record. The digitalization of diverse pictorial information in medicine (ECG,EEG, pathology,...) needs special attention. The purpose of this paper is to describe an approach to the development and implementation of the 2nd generation of a H.I.S. based on an architectural plan in the university hospital of the VUB.

I.   1ST. GENERATION HIS INTRODUCTION

The A.Z.-VUB established in 79 is a full-service. 800 bed university hospital that provides care for 23.000 inpatients and supports over 300.000 outpatient visits a year (emergency patients 32.000 a year). The hospital's central information system -which is 24 hours a day on-line (400 terminals) and performs 10.000 transactions per hour during peak periods- runs on an AMDAHL computersystem under the IBM VM/ O.S.. The actual in-house developed Hospital Information System (HIS), is based on a IDMS/R codasyl DBMS, running on an Amdahl mainframe. Our hospital information system was created completely by our own development staff. Using the intrinsic integration experience from our 1st generation of HIS we believe it will be the precursor to tomorrows online medical record , therefore the product we envision for our tomorrow 2nd generation HIS is a direct outgrowth of the path we set in the past,.with our 1st generation HIS. This first generation HIS focused primarily on automating more administrative and managerial tasks. It taught us many lessons towards the development of our second generation HIS based on distributed UNIX systems.

The next generation

In order to optimize the healthcare management system, information management is necessary (essential). Management is to be concieved as a feedback system which controls dailly operations in order to achieve optimal patient care.

The architecture of the next generation of HIS is based on a set of layers, founded on an open software technology. This open software technology is based on operating systems not machines.

Machines are constantly replaced as newer ones render older ones obsolete. A technology based on machines requires successive cycles of reeducation : progression at the price of retrogression. Operating systems evolve continuously. A technology based on operating systems also evolves continuously. We have chosen a culture of continuous progress rather than a series of dead ends. The relation of Man and Machine is fundamentally changed.

After a through analysis of RDBMS available under UNIX, the A.Z.-VUB selected the Sybase RDBMS to run on a Pyramid MIS super-minicomputer using UNIFACE as 4GL, and for other applications an X-windows/OSF -motif/ C++ environment. Sybase DBases contain actually patient files in 3 GB of storage.In the following sections the architecture of our next generation HIS is described.

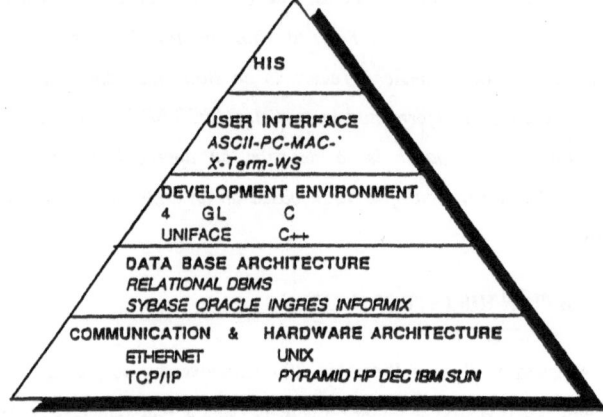

II.   THE ARCHITECTURE OF THE DISTRIBUTED IS

II.1. The data-base architecture

The medical information required to effectively diagnose and treat patients is nowadays largely contained in historical "active paper" medical records and in departmental medical systems. However, without a data consolidation and presentation mechanism bridging these administrative and medical systems, the information does not fulfil the need in offering an integrated patient picture for physicians or an integrated hospital picture for administrators.

The Long Term Database (LTDB).

The primary requisite for a medical record is the registration of a patient's clinical and administrative information from various departments in order to build a longitudinal medical record that ties outpatient and inpatient clinical information in a single patient clinical record. In that way a multimedia LTDBs has been implemented including all inpatients, outpatients, active patients, and previous episodes of care, medical and related administrative data to fulfil that need. Other shared institutional files are also centralized in the LTDB. In fact the LTDB actually consists of a patient identification database, a database holding the read-only dictionaries with relatively static information, a database holding all the scheduled appointments for in- and outpatients, a database holding previous clinical data for each ancillary service. This DB is essential for fulfilment the function of a total historical patient medical record. The LTDB is surrounded by a knowledge layer, who registers metadata as well as some procedural rules concerning the underlying application-clients

The Short Term Database (STDB)

The second objective was to integrate patient appointment scheduling ,ADT, and nursing systems.Nursing is starting to take a strong business orientation in terms of measuring productivity. So the second component are "short-term" data-bases maintained by particular clinical systems (departments) for management of detailed current clinical information for active patients. Access to the database is very carefully controlled, so that only authorized users have permission for certain operations. Sybase stored procedures provide a higher level of security than standard SQL. Medical data becomes available in the LTDB after it has been validated real-time in the STDB rather than as part of a periodic "batch" update. Each of these data bases must have access to, and coordinate with the central LTDB.

II.2 The hardware architecture : Client-Server Networks (C/S)

Not long ago, the choices you had in configuring a computersystem were limited. The speed of processors, the connectivity and software capabilities were all limiting factors.If one thinks of the 60s as the era of batch processing, the 70s as the era of timesharing, the 80s as the era of personal computing the 90s will become clearly the era of the client server architecture and the building of distributed applications to run on such systems.Today, the architecture and its components are being defined more and more by major open consortia and standard bodies rather than by proprietary systems manufacturers. Specialized computers, or servers, "serve" applications to the desktop workstation. True C/S computing involves cleaved applications that split processing tasks between client (PC or UNIX WS) usually on a LAN and one or several servers The user get GUI and application processing at the desktop, along with the benefits of cooperative processing with larger systems. The objective of the C/S model is to offload as much processing as possible to the client, and leave the server with shared information and software for managing it. In the background and less visible to users specialized computers or servers "serve" applications to the desktop. The architecture of the distributed HIS is presented in the next figure.

Components of our networking computing are :

- *application servers* providing computational resources for executing the application (X86 PC's, 680XO Unix WS)
- file *servers* containing multi - media filing systems (Pyramid Unix multiprocessor)
- *A I servers* : expertsystems
- *utility/administration servers* including (X86 PC's, 680XO Unix WS)

- File and print services (such as LAN servers)
- user account servers who mange a global registry that contains user (login) account information
- network management server providing a view of the network environment including resource utilization, available capacity description of resources being used by each user application.
- management facilities : automatically backup, automatic software distribution system updating applications

Workstations and servers communicate via the high - speed fiber optic netwerk. In the past all our applications were processed by two (some times one) mainframes. In order to define a distributed architecture one of the fundamental problems is to decide where to locate software, data and computers all over the network. The decision rules are organisational, economic, functional and technical. All of them change in the course of time. The natural location of application software and data is on a personal host (pc-WS) when dedicated to a single user, on a common host when shared by several (functional) departments.

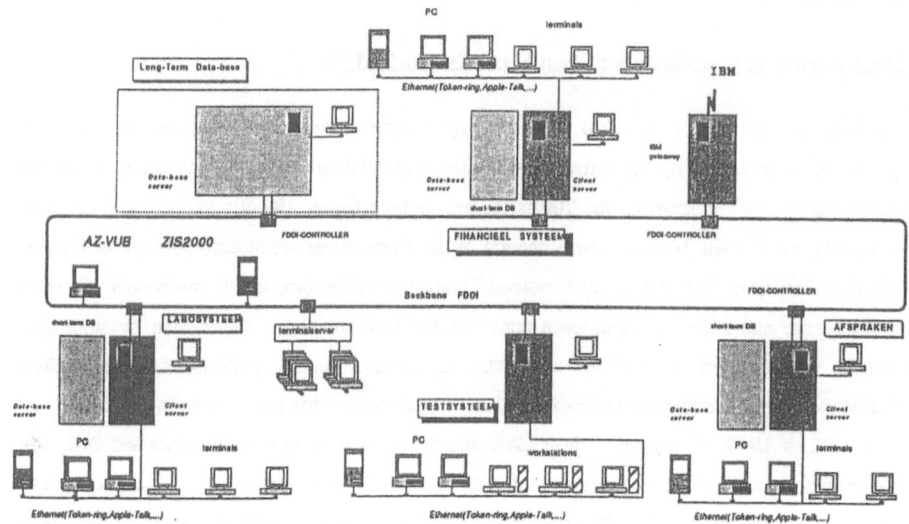

II.3 Implementation scenario

The A.Z.-V.U.B. will not go in one step from a star network to the future network. So the computer centre evolves continuously rather than step by step, towards its ultimate function : providing the heart of the information services and safeguarding the hospital information. Although many tasks of the computer centre are decentralised to local systems, it continues to grow exponentially in computer performance (20. %) and storage capacity (15 %) as a result of common databases expanding and more users who wish to access them.

The implementation scenario for our next generation is phased as follows : first phase : perfect star ---> 1990, next phase : the central system connected to satellites 1990 ---->1992 and finally in the last phase : distributed network (1993) ---->

The benefits and characteristics of this distributed, networked heterogeneous computing environment are : ' distributed : the cost to add (or delete) incremental computing is reduced since the

> environment is comprised of multiple "smaller" elements versus an environment composed of a large computer

> ' networked : enterprise environments are a reflection of a networked society. The technology is scolable so that smale hospitals also benefit.

> ' heterogeneous and dynamic : Computers from different vendors operate and participate in a non-proprietary open system environment.

II.4. The enduser workstation

As physicians, nurses are occasional computer users, who don't like to spent much time to computer education, user training has to be minimized and user productivity optimized through adoption of a consistent graphical user interface.(GUI). The workstation is the window to the environment and to its applications. It presents a graphical metaphor to the user conveying not just the applications available but also the resources of the environment. Pop-up windows, pull-down windows and the use of "pointing" devices were in our opinion necessary and obvious to give it to the user with minimal training. In some application color will been used to achieve this goal. The user workstation question arise what kind of userworkstation we are going to use ? Will it be an ASCII-terminal-PC or MAC-workstation or X-terminal ? The answer is relatively simple : "use the least powerful type of computer ..." The economics are worth discussing it.

*   First we can compare the basic costs (including host ports and network connections)
*   Second we can compare strategies for allocation of the computing budget. A MIP of processing power
*   Third a single CPU with terminal user support is a Von-Neumann machine ; it processes single instruction stream, switching rapidly between users programs to provide service. However a collection of workstations can execute all applications programs in parallel.

So we have chosen to support every hardware platform :

' PC's/MAC's with various software products to provide windows for secretaries, physicians coupled with accompanying cut and paste facilities.

' **Workstations/X-terminals** at the high-end for extensive users, appointment & scheduling. In fact the computer power need to manage and support the user environment of a hospital workstation will be a compact desktop unit with a 16-19 inch screen, a high-resolution colour or monochrome screen (where necessary), a Unix OS, 10 Mips processing power, minimum of 4 MB RAM per user

This processing will come from 386, 486 or 68030 processor offering some DOS-compatibility, or from the latest generation of RISC-processors.

Some users will have X-terminals coupled to shared computing systems rather than workstations

° ASCII-terminals

For other users it may be simpler and more cost effective to meet users' need with a terminal.

10 terminals with a 10 Mips host will probably be more economical and offer better performance than 10 workstations, 90 % of which are idle or underused. Because a lot of users in a hospital don't need the capabilities of a PC/WS it is not cost-effective to install a workstation at places used in a very limited way or used only 10 % of the time e.g.admission clerks, kitchen, inventory-warhouse, data-entry financial, ...For the user the choice of underlying technology will be irrelevant - they will just see their screen, keyboard and mouse.

IV.   REFERENCES

(1)   David R. Vinzant "SQL Database servers" , Data communications International 1 january 1990

(2)   J.E. Toole, S. Campbell, "The decade takes shape : computers in Healthcare for the 90's", Computers in Healthcare, march 1990

(3)   R.H. Richart,"Evaluation of a hospital computers system", M. Collen (Ed) : Hospital Computer Systems, New-York, John Wiley & Sons 1974

(4)   A. Seiver, H. Comerchero, "Clinical information management in Critical care";Intensive & Critical care digest vol. 6, n°4, Dec. 89.

(5)   Moad J., "Maintaining the competitive Edge", Datamation - February 15,1990

(8)   W.G. Smith, "IRM-interview"; Data Base Newsletter VOL 18,1, Jan, 1990

(9)   EEC, "Guide-lines for an informatics architecture", third edition, Luxembourg 1988

THE MEDICAL RECORD LINKAGE PROCESS WITHIN THE DIOGENE HOSPITAL INFORMATION SYSTEM

M. BERTHOUD,   D. GURTNER and J.-R. SCHERRER
Hospital Information Center
Cantonal University Hospital of Geneva
CH-1211 Geneva 4

ABSTRACT

In the DIOGENE HIS (Hospital Information System), all the medical and administrative information about a patient is recorded systematically.   However, despite all the identification checks made when the patient is admitted, readmitted or transferred to one of the outpatient clinics, it occurs from time to time that a patient might be registered more than once.   The present paper gives first an overview of the most frequent conditions of multiple registration of the same patient, and of the following consequences; secondly, it describes and shows the effectiveness of the software tools installed to overcome the problems encountered when dealing with the multiplicity of identification records, from the design stage to its implementation onto an open architecture.

Taking into account the wide variety of cases encountered, the linkage as such is a computer-assisted linkage, that is to say, an interactive application programme that provides for easy consultation of all records selected for each patient and, whenever it is feasible, displays a sound proposal of the best possible linkage for the selected set of records.   The approach chosen for the implementation is decentralised and based upon object-oriented programming using Smalltalk 80.   Considerable expertise has been acquired in representing and manipulating objects of a "linked-list data-base" and of its associate design of a new friendly user interface.

1.   MULTIFOLD IDENTITY OCCURRENCES IN THE DIOGENE HIS

1.1.   The multifold identity occurences and their consequences

The quality of service of a HIS like DIOGENE, since 1 January 1978 [Ref. 1], is strongly dependent upon the quality level of a patients' identification.   A patient previously incorrectly or insuffiently identified may be registered as a completely new patient at the next admission.   It will then generate a duplication of a patient's record and thus create a multifold identity.   We call a multifold identity all the records that represent the same patient.   In the DIOGENE HIS, the number of patients that have been registered, separately, several times is estimated to be only 4% of the total patients on the DIOGENE data-base, and which by November 1990 amounted to 450'000 patient's records.

All these multifold identity occurrencies are each in possession of one history of a mix of collected identities, hospital stays and records. Whatever the record to be selected amongst these multifold identity records might be, all the information and data attached to the other records of the same patient will remain unaccessible and will be considered therefore as missing information. Laboratory data, images, discharge summaries and other relevent information may be "lost" this way. The multifold identity occurrences constitute one portion of the ideal unique record of one given patient. It is in order to meet this ideal requirement that a new software tool has been designed and developed that is able to unify the multifold identity occurrences of one patient into one single record. This software is called Patient Record Merge. As well as this, it also helps to detect and prevent multifold identity occurrences. It may occasionally happen that one duplicated record holds a variety of information issued from different patients. In this particular case it is necessary to operate a segregation of various information back to the rule of one record only for each individual patient. The only difficulty is how to seek the right patient to whom the record belongs or part of the record.

1.2. Detection of multifold identity occurences

There are many ways of detecting multifold identities:

The fortuitous case; when accessing the previous patient record it is discovered that quite a lot of information is missing from within the patient history. Further research will lead to the location of other records holding the missing information required. It follows that the identity profile of one of the records may be modified to such an extent that both records might look alike in order to justify maintaining the link between them. Following this type of approach, 3'000 multifold identities have been detected.

The systematic approach; with software tools the whole data base is checked and records gathered on any look-alike case histories by using the probalistic criteria of "record linkage" [Ref. 2]. However, it is mandatory to thoroughly validate these gathered multifold identities of a given patient in order to avoid false positives as there is still a possibility of two records existing on the same patient in perfect harmony.

2. IMPLEMENTATION

The patient record merger application has been for the DIOGENE HIS a pilot experience for the decentralisation of an application programme dealing with a workstation occurring in a central data base of the former control DIOGENE 1 architecture through a decentralised server. The workstation (SUN) and the programming environment (Smalltalk 80) have allowed the easy use of standard modules of user interface construction with the intention of providing a comfortable user-friendly patient record merge facility.

2.1. The user-interface

In order to make a patient merge record easier to handle all the merge records are regrouped in stacks with a stack for each stage. The user may access one merge record stacked if its stage is known to him/her, and which means getting access to the right stack. If the user modifies the stage of the patient record merge process, the new stage is put in a new stack related to this new stage. The application has a graphic user interface that is a control panel with several windows.(Fig.1.)

2.2. Implementation of the application itself

The decentralised application on a workstation has benefitted by a very short cycle of modification compilation within its own development environment. The patient record merge software is split into four shells. The two first shells are independent of the application. They deal with the following functionalities.

Communication

This communication protocol relates the workstation to the database server constituting a local development that defines a standardised representation of all messages in Prolog format fully instantiated. [Ref. 3]

Data base management system (DBMS)

The way of seeing the centralised DIOGENE 1 database is by thinking of it as fully integrated into the object-oriented philosophy of Smalltalk. It manages a cache or store of data and of the accessed pathways for optimising the communication with the DBMS server. This shell manages the types and values of data: the types are transferred from the centralised DBMS and may be consulted or even enriched through an editor of the DBMS type. The representation and the manipulation of the DBMS are defined within a set of Smalltalk classes. (Fig. 2)

Functionalities of the patient record merge process

All the functionalities of the merge process are defined by a set of Smalltalk classes such as "Patient", "Merge", "Candidate", "Elected", "Stays", etc. (Fig. 3). All the combined values of the DBMS are instances of classes like "DBRecords", or "DBStruct". It is always easy to generate a subclass if it appears convenient to add functionalities specific to a "record" or to a "struct".

The user interface

The user interface is implemented with specific windows: editor of DBMS types, inspection of data values of DBMS, windows for the merge process related to the DBMS content. The development of such an interface has been facilitated by re-using capabilities coming from heritages, instantiation, other interfaces and from widgets.

This DBMS server provides through a general access protocol the same services as the centralised DBMS, based either on procedures or on macros. There are extra-functionalities like the "substitution" capability of an elected record to a candidate record and conversely it manages the delicate manipulation of the different pointers from any data of a merged participant record and to any other data of another participant.

CONCLUSIONS

The patient record merge that has been described here is distinct from the "record-linkage" process. However, the techniques of the record linkage process are used for correlating the records of the patients from different DBMS of various origins. The incidence of false positives or negatives is purely statistical. The merge process often implies research that is difficult to fully automate: further enquiries to the medical services or to the police.

Having at disposal a very user-friendly interface seems to be the most appropriate tool for helping to prepare unmistakably the appropriate patient record merge using all the display tools that are available.

REFERENCES

[1]   J.-R. Scherrer, R.H. Baud, D. Hochstrasser, O. Ratib
       "An Integrated Hospital Information System in Geneva"
       M.D. Comput. 1990; 7(2): 81-89.

[2]   L.L. Roos Jr., A. Wajda, J.-P. Nicol
       "The Art and Science of Record-Linkage Methods That Work
       with Few Identifiers"
       Comput. Biol. Med. 1986; 16(1): 45-57.

[3]   A.Rougé, R.Baud, A.Brisebarre, D.de Roulet, J.-R.Scherrer
       "Diogene 2: A Federated Hospital Information System for the 90's"
       In MEDINFO89, North-Holland, Amsterdam;
       B.Barber, D. Coo, D. Qin and G. Wagner (Ed.), North-Holland Publ.;
       pp. 326-329.

Figure 1   CONTROL   PANEL

Message

Stack of
Linked
Records

Description

Candidates
to Linkage

Data of
Candidates

Status

Comments

Record
Aspects

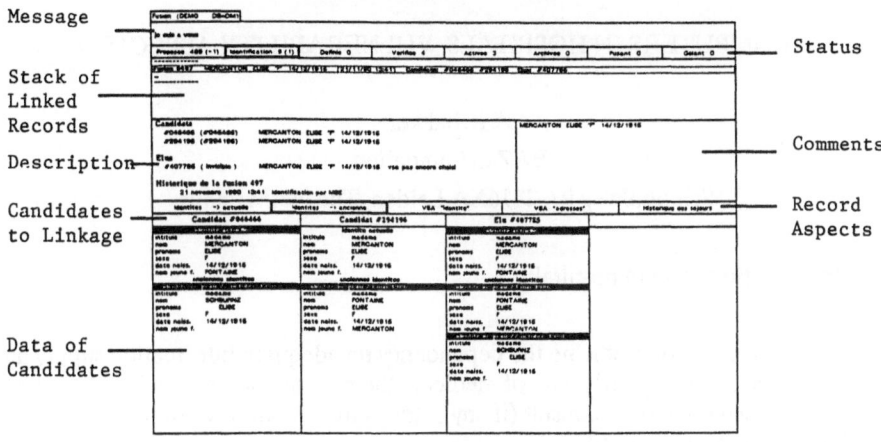

Figure 2   CLASSES FOR MANIPULATION
OF DATA BASE

```
DBtype ('name' )
    DBatomicType ('class' 'example' 'testBlock' 'testBlockSource' )
    DBcomposedType ('fieldNames' 'fieldTypes' )
        DBoccursType ()
        DBstructType ('valueClass' 'valueClassName' )
            DBbankType ()
            DBrecordType ()
            DBvariantType ('variantNumbers' )
    DBfileType ('recordType' 'keyFieldNo' )


DBvalue ('type' 'owners' )
    DBcomposedValue ()
        DBstruct ()
            DBbank ()
            DBrecord ('file' )
        DBvariant ('selectorValue' 'value' )
    DBfile ('name' 'bank' 'keyIndex' 'recordIndex' 'listIndex' 'transactionEntries')
    DBcacheEntry ('file' 'key' 'lock' )
        DBcacheEntryList ('recordList' 'complete' )
        DBcacheEntryRecord ('record' 'inDBMS' 'modified' )
```


Figure 3   CLASSES OF FUNCTIONALITIES OF
THE MERGE PROCESS

```
DBstruct
    DBrecord ('file' )
        DossierFusion ('next' 'previous' 'comment' )
        Passage ('dossier' )
        Sejour ('instant' 'passages' 'dossiers' )
        Patient ('historiqueIdentites' 'vsaOrigine ' 'vsaAdresse' 'historiqueSejours' )
    DateNaissancePatient ()
    Identite ()
    IdentiteResumee ('noPatient' )
    NoTelephone ('printString' )
    ParticipantFusion ('patient' )
        Candidat ()
        Elu ()


DossierFact ('noDossier' 'noPoli' )
Trajectoire ('passages' 'sejours' 'patient' 'estSimulee' )
```

COMPUTERS IN HOSPITALS, VULNERABILITY ASPECTS

A.R.Bakker

BAZIS foundation

Schipholweg 97, 2316XA Leiden, The Netherlands

1. Introduction, data in hospitals

With the advancement of medicine the dependency on adequate information supply has gradually increased. In the early days of medicine the patient had only to deal with 'his' doctor who collected the data himself (if any), stored them in his own brain, where also most of his expertise was stored.

Triggered by the increase of medical knowledge on one side and the diagnostic and therapeutic options on the other side we see in modern medicine a high level of specialisation. As a consequence the care for/treatment of the patient is not longer in the hands of one doctor, the patient is in modern hospitals confronted with ' the medical team'. This team may be spread over more than one department. Besides that the diagnostic examinations are as a rule carried out by special departments (radiology, laboratories). All the people involved in the treatment of the patient need data/information on that patient.

It is not surprising that the potential benefits of application of computers in the hospital were recognised in an early stage. Initially (mid sixties) some isolated computer applications were developed. At the end of the sixties the concept 'Integrated Hospital Information System' (HIS) arose [1].

Although many of the attempts to realise an HIS lead to disappointments and failures, mainly because both hardware and software technology were not sufficiently far developed, we find nowadays some approximation of HIS in most of the hospitals in the western world. Already now they are of great importance for the functioning of the hospital, they can be expected to expand further [2]. In this paper vulnerability aspects will be discussed, hopefully this discussion will be of help in the responsible further development of HIS.

2. Computer applications in the hospital

Computers are used on a wide scale for the storage, retrieval and communication of data, both patient data and logistic data (HIS). Typical applications are: patient registration, admission/discharge/transfer, diagnosis registration, accounts receivable, order entry, meal supply, registration of operations. Often in addition to this some process control or coordination is strived at, e.g. in appointment scheduling, laboratory systems, radiology systems, stock control. Sometimes computers have on-line control over equipment, e.g. in laboratories and in analysis of fysiologic signals (ECG).

Expert systems are not (yet ?) in widespread use in hospitals. However, the 'intelligence' of computer applications is increasing, as is demonstrated by computer support of: checks on drug interaction, dosage prescription, protocols.

The patient data can roughly be divided into medical data and administrative data. Especially the medical data are used for decision support, at present mainly by presenting them in overviews (either on screen or in printed form). These overviews can be used in both diagnosis and therapy/care. Most of the data handled are of the type alpha-numeric. With the advancement of technology the use of computers to handle also digitised images is coming within reach.

3.   The organisation around computer applications

The organisation around the application of computers in the hospital shows a wide variation. As long as the HIS is based on a central configuration we find in general a professional data processing department where the usual measures of separation of responsibilities and written procedures are implemented. When the HIS contains departmental systems linked to the central computer the operations and support activities around the departmental computer are often in the hands of one local 'system manager', often part-time, with limited training. When PC's or PC networks are used to support the hospital the management of such systems is often very weak, 'do it yourself' describes in most situations the working methods best. Although for the main applications the software is purchased from a professional vendor we find in the larger hospitals at least some programming capabilities. The quality control and the acceptance testing of software is rudimental.

4.   Medical data and dataprotection

At the end of the sixties it was gradually realised that application of computers could have harmful side-effects. Westin [3] contributed to the awareness of the threats to privacy. IFIP TC4, (transformed later into IMIA), installed its working group 4 on Dataprotection in Health Information Systems in 1978. It organised several working conferences [4], [5], [6]. The working group is still active in organising workshops during major international medical informatics conferences. Since 1987 the European Federation for Medical Informatics (EFMI) has its working group 2 dealing with dataprotection. In cooperation with the AIM office of the EC this working group organised a working conference in march 1990. Both IMIA WG4 and EFMI WG2 try to cover the full breadth of the dataprotection field, for the medical domain. According to IMIA WG4 the field has to deal with three main topics: the usage integrity (privacy related), the data/program integrity and the availability of the data.

In [5] possible measures to improve protection are considered. These measures need continuous monitoring since the threats and associated risks are dependent on the available technology and the use of the computers in the health care. One of the major messages of IMIA WG4 is: reduction of the risks to zero is not feasible, each organisation has to strike the balance between costs and burdens of protection on one hand and the possible damage on the other.

5.   An HIS case

To give a feeling for the scope of present HIS-ses and the related quantities some data
are presented in this section on the HIS at Leiden University Hospital The Netherlands.
This is a typical European university hospital with 875 beds and over 300,000 outpatient
visits per year. The HIS [7] contains already a broad range of applications.It is organised
around a central databank holding data of over 800,000 patients. Terminals are installed
throughout the hospital, in total over 1000. The heart of the system is a fully duplicated
configuration in a professional environment. The system is operational 24 hours per day,
seven days a week. The number of interactions (CR symbols, after which the HIS has to
react) in the day shift exceeds 800,000. The number of user id's issued exceeds 4000.
Thanks to the full duplication of the central configuration, software provisions for
reconstruction of the database in case of loss or corruption and explicit procedures how
to handle system break-downs, the probability of an interruption of HIS service for
several days is low. The realised availability is 99.8%

6.   Potential harms by information processing in hospitals

When considering potential harms of the use of computers in hospitals we should realise
that the manual way of information handling also implies risks for harm,e.g.
- data often are handwritten, with a risk of misinterpretation,
- data have often to be transcribed; an errorprone activity,
- a paper record is only accesible at one location, so the risk to miss data needed will
  influence the quality of care,
- paper records may rather easily get lost,
- since the same data are recorded in more than one document, so a risk not to dispose
  of the most up to date version,
- handwritten or typed data can't be processed, checks on data quality are not possible.

When computers are applied some of the risks mentioned will reduce in size, e.g.
transcription errors will become highly improbable, the readability of the data will
increase, data will be more up-to-date when retrieved from a central databank, there will
in general be safe-copies of the data. On the other hand new risks will be introduced.
The new risks will be considered in the sequel in relation to the three main topics of
IMIA WG 4: usage integrity; data/program integrity; availability.

7.   Potential harms of unauthorised access to medical data

Storage of medical data in a databank is done amongst others to improve the
accessibility of the data. The data can be accessed quickly from many terminals. The
systematic selection of data is made possible. The advantages of this new facility are
evident, the dangers as well: medical data are often highly sensitive, when known to
unauthorised persons they may harm the patient e.g. in his career, social functioning,
insurance. In health care absolute privacy is not possible, to be able to function, the
members of the health care team need data on the health status of the patient. This
principle of 'need to know' should first be made explicit in regulations and next
supported by both software and organisational measures.

The potential harms indicated here were recognised rather early. The Council of Europe issued its "Recommendation on Automated Medical Data Banks" in 1981. Although the implementation of legislation is proceeding slowly, in most of the western countries we find nowadays a dataprotection law.

However, in practise there is still a lot to be done. Even for this aspect of dataprotection (privacy), that attracts most interest in medical informatics conferences, the awareness amongst the users is limited. The measures implemented can only be fully effective when this awareness in increased.

8   Potential harms related to quality of data and programs

When data would be corrupted or lost this may harm the patient directly since wrong data may trigger wrong decisions. Whereas errors in the manual situation in general will effect only one patient, when using computers we may expect both incidental errors and systematic errors. The latter category may effect large groups of patients. E.g. errors in 'knowledge' in general will have an effect on many patients. Since software is a representation of knowledge, errors in software are a specific point of concern. To give a few examples of what can happen:

- An error in a radiotherapy system caused, when the system was used in a specific way, a much too high radiation dose. The effect was that two patients died.
- An error in a dosage prescription program caused for a special combination of input data a patient to get the dosage prescribed for the previous patient. This lead in one reported case to bleeding, that fortunately had no serious consequences.
- A modified interface of a text module lead sometimes to loss of the first character of the report of histology. This in some cases changed the meaning completely. Fortunately no wrong clinical decision was made on this misleading information. Besides harm to the patient, software errors may lead to corruption of the databank that can not easily be recovered, because the software error itself may cause the users to enter mutations that otherwise would not have been generated.

9.   Potential harms related to the non-availability of the system

Although the introduction of computers in hospitals has not proceeded as rapidly as initially expected, we have arrived now at a stage where their proper functioning becomes vital for the functioning of the hospital as a whole. Assuming the availability of support of the information systems the hospital organisation has adapted its working methods and staff levels. Although for some vital functions manual back-up procedures may be available, this will not prevent significant problems in situations where the computer support would not be available, e.g.:

- Retrieval of data from the databank will not be possible, the paper medical record will have to be the back-up.
- Supply of medication will have to be done manually; checks on possible interactions will not be applied.

- The diagnostic support departments (laboratories esp.) will be able to process only a limited percentage of the normal production. Only urgent tests will be done manually.
- Appointment scheduling facilities will not be available, patients will have to be asked to make their appointments later (when the system is operational again) by telephone.
- For meal supply there will hopefully be a manual back-up procedure with reduced choice options for the patient,
- Stock control will not take place, departments will run out of stock for some supplies.

When such a situation would last for a few hours it would already be a nuisance. When lasting longer it would be a disaster. It is surprising that this dependency of the hospital on the proper functioning of its information processing has not received much attention till now. It is absolutely necessary to pay more attention to this problem and come to some guidelines on the acceptable level of availability and the measures to implement.

10   Concluding remarks

The primary problem with dataprotection in health information systems is the lack of awareness. Without awareness of the risks, measures to reduce them will hardly be accepted or taken seriously. The medical informatics community has the responsibility to make clear the growing risks that exist. In addition to that measures should be designed in dialogue with hospital management and the health care professions. Software errors may cause situations that are a direct threat to the health of the patient or the functioning of the institution, e.g.when the administration of drugs is supported, or when results of diagnostic tests are reported, or when the logistic process of the hospital is supported. The present attitude towards quality control of software to be used for medical applications is absolutely inadequate. This holds not only true for PC software. Regulations for certification of software (similar to those for pharmaceuticals) are needed. A quality control policy on software development should be mandatory; perhaps a task for EFMI in conjunction with IMIA together with the WHO. With the maturation of Hospital Information Systems, a complete break-down for a period of several days would lead to a chaos in the hospital. More attention is needed for back-up facilities and other measures that reduce the risk of such a break-down.

References

[1] Collen, M.F., HIS Concepts, Goals and Objectives. In Bakker, A.R. et al (eds.) (1988), Towards New Hospital Information Systems. North-Holland, Amsterdam, ISBN 0-444-70502-3. pp 3-9.
[2] Bakker, A.R. et al (eds.) (1988). Towards New Hospital Information Systems. North-Holland, Amsterdam.
[3] Westin, A.F. (1976). Computers, Health Records and Citizen Rights. Nat. Bur. Stand. (U.S.), Monograph 157.
[4] Griesser, G.G. (ed.) (1977). Realisation of Data Protection in Health Information Systems. North-Holland, Amsterdam.
[5] Griesser, G.G. et al (eds.) (1980). Data Protection in Health Information Systems, considerations and guidelines. North-Holland, Amsterdam.
[6] Griesser, G.G. et al (eds.) (1983). Data Protection in Health Information Systems, where do we stand ?. North-Holland, Amsterdam.
[7] Bakker, A.R. (1990). An Integrated Hospital Information System in The Netherlands. Clinical Computing Vol.7, No. 2, pp 91-97

NURSING INFORMATIONS SYSTEM - A STATE OF THE ART STUDY

P.R.B. Heemskerk - van Holtz, H.B.J. Nieman
BAZIS, Central Development and Support Group HIS
P.O. Box 901, 2300 AX Leiden, The Netherlands

This paper describes the approach and results of an exploratory study on the
state of the art with respect to nursing applications in European hospitals.
The study consisted of a questionnaire based survey and a literature review.

1. INTRODUCTION

This paper describes the results of a study on the state of the art with respect to
nursing applications in European hospitals. The study was undertaken by BAZIS
within the RICHE-project (Reseau d'Information et de Communication Hospitalier
Europeen) which is partially funded by the ESPRIT-program of the CEC. The state of
the art study consisted of two major activities: an exploratory survey on the
current use of computer applications by nurses at clinical wards, and a literature
review based on the major medical/nursing informatics conferences of the past five
years. Chapter 2 describes for both the survey and the review the approach taken;
chapter 3 gives for each a summary of the results.

2. STATE OF THE ART STUDY - APPROACH

2.1 Exploratory survey

Goal of the survey was to get an insight into the current situation in Europe with
respect to the use of presently existing clinical nursing applications and
developments expected in the coming five years. The survey was carried out by means
of a questionnaire as it was not feasible to actually visit all major hospitals and
vendors throughout Europe.

The questionnaire focussed on the actual use of computer applications by nurses
themselves. As we felt that the ward was one of the last places in the hospital to
be automated, we included questions on both the degree of automation at the wards,
and the degree of automation in the hospital in general. The degree of automation

in the wards concerned both the equipment and training facilities available, the percentage of nurses with usernumbers and the actual use of (groups of) applications by nurses. The degree of automation in general concerned the HIS-architecture, the budget hospitals are spending on EDP and their HIS-usage statistics. Other topics we thought of relevance are the use of applications by patients themselves and the developments currently taking place in the area of Nursing Information Systems (NIS).

The questionnaire was sent to 51 addressees, including a.o. the European members of the International Medical Informatics Association (IMIA) working groups 8 (Nursing Informatics) and 10 (Hospital Information Systems) and others who were known to be active in the field of nursing informatics.

2.2. Literature review

The literature review has been performed by counting the number of publications per country on nursing systems in proceedings of the major international conferences on medical informatics over the past five years:
- the MIE congresses of 1987 (Rome), 1988 (Oslo) and 1990 (Glasgow), organized by EFMI
- the MEDINFO congresses of 1986 (Washington) and 1989 (Singapore/Beijing), organized by IMIA
- the second and third International Symposium on Nursing Use of Computer Applications and Information Sciences "Nursing Informatics" in 1985 (Calgary) and 1988 (Dublin), organized by IMIA working group 8.

Finally we studied the program of the oncoming (fourth) symposium "Nursing Informatics '91", to be held in Melbourne, Australia.

To structure the processing of results we divided the application domain into the categories Clinical, Administrative, Research, Education and Other (dedicated or ward specific) Applications, and we identified categories of aspects: Development (or technical), User and Patient oriented and Others.

3. SUMMARY OF RESULTS

3.1. Exploratory survey

The survey has been done with limited means and does not cover all European countries. Table 1 shows the distribution and coverage of the survey among different European countries (number of questionnaires sent and received, number of hospitals covered and percentage of hospitals covered within each country).

For some countries only a very small percentage of hospitals has been covered. The results of this questionnaire alone should therefore not be considered to form a comprehensive survey, but merely giving a global indication in the present use by nurses of computer applications at clinical wards. Taking into account though that the questionnaire was sent to institutions who are known to be the most active in the field, one can only assume that in general the degree of automation in clinical wards is even lower in the hospitals not covered by the survey.

Table 1 Distribution and coverage of questionnaires

Country	# sent	# received	covered
Netherlands	13	16	25 (25%)
Belgium	3	4 + letter	– (26%)
France	4	4	12 (3%)
Germany	6	2	2
UK	6	12	12
Norway	2	0	0
Sweden	1	1	6
Denmark	3	1	– (75%)
Finland	4	3	3 (4%)
Switzerland	1	0	0
Portugal	1	1 + letter	all
Spain	2	3	3
Italy	4	2	32
Yugoslavia	1	0	0
Total	51	49	

Some remarkable results of the survey are:
- General patient administration functions and general applications (e.g. word processing) are the most frequently used applications. Nursing applications like care planning and vital signs, together with medication applications have the lowest frequency of use (see also table 2). There are no complete integrated NIS'ses in operation in Europe.
- Nurses' use of HIS applications is often indirectly (by means of print-outs and filled-out forms, that are entered in the HIS by clerks at another place).
- More than half of the wards have no terminals or printers at all (fig. 1). The location of the terminals is almost invariably the nursing station.
- 40% of the respondents indicate that all nurses are enabled to access the HIS/PC, either with a shared usernumber or a usernumber of their own. Relatively often one shared usernumber per ward is found.
- Nursing training in computer use is mainly informal and do-it-yourself.
- Nurses' involvement in automation projects is rather high with respect to the decision to automate but rather low with respect to the actual design and implementation.
- New developments mainly deal with 'isolated' NIS/HIS applications. In three cases an integrated NIS development is taking place.

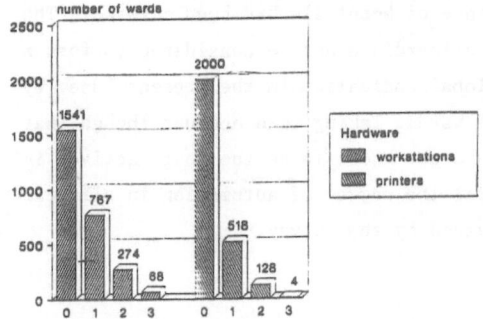

Figure 1. Hardware at clinical wards

Some remarkable results with respect to HIS in general are:
- The most frequently found system architecture is that of one (or more) central computer(s) with terminals.
- Daily system back up is most common. 19% of the respondents indicate a situation in which there are no back up facilities in case of break down; in almost all cases there are no back up facilities at another location than the central system.
- Most delicate/difficult questions turned out to be the ones on the budgettary investments in NIS applications and the questions on the use of the HIS in general. No clear picture could be obtained of the degree of automation in hospitals in the different European countries.

The exploratory survey also demonstrated the need for clear definitions of notions like 'nurse', 'bed', 'hospital' and the need for units to describe and measure the degree of automation in hospitals.

Table 2 Relative scores of countries per application area
    + relative high score
    o relative average score
      relative low score

	PATNT ADMIN	NURSING CARE	ORDER ENTRY	RESULT ENTRY	MEDI- CATION	LAB	MANA GMNT	GENE- RAL
NETHERL	+			+		o	o	+
BELGIUM	+	o		+	+	+		+
FRANCE	+		o			+		+
GERMANY	o				o	o	o	o
UK	+	o		o		o	o	o
SWEDEN	+					+	o	o
DENMARK	o		o	o		o	o	
FINLAND	+	o				o	o	+
PORTUGAL								
SPAIN	+	o	o		+	+	o	
ITALY	+		+		o	+		

3.2. Literature review

The literature review covered 409 publications on nursing informatics. It showed an increasing interest in Nursing Informatics, as the number of publications at the nursing congresses is rising rapidly (CIN'85: 48, CIN'88: 115, CIN'91: 167, even though the number is diminishing at the MIE and MEDINFO congresses). However the review showed that the USA is more active with publishing than Europe: 46% of all publications originate from the USA (see figure 2). Partially this may be due to a more publicity oriented way of working in the USA, but it also suggests that the USA puts more efforts and/or plays a more leading role in nursing informatics than Europe. European "topscorers" are the UK (11%) and The Netherlands (6%).

Figure 3 shows the number of publications per category. It shows that there is not a large difference in interest between the application areas (clinical, administrative, research, education and others), and that user oriented aspects are of more interest than technical or other aspects. When taking a closer look at each of the topics distinguished, it becomes clear that administrative and clinical systems, together with user oriented aspects, are the areas of the most common interest. Research systems are only published about by six countries. Some remarkable findings for the 'top 5' of scoring countries related to the different areas are:
- Research is a relatively popular area in the USA: 69% of the publications are from the US (again 49% of all publications).
- The UK has a relatively high interest in community care (district nursing, WAN's) but no publications on technical aspects.
- Canada scores relatively high in the educational systems and the user oriented aspects.
- The Netherlands show a high interest in clinical systems but has no publications on research systems.
- Australia scores relatively high in administrative systems but not at all in research and educational systems.

Looking at the number of publications per category for each conference, it seems that over the years there is a slightly decreasing interest in research applications and an increasing interest in technical aspects.

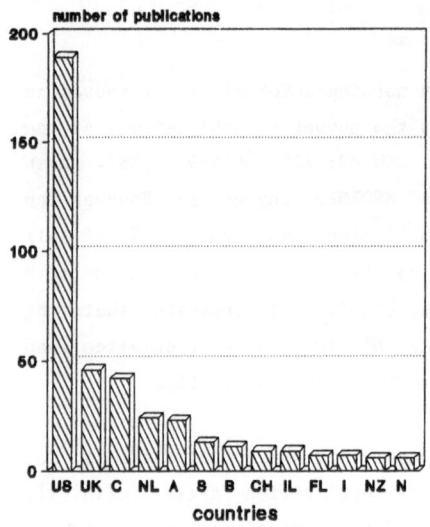

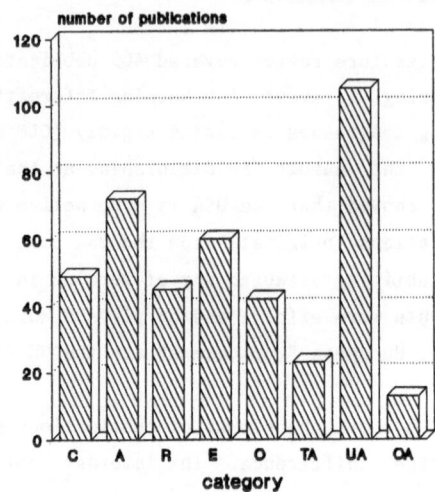

Figure 2. Publications per country   Figure 3. Publications per category

4. CONCLUSIONS

The overall conclusion is that the area of Nursing Informatics is still in its infancy in Europe, but has started to grow rapidly. This is indicated by developments such as in the RICHE-project, the founding of an EFMI working group on Nursing Informatics, and the rapidly growing number of publications with respect to Nursing Informatics.

REFERENCES

Nursing Information Systems - State of the Art,
RICHE-WP5 report BA-10-0500-001, BAZIS, The Netherlands

CONVERTING AMERICAN SOFTWARE FOR EUROPEAN HIS REQUIREMENTS

RONAN HERLIHY

GERBER ALLEY INTERNATIONAL

SUPERQUINN HOUSE, SWORDS, CO DUBLIN, IRELAND

INTRODUCTION

Having participated in two projects where American software was converted for use in international markets practicing socialised medicine, this paper considers the merits of using existing software rather than bespoke solutions. Work on these projects, involved research and analysis of work methods and management practices in two medium sized US hospitals, two Irish hospitals, and three Australian hospitals. Other sources of reference included statements of requirements from hospitals in Oman, Hong Kong, England and Italy. Methods used involved interviews with key departmental managers and were followed by questionaires for more detailed analysis. Supporting documentation and reports were gathered to verify the information provided at the time of interview.

Experience from these projects has validated the view that using existing software, going through a conversion and modification phase, is a faster approach to successfully implementing Hospital systems.

CHARACTERISTICS OF AMERICAN HOSPITAL SYSTEMS

The immediate reaction by Europeans to American software is dissatisfaction, and a belief that it could not satisfactorily be changed for European requirements.

In the first instance, there is a predominance of financial and insurance data. Secondly, the presentation of screens and terminology is undesirable and thirdly, there is an absence of functionality in terms of Out Patient services, Waiting List management and Community Care support.

Items of presentation include the use of #, S, Zip Code, Address format, Nursing Station and date layouts. Reimbursement data is abundant and Guarantors while existing in concept in European hospitals are not immediately understood. In addition there are stringent Medical Record audit and completion requirements.

Work practices are different, there are a greater number of support staff in the United States, particularly Ward Clerks, consequently data entry of patient transactions are up-to-date.

CHARACTERISTICS OF THE INTERNATIONAL HOSPITAL

The following is a list of the functions which are required internationally and not usually provided in American products:-

Patient identification issues such as the use of soundex and providing search facilities by alias. The Social Security Number is a more definite identification in America and such a number is not always used internationally.

High Bed occupancy rates, choice of doctor, and waiting lists are particular to our Health Service. Many transfers take place while in hospital between beds, specialties, and doctors. Tracking and reporting of such transactions is required.

Treatment of patients on an Out Patient basis as well as follow-up care within community services is common in European Health Systems.

There is less experience of automation at ward level with consequent high initial level of training required for all staff.

Investment in Administrative and Management staffing has been relatively low and functions such as Medical Record coding are not well supported.

Case Mix is seen by most as a more desirable method of funding for hospitals and both local management and funding authorities are eager to implement this. However, considerable work has to be undertaken to arrive at a standard cost model.

DISCUSSION

The acquisition of Hospital systems in Europe is a difficult process because of Health funding shortages. Justification for purchasing systems is based on improved service to the patient, efficiency within departmental systems and improved management information leading to a more cost effective service. While these are valid justifications, most Funding Agencies require confirmation of benefits to be achieved from implementing such systems.

The question is, why do medium sized American private hospitals spend a higher percentage of their operating budget on systems? And why, if you look at private hospitals around the world are the requirements for patient data so similar to the standard American product?

The reason is that these systems are vital for the capture of data to support the reimbursement requirements and also to identify clearly whether the business is failing or succeeding. It is an accepted fact that such systems are required and there is less emphasis on reports for cost benefit analysis when a hospital decides to replace a system.

The introduction of Case Mix based funding within Europe will lead to the same reliance on accurate data collection and investment in staffing to support such functions. When funding is based at patient level and a Third Party is responsible for remunerating the hospital for each patient visit, then all the regulations and audit requirements quickly come to bear. The concept of a Guarantor, may be a person, a Doctors practice, or a Health Authority responsible for paying for hospital services. Full accountability for all patient transactions can be expected and Debt collection will be a reality either because of invalid data or simply Bad Debtors.

Many of the accounting functions of American systems are seen purely as billing requirements and are quickly dismissed as inappropriate simply because of the title "Billing". Examples of such redundancy include establishing tables of charges for patient services and commodities. Such data is also necessary to accumulate patient treatment costs to support Case Mix even if an external Authority is not responsible for the cost of the patients stay. The degree to which a hospital is prepared to maintain current or standard costing methods also has to be considered.

IMPLEMENTATION

European implementations are more difficult because they are frequently first time installations. There is a greater involvement of Doctors and Nurses in data entry, and data accuracy is more difficult to achieve. Consequently the following considerations are critical for successfully converting and installing American Software:
- Changes in terminology to reflect local practices.
- Provide applications to support Out Patients and Wait Lists.
- Improve patient identification with Soundex and Alias searches.
- Allow for a Regional Patient Master Index and the development of the system to support Community Services.
- Provide computer assisted training for the high volumes of Doctors and Nurses who will be using the system.
- Do not dispose of the Accounting functionality even if hospitals are not yet at that level of accountability.
- Allow time for educating middle management of their roles within the total service of the hospital and develop their skills in using management information.
- Screens need to be designed for use by staff who will have little time for training.
- Statistical reporting needs modification to support recording of activity by Medical episode, length of stay analysis for multiple Doctors per episode, and external reporting.

CONCLUSION

At the centre of a Hospital System is the PATIENT, and it is logical that details of the patient will be stored along with the treatments they have had, and who treated them. These features are common in all countries and do not pose any fundamental difficulty in converting software. European hospital management is advancing towards greater sophistication and its information requirements, and the accounting and reporting functions of American software are becoming more relevant. Recognising the characteristics of international health care, both now and in the future is the key to successful translation. The process of making changes to software written in Fourth Generation languages provides an easy conversion process and will save considerable time compared with writing a system from the start.

REFERENCES

M. Koens, Logistics Management in Health Care:
Evolution or Revolution MIE 90 proceedings, Glasgow

D Moriarty, Strategic information systems:
An opportunity for Health Service Providers.
MIE 90 proceedings, Glasgow.

DEPARTMENTAL INFORMATION SYSTEMS

The Concept of a Ward Information System

R. Baud[1], J.-R. Scherrer[1], J. Coignard[2], L. Lucas[2]
P. Degoulet[3], F.-C. Jean[3], M.-C. Jaulent[3]
A. Springub[4], U. Engelmann[4], H.-P. Meinzer[4]

[1] University State Hospital of Geneva, Switzerland
[3] Broussais University Hospital and [2] CAP-SESA Tertiaire, Paris, France
[4] German Center for Cancer Research, Heidelberg, Germany

Abstract

The Ward Information System (WIS) is certainly a goal to be reached before the end of the current decade, and quite a number of medical software designers are working on this subject. This paper offers some basic objectives, based on a long experience with a Hospital Information System (HIS) and expresses what is thought to be the essential users' requirements. A taxonomy of the WIS functions is then proposed in a three by three grid, totalizing to 46 functions, each more or less independent of the others.

Considerations are also presented about the WIS "look and feel", as the resulting implementation of a prototype of a WIS environment. This work was carried out within an AIM project of the CEE, under the name of HéLIOS [Dego90].

The WIS actors

First of all, it should be made clear that WIS , in the authors opinion, is definitely a system to be shared by physicians and nurses. This is a necessary requirement, because these two groups of actors share a vaste amount of common information, i.e. data as well as knowledge. There is no real possible computer solution without the complete involvement of physicians and nurses. Needless to say, the reluctance of one of the groups to be part of the WIS design process would certainly result in a failure!

Furthermore the patient is a very important actor, certainly not as a terminal user, but as the source of basic information and as the object of a large number of actions. From this standpoint we can define three major levels acting in the Ward Unit:

- patients

- physicians

- nurses

The three levels are closely related within WIS. The major benefits of such a system will result from a careful integration of common information. Special care should be taken, during the design phase, not to favour one entity against the others. A perfect symmetry is strongly recommended.

The WIS objectives

The set of objectives presented herewith for the WIS should be understood as the fundamental requirements of health care providers. In fact not all the objectives are directly
expressed by nurses or physicians, but they are all thought to be necessary for a safe
implementation of the WIS. They should be considered as guidelines for further analysis
[Heli89].

- **to maintain the equilibrium between nurse, physician and patient levels.**

- **to preserve the specificity of the WIS against other Information Systems.**

- **to warranty the unicity of input and the multiplicity of output.**

- **to be careful about integration needs for data from different sources.**

- **to allow foolproof multi-user access to the WIS.**

- **to provide the actors with interactivity and conviviality.**

The WIS taxonomy

Having recognized three groups of actors in the WIS , we are now in a position to distinguish three ward activities, in a very basic schema, as follows:

- **Care providing activities:** directly related to the patient care process.

- **Data acquisition activities:** input of data from physicians and nurses.

- **Presentation activities:** display of data, including search and browsing.

The above distinctions of three kinds of actors and three categories of activities lead
to a three by three taxonomy of the WIS. The main functions are placed within this grid:
this list is certainly not exhaustive. Figure 1 sketches 46 WIS functions.

Specification and detailed analysis has been started for the **HéLIOS** project. However
it should be clearly understood that the global task of designing a WIS cannot be achieved
in a couple of men-months. A rough estimation is 10 to 20 men-years for analysis purposes,
and 50 to 100 men-years for realization of the whole project.

The WIS "look and feel"

Aparts from the design decisions and implementation constraints, a large Information
System like WIS should have a clear definition of style. It is desirable to explicitly
state from the beginning what the WIS "look and feel" is. The main reason for such an
action is to provide a kind of unicity to the whole concept, in order to make any user of
the system confortable, without having the impression of travelling in different countries
each time he/she switches from one activity to another. A good environment provides
an adequate linkage between components and basically ensures data reusability between
WIS applications developed by different programmers. The main constraint for WIS is

Levels	Care Providing	Ward Activities Data Acquisition	Presentation
Patient	patient care plan drug distribution dietary activities patient agenda specimen collection medical orders	vital signs collection drug consumption dietary information administrative data patient history patient examination	vital signs chart administrative data care status HIS data drug chart
Nurse	care plan strategy care plan per nurse drugs preparation sample collection load levelling	patient load staff availability supply orders medical orders nurse appraisal	ward load staff time-tables nursing notes HIS procedures
Physician	medical orders consultation visit schedule alarms processing	case discussion diagnosis encoding treatment, therapy progress notes discharge summary	medical record MEDLINE access case queries help procedures Decision Support card paging system

Figure 1: The 46 main functions of WIS.

that the final product – as a whole – must be operational in a unique environment, and totally accessible from a user workstation located in the ward unit. Such a constraint is certainly a burden for a software product to be developed over a number of years, some parts of which are inherited from existing Information Systems like HIS. Nevertheless, it is highly desirable to provide a maximal effort in this direction, because a discrepancy in this respect could clearly result in the failure of the whole system.

Data integration is certainly one of the basic conditions for a successful WIS. Conceptually a unique database is needed. Whether it is physically centralized or distributed is another problem. The designer will try to avoid redundancies within this database (exept perhaps for performance reasons). This means that each datum is uniquely represented and all activities must share it, using, for this purpose, the mechanisms of a transaction system.

However, data integration is not achieved easily. The WIS is a programming task of 50 to 100 men years or more, and will be developed over a long period, i.e. 5 to 10 years, thus, the coordination of developments over such a long period is very difficult. Even during a short period, the coordination of different people requires the definition of certain standards, and an active enforcement mechanism. Even so, this is not sufficient to guarantee success, because human beings prefer to follow their own individual ideas rather than be disciplined. This is especially true amongst programmers.

What are the main components which make up the definition of a WIS environment?

The first one concerns the identification of the end-user. The rights of access are certainly very sensitive in the WIS, and the need to finely tune the system on a customer basis is clear. Different tasks must be defined for identification, validation of access right, control and delegation. The care providers assume numerous tasks, and strict control is necessary in the ward unit. The greater the transparency of the component, the more efficient it will be.

It might prove difficult for a new employee to find his/her way around in a large WIS. Formation and education of the end-user therefore, is very important. However, there will always be a problem of users getting lost, so some on-line help facilities are necessary. It is certainly a task of the WIS environment to provide information in such cases. Therefore, at all times, the WIS should be able to locate the user and to know what he/she intends to do, and what is his/her right of access.

The WIS workstation architecture

From the above list of requirements, it is now possible to draw up the architecture the future Ward Unit workstation [Sche89,Baud90,Sche91]. The fact that no fully operational WIS will be available before 1995, has been taken into accounts as well as the fact that the computer market will be really different from what it is today. The major trends are known, and the related costs can be anticipated. It would thus be totally erroneous to build a WIS architecture on the grounds of today's hardware and software! The near future will certainly be dramatically different, just as the configurations now are different from those of the mid-eighties, when the PC was not yet in widespread use!

The architectural aspects related to user interaction are as follows:

- **Graphical colour workstations:** a bitmap screen with a 1000 by 1000 pixels resolution and colour are necessary, depending on the quantity and quality of information displayed either textual or graphical.

- **Multiple windows:** a way to handle multiple tasks evolving in parallel.

- **Simultaneous multiple users:** to handle the fact that an interrupted session for one user should not prohibit the use of the station by another user; and later the first user can resume his/her own session.

- **Pointing devices:** the preferred input means from the health care professionals, when textual information is not necessary.

- **Excellent response time:** this is the most fundamental requirement; no WIS would be acceptable with a waiting time of more than 2 seconds in common situations.

- **Immediate availability:** the number and localization of workstations should be adequate to accomodate all users' needs; one workstation for five patient beds seems a reasonable figure.

- **High conviviability:** this means that the system may be used more or less without instruction of the users; this also means the presence of a permanent team of helpers, to guide any lost users!

A working prototype [Heli90] of such an environment has already shown how appropriate the above targets are, concerning the needs of health care professionals. Despite the high level of requirements, these targets would seem to be more or less a set of minimal conditions. Economically, it would seem feasible that the architecture presented above be achievable by 1995 at an investment cost of three thousands dollars per patient bed! With a redemption period of four to five years, this means about 600 dollars per patient bed, per year. The software development and maintenance costs are not included.

Conclusion

The WIS is definitively a large set of functionalities sharing common information in the Ward Unit. A sound approach to this system necessitates a global view of all the components, an adequate state-of-the-art architecture, a sharply designed environment and a sufficient amount of men-years in computing resources.

Acknowledgements

The development of HéLIOS has benefited from the financial support of the Commission of European Communities (contract CEC/AIM 1004), and the CERS for the EFTA country. Additional support was available from Digital Equipment, Ingres and Servio-Logic.

References

[Baud90] Baud R. **Software Technology Assessment for Future HIS** in proc. IS-TAHC/IMIA/ENSP Joint Working Conference on Assessment of Medical Informatics Technology, oct 1990, Montpellier, France, ENSP edition.

[Dego90] Degoulet P. & al. **The HéLIOS European Project on Software Engineering** in proc. IMIA Working Conference on Software Engineering in Medical Informatics, oct 1990, Amsterdam, the Netherland, Elsevier publ.

[Heli89] HéLIOS Deliverable D2 **Report describing the Requirements and functional Specifications of the WIS Application**, dec 1989, by the authors.

[Heli90] HéLIOS Deliverable D9 **Detailed Specifications of a Ward Information System (selection of specific activities)**, dec 1990, by the authors.

[Sche89] Scherrer J.-R, Rougé A, Assimacopoulos A, Baud R. **L'unité de soins informatisée dans DIOGENE 2** in: Informatique et gestion des unités de soins, june 1989, Springer-Verlag, Paris.

[Sche91] Scherrer J.-R. **Nouvelles architectures destinées à des réseaux d'ordinateurs hospitaliers ouvrant le monde médical à plus de facilités de communications de tous ordres** in: Schweizerische Medizinische Wochenschrift, SMW Nr. 49, 204, 1991.

DAMS—SOFTWARE PACKAGE TO SUPPORT THE DAILY ACTIVITIES OF A HOSPITAL WARD

T. Obradović, J. Mihaljev[1], D. Obradović, B. Perišić, S. Latinović
Computers, Control and Measurement Institute
[1]Institute for Neurology, Psychiatry and Mental Health
University of Novi Sad

ABSTRACT

A structured system analysis was applied to study the daily activities of a hospital ward. On the basis of the results obtained, the DAMS software package was developed. DAMS supports: (a) reception of a patient into a ward (by recording the patient data in the database); (b) recording of the services given to a patient in the course of diagnostic/therapeutic treatment; and (c) transfer and/or release of a patient.

I. INTRODUCTION

A hospital ward covering specialized medical activities represents a fundamental unit of a hospital. Basic functions of a ward are:

- reception of a patient
- diagnostic and therapeutic treatments
- transfer and/or release of the patient.

In the process of patient reception, based on a regular or urgent referral form, some administrative procedures have to be followed. On the basis of the referral form, the patient is assigned to the ward and the diagnostic and/or therapeutic activities are performed, which requires also a lot of administrative work. In the process of transferring patients to another ward or clinic of the hospital or releasing them from the hospital, there is again administrative work to be performed.

As is well known, such administrative procedures are usually carried out by the medical staff, especially by nurses, whose time to be devoted to the patients is accordingly reduced. In order to free the medical staff from excessive administrative work, the DAMS program package was developed.

II. METHODOLOGY EMPLOYED

In order to develop the DAMS programming system, a structured system analysis was applied [1]. The results of the analysis are:

- data flow diagrams and data flow dictionary
- description of the processes (algorithm) involved
- elementary data dictionary
- data files description.

Data flow diagram and dictionary represent a graphic presentation of the information flow and a description of interactions between data files and the environment.

The top level of data flow diagrams is the CONTEXT DIAGRAM, whose main goal is to portray all the net inputs and outputs of the system, without any more detailed decomposition. The context diagram for the DAMS system is shown in Fig. 1.

The next step in drawing data flow diagrams is the DIAGRAM 0 whose purpose is the definition of organizational subsystems. For DAMS, this is shown in Fig. 2.

To illustrate further decomposition of the data flow diagrams "bubble" 2 (RECEPTION, TRANSFER and RELEASE of patients) is considered. The other two "bubbles" (macro processes) are not explicitly decomposed for two reasons: macro process 1 is a standard set of procedures for catalog maintenance, and its decomposition is rather obvious; on the other hand, the decomposition of macro process 3 is not as obvious, but as a result it would only give us relatively simple processes for adding records to a file, or for printing various reports. Therefore we will stick to process 2 the decomposition of which gives us the diagram shown in Fig. 3.

Following this procedure, according to [1], we will arrive at the primitive processes.

The processes are presented in a formalized way using a structured lan- guage which can easily be transformed into the programming language to be used.

The elementary data dictionary is sorted in alphabetic order including the elementary data name and the description of possible data values.

Data files are described by names, data structures and the record type.

On the basis of these results, data models are obtained in the first normal form. The data structure is shown in Fig. 4. Notations are standardized, with the following meanings:

- a rectangle represents the record type
- an arrow represents a relation of the one-to-many type
- letter C with an angular arrow identifies the record types with direct access (calc key).

A brief look at the data structure tells us that it is given for the most part in hierarchical form, representing a typical situation of a hospital. An important exception is the record type of SERVICES GIVEN which is relational record for the record types of PATIENTS and SERVICES where the relation is of the many-to-many type.

III. SOFTWARE PACKAGE CHARACTERISTICS

On the basis of system analysis described above, the software package DAMS is developed for personal computers (IBM XT/AT or compatibles) using the software tool FoxBase. The user communicates with the package via four segments. The first segment offers a choice of the functions to be exploited by the user. The second segment covers input to data files or modifications. The third segment represent warnings about possible errors and explorations of help functions. The fourth segment offers output reports.

In the beginning the user may choose one of the following functions:

- interaction with the basic catalogs
- reception of patient on the ward (recording the patient)
- services to the patient in the course of his or her presence on the ward.

The layout of the main menu is given in Fig. 5.

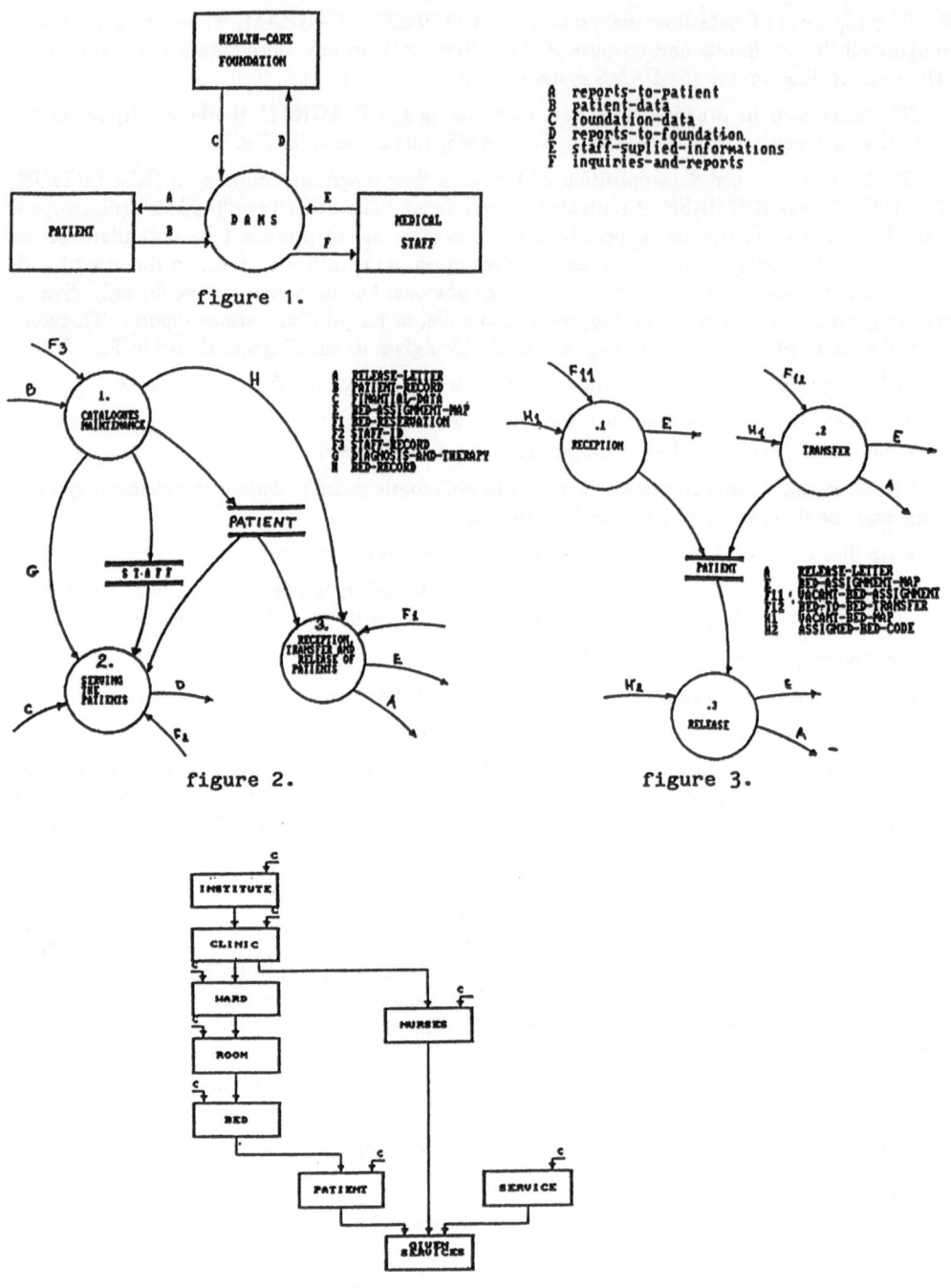

figure 1.

A   reports-to-patient
B   patient-data
C   foundation-data
D   reports-to-foundation
E   staff-suplied-informations
F   inquiries-and-reports

figure 2.

A   RELEASE-LETTER
B   PATIENT-RECORD
C   FINANCIAL-DATA
D   BED-ASSIGNMENT-MAP
F1 BED-RESERVATION
F2 STAFF-ID
F3 STAFF-RECORD
G   DIAGNOSIS-AND-THERAPY
H   BED-RECORD

figure 3.

A   RELEASE-LETTER
D   BED-ASSIGNMENT-MAP
F11 VACANT-BED-ASSIGNMENT
F12 BED-TO-BED-TRANSFER
H1 VACANT-BED-MAP
H2 ASSIGNED-BED-CODE

figure 4.

By choosing one of these functions via menu, the other appropriate functions are automatically offered. In this way, the DAMS program allows accepting a patient, bed assignment, transfer of patients within a ward or from one ward to another, permanent recording of the services, therapies, etc., given to patients. Corresponding reports are also prepared (on screen or as hard copy).

A sample of the data entry screen is shown in Fig. 6.

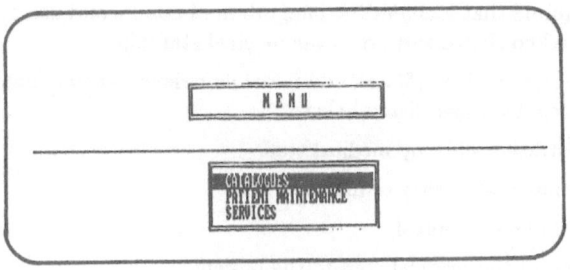

figure 5

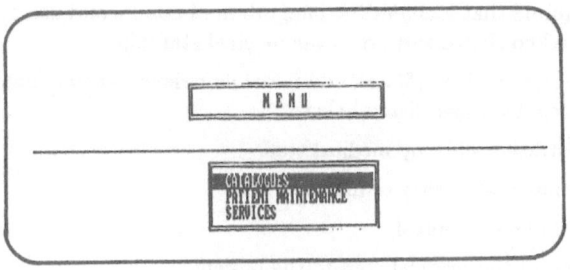

figure 6

IV. CONCLUSION

The DAMS software package is a subsystem of a hospital information system [2,3] which is operating at the Clinic for Neurology of the University of Novi Sad Medical Faculty with the main aim of following the daily activities within a hospital ward.

The fundamental idea for the development and application of the DAMS program package is based on the understanding that efficiency represents the process of transforming investments into products minimizing the price/performance ratio or, in the field of health care, the art of employing available resources to satisfy the set goals [4]. To maintain the required efficiency, an integral approach is required that includes the integration of donors and users of services, as well as the integration of the knowledge and art of the medical staff [5].

Using a well-known methodology [6] and additional experience, the application of the DAMS program package has the advantages listed below:

- reduction of administrative work by medical staff
- extension of the volume and quality of medical data
- possibility for overall quality control
- more human relations of the medical staff to the patients.

REFERENCES

[1] T. DeMarco. Structured Analyses and System Specification. Prentice-Hall, New Jersey, 1979.

[2] B. Perišić, D. Obradović, M. Tasić, S. Živojinović. DMIS—Distributed Medical Information System Concept and Structure. System Science, Vol. 13, No. 1-2, 1987.

[3] T. Obradović. Information System of a Hospital Ward. Faculty of Technical Sciences, Novi Sad, 1990 (in Serbo-Croatian).

[4] M.S. Feldstein, A.O. Taynor. The Rapid Rise of Hospital Costs. Medical Technology and Health Care Systems. National Academy of Sciences, Washington, 1979.

[5] J. Mihaljev-Martinov, D. Obradović. Rationalization of Diagnostics in Neurology. Chapter: Technological Achievements in: Neurologija, Vol.37, 1988, 119–125.

[6] J.P. Glaser, N. Drazen, P. Erica, N. Cohen. Maximizing the Benefits of Health Care Information Systems. Journal of Medical Systems, Vol. 1, No. 1, 1986.

THE FEBE PROJECT: DESIGNING A CLINICAL INFORMATION SYSTEM

Romilly C. Gregory[1], Mark S. Leaning[1], John A. Summerfield[2], Jonathon Browne[2], Deborah Wilkinson[2] and Anthony McGrath[2]

[1] Clinical Operational Research Unit, University College London, Gower Street, London, UK.
[2] St Mary's Hospital, London, UK.

Abstract

Systems design is critical to the success of clinical information systems. On the FEBE ('Fluid Electrolyte Balance Estimation') project a bedside workstation is being developed which aims to improve the management of fluid, electrolyte, acid-base and nutrition therapy. Working in close co-operation with a team of doctors and nurses a prototype has been built which incorporates design principles of wider applicability to the development of clinical computer systems.

Introduction

The FEBE project was set up to address the clinical problem of the frequent poor management of fluid, electrolyte, acid-base and nutrition therapy in the critically-ill patient and the demands on nursing resources required in maintaining the present paper records [1]. The goal is the development and clinical testing of a bedside workstation to manage the data required for these therapies and to provide therapy advice. The objective is to test the hypothesis that such a system leads to an improvement in the standard and outcome of this therapy.

Despite the potential value of computer systems for clinical data management, many systems have proved unacceptable in practice. Two of the main reasons for this are unreliability and the time and effort required by busy medical staff to use them. The FEBE system addresses these problems: data reliability is enhanced by using a commercial relational database management system; the system is made easy to use (and less time-consuming) with a high quality direct manipulation graphics interface. Most importantly, users have been involved from the start in the design of the system.

Method

A user centred approach has been adopted to system development, the main techniques being process and data modelling [2] and iterative prototyping [3]. The models and prototypes have been developed at the Clinical Operational Research Unit (CORU) in close collaboration with the team of clinicians and nurses at St. Mary's Hospital. We started by developing process models of the major clinical and nursing processes performed in the management of fluid therapy [4]. These models were helpful in providing an explicit understanding of the tasks carried out and in delimiting at a strategic level the boundaries of the proposed system and its scope (e.g. showing the dataflows between the system, the ward, the labs, etc.). However, in general the medical team found the formalisms confusing and the detailed process models hard to comment on. The models were thus not as useful as we would have liked at eliciting user feedback. They did not easily assist with systems design, apart from capturing the main processes the system had to perform. The data model has ultimately proved to be more use to the technical team, although the users still found the formalisms difficult.

Ideas for the system have been prototyped in various ways since the beginning of the project. The first prototype was a set of screens developed on an Apple MacIntosh which were used to test users' response to computerised charts - paper look-alikes. The response was very positive. Specifically, the paper look-alike screens were found to be intuitive to use. Of course, this initial prototype had limited functionality for data handling. The second prototype was developed on a Sun workstation using a relational database management system. In this prototype, the existing paper charts were emulated as closely as possible, although the underlying data tables were not based on the data model. Using these screens led to a wealth of ideas and information from medical staff about features they would like the system to have. For example graphical data entry screens were suggested as a more rapid means of entering observations (eg weight and temperature). In addition to other design priniciples now adopted (see below), the clinical team also suggested how the handling of fluid and electrolyte data could be extended to include nutritional balance data. This has now been incorporated.

The third prototype is a re-implementation based on the data model and incorporating many of the design ideas that have arisen during prototyping. This prototype is intended to evolve into the final system to be used on the ward. In retrospect, it would have been beneficial to have completed the data model earlier, before the second prototype was developed (i.e. at the time that a relational database system was introduced for data management).

Design and HCI issues

To achieve the aim of developing a system which both looked like and had the same flexibility and ease of use as the present paper system we decided to use a WIMP interface. The following important design principles were adopted: crucial information should be immediately available; not too much information should be displayed at one time; navigation around the system should be simple. For these reasons we decided to employ a default screen with the crucial summary information, with pop-up windows for additional displays and data input charts. The pop-ups are called from a control panel which is always visible. They are designed to be temporarily displayed, then exited. No further windows can be called from the pop-ups. In other words the interface is as 'flat' as possible.

Version 3 of the prototype has been built based on this design concept (Fig. 1). However, the ideal user interface development environment which would enable the prototyping of a WIMP interface and a relational database is not currently available. The software we used did not support WIMP and we have had to add some WIMP functionality.

The main screen displays summary information for the current patient for the current day. In order to achieve the small pop-up windows the original large data input charts have had to be redesigned. The principle we have adopted is that the pop-up window displays one record. It is possible to scroll backwards or forwards through the other records. The graphic displays enable users to get a quick overview of data in the database, such as fluid and electrolyte balances. The long term aim is to enable users to customise their own graphical displays of whatever variables they choose.

The system has been built on a Sun 3/80 workstation running the X Window System and an Oracle relational database (Fig. 2). The forms have been built in Oracle's 4GL, SQLforms with additional C programs performing basic fluid, electrolyte and nutrition calculations and balances. The graphics tool-kit is written in C and Xlib.

Ward Testing

The current prototype has completed a week of ward testing. The aim was a preliminary evaluation of the system, in terms of its accuracy and completeness of data handling, and of the users response to it, including their assesment of its clinical value. The system was able to handle the fluid, electrolyte and nutrition data of three critically ill patients and to produce accurate balance data. The doctors and nurses found the interface easy to understand, though less easy to use because of the limitations of the current partial WIMP implementation. They found the system valuable particularly in its better presentation of summary data, the extra electrolyte and nutrition data and the graphical displays.

We are currently reimplementing the system in the next version of the SQLforms software, which does fully support WIMP and incorporating the enhancements suggested by users during ward testing. We will also add the therapy advisor and acid base modules. This prototype will then be tested in extensive ward trials.

Conclusions

The approach we have adopted of a high degree of user involvement in both modelling and iterative prototyping contrasts strongly with the way many clinical information systems are being introduced into hospitals. Usually a complete system

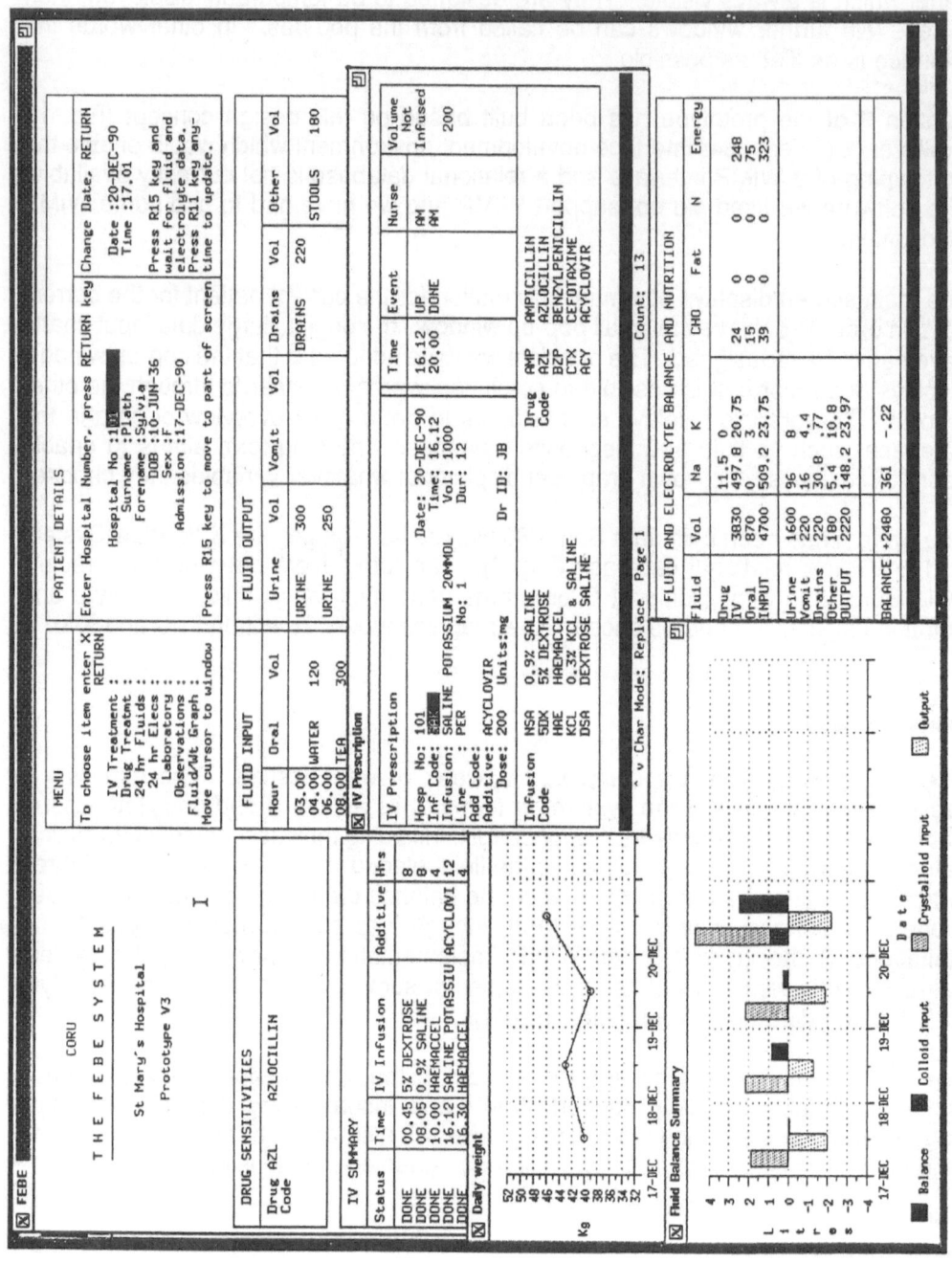

Fig 1. The FEBE Prototype, Version 3.

94

is delivered and the users must learn to adapt to it. Our approach attempts to ensure that the system addresses the clinical problem it was designed to solve in a way that the users accept. It has also led to the development of design principles such as the use of a 'flat' WIMP interface displaying forms based on familiar charts, but with improved summary and graphical displays which are likely to be valuable for other clinical information systems.

Fig 2. FEBE Software Architecture

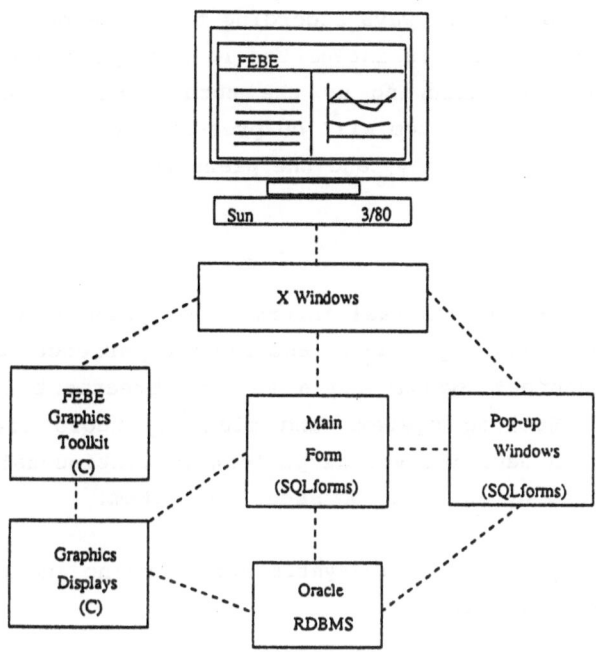

References

1. Leaning M, Summerfield J, "Microcomputer-Based Management of Fluid and Electrolyte Balance in Hospitalised Patients", MEDINFO 86, 1986.
2. Martin J, Maclure C, "Diagramming Techniques for analysts and Programmers", Prentice Hall, 1985.
3. Dearnley P, Mayhew P, "In Favour of System Prototypes and their Integration into the Systems Development Cycle", The Computer Journal, Vol 26, No 1, 1983.
4. Gregory R, Leaning M, Summerfield J, "The FEBE Project: Modelling a Clinical Information System", MIE 90,1990.

Acknowledgements

This work is supported by the Medical Research Council and the Dept. of Health.

A WARD NURSING SYSTEM INTEGRATED IN A COMPREHENSIVE HIS

Marian Thygesen
Kommunedata I-S, Center for Hospital Information Services
P. O. Pedersens Vej 2, 8200 Aarhus N - Denmark.

The Ward Nursing System presented in this paper is a flexible system which can be used in different ways according to the taxonomy of the ward using the system. The system is integrated in a comprehensive HIS which gives possibilities of following up the total activity concerning a patient. The ward nursing system will be presented with emphasis on the way the system can be used today, and the plans for the system's further development.

Introduction

DANHIS is a dialogue based hospital information system with integrated user guidance for both the experienced and the inexperienced user. DANHIS has a Patient Management System and a Patient Treatment and Services Management System. Booking systems and planning tools are included. Comprehensive data on each individual patient is continuously collected and data is protected by an advanced security system.

Integrated in this system is a sub-system for planning and following up nursing activities in wards.

The Ward Nursing System

In Denmark several experiments have been carried out with manual registration of different Ward Nursing Systems (inspired by for example GRASP or RUSH) in order to be able to document the work load and to follow up quality compared to the ward's objectives. The benefit however rarely matches the extensive manual calculation involved. Only with the use of advanced EDP-tools is it possible to develop work routines which fulfil the objectives of these experiments. The DANHIS Ward Nursing System was developed by Kommunedata in cooperation with a large hospital in Copenhagen. A working group was set up at the hospital composed of matrons, staff nurses and a representative from the senior nursing management. Experimental techniques have been used during system development. Among other things the working group was shown prototypes before the final design of the system was determined.

Our interests went beyond this specific collaboration. We put resources into developing a system which was to be used by many different hospitals and for different nursing systems. The system had to be flexible, and the individual hospitals or wards had to be able to decide the level of ambition as regards planning and following up.

Therefore the system was developed as a tool giving the hospital the possibility of tailoring the system so that it exactly meets the needs of the ward.

The Ward Nursing System consists of 3 parts - a classification part for defining the basic taxonomy for nursing activities, a data entry part which enables the nursing situation in the ward to be recorded, and an information part delivering aggregated information which is the basis of planning and following up.

Classification

Using the classification part, the hospital itself builds up a classification of the nursing activities which are used in planning and following up. A code with associated text is established for each nursing activity. Codes are grouped into chapters. The classification is for the whole hospital and can consist of any number of chapters and codes. A code can represent a specific nursing activity or a patient category, according to the taxonomy of the hospital/ward. A code could also be a nursing diagnosis.

Each ward creates its own catalogue, which is a subset of the classification. The catalogue contains only those codes which the ward will use for registering. The ward selects the relevant codes from the classification, allocates points to each code and, maybe, a description.

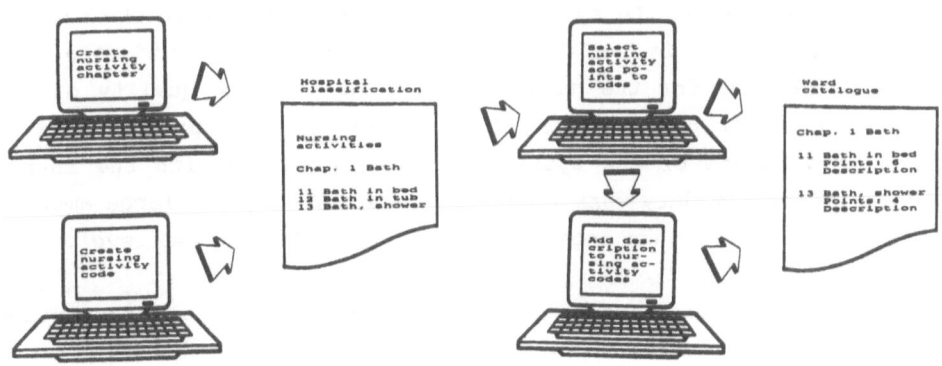

Registration

When the catalogue is built up, the ward can use the system for recording the activity of the ward.

It is possible to register nursing activities, using these codes, for each patient on the ward. When registering, the nurse can select one or more codes from a pop up window where the catalogue codes with text are listed. The selected codes will be transferred with text and points to the panel where the nurse will confirm the registration. So the nurses do not have to memorize the codes. The expected and/or actual nursing care can be reported in the system, expressed by one or more codes per patient. According to the codes, a total point sum per patient is calculated each day as an expression of the work load needed for each patient.

The system is constructed with comprehensive help facilities so that data entry becomes easy and quick, even though the department chooses to report very detailed information.

Furthermore the system allows the registering of indirect nursing care, that is activities which are not directly related to a specific patient.

Information part

Many different types of information can be retrieved from the system, which describe in different ways the situation in the ward. For example there is the possibility of following up expected nursing activities compared to actual nursing activities and of showing the distribution of the work load between ward nursing groups, per day and month.

Use of the system

Today one of the largest hospitals in Denmark is using the nursing system. In order to use the system, some preliminary work in the ward is needed. This in itself is useful, as it results in a common understanding of a basic taxonomy for the nursing activities and the quality of the nursing care - ultimately for the benefit of the patient. Early experiences with use of the system uncovered problems with the rather comprehensive preliminary work required, together with the large amounts of data to be entered when registering at the most detailed level.

In other words motivation of the nurses who are going to use the system is an aspect which should not be underestimated.

The system has a flexibility which allows its use in a large number of ways, for example:

- Reporting once or twice a week of actual nursing activities, as an overview of the tendencies in the ward.
- Detailed and intensive reporting of both expected and actual nursing activities for a short period and repeated some months later. E.g. with regard to adjustment of goals and quality of the ward.
- Reporting only expected nursing activities the use of planning and resource distribution.
- Reporting only actual nursing activities in order to document the work load.
- Daily reporting of both expected and actual nursing activities in order to evaluate quality of work compared to objectives, and as a documentation of the work load and for planning purposes.

The system is sufficiently generalised for other staff groups to be able to use it for planning and following up their activities. There have already been tests with occupational therapists.

The future

The Ward Nursing System today is used only by nurses. In a later phase it will be extended to incorporate a care plan, worked out in cooperation between patients and nurses. It is planned to provide word processing facilities, so that the system will become a computerized Kardex. Also information about the available staff resources will be an integrated part of the total Ward Nursing System, which again is an integrated part of the whole HIS.

DANHIS already has other functions for registering, for example, the patient's degree of self-care and for categorising patients. The collation of data from these parts of the system, from the Ward Nursing System and from other parts of DANHIS, (for example diagnoses and services such as operations, examinations and treatments), gives new possibilities for registering the total activity concerning a patient. This will allow the effect and quality of nursing care and treatment received during a period of care to be compared with the intended goals.

References

1. Ole Mikkelsen: "Changing from red to green" in "Software Report 4/88" - 1988.
   Article describing the development of the "Green System", the Danish version of DANHIS.

2. Nils Birkegaard: "User Authorisation in Distributed Hospital Information Systems" - March 1990.
   Paper presented at the AIM Conference on Data Protection, Brussels.

3. Jørgen Bagge Pedersen: "What is a guiding system?" - 1988.
   English translation of a prize-winning paper presented at the 1988 NordDATA conference.

4. Preben Etzerodt: The Administrative Information Systems of the 90'ies.
   Paper presented at the 1989 NordDATA conference. (in danish).

5. Preben Etzerodt and Svend Gylling: "The Green System" in "Tidskrift for danske sygehuse 8/1989" (in danish).

6. Karin Dørum: Patient Classification - Ressource Management in Nursing, Danske Sygeplejeråd 1984 (in danish).

7. DISS: Nursing Work Load. Patient Classification and Nursing Workload Measurement, 1984 (in danish).

A distributed system for the integrated management of general and subspecialist pediatric outpatient clinic [1]

Antonio Bernabei*, Vincenzo Currò‡, Alessandro D'Atri*, Giovanna La Cava‡

‡ Ist. Clinica Pediatrica, Università Cattolica S. Cuore, L. Gemelli 8, I-00168 Roma
* Dip. Ingegneria Elettrica, Università di L'Aquila, I-67100 L'Aquila

Abstract ARPIA II is a system for handling, on a local area network, a distributed enviroment of pediatric outpatients clinic. The main user requirements, standardization aspects and functionality taken into account in designing this system are presented.

1 Introduction

Working in an outpatient clinic implies that the physician must face complex problems such as handling a great amount of clinical and laboratory data, making diagnostic and therapeutic decisions in the short time of a visit and writing down concise but detailed reports of the physical examination. The more coordinated are the connections between the administrative structures, the medical services and the various specialists the more efficient is the outpatient clinic work. If the physician in the outpatient clinic has direct access to the diagnostic information available in the whole organization where he/she works, the patient will have the opportunity to quickly arrive at the end of his/her diagnostic iter. Furthermore, the outpatient clinic represents the link between the outside environment and the hospital wards, a consequence is that the patient plays a double role: both a person to care for and a social entity for epidemiological analysis. For these reasons, the variety of tasks to be carried on in ambulatory care requires an automation of both administrative and medical activities.

The introduction of information and telecommunication technologies to assist the health-care workers in pediatric outpatient clinics is the first issue taken into consideration in our research. Moreover most of the results we obtained can be easily extended to other kinds of outpatient care.

An efficient distributed computer system is needed to link the primary care community pediatricians with (general and specialistic) pediatric hospital departments (secondary care organizations). To reach these goals it is important to define and use a Minimum Basic Data Set for AmbulatoryCare (MBDS-AC), as suggested by the EEC [6].

Additional requirements for a system to be well accepted in the outpatient framework are: medical procedures must not be interrupted or delayed; it must be centered on the patient's data that must be available during the clinical examination; it must

---

[1]This work has been partially supported by the CNR strategic project on "Information systems for biomedicine".

take into account the needs of several users (physicians, nurses and patients), not accustomed to computer systems and having different levels of experience, and different roles in the health care system.

The research results described in this paper cover some aspects of the study, the design and the validation of a distributed system for the management of outpatient clinical records. The prototype we developed is devoted to the integration of general and subspecialist pediatric outpatient care by means of computer aided procedures.

2 From ARPIA I to ARPIA II

The modular development of a complex system, such as an outpatient clinic information system, requires a unique and integrated database. It is in fact necessary to divide data from procedures: data have common characteristics from the user's point of view and are stable in time, whereas there are a lot of distinct procedures for the several activities to be computerized.

The main previous result of our research on this topic was the ARPIA system (Ambulatory and Research in Pediatrics by Information Assistance), for computer aided ambulatory care [4]. The first version of the system, termed ARPIA I, was run on a personal computer and was composed of:

- a relational database of outpatient clinical records;
- a predefined set of computer assisted procedures to carry on the main medical activities, corresponding to database operations of different complexity;
- some advanced, user friendly, flexible and fast human computer interaction techniques to activate such procedures.

After one year of usage, ARPIA I had shown some limits in the fields of coding, organization and communication of data:

- the system was devoted to a single and autonomous outpatient clinic of general pediatrics, without considering its integration either in a more complex hospital information system, or in the enviroment of a pediatric outpatients clinic;
- the clinical record was composed of an excessive number of items, some having a greater and some a minor relevance, referring to the several aspects of a child's medical history, not taking into account the concept of MBDS-AC;
- the ARPIA I procedures, although conceptually correct and didactically valid, were unsuitable for the on-line usage of the system during the physical examination. Data input was done by means of very rich rigidly structured windows;
- the storage of data on magnetic devices used non-standard codes, without taking into account national and international standards. For this reason, exporting data was a very difficult task.

Hence a prototype version of a new system (termed ARPIA II) has been implemented. ARPIA II works on a local area network of personal computers to support activities of an outpatients clinic. It enables both an easy information exchange, and a modular insertion within a more complex health care information system, where inpatient and outpatient structures are supposed to coexist.

The more a doctor knows about the clinical life of his/her patient, the more correct is the diagnosis and the choice of therapies. But the clinical life of a person is characterized by clinical data (diagnostic tests, physical examinations, courses of disease, etc.) obtained at different times and places by different health care operators: to have an information system dealing correctly with such data, it is compulsory for data of the same kind to have common characteristics. As in our system we are mainly concerned about the physical examination, we devoted a great deal of attention to defining and using for every examination recorded a minimum and meaningful set of data: for example it is necessary to identify and group together enconters which are casually related. So the MBDS-AC must contain information about patient, pediatrician, payer, episode reference, health plan, encounter date, location, results achieved, problems and diagnoses, services provided and goals to be achieved.

The free usage of natural language is inadequate for the exact characterization of medical events composing a computerized medical record because of ambiguity which mainly depends on the context sensitivity and on the speaker; hence a more formal representation (codification) is needed. In ARPIA II codes were designed according to the following recommendations[2]: the user interface must display each code in natural language, physicians and nurses must be motivated and share interest in the data entry process, common standards are needed to store health care information, the system must automatically generate reports about diseases and causes-of-death, which are requested from central national and international health care organizations.

3   Some functionality of the developed prototype

The developed prototype is now working on a local area network between two pilot applications: the outpatient clinics of pediatrics and of strabismology, both at the Policlinico A. Gemelli of Rome. The system handles the data of each clinic and the data common to both, and it is used by both physicians and nurses working in the two clinics. Procedures available in ARPIA II can be classified in this way:

- Primitive procedures. These procedures support a single task such as data entry or data display. They are non intelligent atomic procedures and they allow the user to change, insert or read data. There have been several changes and enhancements as regards the corresponding procedures in ARPIA I. Most of the changes are aimed at increasing the friendliness of the system with new human computer interaction techniques.
- Complex procedures. These procedures are devoted to the implementation of multiple step tasks, following a suitable interaction protocol. Examples of complex procedures in ARPIA II are: a developmental screening test, a calendar of immunization, a set of telephone consulting protocols, a drug database and an appointment list.

The local area network permits the quick exchange of information about the patients regardless of the place where it is inserted. For example "electronic reporting" saves time in a specialistic consultations. In the system the physician can have his/her request shown on the specialist's monitor and the latter can give his/her answer directly in real time.

The ARPIA II database is organized in:

- the shared database, accessible to all the workstations and stored in a common secondary memory device. This database is composed of: general case histories, database administration items and data for the management of "electronic reporting";
- the private database of each outpatient clinic, inaccessible to other clinics and stored in the private secondary memory device of each workstation. This database is composed of the specialistic history data and the physical examination data (customized for each clinic).

The presentation style of the retrieved data depends on the type of the data :

- case histories data are displayed in the most talkative way;
- historical access (time-evolution of a clinical value) is displayed by a flowsheet form with values in chronological order;
- a data value of a single exam is displayed by the same form used for its input.

When the infomation to be inserted is not composed of a single item, the system enables the user to choose those of interest without filling an exhaustive form. The ARPIA II data structure that collects medical knowledge, which is in continual evolution, is easily accessible to the user. Such a structure is a tree because medical knowledge can be hierarchically organized into several levels of refinement, from more general to more specialized concepts. By using a suitable environment of ARPIA II, it is possible for the user to visit the tree and change its organization and contents.

Another goal for data input was to reduce free text in natural or artificial languages. This is obtained both by introducing standard data items and by providing all reasonable selection mechanisms supported by advanced input devices (such as a touch-screen).

Coded data have been classified into those coded only to save space in the mass storage devices, and those coded also for exporting them. In both cases codes are grouped in homogeneous lists and are displayed by means of dynamic windows. In the first case the window contains all possible values and one of them can be selected either by a pointing device or by a keyboard. In the second case the window displays, by levels, the codification tree described above, where a deeper level corresponds to a more detailed description. The user can only see the decodification in natural language of the medical data which is associated with each node: by means of easy interaction primitives the system permits navigation through the tree in order to reach the leaf-item of interest.

4   Discussion

The first requirement we considered in designing ARPIA II was that the database must give a meaningful and concise view of the clinical status of a patient. Hence it was necessary to use a minimal data set for outpatient care, according to international standards[6]. The MBDS-AC is one componnent in an extensible structure of Data Set for Ambulatory Care. The encounter is the only level for data collection, but the provision of outpatient care is potentially a complex process. The health plan, a planned health care process, consists of data from each encounter and may be clustered in an episode. An episode is a completed health care process, comprising one or more health plans. So a hierarchical model of the outpatient care process can be developed.

As the starting point of the classification used in ARPIA II, we took into consideration the ICD-9-CM [5]. Starting from this classification other digits can be added for clarity when considered necessary by the physician [7] [1]. In this way pediatric codifications can be evalueted, according to one of the goals of our research, and at the same time it is possible to obtain data aggregation by suppressing digits at the end of the code itself.

Since the main requirement taken into consideration in the design of the system (although not described in detail in this paper) is that the latter must be oriented towards people with little experience of informatics, the prototype design required the most recent and technologically advanced dialogue techniques, interaction environments and computer assisted communication languages. In particular we considered user interface management systems based on graphics, visual languages based on icons and direct manipulation, and i/o devices which are innovative for the medical field (some preliminary results can be found in [3]).

Finally we note that the design and the implementation of other modules, corresponding to distinct pediatric and non-pediatric specialistic outpatient clinics, becomes an easy task: this work has to be devoted only to develop ad hoc procedures and to add data of specialistic medical history and physical examination.

References

[1] A. Assimaculopolos, C. Le Coultre, V. Griesser, J.R. Scherrer: Nomenclature or classification? Proc. MEDINFO'86, Elsevier Science Publishers, 1986; 865-869.

[2] R. A. Cotè, D.J. Rotwell: The classification nomenclature issues in medicine: a return to natural language. Med. Informat. 1989; 14: 25-41.

[3] V. Currò, A. D'Atri, F. Prosperi Porta, L. Tarantino: A graphical multiwindow interface to an ambulatory information system. Proc. Computers in Medicine and Health Care. 1990; 206-210.

[4] P. Di Felice, A. D'Atri, and V. Currò: Functionality of the ARPIA ambulatory information system. Comput. Programs Biomed. 1990; 31: 125-137.

[5] ICD-9-CM. International Classification of Diseases. 9th Revision. Clinical Modification. U.S. Department of Health and Human Services (DHHS), Washington, 1980.

[6] Proceedings of the European Community Workshop on Data sets for Ambulatory Care. CHIC/WP3.3/A053. CEC DG XIII-AIM Project A1009 and A1026. April 18, 1990.

[7] F.H. Roger, M. Joos, P. Servais, Y. Legrain: International classification of diseases extensions: lesson from experience in Belgium. Proc. MEDINFO'86, Elsevier Science Publishers, 1986; 355-357.

Experiences with PATSY

An Information System for Pathology

A. W. Zaiss, Schaefer H.-E.[*], Klar R.

Department of Medical Informatics
Institute of Pathology[*]
University Hospital Freiburg
D-7800 Freiburg, F.R.G.

Abstract

The Institute of Pathology deals with more than 36.000 histological, cytological and autoptic reports each year. Furthermore it has to accomplish quite different tasks like patient care, research, teaching, management and tumor registry. Computers are used in all these fields. Thus the Institute a baseline organisation system for pathology has been installed since 1988. This system runs now for more than two years with any serious trouble like hardware failures or lost reports or inconsistency of the database. The system is upgraded to a large system with more than 60 terminals this year. PATSY software is written completely in MUMPS and supports all necessary tasks of the Institute. This paper describes the structure of the hardware and software in detail and discusses the advantages of our solution with regard to other published papers dealing with organisation systems for pathology.

Introduction

The Institute of Pathology and the Department of Medical Informatics installed a baseline system of PATSY (DSE-Company, Korschenbroich, F.R.G.) in december 1988 using a MicroVAX II minicomputer with 9 MB RAM, 460 MB winchester disk space and 16 asynchronous lines (10 videoterminals and 4 printers). The system runs under the VMS operating system and uses VAX DSM (Digital Standard MUMPS) as database system and programming language. Only the registration of order entries and report writing and all necessary management facilities have been implemented in this first step. With regard to the good experience and the very good acceptance by the user the baseline system will be expanded to a complete information system for pathology serving all important tasks of the institute (patient care, research, teaching, tumor registry, ...). This upgraded system handles more than 36.000 histological, cytological and autoptic reports per year. In the last two years there was no serious trouble with hard- and/or software. The new system will be ready to run during march 1991 and is described in this paper.

Hardware

The new central minicomputer is a DEC VAX 4000-300 model with 32 MB RAM, two RF72 winchester disks with one GB each, a magnetic TK70 tape for software maintenance and a 1.2 GB DAT drive to backing up the database (Pic. 1). All peripheral devices are connected via an ethernet LAN with one multiport repeater and terminal servers on each floor and also in an adjoining building. Personal computers are integrated directly into the LAN using ethernet adapters and DEC's PCSA-Software, a part of DEC's Network Application System. Thus it is possible to use the VAX 4000 computer as network server for MS-DOS disks, files and printers. Furthermore all PCs emulate a VT320 terminal for the use of PATSY. The system has a X.21 link through a LAN bridge to the department of Medical Informatics to maintain the system. In addition the system is connected by this X.21 line with the Siemens H90 (BS2000) mainframe computer of the clinic computer center for mailing pathologic reports to the stations of our hospital electronically. This slow X.21 (64 KB/s) line will be replaced by a fiberoptic high speed network for the entire university hospital some years later.

System Software

The VAX computer is running under the VMS operating system version 5.4. The database system and programming language is VAX DSM (Digital Standard MUMPS) version 6.0. Furthermore DECnet, VMS-Services for MS-DOS and FTSIE are installed. FTSIE is used to transfer and postprocess files between PATSY and the Siemens mainframe in both directions synchronously and asynchronously. FTSIE uses VOTS (VAX OSI Transport Services) on level 4 of the ISO norm. With the aid of VOTS it is possible to do interprocess communication between the departmentsystem PATSY and an OSI application on the Siemens mainframe computer. Thus it is possible to read directly patient data from the central administration ADABAS database (1) on the Siemens host computer into the MUMPS database of PATSY and vice versa.

Application Software

The application software PATSY is completely written in MUMPS and supports the following tasks of a pathological institute:

- **Order entry registration:** Acquisition of the patients data, the kind of specimen and the address of the sender. Record linkage to prior examinations of specimens of the same patient is provided automatically. (4 terminal, 1 printer).

- **Microscope working places:** Each microscope working place has a terminal to read former reports of the actual patient quickly and easily. Furthermore it is possible to setup, start and evaluate scientific retrieval queries. (17 terminals, 4 PCs, 2 printer).

- **Report writing:** This is the most important working place. More than 36.000 histological, cytological and autoptic reports must be handled each year. The writers complete order

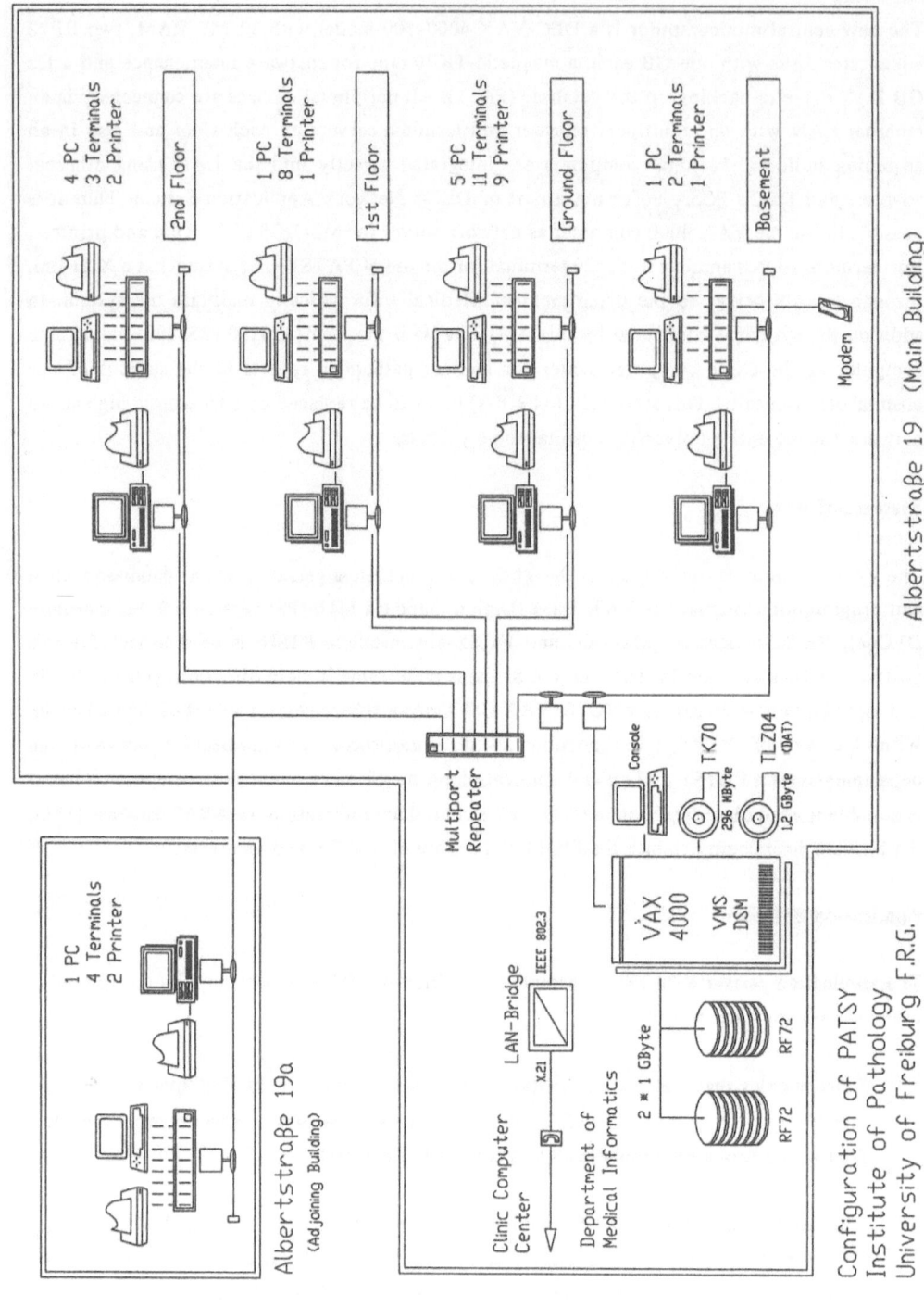

Configuration of PATSY
Institute of Pathology
University of Freiburg F.R.G.

entry data if necessary. Then the reports are written from dictation using the PATSY word processing facility. This can handle abbreviations, word modules, automatic syllabification, spell checking with a self learning thesaurus of pathological words and other important word processing features all well known from PC based word processing systems. At the end of each report the examined organ, the diagnoses and in addition keywords are acquired for the quick scientific retrieval.

- **Report mailing:** This is done conventionally until now. In future the reports of inpatients of the university hospital shall be delivered by electronic mail using the above mentioned file transfer and postprocessing product FTSIE to the Siemens host computer of the clinic computer center and to an ISDN based PBX system.

- **Billing:** PATSY provides different modes for private patients, inhouse patients and other patients. Furthermore an interface to the administrative applications software SAP will be implemented.

- **Scientific Retrieval:** This module provides different standardized queries using a variety of selection masks. Patients can be selected due to their age and sex. Specimens can be filtered by a registration number interval and/or the investigating laboratory. The interesting reports can be searched by the examined organ and words or word fragments of the diagnosis. In the case of malignacies it is also possible to use the ICD-O-DA code. Furthermore free text retrieval is also possible with any logic combination of whole or fragmented words over a preselected set of reports. Free text retrieval is more time consuming than structured retrieval and therefore this jobs must be submitted to the batch queue. The queries and the results can be stored permanently. For individual and seldom used queries we use the standard SQL-interface of the DASL (DEC System Applications Library).

Experiences and Discussion

Data processing in pathology is mostly concerned with the administration of order entries and the pathology report. The first function is a database problem the second one a word processing problem. With the aid of the programming and database language MUMPS it was possible to built the integrated system PATSY which was bought (DSE Company) and adapted to our purposes. An other advantage of MUMPS is the very good portability and the very good performance. MUMPS is available from PC up to mainframes. In general the database accesses are twice as fast as with relational databases. During the last two years we had not a single inconsistancy of the database. Furthermore the programming and string processing features of MUMPS allow the implementation of a very comfortable word processing system. The structured order entry data and the corresponding reports are integrated in one database. In view of the good experience with the baseline system during the last two years the system is now expanded to a complete information system for the institute of pathology providing modules for all main tasks of the institute (2, 3, 4). The VAX system architecture and DEC's network application support allow us to install a department system with a central database. Thus the reports are not splitted over different PCs. Each patient with all its registered reports can be accessed from any terminal by the registration number or by its name, prename and date of birth. On the other side PCs can be integrated into the network using DECs PCSA software. Files can be exchanged easily between PCs and the VAX computer. Furthermore it is possible to connect the VAX computer with our Siemens H90 mainframe using ethernet and OSI standard protokolls. The patients data and the completed reports of inhouse patients can be transferred easily by this way.

With this features PATSY fits very well in the general concept of the Freiburg hospital information system (2). Our system fulfils also the properties of the different types of computer systems as mentioned by Loy (1). The new PATSY system is also able to serve and integrate future tasks like workstations (5) and a pathology PACS (Picture Archiving and Communication System). During the last two years there was an excellent cooperation between the institute of Pathology and the department of Medical Informatics. Planning, project management, installation and maintenance of hardware and systemsoftware was done by the department of Medical Informatics. PATSY is maintained by the Institute of Pathology.

References

(1)   Klar R., Zaiss A., Timmermann U., Schrader U.: The Information System of the Freiburg University Hospital (See these proceedings).

(2)   Loy V.: Large Scale Data Processing in Pathology. The Information System of the Institute of Pathology, Klinikum Steglitz. Proccedings of 7th International Congress on Medical Informatics Europe 1987 in Rome, 347-351.

(3)   Richter H.A., Heinrich J., Mittermayer Ch.: Archivierung von Patientenstammdaten und Befunden per Datenverarbeitung im Pathologischen Institut. Schriftenreihe Medizinische Informatik 1984, Oldenbourg Verlag Wien, 143-146

(4)   Rupp W.: Computereinsatz im Pathologischen Institut, Erfahrungsbericht. Der Pathologe (1984)5:119-127

(5)   Ginneken A., Jansen W., Smeulders A., van der Lei J., Baak J.: A Method for the Acquisistion of Formalized Knowledge in Pathology.

Low-Cost Hospital Informatics in Africa:
The Ile-Ife Experience

R.O.A. Makanjuola
O.A.U.T.H.C.
P.M.B. 5533
Ile-Ife, Oyo State
Nigeria

O.A. Daini, H.A. Soriyan
Computer Science Department,
Obafemi Awolowo University
Ile-Ife, Oyo State
Nigeria

M. Korpela
Computing Center
University of Kuopio,
PL 1627, SF-70211 Kuopio,
Finland

A joint Nigerian-Finnish project has developed a low-cost multiuser system for the basic Medical Records functions of a teaching hospital, based on a standard microcomputer. Public-domain software from the USA was used as the basis and adjusted to local requirements. A four-user system costs about the same as two family cars.

Although the technology was found highly suitable, it is claimed that the successful establishment of a network of support activities is even more important to the viability or otherwise of computerized information systems in Africa.

Introduction: Health informatics in Africa

African voices in MIE or MEDINFO have been almost non-existent. Even in the only scientific conference this far dedicated to health informatics in Developing Countries [Fernandez Perez de Talens & al. 1983], just one paper and four participants represented Sub-Saharan Africa. This reflects Black Africa's weak position in world technological markets: 0.2 % in value of general purpose computers in 1980 [Kluzer, 1990].

One may even ask if it is decent to use computers in countries where simple diseases like measles are the main causes of morbidity. The ethical issues have been discussed in detail elsewhere [Korpela & Soriyan 1991], so it suffices to remind that there cannot be double standards. If computers are considered highly beneficial in Europe, then why not in African health care which is directly concerned with a basic need of the population?

If legitimacy is not an issue, finding suitable systems still is. As Forster [1990] points out, medical informatics (clinical decision support, imaging, etc.) is in general less relevant to African countries than health informatics in the broader sense (epidemiological, administrative, etc.). Systems designed for the industrialized countries do not suit the developing countries without considerable adjustment [Agbalajobi 1983].

Most developing countries are now embarking on a health care policy based on Primary Health Care (PHC), but within continued development and support of secondary and tertiary facilities [Adeyami & Petu 1989]. Computerization would be of questionable value on the field level of PHC, bearing in mind the degree of sophistication. Computerization would be more relevant to the central coordination of activities and data collection in PHC. This direction is currently being embarked upon by the Nigerian Federal Ministry of Health.

It is at the secondary and in particular the tertiary level that computerization would be most directly relevant to Health Care Delivery per se. Hospitals in developing countries are organized in just the same way as those of industrialized nations. The information procedures in these hospitals are often well organized and staffed but employ a manual system of storage and retrieval. Such systems are ripe for computerization, and can form a basis for coordination centres serving the PHC also, provided the costs can be kept low.

Microcomputers have opened up new opportunities for health informatics in Africa [Byass 1987 & 1989, Woelk & al. 1987]. In the project described here, non-expensive microcomputer technology is being used for supporting the basic Medical Records functions of a teaching hospital in Ile-Ife, Nigeria.

The Joint Project for Computerized Medical Records at OAUTHC, Ile-Ife

In 1988 the Obafemi Awolowo University Teaching Hospitals Complex (OAUTHC) decided to purchase computer systems for its Accounting and Medical Records Departments. At the same time, the Computing Center of University of Kuopio, Finland, established an experimental research project on health informatics in Africa. These developments merged during a Finnish researcher's stay at the Computer Science Department, OAU, in 1989.

OAUTHC comprises two hospital units, three health centers and a dental hospital in three nearby towns. It was decided that in the first phase the computer system should focus on the specialist in- and out-patient activities of the main hospital in Ile-Ife. Ife State Hospital (ISH) has a well established Medical Records Department in charge of the health information collection, processing, and delivery. More than 100,000 Case Note Folders are in the archive. The card boxes for the Master Name Index take up several square metres of space.

The Medical Records Department produces the daily Bed Statistics and Appointment

Lists. Moreover, diagnostics (ICD-9) and operations codes are extracted from the in-patients' Discharge Summaries filled by the consultants. Statistics for the Federal Ministry are kept about cases per code per month and year, using another large cabinet of cards. While OAUTHC is a teaching institution, the Medical Records staff often needs to find the Case Note Folders for patients with a given diagnosis for resident doctors doing research.

University of Kuopio has long experience with the public-domain software developed by the U.S. Department of Veterans Affairs (VA). The VA Admission-Discharge-Transfer package was compared with the requirements of ISH, and within a couple of weeks of programming it was adapted to reflect the existing manual practice.

The basic functions of the system are represented in figure 1. Besides that, there are the statistical and systems management functions. It is entirely menu driven, plain language oriented, and incorporates powerful data retrieval facilities

```
1    Inquire to patient data
2    Register patient
3    Admit a patient
4    Transfer a patient
5    Discharge a patient
6    Enter discharge summary
```

Figure 1: The basic functions.

for the advanced end user. The information contents and concepts are familiar to the Medical Records staff — for example, the Patient Inquiry display (figure 2) imitates the form on the inner cover of the Case Note Folder. Consequently, the staff adopted the system easily.

The VA software, besides being easy to use and available at a nominal fee, has one big advantage [Houser 1985]. It is portable from big mainframes to personal computers and, because of the MUMPS programming language, it makes a standard single-user micro into a true multiuser system. Using MUMPS and the VA software, today's powerful "personal" computers can serve from eight up to thirty display terminals connected to them.

After many comparisons, discussions, and a host of typical problems [Korpela 1990], it was found out that the hospital had funds for one microcomputer only, besides three terminals, cables from the computer room to three Medical Records offices around the hospital, a printer, and an uninterruptible power supply (UPS). One micro cannot run both MUMPS and some

```
TESTCASE,TUNDE FEMI                                          No:      124589
71 MOORE STREET             65 ONDO BY-PASS                  M 45 yrs  Marr.
ILE-IFE                     MODAKEKE, ILE-IFE                Born: 11/05/1945
OYO State                   OYO State                        X-ray:

Next of kin: TESTCASE,YEMISI ADELOLA (WIFE)
             Same address

Place of origin             Ethnicity       Occupation          Religion
IMESI-ILE/OYO               YORUBA          CARPENTER           CHRISTIAN
```

Figure 2: The patient inquiry display, imitating the Case Note Folder's inner cover.

other system simultaneously, so the Accounting system had to be temporarily postponed.

Key to success or failure: Network of support activities

The four-user hardware described above cost roughly equal to two Nigerian-assembled Peugeot 504s. Is it cheap or expensive? Compared to minicomputers or European health technology investments, it is very cheap indeed. But compared to the OAUTHC budget, it is still not a minor thing. In order to justify itself, the computer has to provide tangible benefits.

The system is still in its infancy. Now that the basic investment has been made, there are a lot of good uses for it. It has been planned that information from the laboratories, radiology and pharmacy will be incorporated gradually. No hardware expansions would be needed but the covering of relevant information would be significantly improved. Accounting applications have already been mentioned. An Inventory Control program for the Pharmacy and General Stores would enable better control of scarce resources. With the VA out-patient scheduling package also installed, all the data for a Billing System would be there, removing the need for patients to queue at several counters for different payments as today.

As the number of functions and users increases, the MUMPS based system can be expanded in small steps, adding more terminals and networking more micros. There seem to be exciting potentialities everywhere. But can they be materialized?

Alain Wisner [1983] has pointed out that successes and failures in technology transfer are related to whether the *totality* of the technology is transferred, including organizational and maintenance aspects, and so on. What matters is that a network of supporting activities is found or established. Engeström [1987] gives a useful, though tedious, framework for studying the development and interrelations of work activities. Without going into details we just point out that two support activities — hardware maintenance and systems development — are crucial for a computerized Medical Records activity.

Computer hardware maintenance is not too well established in Africa, but by sticking to the most popular manufacturer and model one can cope. Systems development activities are even less mature. Commercial enterprises which need just text processing and spreadsheets, can do with rather elementary systems support, but Medical Records applications can hardly be found off the shelf, and certainly cannot be expanded without Systems Designers.

The Computer Science Department, OAU, therefor decided to establish a MUMPS Group for developing the hospital system and installing it to other sites. The Department has also embarked on developing accounting applications with this low-cost technology.

Conclusion: Whither health informatics in Africa?

There are a lot of fruits to be picked for health informatics in Africa [Okeke 1989], and suitable technology is available. It is easier to use a modern computer system than to keep up a 100,000 card index box. Maintenance and electricity are problems, but not unsurmountable. The critical factor is systems development. What is needed is involvement of indigenous systems developers and cooperation between health care institutions.

A few teaching hospitals in Nigeria have seen the need for computers. The problem facing all of them is whether they get what they wanted. In that respect, the cooperation of the Computer Science Department and the OAUTHC is a model worth being regarded. We in the Joint Project wish to learn from others working with African health informatics, and to share our experience with them. Therefor we are planning to arrange a *Symposium on Health Informatics in Africa* in Ile-Ife next year.

References

Adeyami, K.S. & Petu, A.O. (1989): A health strategy for Nigeria. *Long Range Planning*, 22:6, p. 55-65.

Agbalajobi, F. (1983): Indigenisation of health informatics through adaptation. In: Fernandez Perez de Talens 1983, p. 173-180.

Byass, P. (1987): Computers in Africa: appropriate technology? *Computer Bulletin*, June 1987, p. 17.

Byass, P. (1989): Choosing and using a microcomputer for tropical epidemiology. *Journal of Tropical Medicine and Hygiene*, **92**, p. 282-287 & 330-337.

Engeström, Y. (1987): Learning by Expanding: An activity-theoretical approach to developmental research. Orienta-Konsultit.

Fernandez Perez de Talens, A. & al. (ed., 1983): Health Informatics in Developing Countries: Experiences and viewpoints. North-Holland.

Forster, D. (1990): Health Informatics in Developing Countries: An Analysis and Two African Case Studies. Dissertation. University of London.

Houser, W.R. (1985): Riding the VA MUMPS Underground Railroad: The evolution of the Veterans Administration Decentralized Hospital Computer Program. *MUG Quarterly*, 14:4, p. 3-18.

Kluzer, S. (1990): Computer diffusion in Black Africa: A preliminary assessment. In: Bhatnagar, S.C. & Bjørn-Andersen, N. (ed.): Information Technology in Developing Countries, p. 175-188. Elsevier.

Korpela, M. (1990): The Ife Project - Report 1989. University of Kuopio.

Korpela, M. & Soriyan, H.A. (1991): Health Informatics in Africa - Appropriate or Not? Poster presented in the International Symposium on Technology Assessment in Health Care, Helsinki, 23-26 June 1991.

Okeke, A.N. (1989): The role of computers in effective management of medical records. Paper presented at the 19th Annual Seminar/Workshop of the Nigerian Health Records Association.

Wisner, A. (1983): Ergonomics or anthropotechnology: a limited or a wide approach to working conditions in technology transfer. In: Shahnavaz, H. & Babri, M. (ed.): Proceedings of the First International Conference on Ergonomics of Developing Countries, p. 30-49. Luleå University.

DATA MODELLING FOR INTENSIVE CARE WITHIN THE INFORM PROJECT

Claire E. Yates[1], Mark S. Leaning[1], David L.H. Patterson[2],
Claudio Ambroso[3] & Seppo T. Kalli[4]
[1] Clinical Operational Research Unit, University College London, London,
UK. [2] Whittington Hospital, London, UK. [3] SOGESS, Milan, ITALY
[4] Technical Research Centre of Finland, Tampere, FINLAND

Abstract

The paper describes a data model for intensive care which embraces clinical data, operational management and strategic information about care evaluation, cost-effectiveness and planning. The model has been developed to specify database requirements for a new generation of ICU computer system as part of the AIM INFORM project. It may also contribute to the development of a common medical record structure for intensive care.

Introduction

The INFORM project [1] is concerned with the development, implementation and evaluation of a new generation of computer system for intensive care and other high-dependency environments (HDE). In this paper we describe the model of ICU clinical and unit management data which has been developed in conjunction with process models of ICU decision-making and tasks [2]. The model provides a detailed technical statement of database requirements for the INFORM system; no assumptions have been made about what type of database management system will be used. It has been developed in collaboration with clinical and technical groups in 5 European countries with the intention of specifying a system with European wide applicability (if not international).

The objectives of INFORM are to improve the quality, efficiency and cost-effectiveness of patient care in the ICU. To achieve these goals there are 3 conceptual data groupings that the system requires: clinical patient data; operational ICU management (administrative) data; strategic data concerning quality of care, effectiveness, etc. each supported by reference data, for example standard protocols, drug information, reference ranges for monitored variables and itemised costing data.

The methodology used for data modelling is an object-oriented extension to "entity-

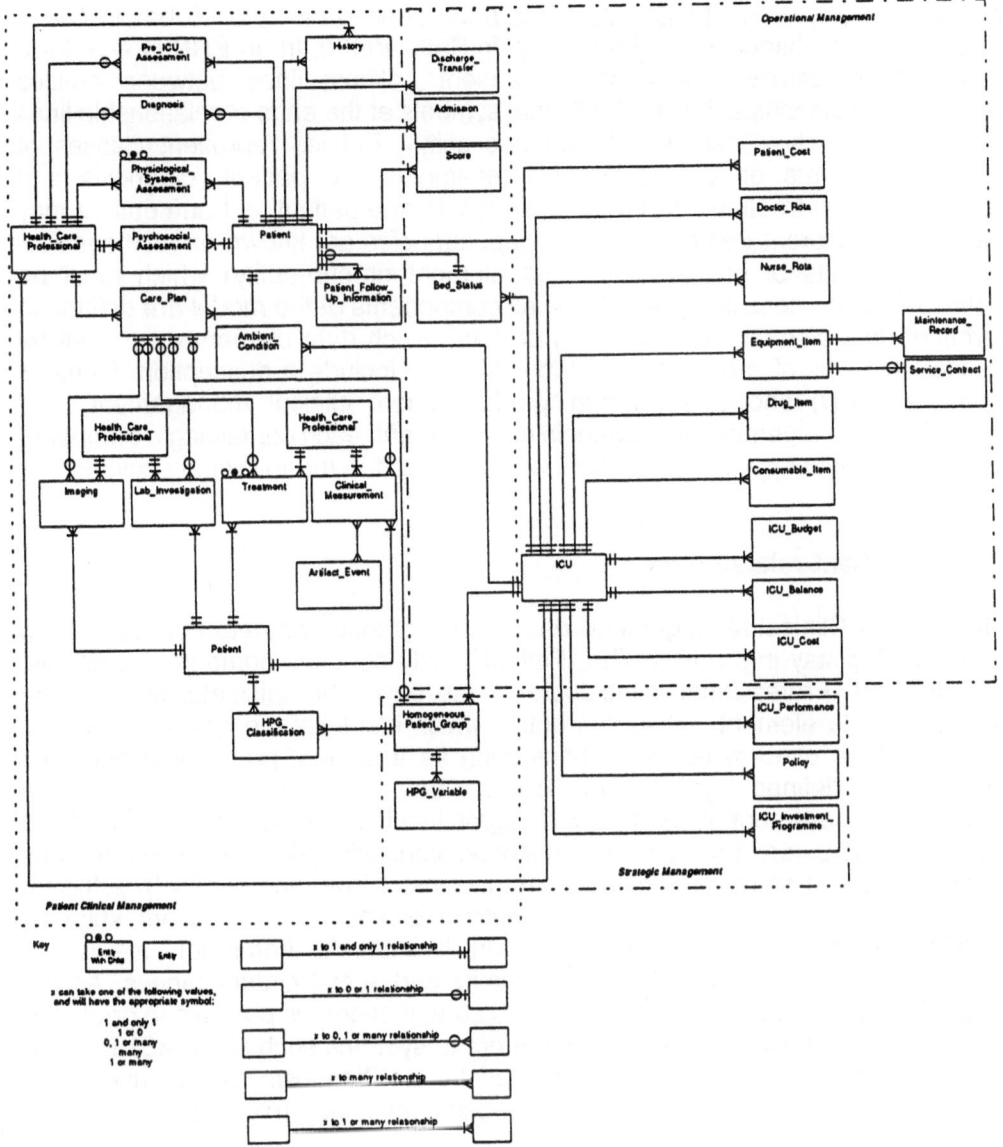

Figure 1. Data model for intensive care.

117

relationship diagrams" (ERD) which has been applied using a PC based CASE tool, System Architect (Trade Mark, Popkin Software)[3]. In an ERD [4 & 5, for a standard presentation] rectangles represent entities; lines between entities represent relationships (Fig.1). Additional symbols at the ends of relationship lines denote cardinality ("many-ness" and necessity). Entities represent classes of objects, concepts or events. Medical examples are patient, diagnosis and treatment. Each treatment will relate uniquely to one patient, but one patient may have many different treatments. Such dependencies are known as relationships. Entities consists of components (data element or sub-entity) which must be defined. This process is repeated until all components of the model are defined in terms of data elements (single items of data). Each data element must itself be defined in terms of a number of attributes which include a description. Figure 1 (top-level ERD) shows the groupings for patient clinical management, ICU operational management and strategic management; each containing a number of entities. Individual parts of the model are discussed in the following sections.

Clinical patient-related data

The "Patient Clinical Management" data grouping concerns data entities relating to a patient's stay in the ICU. The "Patient" entity contains demographic details. "Health_Care_Professional" is the doctor, nurse, physiotherapist, etc. caring for the patient. A data element, within this entity, which identifies the type of staff (e.g. doctor) will be used to restrict actions such as treatment prescribing and data access to defined groups of users. Before entry to the ICU, a "Pre_ICU_Assessment" is made of the degree to which the patient needs and can benefit from ICU care, i.e. intensive monitoring, ventilation, dialysis and other forms of life support. In some circumstances (e.g. transfer from another ICU), sufficient clinical data may be available to compute a disease severity score such as APACHE II on which to base the admission decision. At "Admission" a "History" is taken of recent medical illness and family and social circumstances. As the patient is monitored and treated during ICU care, it becomes possible to grade the severity of disease in a "Score", which refers to systems such as APACHE II and TISS. The patient is further characterised by a "Diagnosis" of the underlying medical condition, usually expressed as a taxonomic code (e.g. ICD-9 or Read).

During care, "Physiological_System_Assessment" and "Psychosocial_Assessment" are made repeatedly to assess the patient's state, problems, response to treatment and the opportunity for "Discharge_Transfer". Assessment data may come directly from the doctors and nurses, and also be generated by the decision-support functions of the INFORM system.

Treatment and monitoring plans are made in the form of a "Care_Plan". As a result of the care plan, specific "Treatment" will be ordered and administered. We distinguish between the plan and the actual order/record. The model has been designed so that "Treatment" can be ordered in the absence of a "Care_Plan". Following discharge, "Patient_Follow_Up_Information" may be obtained about survival and quality of life as a means of monitoring the effectiveness of intensive care.

Each of the following entities: "Treatment"; "Lab_Investigation"; "Imaging"; "Clinical_Measurement" is a combination of a prescription/order/request event and a record/result event. "Lab_Investigation" of urine, blood and other specimens is done by the diagnostic laboratory services and, to a limited degree, in the ICU itself. "Imaging" refers to X-ray, CT scan, MRI and ultrasound investigations. "Clinical_Measurement" is the measurement of the patient made by automatic means (monitors and treatment equipment) and manually by the bedside. Its data items include sampling rates, alarm settings, the raw data, alarms, and trended values.

Operational ICU management

This section of the data model (Fig. 1) deals with day-to-day aspects of ICU management or adminstration. Stock levels, costs and medical details are required for "Drug_Item" and "Consumable_Item". Treatment, monitoring and other equipment and their service plans and maintenance record are represented in "Equipment_Item", "Service_Contract" and "Maintenance_Record". Costs are calculated for "Patient_Cost" and overall "ICU_Cost", both of which are further divided into directly-attributable costs (procedures and drugs) and indirect costs (labour and other overheads). Budgets are set and monitored in the "ICU_Budget" and "ICU_Balance". "Doctor_Rota" and "Nurse_Rota" keep information on duty times of staff members. These will interact with the wider hospital systems. "Bed_State" holds information on bed occupancy and special equipment facilities offered at each bed.

Care evaluation, cost-effectiveness and planning

The following describes a methodology for patient classification which has been developed to allow cost-effectiveness assessments of ICU care to be made. Each patient receives an "HPG_Classification". An HPG is a "Homogeneous_Patient_Group" which contains all patients with similar diagnosis and disease severity. The "Homogeneous_Patient_Group" entity contains classifying information for an HPG and some statistics relating to the patients who have been classified as belonging to that HPG. Associated with each HPG are the statistics of a number of "HPG_Variable" such as survival, length of stay and costs. Each "HPG_Variable" entity contains a variable relating to a particular HPG together with the mean, variance and distribution of the variable for patients in the ICU concerned, and the values of these parameters in some other population to which the ICU is being compared. Such a concept will provide a platform for inter-unit comparisons, over comparable patient populations, of cost-effectiveness, outcome and quality of care. Other strategic issues associated with the ICU are "Policy", "ICU_Performance" and "ICU_Investment_Programme".

Conclusions

Future work on INFORM will include further analysis and design, prototyping and finally clinical testing. It is likely that the database will be implemented in a relational database management system initially. This will require normalisation of the model in Fig.1., eliminating repeating elements etc.. While object-oriented databases (OOD) have the advantage that the model could be implemented directly, currently, commercially available OODs do not have the performance of relational systems and there is no OOD standard comparable with SQL. Physiological and psychosocial assessment of patients plays a key role in deciding management, whether to discharge and when to withdraw care in the terminally ill. These aspects, and care plans themselves, have been difficult to analyze and structure, and still require substantial work. Although the model has been developed for general, adult ICUs it will be applicable to other HDEs after modifications and additions, but a complete data analysis will not be necessary. Similarly the model may be applicable to other areas of hospital care.

References

1. Bowes CL, Kalli S, Hunter JRW, Gilhooly K, Ambroso C, Leaning M, Carson ER, Groth T, Chambrin M-C & Cramp D. INFORM: Development of Information Management and Decision Support Systems for High Dependency Environments. In: O'Moore R, Bengsston S, Bryant JR, Bryden JS. eds. Medical Informatics Europe '90 Proceedings. Springer-Verlag Berlin Heidelberg, 1990:25-28.
2. Kalli S, Ambroso C, Gregory R, Heikelä A, Ilomäki A, Leaning M, Marraro G, Mereu M, Tuomisto T & Yates C. INFORM: Conceptual Modelling. International Journal of Clinical Monitoring And Computing 1991 (To appear).
3. Leaning MS, Yates CE, Patterson DLH, Ambroso C & Kalli ST. A Data Model for Intensive Care. International Journal of Clinical Monitoring And Computing 1991 (Recently submitted).
4. Chen P. The Entity-Relationship Approach to Logical Data Base Design. Q.E.D. Monograph Series on Data Base Management, no. 6. Wesley, MA: Q.E.D. Information Sciences, Inc., 1977.
5. Martin J & McClure C. Diagramming Techniques for Analysts and Programmers. Prentice Hall, New Jersey, 1985.

Acknowledgements

This work was partially supported by the CEC in its AIM programme (Project A1029). The Clinical Operational Research Unit is supported by the U.K. Department of Health. We would like to thank our project partners for their contributions to the model: Kontron Instruments Ltd., UK; Aberdeen University, UK; City University, UK; Uppsala University, Sweden; and INSERM U279, France.

A TEMPORAL DATABASE MANAGEMENT FOR
MEDICAL AND HEALTH CARE SYSTEMS

Ling DHO, Bell DA, Young IR

Dept. of Information Systems

University of Ulster, Jordanstown

Northern Ireland, U.K., BT37 0QB

ABSTRACT

This paper describes a new architecture (based on the relational data model) for the handling of time-varying data which is well suited for medical applications. This model also provides a heterogeneous distributed capability such that current and historical data may be stored on a network of different computing facilities. We have prototyped such a temporal data management system under the UNIX operating system using the C programming language which interfaces with the commercial relational database management system - Ingres.

INTRODUCTION

Time is increasingly being perceived as an important aspect in medical applications and yet is not fully supported in currently existing database or file-handling systems. Most existing database systems maintain only data or information about up-to-date current-views of the real world. Old data in database systems is normally overwritten by a new incoming data. Hence information about the past is lost. Generally there are two main methods of capturing the historical data: either by adding additional time field(s) to the database schema or by using a temporal system. The former method provides simple ad hoc time-varying values to be associated together these can be handled by the existing database systems. However, one of the serious limitations of this approach is that temporal (or historical) data may not be manipulated automatically by these systems; often end-users have to interpret the temporal results themselves. The latter method attempts to automate the manipulation of the temporal data by the system and hence improve the query processing capabilities. This paper addresses the latter approach. (Readers who are interested in the taxonomy and bibliography of temporal/historical databases can refer to [1,2] and [3] respectively).

We describe a new architecture (based on the relational data model) particularly suited for handling of time-varying data in medical domains. The proposed architecture for the temporal model overcomes several weaknesses of currently developed historical models (more detail can be found in [4]). This model also provides a heterogeneous distributed capability such that current and historical data may be stored in a network of different computing facilities.

One of the main features, apart from automated processing/archiving temporal queries/data, of our model is the ability to distinguish between the *corrective* and *progressive updates*. The *progressive update* implies that a more recent value supercedes its older value whereas the *corrective update* indicates that a value can be either incorrectly entered into the system or an external domain related error. Consider a patient attending a clinic who was diagnosed as having an eczema and treated with steroids. A few days later his condition was worse. Upon careful examination it was confirmed that he should have been diagnosed as having tinea, and be treated with antifungal agents all the time. Most temporal systems (e.g. [5,6,7,8]), which provide the progressive update mechanism only, would fail to record such common occurrences in the medical realm correctly. We argued that semantically it is important to distinguish between the exact status of updating data values (see next section).

OVERVIEW OF SYSTEM CONCEPT

Our temporal model is based on the relational approach and is similar to the multi-database approach for distributed databases [9]. The main difference between our temporal system and existing DataBase Management Systems (DBMSs) is that time related attributes can be stored, processed and manipulated automatically by the temporal system itself. Time related (or varying) attributes are represented in the same way as the other allowable data types. However each time related attribute *value* is associated with a three-field element: *status-kind, logical-time* (time when an event occurs), and *physical-time* (time when an event is processed by the computing facility). The *status-kind* field provides information which depicts the reason(s) for associating with its *value*. Once a value is stored in the computing device(s) it can not be erased. Therefore we use the surrogate key (a key generated by the system) concept for ensuring the uniqueness of tuples in the temporal database.

Consider the patient-treatment scenario again. (For simplicity, let us ignore the *physical time* and consider only the *logical time* with no intervals) The first entry for the patient, say, Mr. Brown, may look like:

PATIENT RELATION

PATIENT-NAME	DIAGNOSIS	TREATMENT	TIME
Brown	Eczema	Steroid	T1

A few days later, when time = T2, the temporal systems without the corrective update mechanism will become either:

PATIENT RELATION

PATIENT-NAME	DIAGNOSIS	TREATMENT	TIME
Brown	Eczema	Steroid	T1
Brown	Tinea	Antifungal agent	T2

or

PATIENT RELATION

PATIENT-NAME	DIAGNOSIS	TREATMENT	TIME
Brown	Tinea	Antifungal agent	T1

Clearly neither of these semantics is correct. In our temporal system such scenario is captured as:

PATIENT RELATION

PATIENT-NAME	DIAGNOSIS	TREATMENT	TIME	STATUS-KIND
Brown	Eczema (*2)	Steriod (*2)	T1	incorrect diagnosis
Brown	Tinea	Antifungal agent	T2	correction

note: (*2) - external domain related error with logical time = T1.

Therefore the *status-field* field plays an important role in temporal databases and is handled by our system.

SYSTEM ARCHITECTURE

Our model is pragmatic and therefore the system is loosely-coupled with existing DBMSs. This provides an additional advantage of flexibility for integrating with other pre-existing file handling or database systems. For easy management, we apply the multi-database philosophy [9] of data distribution to temporal distribution; i.e. we divide the temporal system into the Global Temporal Module (GTM) which coordinates and initiates a user's query, and four passive sub-modules. The Future Management Module

(FMM) records the future data. This is applicable to medical applications; e.g. a patient may be required to be under observation for a treatment over the next six weeks and hence he/she will have to make appointments in advance of current time. The Current Management Module (CMM) translates global temporal queries into appropriate requests and then submits these requests to the local DBMS. Results derived from the DBMS will then be sent or routed back to the GTM (note: each sub-module will contain a communication layer for routing information through the network. See FIG 1). The Historical Management Module (HMM) stores all historical data. The Auxiliary Management Module (AMM) records the data not normally available in other bases. Many potential hypothesis and their preliminary findings can be recorded here.

When a request is made at the GTM, its query processing layer will then decompose the temporal query into appropriate sub-queries and send to the appropriate sub-module(s) for results. All intermediate results will then be concatenated and further processed to form a final result at the GTM site.

The layered system architecture coupled with the multi-database approach provides a good software engineering approach with minimium implementation effort and also flexibility in allocation of historical data over dispersed computing devices linked via communication network. To this end it is possible to allocate different storage device media (e.g. magnetic tape/disk, optical disks, etc) to different bases according to its needs and characteristics of data. A possible configuration of the system is shown in FIG 1.

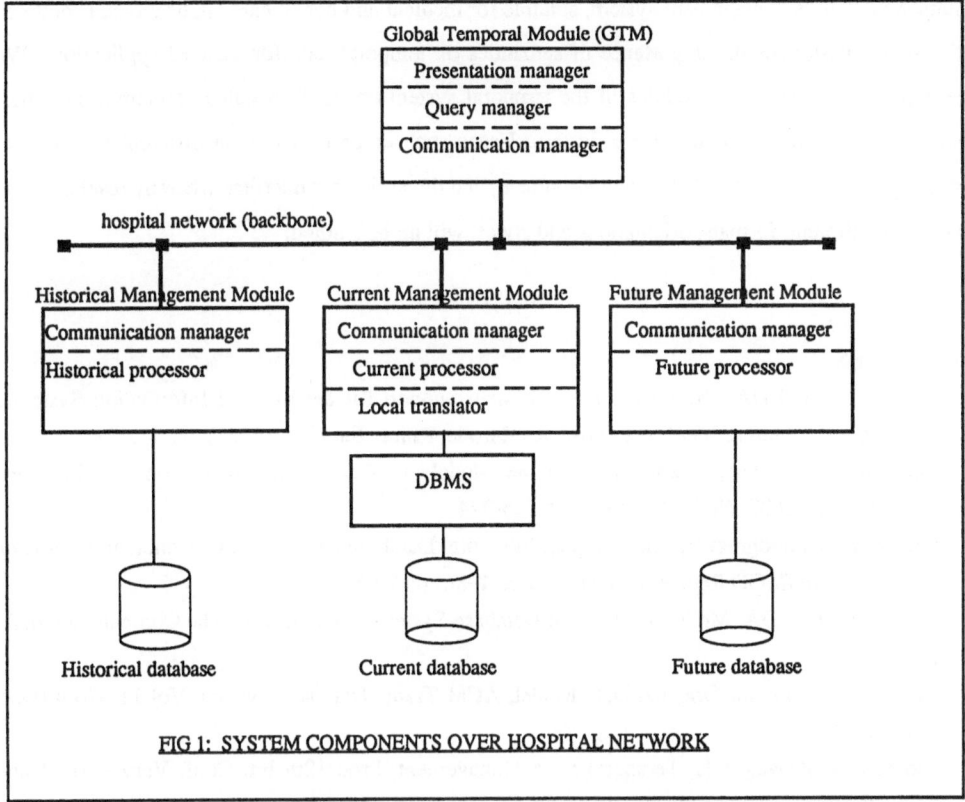

FIG 1: SYSTEM COMPONENTS OVER HOSPITAL NETWORK

IMPLEMENTATION

We have implemented the Global Management Module, Current Management Module, and Historical Managment Module, to demonstrate the feasibility, functionality, and capability of our temporal model, on SUN workstations and the DEC MicroVax computers linked via the Ethernet cable with the TCP/IP communication protocol. Both machines run on the UNIX operating system. Most of the software modules are coded in C programming language. All temporal data are held on-line using the magnetic disks.

Temporal queries are posed to the system using the extended SQL language. The system provides a range of possible temporal queries to be addressed [10]. These include the notion of NOW (e.g. SELECT NOW will return the system clock time) and complex temporal queries which may involve *temporal project, temporal select, and temporal join* opeations on multiple tables/relations (note: these operations are not the same as the classical relational select, project and join).

CONCLUSION

A temporal database management system, suitable for medical and health care applications, is outlined in this paper. It stresses the importance of semantics on temporal data for medical applications. We have implemented the main modules of the temporal system on the distributed computing facilities. More research is need to improve the system. Issues such as perfomance on different disk media, processing strategies in the distributed environment, and dynamic user interface whereby results can be displayed in different formats, orientations and styles, will all be studied.

REFERENCES

[1] Ling DHO, Bell DA, Young IR, Time Domain Support for the Medical Information Systems, Proc 7th Int. Congress Medical Informatics Europe, Rome, Italy (Sep 1987), pp 545-551.

[2] Ling DHO, Bell DA, Taxonomy of Time Models in Databases, Information and Software Technology, Vol 32, No 3 (Apr 1990) pp 215-224.

[3] McKenzie E, Snodgrass R, Bibliography: Temporal Databases and Research Concerning Time in Databases, SIGMOD Rec. Vol 15, No 4 (Dec 1986) pp 20-52.

[4] Ling DHO, Bell DA, Modelling Time in Database Systems, to appear in The Computer Journal, 1991.

[5] Ariav G, A Temporal Oriented Data Model, ACM Trans. Database System, Vol 11, No 4 (Dec 1986) pp 499-527.

[6] Shoshani A, Kawagoe K, Temporal Data Management, Proc 12th Int. Conf. Very Large Data Bases, Kyoto, Japan, (Aug 1986) pp 79-88.

[7] Snodgrass R, Ahn I, A Taxonomy of Time in Databases, Proc ACM-SIGMOD Int. Conf. Management of Data, Austin, USA, (May 1985) pp 236-246.

[8] Segev A, Gunadhi H, Event-join Optimisation in Temporal Relational Databases, Proc 11th Int. Conf. Very Large Data Bases, Amsterdam, The Netherlands (Sep 1989) pp 205-216.

[9] Bell DA, Grimson JB, Ling DHO, Implementation of an Integrated Multi-database-PROLOG system, Information and Software Technology, Vol 13, No 1, (Jan 1989) pp 29-38.

[10] Ling DHO, Query Execution and Temporal Support in a Distributed Database System, PhD Thesis, University of Ulster, Jordanstown, UK (Jul 1988).

SYGMA: A General Object-oriented Medical Application Development System

M. Madjaric, G. Gell
Department of Medical Informatics, Statistics and
Documentation, Graz University Hospital, Austria

0. Abstract

The authors are describing SYGMA, a general object-oriented medical application development system, which was built during 1990 in the Department of Medical Informatics, Statistics and Documentation of the University Hospital Graz, Austria. The system is intended to replace most of the existing applicative software for processing general medical data in the departments of diagnostic radiology, pathology, radiotherapy,etc.

In the introduction the authors are giving a brief outline of object-oriented programming, applied to medical application development. The authors describe the existing medical documentation system with its advantages and disadvantages, as well as the goals to be obtained with the new system. A brief specification of the pilot area (a radiology information system) for the new development is also presented.

SYGMA, a **SY**stem for **G**eneral **M**edical **A**pplications, consists of a stand-alone program for performing common medical data processing functions in an object-oriented manner. The general mechanisms and concepts are defined in the SYGMA program, but their behavior and the interaction with the outside world are described in the environment. This allows building the applications without changing the program itself, but rather by customizing the application environment (screen layout, parameters, control files).

Finally, the authors discuss the experiences with building and using the SYGMA system as well as intended future developments.

1. Introduction

In the 1990s software development lags behind the computer hardware capabilities, and the lag is increasing (1). Although the hardware requirements for an integrated hospital information system (HIS) are enormous, the previous statement can be applied especially to this area. Worldwide HIS experience shows very high costs for application software development and maintenance.

At the University of Graz, a set of departmental medical information systems based mainly on free text has been developed and used for more than twenty years (AURA) (2,3). Those systems are written in conventional structured programming technique and based on a flexible record structure and index-sequential files. The solutions chosen are well adapted to user needs and proven and accepted in clinical routine. However, as described above, the cost of programming new applications and maintaining and updating the existing ones became too high. Therefore we decided to develop new and more flexible software, following the objected-oriented approach.

The prototype of this new system - SYGMA - was used to implement a part of a new Radiology Information System (RIS) with the following features:

- patient admission including retrieval of previous reports;
- patient management, i.e. routing of patients to the different examination rooms, where the radiographer selects the next patient from a list on the terminal;
- recording of different examination-specific parameters (films, dose, time, drugs, contrasts, etc.), including data for specific fields (i.e. mammography);
- direct output of patient data to the film development machines for film identification;
- reporting.

The system streamlines department operation and gives all kind of management information (waiting and examination times, actual state of all examinations, billing etc.).

2. SYGMA system design

SYGMA system design is schematically presented in figure 1. The executable program SYGMA.EXE is developed in the Fortran programming language and intended to be run on DEC VAX computers under the VMS operating system. This program can access the needed number of indexed files organized by DEC's Record Management Services (RMS). Program execution is controlled by a set of parameters which are defined in the program environment. These environment parameters are placed in the DEC Forms Management System (FMS) description, such as FMS Screens, FMS Named Data and FMS User Action Routines (4), as well as in the VMS symbols and control files.

The SYGMA concept has been developed according to the earlier author's experiences in the general applications software building (5).

From this brief system design description we can see that the SYGMA system is a kind of interpreter, because the compiled program interprets during the execution time different external parameters which describe the application.

This approach allows several advantages in the application development process:

- only one (or some) compiled program(s);
- costs, efforts and complexity for the development of application instance are substantially reduced;

- high flexibility for adjusting the system to the specific user needs and environments;
- unique end-user application interface for different applications.

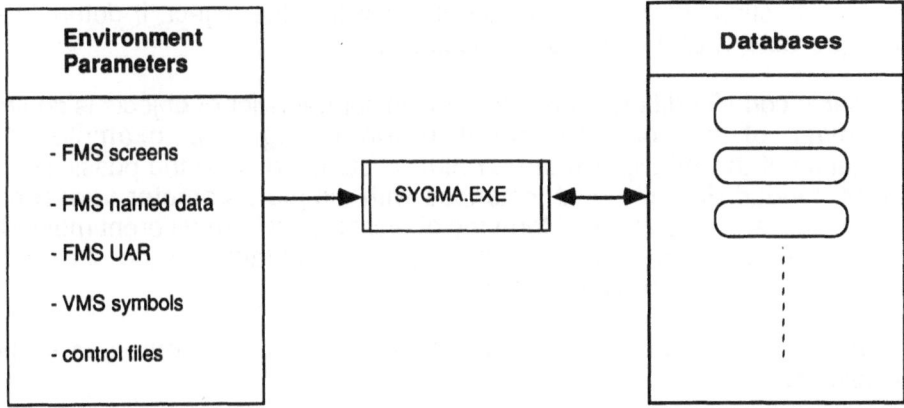

Figure 1: SYGMA system overall design

One of the most important characteristics which we had in mind when designing the SYGMA system were the issues of software quality. All of the quality elements applied to software products according to (6) are strictly obeyed:

- **correctness** and **robustness**: substantially easier to achieve than in hundreds of different application programs;
- **flexibility** and **generality**: FORTRAN programming is applied to the class (the application instance is programmed with parameters);
- **compatibilty**: proven in our new RIS by SYGMA cooperation with the existing system.

3. Object-oriented SW rules applied

Defining the application parameters in the SYGMA system is some kind of programming. With these parameters the application programmer defines field attributes, screen and field sequence, data conversion and transfer, stored information retrieval, data related checks and actions etc. Although all of these actions could be considered as procedures, we defined them in a rather object-oriented way as objects. We followed the object orientation as far as possible, applying the rules of the basic mechanisms, key concepts as well as the related technical terms defined in the object-oriented SW rules (1). The objected-oriented concepts have been translated "manually" into screen descriptions, parameters and control files.

The basic mechanisms of object orientation, that is the object, message and method, class and instance as well as the inheritance principle have been used to implement SYGMA. For example, we consider the screen (or the form) as an object: it contains both the data about screen layout, but also the instructions that operate upon those data (fields sequence). Of course, the screen object is a composed one, consisting of several elementary objects.

The set of instructions or the method is defined within the object. It determines how the object acts when it receives the message.

Using reusable code for different instances of similar behavior of objects is central to the power of the object-oriented programming. For example, the implementation of this principle in the SYGMA system led us to the possibility of defining all needed data retrieval instances with simple parameter variations. Thus, all instances of data retrieval form the object class, where different methods of data retrieval are defined. That shows the implementation of the class and inheritance principle in the SYGMA system.

All the four key concepts of object orientation are to some extent used in the SYGMA system:

- **encapsulation**: data access only through the object's own procedures;
- **abstraction**: common behavior (such as check mechanisms, data retrieval, and so on);
- **polymorphism**: interpretation of the same message depends upon the object;
- **persistence**: temporary and permanent object data in the storage.

Finally, some of the object orientation related technical terms or tools are implemented in the SYGMA system (such as dynamic binding, trigger mechanisms, agents), but others have no sense in an interpretative environment (BLOB) or need other user interfaces (visual programming).

4. Discussion and Experiences

The development of the SYGMA prototype needed about 4 man-months. Using the prototype to build a fairly complex actual application needed about 10 man-weeks, including user training as well as writing user documentation from scratch. The second figure is to be considered carefully: it was the application programmer's first contact with such a product, needed new SYGMA features were programmed continuously and there was no application programming documentation. We expect that the development of future applications shall need a substantially shorter period of time.

Despite of the additional difficulty that SYGMA had to cooperate and share data with an existing system, the expected benefits could be fully achieved. After relatively little initial testing no severe errors have been reported during the operation. The presumed advantages in the flexibility domain showed up very soon: the field specific only to one examination room (out of about 15) omitted in the analysis phase was added to the application (on the screen and in the data file) in a few minutes! The flexibility of the SYGMA system allowed also to the application programmer to tailor the user interface interactively in cooperation with the radiographers (the main end users).

5. Future

Further development of the system are planned as follows:

- replace the existing software in Radiology, Pathology etc. by SYGMA;
- new application areas completely made from scratch using SYGMA;
- new application programming interface, including also object oriented consistency and terminology ;
- new screen interface (DEC Forms);
- new reporting module (list and form capabilities);
- try to build a new "programming language" for the medical area to describe the application instance;
- new file access system to avoid Fortran RMS constraints and to allow the comunication with relational databases (RDB, INGRES);
- including new application functions in the system (for instance   patient scheduling).

6. References

1. Winblad, A. L. et al.: Object-Oriented Software, Addison-Wesley, 1990.
2. Gell, G., H. Becker: Computer in der Pathologie: Die Dokumentation von Autopsiedaten, First Int. Congress of Yugoslav Pathologists, Zagreb, 1969, Acta Facultatis medicae Zagrebiensis 18 (1970) Suppl. 1, 905 - 913
3. Gell, G.: AURA: Routine Documentation of Medical Texts, Meth. Inform. Med. 22 (1983) 63 - 68
4. - : VAX-11 FMS; Introduction; Utilities reference manual; DEC 1983
5. Madjaric, M; Kummer,Z: General Application Software, Proceedings of the Symposium "Community Information Systems", Zagreb, Yugoslavia 1984.
6. Meyer, B.: Objektorientierte Softwareentwicklung, Prentice Hall Int., 1990.

What *Should* We Mean by 'An Electronic Medical Record'?

S. Kay, A.L. Rector, W. A. Nowlan, C.A. Goble, B. Horan, T.J. Howkins
and A. Wilson

Medical Informatics Group, Department of Computer Science
University of Manchester,Manchester M13 9PL
+44-61-275-6133/5719 Fax: +44-61-275-6236

Abstract

Development of the PEN&PAD prototype patient care workstation[1] has made us acutely aware of the need to re-examine and analyse the basic requirements of the medical record. We present the work emerging from this analysis which we believe applies to any 'electronic medical record', and argue that the principal purpose of the medical record is to support *direct patient care*[2]. This is a fundamentally different position to many existing medical record systems whose designs derive, explicitly or implicitly, from the need to use aggregated data. Furthermore such a view has important implications for the standardisation of the electronic medical record. The goal is to create an architecture for the medical record which is faithful to the process of patient care and useful to and usable by clinicians.

Basic Requirements of an Electronic Medical Record

The current medical record has many well documented failings, but it has merits which are often overlooked: a) It is accessible to all clinicans; b) It is also readable (more or less), in precisely the same form as the author intended it. The organisation, style and layout of the recorded statements convey details often not expressed directly in the content. The adequacy of the record for the purposes of clinical care is directly related to its richness and its capability to assist the clinician to interpret the data and form a model of the patient. Its utility lies as much in what is left unsaid and in the relationships between what is said as in the raw recorded facts. These last points emphasize the individuality of the observer (and/or author) which is an important characteristic of today's record.

By contrast, current electronic records reduce a semantically rich original to a poor subset which is all but anonymous. This `shadow' can be readily accepted by current data processing systems, but much of the context and value are lost; a future record architecture should improve the record it seeks to replace, not impoverish it.

Electronic Documents require Comprehensive Structure

It follows from this that the first requirement of any electronic document is that it must be structured. This is a common requirement across application sectors[3] but of critical relevance to medical documentation in general and to the medical record in particular[4].

All clinically significant information must exist in a structured form if they are to be interpreted and used effectively by the system. Fundamentally, it does not matter whether the source of the structured information was pre-coordinated input (e.g. a forms interface) or a natural language processing system. (We would contend that pre-coordinated data, captured via systems of forms augmented by simple automatic encoding of phrases, is almost always preferable clinically, since it provides the clinician with cues which improve the completeness and consistency of data collection and help to avoid clinical errors. What is essential, however, is that ultimately the system has a structured model of the information.)

Faithful to the process of patient care

The major requirement which is unique to the medical domain is that the record be faithful to the process of patient care. Paradoxically, the chief consequence of this requirement is that the medical record is not about what was 'true' of the patient but about what was observed and believed by clinicians. Inferences about what was 'true' may be made on the basis of what was observed and believed, with greater or lesser confidence depending on the circumstances, but they remain inferences.

Furthermore, in this view the model of the medical record must be *descriptive* rather than *prescriptive* [5] The medical record is a faithful account of what was observed; what actually happened cannot be constrained to fit within a predefined view of what *ought* to have happened.

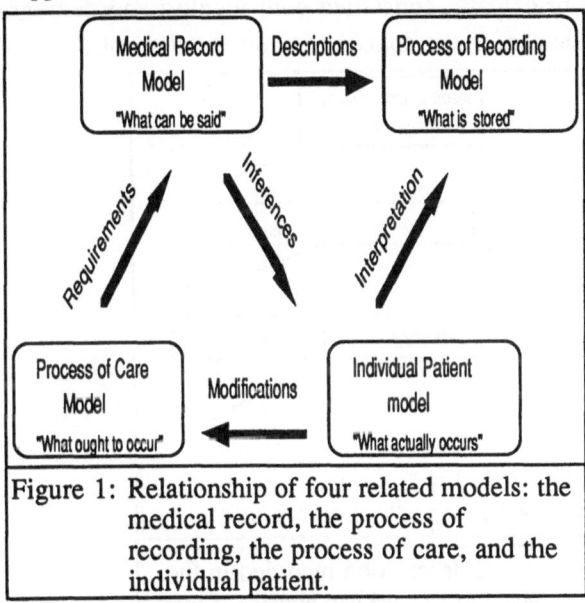

Figure 1: Relationship of four related models: the medical record, the process of recording, the process of care, and the individual patient.

We therefore distinguish the four different models shown in Figure 1: that a patient can have repeated measurements of blood pressure is part of the model of the medical record; how these repeated measurements are entered into the physical record is part of the process of recording; that patients ought to have their blood pressure taken repeatedly is part of the model of the process of care; that a patient can only have a single blood pressure at any given moment in time is part of the model of the patient. The paper focusses specifically on the medical record model and the process of its recording as these are both necessary to maintain a faithful record of the process of care.

The Medical Record Model: Statements and Meta Statements

The medical record is based on observations but contains much more than just the raw observations. It contains information on how decisions were made, how doctors viewed the observations, and how the various statements fit into the complex medical dialogue amongst the clinicians caring for the patient. To maintain this view and yet remain faithful to the whole process of care, the medical record must be considered as containing two levels of statements (see Figure 2) - statements of observations about the patient (level 1), and meta statements relating those observations to the decision making process and clinical dialogue (level 2). We argue too that the record must be *attributable, permanent and authentic* and that these properties apply to both levels of statement.

We concur with the EWOS categories of data and regard non-clinical statements as being those which are principally concerned with identity and demographic data[6]. Here we restrict the arguement to the domain of clinical statements.

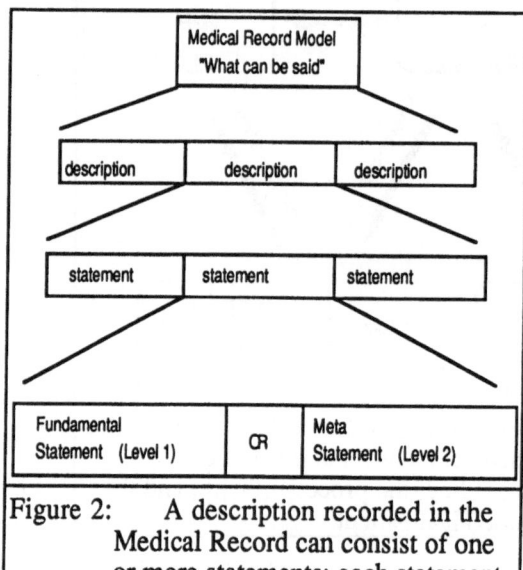

Figure 2: A description recorded in the Medical Record can consist of one or more statements; each statement is either a level 1 or level 2 statement.

The first level: Faithfulness to the observations

At the first and most fundamental level, the medical record consists of statements of observations of what clinicians (or other 'agents') have heard, seen, thought or done with direct regards to the patient. Examples of the Attributable, permanent and authentic properties of the record at this level include:

Attributable - Observations must have been made by an observer at a particular place and time.

Permanent - The fact of an observation is unalterable. Subsequent observations may show that the first observation was an error, but the fact of the observation remains unchanged.

Authentic - the record must reflect the clinician's process of observation accurately. Further requirements resulting from this property are discussed in detail in [7].

The Second Level: Faithfulness to the decision making process and clinical dialogue

The characteristic features of meta statements is that they can be altered without changing the underlying statements. For example, the choice as to whether the observations of 'chest pain' and 'swelling of the ankles' relate to one problem or to two separate problems does not alter the fact of the initial observations.

As an example, we identify two sets of decision making statements. The first set is used to group observations together with respect to problems, episodes, complaints and plans. These statements describe how the clinician viewed the basic observations. Note that on this view 'problems' are not themselves primary observations, but statements about observations. The second set of statements describes the reasoning process itself - the *justifications* for various conclusions. Clinicians' reasoning and justifications are vital information both for clinical care and for later audit[8], and are essential for many decision support systems. The three properties of the record model are also applicable to level 2 statements:

Attributable - Faithfulness requires that the time place and agent recording the information, as well as the observer, be recorded, since this may affect the confidence placed in the information.

Permanent - That a decision has been made or not made is permanent; it may of course be changed later but both events are audited.

Authentic - To adequately understand the clinicians actions, there is a need to capture the context.

The Process of Recording Model

The separation of the Medical Record Model from the *model of the process of recording* enables us to identify issues which are often confused due to their close association. The Medical Record Model is about what it is reasonable to say for the purposes of direct patient care. It follows naturally from this that such statements should be recorded faithfully in the physical record; i.e. that the authentic property of the conceptual model should be instantiated physically. The Medical Record Model, not the Process of Recording Model, should determine the actual content of the patient's record. By identifying the latter model it is possible to understand the practical implications of the medical record model and to expose the results of any mis-match between intention and practice. For example, if one equates the Medical Record Model to a classification system then the resulting record may degenerate into a collection of unrelated codes which violates a basic requirement i.e. that the clinician's understanding should not be distorted by the recording process, e.g. by being forced to code an overly precise diagnosis.

By contrast, the Medical Record Model described here has properties which require the recording process to be achieved in a principled way allowing, for instance, descriptions to be recorded to an arbitrary level of detail whenever it becomes necessary to do so. The distinction between the two models explicitly recognises that the difficult translation of psychological terms into physical ones has to be "addressed in the design, analysis and use of systems"[9]. Particular attention must be applied to the HCI issues if the role of the "Computer as Filter" is not to distort or even invalidate the information recorded.

Standardisation

The purpose of the 'process of recording model' is not to dictate specific details of how proprietary systems should be implemented. This is properly the domain of the systems suppliers. Rather, its purpose is to provide a conceptual reference to ensure that the stored information is faithful to the record model.

This issue is critical at a time when there is increasing activity towards standardisation of electronic medical records[6][10][11]. All these initiatives recognise the principle of 'openess'; the needs of both user and supplier within the market place. It is important, however, that neither the market place nor the technology determines the content of the medical record. We recognise the urgent requirement for standards now but believe it is essential that standardisation is at the appropriate level to permit extensibility[6]. The key to this with respect to the medical record is to do with the structure and granularity of the information, best illustrated by the following discussion on the use of aggregated data.

Aggregated Data

We have argued that the principal purpose of the medical record is to support direct patient care, that the requirements for security, confidentiality and analysis of aggregated data follow, as a matter of course, from the features needed to represent direct patient care faithfully and comprehensively. The greater become the demands to use the same information for many different purposes, the more important becomes the requirement that the underlying models of that information accurately reflect the nature of the information.

The approach described here must accomodate the important requirement for aggregated data if it is to be accepted by the user community. The use of aggregated data depends, fundamentally on the comparability of the data collected. The demand for a structured record is the first pre-requisite - without structure there is little hope of comparability. However, it is not sufficient. If two doctors use different criteria for the same sign, symptom or diagnosis, then their data will not be comparable regardless of how well it is structured. The natural demands of clinical expediency will always be, to some degree, in conflict with the needs of aggregating data for later use.

We would respond to this objection in three ways. Firstly, that the criteria for a given item belongs not to the medical record model but to the model of the process of care. The framework presented here makes it possible to separate the two issues and therefore to express the criteria and discuss them explicitly. In many situations, epidemiologically sound data can only be collected after careful clinical consensus. The medical record should be able to record that consensus, but to build it into the structure of the medical record would be to distort the actions of other clinicians outside the consensus group. Secondly, the fundamental limitation on collecting data for later aggregation is the willingness of clinicians to collect it. Structures which are faithful to clinical care are are more likely to be recorded faithfully. Thirdly, premature classification for one purpose reduces the capacity to reaggregate the data for other purposes. It is easier to regroup information and view it flexibly from different angles if it is collected in more detail at a finer grain size.

Discussion

In the light of these arguments, how can we answer the question posed in the title of this paper? Too often there has been a tendency to assume that 'electronic is better' while ignoring the question of whether or not users' underlying requirements were satisfied.

Our User Centred Design process in PEN&PAD [12] has shown the positive attitudes of clinicians towards using the medical record for direct patient care. The strategic importance of this approach is supported by a recent study of computerised nursing records conducted by Garber and Fitter[13].

Indeed, many of the requirements cited above correspond to those cited by others for the use of the record as a legal document (permanence, attributability), as a basis for decision support (recording of plans, expectations and justifications), or for purposes of communication(structuring of requests and responses). The other major uses of the medical record as sources of aggregated data have long been championed. Here we present a unifying, model-based architecture which in its prototype stage is seen by many to satisfy the complex and sometimes conflicting requirements of the electronic medical record.

On a broader front, the requirement for comprehensive structure leads to the requirement for a comprehensive model of medical semantics and medical language. Recent work by ourselves [14], Rossi-Mori [15]and older work by Méry et al [16] indicate that this is now possible. A practical model based on these criteria and encorporating a semantic structure of a significant subset of medical language has been formulated during the PEN&PAD project. The signs are that the prototype will scale up smoothly to a comprehensive system, but definitive proof must await the outcome of the next phase of the project.

References

[1]   Howkins TJ, Kay S, Rector AL, Goble CA, Horan B, Nowlan WA , Wilson A (1990). An Overview of the PEN & PAD Project *in* R O'Moore, S Bengtsson , JR Bryant & JS Bryden (eds), *Medical Notes in Medical Informatics no.40 MIE 90* , Springer-Verlag, Berlin, pp 73-78.

[2]   Rector AL, Goble CA, Horan B, Howkins TJ, Kay S, Nowlan WA, Wilson A (1990). Shedding Light on Patient's Problems: Integrating Knowledge Based Systems into Medical Practice, *in* L Aiello (ed), *Proceedings of the Ninth European Conference on Artificial Intelligence, ECAI 90,* Pitman Publishing, pp 531-534

[3]   Bryan M. SGML an Author's Guide to the Standard Generalized Markup Language(1988) Addison-Wesley Publishers Ltd.

[4]   Dvergsdal P, Hannemyr G, Hanseth O, Larsen H (1990). An ODA Based System for Standardized Exchange of Medical Documents. *in* R O'Moore, S Bengtsson , JR Bryant & JS Bryden (eds), *Medical Notes in Medical Informatics no.40 MIE 90* , Springer-Verlag, Berlin, pp 73-78.

[5]   Rector AL, Kay S (1989).Descriptive Models for Medical Records and Data Interchange, *in* B Barber, D Cao, D Qin, G Wagner (eds), *Proceedings of MEDINFO 89*, North Holland, Amsterdam, pp 230-234.

[6]   European Workshop for Open Systems (EWOS PT007 Medical Informatics). Study and Investigation of Problems Related to Standardisation & the Relevance of Open Systems Standards in Medical Informatics. Final report (1991)

[7]   Rector AL, Nowlan WA, Kay S,(1991). Foundations for an Electronic Medical Record. accepted for publication.

[8]   van der Lei J, Westerman RF, Mosseveld BMTh (1990). Critiquing based on Automated Medical Records: An Evaluation of HYPERCRITIC,*in* R O'Moore, S

Bengtsson, JR Bryant, JS Bryden (eds) *Lecture Notes in Medical Informatics no.40, MIE 90,* Springer-Verlag, Berlin, pp 369-374.

[9] Norman DA. Cognitive Engineering in DA Norman and SW Draper (eds), User Centered System Design(1986) Lawrence Erlbaum Associates pp 31-61.

[10] European Standardisation Committee(CEN). Directory of the European Standardisation Requirements for Healthcare Informatics and Programme for the Development of Standards.draft version 1.0(1991)

[11] Read JD (1990). Computerising Medical Language *in* H de Glanville and J Roberts (eds) *Current Perspectives in Health Computing HC90,* British Journal of Healthcare Computing, Weybridge, pp 203-208.

[12] Kay S, Horan B, Goble CA, Howkins TJ, Rector AL, Nowlan A, Wilson A(1990). A Consulting Room System with Added Value. *in* R O'Moore, S Bengtsson , JR Bryant & JS Bryden (eds), *Medical Notes in Medical Informatics no.40 MIE 90 ,* Springer-Verlag, Berlin, pp 73-78.

[13] Garber B, Fitter M,(1991). Who benefits from computerised community nursing records: a stakeholder analysis *in* B Richards and H MacOwan (eds) *Current Perspectives in Health Computing HC91,* British Journal of Healthcare Computing, Weybridge, pp 203-208.

[14] Rector AL, Nowlan WA, Kay S (1990). Unifying Medical Information using an Architecture Based on Descriptions *in* RA Miller (ed), *Proceedings of the Symposium on Computer Applications in Medical Care, SCAMC 90,* Washington, pp 190-194.

[15] Rossi-Morri A, Thornton AM, Gangemi A. An Entity-Relationship Model for a European Machine-Dictionary of Medicine. in *Proceedings of the Symposium on Computer Applications in Medical Care, SCAMC 90,* Washington, pp 185-189

[16] Méry C, Normier B , Ogonowski A. (1987). "INTERMED": a medical language interface. *in* J Fox, M Fieschi and R Engelbrecht (eds). AIME-87: European Conference on Artificial Intelligence in Medicine. Springer Verlage, Berlin. pp3-8.

Requirements for a Medical Workstation using User-Centred Design

R. Engelbrecht , M. Fitter [+] , A. Rector [*]

GSF-Medis Institut, München , SAPU, University of Sheffield[+] , MIG, University of Manchester[*]

Abstract

The development of medical information systems which can be used in the consulting room has led to independent solutions which are dedicated to specific tasks. Integrating users in the development process is a prerequisite to find the correct solutions to the medical problem and acceptance of the system. The PRECISE-CRS Project tested and enhanced the method of "User centered Design" to gather requirements for a medical workstation. This was done in specific European workshops with physicians from three countries for analysing and assessing human factors, requirements, and variations in scenarios and consultation simulations of different system prototypes.

Introduction

Information processing in medicine has matured to a point where many support functions in medical care and research are available. These systems, however, have been developed independently , resulting in widely varying operating systems, datastructures, interfaces, styles and technologies. In the clinical and research environment of today, the usefulness of these systems depends critically on the possibility of their integration: dataprocessing systems must be coupled transparently to each other and to information systems.

The advent of powerful graphical workstations poses the challenge to build a workstation that offers user friendly access to information systems and dataprocessing software in a clinical environment. This requires both a high level of integration and user-friendliness.

The project PRECISE (PRospects for Extramural and Clinical Information System Environment) concerned an AIM exploratory feasibility study and aimed at developing medical workstations for different medical professionals in different health care areas and explored different methods to gather information on the necessities of medical workstations.

Three different complementary approaches to the topic "medical workstation" covered all main functions necessary:

- the physician in his/her consultation situation
- the nurse in his/her office or at the bedside
- the researcher physician
- the patient

PRECISE could specify the major requirements for the design of a European Consulting Room System as well as a Hospital and Ward Information System. These specifications will provide the basis for industrial and research exploitation [1,2,3,4,5].

PRECISE CRS Subproject

Consulting Room Systems (CRS) are part of the European Community's exploratory action on Advanced Informatics in Medicine (AIM). These are steps towards developing systems for use in doctors' surgeries and consulting rooms across Europe. It's main objectives are:

- Testing of user centred methods for analyzing requirements and variations

- Analysis of the requirements for Consulting Room Systems
- Development and testing a style of user interface for a consulting room system

The fundamental hypothesis underlying the CRS-subproject was:

- If a European Consulting Room System is to succeed it must fulfill three criteria:
- It must be compatible with administrative and organisational features of the health care system in each country.
- It must be perceived to be useful and usable by clinicians in each country and each relevant clinical situation.
- It must be technically sound and compatible with the telecommunications and other information technology infrastructures in each country.

Two workshops were held to approach these issues, the Human Factors Assessment Workshop in which potential users were involved in the capture of requirements and the evaluation of the prototype in an iterative design-evaluation cycle and the Designers' Technical Workshop that focussed on technical and organizational issues.

The combined aims for the two workshops were:

- To demonstrate that user centred design workshops are feasible and valuable

as part of the design/evaluation cycle for AIM

- To apply the methology of the user centred design workshops to a range of

systems not developed locally.

- To gather information needed for a European design for a consulting room system.

The Human Factors Assessment Workshop

With the development of advanced technologies the time between the initiation of a new idea and its emergence as a product in the health care domain is increasing steadily. It is not uncommon for an advanced informatics product to take more than five years to get to a full field trial.

Establishing user requirements for innovative systems is difficult. Since the systems are radically different from the systems that the users have experienced, by definition, they cannot specify how they should best be used. In addition, health services and health care practice changes rapidly, so that there is a rapidly moving target.

The Human Factors Assessment methodology aims to support the development of advanced medical informatics systems to ensure that, as far as possible, the prototype or products developed meet the needs of the end users. To this end, it is based on a user-centred design and assessment process which provides supportive feedback to the system design team. However, the methodology can also be used to provide evaluative feedback to end users, project funders and other stakeholder groups involved in the development programme.

The methodology is particularly useful in contexts where the system will be used by clinicians during their consultations with patients. A major part of the methodology includes an assessment of prototypes in a laboratory simulation of the real environment, the authenticity of which depends on the resources available to recreate that environment. The focus of the formative assessment is on the following criteria:

- Functionality.
- Usability.
- Acceptability.
- Clinical impact.
- Social and organizational impact.

A comprehensive strategy for the evaluation of Knowledge Based Systems designed to support clinical consultations requires at least four levels of analysis: Verification, Validation, Human Factors Assessment and Clinical Assessment.

Verification refers to the comparisionn with the system's specification and internal static checks on the knowledge base which can be performed without test cases.

Validation refers to tests performed to check the accuracy of the results given by the system. Normally validation must be performed both at the level of the individual module
'Does the module produce the results intended when used in isolation and at the level of the integrated system
'Do all of the modules working together produce the intended results?'.

Human Factors Assessment refers to the assessment of human factors and organisational issues i.e. it addresses questions such as, whether the system is useful and usable, whether the system will meet other external health system and/or user requirements.

Clinical Assessment refers to testing via simulations or field tests whether the use of the knowledge based system in its intended environment is effective in improving the process and outcome of clinical care. Normally, it is a test of a system plus a user compared with either an unaided user or a user aided by an alternative system.

The function of the Assessment Workshop is to allow users to use a prototype system in as realistic a situation as possible, to comment on the system, and then to disuss both the system itself and broader issues raised by their experience with the system. Doctor-Patient Role Play with the system is used to enable as realistic a simulation as possible. Thus, the Human Factors Assessment Workshop will normally contain the following types of activities; which are organized in the following sequence:

. Introduction to the goals and steps of the workshops

. Training Sessions on the prototypes

. Simulations. Role play Using Scenarios developed by the design team in conjunction with the assessment team, the users simulate a Doctor-Patient consultation with the system: one user playing Doctor, the other the patient.

. Questionnaires After Role-Play, users fill out questionnaires on the software ergonomics and interface features of the system, the functionality of the system and other issues such as role playing technique and training. Normally, the users also fill out a questionnaire about their experience with computing.

. Small Group Discussions are held to discuss the detailed software ergonomics of the system. The discussions are moderated by the observers.

. Large Group Discussions are then held to discuss wider issues. The discussion is moderated via a senior member of the assessment team and the discussion topics are selected in advance. The design team may participate in these discussions.

. Immediate Feedback to the Design Team

The workshop activities constitute the part of the overall workshop in which the users are directly involved.

The function of assessing a prototype is to extrapolate from the prototype to the eventual system. By definition, the prototype lacks features and functionality of the eventual system - otherwise it would not be a prototype. The key to effective use of prototypes is understanding, and being explicit about, the remit of the prototype, i.e. to answer the question: "What extrapolations will be made from the assessment of the prototype?". The prototype is normally meant to emulate only certain parts of the eventual system's performance. Four important levels of prototype may be distinguished:

. User Interface Prototypes

. Human Factors Prototypes (Or Human Computer Environment Prototypes)

. Deep Human Factors Prototypes

. Functional or Architectural Prototypes.

The purpose of the prototyping is to extrapolate to the eventual system. User interface and human factors prototypes as defined above are by definition limited. The assessment attempts to focus on aspects of the design which are expected to carry over into the eventual design. However, inevitably, users sometimes become involved in minor features of the prototype which are of little long term interest. Doctors primary interest is in clinical questions. The choice of clinical scenarios and clinical information is therefore vital, since doctors can easily be diverted by minor clinical flaws.

The CRS workshops took place in Manchester February 1990. It was an experiment in extending the above described methodology for user centred design developed seperately at one of the sites (Manchester University) to systems developed at other sites and in other countries. It was also an experiment in involving clinical users from countries outside the United Kingdom.

Potential users and physicians from three different countries (Finland, Great Britain, Germany) participated in the evaluation of four different prototype systems during this workshop.

All of the four systems had been developed by other projects and loaned to the organizers. They had been designed to demonstrate different approaches and styles. The four systems were:

- the Pen/Pad system from MIG,
- the MEDAIS-Drug Information system from Germany,
- the Diabeta-System from St. Thomas's Hospital in London and
- the Oxford System of Medicine (OSM) from Imperial Cancer Research Fund London.

In addition there were a number of other systems being demonstrated but not formally evaluated. Both users and designers were encouraged to see as many systems as possible before the main joint plenary session.

User panels examined the systems, not to produce a formal comparison but simply to assess the usability of the interface and its functionality. The results of the assessment of each prototype were reported in four sections:

- functionality: What the system does
- Review of the System in Use: How the users interacted with the system overall
- Overview of Findings: General impressions and useful qualitative information
- Human factors:The ergonomic details and acceptance requirements

The specific issues relating to the software ergonomics of the user interface have been organised using criteria like visual clarity, informative feedback, flexibility, consistency, compatibility and explicitness.

The use of the contrasting systems served to stimulate discussions of the features needed to make a consulting room system effective. Combined with the observation they allowed the team to identify the requirements summarized below:

- the system should save time and/or enable the GP to provide a better standard of health care for patients.
- the system has to be flexible enough to support different consultation styles, because GPs across Europe have a great deal of autonomy in the way in which they conduct consultations with patients.
- graphical representation in particular time-related data, was seen as an important requirement for a CRS.
- a European CRS would need to cope with differences, like e.g. the administrative or medical-legal requirements or the symptomatology in the different countries.

In order to identify major requirements for a European CRS discussions were held about major design issues and the major administrative and cultural obstacles in the Designer's Workshops. Here, specific workshops investigated the similarities and differences between the medical systems in European countries and the problems that this is likely to bring to system designers.

There were four main areas of discussion, and each discussion consisted of pre-prepared oral presentations followed by a general discussion and production of report. The report was then presented at a plenary discussion to all participants.

The most striking result was the strong support for the idea of an integrated Consulting Room System (CRS). There was a high degree of commonality amongst the clinical functions needed in the consulting room situations in the various countries despite differences in administrative and financial arrange - ments. The following major requirements could be identified:

- the system should save time and/or enable the GP to provide a better standard of health care for patients.
- because GPs across Europe have a great deal of autonomy in the way in which they conduct consultations with patients.
- graphical representation in particular time-related data, was seen as an important requirement for a CRS.
- a European CRS would need to cope with differences, like e.g. the administrational or medical-legal requirements or the symptomatology in the different countries, and above all:
- the system has to be flexible enough to support different consultation styles.

Reports from the workshops produced recommendations for the CRS which were submitted to the Commission as Deliverable 3 of the PRECISE project [1].

Recommendations

The range and importance of the issues raised during the workshops indicated that such Human Factors Assessment Workshops will be essential to achieve an effective design for a European- Consulting Room System. The experience of this workshop provides strong support that such workshops can be standardized on a European scale.

The subproject CRS will establish means and procedures to ensure user centred system development and application. This can take the form of a central facility to assist with user centered design which might also sell its services more generally to the health information industry, incorporating user centred design techniques into programmes developing health care informatics

References:

[1] Engelbrecht, R., Fitter, M., Newton, P., Rector, A., Robinson, D., Sneath, L., PRECISE/CRS: Re- port on User Workshop, Deliverable 3 of AIM Project PRECISE, nr. A 1043, June 1990.

[2] Ahonen, J., Koskivirta, M., Saranummi, N., PRECISE/CRS: Report on State of the Art of Key Technologies and Emerging Technologies, Deliverable 2 of AIM Project PRECISE, nr. A 1043, June 1990.

[3] Langhout, A., de Leao, B.F., van Mulligen, E.M., Timmers, T., Gill, H., Ahlfeldt, H., Wigertz O., Generali, G., PRECISE/MW2000: Overview of results of MW2000; Deliverable 5 of AIM Pro- ject PRECISE, nr. A1043, June 1990.

[4] Heemskerk - van Holtz, P.R.B., Kraamer, K., PRECISE/BAZIS: The Use of Computer Applica- tions by Nurses at Clinical Wards in European Hospitals - An Exploratory Survey; Deliverable 6 of AIM Project PRECISE, nr. A1043, June 1990.

[5] Heemskerk - van Holtz, P.R.B., Nieman, H.B.J., PRECISE/BAZIS: Global Report on WIS-Con- cepts; Deliverable 7 of AIM Project PRECISE, nr. A1043, June 1990.

The Use of a Touch-screen Computer for Dental Charting

B. Richards and D. Khoury

Department of Computation, UMIST, Manchester, England

Abstract

This paper describes a computer software package which enables a dentist to maintain a database of patient records and to chart a patient's teeth directly into the computer via a touch screen. The monitor screen can display all 32 adult teeth at once, or any of the four quadrants, or a single tooth. In this way it is possible to replace completely the usual paper records. However, at any given time, it is possible to obtain a print out of the patient's dental chart and the other patient details, eg age, NHS number etc, at the touch of a key.

Introduction

With the almost universal use of computers in the service industries, it is not surprising that dentists are following the doctors and using the computer for patient records. In dental practice, a patient record will consist of patient identification details, a current dental chart, and a record of all work done by the dentist. Whilst the first and last of these three can be entered via the keyboard, a dental chart is essentially a graphic display of the arrangement of the teeth within the mouth. Whilst one might add to the graphic display of a tooth using the keyboard, or a mouse, the ability to modify the display using a touch-screen proves to be far more efficient and user friendly. What follows will describe a database built around a touch-screen computer system, one which is both efficient and user-friendly, and one which will enable the dentist to chart a patient without the assistance of a second pair of hands provided by his assistant.

A by-product of such a computer system is the possibility of the database being used in the Dental School for the training of the dental students. This too will be illustrated below.

The Computer System

A Hewlett Packard HP150 was chosen for this exercise as it has a touch-screen which can easily be programmed in BASIC and supports a large fixed disc. The philosophy throughout the design of the software system was that the touch-screen should be used instead of the keyboard whenever possible.

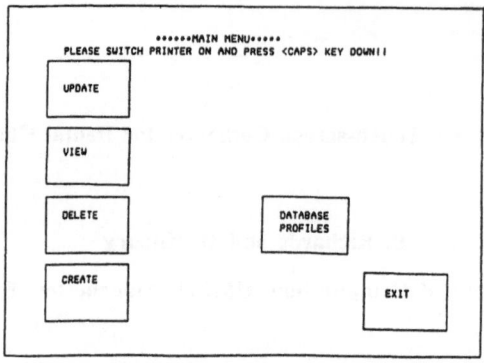

```
******MAIN MENU******
PLEASE SWITCH PRINTER ON AND PRESS <CAPS> KEY DOWN!!

UPDATE


VIEW


DELETE                    DATABASE
                          PROFILES

CREATE
                                              EXIT
```

Figure 1:   The Main Menu

Therefore, having initiated the system from the keyboard, the dentist (the User) will be confronted with the Main Menu, see Figure 1. This gives the User two distinct modes of progression, identified by the four boxes in the left-hand side of the screen on the one hand and the single box, right of centre, on the other. The four boxes on the left enable the User to deal with an individual patient record, whilst in the other mode the User can profile the whole database.

The Main Menu gives access to the patient record. The User will usually select the CREATE Record option first and then enter the necessary information. Subsequently he can UPDATE (amend) the record during each patient visit. Occasionally, the Dentist might simply wish to check through the patient's record. This he can do by selecting the VIEW option whereby he will be able to view on the screen the various pages comprising the record. The DELETE option will be useful when one is setting up a fictitious database, as for example, when one is teaching dental students.

At the close of a day, the Dentist will terminate the use of the dental database system by pressing the screen on the EXIT square. He will no doubt then use the computer for his accounts.

The Patient Record

The Patient Record consists of one Identification (ID) screen and one Dental Chart screen.

The blank ID screen is shown in Figure 2 ready for data entry. The User will enter the required data via the keyboard (the only occasion when the keyboard is used). The data required comprises the patient's name and address, age, sex, marital status, and, in the case of females, whether pregnant or not. (In the UK, patients who are pregnant receive free dental treatment). The User can enter the date of the next visit and any general remarks or reminders. Figure 3 shows a patients' ID screen with the fields filled in. The boxes at the bottom of the screen can be pressed to move on. The User will normally press the box marked TEETH.

For a new patient, the Dentist will then be presented with a blank dental chart on the screen. If the patient is an adult (as determined by the computer from the patients' age), a full set of 32 teeth will be displayed. If the patient is an infant, the dental chart will display 20 teeth.

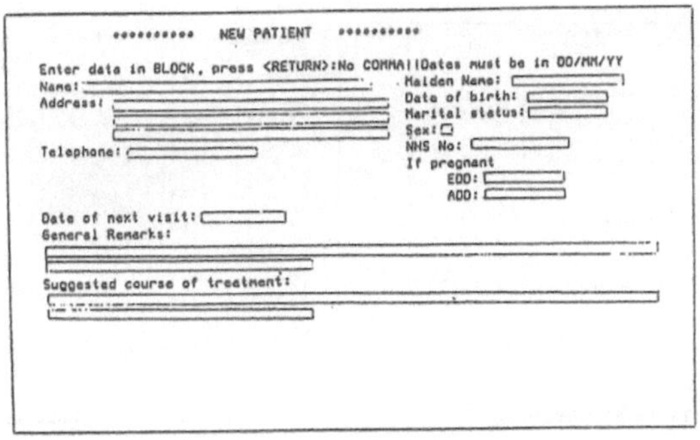

Figure 2: The Patient's Identification Screen (Blank)

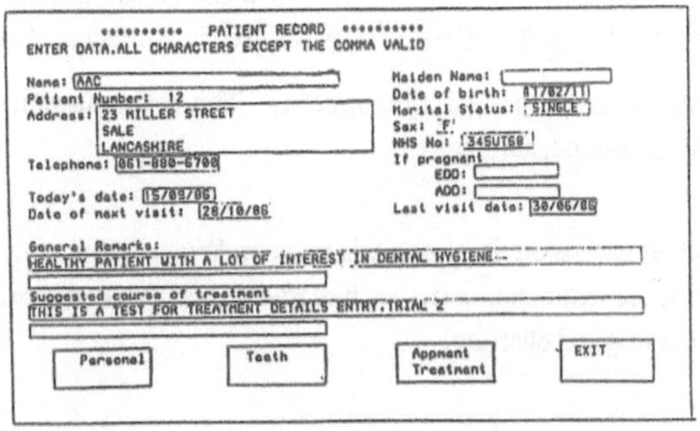

Figure 3: A completed Identification Screen

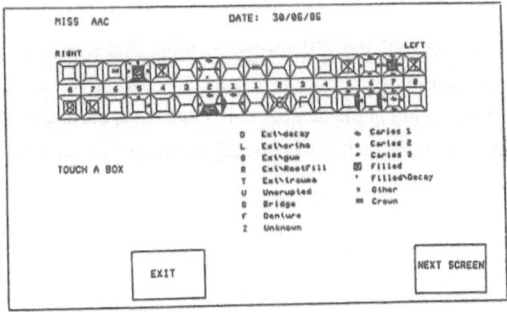

Figure 4: The full Dental Chart

The screen shown in Figure 4 displays the dental chart after the patient has been charted. This would not be the screen used for the actual charting as the teeth are too small to allow the up-dating by touch. A much larger representation is needed. When the dentist touches the box NEXT SCREEN, he is presented with a menu (Figure 5) which gives him the option of viewing the chart of one of the four quadrants (8 teeth). This chart is there for him to select one tooth for detailed display, a tooth now being the size of his finger tip, 2cm square. Thus, he finally arrives at one individual tooth, see Figure 6. He will now select, by touching, a box indicating the condition of the surface he has just examined, or filled. He will follow this by touching that surface of the tooth which is to be updated (in the computer) with the "condition" just chosen.

147

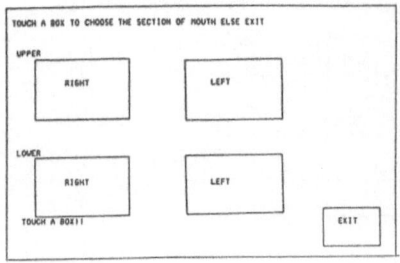

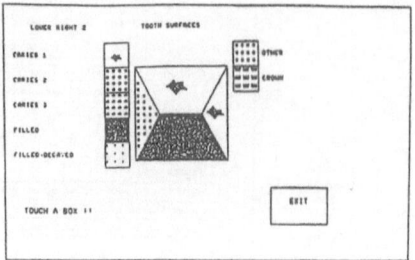

Figure 5:   The Sub-menu for Charting   Figure 6:   One tooth, Lower Right 2

The tooth shown in figure 6 has previously been filled on the buccal (outer) surface. It has grade 1 Caries on the Lingual (tongue) surface and on the Mesial surface. Caries Grade 1 indicates a surface cavity which needs coating to prevent further decay. The chart shows a Caries 2 cavity (which needs filling) on the Distal, left-hand, surface.

The dentist will chart each tooth in turn in this manner. When he has completed the whole set of 32 teeth, he can then commence treatment. After each tooth has been treated, the record will be updated in a manner analogous to the original charting.

Profiling the Database

The User selects DATABASE PROFILES by touching that square on the Main Menu (Figure 1). This in turn leads to the Sub-menu shown in Figure 7. This gives the User the choice of nine different tabulations of the information in the database. In each case, the age of the patient will be one of the variables in the two-way table which will subsequently be output on the printer.

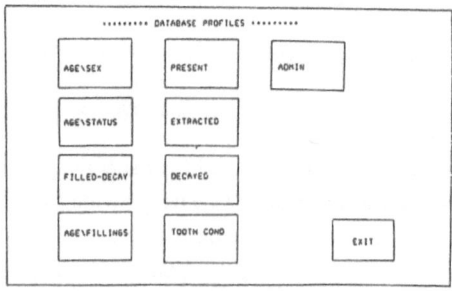

Figure 7:   The Sub-menu for Profiling

148

Use in Training

In the Dental Schools the tutor can set up a database of fictitious patients with teeth in various stages of decay. The dental student will be given the database on his computer and be asked to "treat" the patients. The student must go through each surface of each tooth and carry out the appropriate treatment, amending the chart when he has done so. The treatments will include fillings, crowns, bridges etc. However, in some cases the student will be expected to note the patients social conditions and the distance to and from the surgery. A pregnant lady with three children in tow is not likely to make frequent visits walking from a home several miles away.

At the end of the exercise, the tutor can examine the student's disc containing the revised database, and see what actions the student has taken.

Conclusion

What is unique about this system is that the dentist can chart a mouth merely by prodding the screen with the pick that he has been using to explore the tooth itself. The whole mouth can be charted without the need to touch the keyboard or to write anything down on paper. Yet, at the end, the dentist can obtain an accurate printed copy of the patient's chart.

The system is easy to use, efficient in storage, and a great time-saver. It can cope adequately with a normal size practice. A sensible extension would be to link the treatments, entered into the database, with the list of work done which has to be sent to the Dental Estimates Board to initiate payment to the dentist.

A.RE.S.:An Interface for Automatic Reporting by Speech

G. Antoniol (*), F. Brugnara (*), F. Dalla Palma (**),
G. Lazzari (*), E. Moser (**)
(*) I.R.S.T. - Istituto per la Ricerca Scientifica e Tecnologica
38100 Trento - ITALY
(**) Istituti Ospedalieri S. Chiara, Radiology Dept.
38100 Trento - ITALY

1 Abstract

The project and the first prototype of an interface for dictating, recording and printing radiological reports is presented. The most important feature of this interface is multimodality. The radiologist may choose among speech, keyboard and mouse to generate a report. If he is busy with hands and eyes, he can dictate most of the report, when holding and analyzing the radiographs. He can type the text and select some actions from a menu or click some meaningful icons when he has his hands free. The choice of the input modality depends on the "freedom" of the radiologist and the easiness and quickness of communication. The motivation for such a project, and the study of the impact of this system on the organisation of the radiologic department in terms of possible improvements on the reporting service, are also presented. The constraints on the radiologist-computer speech communication are analyzed. The interface has been tested with the speech modality. The speech recognizer has been trained on two main dictionaries obtained by processing chest and US reports. Four users pronounced 100 chest and 20 US reports, that have been used as a speech data-test for the automatic speech recognizer. The recognition rate of the speech recognizer, on the two dictionaries, has been 98% in the best case (speaker SP4) and 93% in the worst case (speaker SP1).

2 Introduction

High interactive user-computer interfaces, allowing the user to choose among different communication modalities, are now available. Speech recognition technologies, on the other hand, make feasible the development of high performance speech recognizers if the user follows some constraints in the communication process with the computer and when the application or the task fits some language requirements [1]. Isolated word pronunciation, speaker dependency and medium size vocabulary (2000-5000) are necessary constraints on user communication when high performances are required by automatic speech recognizers (ASR). The performances fall immediately when one or more of these constraints (i.e. multispeaker, continuous speech or large vocabularies) are relaxed. The "performances" of an ASR are normally related to "laboratory tests" run on a collected data base of speech samples recorded in a quiet environment. High performances in ASR are also related to the kind of language used in the communication process. It is well known that the probabilistic approach to speech recognition is the most widely diffused today [8]. An important component of the recognizer is the probabilistic language model. It can enhance the performances by 15-20%. Given a task or an application (i.e. report generation), the more specialized the language, the less complicated its modelling. An "artificial regular language " can be a lowest boundary in this case. The report generation language is characterized by a simple sentence structure, mostly telegraphic, consisting of complex noun phrases and a rich vocabulary [3] [4]. Once language requirements and communication constraints are defined, it is very important for the outcome of the system to study and thoroughly understand the role played by the speech recognizer in the interface. Therefore the purpose of the project shifts from the design of a speech recognizer to the study of a radiologist-computer multi-modal interface [5]. This is a key point: all the systems available suffer from this problem. This type of application is normally designed with only the ASR performances in mind. Changing this stand-point becomes a necessary condition for the outcome of voice activated radiologic reporting, and in general of all the applications involving speech recognition [6].

3 The Report-Generation Task

The radiologic department of S. Chiara hospital, Trento, produces, every year, an average of 80.000 reports, about 40-50% of which are 'negative'. The report generation task is organised in three different ways. Most reports are first dictated onto a tape recorder and later typed on a typewriter. In normal working hours, the emergencies are dictated by a physician to a typist. After hours the radiologist has to write or type these emergencies by himself. The average reporting time when the radiologist dictates an emergency report to a typist is about 2 minutes. This is a comparison boundary with every automatic dictation system. The most frequent radiological fields of reporting are: emergency, chest, osteoarticular, US and CT examinations. Altogether they cover about 90% of the work. It is well known that the estimation of a probabilistic language model needs a large amount of data. A choice has been made between modelling a general reporting language [7] or a set of sublanguages corresponding to different reporting methods. The later solution has been selected for two main reasons. First of all, it gives a more accurate estimation of the 'real' language used by the physician. Moreover, it gives the possibility to build a system incrementally, allowing a soft introduction of the new technology and better testing conditions. In order to collect data, two main activities have been planned. First, to collect as much data as possible in the short term in order to get an initial estimation of the languages chosen for the first version of the system, i.e. chest and US. Second, to substitute the typewriters with personal computers provided with a powerful word processor and an interface designed for a multimodal interaction. At present, about 2 million words have been collected, half of which acquired with a scanner system and an OCR (Optical Character Recognition) program. A PC has been installed and two other PCs will soon be available to complete the language collecting system.

4 A Multimodal Interface

The report generation task is very well suited for a multimodal interface and especially for introducing speech technology [2]. Most of the time, the radiologist is busy with hands and eyes, therefore using voice to dictate the report is more convenient. The main reason is that voice is the most common modality of reporting. In fact, the physician dictates onto a tape recorder his report, avoiding some typical errors due to changing modality. The radiologist can focus his attention on the radiographs instead of sharing it with other activities (typing or looking at the screen). Having discussed the reasoning behind our research we may now summarize the purposes of the project and the features of the first prototype. The purpose of the project is the development of a workstation equipped with a multimodal interface.

The workstation is characterized by four main features:

- automatic report generation by a physician without intermediate steps;

- better average time reporting (more or less the average dictation time of the report);

- reports and radiographs managed by a relational data base with data retrieval on line;

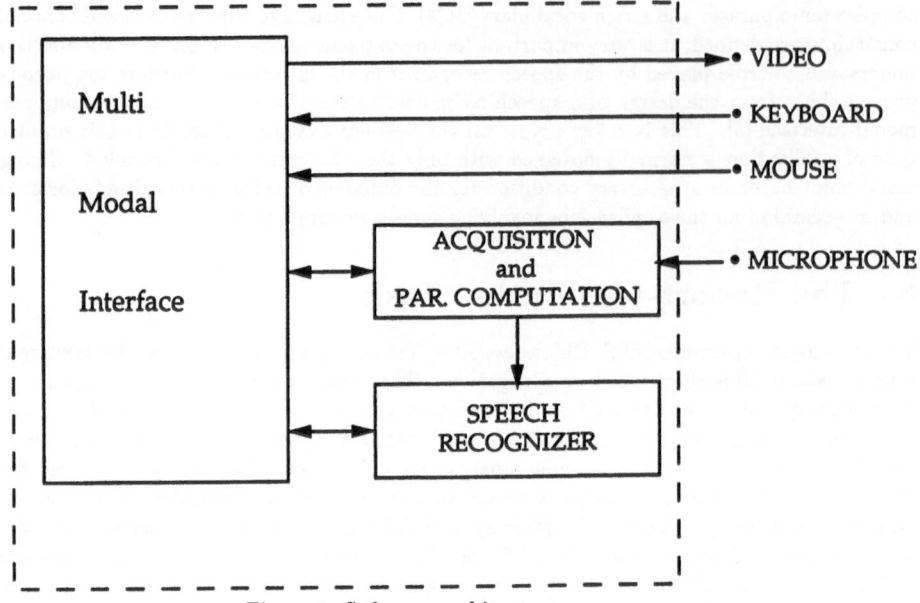

Figure 1: Software architecture

- connection to hospital information system for user's data and requests.

The multimodal interface, in the first prototype, allows the following operations :

- free dictation of the reports related to chest and US examinations with a small pause in between words;

- a short training procedure for adapting the recognizer to the radiologist's voice;

- recognition of medium size vocabulary (2500-5000 words) with the possibility to upgrade the vocabulary run-time;

- typing the report instead of dictating;

- use of function keys or keywords for generation of the negative reports;

- report retrieval by a simple data base.

5   Software Architecture

The multimodal interface is based on three main modules: the first is devoted to voice acquisition and parameters computation. The second, the speech recognizer, outputs a list of hypotesized words ordered by a likelihood score. The last module manages the multimodal user interface: it starts the acquisition, calls the speech recognizer, interprets keyboard and mouse commands and supervises all the user interactions. The first two modules have been implemented on two LSI DSP 32C boards, that mounts each a DSP 32C Digital Signal Processor. The programs have been written on a C and assembly language of the DSP 32C processor. The third module, written in C language, runs on a 486 or 386 PC under Unix operating system and X-window.

ACOUSTIC MODELING:	51 units extracted from 5 repetitions of a 1000 words dictionary pronounced by speaker SP1.
TUNING MATERIAL:	8 radiological reports pronounced by speakers SP2, SP3, SP4.
DICTIONARIES:	2500 words CHEST Dictionary (CD)
	3900 words US Dictionary (USD)

SPEAKER	MATERIAL TEST	DICTIONARY	TUNING	REC. RATE
SP1	30 chest	CD	NO	93 %
SP2	35 chest	CD	YES	95 %
SP3	35 chest	CD	YES	94 %
SP4	20 US	US	YES	98 %

Figure 2: Training material and recognition tests of first prototype

6 Experimental Results

Building an interface for automatic radiological reports is a process that we planned in different steps: developing a baseline system, testing the first prototype off-line, testing the system in an hospital environment. In order to develop the speech recognizer of the baseline system and test the first prototype, we have collected a text data base of radiological reports, as we already stated, and various speech data bases. The baseline recognition system, has been trained on the first five repetitions of a 1000 words dictionary (D1) pronounced by speaker SP1 (Moser) and a speaker-dependent isolated word interface. It gives a recognition rate of 94% on the sixth repetition of D1 and a recognition rate of 75% on the 5000 more common words of the text data base. In order to improve this recognition rate, a language model (LM) has to be used. The language models considered, based on the frequencies of the couple of words, were extracted from the corpus of radiological reports divided into chest and US examinations. Recognition tests and errors rates are summarised on Figure 2.

7 Conclusion

The first results provide two main considerations. The mean time for producing chest reports is about 1.5 min. and the mean time for US is 2.5 min, less than the time needed for typing the same text. Since the negative reports are at least 40%, there is no reason for spending physicians' time in dictating a predefinite negative text. Most of the errors of the recognizer are confusions between singular and plural. This does not affect the meaning of the reports and can be removed for the Italian language using high level linguistic knowledge. Future work will include several activities. An exhaustive testing on the LMs with more speakers and a first testing of the system in the hospital environment has to be done for assessing the global performances of our system and the impact of the new technology on the department organization. One of the main research activities in speech recognition systems is aimed at relaxing the constraints imposed on the users. The final goal of our system is aimed at removing the insertion of the short pause between words, allowing continuous speech.

8 References

1. G. Lazzari, "Riconoscimento del parlato: nuovi problemi e prospettive di ricerca",*Sistemi di Telecomunicazione*, June 1989.

2. A. Robbins, D. Horowitz, et al., "Speech-Controlled Generation of Radiology Reports",*Radiology*, 164, n. 2, pp. 569-573.

3. Medical Applications of Voice Response Technology Proceedings, Pittsburgh (PA), December 5-6, 1989.

4. G. Dunham, "The Role of Syntax in the Sublanguage of Medical Diagnostic Statements",*Analyzing Language in Restricted Domains*, LEA, London, 1986.

5. L. Hirschman," Discovering Sublanguage Structures", *Analyzing Language in Restricted Domains*, LEA, London, 1986.

6. G. Antoniol, F. Dalla Palma, G. Lazzari, E. Moser "Un Sistema per la Dettatura Automatica di Referti Radiologici", Proceedings of AIIM 90, Ed. Franco Angeli, pp. 21-28.

7. P. Alto, M. Brandetti,M. Ferretti, G. Maltese, F. Mancini, A. Mazza, S. Scarci, G. Vitiliano, "Adapting a Large Vocabulary Speech Recognition System to Different Tasks", Proceedings of EUSIPCO 90, pp.1379-1382.

8. L.R. Bahl, F. Jelinek, R.L. Mercer, "A Maximum Likelihood Approach to Continuous Speech Recognition", *IEEE Transactions on PAMI*, vol. 5, no.2, 1983, pp.179-190.

HOSPITAL COMMUNICATION
NETWORKS AND
PACS

THE NHS INTEROPERABILITY TESTING FACILITY (ITF)

P S Athwall and S A Mason
NHS Information Management Centre
19 Calthorpe Road, Birmingham, B15 1RP, England (U.K.)

The data communication services used by the UK National Health Service (NHS) have increased considerably during the last few years. The availability of good quality data communications services is recognised as a key factor in the successful implementation of the changes proposed in the recent government legislation. The NHS already has a considerable number of data communication networks, supporting many different manufacturers' systems. This paper briefly explains the role of interoperability testing, to ensure that users get systems that work, and the service offered by the NHS Information Management Centre.

1. The NHS Review - Data Communication Services

Implementing many of the changes brought about by the UK Government's review of the NHS will require the use of efficient data communication services. One major change in particular, namely moving the NHS into a more commercial arena - where buyers and providers of services need to exchange large volumes of information - will have a very significant impact. It will increase dramatically:

* The volume of data transmitted/received.

* The number of systems inter-connected.

* The range and type of systems that need to inter-work.

* The number and different types of access points.

In addition, several other areas take on a more significant role:

* The right degree of Security, Privacy and Integrity will have to be implemented on all network services.

* Approved audit procedures will have to be implemented.

Getting an application developed on one supplier's machine to run on another supplier's machine is difficult enough. Add to this the need to get all these different machines to interwork over a data communications infrastructure and it is clear that the NHS is presented with a very formidable task.

2. Interoperability Testing

For the last ten years, one of the main topics in the IT world has been Open Systems Interconnection (OSI). The aim of OSI developments is to provide the necessary international standards that will enable interworking between IT products from different suppliers. For such goals to be attained suppliers have to adopt the relevant standards and it is only of late that most suppliers are actually producing IT products conforming to internationally agreed standards. Suppliers can get their products tested for conformance at special approved test centres.

The creation of an International Standard is a lengthy and expensive process. It requires agreement by many international and national organisations and this is extremely difficult when there is so much at stake. As a result, the eventual international standards contain many optional features, so many in fact that a supplier can produce an implementation that conforms to the standard that will not work with another supplier's implementation that also conforms to the same standard.

In order to aid the development of OSI products to meet the needs of a user community, functional profiles have been developed. The early European work on functional profiles was carried out by the Standards Promotion and Application Group (SPAG). Currently the development of International Standardized Profiles (ISPs), is being undertaken through ISO. A functional profile narrows the options and parameters available in base standards. In the UK, the Government OSI Profile (GOSIP) has been developed by the Central Computer and Telecommunications Agency (CCTA) to meet the administrative needs of U.K. Government Departments [1]. The NHS has aligned its functional profile with GOSIP specifications.

To try to ensure interworking of communication systems, two levels of testing are required: conformance testing and interoperability testing.

a) Conformance Testing verifies whether the implementation meets the formal requirements defined in the profile to which it claims to conform. Conformance testing is therefore clearly defined by being limited to the protocol behaviour specified in the base standard.

b) Interoperability testing verifies whether the product in fact is able to interwork with other products and systems based on the same standard(s), and conforming to the same functional profile. Testing at this level is performed in an environment that maps, as closely as possible, to the real user environment for which the product is intended.

The existing conformance testing laboratories set up under the European Commission's CTS Programme do not provide exhaustive testing. For example, the conformance testing of FTAM (File Transfer, Access and Management) involves some 600 abstract test cases, whereas over 4000 test cases would be required for exhaustive testing.

Conformance testing is always the first step and interoperability testing the second step in the testing process. Neither testing level can replace the other[2]. International standards for conformance testing are now reaching maturity (ISO 9646)[3]. In the area of interoperability testing, there is very little national or international standards activity; here the work is undertaken on an *ad hoc* basis and is mainly user led.

To ensure that "applications" will successfully interwork, it is essential first to verify that the data communications systems are fully interoperable. This requires the behaviour of both cooperating communications systems to be fully acceptable to each other, including the handling of the possible error conditions that may occur. To examine an implementation's behaviour to all possible error conditions that could arise in such circumstances requires extensive testing using sophisticated tests and test equipment.

3. Current International Scene

The need for interoperability testing was identified by IT suppliers and manufacturers who wanted to demonstrate their capability of interworking with other suppliers at various exhibitions. This was a purely *ad hoc* arrangement; however, more formalised methods for interoperability testing are beginning to emerge:

* In Europe the collaboration agreement between SPAG and EurOSInet.

* Internationally, the newly launched US based initiative, OSI^{one}, is providing world-wide collaboration on interoperability testing methodologies.

The OSI^{one} initiative aims to provide worldwide coverage of interoperability testing services and a mechanism by which testing and test results can be recorded. In practical terms this should result in agreements on interoperability testing specifications [4].

During 1990, EurOSInet in Europe and OSInet in USA, were joined by similar organisations in Japan, Singapore, Hong Kong, Australia and Italy. They agreed to collaborate with OSI^{one} in producing and agreeing interoperability test suites. This will provide comparable interoperability testing facilities on a global basis.

All the test suites used by the respective national organisations are approved by the other member organisations.

At the beginning of 1991, SPAG initiated a major work programme entitled "Process to Support Interoperability (PSI)". PSI is a multivendor quality code of conduct aimed at securing user confidence in open systems and stimulating product development. The award of a SPAG trade mark is achieved through several steps: profile selection, conformance testing, interoperability evaluation and possibly conciliation.

4. The scope of the NHS ITF

With all the activity that's taking place internationally, why has the IMC created its own interoperability testing facility (ITF)? To answer such a question one needs to look at the aims of the international testing services, such as EurOSInet, and its members. Firstly, over 90% of members are suppliers whose prime concern is increased marketing by demonstrating interworking with other suppliers. Secondly and looking specifically at X.400, of the 90 or so tests available, a supplier has only to perform the 5 mandatory tests to claim interoperability; the rest are optional. IMC experience has shown that, to prove successful interoperability requires in the region of some 100 tests. Obviously, performing this number of tests is not only time consuming but also expensive. This degree of testing also requires much greater cooperation by the suppliers involved and can these suppliers agree on their potential customer's requirements?

Development and operation of interoperability testing facilities is a very expensive business. The specialist skills required are scarce. The NHS is a very large organisation with several hundred constituent bodies. To have testing facilities replicated by different parts of the NHS would not only be impossible but a very inefficient use of valuable resources. The results of a feasibility study recommended the establishment of an NHS central facility which would provide the interoperability testing service and also develop and maintain staff with the skills that are needed to carry out and interpret the test results.

The NHS Information Management Centre has, with the assistance of the National Computing Centre (NCC), set up facilities that enable testing of the OSI "Upper Layer" services. Interoperability testing is provided for Message Handling Service, X.400 (1984) and File Transfer, Access and Management (FTAM), ISO 8571.

The international interoperability testing service available is described as "passive", that is monitoring instances of communication between implementations to determine behaviour. "Active" testing, the injection of error conditions into the communication in order to drive the communication through a define state/event, is not available from EurOSInet or the OSI^{one} initiative.

The IMC ITF offers, to Health Authorities and other NHS bodies, full interoperability testing, "passive" and "active", of both Message Handling Service, X.400 (1984) and FTAM. The test service can be accessed using British Telecom's X.25 based Packet SwitchStream (PSS) network or locally over the LAN (ISO 8802-3) at the IMC offices in Birmingham.

The interoperability testing does not repeat any conformance tests. To determine whether or not two implementations are likely to interwork, the first phase of interoperability testing is the examination of each implementation's completed Protocol Implementation Conformance Statement (PICS). For implementations that conform to the agreed functional profiles, the next stage is to agree those optional facilities that are not implemented so the relevant test can be excluded. The implementation under test is then subjected to the agreed test suite. Figure 1 shows a schematic of the interoperability testing facility. The results of each test are recorded in a formal report. This report not only records the test results but also lists the tests not included and specifies the environment in which the implementations where tested.

Figure 1: Interoperability testing facility schematic

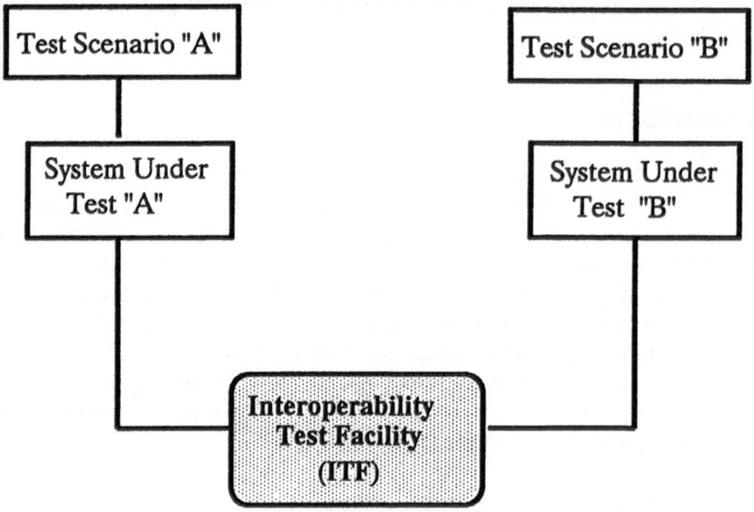

The outcome of the various tests that are performed on each implementation are monitored and recorded by the IMC system. This system consists of a Sun Series 4 Workstation which runs the NCC OsmOSIs software. The NCC software acts as a relay through which all signals have to pass. This enables the monitoring of the signals that flow through the upper layers stack and between each implementation. To ease the test operator's task, specific test files and messages have been created. These files, together with script files that assist in the tailoring of the test files for specific operating environments, enable the test operator to quickly create the data necessary for any specific test. Documentation is available covering all aspects of the ITF service:

(i)   The test purposes for each upper layer application that interoperability testing can be performed.

(ii)   Test procedures manual for each application tested.

(iii) The available test suite for each application.

(iv) Sample test Reports.

5. The Future

The IMC has started the implementation of an X.500 Directory Service and plans to create an "NHS-wide" Directory. The MHS service will be upgraded to the 1988 version of X.400, supporting added security features and a Message Store. The IMC is undertaking preparatory work to establish an NHS Registration Authority for network addressing and X.400, originator and recipient names.

It is unlikely that there will ever be an interoperability testing service that will completely cover all possible combinations of different suppliers' products. Large organisations, like the NHS, will have to review the results from interoperability testing and subsequent operational use. The enhancement to implementations previously tested will necessitate periodic reviews of their continued interoperability with both new and old implementations.

Currently, very little "active" interoperability testing is performed. However, this is likely to increase and may need to address issues and "real effects" which are outside the scope of the base standards.

References

1. --, U.K. "Government OSI Profile (version 3.1)", HMSO, London, January 1990.

2. Lamb N, "User requirements for Conformance Testing and Certification", Proceedings of the European Conference on Conformance Testing & Certification in IT&T, European Commission, Brussels, June 1990.

3. --, "OSI Conformance Testing Methodology", ISO 9646, International Standards Organisation, 1987.

4. Read C, "GLOBAL HARMONY: The Delivery of Proof", Proceedings of the 6th International Conference on the Application of Standards for Open Systems, IEEE Computer Society Press, Los Alamitos, USA, October 1990.

PC NETWORK FOR HOSPITAL INFORMATION SYSTEM
A really distributed, challenging approach.

Dr. Nandor BALOGH

Hungarian Institute of Cardiology   Budapest
Head of Department of Medical Informatics
E-Mail: h1536bal@ella.UUCP
Fax: +36-1-1137067   **Tel:** +36-1-1131220

<u>Keywords:</u> **LAN, HIS, PACS, MIS**

ABSTRACT

It was my intention to go toward an **integrated HIS** that covers both the whole clinical operations and the management information system.
However the importance of integration was realised neither by department head physicians and economic people nor by the top management -so we started to develop and purchase **local** (departmental) LAN-based **systems** since 1988. I tried to use homogeneous tools (network hardware/software, database formats e.t.c) to make more easy the forthcoming integration though. Presently about 50 PCs (with common user menus) are cabled together across our 250 bed hospital.
At the **clinical side** we started with the admission department, chemical laboratory, pediatry cardiology systems; followed by the ergometry and holter lab system, the heart surgery complex (including intensive care unit and post operation follow up), the animal research department, the cath lab, the cardiomyopathy lab. Then we replaced with own development the chemical lab system, and partly the cath-lab, the pharmacy system followed soon and the new pediatry cardiology system under beta test by now.
Our institute was the first in Eastern-Europe to have online connection to US data networks (for heart wall motion analysis study in 1977), and last year we joined the X.25 network in Hungary for cardiology cooperation.
At the **management side** we started with personnel administration and salary (payroll) system, continuing with financial department(general ledger) and equipment & material stock register system. However to use real business principles in the two stage production process of a hospital we need more serious department cost analysis and product line analysis.

For the **technical side** I've selected multiserver <u>Novell</u> 3.1 LAN with Arcnet, MS-DOS 3.2 based desktop stations and palmtops (Poquet) for bedside data collection and decision support. The applications we developed in <u>Clipper</u> and Microsoft C. For medical statistical analysis we developed bigger databases in PC Oracle on local 386 based computers hooked to the network. For the management information system we'll follow this approach to, probably changing from DOS to UNIX but remaining at the same SQL with graphical user interface as front-end.

As we've got at the cath-lab a DSA that real time stores movie sequences of the biting heart on hard disk we've started to develop an Ethernet based **Micro PACS** as part of our HIS. I named it micro because it'll store preselected cardiac images from DSA sequences, from digitised ultrasound and from gamma camera (SPECT) only, and because it'll consist of (super) microcomputers only.

For **archiving** of alphanumerical and image data we try to use a multifunction drive that can handle both WORM (for mandatory long time storage) and magneto optical media (for security backup).
Introducing new information law in Hungary and 2Mbyte optical **patient cards** at admission/dismission departments the archiving/retrieval philosophy should be modified.

INTRODUCTION

The need for higher hospital throughput, the need for medical standards, the need for flexibility; the growing waiting lists for higher level cardiac care and heart surgery, the rising demand for quality assurance supported by research, the drastical financing/budgeting changes in Eastern-Europe (financial restrictions and more cautiousness) **urged** the work done; on the other hand the decreasing price/power ratio of MS-DOS based personal computers and the step-by-step technical approach possibility via LAN **gave the chance** to start the project.The complexity of Hospital as an organisation, the diversity and intensity of medical work, the lack of standards and protocols in medical terminology, the big differences in phisical displacements of laboratories/departments, the different machinery, the different working processes, the different size and different number of patients in hospitals, the revolutionary development of computer hardware and software, the lack of management skill, the different level in informatics and in English of hospital staff, the unpredictable reimbursement system and financial changes in our countries all make **the work very difficult.** Our independent hospital specialised only to cardiology problems, we have 4 open heart surgery theatres with all laboratories and departments necessary to them. We are the methodology centre for cardiology in Hungary and we are the faculty of Cardiology of the medical university in Budapest. For my initiatives the Collegium of Hungarian Cardiologists (that consist of the top cardiologists of all academic and district hospitals in the country) decided to form a foundation called **HUCINS** (HUngarian Cardiology Information Network Structure) to concentrate the financial and human resources for computerisation in cardiology [1]. Our Institute is the main pilot site for HUCINS.

DISCUSSION

1. Information analysis

On the top of the well known organisation **pyramid** is <u>strategic planning</u>, below is the <u>management control</u> followed by the <u>organisation control</u> at the bottom. I deal with the last two layers. For the management we need management information system (MIS), for the daily operation of the hospital we need clinical information system (CIS).

The **CIS** is a transaction oriented system that should have fast response time for a specific problem (normally for one concrete patient), and used continously in a hospital, so it is a critical key factor in the institute for the routine work.
The **MIS** should be a very complex system, working on huge amount of aggregated (generally archived by CIS) data with complex and flexible query and graphical representation facilities. Because it is used ad-hoc and not routinely, the response time is not very critical. However the successful leading of the hospital both internally but especially toward the external world very much depend on MIS so it is a critical success factor in the institute.

Under **HIS** I understand the symbiosis of MIS and CIS, some level of integration but definite interfacing of the two. For HIS few people understand CIS that historically based on medical records, chemical lab system, general ledger and payroll systems, where the last items regarded as MIS information. This (mostly mainframe oriented) systems often have two problems, they are
- medically not detailed and technically not friendly enough to attract doctors
- they give raw data instead of real (friendly and easy understandable) information to managers, so hospitals sometime use separated case mix reporting systems and separated procedure costing systems.

The HIS should follow the **improvements** toward two directions, be <u>medically detailed</u> enough to cover the operation of the department and be sophisticated enough to give <u>real information</u> to the questions of different level <u>management</u>.
Combining this two (in a user friendly way) in one central system and integrate PACS with it is extremely difficult.

Since clinical subsystems too colourful to go to detail, underlining tho importance of the nursing system there, I'll focus on general planning and on a more fashionable **management aspects**.
Designing an automated (computerised) information system one shouldn't avoid making <u>information plan</u> (IP), <u>information strategy plan</u> (ISP), and <u>business area analysis</u> (BAA) as blueprints for develop the system.

The aim of a MIS to apply sound <u>business principles</u> (responsibility centres, marginal costing, variance analysis e.t.c) and advanced information technology to a hospital's planning and management control needs. To use these principles it is necessary to view **hospital activity as a two-stage production process**.

In the **first stage** hospital resources are converted into "intermediate products", which are the procedures and services provided in the patient-care process, such as X-rays, lab tests, nursing hours, operating room time e.t.c.

In the **second stage** of the hospital production process, these intermediate products are grouped to produce the "end product", the treated patients or cases. These products are typically defined according to DRGs (like in Hungarian hospital experiments [2]), but may also be defined according to any classification scheme deemed appropriate (ICD-10, ICD-9-CM e.t.c).

The two stages need two types of analysis: **department cost analysis and product line analysis.**

Because the two production stage controlled by different persons (the first by the department manager, the second by the physician) it is crucial that hospitals be able to fully integrate clinicians into the management process to improve the patient care process and at the same time optimise hospital resource utilisation.

So hospitals need clinical assessment tools that bring together quantitative and qualitative measures that clinicians and administrators can use to ensure that the highest quality care is delivered most costeffectively.

2. Technical review

The hospital is one of the most complicated environment that needs the complete scale of information technology (word processing and mail, spreadsheet, data base management, expert systems, medical and economical statistical analysys, signal processing, image processing e.t.c).

I tried to encourage head physicians to buy MS-DOS compatible equipments and LAN based applications -sometime with little success.

I also suggested to prefer own developments by expanding the department because it was much cheaper, the results were more modifiable and maintainable applications. (I realised that HIS development is a never ending process). Beside that it is very difficult to adopt a general HIS to our very specialised institute. The topology of our HIS can be seen on Fig. 1.

The modules I mentioned at the Abstract so here I underline only some feature. The most commonly used self developed system is the **chemical laboratory** one [3]. Inquiries for tests can be done directly from the requesting departments, test results can be seen or printed there too(after verification at the lab). So there is no paper movement between the lab and the departments. The Hitachi 704 lab. automata and the Medicor hematology **automats directly connected** to the local, networked PC, requests and results automatically controlled by it.

At the **Cath-lab** we connected a PC and can online retrieve the data from

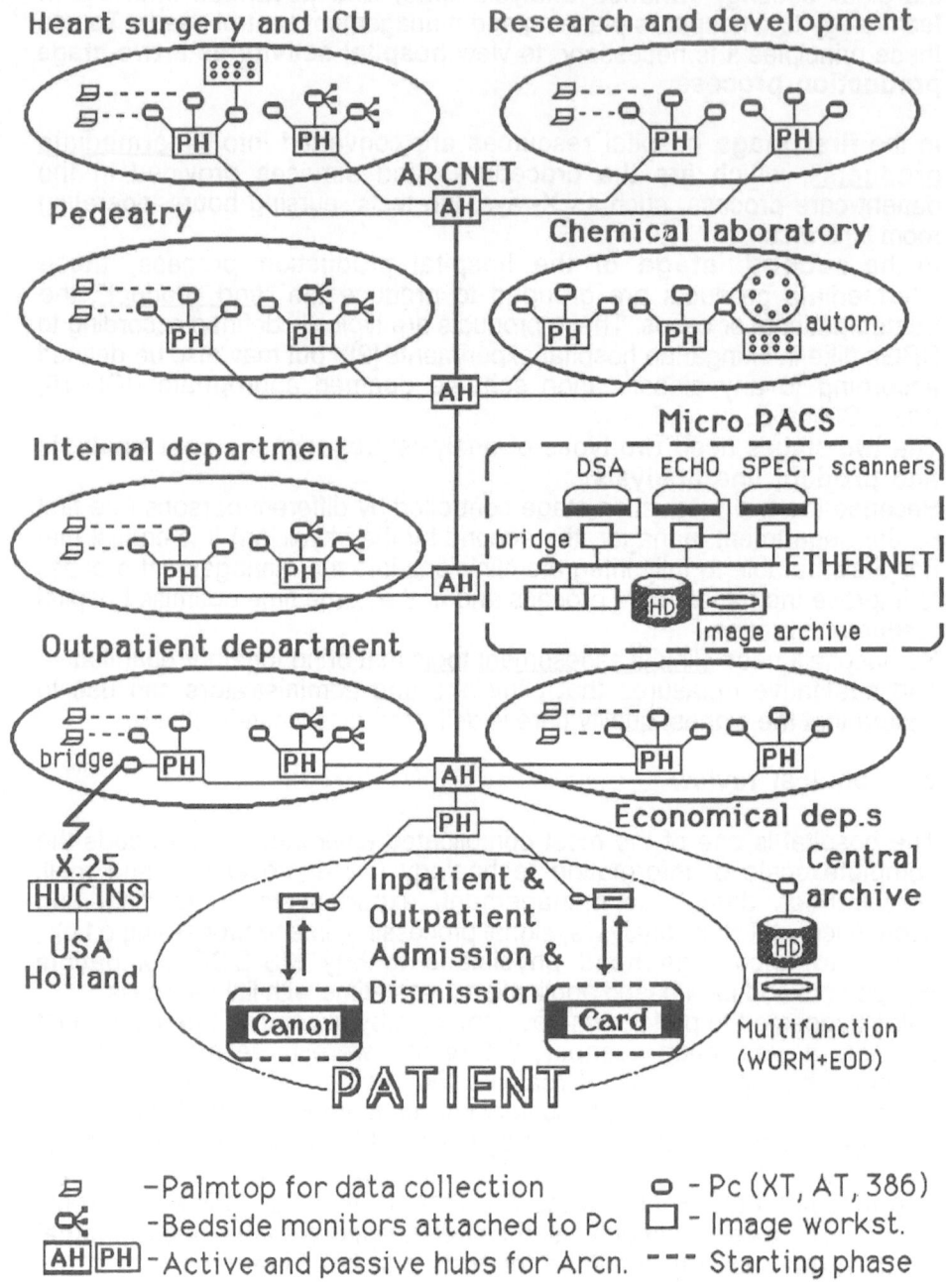

Heart surgery and ICU

Research and development

ARCNET

Pedeatry

Chemical laboratory

autom.

Internal department

Micro PACS

DSA   ECHO   SPECT   scanners

bridge

ETHERNET

Image archive

Outpatient department

bridge

X.25
HUCINS
USA
Holland

Economical dep.s

Central
archive

PH

Inpatient &
Outpatient
Admission &
Dismission

Canon   Card

PATIENT

Multifunction
(WORM+EOD)

🗒 –Palmtop for data collection   ⊙ – Pc (XT, AT, 386)
✂ –Bedside monitors attached to Pc   ☐ – Image workst.
AH PH –Active and passive hubs for Arcn. --- Starting phase

Fig. 1. Network topology

the Siemens Sicor/Micor system there to our LAN based cath-lab system. At the departments where there are bedside monitors (e.g. **ICU**) we collect the data from the monitors online to the local PC there via A/D cards. Normally we need to monitor the patient on PC screen there so we embedded C and assembly routines into Clipper. (e.g. for blood pressure curves). At the normal bedsides we collect data via palmtop computers. We developed some application and tried it on Poqet PC, but for massive use we're waiting for it's decreasing price.

We recently started an experiment with the 2Mbyte Canon optical card at our inpatient and outpatient **admission** and dismission department by self developed applications. However the wider use of the card is a multiparty project with slow decision making.

At the **image scanning labs** we try to build up an experiment for selected images. During the normal scan/digitalisation or at quick playback the physician selects those images that best describe the problem.

For better and more complex heart analysis new scanning modalities can be emerged [4]. We plan a consilium/teaching viewing (multidisplay) station, where all the relevant data for a patient can be seen at the same place, that is the selected DSA/Ultrasound/SPECT images and interpretations, the ECG waves and their's interpretations from the central ECG archive, the chemical lab results, operating reports e.t.c. Even the heart sounds can be stored for teaching purposes on these multimedia workstations.

For **archiving** we try to use homogeneous hardware and media. That's why we selected the multifunction drive because it seemed to be good for both long term and security archive and for image and traditional data. It can be used for Novell and for Mac II-s too. However optical storage is still a very sleepy road.

We joined last year the experimental **X.25 network** of Hungary via X.25 card put in a PC as a bridge. Multiply outside connections can be made from the LAN workstations. We plan to use this facility toward other hospitals, suppliers of products, Insurance companies, banks, public authorities perhaps to pharmacists and GPs later. We developed some PC based (bilingual -Hungarian English) application that can be reached from outside. These applications covers our cardiac library, a data base that covers patients with cardiomyopathy, and several huge databases with different epidemiological studies. The improving teleprocessing infrastructure gives some more chance for such developments and cooperations [5,1]. I convinced in the symbiosis of the patient cards (for routine) with the network (for research and teaching).

CONCLUSION

The pioneer role of introducing the first automated system in a highly unstructured hospital environment is very unhonoured. After my two years effort we recently formed a comitte for standardisation the content of our HIS. I was a bit skeptical at the beginning concerning a PC only HIS, but even at that time the Netware for VMS was an escaping facility. During this three years the capacity and speed of storage medias increased rapidly, introducing new power-user machines (like i486/i860 EISA based servers) and brilliant multimedia workstations (like NeXTdimension) with good connectivity (like Netware for MAC) and image databases (like 4-th Dimension) gives the chance for small/medium sized hospitals to remain at the "micro" computer basis even for PACS using the emerging FDDI technics. Palmtops like Poqet or PenPoint give chanche for bedside data collection. New releases of Netware and LAN Manager gives horse power for the manager of HIS by offering different servers (technical servers like file server, mail server, fax server, compute server; or functional servers like departmental servers or ECG server, image server). The database management systems however don't follow the hardware and system software rush. SQL based client/server facilities don't gives the possibility for real multiserver applications yet. The tables belonging to one application can't be physically at different sites managed automatically by the kernel. Till that happens data integrity gives lot of organisational problems for the LAN supervisors. Still, I convinced these systems can be fast enough by cleverly separate and organise some central (medical and managerial) task to powerful workstations, the increasing reliability of PCs and networks give the chance to build a multifunction HIS at these platforms interconnecting departmental systems and medical instruments via standard interfaces (like HL-7).

REFERENCES

1. N. Balogh: "Novell LAN for the Hungarian Institute of Cardiology", Computers In Cardiology 1991, Venice (under press)
2. A. Javor, I. Bordas, J.Nagy: "Introduction of DRG system in Hungary", MIE'90, 1990 Glasgow.
3. G. Kovacs, E. Maklari, N. Balogh: "Labor info System for HIC", International conference on lab equipments, 1990 Budapest
4. N. Balogh: "3D coronary anatomy analysis with parallel processing", Medical Informatics 1991 (manuscript sent in August 1990)
5. N. Balogh: "Computer networks and their telecommunication and computer background in the developed countries and in Hungary", Doctoral thesises 1980, University of Economics, Technical University of Budapest.

A Hospital Communication System based on CON-NECT - Medical User Interfaces

B. Wentz, G. Hergenröder, L. Horbach, H. Seibold, F. Wolf

Rechenzentrum der Medizinischen Fakultät

Universität Erlangen-Nürnberg, Martensstraße 1, D-8520 Erlangen

1 Summary

The data communication system of the university hospitals in Erlangen uses the office communication system CON-NECT which is based on the database system ADABAS. The first version has been implemented for the dermatological hospital. It was installed in March 1991 and is being tailored to their particular requirements. The communication between the hospitals, institutes, and subsystems in Erlangen will be based on the message handling system X.400, using a private X.25 network which will be replaced by an FDDI ring.

2 Introduction

The communication system of the university hospitals in Erlangen is intended to support medical documentation, patient data transmission, and message passing [2]. It should support the routine operation of the hospitals and simplify the evaluation of medical data for scientific purposes by making this available in databases [4,5]. The powerful database system ADABAS and the forth generation language NATURAL from Software AG Darmstadt (SAG) have been used in Erlangen since 1982. This led us to investigate whether the office communication system CON-NECT, which is also from SAG and is based on ADABAS and NATURAL, should be used for communication in the hospitals [3]. Similarly we decided to evaluate MEDIK, a program for medical documentation in hospitals from Gesellschaft für

Systemforschung und Dienstleistungen im Gesundheitswesen (GSD) in Berlin, which is also based on ADABAS and NATURAL.

3 Hardware and software requirements

Mainframe computers from SIEMENS with the BS2000 operating system act as database servers for the ADABAS-NATURAL development system, CON-NECT, and MEDIK. The clients are computers running MS-DOS, OS/2, and UNIX (SINIX). These computers are temporally connected via Ethernet for testing. The network protocols defined in the ISO layered model are used (ISO-IP with TP4) [1]. During 1992 FDDI (Fiber Distributed Data Interface) will be installed in the university hospitals which are dispersed throughout Erlangen. This will be funded by a network investment program (NIP). Ethernet will be used for cabling inside the individual buildings. A private X.25 network will be used for the communication until the FDDI network is available [1].

ADABAS, NATURAL, CON-NECT, and MEDIK run on mainframe computers from SIEMENS, IBM, and DEC , and are currently being ported to the UNIX and OS/2 operating systems.

4 The implementation of medical functions in CON-NECT

CON-NECT is an object oriented office communication system. It provides an application programming interface (API) in which functions specific to the hospitals (methods) can be implemented. Extensive software tools are provided to facilitate the implementation. Standard objects in CON-NECT are folders, files, documents, etc.; these provide an electronic representation of the organisation of an office. Some standard functions of CON-NECT (diary, appointments, messages, notice board) can be used in the routine running of the hospital. Other functions can be implemented by using the variable CON-NECT interface. Offices are implemented in CON-NECT for wards, stations, and laboratories; these contain folders for patients, incoming post, and outgoing post. User objects are defined for patient personal data, requests, reports, and medical documents. CON-NECT methods are programmed using the functions of the application programming interface.

The patient admission function provides the interface to the patient administration system and to the central patient database in which the personal data of over 200 000 patients are maintained.

The forms, lists, and mailboxes described in the request and report system are electronic representations of the organisation of the hospitals. For example a laboratory request can be selected from a list of forms at a ward, and the required patient is selected from the list of patients. Thus the most important data (patient data, date, time, name of ward) are automatically assigned. Further information can be entered by the hospital staff and the request can be placed in the outgoing post basket of the ward.

```
                            DERMATOLOGIE

    Laboranforderungen RIA-Labor                    Station:   STATION1
      ADAM,ANNA 19.12.1913 W 1587893895

    Klin.  Befund :  V. a. Lues_____  Editor  _
    Fragestellung :  _____     Editor  _

           x TPHA (Luesserologie)      _ VDRL
           _ FSH/LH                    _ Testosteron
           _ Prolactin                 _ GnRH-Test
           _ Cortisol                  _ Cortisoltagesprofil
           _ Kryoglobulin /-fibrinogen _ Gonokokkentypisierung
           _ Gesamt-IgE                _ RAST (spezifisches IgE)
           _ Phadiatop


           _ Sonstiges   _____

     18.09.90     10:29:50 Uhr      verantwortl. Arzt:  Dr. Diepgen_____
    Enter-PF1---PF2---PF3---PF4---PF5---PF6---PF7---PF8---PF9---PF10--PF11--PF12---
         HILFE        ENDE
```

Figure 1. Display mask of an electronic request form

The doctor in the ward is authorised to alter the form and to send it to the required laboratory. A copy of the request sent is automatically placed in the appropriate patient file at the ward.

The electronic report is generated at the laboratory as follows: first the request is selected for which the report is to be made. Important data (name of request, patient data, date, time) are transferred to the report so that it is only necessary to enter the actual laboratory data. The completed report is placed in the electronic outgoing post basket. The doctor responsible is authorized to alter the report if necessary, to approve it, and to return it to the ward. Processed requests and copies of transmitted reports are archived at the laboratory in appropriate folders.

When the laboratory report has been read in the incoming post basket at the ward, it is automatically placed in the file of the patient.

After the patient has left the hospital those documents which are of medical interest are stored in the central patient archive. A semi-automatic short letter from the doctor is included. A final diagnosis is also input; this is transmitted electronically to the central hospital administration. Programs are available which allow the system manager to administer the electronic forms. These are used to create new forms or change existing forms without delay and without interfering with the running of the system. The system manager can generate individual lists of forms for each station. In addition there are programs which control access and monitor the performance of the system.

5 Integration of subsystems

Subsystems should normally be connected via the message handling system X.400, since the new version of CON-NECT supports X.400 [6]. It is intended that the institutes of pathology, microbiology, and radiology should be integrated into the hospital communication system. The central laboratory is currently connected directly to the BS2000 computers via a special interface. This will be replaced by the standardised file transfer method FTAM. International standards (EDIFACT, ODA/ODIF, MEDIX) will be used to standardize the contents of the files transferred.

Some non-standard implementations of particular hospitals in Erlangen create problems as they do not conform to national or international standards. It is impossible to say which of these systems will be connected to the hospital communication system, since such systems require special interfaces.

6 Conclusion

The provisional system which has been implemented shows that by using CON-NECT it is possible to construct a hospital communication system with a predictable amount of programming effort. The flexibility of the standard CON-NECT interface, the powerful programming interface, and the many auxiliary functions, combine to make CON-NECT a highly efficient product [3].

CON-NECT is currently only available on mainframe computers but it will soon be ported to UNIX systems and PC networks. MEDIK can be integrated into the hospital communication system in Erlangen and provide support for medical documentation. Its practical application is currently being evaluated in conjunction with the hospitals. The first practical test has been running since March 1991 in the dermatological hospital, one of three hospitals selected for testing the system. It is currently beeing prepared, in intensive cooperation with doctors and nurses, for its first live use.

7 References

1.	Bauerfeld W, Holleczeck P (1989) Global Connectivity. North Holland Computer Networks and ISDN Systems 17 (4,5) : 300-304
2.	Engelbrecht R, Schlaefer K (1986) Information und Kommunikation im Krankenhaus. S 29-32, Ecomed Verlag, Landsberg, München
3.	Hergenröder G, Wentz B, Horbach L, Wolf F, Seibold H (1990) Entwurf des Pilotprojektes Klinikkommunikation Erlangen. Zbl Haut 158: 406
4.	Horbach L (1988) Deutsche Gesellschaft für Medizinische Dokumentation, Informatik und Statistik. In: Handbuch der Medizinkommunikation, S 115, Deutscher Ärzteverlag, Köln
5.	Reichertz PL, Schmeetz HD (1983) Möglichkeiten und Grenzen von DV-Verfahren. Das Krankenhaus 10: 425-430
6.	Schicker P (1988) Mitteilungssysteme. In: Datenübertragung und Rechnernetze, S 221-250 , B.G.Teubner Verlag, Stuttgart

MIDAM - A GENERALISED SYSTEM FOR INTEGRATING MEDICAL IMAGES AND PATIENT RECORDS

I.R. Young, D.H.O. Ling, D.A. Bell

Dept. of Information Systems, University of Ulster, Jordanstown

Newtownabbey, Co. Antrim, Northern Ireland. BT38 0QB

ABSTRACT

There is a need to integrate image data held in digitised format in radiological departments with the textual data concerning patients which forms part of a computerised hospital information system. Currently multidatabase systems allow record-based textual data from different locations to be integrated. This approach is extended in the MIDAM system, the architecture of which is presented in this paper.

INTRODUCTION

Computerised hospital information systems have been around for a number of years. More recently the concept of integrating data from a number of databases within a hospital using a distributed database or multidatabase management system [1] has been proposed. This allows the integration of structured text, which may take the form of patient administration records, medical treatment records etc.

Much work has recently been published on the storage and retrieval of medical images, such as X-rays and other modalities, in a digitised format [2,3]. These Picture Archiving and Communication Systems (PACS) are concerned with the practical issues such as the high volume of image data to be stored, the design of appropriate workstations allowing clinicians to view and compare medical images for disgnostic purposes and the development of networks with high data transfer rates. In first generation PACS systems however, the problem of integrating distributed multi-modal data, which is heterogeneous in terms of languages and equipment, has not been fully solved.

An important feature of the second generation PACS approach is the provision of access for the radiology information system (RIS) module of the HIS to textual data in conjunction with the corresponding image data (Fig.1). It has been suggested that a generalisation of the multidatabase approach be used for handling information which is multi-medium, multi-modal and multi-site [4]. A pilot scheme involving a specific link between digitised patient records and their corresponding medical images demonstrates the feasibility of the integrated approach [5]. What is described in this paper is a generalised multimedia approach employed by EDDS (Experimental Distributed Database System) [1,4].

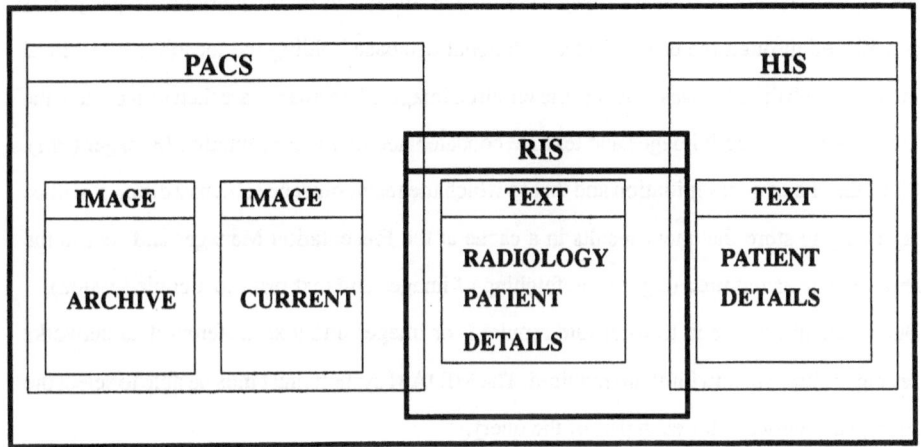

FIG.1: SECOND GENERATION PACS

MIDAM Approach

The MIDAM system uses an extension of the multidatabase approach to allow for handling of multimedia data, in this case text and image [1,4]. The multidatabase approach originally used in EDDS and described in detail elsewhere [1] uses the well-accepted relational model. The system has a global transaction manager (GTM) which allows users to pose queries over an HIS using a single global query. This means that as far as the user is concerned, the various underlying and geographically distributed databases are a single centralised database. This is achieved through decomposition of the global query into subqueries which are then passed to the local databases under the control of local data managers which translate as required from the global query representation to the local database query language and return the sub-results to the GTM where they are concatenated to give a single global result.

The MIDAM approach is an extension of the multidatabase approach whereby the global query is first decomposed according to medium (i.e. image or text). The textual part of the query is handled as mentioned above and the image part is decomposed globally according to image type and image database location. This is achieved by the Global Image Manager (GIM), which produces a number of subqueries which are then sent across the communications network to the appropriate local image handling modules. Each image base has a local image handling (LIH) module responsible for interfacing with the local image base to retrieve the appropriate image or set of images required as an answer to the query or subquery. This is achieved through the use of a local relational database holding the locations of all local images which the LIH uses to locate the required images. The images are then sent back to the global site where both images and text are concatenated by the Presentation Manager (PM). Since the site of query initiation and that to which the result must be sent may differ, it will be necessary to store the query results in a cache at the Presentation Manager and sent to the required site as required (e.g. for prefetching of images and text prior to a clinic session).

Due to the difference in transfer rate required for images and text, different data networks having different bandwidths are required. The MIDAM system must thus be able to select the appropriate network for each part of the query.

It can be readily appreciated that the general architecture, as shown in Fig.2 and outlined above, covers the multi-media and multi-modal requirements for medical information handling. A prototype system on SUN and Microvax workstations have demonstrated the integration of image and text [4]. Our next step is to implement a generalised multimedia database system using the MIDAM architecture.

The important issues of this system are those of harmonisation, integration, representation, interrogation and performance. Such a system addresses the harmonisation and integration using an extension of the multidatabase approach. All system objects are represented in a relational form with pointers being used to give the location of non-textual data. Interrogation

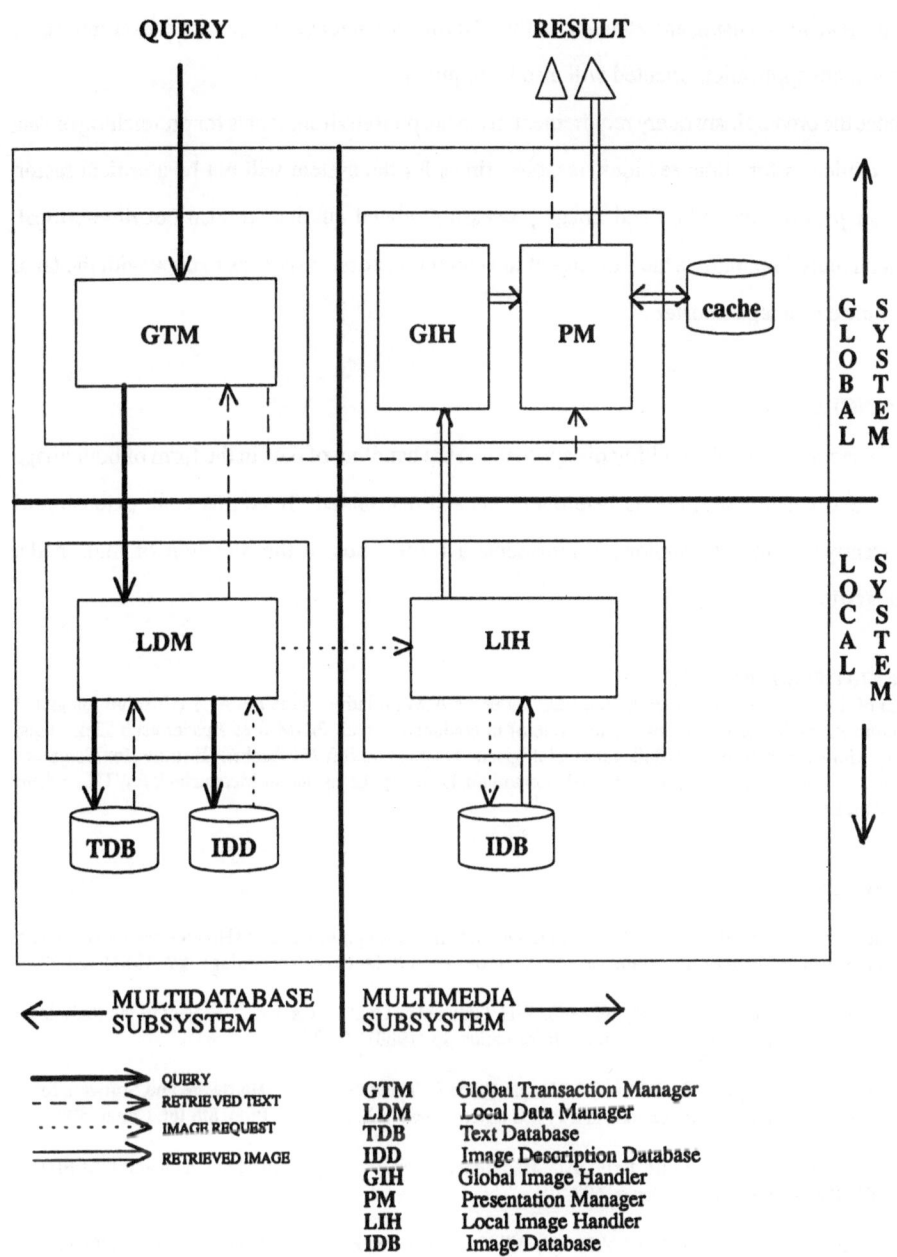

FIG.2 MIDAM SYSTEM ARCHITECTURE

will be achieved using an extension of the SQL query language. Higher level user interfaces which are application oriented will also be required.

Since the predominant query requirement in the hospital environment is for prefetching of data by clinicians for clinic sessions, response times for the system will not be a critical factor. Other pattern recognition and image processing related queries are also not time-critical. Much more important is the capacity of the communications networks to cope with the large volumes of image transfer.

CONCLUSIONS

This paper outlines the multimedia approach to the handling of data in the form of both image and text, where both may be heterogeneous and distributed. Since this is an extension of currently accepted technology it represents a further step in the direction of multimedia integration.

ACKNOWLEDGEMENTS
Part of this work was supported by the EEC under the AIM initiative as the HIPACS (Hospital Integrated Picture Archiving & Communications System) in conjunction with PRIMIS & Academisch Ziekenhuis, Vrije Universiteit Brussel; Klinik fur Radiologische Diagnostik, RWTH Aachen; Institute for Computer Science, Crete; Philips GmbH Forschungslaboratorium, Hamburg; Lehrstuhl fur Messtechnik RWTH,Aachen; BAZIS, Leiden.

REFERENCES

[1] Bell DA, Grimson JB, Ling DHO. EDDS - A System to Harmonise Access to Heterogeneous Databases on Distributed Micros and Mainframes   J. Information & Software Technology $\underline{29}$ (1987) 362-370

[2] Becker M, Gell G, Wiltgen M, Schneider GH, Greinacher CFC.   The PACS Project in the Radiology Department of the LKH-Graz   Med. Informatics $\underline{13}$ (1988) 249-253

[3] Mattheus R, Lupyaert R, Osteaux M, Van de Velde R, Temmerman I.   Hardware and Software for Integrating Special Applications in a PACS environment   MIE 1988 - Proc. 8th Int. Congr. 538-542

[4] Abul-Huda BAH, Young IR, Bell DA.   Handling Multimedia Objects In Medicine using KALEID   MIE 1988 - Proc. 8th Int. Congr. 697-701

[5] Lodder H, van Weperen JH, de Valk JPJ, Bijl K, Bakker AR, Helder JC, Scharnberg B.   HIS-PACS Coupling: First Experiences   SPIE $\underline{914}$ Medical Imaging II (1988) 1141-1146

THE INTEGRATION OF PACS, DIGITAL RADIOGRAPHY, NUCLEAR MEDICINE AND ULTRASOUND DEVICES: AN OPPORTUNITY AND A CHALLENGE FOR THE GENERAL HOSPITAL.

B. Bagni, M.D., *P.N. Scutellari, M.D., C. Orzincolo, M.D.

Department of Radiology and Nuclear Medicine - S. Anna Hospital,
*Institute of Radiology - University of Ferrara, Italy

Introduction

Today, PACS installations in Europe are at least twenty, most of which are commercial. In Italy, eight PACS sites are activated, and in four cases they are connected to a digital radiography system (PCR).

As a part of a project funded by the Regional Authority, an archiving and communication system has been implanted in the S. Anna Hospital of Ferrara, Italy, and is connected to a digital radiography set as well as to each other diagnostic devicde in use in the Imaging Department. It utilizes both Philips and AT&T equipment. The PACS structure is detailed in Fig. 1, while Fig. 2 summarizes the principal connections between imaging facilities and data acquisition and retrieval modules.

Fig. 1

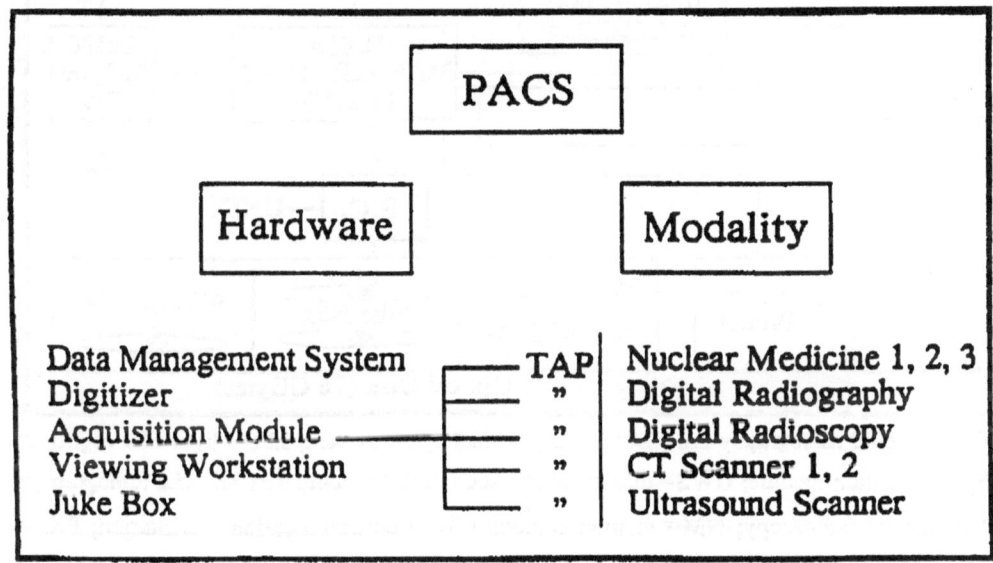

Methods

The essential aim of the project is to create a common image archive and patient database, while making the image electronically available to each display workstation (DWS) installed at different sites inside the Imaging Department.

The PACS is connected to a digital radiography system that uses photosensitive, solid-state plates instead of normal radiographic film. Other devices (gamma cameras, CT scanners, digital radioscopy, ultrasound scanners) are connected to an optical fiber network via analog-to-digital converters. An International Radiology Information System (IRIS) is also available on line through an ORACLE relational database that links images to patients' data, thus realizing an integrated retrieval system. Diagnostic viewing stations are situated in each remote site ad use high resolution catode tube displays (1024x1024x8 bit depth). In the operating and viewing room (the central site), a laser reader and a laser hard copy unit are available for digitizing and printing images coming from different peripheral devices. Using only one digital radiography unit (35 images/hour) the system capacity is 4500 images in the hard disk of the Data Management System; the maximum capacity of the juke box is 12,500 x 3 compressed radiographic images. For images coming from other devices the ratio is 1/12. The transfer time from the digital radiography unit to the display workstation is 15:30 sec/frame and is faster from other modalities.

Fig. 2

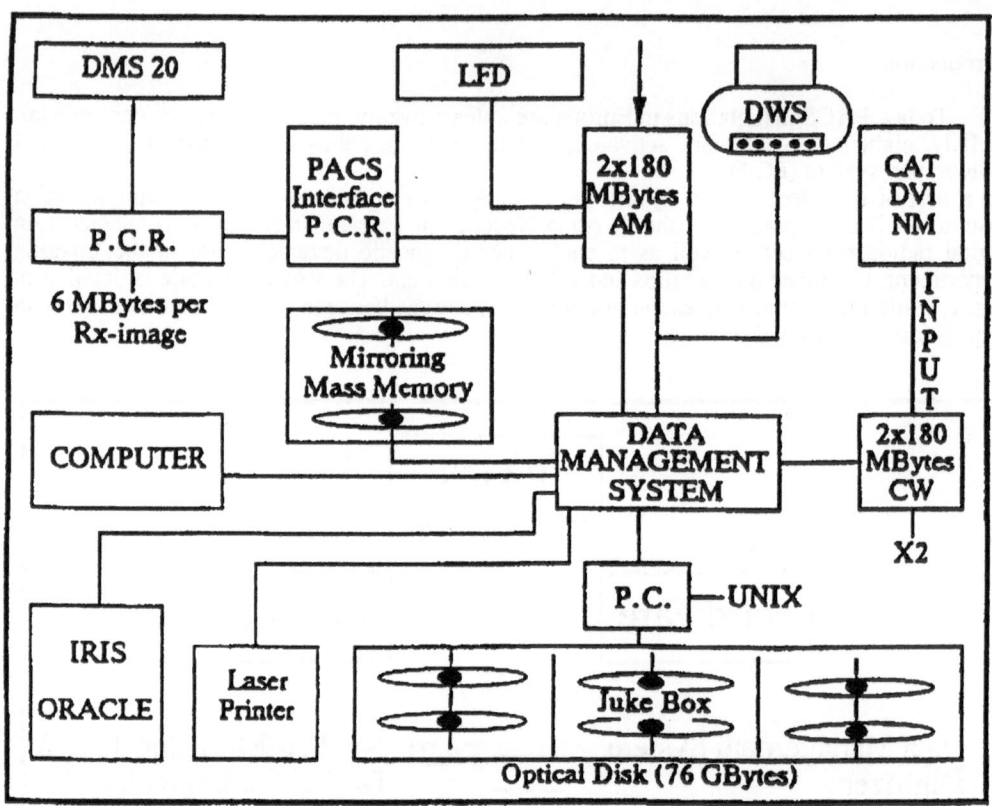

P.C.R.= digital radiography unit; DMS = digital managing system; LFD= light film digitizer; AM= acquisition module; DWS= display workstation; CAT = computerized axial tomography; DVI= digital radioscopy; NM= gamma camera; CW = communication workstation; P.C.= personal computer.

The current first phase of the project is devoted to the analysis of the consequences of "switching" from analogic to digital radiology with data transmission to PACS. In this first phase of the projects, the productivity and diagnostic implications of the introduction of PACS in the Department of Radiology along with a cost/benefit analysis of digital mammography (50 examinations per day) are under investigation.

Results and Discussion
At the moment, only one-way data transfer is possible, since the NCR NEMA interfaces are not yet in use. Soon, bidirectional image transmission will make possible to process rough

incoming data from the various peripherals.

Hence, the second phase of the project will investigate the consequences of hospital database and digital archive integration. A preliminary remark is possible today on the limitation represented by the availability of monitors that simultaneously display only four low-resolution images of compatible format, thus hampering a real time comparison of high-resolution images of different formats.

Based on the first months of experience, it appears that the integration of the whole diagnostic devices currently used in an Imaging Department of a General Hospital is a unique opportunity for improving the productivity and the diagnostic efficiency, but is still a highly costly and difficult task to achieve.

Advantages and limitations of PACS in the present configuration are finally analyzed.

The former ones involve: better efficiency of already available functions (e.g. CT and US backup; availability of new functions (e.g. immediate access to images). The limits concern: operational overhead (operational drawback); operational complexity of some functions (reporting drawback); reduced number of simultaneously viewed images (reporting drawback); small image size (teaching drawback).

References
1. ARENSON RL, CHAKRABORTY DP, SESHADRI SR, KUNDEL HL:
   The Digital Imaging Workstation
   Radiology (1990), 176: 303-315.
2. DALLA PALMA L, UKOVICH W, STACUL F, CUTTINI-ZERNICH R, CARBI N,
   GIRIBONA P,: Sistema PACS a progetto modulare.
   RAD MED (1990), 80:9-23.
3. HUANG HK, KANGARLOO H, CHO PS, TAIRA RK, HO BKT, CHAN KK: Planning a
   Totally Digital Radiology Department.
   AJR (1990), 154:635-639.
4. LEMKE HV: Europeans begin to close PACS technology gap.
   Diagnostic Imaging International (1990), 10:38-43.
5. SCHMIEDL UP, ROWBERG AH: Literature Review: Picture Archiwing and Comunitaion
   System.
   Journal of Digital Imaging (1990), 3:178-194.

Modular Development of a Hospital Wide Picture Archiving and Communication System (PACS)

Osman Ratib, Yves Ligier, Matthieu Funk, Denis Hochstrasser, Jean-Raoul Scherrer

Digital Imaging Unit, Center of Medical Informatics, University Hospital of Geneva

1211 Geneva-4, Switzerland

Abstract

The PACS under development at the University Hospital of Geneva is a hospital-wide Image Management System for radiological as well as non-radiological medical images which is part of a one of the widest hospital information systems (HIS) in Switzerland (Diogene system). It is based on a multi-vendor open architecture and a set of widely available industry standards, namely: Unix as the operating system, TCP-IP as network protocol and an SQL-based distributed database (INGRES) that handles both the PACS and the HIS. The PACS is based on a distributed architecture of servers of two types: the Archive Servers connected to the sources of images and equipped with large optical disk libraries (Juke Boxes) and Display Servers distributed over the hospital. A standard image storage format was developed based on the ACR-NEMA standard. This file format called the PAPYRUS format, allows to store sets of images as a sequence of ACR-NEMA messages in an "encapsulated" file structure. In order to provide a more uniform user interface on a variety of different workstations a common platform for image display and manipulation called OSIRIS is developed based on X-11 windowing system and OSF/Motif extension. Such a platform is designed to be portable to any computer running Unix and equipped with a graphic display system running X-11. Also because this software is written in the object oriented language C++, it is easily expandable and easily adaptable to different needs and requirements.

1. General Architecture

The University Hospital of Geneva has initiated a hospital-wide PACS project that officially started the third quarter of 1989. The aim of this project is to develop an integrated Image Management System for radiological as well as non-radiological medical images. The main characteristic of this PACS is that it is directly part of a large scale Hospital Information System (HIS). Since 1975, the Medical Informatics division of the hospital has developed one of the widest hospital information systems in Switzerland, called the Diogene system [1]. The evolution of the Diogene HIS from a centralized system to a distributed architecture has promoted the concept of the integration of the PACS directly as a part of the HIS. In this architecture the images are viewed as another type of information to be handled by the HIS. This leads to a new concept of Ward Information System (WIS) where physicians and nurses could review and update their patient's medical record directly in digital form.The Geneva PACS is based on an open architecture with heterogeneous systems and multi-vendor equipment. It is built around a set of widely available industry standards, namely: Unix as the main operating system of all computers, TCP-IP as network protocol currently implemented on Ethernet networks but soon supported transparently by high speed networks as well and an SQL-based distributed database (INGRES) that handles both the PACS and the HIS. The PACS is based on a distributed architecture of large number of servers. Two main types of servers are designed: the archive servers connected to the sources of images and equipped with large storage capacity using optical disk libraries (Juke Boxes), and display servers distributed over the hospital for temporary storage of images of current patients (see figure 1).

A special file transfer management software is developed for the distribution of the images to predefined display servers where images can be accessed by the users. Images can thereby be distributed to several Display Servers simultaneously to be available at different locations in the hospital such as the radiology reading room and the medical ward for example. Images from previous examinations are extracted from the image database and sent through the same path either together with the current images or in advance prior to the requested examination (using a "prefetch" algorithm).

Display servers are equipped with magnetic or opto-magnetic disks for temporary storage of images. One server will support a cluster of several display workstations. The user of a given workstation can only access the images available on the corresponding Display Server. If the user requires an image that is not available on the local Display Server, provided he has the proper privilege to access these images, a special request can be posted from the workstation to the archive server through a query to the PACS database. The corresponding images are transferred from the Archive to the Display server in batch mode according to priority schemes and depending on the network load. The user is notified when the requested images are available on his local server. A queueing system allows to control the network load at all time and avoid excessive traffic due to large number of simultaneous requests that may be submitted to the Archive Servers.

Different types of workstations are required for different usage in a hospital-wide PACS. High performance workstations equipped with multiple high-resolution displays are needed for review and primary diagnosis by the radiologists. Multipurpose workstations for accessing images and other clinical information are to be designed to support the WIS. Finally there is an increasing demand for more quantitative analysis workstations, for image processing and computer-assisted image interpretation.

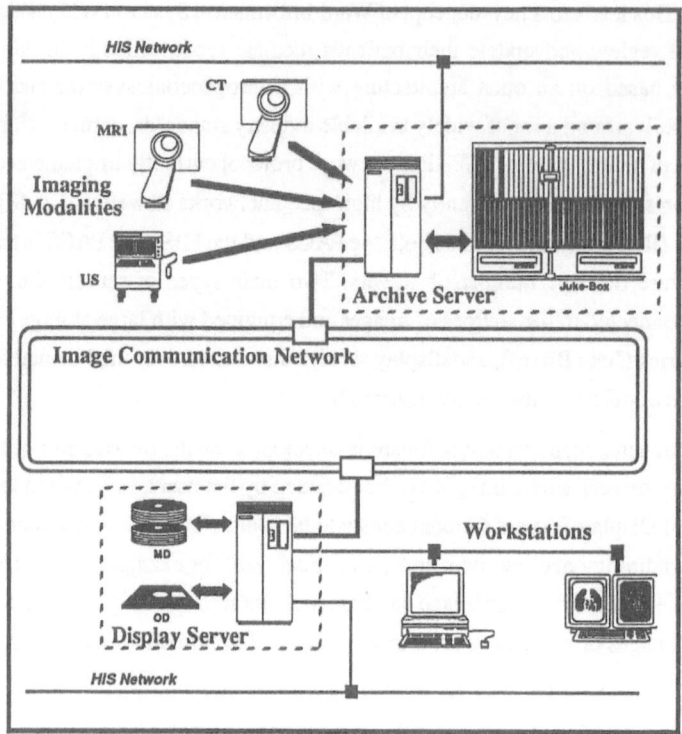

Fugure 1: Schematic diagram of the general architecture of the PACS in Geneva. Two types of servers are implemented: Archive Servers for acquisition and long term storage of images and Display Servers for local storage of images to be accessed by several workstations.

In order to provide a more uniform user interface on a variety of different workstations we elected to develop a common platform for image display and manipulation that can be ported on different workstations. A software called OSIRIS is currently being developed based on X-11 windowing system and OSF/Motif extension [2]. Such a platform is designed to be portable to any computer running Unix and equipped with a graphic display system running X-11. Also because we develop this software in the object oriented language C++, it is easily expandable and easily adaptable to different needs and requirements.

Part of PACS development, a portable software called OSIRIS for the display and manipulation of images is being developed. In the design of the OSIRIS program special care was taken to provide a very consistent approach with the different image processing tools. The way the different tasks are performed are always very similar allowing the user to rapidly become familiar with the operation of all the features of the program. The OSIRIS software is developed under X11 and

OSF/Motif windowing environment to ensure its portability to any UNIX platform.

A standard image storage format was developed based on the ACR-NEMA standard of image communication [3]. This file format, called the PAPYRUS format, allows to store sets of images as a sequence of standard ACR-NEMA messages in an "encapsulated" file format [4]. A "folder" structure allows to keep a directory of related images in a single file or in different files. All images obtained from different modalities are converted to the PAPYRUS format prior to archiving.

2. Current implementation

As mentioned earlier the Geneva PACS is designed by a development team that is in charge of the development and implementation of the different components of the PACS. A modular development of the hospital-wide PACS will allow to develop clusters of sub-PACSs in different sections of the hospital. The general architecture is based on sets of archive servers, each of them supporting a groups of image sources. Images are then distributed to display servers each of them supporting one or several workstations.

The current status of the project includes the following sections: 1) A software development laboratory equipped with a variety of workstations for the development of software tool for image management and communication as well as the OSIRIS image manipulation software. 2) The first PACS module currently implement consist of a cluster regrouping two CT scanners, and MRI scanner and an Ultrasound unit. All the images from these imaging units are stored on the same archive server consisting of a sun 4/490 server and a Cygnet Jukebox with ATG optical disk drives for 6.4 GByte platters for a total capacity of approximately one TeraByte. 3) A prototype project for implementation of multimedia workstation in intensive care unit. This project developed in collaboration with Hewlett Packard will focus on the development of workstations where the data obtained from patient monitoring systems can be reviewed together with the laboratory results, medication, nursing observations and the radiological images. It is a first step toward a completely integrated bedside workstation for a ward information system.4) A laboratory for acquisition and analysis of non radiological images such as autoradiography, electrophoresis and histological images. This lab is equipped with a high resolution laser scanner and a table-top phosphor plate computed radiography system and several workstations for image display and analysis. Clinical images obtained from this laboratory will be incorporated in the PACS database as well. 5) A special laboratory for development of image analysis software and artificial intelligence tools is also implemented

3. Future Planing

The choice of a very modular architecture with clusters of archive and display servers allows for a progressive planning of the PACS implementation on a hospital-wide scale. Different PACS modules will be progressively implemented. After the completion of the first module for cross sectional images (CT, MRI and US) expected in the middle of 1991, the following modules are planned (in chronological order):

- PACS for intensive care units
- PACS for Emergency room
- PACS for molecular biology images
- PACS for Nuclear Medicine
- PACS for digital angiography
- PACS for Cardiology

All these modules will be developed on a similar architecture even if the hardware choices may differ depending on the availability of new and more performant equipment. A distributed database allow to access all the images from the different modules. Prefetch algorithms are being developed to anticipate the needs and regulate the traffic of images between the archive servers and display servers.

Also a pilot project for teleradiology and remote consultation is currently underway as part of the European TELEMED project. This projects includes developments of videoconferences and remote expert consultation systems, establishment of a radiology reference image database and PACS to PACS communication systems. The University Hospital of Geneva will be able to test high speed communication lines (2 Mbits/s) for the transfer of images with other partners of the TELEMED project in Europe (Sweeden, Norway, Germany, France, Spain, Italy and Greece). The PAPRYUS image file format proposed by Geneva was adopted as a standard file format for image communication in this project..

References

1. Scherrer JR, Baud R., Hochstrasser D., Ratib O.: An Integrated Hospital Information System in Geneva. M.D. Computing, vol. 7, No. 2: 81-89, 1990.

2. Ligier Y., Funk M., Ratib O., Perrier R., Girard C.: The OSIRIS user interface for manipulating medical images. Proc. of NATO ASI meeting on "Picture Archiving and Communication System (PACS) in Medicine". Evian, 1990.

3. ACR-NEMA standard publication. "Digital Imaging and Communications". #300-1988.

4. Ratib O., Appel R., Scherrer JR: PAPYRUS: A multimodality Image File Format for PACS and Teleradiology. Radiology, vol 177(p): 320, 1990.

5. Ratib O., Huang HK. CALIPSO, an Interactive Software Package for Multimodality Medical Image Analysis on a Personal Computer. J. of Medical Imaging, 3: 205-216, 1989.

PLANNING A LARGE SCALE PACS: THE VIENNA SMZO-PROJECT

Hans Mosser[1], Wolf Rüger[2], Michael Urban[1], Walter Hruby[1]

1) SMZO Hospital, Langobardenstraße 122, A-1220 Vienna, Austria
   (Chairman Radiology Dept.: Univ.Doz.Dr.W.Hruby)
2) SIEMENS Medical Group, Erlangen, Germany

Abstract: Goal of this paper is to present a large scale PACS project, as planned for the SMZO Hospital in Vienna, Austria. This 1400-bed teaching hospital will start its operation in early 1992. Since 1988 a team of radiologists and computer engineers has been planning the design and the operational structure of this all-digital radiology service. The goal of this project is to optimize the service by improving communication within the radiology department and with other departments and to increase the accessability of radiological images. In this paper the major considerations in the planning and development phases are outlined. An overview of the physical structure of the system will be given according to the current plans, which still are open to changes if necessary as planning progresses, in line with further technological development.

Keywords: SMZO, PACS, HIS, RIS

Introduction:

At the turn of the century the larger part of radiologic images is assumed to be operated with digital modalities and manipulated within a Picture Archiving and Communication System (PACS), in particular as soon as digital images will account for more than 40 to 50 percent of all imaging (1 - 6). The implementation of PACS is expected to improve patient care, education, teaching and research (7 - 10) and to support administrative tasks in connection with Radiology and Hospital Information Managment Systems (RIS, HIS), thus improving the efficiency not only of the radiology department but of the whole hospital as a whole

The term "large scale PACS" refers to a hospital-wide and all imaging modalities covering PACS, associated with a RIS and HIS. To our knowledge, currently there are worldwide four large hospitals planning such a total PACS: The Madigan Army Hospital in Tacoma, Washington, the Hokkaido University Hospital in Japan, the Hammersmith Hospital in London and the SMZO Hospital in Vienna.

The SMZO Hospital:

SMZO stands for "Sozialmedizinisches Zentrum Ost", meaning "Social and Medical Center East".
It is a complex patient care system, in which health care is supported by social services. In detail, the SMZO encircles:

* a nurse training center operating since 1978,
* a 400 bed geriatric medical center since 1982 for geriatric and long term diseases,
* housing facilities.
* The last and largest part of the project is the 900 bed teaching hospital, which is under construction since 1985 and -with its major part- will start operation in 1992.

Medical planning aspects: The objective of the planning activities for the SMZO-Hospital, which started in 1979, was to achieve the optimum medical care for the patient; with this in mind, it had to live up to the latest developments of science, and in this sense there were primarily medical aspects which determined its constructional design, its outfit and its organisation (11).

SMZO-PACS: Planning phase:

Detailled planning for the radiology department started 1988, as soon as the designated chairman was appointed. In order to avoid obsolescence right from the start, in planning a new hospital it is necessary to take into account the emerging technologies concerning the application of computer- and information-sciences in radiology. A project team of computer scientists, engineers and radiologists investigated the potential benefits of these technologies, in particular of Digital Radiography (DR), PACS and information managment systems. These investigations showed that PACS is feasible, and that it offers medical benefits resulting from improved access to images as well as increased communication. Additional benefits are based on the support of administrative tasks.

PACS vendor selection:

Having the plan to implement a large scale PACS in a new hospital without own PACS research- and development facilities, leaves one at the current technological situation only with the alternative to contract potential PACS vendors. Considerations like project responsibility, standardization, compatability, consistent user surface, easy upgrading and updating, service and maintenance, and last not least budget criteria have led to the decision to contract one single major vendor. On a tender basis and after competitive bidding, SIEMENS, Erlangen has been selected as this PACS manufacturer. A multidisciplinary PACS planning team, together with staff members of the vendor has been formed within the project organisation. This collaboration proved to be of vital importance, and is regarded as a prerequisite for the successful planning and implementation of a PACS (1,2,12).

SMZO-PACS: System's overview:

The radiology department consists of 25 examination rooms (table 1). Emphasis has been placed on the multifunctionality of these rooms in line with the system failure concept.
The PACS architecture for the radiology department (Fig. 1) and the associated Trauma Center (Fig. 2) is based on a modular concept, designing the various modules according to their specific tasks.
The high performance of the system is based on
* FDDI networking

* Direct connection of archives and workstations to the FDDI network, which reduces image transfer times to acceptable values (e.g. transfer-time of a CT exam of 30 images (512x512 matrix, i.e. 15 MByte) from archive to workstation: 5 seconds).

* Allocation of archives to dedicated modules: optimized network architecture combining the advantages of star- and ring-topology.

* Planned direct connection of most of the imaging equipment to the FDDI network.

* Multifunctional workstations for primary diagnosis.

Interfaces, databases and networks are based on the ACR-NEMA standard and SPI-specifications. For diagnostic and consulting purposes many workstations with interactive manipulation possibilities will be installed in the radiology department. Additionally numerous remote viewing stations with limited manipulation capabilities on a PC basis will be located in specific sites of the hospital (mainly image dependent clinical departments). The necessary number of diagnostic reporting consoles and viewing stations is still to be determined. The workstation´s monitor requirement depends on its primary task. For those screens, where primary diagnosis of high-resolution images like chest is performed, the minimum monitor´s spatial resolution is required by the radiologists to be 2K x 2K. For images with less resolution like CT or MR, or for reviewing sessions with clinical collegues, 1K monitors will suffice.

P A C S - R I S - H I S : The RIS used in the SMZO radiology department is the SIMEDOS ® (SIEMENS, Erlangen), which is adapted by radiologists to the specific needs and requirements of the SMZO. An overview of the different tasks and the data flow between these subsystems is given in table 2.

PACS as a stand alone system, without the connection to a RIS, is unacceptable for routine operation in a clinical setting. Therefore the integration of these subsystems is a prerequisite and will determine user acceptance.

D a t a   v o l u m e : The overall daily data volume to be handeled for the first two years of operation - having in mind the "worst case" - is estimated at about 13-15 GByte. The analysis of the workload in regard to the different image matrices with the resulting digital values is summarized in table 3.

Perspective and conclusion:

The top priority of PACS is improved patient care, with medical grounds clearly ranking first in considering the implementation of such systems in a new hospital. Medical justification must precede economic justification without, however, disregarding the latter. Reducing the enormous amount of cost for film and for archival space, as well as increasing the efficiency of administrative tasks are important figures in this regard.

The radiologist´s involvement in PACS implementation is necessary from the earliest planning stages, to keep the practical orientation of such a project. And it is the radiologist who determines the importance and the benefits of PACS for patient care, teaching and research, by the way he employs these new technologies.

Table 1: Radiology dept.: examination rooms:

• MR 1	• Skeletal 1
• MR 2	• Skeletal 2
• CT 1	• Conv. Tomography
• CT 2	• Multifunct. uroradiol. exam room
• Cardiolog. Angiography	• Integrat. digital chest unit
• Angiography	• Pediatric examination room
• Interventional exam room	• Mammography
• Fluoroscopy 1	• 6 x Ultrasound
• Fluoroscopy 2	
• Trauma center (4 rooms)	• (7 Mobiles)

Table 2: Communication and data flow PACS/RIS/HIS:

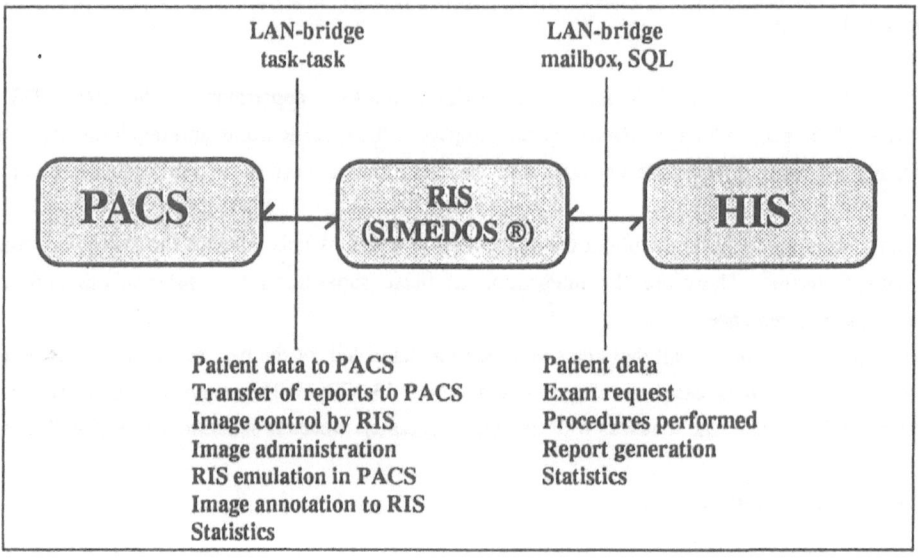

Table 3: Data production per day in regard to matrix size

Matrix	Imag./ day	MByte
512x512	4.900	2.548
1024x1024	695	1.459
2048x2048	1.100	9.233
		13.240

Figure 1: PACS Overview of the Radiology Dept.

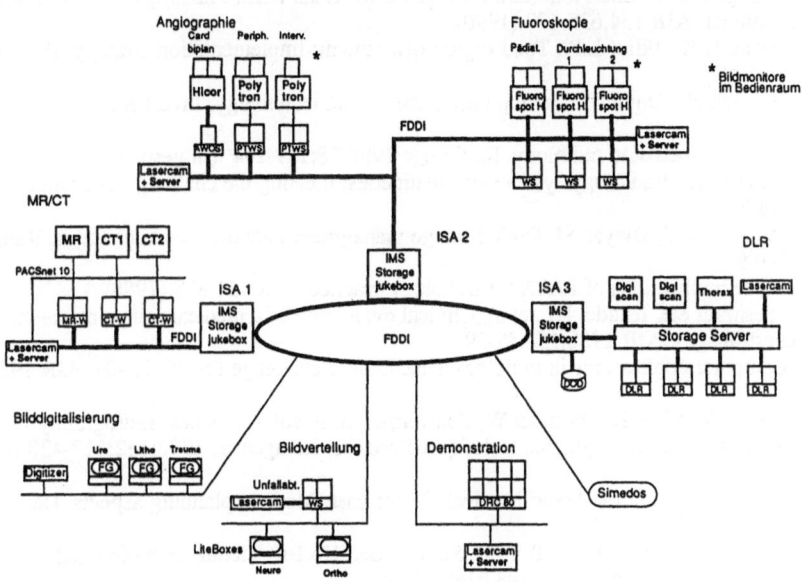

Figure 2: PACS overview of the Trauma Center:

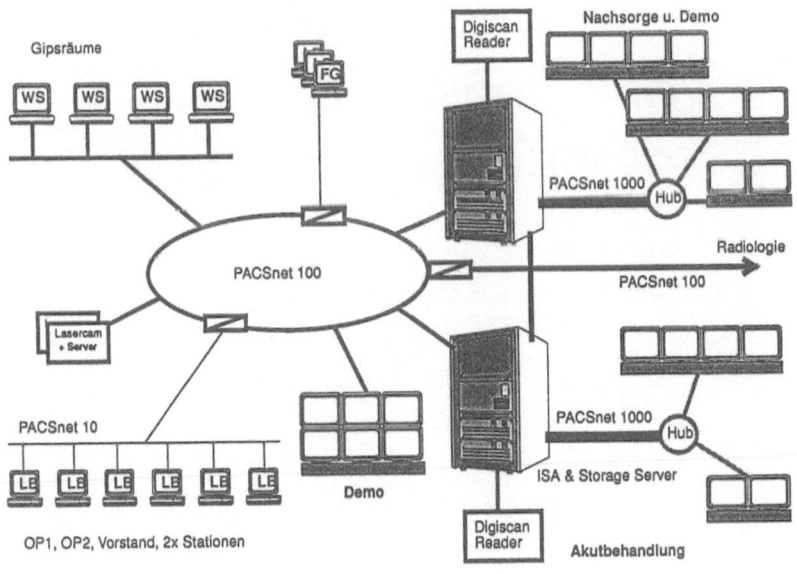

References:

1. Huang H.K., Kangarloo H., Cho P.S., Taira R.K., Ho B.K., Chan K.K.: Planning a totally digital radiology department. AJR 154,635-639 (1990)
2. Mun S.K., Benson H.K., Elliot L.P.: Total digital department: implementation strategy. Proc SPIE 1093,133- 139 (1989)
3. Jost RG, Mankovich NJ. Digital archiving requirements and technology. Invest Radiol 1988;23:803-809
4. Lemke HU. Computer-assisted radiology. Radiologe 1988;28:189-194 (in german)
5. Lodwick GS, Taaffe JL. Radiology systems of the nineties: meeting the challenge of change. J Dig Imag 1988;1:18-23
6. Templeton AW, Cox GG, Dwyer SJ. Digital image managment networks: current status. Radiology 1988;169:193-199
7. Mezrich R.S.: The implications of PACS for radiology practice. AJR 151,828 (1988)
8. Arenson RL, Seshradi SB, Kundel HL, et al. Clinical evaluation of a medical image managment system for chest images. AJR 1988;150:55-59
9. Tessler FN. Computer applications in radiology education: a challenge for the 1990s. AJR 1989; 152:1169-1172
10. Witte G, Bause HW, Maas R, Pothman W, Schwermer B, Nicolas V. Chest radiography in intensive care by a digital radiographic technique. Fortschr. Röntgenstr. 1990;152:417-420 (in german)
11. Tragl, K.H.: The hospital in the Socio-Medical Center east: Medical planning aspects. Der Aufbau 10 (1987) 491-493
12. Huang HK, Mankovich NJ, Cho PS, Taira R, Stewart BK, Ho BK. Picture archiving and communication systems in Japan. AJR 1987;148:427-429

DRUG INFORMATION AND DECISION SUPPORT SYSTEMS

DRUG INTERACTIONS IN PRIMARY CARE - A RETROSPECTIVE DATABASE STUDY

Rolf Linnarsson
Dept Med Informatics, University, Linköping and
Kronan Health Centre, S-172 83 Sundbyberg, Sweden

Abstract

In a retrospective study all drug prescriptions in a primary health care centre during a four year period were analyzed concerning potential drug interactions. The analysis was done using a query language on an automated medical record database. The study shows that 1.9 % of all drug prescriptions result in a potential drug interaction. Based on the results of the study a decision support system for drug prescription in primary care has been developed. The system is data driven and integrated with the automated medical record. A knowledge base, comprising clinically relevant drug-interactions, is the core of the decision support system. The factual medical knowledge is represented as a semantic net, and the critiquing knowledge in a standard frame-like representation.

Introduction

In primary care drug prescription is the most commonly used therapeutic procedure. However, pharmacotherapy also may contribute to morbidity, especially in elderly people who have multiple illnesses and need multiple drugs. Different types of drug interactions may result in adverse drug effects. The frequency of drug interactions rises with the number of drugs prescribed. Clinically important interactions may occur in about 6 percent of patients at risk [1]. The use of automated medical records has increased the interest in retrospective studies. Large databases and query methods have made it possible to analyse medical data from thousands of patients in short time [2]. The aim of this study was to investigate the occurrence of potential drug interactions in primary health care, and to use the results for developing a drug-prescription decision-support system.

Methods

The study was conducted using the automated medical record at Kronan health centre in suburban Stockholm. The practice includes 6 general practitioners and 2 physicians on vocational training. The information system is a problem-oriented medical record, Swede-star [3], originally based on

COSTAR [4] and it serves as the sole medical record for the physicians at the health centre.

The collection and analysis of prescription data were done with a query language, MQL [5]. Each prescription done during a 4 year period, 1 Nov. 1986 - 31 Oct. 1990, was analysed concerning potential interactions. In order to determine if two drug prescriptions were concurrent, the frequency, quantity, and refills of the prescriptions had to be considered. A potential interaction was defined as the occurrence in the patient database of concurrent prescriptions of two drugs that have a reported interaction according to the Swedish drug catalogue. The drug catalogue contains 368 different drugs and 4942 different drug pairs with potential interactions. Concurrence was defined as overlapping prescriptions: prescription of drug #1 on date t1 and prescription of drug #2 on date t2, where the interval t2-t1 is maximum one year and where the quantity of drug #1 is sufficient to cover the interval t2-t1.

The drug interactions found in the database are potential, which means that they might produce an adverse drug reaction. Several factors influence the drug effect, such as diseases, doses of drugs, routes, duration of administration, renal and hepatic status. The drug interactions have been assigned to one of three categories (major, moderate and minor) of clinical significance according to Hansten-Horn [6]. The rating is based on the severity of the potential interaction, the predictability of the adverse consequences, and the documentation available. Since the study considered all interactions found in the Swedish drug catalogue, some of them were impossible to classify in this way.

Results

During the study period 16177 patients visited the health center. At least one drug was prescribed to 11945 patients (73.8 %) and 695 of these (5.8 %) got drugs with one or several potential interactions. Elderly people (>=65 years of age) used drugs to a greater extent: 24.8 % of all patients were elderly, while 29.6 % of patients getting drugs were elderly. As much as 80.1 % of the patients having potential drug interactions were elderly.

In total 55649 drug prescriptions were analyzed concerning potential drug interactions. Of these prescriptions 16.8 % were cardio-vascular drugs. There were 1074 cases of potential drug interactions in the database, distributed among 93 different drugs and 217 different drug pairs. Each case represents a drug pair, hence 1.9 % of all drug prescriptions result in a potential drug interaction. Cardio-vascular drugs were represented in 84.5% of the cases. Table 1 shows the clinical significance of the cases.

Hansten-Horn [6] includes 37 different groups of major drug interactions. Ten of these (27%) were found in the database. These 10 drug-pairs are: amiloride -- potassium, antacids -- tetracycline, anticoagulants -- salicylates, anticoagulants -- sulfonamides, anticoagulants -- thyroid hormones, antidiabetics -- beta-adrenergic blockers, cimetidine -- theophylline, digitalis glycosides --

amphotericin B, digitalis glycosides -- quinidine, and spironolactone -- potassium.

Table 1

Potential drug interactions by clinical significance

	Cases	%
Major clinical significance	129	12
Moderate clinical significance	614	57
Minor clinical significance	155	14
Not classified	176	16
Total	1074	99

Computer-based drug prescription

The computer-stored medical record system used at the Kronan health centre [3] has been further developed to include a module for computer-based drug prescription. Drugs are prescribed by the physicians on video terminals in their offices and electronically transferred to the computer used in the local pharmacy. The drug prescribing system includes decision support on several levels: 1) on-line access to part of the Swedish drug catalogue with data on drugs, trade names, size of drug packages, doses and routes; 2) on-line access to the medical records with information about the problems of the patients, and about previous drug prescriptions; 3) on-line recommendations from the local drug committe on choice of drugs and trade names; 4) on-line information about the local therapy tradition with recommendations on choice of drug therapy for different diagnoses; 5) data-driven reminders about potential drug interactions.

The decision support system is based on the integrated function of three basic components: the clinical patient database, the medical data dictionary and the knowledge base. The first two components have been described in detail elsewhere [3,7]. The third component, the knowledge base, has two kinds of knowledge: 1) factual medical knowledge represented as a semantic net, and 2) critiquing knowledge represented in a standard frame-like representation.

The semantic net has nodes and links, which denote objects and their relations. Possible nodes are medical concepts expressed as medical terms in the controlled vocabulary of the system, the data dictionary. The possible links constitute a set of defined relations between those medical concepts. The following example shows the structure of the representation:

drug #1 --> INTERACTS_WITH --> drug #2

Here "interacts_with" is the link and "drug #1" and "drug #2" are the nodes. These nodes correspond to elements in the data dictionary. The network was primarily defined with the following links: "treats", "contraindicates", "interacts_with", "has_adverse_effect", and "is_a". Each link has its inverse: "is treated with" is the inverse of "treats". There are some constraints regarding how different nodes may combine with the links. The link "contraindicates", for example, must have a diagnosis as starting node and a drug as ending node.

The representation of the critiquing knowledge (the data-driven reminders) is more complex. It is a frame-like representation in modules according to the so-called Arden syntax [8]. The modules are called MLM (medical logic modules), and broken into slots in three categories: maintenance, library, and knowledge slots. The knowledge category contains those slots that really specify what the module does. The following example shows the knowledge slots of a sample MLM, whose purpose is to remind the physician, prescribing verapamil to a patient, which is on digoxin, of the potential interaction between the two drugs:

type: data-driven;

data: let *dig* be read

{input patient; set [current_meds]=null; when code=digoxin; set [current_meds]=digoxin};

let *ver* be read {verapamil prescription};

evoke   on storage of {verapamil prescription};

logic   if *dig* and *ver* then conclude true else conclude false;

action   store "Caution: potential drug interaction digoxin-verapamil. Consider reduction of digoxin dose or check serum level of digoxin.";

Those parts of the MLM that are enclosed in curly brackets - "{...}" - are institution-specific references to the patient database. Such a reference may be a query {input patient ...} or may refer to the storage of data in the database {verapamil prescription}.

Discussion

The study shows that potential drug interactions occur in 5.8 % of patients at risk (those receiving drugs), and that 1.9 % of all drug prescriptions result in a potential drug interaction. The results are comparable to those reported by others, although the rates are slightly lower. The very high rate of elderly patients among those having potential drug interactions implies that adverse drug reactions may be a serious health problem among the elderly.

The study results have several implications for the design of a drug-prescription decision-support system. It is obvious from the results that there is a need for decision support. New drugs are constantly introduced and it is impossible for physicians to keep in mind all interactions described in literature. Computer reminders have been proven by others to be successful in preventing irrational drug prescription [9]. However, it would not be wise to give alerts to the physicians too often. Too many alerts could in the long run reduce the attention to the reminders. An acceptable level probably would be to give one alert in every 75 drug prescriptions. According to the study results, this corresponds to giving alerts for all major and moderate drug interactions.

Based on the experiences of this study, we have developed the first part of a decision support system for drug prescription in primary care. The system is data driven and integrated with the Swede-star automated medical record. A knowledge base has been developed in which the factual medical knowledge has been separated from the critiquing knowledge [10]. The factual medical knowledge covers all drugs and their potential interactions, while the critiquing knowledge has been focused on the real needs of the prescribing physicians according to the results of the database review.

The full implementation of the decision support system within the medical record system requires the creating of several program modules to interconnect the patient database, the data dictionary, and the knowledge base [11]. In the first version of the system, the MLM has been implemented using the query language of the system as interconnecting module.

References

[1] Lamy P.P.: Pharmacotherapeutics in the elderly. Md Med J 38 (1989) 144-148.
[2] Dambro M.R., Kallgren M.A.: Drug interactions in a clinic using COSTAR. Comput Biol Med 18 (1988) 31-38.
[3] Linnarsson R.: Development and evaluation of a complete computerbased problemoriented medical record system for primary care. MIE 87 Proceedings (1987) 209-214.
[4] Barnett G.O.: The application of computer-based medical-record systems in ambulatory care. NEJM 310 (1984) 1643-1650.
[5] Webster S., Morgan M., Barnett G.O.: Medical Query Language: Improved access to MUMPS databases. Proceedings of the 11th Annual Symposium on Computer Applications in Medical Care (1987) 306-309.
[6] Hansten P.D., Horn J.R.: Drug interactions. Lea&Febiger. Philadelphia-London 1989.
[7] Linnarsson R., Wigertz O.: The Data Dictionary - a Controlled Vocabulary for Integrating Clinical Databases and Medical Knowledge Bases. Meth Inform Med 28 (1989) 78-85.
[8] Hripcsak G., Clayton P.D., Pryor T.A., Haug P., Wigertz O.B., Van der lei J.: The Arden syntax for medical logic modules. Proceedings of the 14th Annual Symposium on Computer Applications in Medical Care (1990) 200-204.
[9] McDonald C.J., Wilson G.A., McCabe G.P.: Physician response to computer reminders. JAMA 244 (1980) 1579-1581.
[10] Van der Lei J., Musen M.A.: Separation of critiquing knowledge from medical knowledge: Implications for the Arden Syntax. Proc. IMIA Working Conference on Software Engineering in Medical Informatics. Amsterdam 1990.
[11] Magyar G., Arkad K., Ericsson K.E., Gill H., Linnarsson R., Wigertz O.: Realizing Medical Knowledge in MLM Form as Working Modules in a Patient Information System. Proc. IMIA Working Conference on Software Engineering in Medical Informatics. Amsterdam 1990.

DRUG UTILIZATION MONITORING IN THE CLINICAL HOSPITAL CENTER-ZAGREB

Višnja Lovrek[1], Josip Čulig[2]
Clinical Hospital Center Zagreb
[1]Informatics Division, [2]Department of Medicine Rebro
41000 Zagreb, Šalata 2, Yugoslavia

ABSTRACT

A fifteen-year period of experience in the monitoring of drug consumption and drug utilization in a clinical hospital is described. The drug classifications and the methods used in drug monitoring are explained. The drug utilization program was created in order to improve drug prescription and the possibilities of predicting drug consumption in the hospital.

1. INTRODUCTION

In the Clinical Hospital Center Zagreb (CHC), drug utilization has been monitored by the use of a computer since 1977.

In the first phase, only limited information on drug use was obtained as there was nothing but inventory monitoring and stock control of the hospital pharmacy. These reports did not reflect the link between drug consumption and the duration of a patient's stay in the hospital, nor any other relevant parameter on the patient.

In 1981, a comprehensive database on drugs was created to carry out not only the administrative tasks for the hospital pharmacy and various hospital wards and departments (calculating treatment costs and processing administrative, pharmaceutical, and economic data), but also to provide scientific information to physicians and pharmacists. This database and the system has now already been in use for ten years, and it is constantly being extended and adapted.

2. METHODS

The goal of this project is to support the professional aspects of the hospital pharmacists and research projects of clinical pharmacologists. Accordingly, the database on drugs comprises two parts. One presents information on the drug stock available in the hospital pharmacy and its distribution to the various hospital departments and wards. The hospital pharmacy subsystem supports stock control and management within the hospital pharmacy. All administrative functions in the system, such as purchase and stock administration, use the descriptive part of drug information. The main functions are as follows:

- receiving the goods from the supplier;
- drug distribution to the hospital departments;
- on-line stock control and price calculation;
- printing of documents: products, suppliers, consumption;
- connection to the other subsystems and applications.

The database contains all data concerning the drug, such as trade name, local code, generic name, strength, dosage form, route of administration, various classifications, defined daily doses, price information, etc. The drugs are classified into therapeutical groups according to the Yugoslav drug classification.

In order to obtain comparative data on drug consumption between different countries, a common basis of analysis, i.e. a common drug classification system, should be applied. Therefore we recently introduced the anatomical therapeutic chemical classification system (ATC). The ATC system has proved suitable for drug utilization studies at different levels and it contributes to a further standardization of the basic material in national and international drug utilization statistics.

The defined daily doses (DDD) method is used in drug monitoring to allow comparative analysis of different samples. Our hospital has ten years of experience in using DDD. The defined daily dose for a drug is established on the basis of the assumed average dose per day for the drug used in its main indication in adults. It is a technical unit of measurement which provides possibilities of comparing the consumption of various drugs, both nationally and internationally. The number of DDDs is given per 1000 inpatient bed days.

There is a link between drug prescription as an input to the hospital pharmacy and data on the patient as an output. For each patient drug medication history at the hospital ward (about 60000 inpatients per year for the entire hospital), there is also information concerning other data on the patient (name, sex, age, physician, ward, etc.) as well as diagnosis, country or region. As a result, various reports such as a dosage monitoring system related to age or to the diagnosis and a comparison of other significant parameters in the patient's treatment, all expressed in defined daily doses, can be obtained.

One of the disadvantages we have encountered in this project is the lack of a computerized national drug file, so that each hospital has to build up one of its own.

In 1976, the Division of Clinical Pharmacology within the Clinical Hospital Center Zagreb was founded. A few years later, the Hospital Drug Committee was formed as well. The Drug Committee publishes the monthly "Drug Bulletin", containing sundry information on pharmacotherapeuticals, letters to the editor and periodical comments on drug utilization in the hospital. The drug utilization data are delivered from the Hospital Drug Program in cooperation with the Informatics Division of the CHC (all cited above).

3. DISCUSSION

It has been shown that there are differences in the pharmacotherapy of the same disease between countries, regions, hospitals, and individual physicians [2]. There is a need for drug utilization monitoring and permanent activities to improve drug prescription. Computerized monitoring shows the possibility of predicting the consumption of certain drugs [6]. It allows the planning of drug distribution as well.

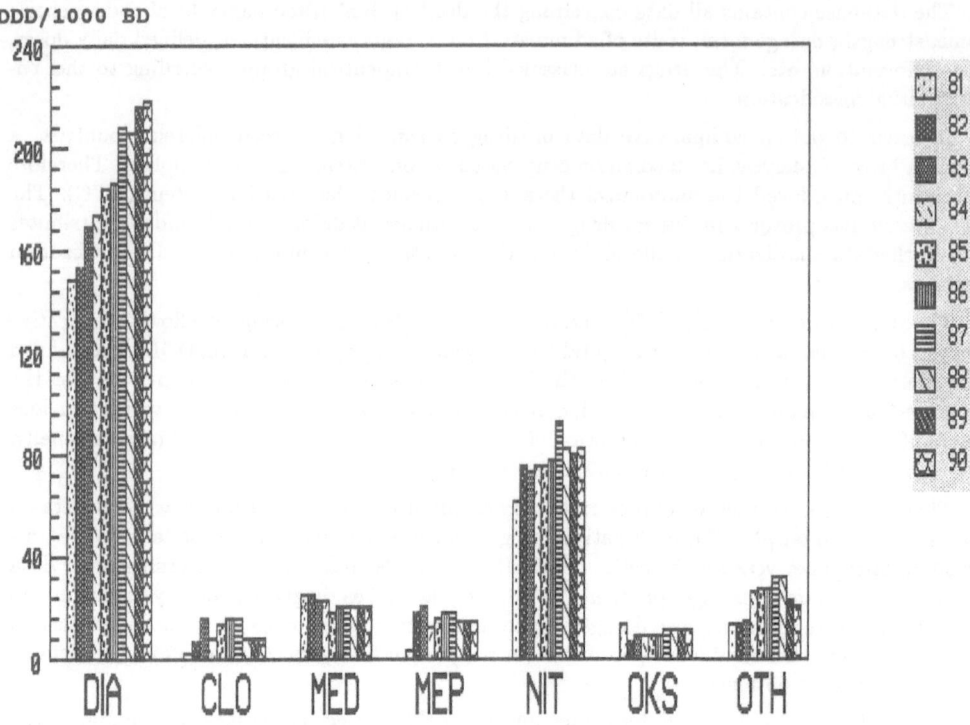

Fig. 1: Utilization of Anxiolitic drugs in CHC - Zagreb (1981–1990)

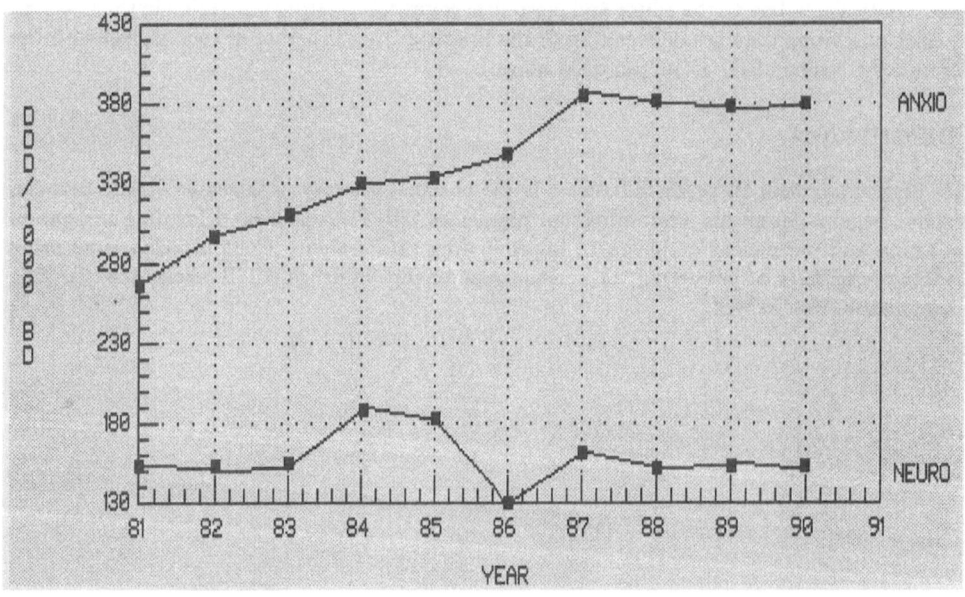

Fig. 2: Utilization of Anxiolitics and Neuroleptics in CHC (1981–1990)

The permanent informative activities, such as the bulletins, lectures, round-table discussions in pharmacotherapy, are partially successful in improving the rationality in therapy [5]. As an example, it has been shown that the consumption of neuroleptics in the CHC decreased from 1984 to 1990 (180.9 vs. 145.3 DDD per 1000 bed days), but in the same period there was an increase in benzodiazepine consumption (330.2 vs. 379.2 DDD per 1000 bed days) D Fig. 2 [7].

On the other hand, the establishment of the local drug list and the List of Reserve Antimicrobials has a much stronger influence on drug utilization in the CHC [5], which indicates an improvement in pharmacotherapy. Rational therapy does not always mean a less expensive therapy. It confirms the previous statement about many different influences on drug prescription, i.e. drug pharmaceuticals marketing, research activities, clinical trials activities, the personality of the prescribing physician, and others [5]. In order to improve drug prescription, the drug utilization program in a hospital should involve various participants who are involved with the drugs and the computerized drug program should be the basic element of the entire system.

BIBLIOGRAPHY

[1] I. Baksaas Assen, P.K.M. Lunde, M. Halse, I.K. Halvorsen, T.J. Skobba, B. Sromnes. Drug Dose Statistics. List of Defined Daily Doses for Drugs Registered in Norway. Norsk Medisinal Depot, Oslo, 1975.

[2] U. Bergman, F. Sjoqvist. Measurement of Drug Utilization in Sweden. Methodological and Clinical Applications in: Acta Med. Scand. Suppl. 683: 15-22, 1984.

[3] E. Weber. Why To Assess Drug Utilization? Drug Utilization Studies in Hospitals. Eds.: M. Hollman, E. Weber, F.K. Schattauer-Verlag, Stuttgart, 1981.

[4] A.A. Van Sorge, N.F. Muller et al. Computer Assisted Drug Dispensing in Hospital Pharmacies. Medinfo 83 Proceedings, ed. by J.H. van Bemmel, M.J. Ball and O. Wigertz, North Holland, Amsterdam, 1983.

[5] J. Čulig. Drug Utilization Analysis in a Clinical Hospital. Master of Science Thesis, Medical School of the University of Zagreb, 1985.

[6] J. Čulig, F. Plavšić, B. Vrhovac. Prediction of Drug Utilization by a Computer Model. III World Conference on Clinical Pharmacology and Therapeutics, Stockholm 1986. Acta Pharmacologica et Toxicologica 1986, Supp. V: 1572 p.

[7] J. Čulig, C. Dohoczky, V. Lovrek. Use of Neuroleptics and Anxiolytic Drugs in CHC Zagreb 1983-1988. Proceedings of the 9th Congress of Yugoslav Physicians, Ohrid, Makedonski Medicinski Pregled, 1990 (Supp.7), A3.48.

[8] J. Čulig, A. Frković, A. Knežević, B. Vrhovac. The Pattern of Antimicrobial Use in the CHC Zagreb 1977-82. Proceedings of the 9th Congress of the Yug Pharmac Soc, Belgrade 1985, Yugoslav Physiol. Pharmacol. Acta 21 (Suppl. 3) 55.

Knowledge-Based Galenical Development of Drug Products: An Overview on the Design of the Galenical Development System Heidelberg

R. Haux[1], T. Wetter[2], H. Stricker[3], J. Flister[1], G. Mann[1], L. Oberhammer[1]

[1] Universität Heidelberg, Institut für Medizinische Biometrie und Informatik, Abteilung Medizinische Informatik, Im Neuenheimer Feld 400, W-6900 Heidelberg
[2] Wissenschaftliches Zentrum der IBM, Institut für Wissensbasierte Systeme, Wilckensstr. 1a, W-6900 Heidelberg
[3] Universität Heidelberg, Institut für Pharmazeutische Technologie und Biopharmazie, Im Neuenheimer Feld 366, W-6900 Heidelberg

Abstract

The intention is to provide information about knowledge-based galenical development of drug products. As result from a systems analysis, types of knowledge needed in galenical development will be presented. The *Galenical Development System Heidelberg* (GSH), currently under construction, aims at reducing time and material needed for the galenical development of drug products by carrying out 'theoretical experiments' by the computer using such galenical knowledge before testing drug products in practical experiments for the sake of the pharmacist and ultimately for the sake of the physician and the patient as well.

1 Introduction: Information Processing in the Galenical Development of Drug Products

1.1 Galenical Development of Drug Products

The development of a new drug product starts with a drug substance. When introduced into special compartments of an organism in a certain concentration, a drug substance is intended to cause certain effects.

A *drug substance* has a set of drug substance properties, e.g. the aggregate state, which describe the drug substance itself, its interactions with other chemical substances, and its behavior in different environments. The developed, applicable drug product also exhibits certain properties, e.g. the recommended concentration of the drug. These properties are determined by the target localization in the organism (e.g. the intestine), by the way to the target localization in the organism (e.g. through the stomach) and by the method of application (e.g. enteral or parenteral). It also has properties determined by legal limitations, e.g. the cleanness and the lifetime of the drug product.

Galenical development of a drug product (cf. [4]) serves to develop a drug substance by adding respectively applying *excipients* or *technical processes*. Excipients are substances without relevant physiological effects, which cause known modifications of one or more drug substance properties. The aim of galenical development of a drug product is to find a *manufacturing instruction*, i.e. a complete, stepwise specification of a sequence of excipients and technical processes, in order to obtain a drug product with certain, initially specified *desired properties* (figure 1).

Determining a manufacturing instruction is also a step-by-step process. After having specified a manufacturing instruction either partially or completely, the corresponding drug products of the intermediate states or of the final state are applied in a *practical experiment*. The *observed properties* of the drug products of the intermediate states and/or of the final state that result from practical experiments are then compared with the specified desired properties, especially for the final drug product. If observed properties and desired properties are not 'sufficiently equal' the galenical scientist tries to improve the first manufacturing instruction, etc., in order to develop an applicable drug product. After their galenical development, drug products may then be evaluated with well known procedures such as controlled clinical trials.

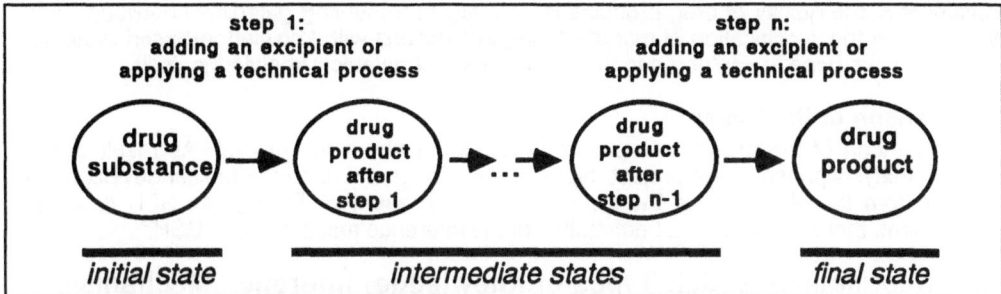

Fig. 1: Galenical development of drug products: manufacturing instruction as a stepwise sequence of adding excipients or applying technical processes.

1.2 Information Processing Problems in Galenical Development

The foundation for galenical development is the developmental knowledge of the galenical scientist, briefly denoted here as *galenical knowledge*. Galenical knowledge consists of knowledge obtained through individual experience, knowledge from preformulation studies (special experiments in order to obtain knowledge e.g. about the behaviour of excipients in the process of galenical development) and knowledge from galenical literature.

Currently, the amount of time and material as well as the cost for the galenical development of drug products is steadily increasing, mainly for the following reasons:

- The requirements for a drug product, and with it the number of properties considered, increase.
- Galenical knowledge is also increasing considerably. Today, e.g., there are several thousand excipients with a growing number of known properties.
- Certainty and completeness of the galenical knowledge used is often not defined.
- The desired drug products are becoming more and more complex.

However, the number of practical experiments in the development of a drug product can be reduced by intensively using galenical knowledge and by 'simulating' the above mentioned practical experiments by *theoretical experiments* on the basis of this galenical knowledge.

2   The GSH Project

2.1 Aim of the Project

In the viewpoint of the authors, time and material needed for the galenical development of drug products can be reduced considerably by carrying out such theoretical experiments before testing drug products in practical experiments, especially before testing the first manufacturing instruction. Theoretical experiments derive proposals for manufacturing instructions by using formally represented galenical knowledge. The represented galenical knowledge should obviously be as complete and as up to date as possible.

Such theoretical experiments can appropriately be done by computer using knowledge-based systems (cf. [3], [6] or [1] concerning medicine). For this reason, the authors agreed to develop the so-called *Galenical Development System Heidelberg* (GSH). GSH shall have the following properties:

For the galenical scientist as user of GSH:
- Simple access to galenical knowledge.
- Deriving proposals for manufacturing instructions by using galenical knowledge.
- Improving manufacturing instructions by changing single steps of the sequence of processes, either by the galenical scientist or by GSH.
- Documentation and explanation of each step of the manufacturing instruction.

For the galenical expert scientist as knowledge engineer of GSH:
- Possibilities for easily adding and correcting the represented galenical knowledge.

As mentioned above, we see the need for such a system and expect a considerable reduction of time and material (as well as a reduction of cost) for the sake of the pharmacist and ultimately for the sake of the physician and the patient as well. We also expect an improvement of the quality of drug products by formally representing galenical knowledge and by supporting the specification of manufacturing instructions with knowledge-based systems. Additionally, we hope to contribute to the improvement of galenical knowledge itself.

2.2 Intention of the Paper

The intention of the paper is to provide information about the project. As result of the systems analysis phase of the project, types of knowledge needed in galenical development (at least from the viewpoint of the authors) will be presented. Finally, as GSH is under development, there will be only a brief outline of the inference mechanism of GSH.

3　Informatical Model: Types of Knowledge, Inference Mechanism

3.1　Types of Knowledge

3.1.1　Introduction

In this section the galenical knowledge needed for the galenical development of a drug product will be described. This knowledge forms the basis for the inference mechanism, outlined in section 3.2.

The individual galenical knowledge of a galenical expert is represented in the following ways:
- Description of interactions between drug substances and excipients and their combination.
- Definition of a hierarchical order of technical processes and excipients after their preference by the galenical expert. This order is represented by the rank, depending on the desired application form.
- Specification of the confidence of the galenical expert. The confidence is represented by a certainty value, ranging from 1 for the lowest confidence to 10 for the highest.

Let us first define some general elements for the knowledge types used. If not mentioned otherwise, the cardinalities of the sets are ≥ 1. Examples will be given in sections 3.1.2 and 3.1.3.

Let $\underline{D}$ denote the set of **designations**.

A **property** P, say, of a drug substance, an excipient or an interaction is defined as
$P := (K_P, V, C)$, where
- K_P denotes the kind of property,
- V denotes the value of property and
- C denotes the certainty of information.

Let $\underline{P}$ denote the set of all such properties P.

A **property of a drug product** P, say, is defined as
$P_{DP} := (K_{DP}, DV, LV, HV)$, where
- K_{DP} denotes the kind of property,
- DV denotes the desired value,
- LV denotes lowest possible value and
- HV denotes the highest possible value.

Let $\underline{P}_{DP}$ denote a set of such properties P_{DP}.

Excipients and technical processes are used in different steps of galenical development. Such a **use of application** UA, say, is defined as
$UA := (K_{UA}, R)$, where
- K_{UA} denotes the kind of use and
- R denotes the rank, specifying the preferred use by the galenical expert.

Let $\underline{UA}$ denote the set of all such uses of application UA.

3.1.2 Types of Knowledge Specified by the User

A **drug substance** DS, say, is defined as
DS := $(\underline{D}_{DS}, \underline{P}_{DS})$, where

- $\underline{D}_{DS} := \{D_{DS_1}, D_{DS_2}, ...\}$ denotes the set of designations for DS, $\underline{D}_{DS} \subseteq \underline{D}$, and
- $\underline{P}_{DS} := \{P_{DS_1}, P_{DS_2}, ...\}$ denotes the set of properties of DS, $\underline{P}_{DR} \subseteq \underline{P}$,

e.g. ({glucose,sugar,...},{(aggregate state,firm,10),...}).

A **drug product** DP, say, is defined by
DP := $(\underline{D}_{DP}, \underline{P}_{DP})$, where

- $\underline{D}_{DP} := \{D_{DP_1}, D_{DP_2}, ...\}$ denotes the set of designations for DP, $\underline{D}_{DP} \subseteq \underline{D}$, and
- $\underline{P}_{DP} := \{P_{DP_1}, P_{DP_2}, ...\}$ denotes the set of properties of DP as mentioned above,

e.g. ({solution of glucose,...},{(concentration, 10 %, 8 %, 15 %),...}).

3.1.3 Types of Knowledge Specified by the Galenical Expert

An **excipient** EX, say, is defined as
EX := $(\underline{D}_{EX}, \underline{UA}_{EX}, \underline{P}_{EX})$, where

- $\underline{D}_{EX} := \{D_{EX_1}, D_{EX_2}, ...\}$ denotes the set of designations for EX, $\underline{D}_{EX} \subseteq \underline{D}$,
- $\underline{UA}_{EX} := \{UA_{EX_1}, UA_{EX_2}, ...\}$ denotes the set of uses for EX, $\underline{UA}_{EX} \subseteq \underline{UA}$, and
- $\underline{P}_{EX} := \{P_{EX_1}, P_{EX_2}, ...\}$ denotes the set of properties of EX, $\underline{P}_{EX} \subseteq \underline{P}$,

e.g. ({H_2O,water,...},{(medium for solution,1),...},{(aggregate state,fluid,9),...}).

A **technical process** TP, say, is defined as
TP := $(\underline{D}_{TP}, \underline{UR}_{TP}, \underline{E})$, where

- $\underline{D}_{TP} := \{D_{TP_1}, D_{TP_2}, ...\}$ denotes the set of designations for TP, $\underline{D}_{TP} \subseteq \underline{D}$,
- $\underline{UA}_{TP} := \{UA_{TP_1}, UA_{TP_2}, ...\}$ denotes the set of uses for TP, $\underline{UA}_{TP} \subseteq \underline{UA}$, and
- $\underline{E} := \{E_1, E_2, ...\}$ denotes the set of effects of TP,

e.g. ({move,...},{dissolve,1),...},{increase of solubility,...}).

An **interaction** I, say, i.e. an effect between drug substances, (intermediate) drug products and ajduvants and their combination, is defined as
I := $(\underline{D}_I, \underline{ES}, \underline{P}_I)$, where

- $\underline{D}_I := \{D_{I_1}, D_{I_2}, ...\}$ denotes the set of designations of the drug substance or of the excipient, which is modified, $\underline{D}_I \subseteq \underline{D}$,
- $\underline{ES} := \{ES_1, ES_2, ...\}$ denotes the set of substances which cause the effects, and
- $\underline{P}_I := \{P_{I_1}, P_{I_2}, ...\}$ denotes the set of properties which are modified, $\underline{P}_I \subseteq \underline{P}$,

e.g. ({NA_2HPO_4,...},{KH_2PO_4,...},{(cleanness,unclean,7),...}).

A **method** M, say, is defined as
M := $(\underline{D}_M, \underline{IP}, VR, MF)$, where

- $\underline{D}_M := \{D_{M_1}, D_{M_2}, ...\}$ denotes the set of designations for M, $\underline{D}_M \subseteq \underline{D}$,
- $\underline{IP} := \{IP_1, IP_2, ...\}$ denotes the set of input parameters,
- VR denotes the value of the result and
- MF denotes the mathematical formula.

3.2 Outline of the Inference Mechanism

The inference mechanism is based on frames and scripts (e.g. [2]). At first, two frames will be generated: one for the drug substance, one for the drug product. New properties can be calculated from basic properties by applying methods introduced above. If the value of a property of the drug substance frame is outside of the limits of tolerance of the target frame, the system activates a script for this property. An activated script searches a technical process or an excipient in order to appropriately change the value of the property, etc..

Within the inference mechanism we can distinguish between two levels of abstraction and between different phases within each level. On the first level of abstraction, the following phases of inference exist: solubilization, stabilization, mixing, isotonization, filtration, sterilization, packaging, storage, lyophylized product, optimization.

Within each phase, appropriate scripts are activated as mentioned above. 'Optimal' results of a phase may be suboptimal after a next phase and may be rejected and lead to repetitions within the inference process. The inference mechanism will use information on ranks and certainty values in order to find an 'optimal' drug product.

4   State of the GSH Project

Currently (April 1991), the systems analysis for GSH - especially the specification of the types of knowledge needed - has been finished. A first prototype on an IBM 6150 RISC machine running under AIX is under development. At the moment, however, we consider only fluid drug products.

5   Discussion

Details of GSH concerning pharmaceutical aspects can be found in [5].

The types of knowledge in section 3.1 describe qualitative knowledge occuring in drug product development, e.g. principal possibilities for using excipients, technical processes, etc. in order to obtain certain properties of a drug product. In addition there are numerical relationships, describing the strength of effects (dose-response characteristics) of the excipients used or processes applied. Their use is subordinate to the use of qualitative knowledge, but also necessary for the inference process as outlined in section 3.2.

If the inference process is understood in terms of a state space, whose states are the intermediate results of developing a drug product and steps are defined by excipients or processes available, it is obvious to conclude that the graph is well known locally (the isolated effect of a process or excipient can be predicted more or less accurately), but that it is unknown as a whole (complex interactions between treatments may only become apparent after several other treatments). For this kind of problem, best-first search lends itself and will be applied here.

In the systems analysis of the project we found that the success of GSH has to consider among others the following two aspects. The first one is the terminology of pharmacy, with its partially non-unique designations, especially for excipients. The second one is the high quantity of properties of drug substances, excipients, etc., which together with the not polynomially bounded complexity of the inference mechanism may lead to run-time problems, if no effective reduction of the state space can be found.

However we have the advantage that for knowledge-based galenical development of drug products there exists a clear aim of the inference process: finding an appropriate manufacturing instruction, resulting in a drug product with clearly specified properties.

Acknowledgement

The GSH project is supported by IBM Germany.

References

[1]   HAUX R, MANN G (1991): Wissensbasierte Systeme in der Medizin und ihre Integration in Informationssysteme. To appear in: Guggenmoos-Holzmann I (ed.). *Proc. 35. Jahrestagung der Deutschen Gesellschaft für Medizinische Dokumentation, Informatik und Statistik.* Berlin: Springer.

[2]   MYOPOULOS J, LEVESQUE H (1983): An Overview of Knowledge Representation. In: NEUMANN B (ed.): *GWAI-83,* 143-157. Berlin: Springer.

[3]   RICHTER MM (1989): *Prinzipien der Künstlichen Intelligenz.* Stuttgart: Teubner.

[4]   STRICKER H (ed.) (1987): *Physikalische Pharmazie.* Stuttgart: Wissenschaftliche Verlagsgesellschaft.

[5]   STRICKER H, HAUX R, WETTER T, MANN G, OBERHAMMER L, FLISTER J (1991): Das 'Galenische Entwicklungs-System Heidelberg' (GSH). To appear in *Pharm. Ind..*

[6]   WATERMAN DA (1985): *A Guide to Expert Systems.* Reading, Ma.: Addison-Wesley.

DEVELOPMENT OF AN EXPERT SYSTEM FOR THE DETECTION OF ADVERSE DRUG REACTIONS

O. Juan-Babot *, P. Ferrer-Salvans *, L. Alonso-Vallès *, I. Ferrer-Salvans *, C. Castells-Nat *, Vidal-Casas E. *, R. Rubio-García **
* Hospital Duran i Reynals
Unitat de Farmacologia Clínica. Ciutat Sanitària de Bellvitge.
Autovia Castelldefels Km 2.7, 08907 L'Hospitalet de Llobregat
Barcelona, Spain
** Andersen Consulting. Madrid. Spain.

Abstract
The development of an expert system for the detection of adverse drug reactions based on the epidemiological approach and careful monitorization of a random sample of inpatients is proposed. Clinical parameters at the time of admission to hospital are taken as a starting point to assess new manifestations appearing during hospitalization. The newly developed signs and symptoms are sequentially introduced in a data base and analyzed using causality algorithms and statistical tests. Any statistically significant observation made or causality association established are entered into a medical knowledge data base. The expert system proposed may be used as a consultation tool or therapeutical decision aid.

Introduction

An adverse drug reaction is defined as 'every nondesired effect, bad for the patient, that appears after the administration with diagnostic, prophylactic or therapeutic purposes, of a form of titration of a medicine, used in a correct dose and indication'. This definition excludes therapeutic failures and intoxication by overdose (1).

In a study carried out in our country (2), adverse drug reactions caused 4% of emergency room admissions and 5% of the total number of admissions to hospital; in addition, they occurred in 18-30% of inpatients with a mortality rate of 0.5%. Based on these findings a special program for detecting adverse drug reactions at our institution was developed.

Methods

Following the policies for hospital accreditation of the 'Generalitat de Catalunya' a program for detecting adverse drug reactions at our hospital was designed. It included the analysis of, a) adverse drug reactions recorded in clinical records; b) reports of emergency admissions caused by adverse drug reactions; c) adverse drug reactions recorded by the hospital pharmacy in the unit dose dispensation protocols; and d) a special prospective follow-up program was implemented in a random sample of hospitalized patients.

In this special prospective follow-up program, information related to clinical manifestations, results of laboratory tests, and drugs administered is collected and introduced in a data base. Each file of the data base covers a specific clinical area, i.e. gastroenterology, biochemistry, etc., for a total of more than 200 items referring to commonly observed events in daily clinical practice and main laboratory parameters, codified as 'closed' questions. Fields for recording other events free questions are included in the files. From this data base a statistical analysis using the SPSS program is carried out. These procedures are illustrated in Figure 1.

THERAPEUTICAL PRESCRIPTION   **FOLLOW-UP**

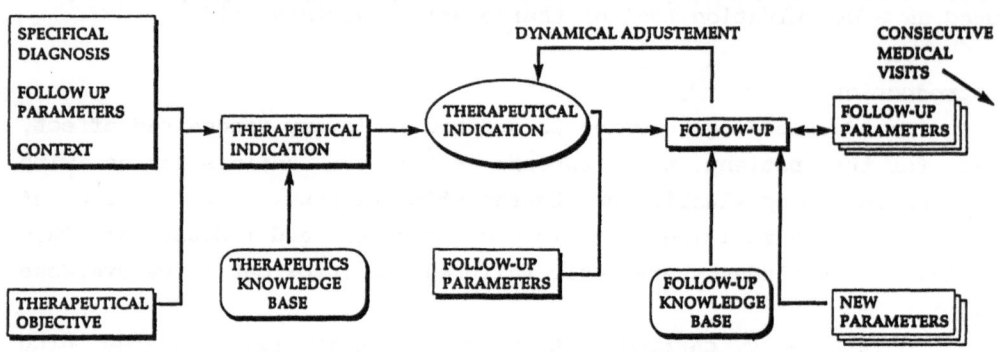

Fig. 1

Results

Preliminary results (3) of adverse drug reactions recorded in clinical records revealed an incidence rate of 4 for 1,000 (61% men, 39% women). Pharmacological agents and organic systems most frequently involved are referred to in Tables 1 and 2. The corresponding figure for reports of emergency admissions caused by adverse drug reactions was 6 for 1,000 (42% men, 58% women) (Tables 3 and 4).

Table 1. Drugs most frequently involved in adverse drug reactions recorded by physicians in inpatients' medical records.

Therapeutic category

Anti-inflammatory, analgesic	24%
Antineoplastic, immunosupressant	20%
Cardiovascular	14%
Antimicrobials	11%
Polypharmacy	8%
Endocrine, metabolism	6%
Nervous system	4%
Hematologic	4%
Gastrointestinal	2%
Miscellaneous	7%

Table 2. Organic system most frequently involved in adverse drug reactions recorded by phisicians in inpatients' medical records.

System or Apparatus

Gastrointestinal tract	29%
Hematologic	24%
skin	12%
Cardiovascular	7%
Endocrine	7%
Renal	6%
Nervous	4%
Respiratory	2%
Metabolism	2%
General disturbance	2%
Miscellaneous	5%

Table 3. Drugs most frequently involved in adverse drug reactions recorded in emergency admission records.

Therapeutic category

Polypharmacy	21%
Antimicrobials	19%
Anti-inflammatory, analgesics	17%
Cardiovascular	10%
Miscellaneous	10%
Endocrine, metabolism	6%
Nervous system	5%
Hematologic	3%
Respiratory	3%

Table 4. Organic systems most frequently involved in adverse drug reactions recorded in emergency admissions.

System or Apparatus

Skin	37%
Gastrointestinal tract	27%
Nervous	9%
Cardiovascular	8%
General disturbances	8%
Eye	4%
Hematologic	3%
Respiratory	2%
Miscellaneous	2%

Discussion

The use of indicators such as adverse drug reactions recorded in clinical records and reports of emergency admissions caused by adverse drug reactions show a low sensitivity as compared with indexes published in literature (4,5). The imputability or cause-effect relationship constitutes the main problem that arises when assessing drug-associated reactions. Different causality algorithms have been proposed as those described by Naranjo et al.(6), Kramer et al.(7), Venulet et al.(8), and Karch and Lasagna (9). All of them consider a) the temporal sequence of events, b) the fact that the adverse effect should be sufficiently documented in the literature, c) the reappearance of the effect when the drug is readministered, and d) the absence of an alternative causal explanation.

Because many cases of suspected drug-associated reaction remain unsolved, an epidemiological approach is suggested. Instead of analyzing each case individually, we propose to study all cases as a whole using statistical methods for pattern recognition and grouping of similar cases. Based on this information the final objective is to develop an expert system for the evaluation and follow-up of adverse drug reactions using artificial intelligence techniques (10,11). The methodology developed for the AEDMI program (12) (An Epidemiological Approach to Computerized Medical Diagnosis) can also be applied for this purpose. From an initial diagnosis and subsequent therapeutic indication, three possible time-courses can be defined, 1) the abnormal symptoms disappeared, 2) some criteria of improvement are achieved, 3) some kind of alleviation referred to the starting point is achieved. If the time-course is not foreseeable, i.e. the patient's condition is not changing as the physician expects, a lack of response is considered. The new parameters should be evaluated in order to dilucidate, a) if there is an evolution of the underlying condition, b) an event that requires a clinical diagnosis, and c) a complication in medical care or iatrogenic event of pharmacological origin that makes necessary therapeutical knowledge. The newly developed signs and symptoms are sequentially introduced in a data base and analyzed using causality algorithms and statistical tests. Any statistically significant observation made or causality association established are entered into a medical knowledge data base.

The aim of this approach is to develop an expert system as an aid for the control of adverse drug reactions asssisted by the use pharmacological data bases. The expert system proposed may be used as a consultation tool or therapeutical decision aid.

Acknowledgments

This work is receiving the grant from FISss 90/0403
The authors would like to thank the mangement authorities of Bellvitge Hospital, Dr. Eng. F. Moreu, Dr. C. Serra, and Dr. F. Ramos for their support to the different research lines of AEDMI Project.

References

[1] Karch FE, Lasagna L. Adverse drug reactions. JAMA 1975;234:1236.
[2] Pintado V, Martin A, Guiard MV, et al. Reacciones adversas a medicamentos. Medicina Integral 1990; 15: 89-96.
[3] Alonso L, Castells C, Ferrer I, Ferrer P, Juan O, Matud C, Pereiro J, Rubio R, Valiño J. Programa de farmacovigilancia: nueva metodología. IX Reunión científica del FISss, Barcelona. 1990;111.

[4]   Caranasos GJ, May FE, Stewart RB, Cluff EC.   Drug-associated deaths of medical inpatiens. Arch Intern Med 1976;136:872-5.

[5]   Martinez B, González de Suso MJ, Mota C, et al. Estudio de las reacciones adversas causadas por medicamentos en pacientes encamados en un hospital universitario.   Rev Clín Esp 1986; 179:73-6.

[6]   Naranjo CA, Busto U, Sellers E, et al. A method for estimating the probability of adverse drug reactions. Clin Pharmacol Ther 1981; 30:239-45.

[7]   Kramer MS, Leventhal JM, Hutchinson TA, Feinstein AR. An algorithm for the operational assessment of adverse drug reactions(I). JAMA 1979; 242:623-32.

[8]   Venulet J, Ciucci A, Berneker GC. Standardized assessment of drug-adverse reactions, rationale and experience. International Journal of Clinical Pharmacology, Therapy and Toxicology 1980;18:381-8.

[9]   Karch FE, Lasagna L. Toward the operational identification of adverse drug reactions. Clin Pharmacol Ther 1977; 21:247-54.

[10] Roach J, Lee S, Wilcke J, Ehrich M.   An expert system for information on pharmacology and drug interactions. Comput Biol Med 1985; 15:11-23.

[11] Smeets R.P.A.M., Talmon J.L., Lugt P.J.M. van der, Schijven R.A.J.   The development of a knowledge system for surveillance of anti-epileptic medication. In AIME 89 Lecture Notes in Medical Informatics. (Hunter J., Cookson J. and Wyatt J. eds.) 1989 Berlin. Springer-Verlag. 14-23.

[12] Ferrer Salvans P, Alonso Vallés L. An epidemiological approach to computerized medical diagnosis: the AEDMI program. Comput Biol Med 1990; 20:433-43.

INFORMATION SYSTEMS AND
DECISION SUPPORT

ADVICE AND WARNING WITHIN HIOS+

Francois M.H.M. Dupuits, Arie Hasman, Erik M.J.J. Ulrichts
and Jeroen J.M. Valkenburg
University of Limburg, Dept. of Medical Informatics
P.O. Box 616, 6200 MD Maastricht, The Netherlands
Telephone: +3143888412

Abstract

In this paper, HIOS+ Advice and Warning is described. HIOS+ is a decision support system for medical purposes. Its AW module functions as an inference engine, and as such generates advice and warnings concerning medical diagnoses and treatments. In order to be able to do so, HIOS+ AW makes use of models stored in the model base of HIOS+ MM and actual patient data stored in the data bases of the registration system HIOS. Although the development of AW has been initiated only recently, actual reasoning is already being performed in the filter items part of several protocols. Reasoning situations which can be distinguished concerning filter items (findings) are: a GP or medical specialist (1) adds new data to or changes existing data in the HIOS data bases, (2) requests advice, (3) requests information about findings of which outcomes have not yet become available, (4) requests explanations about the reasoning of AW, and HIOS+ AW automatically (5) presents reminders, advice and/or warnings. The heart of HIOS+ AW is a patient/protocol dependent file called MISHITS which enables the actual reasoning process. In this file 'hits' and 'misses' are recorded when checking filter items of a protocol against actual data of a patient.

Keywords are: Decision Support, Inference Engine, Medical Protocols, Reasoning.

Introduction

At the end of 1988 and the start of 1989, a poll was held among GPs to determine their

217

need of automated decision support. The outcomes of the poll and a request of internists at the University Hospital Maastricht instigated the development of Decision Support System (DSS) HIOS+ within a project called 'Decision Support System in Health care' (DSSH). General information about DSS is given in [7]. HIOS+ consists of the modules Information Facility (IF), Model Maker (MM) and Advice and Warning (AW) and makes use of the HIOS data bases in which basic and medical data of patients are stored. IF provides additional information on diseases. Diagnostic and therapeutic models (protocols, standards and/or work agreements) are constructed with MM. AW generates advice and/or warnings about possible diagnoses or treatments. In figure 1, the structure of HIOS+ is shown.

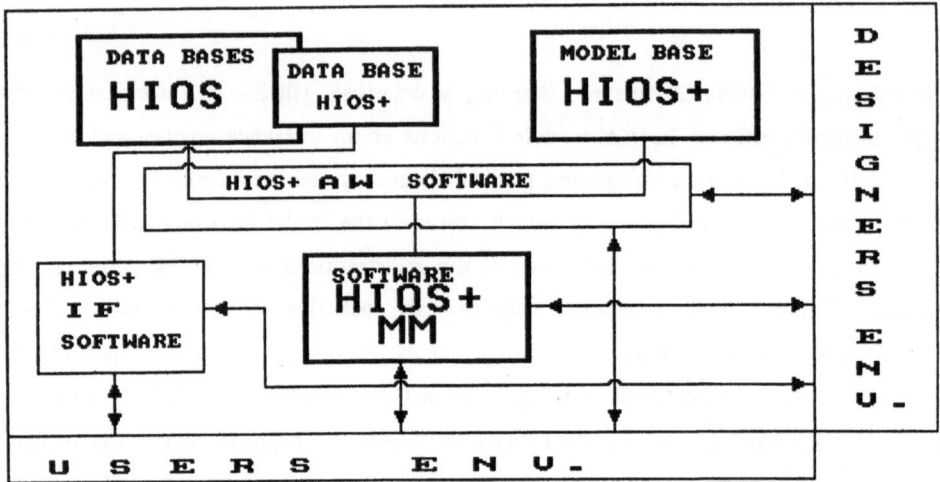

Figure 1. The structure of HIOS+

Development environment of HIOS+

Several information system development methods and techniques are being used in the design process. Evolutionary prototyping and iterative design for instance are being applied in combination with an in-house developed Phased Development Method. This Method involves the development of several versions, from system 0 up to and including system X. Each new version signifies a further, more sophisticated evolution in the development of HIOS+ or one of its components. The check list concerning wishes and demands of users preferably should not contain any items immediately after system X has been developed. Future developments might cause a user to add wishes and/or demands to the check list. These will be evaluated and proper action taken. A detailed description of the HIOS+ design environment is given in [2] and [6].

HIOS+ Advice & Warning: the Reasoning Process

The Advice & Warning (AW) module is the most important decision support facility within HIOS+. In order to be able to give advice and present warnings, the inference engine HIOS+ AW makes use of models stored within the model base of HIOS+ MM and actual facts stored within the HIOS data bases.

In the summer of 1991, HIOS+ AW is expected to become available as system 0. Although the development of HIOS+ AW has been initiated only recently, some preliminary results can be reported because of the fact that actual reasoning is already being performed within the filter items part of several protocols. The authors of [4] and [5] deal with reasoning processes in medical environments; while reasoning in general is described in [8]. Within the reasoning process applied in the filter items part of HIOS+ (concerning findings), several situations can be identified: - a medical user adds new data to or changes existing data in the HIOS data bases; - a medical user requests advice; - a medical user requests information about findings of which outcomes have not yet become available; - a medical user requests explanations about the reasoning of HIOS+ AW and - HIOS+ AW automatically presents reminders, advice and/or warnings. When working ·with HIOS+, the first situation often occurs. Because of the fact that all entries within HIOS+ AW will be stored within the HIOS data bases, often new data are added to or existing data are changed within an automated medical record of a patient. Every alteration of facts stored within the HIOS data bases has its impact on a file called MISHITS and vice versa. In this file 'hits' and 'misses' are recorded when checking filter items of a protocol in the filter items part of HIOS+ MM against actual data of a patient. It is this patient/protocol dependent file which in fact constitutes the heart of HIOS+ AW and which enables the actual reasoning process about diseases. In the second situation, a user requests advice. Then, all items within the MISHITS file for a certain protocol on which no information is stored in the HIOS data bases are presented. In figure 2, an advice is given on a specific patient with regard to a certain protocol. In the third situation, a user requests

```
VERSION 010291  HIOS+ ADVICE AND WARNING  05-04-91 13:11:12  (MI&S)
MIS 010885 Mr.  ERT   Medical Informatics -              Example
Annalaan 60           6417 KC Maastricht    Male Single  5
         ADVICE ABOUT FILTER ITEMS MARKED AS MISSING
Which signs and symptoms are present?            (Y/N)
Clammy hands                                       Y
Eyes red                                           N
Loss of weight                                     Y

Which diagnoses are present?                      (Y/N)
Exophthalmus                                       Y
Hyperkinesis                                       N

Which therapy or treatment is followed?          (Y/N)


```

1:HELP 2:SEARCH 3:IF

Figure 2. Advice on filter items

information about findings of which outcomes have not yet become available. Then, this user is presented all previously requested items of which results are not yet present. In the fourth situation, a user requests explanations about the reasoning of HIOS+ AW. Then, an overview is presented showing the total of points actually scored and the number of points necessary to be reached for the protocol network to get activated. Confirmed, denied and requested findings are also presented. In the fifth situation, HIOS+ automatically presents reminders, advice and/or warnings. Reminders may deal e.g. with data about the follow-up of patients suffering from a certain disease. Advice presented deals with recommendations concerning diagnoses and therapies of diseases. HIOS+ automatically presents a warning when a user is about to act in violation of a protocol. The automatic review also lists items of which the results ought to be available. Future AW developments will involve the construction of learning and priority algorithms. When determining priorities between items, priority algorithms will have to be able to take into account certain aspects like: predictive value, costs involved and delivery time of results. The presentation of alternatives to users in such a way that the most likely one is listed first, is a striking characteristic of a DSS. In HIOS+, items are also listed according to this phenomenon. A user can choose one of the listed items or activate an escape facility. HIOS+ guarantees flexibility of usage to users: a user is always given the opportunity to overrule the system.

Conclusions about HIOS+

Although the development of HIOS+ is still in progress, we are certain that this DSS will be of enormous value to GPs and medical specialists. It supports its users in their decision making concerning diagnoses and therapies of diseases. HIOS+ AW and HIOS+ IF are the most important decision support facilities within the system. HIOS+ AW generates advice and warnings concerning diagnoses and therapies of diseases. It furthermore advises in the follow-up of patients suffering from chronic diseases. It might be possible to avoid a disease from (re-)developing within a patient or to avoid a deterioration of a patient's condition. General information on preventive measures is given in [3]. With HIOS+ IF a user can consult medical textbook information. Although HIOS+ AW provides diagnostic and therapeutic decision support, it would not be able to do so without HIOS+ MM and HIOS. HIOS+ MM enables a user to create and store models. HIOS is a tool for storing basic and medical data. The purpose and scientific value of HIOS+ is described in [1].

References

[1] Dupuits FMHM, Hasman A, Schoonbrood GGM. Decision Support in a General Practice. In: O'Moore R, Bengtsson S, Bryant JR, Bryden JS, eds. Lecture Notes in Medical Informatics - Medical Informatics Europe '90 Proceedings - MIE 90, Glasgow, Scotland, 20-23 August 1990. Berlin Heidelberg: Springer-Verlag, 1990: 40, 231-235.

[2] Dupuits FMHM, Hasman A, Ulrichts EMJJ. The Designing of HIOS+. Software Engineering in Medical Informatics (SEMI), Amsterdam The Netherlands 8-10 October 1990.

[3] Gray M, Fowler G. Preventive medicine in general practice. Oxford: Oxford University Press, 1983.

[4] Haux R. Knowledge-Based Decision Support for Diagnosis and Therapy - On the Multiple Usability of Patient Data. Meth. of Information in Medicine 1989; 28 (2), 69-77.

[5] Keravnou ET, Johnson L. Towards a generalized model of diagnostic behaviour. Knowledge-Based Systems September 1989; Vol. 2 No. 3: 165-177.

[6] Senyk O, Patil RS, Sonnenberg FA. Systematic Knowledge Base Design For Medical Diagnosis, Hemisphere Publishing Corporation, 1989: 165[249]-190[274].

[7] Turban E. Decision Support and Expert Systems - Managerial Perspectives. New York U.S.A.: Macmillan Publ. Co., 1988.

[8] Winkelbauer L, Markstrom S. Symbolic And Numerical Methods In Hybrid Multi-Criteria Decision Support. Laxenburg Austria: International Institute for Applied Systems Analysis, 1989.

Strategies for Efficient Implementation of the Arden Syntax for Medical Decision Support.

Gabor Magyar, K. Arkad, X. Gao, H. Gill, O. Wigertz, H. Åhlfeldt.

Dept.of Medical Informatics,
Faculty of Health Sciences, Linköping University,
S - 581 83, Linköping SWEDEN.

Abstract

Together with other medical centres we are working on a common language, called Arden Syntax to present medical knowledge, that can be used for knowledge exchange between different institutes. The form of the language has evolved during the last eighteen months and work is still going on to improve the expressiveness and implementability of the language. In this paper some of our experiences, both in connection with the language and in connection with the operating environment are described. Properties of operating environments and medical information systems that may facilitate integration of medical logic are described.

Introduction.

In this paper we give a short description of the experiences achieved during the implementation work of the MLM language. We specify some useful tools to improve the productivity of the MLM-type knowledge description. We also discuss possible extensions and alternatives to the syntax, preserving its simplicity and extending its usability. We also make an attempt to find frequently used logical structures, which are usually necessary to use in case of a decision support system with a complex medical thesaurus and a detailed patient information system. The usage of these structures could be helpful when planning and modifying a medical information system.

The most important parts and the main components of a medical information system are

- the patient data base (PD) in which all patient records are stored
- the data dictionary or the medical entity dictionary (MED) which includes all the terms that are used in the application area and arranged in a logical and work environment oriented way
- the knowledge base (KB) in support for data interpretation and patient management decisions.

Other technical components and subsystems are also important but they are coming and going on the market with rather short life-times especially regarding the vendors. It is therefore important that the three main components mentioned above, are as <u>independent</u> as possible regarding systems technique, software and hardware.

We are using a proposed knowledge representation language called the *Arden Syntax* and using the Arden syntax as a language we create *Medical Logic Modules*

[MLM89,Hri90]. This syntax is developed at the University of Utah, the Columbia University in New York, the Erasmus University in Rotterdam and the Linköping University.

The concept of the Medical Logic Module (MLM) is an emerging standard with the purpose of allowing multiple users to create, criticize and share pieces of medical knowledge *[Wig89,Cla89-90]*. The use of such a standard does not only have medical motivations, but also economical because the construction of extensive, accurate knowledge bases is a very time and cost consuming task. The main goal of the project is to make it possible to send pieces of knowledge between institutes, which means also that the formalized knowledge is not supposed to be very complicated neither very specific. The MLMs are supposed to contain small and well defined rules, which can be controlled easily. The Arden Syntax also contain different control structures to gather information and to produce a time scheduled behaviour.

We have reported a proposed system design for the realization of Medical Logic Modules as working modules in a patient information system *[Ark90,Mag90]*.

DATABASE ISSUES TOWARDS A COMMON DECISION SUPPORT

THE MEDICAL ENTITY DICTIONARY

The Medical Entity Dictionary (MED) referred to here can be looked upon as a system catalogue (data definition catalogue). A definition of the MED might be: - A set of medical terms with their properties and relationships organized according to the needs of the patient database (patient record database /PD/) and the medical knowledge base (KB).

The basic concept of the MED is the *medical term*. The medical terms used in a patient database or a medical knowledge base form a subset of the entire medical nomenclature. The concrete structure of the MED is imbedded into the database through relations and structured statements (MAPPING & PROCEDURES). The medical terms have different attributes like KEY, NAME, SYNONYMS, MAPPING, DOMAIN, MODULE and PROCEDURE. The attributes KEY and NAME are unique designations of a medical term. The MAPPING attribute maps the term to appropriate classifications and places it in zero or several hierarchies. DOMAIN defines the type of data that may be linked to the term when it is stored in the patient's database. The DOMAIN attribute may also include references to other medical terms. PROCEDURE represents specific procedures that control the entry and retrieval of the term and its attributes in the database. MODULE represents those medical facts in the knowledge base in which the term is used as a variable. MAINTENANCE contains information about when and by whom the term is created or edited and also a reference and comment. These attributes define the position of the medical term in a very variable and elastic data base. This elasticity and variability allow to use the different categorisation systems of the medical practice, thought it's effect for the performance requires further research and fast data base handling algorithms. *[Lin89]*. The procedure, module and maintenance attributes are the predecessors of an object-oriented approach. The medical terms including the attributes, mentioned above are fitting well into an object-oriented approach and the object-oriented approach is one of the most natural realization of a medical term dictionary.

THE PATIENT DATABASE

The Patient Database (PD, we use this abbreviation for the entire database which contains individual patient records) itself is the first component of a complex clinical information environment and although we don't deal with this part in details, we find it important to mention some properties, which are necessary for the data base management applications. Generally a PD application is a running process in a computer environment, whose task is maintenance, retrieving, producing results, etc. The PD programs should keep contact with the KB-processing part of the information system *[Pry88,Ste88]*. The communication between the PD-applications and the decision support parts of the system is taking place through a message sending mechanism, where intermediate interface modules are responsible for the appropriate execution or the scheduling of the requests.

Another, and better solution is to use object-oriented databases for the storage of the patient data, and in this case the defined objects are able to send messages without the need of modifying the application programs. We suppose moreover, that the description of the PD structure is available through the MED, and the KB frames are able to extract it from there.

UTILITIES TO IMPROVE THE WRITEABILITY OF THE KNOWLEDGE MODULES

THE MLM EDITOR

The MLM editor is one of the most important development tools of the MLM based medical information system. The editor makes it possible to choose an appropriate module or group of modules to work with. It automatically checks the possible relations between different modules and sends an error messages in case of a discovered contradiction. With help of the editor the user gets the possibility to be familiar with the Arden syntax and it contains a tool for browsing the Medical Entity Dictionary. There is an essential question what the MED should contain and how to share the MED into logically separated subcomponents. The nature of the MED is at least twofold. The medical entity holds information about itself by placing it into a hierarchy and holds information about the method of its retrieval from a patient database. The second attribute is more technical. In a strict sense we don't bother with the technical details of the MED, however the knowledge of the particular properties of a medical entity can have a very essential effect on the performance of the system.

The main functions of the editor are the syntax directed creation of a new MLM, to produce standard format MLM lists, managing the source KB as deleting, modifying and adding new MLMs, checking the names and preventing contradictions, on-line help to retrieve and incorporate medical terms from the MED (help for choosing an existing medical term).

THE MLM PRETTY-PRINTER

To improve the writeability of the knowledge modules we also give another possibility which allows a minor deviation from the Arden syntax in a reversible way. In case of the user has no access to an MLM editor she can still use a plain text editor to create MLM-text. It can be a restriction that by the Arden syntax the form and the sequence of possible slots are strictly determined and from the individual user's point of view it seems to be redundant. With help of our pretty printer the developer can concentrate on the definition of those slots which carry information beside an institution standard. This means that the developer uses a template with the administrative and identification slots and she can concentrate on the essential *library, data, logic, evoke and action* slots. The pretty-printer, parametrized the proper way does the rest of the work.

THE MLM COMPILER

The MLM compiler translates the source knowledge base into an intermediate form. The compiler's task is also to compile MLM text into the knowledge base and to make a syntax and compatibility test (compatibility with the KB and with the MED). The compatibility control is highly simplified in case of an object oriented medical term database, because the integrity and interrelating dependencies are imbedded into the database. Summarizing the tasks of the MLM compiler, it must check the syntax of the MLM texts, check the variables and consistency with the MED, and the KB, generate code (fast interpretable code).

The result of the MLM compilation is a new object, which contains a list of codes about the activities of the MLM in the form of a pseudo code, or coded series of messages, a list of MED objects referenced in the MLM and a control structure for a C++ supervising program with imbedded database handling statements. The advantage of storing the compiled MLMs in a database is handsome, and there is the opportunity to use the facilities of the database management system for the recording and maintaining the knowledge base administration.

The access of different databases takes place through imbedded database handling statements, while the control functions, mathematical computations, communications with the operating system and between the different programs are carried out via C++. The nature of the database handling statements can vary depending on the realization of MED and PD.

THE MLM MANAGER.

The MLM manager is a mixture of a linker and a library maintenance program, known from the practice of traditional programming languages. The tasks of the manager are adding, deleting and replacing an MLM in the interpretable KB, maintaining the inverted lists corresponding to the changes, resolving the unresolved external references to other MLM-modules and medical terms remaining after compilation, listing of the loaded MLMs and different kind of cross-reference tables, creating a subset of the KB with user selected content, joining and projecting knowledge bases and checking the integrity of KB.

POSSIBLE EXTENSIONS OF THE ARDEN SYNTAX

Working with the MLM compiler we found it important to allow a possibility for supporting more complex logical decisions in an easier form. In our local version we allow the use of the case-statement and we also proposed for the standard of the Arden syntax. The form of the case statement is borrowed from the SQL-standard. The statement has the form

CASE

WHEN logical-expression statement

...

END CASE

In our version we use a filter which forces the pretty-printer to convert the CASE statements to an IF-THEN type equivalent program text to keep the compatibility with the original MLM-standard.

Another important change is that we don't use imbedded database search instructions in the modules, but we have a separate metadatabase (which is not necessary in case of an object-oriented database) integrated with the MED which holds the particular database search statements to retrieve the required data. This solution has the advantage that *we don't need to change the MLM part if there is a change in the database structure*. This means another step towards a database structure independent knowledge base.

SUMMARY

In this paper we shortly introduce the ideas behind the Arden Syntax concept, the main components of a medical information system with decision support. We conclude that the tendencies behind the evolution of the decision support and medical data dictionary techniques lead to an object oriented approach. It follows both from the evolution of the medical data dictionary term concept, as well.as from the structure of the patient data and the development of the knowledge base components. We also introduce some useful utilities which can help in the management of the MLMs. We make suggestions to improve the flexibility of the Arden Syntax preserving the principles of the agreed standard.

REFERENCES

(Ark90) Arkad K, Ludwigs U, Shashavar N, Gao Xiao-Ming, Wigertz O. Medical Logic Module representation of knowledge in a ventilator treatment advisory system. Proc 11th Int Symp Information on Technology in Anesthesia, Critical Care and Cardio-pulmonary Medicine.Rotterdam 1990.

(Blu86) Blum B. Clinical information Systems - A Review. The Western J. of Medicine, (1986) Vol.145. No.6.

(Cla89) Clayton PD, Pryor TA, Wigertz O, Hripcsak G. Issues and structures for sharing medical knowledge among decision making systems. SCAMC 1989, pp.116-121.

(Cla90) Clayton PD, Hripcsak G, Pryor TA. Emerging standards for medical logic. SCAMC 1990, pp.27-31.

(Deg90) Degoulet P, Coignard J, Jean FC, Jaulent MC, Lucas L, Ben Said M, Meinzer HP, Engelmann U, Springub A, Baud R, Scherrer JR. The HELIOS European project on software engineering. SEMI 1990, 16p,

(Hri90) Hripcsak G, Clayton PD, Pryor TA, Haug P, Wigertz OB, van der Lei J : The Arden Syntax for Medical Logic Modules. 1990 SCAMC proc.

(Lei90) van der Lei J and Musen MA: separation of critiquing knowledge from Medical knowledge: Implications for the Arden Syntax. 1990 SEMI proc, Amsterdam.

(Lin89) Linnarsson R, Wigertz O. An Infological Model of an Integrated Medical Information System. MEDINFO 89, Vol 1.,(1989) North-Holland.

(Mag90) Magyar G, Arkad K, Ericsson K-E, Gill H, Linnarsson R, Wigertz O. Realizing medical knowledge in MLM form as working modules in a patient information system. Proc IMIA Working Conf on Software Engineering in Medical Informatics. Amsterdam 1990.

(MLM89) MLM. Arden syntax 1.1 - User Manual; November 21, 1989. Arden House, New York.

(Pry88) Pryor TA. The HELP Medical Record System. M.D. Computing (1988) Vol 5. No.5.

(Pry88) Pryor TA, Warner HR, Gardner R. The HELP System Development Tools. In. H.Orthner and B. Blum (eds.), Methods for Developing Clinical Information Systems. New York. Springer Verlag, Inc., 1988.

(She90) Sherertz DD, Olson NE, Tuttle MS Erlbaum MS: Source Inversion and Matching in the UMLS Metathesaurus, 1990. SCAMC proc.

(Ste88) Stead WW, Hammond WE. Computer-Based Medical Records: The Centerpiece of TMR. M.D. Computing (1988) Vol 5. No.5.

(Wig89) Wigertz O, Clayton PD, Hripcsak G, Linnarsson R. Knowledge representation and data model to support medical knowledge base transportability. Proc Systems Engineering in Medicine, March 1989, Maastricht. Springer Verlag.

Development of a computerized neurological decision support system

W. Ken Redekop, Donald W. Paty

Multiple Sclerosis Clinic
G-33, ECU
University Hospital, UBC Site
2211 Wesbrook Mall
Vancouver, BC, CANADA
V6T 2B5

Abstract

The value of computerized data storage in clinical medicine is well recognized. Such a tool enables rapid, comprehensive, and efficient data retrieval. Yet to be recognized for their full potential in this field are decision support systems. Moreover, the integration of database systems with decision support systems offers great potential. At our clinic, a modified computerized medical record system (MS-COSTAR) for research in multiple sclerosis (MS) has been in place for a number of years. We are not only working to maintain and improve the storage of clinical information but we are also focusing on developing decision support systems to work directly with the data in the system. Reliable measurement of disability has been our focus up until now. This is valuable for many studies dealing with the descriptive epidemiology of MS and it is vital for any drug efficacy trials that are undertaken. Other systems such as one for diagnostic support are being developed. Since many centres in the world are adopting the same information system, any decision support system that works with this system can easily be implemented in multiple sites. This allows for improved data pooling, a useful tool for disease etiology studies and multicentre drug efficacy trials.

1. Introduction

The advent of computer technology has brought with it many new tools for use in medical research. Two such applications are computerized information systems and decision support systems. Computers can be used to maintain large information systems which enable fast and comprehensive retrieval. As systems for decision support, computers can assist researchers and clinicians alike by performing complicated and time-consuming analyses without fatigue and without errors. At the Multiple Sclerosis Clinic at the University of British Columbia, we have focused on both of these areas. Development of tools for the support of epidemiological and clinical research is ongoing at this clinic.

2. MS-COSTAR

The system used at our clinic (MS-COSTAR) is a modification of a computerized medical record system (COSTAR, Computer STored Ambulatory Record) that was created at the Massachusetts General Hospital (1) to support clinical, research, and administrative functions. The MS-COSTAR system was developed by personnel at the UBC Multiple Sclerosis Clinic and has been in operation at UBC for more than five years. The system presently contains more than 2800 patient records and includes data on patients' medical histories, neurological and ophthalmological examinations, and laboratory results. Actual results from neurological examinations are entered in a standardized format, thereby avoiding two types of potential problems: first, the need to examine "raw" examination data that was not entered and, second, the problems that result when data is not collected in a standardized manner. MS-COSTAR has already been installed at 8 other MS clinics in Canada (2). It has been accepted by the U.S. MS Society and the Consortium of MS Centers as the standard system for MS clinical research computer systems for all of North America and is presently being used in 9 centres in the United States. One clinic in the Netherlands is now using MS-COSTAR and several other European and Japanese MS centres have also expressed interest in this system. The establishment of such a network of clinics with the same computerized medical records system is considered to be quite unique in clinical medicine. A common computerized system supports the need for gathering data from different sites by minimizing the time and energy required to pool and analyze the data. Its existence enables fast and efficient data pooling, valuable for the support of various research activities including the coordination of multicentre drug evaluation trials. Multicentre trials are very important in a disease such as MS where the course of disease is highly unpredictable and large numbers of suitable patients are required in order to demonstrate a statistically significant treatment effect. Such a coordinated system is useful, for example, in matters of patient selection where the identification of suitable candidates for drug trials involves the examination of many different patient attributes. For research in descriptive epidemiology, data pooling enables standardized methods for evaluating large groups of patients. Such analyses can help in the development of new hypotheses regarding disease etiology.

3. Decision support systems

Our work on decision support systems has up to now centred around the fact that, in multiple sclerosis, there is no unequivocally accurate method of evaluating neurological impairment. This is a major problem since measurement of impairment in MS (as with many diseases) is valuable for the description of the clinical course and as a measure of treatment efficacy. Scoring systems created by J.F. Kurtzke (Functional Systems (FS) and Expanded Disability Status Scale (EDSS)) have been most widely used (3). Use of these scales produces scores based on neurological examinations. The rules for assigning impairment scores are not easily applied; the result is inconsistency in scoring by one clinician and between clinicians. Changes in recorded impairment sometimes have less to do with actual changes in the patient and more to do with these inconsistencies. To resolve some of the problems involved with the use of these scales, computer assignment of these scores is being developed. Computerized scoring assignment eliminates the inconsistencies in scoring by an individual neurologist and between neurologists by enabling a standardized method of scoring.

In the scoring of impairment, a summary score (EDSS) is created on the basis of both the ability to ambulate and the scores for impairment in different systems in the body (FS scores). Through consultation with a neurologist (D.W. Paty), computer programs were designed that compute scores (FS scores) for different systems in the body based on actual neurological examination results (such as visual acuity, muscle weakness, etc.). Computer programs were also created that automatically calculate EDSS scores based on FS scores. This enabled automatic conversion to computerized EDSS assignment directly from neurological examination results.

To examine the effects of the computerized scoring method, the results of the most recent examination of each patient diagnosed as having definite MS (clinically definite or laboratory supported definite) were used to calculate computerized EDSS scores. Figure 1 shows the distribution of computerized scores as well as the distribution of scores assigned by the neurologists ("manual scores"). Table 1 is a cross-tabulation of manual scores versus computerized scores. The distribution using computerized scores differs from that using manual scores because certain problems with the manual EDSS have been rectified. (The heavy influence of ambulation on EDSS scoring has been removed to allow this summary score to be more sensitive to the degrees of impairment in other functional systems in the body.) In the distribution of computerized EDSS scores, the large peak at 8 likely represents a true peak and not an artefactual one.

Figure 1. FREQUENCY DISTRIBUTION OF EDSS

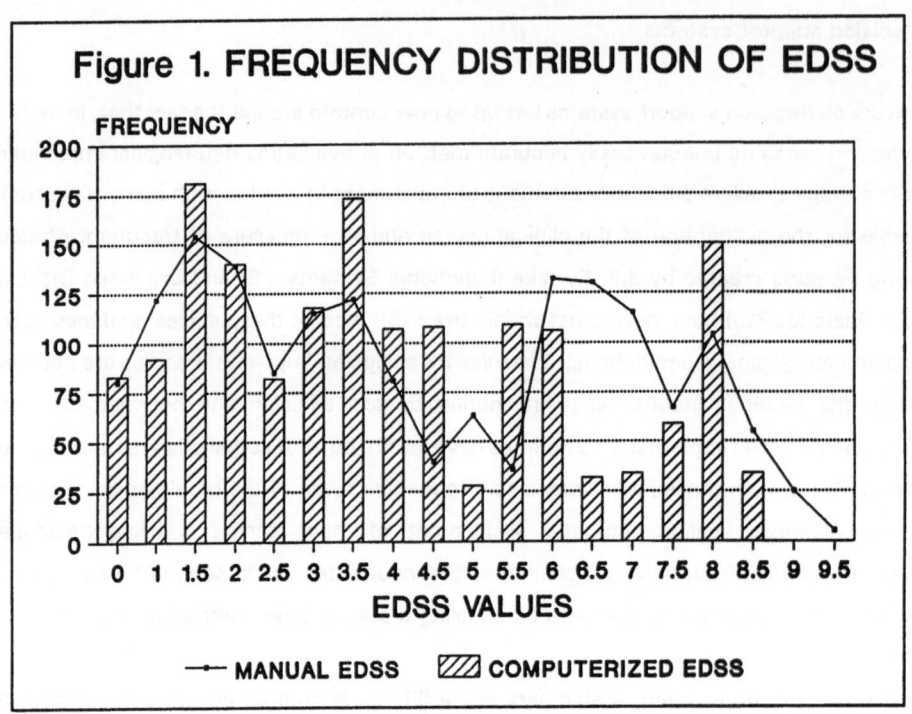

Figure 1. FREQUENCY DISTRIBUTION OF EDSS (MANUAL EDSS, COMPUTERIZED EDSS)

Table 1. CROSS-TABULATION OF MANUAL EDSS VS. COMPUTERIZED EDSS

COMPUTER EDSS	\ MANUAL EDSS → 0	1	1.5	2	2.5	3	3.5	4	4.5	5	5.5	6	6.5	7	7.5	8	8.5	9	9.5	TOTAL
0	(78)	4	1																	83
1	2	(89)	1																	92
1.5		25	(149)	6	1															181
2		2	3	(115)	17	1														140
2.5				6	(62)	10	1			1	1		1							82
3				7	5	(62)	24	7	3	2	2	3	3							118
3.5				1		25	(70)	26	10	11	3	20	5	2						173
4			1			7	18	(22)	9	14	10	15	6	4	1					107
4.5	1		1			4	2	9	(11)	16	3	23	22	10	2	3		1		108
5								1	1	(1)	1	11	6	4	1					28
5.5	1		1	1	2	2	3	2	4	(4)	19	25	18	15	6	5	1			109
6							4	10	4	11	8	(22)	25	14	4	1	1	2		106
6.5		1		1			3				3	3	(5)	9	4	2	1			32
7			1				1		1			3	10	(6)	5	5	2			34
7.5									1		1	9	12	21	(7)	6	1		1	59
8												1	5	20	24	(64)	33	1	2	150
8.5														3	1	14	(8)	8		34
9																		(0)		0
9.5																				0
TOTAL	80	122	154	139	85	115	122	81	40	63	36	132	130	115	67	104	55	25	5	1636

MANUAL EDSS

Computerized EDSS scoring removes some of the subjectivity noted in the scoring of impairment. Reliability in score assignment can be greatly improved through computerized scoring. Since a proper and reliable assessment of impairment in a disease plays a key role in learning more about the disease (such as its natural history), these computer programs comprise a very important decision support system.

4. Decision support systems with computerized information systems

Utilization of computer systems for decision support (such as the computerized scoring system described above) is complementary to the use of a computerized medical record system such as MS-COSTAR. Moreover, widespread use of the same information system facilitates widespread implementation of any decision support system oriented toward that information system. If a scoring system such as the one discussed above is implemented in such a database, the time required to calculate scores for each patient visit is minimized while the accuracy is maximized. In addition, if the time required to try out new scoring methods or computerized diagnostic support systems is minimized, researchers may be more likely to examine them to evaluate their usefulness.

Future work at our clinic will focus on further developing this and other decision support systems to perform neurological and epidemiological studies in multiple sclerosis. For example, algorithms to support diagnosis in multiple sclerosis are being developed. Currently, the programs described above are being used to re-assess results from a completed drug trial conducted at UBC. Changes in impairment of patients in the clinic population will be examined, comparing the computer scores with the scores assigned by neurologists. Application of the computerized scoring programs would be useful in terms of predicting the prognosis (i.e., degree of impairment) of individual patients given the observed association in the clinic population between the status of certain factors (such as sex, age at onset, etc.) and a poor or good prognosis. In multiple sclerosis, as with many diseases, there is a need for a greater understanding of its natural history.

The lessons learned through the MS-COSTAR project are of value not only in MS research but also in other areas of clinical research. The creation of decision support systems and the utilization of sophisticated information systems such as MS-COSTAR can be of enormous value in many aspects of medical research. While information systems themselves have become widely recognized as useful, their use in tandem with decision support systems remains full of potential. Furthermore, even greater benefits to clinical, epidemiological, and other areas of research can be realized with the coordinated use of the same computerized information system in multiple sites. The development of decision support systems for use with information systems found in multiple sites can significantly facilitate multicentre drug evaluation trials as well as coordinated efforts to study the epidemiology of a disease.

References

1.   Barnett, G.O., Justice, N.S., Somand, M.E. et al. COSTAR: A computer-based medical record system for ambulatory care. Proc. IEEE, 1979; 67: 1226-37.

2.   Studney, D.R., Paty, D.W. Linking and pooling national and clinical research data. In: Barber, B., Cao, D., Qin, D., Wagner, G. eds. MEDINFO 89. Amsterdam: Elsevier Science, 1989: 1117-20.

3.   Kurtzke, J.F. Rating neurological impairment in multiple sclerosis: An expanded disability status scale (EDSS). Neurology, 1983; 33: 1444-52.

ProtoVIEW : a workstation for the use of clinical algorithms

PFHM van Dessel(1), A Hasman(1), CJ van der Linden(2).

(1)Dpt of Medical Informatics and Statistics, University of Limburg, PO Box 616,

6200 MD Maastricht (the Netherlands)

E-MAIL : MFMISPAS@HMARL5.bitnet

(2) Surgical Department, Maastricht University Hospital,Maastricht.

Abstract

In this paper a prototype of a clinical protocol supporting information system called ProtoVIEW is described. The system was evaluated in a non-clinical setting by 13 surgeons. Although many issues concerning protocol presentation and retrieval still have to be resolved, it is concluded that a computerized protocol management system can be of use for surgeons in clinical practice.

Introduction.

Protocols are powerful tools for structuring medical policy. Clinical algorithms are often used to portray the complex branching structure of therapeutic and diagnostic strategies and to reflect the expert opinion regarding specific medical problems [1]. Protocols allow clinicians to transfer knowledge about diagnostic and therapeutic procedures to other institutions. Furthermore using uniform guidelines is a very efficient way to introduce consistent medical behavior in a clinical department [1,2]. Despite these advantages, clinical protocols seem to suffer from several limitations when used in a static medium like paper workbooks. We have investigated ways in which these limitations might be overcome by presenting the relevant protocols to the surgeons and residents of the Surgical Department of the Maastricht University Hospital in a more dynamic way using the information system ProtoVIEW.

Importance of protocols for clinical practice on the Surgical Department.

Protocols have been used successfully for years to overcome the discrepancies between textbook knowledge taught during the medical study and knowledge about clinical practice that is needed at the bedside [2]. Propagation of this kind of knowledge throughout the Department however is complicated by a number of factors. First of all surgical insights tend to change rapidly. Secondly, dissemination of treatment consensus is hindered by the short stay of most assistants and junior staff members in the Department. Thirdly, therapies are becoming more and more complex due to multicentered and multidisciplinary approaches. The main objection against (paper) protocols is that they are being little flexible in their use. Therefore they are hard to keep up to date. Furthermore, protocols collected in a paper workbook are not easily accessible for retrieval of information and do not allow the user to retrieve additional information in an associative and natural way. Therefore numerous attempts have been made to computerize protocols. Because the technological state of art has improved ever since [3,4,5], we have started the development of a algorithm processing software package that will offer the user a broad scope of 'desk-top knowledge'.

A description of ProtoVIEW.

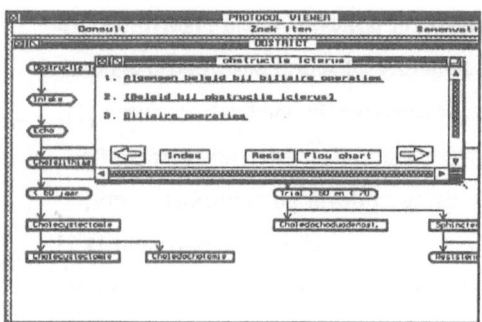

Fig. 1 Example of ProtoVIEW

ProtoVIEW is a prototype of an object-oriented software package - written in Turbo Pascal 5.5 for the MS-DOS operating system. The knowledge contained in the system is divided into separate units of information, called knowledge topics. Knowledge topics are stored in a variable record length database using the Novell BTRIEVE Record Manager. The information system is provided with a hypertext-oriented graphical interface (

Fig 1.) which allows the user to browse through the knowledge topics in an associative way. Two kinds of hypertext links are available : (1) explicit links, defined by the protocol author which jointly form the procedural knowledge of the protocol and (2) implicit links. Implicit links are not predefined. They allow the user to consult knowledge topics not strictly belonging to the protocol but possibly containing additional information. The knowledge base can be consulted in four different ways. Firstly, the user can consult the system by following the protocol steps sequentially. Secondly, information can be retrieved by searching the knowledge base directly using a search key. Thirdly, the structure of the protocol can be displayed as a graphical flowchart from which the user can select a protocol topic. Fourthly, the user can select a word at random from the text that is presented to him; the system will generate a link if further information about that topic is available (implicit linking). During consultation the system keeps track of the state of the patient. At any time a synopsis of the clinical state of the patient can be inspected. In the future the system will be linked with other knowledge sources like the Unified Medical Language System (a semantic net for medical taxonomy) and the MEDLINE literature database.

Evaluation of the system

Main objective of this evaluation procedure was to establish the appropriateness of the hypertext related approach we had chosen. The surgeons created a questionnaire about 16 case histories. Ten residents and five staff members were invited to answer the questions with and without the aid of the information system. First a brief tutorial instruction about ProtoVIEW was given. Next the surgeons were asked to answer questions about the case histories without the aid of computerized protocols. The answer forms were taken in and the surgeons started working with the information system. Registration of the user's searching behavior took place by "event logging" which means that the number of steps through the protocol, the order in which the steps were taken and the time needed for each topic to be found were stored by the computer. The participants again filled in the answers they found on a registration form. Finally, the participants were supplied with an evaluation form in order to evaluate the appreciation of an event- driven user interface, the appropriateness of hypertext for presentation of protocols, the search facilities the information system offered and the estimated impact the information system might have on their clinical behavior when the system would be introduced on the ward. At the time of analysis 2 out of the initial 15 participants were removed from the evaluation since they had not been present during the introductory tutorial. Without the information system 205 case histories were solved as opposed to 114 case histories solved with the aid of the computerized protocol system. To each answer a value ranging from 0 to 1 was assigned, indicating the level of correctness of the answer. Paired analysis of the scores for each answer revealed a small non-significant difference (mean 0.05 , standard error of mean (SEM) 0.05) in favor of problem solving without protocol aid. The appreciation aspects of the software package were divided into three groups : user interface aspects, program facilities and expected "clinical" value. All questions were assigned a value between 4 (judged positively) and -4 (judged negatively). Despite the non-evident "clinical" benefit of using the computer system, the system ranked quite well in terms of acceptance by the user (mean 1.9, SEM 1.1). The question whether computerized protocol processing will mean any difference for their clinical behavior in the future was also answered neutrally (mean -0.46, SEM 0.52), although they expect to use it regularly (mean 1.62, SEM 0.68).

Discussion

Evaluation of the ProtoVIEW prototype protocol processing system was hampered by several factors. First of all, a tutorial of 15 minutes appeared to be too short for introducing the participants properly in the use of the program. Secondly, most of the case histories appeared to be inconsistent with the protocol, meaning the data presented about the cases seemed to be collected out of order with respect to the algorithms they were supposed to test. This made it difficult for the physicians to apply the protocols to the case histories. Thirdly, the familiarity with the problem domain the protocols were dealing with appeared to be quite large (over 60% of the case histories were answered correctly), which made it very hard to demonstrate any advantage of using computers for clinical algorithms. Nevertheless, the basic thoughts behind the program, such as hypertext, and associative retrieval of knowledge seemed to be appreciated rather well. It also seems plausible to assume that when a protocol presenting system will be available in the clinical setting, physicians will start using it.

Although a computerized protocol system offers a great deal of flexibility in using algorithms, patients often do not completely match the protocol. This remains one of the problems in using computerized algorithms. Therefore, in the future the emphasis should be laid on the development of techniques to deal with protocol inconsistent data.

Conclusion

Due to several factors medical problems are getting more and more complex. Consequently, it is hard to keep non-experts who are confronted with these medical problems informed about current insights in the value of specific therapies and diagnostic procedures. Protocols can be very appropriate for formalizing medical behavior and transferral of knowledge. When used in a flexible environment like an information system, clinical algorithms can act as a framework for retrieving background information. Before protocol processing information systems can be taken into use several challenges still have to be resolved. Techniques have to be developed to prevent a user from getting lost in the amount of information that is presented by the information system. Since often data that are collected in clinical practice are out of order with respect to the algorithm a protocol system should be able to cope with this deviant data. Eventually, protocol processing systems can provide a major extension to the currently available decision support techniques.

References

[1] Abendroth TW, Greenes Ra, Joyce EA, Investigations in the use of clinical algorithms to organize medical knowledge, 1988, p. 90-95
[2] Margolis CZ, Uses of clinical algorithms, 1983, JAMA, 249:627-632.
[3] Cannon SR, Gardner RM, Experience with a computerized interactive protocol system using HELP, 1980, Comp Biomed Res, 13:399-409.
[4] MacDonald CJ, Protocol-based computer reminders, the quality of care and the non-perfectability of men, 1976, N Eng J Med, 1351-1355.
[5] Greenes RA, "Desktop knowledge" : a new focus for medical education and decision support, 1989, Proc. Med. Inf. and Ed. , p.90-93.

EXPERT SYSTEMS

DIANA 2 / THE DIAGNOSTIC ANALYZER: DIAGNOSTIC CONSULTATION IN INTERNAL MEDICINE BY PERSONAL COMPUTER

Antonio Muscari

Istituto di Patologia Speciale Medica e Metodologia Clinica
Universita' di Bologna, Via Massarenti 9, I-40138 Bologna, Italy

Abstract

The system here presented is a consultation tool in the field of medical diagnosis. It is based on a program that processes the information present in patient's history in relation to an independent knowledge base. Its potential domain is internal medicine, although the present knowledge base includes 110 infectious diseases only and a dictionary of nearly 3500 terms. After completion of patient's history, the user can request the differential diagnosis suggested by the system and a list of further investigations to discriminate among the diseases in differential diagnosis. The main distinctive features of the system are: 1) The D-LOG language, which has been created to allow sufficient flexibility in disease and patient's history description; 2) Implementation of key-elements of temporal reasoning; 3) Advanced explaination capabilities; 4) Knowledge base consultable as a hypertext. At present, the compilation of a wide and reliable knowledge base remains the most relevant problem to tackle.

Knowledge base and D-LOG language

The expert system here presented is a consultation tool in the field of medical diagnosis. To represent the relevant medical information within the system the D-LOG language has been created. Nine different Types of information are implemented (Table 1), which can be grouped as Data or Attributes. Data are either items of information provided with a primary pathological significance or laboratory-instrumental investigation names, while Attributes are accessory items of information used to localize or specify otherwise the Data, or to describe an investigation result. The names of Data and Attributes are respectively in upper and lower case.

Table 1 - Information Types in D-LOG

A) DATA
1. Simple datum (PAIN, BLOOD GLUCOSE, STANDARD ECG)

2. Alternative datum (CONSTIPATION/DIARRHEA/NORMA BOWEL FUNCTION)

3. Structure (ACUTE PULMONARY EDEMA)

4. Disease (INFECTIOUS MONONUCLEOSIS)

5. Category of data (INFECTIONS, LEUKEMIAS)

B) ATTRIBUTES

1. Simple attribute ([in the] forearm,[in the] epigastrium, [for] ventricular premature beats)

2. Alternative attribute ([of] brown colour/red colour/black colour/etc.)

3. Category of attributes ([in the] upper limb, [in the] abdominal regions)

4. Key-words of Special Procedures

The Key-words of Special procedures (the fourth Attribute Type) are used to perform complex processings, mainly related to temporal reasoning and/or handling of multiple items of information (Table 2).

Table 2 - Special procedures and related key-words

A) GENERAL

1. Sex (male/female)

2. Amount (small-medium/considerable)

3. Result (pos/neg)

4. Side (right/left/centre/bilateral/homolateral/counter-lateral)

B) TEMPORAL

1. Age

2. Daily rhythm (day/night/early morning/morning/afternoon/evening)

3. Seasonal rhythm (spring/summer/autumn/winter/transition seasons)

4. Datum duration and course

5. Episode duration

6. Interval duration

7. Maximum duration

8. Temporal sequence

9. Predisposing

10. Cause (causes/may cause/is associated with)

11. Delay (may persist/retards)

12. Complication (consequence/possible effect/contemporary effect)

13. Necessary phase

A few parameters are associated with each item of information. Some of them are constant and independent of the context in which the information is used, others vary within different contexts, meaning as context the description of a Disease or a less specific complex event (Structure). The most important constant parameter for both Data and Attributes is Specificity, which is an integer ranging 1-4, roughly inversely related to the number of diseases that may present the item of information. A score is associated with each of the 4 Specificity values, which is used additively to attribute an overall score to each diagnostic hypothesis. Other constant parameters include Default status, Cost and Categories of which the item of information is a member. The most important variable parameter is Necessity, which provides a rough estimate of the frequency of association of a given item of information with its context. Its main values are 0 ("sometimes"), 50 ("often") and 90 ("nearly always"). The Necessity value of an attribute indicates the frequency of association of the attribute with its datum. Other variable parameters include Status (pres/abs, neg/pos, incr/decr/norm), Evidence, Attribute inheritability and, for a few special procedures, specification of the temporal intervals allowed. The description of a Disease or Structure profile consists of a list of Data possibly specified by any number of Attributes. Elements of a list may be (and often are) Disease or Structure names, so that the list assumes a multiple-level hierarchical organization. The present knowledge base includes 110 infectious diseases and a dictionary of nearly 3500 terms.

User interface

This consists of a full screen editor-interpreter which allows free insertion of patient's complaints, laboratory and instrumental results, in D-LOG format (i.e. as Data variously specified by Attributes). All the information supplied must be associated with temporal references. If the expression inserted by the user does not coincide with any known term, the system immediately shows the internal dictionary page containing the term alphabetically most similar to the one given. From the dictionary a suitable term may then be easily chosen (several synonyms are implemented) and exported to patient's history. The dictionary can be intentionally called from any section of the program to consult what the system knows about any item of information (constant parameters, synonyms, free-text suggestions or definitions, descriptive lists of Diseases or Structures and related sub-lists in their multiple-level organization).

Differential diagnosis and further investigations

When patient's history is completed, the user may activate the diagnostic process, which produces a list of the most likely diagnostic hypotheses. The diagnostic algorithm may be defined as a "pattern matching", strengthened by a series of routines (the Special procedures) which perform complex evaluations whenever they are called by their corresponding key-words in the descriptive list that is being processed. For each Disease 2 scores are separately computed, which are used to assess the Disease position in Differential diagnosis: the "Pro" score (which is a function of the Specificities of patient's history elements compatible with the disease) and the "Con" score (which is a function of the maximum Necessity value of the disease elements incompatible with patient's history). Together with the differential diagnosis a short comment is also shown to help the user to correctly interpretate the result. Suggestions concerning further investigations, useful to discriminate among multiple diagnostic hypotheses or to test a single hypothesis, may be obtained by the system on request.

Explaination capabilities

The user can obtain detailed explainations concerning system behaviour in relation to any diagnostic hypothesis and any patient's characteristic. First level explainations referred to a given diagnostic hypothesis consist of short messages displayed alongside patient's history elements. Second level explainations consist of more detailed messages (sometimes 2 or more pages) concerning single history elements. For example, after system processing of the hypothesis of Pneumococcal meningitis, the following second level explaination might be associated with the CRANIAL TRAUMA Datum in patient's history: "...CRANIAL TRAUMA was DISCARDED because it occurred on 2/5/1989, while to predispose to PNEUMOCOCCAL MENINGITIS it should not precede by more than 15 days the onset of PNEUMOCOCCAL MENINGITIS (which might coincide with the onset of PETECHIAE, occurred on 18/10/1989)...".

Technical characteristics

The MS-DOS operating system (version 3.0 or higher), a 640 Kb memory and a hard disk are required. For optimum performance a personal computer of AT class is recommended, although not indispensable. The diagnostic program was written in C language and compiled by a Microsoft compiler, with a resulting executable code of 700 Kb. The mean processing time per disease is less than 0.1 seconds. The final disk space occupation, after completion of the knowledge base (nearly 2000 diseases), can be estimated between 5 and 10 Mb. The present system is the evolution of a simpler prototype (1,2) and its overall development has required 8 years of work.

Conclusions

During the last few years several systems have been proposed as consultation tools in the field of medical diagnosis. Among those capable of handling large knowledge bases, Internist/QMR (3,4) and DXplain (5) are especially noteworthy. The system here presented, even though presently provided with a smaller knowledge base, has some affinities with both. For example, they utilize 3 parameters (Frequency, Evoking strength and Import value) to assess the position of each diagnostic hypothesis in the differential diagnosis. The Necessity in DIANA 2 has the same significance as the

Frequency, while the Specificity embodies some characteristics of both Evoking strength and Import value. On the other hand, fewer values are allowed in DIANA 2 for the 2 parameters. Thus, the attribution of values should have been rendered more univocal, reproducible and simple, even though this may have caused some loss in discriminant power. Innovative features in DIANA 2 are the use of Data, Attributes and Key-words of Special procedures in the description of disease profiles and patient's history, separate processing for the items of information and their temporal references, and particularly detailed explaination capabilities. The main problems are presently related to the compilation of a wide, consistent and reliable knowledge base.

References

1. Muscari A. DIANA - Anamnesi & Diagnosi: il personal computer come ausilio all'attivita' diagnostica del medico. Prima parte: strutturazione della base di conoscenza. Medicina e Informatica 4:85, 1987.
2. Muscari A. DIANA - Anamnesi & Diagnosi: il personal computer come ausilio all'attivita' diagnostica del medico. Seconda parte: caratteristiche dei programmi operativi. Medicina e Informatica 4:259, 1987.
3. Miller RA, Pople HE, Myers JD. INTERNIST-1, an experimental computer-based diagnostic consultant for general internal medicine. N Eng J Med 307:468, 1982.
4. Masarie FE, Miller RA. INTERNIST-1 to quick medical reference (QMR): transition from a mainframe to a microcomputer. Proceedings of the Ninth Annual IEEE/Engeneering in Biology and Biology Society. New York, IEEE Society Press, p. 1521, 1987.
5. Barnett GO, Cimino JJ, Hupp JA, Hoffer EP. DXplain: an evoluting diagnostic decision-support system. JAMA 258:67, 1987.

SPES-2: AN EXPERT SYSTEM FOR THE INTRA-OPERATIVE PHASE
OF THE PANCREAS CANCER

M.Rafanelli *, R.Maceratini +

(*) Istituto di Analisi dei Sistemi ed Informatica del CNR, viale Manzoni 30, 00185 Roma, Italy
(+) Istituto di IV Clinica Chirurgica - Università 'La Sapienza', v.le del Policlinico, Roma, Italy

Abstract. In order to support the decision making of the surgeon in the operative room, but also for tutorial aims, a prototype of an expert system is proposed and described in this paper. The medical domain refers to the pancreatic diseases and, in particular, the pancreatic cancer. The system examines the operative risks of the patient, suggests the suitable surgical procedure, follows the surgeon during this procedure (both with regard to the staging phase, and to the properly said surgical procedure), suggesting the appropriate operations by means of pictures and explanatory sentences. It suggests also suitable actions for a large number of surgical complications.

1. Introduction.

In this paper the Authors describe the prototype of an expert system, called Spes-2, able to help a surgeon in the operative room with regard to the surgical therapies of the pancreatic diseases. This prototype considers: 1) the evaluation of the operative risk and the life expectancy and quality; 2) some strategies regarding the surgical procedures to apply in the cases considered by the system. The different databases of the system to manage the Problem Oriented Medical Record (POMR), images (pictures which support the different phases of each surgical act) and texts (in which brief explanations of the phases represented by the previous pictures) is also briefly described. The Spes-2 expert system is part of a complex system which consists of three integrated expert systems (Spes-1 [RA89] refers to the differential diagnosis and Spes-3 to the adjuvant therapies) regarding the pancreatic diseases. The Authors use "classes", "sub-classes" and "objects", each of them with own "properties", to represent the knowledge of Spes-2. The network of objects which represents the knowledge stored, has been segmented in sub-networks, that is: 1) evaluation of the operative risk; 2) evaluation of the life expectancy and standard of post-operative living; 3) surgical planning; 4) pre-operative treatment; 5) surgical staging; 6) surgical procedures and other eventual integrated diagnostic and /or therapeutic procedures. At the end the system carries out the upgraded medical record and suggestion for the post-operative phase.

2. The problems to implement expert systems in the surgical domain.

An expert system in surgery has justified to be useful both for tutorial and for health care purposes in [RA90]. This last case refers to lack of human experts in real time (you can have they, but not within 15-20 minutes), especially for their concentration in defined, specialized health care centers. *Surgery* is "a complex therapeutical system" that is integrated with other therapies much more frequently than other therapeutical systems. The assistance of a consultant acquires a stronger relevance in the operating room, where the decisional time is generally "urgent" (it is not possible to suspend a surgical act to wait the coming of an external expert consultant, admitted that such an expert is available) but not "very urgent" (it is possible to wait some minutes to obtain an opinion in order to use one or more defined procedures). In this case the medical-surgical decision making is founded on two cornerstones of medicine: "scientific" knowledge (insight in problems and processes), primarily gained during medical research, and "empirical" knowledge (experience acquired), which has a phenomenological character. Medical experience appears to be the leading factor in treating patients. An expert system, able to support surgeon in his professional activity, appears more complex than systems developed in other medical areas. This higher complexity depends on the integration "in real time" of diagnostic and therapeutical decisional supports, sometimes multidisciplinary [RA89].

The expert system in surgery implemented, Spes-2, has been divided along the time into three phases:

1) Pre-operative phase; the decisional support for the surgeon has to be performed in order to accomplish more tasks: a) evaluation of the operative risks, which regards also the range of possible surgical procedures, the performance status, the concurrent diseases; b) evaluation of the life expectancy and standard of post-operative living; c) medical-legal evaluation (e.g., the religious precepts, such as the prohibition of blood transfusion for Geova's witness); d) pre-operative management.

2) intra-operative phase; two different aspect are highlighted: a) *staging phase,* in which the system can modify, if necessary, the informations acquired during the first diagnostic phase and acquires the further intra-operative diagnostic informations; b) *surgical act,* in which the system interacts with the surgeon in order to suggests an additional decisional support for the surgical planning and for other eventual intra-operative therapies.

3) post-operative phase; the expert system gives suggestions for the post-operative phase management and the follow-up.

The user can choose the phase in which Spes-2 is divided, selecting an option button (see Fig. 1).

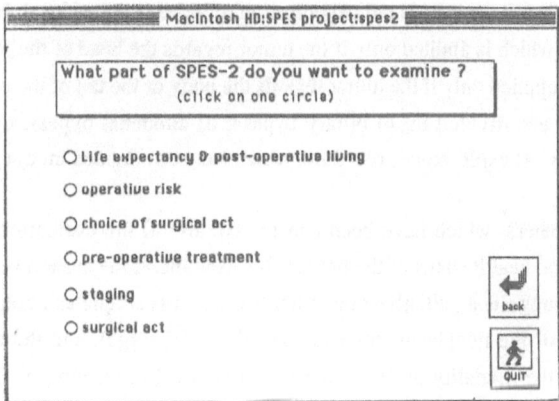

Fig.1

3. The pre-operative phase

In this phase the system before evaluates the operative risks and the life expectancy and post-operative living, in order to suggest the more suitable surgical act, then suggests the more suitable surgical operation.

3.1 The evaluation of the operative risks, the life expectancy and standard of post-operative living

The *operative risk* can be defined as the possibility of an uncertain event to cause a harm. In surgery such an event depends on type of surgical procedure, on the environmental situation (expertise, technical tools, etc.), on the conditions of the patient and on his/her type of reaction. The object "patient" has been split in different diseases which define his/her status of health; each of them is enclosed in a "class of risk" of defined value [RA90]. The method of the "hierarchical groupings" used for the evaluation of the operative risk involves the solution of two sub-problems: 1) to characterize the general conditions of the patient; 2) to define the surgical scenery. For the first point, the different characterization between "innate factor" and "acquired factor" is very important, because the evaluation strategies are quite different; the former (age, sex, blood group, etc.) represents the categorical aspects, with an incidence invariable; for the latter, the possible situations have been split in two classes: acquired factors, linked or to the main disease (in this case, the pancreatic cancer), or to the associated diseases. The main disease is evaluated before respect to its malignant nature, then respect to its extension (tumor staging). The strategy used in the research of the solution [RA90] refers both to the evaluation of the *operative risk,* the *life expectancy,* that is the period that the patient, after the surgical act, presumably will live, and the *standard of post-operative living,* that is the post-operative physical condition of the patient, and, in general, the "quality" of living. Both of them play a very important role both in the decision to operate or not, and in surgical planning.

The diseases considered by the system have been divided in three classes, depending on their importance relatively to the pancreatic cancer. With regard to the life expectancy, five possible time ranges are given, from 1 month to 3 + 5 years (with a little, possible increase).

3.2 The surgical planning

The surgical operation of the adenocarcinoma of the esocrin pancreas presents diversified choice which depends on different parameters. Relatively to the surgical planning, the first parameter considered is the type of operation. The different operations have been divided in four classes: 1) no operation, because the status of the patient advises it against; 2) radical operation (divided in: a) regional; b) total pancreatectomy; c) Whipple procedure (which is applied only if the tumor regards the head of the pancreas); d) distal pancreatectomy (which is applied only if the tumor regards the body or the tail of the pancreas)); 3) palliative operation, which has been divided in: a) biliary bypass; b) duodenal bypass; c) biliary and digestive bypass; d) tumorectomy; 4) exploratory procedure, which has been divided in: a) exploratory laparatomy; b) biopsy.

Other important parameters, which have been considered, are: a) the evaluation of the operative risk, depending on the general health status of the patient (for example, if the system verifies the presence of a high operative risk, it suggests a palliative operation, because it is simple and non invasive); b) the type, the site and the stage of the neoplasm (for example, III or IV stage), and the age of the patient (for example, over 75); c) the modality of execution of the surgical procedure; d) the knowledge and the expertise of the surgical staff; and, finally, e) the available tools.

4. The intra-operative phase and the support to the surgical act

The surgical act can be divided into two parts: staging phase and properly said surgical act . Three sceneries can be thought: 1) All the pre-operative hypotheses formulated at the highest level of probability are intra-operatively confirmed. Investigations or intra-operative therapies are not needed. The intra-operative data, given by the system, will be used as input for the third phase (adjuvant therapies). 2) There is a sufficiently big agreement with the pre-operative hypotheses, with or without of further intra-operative investigations as confirmation or modification of the diagnostic and therapeutic formulated hypotheses, with or without of therapies integrated to the surgery. The system continuously interacts with the surgeon. That is the usual scenery. 3) There is a minimal confirmation of the pre-operative hypotheses. This can happen because of:

a) unreliability of imaging and/or laboratory findings or wrong evaluation of clinical findings; one comes out of the expert system domain; b) insufficiency or unreliability of data in the same domain.

During the intra-operative phase the system, decided the surgical planning, suggests the different phases of the surgical act, proposing alternatively a picture (see Fig.2) and a explanatory text of it (see Fig.3), until the end of the operation. If a change of the situation (for example, a complication) happens, the operator can interrupt the normal procedure and introduce the new situation. Then the system changes own strategy depending on it.

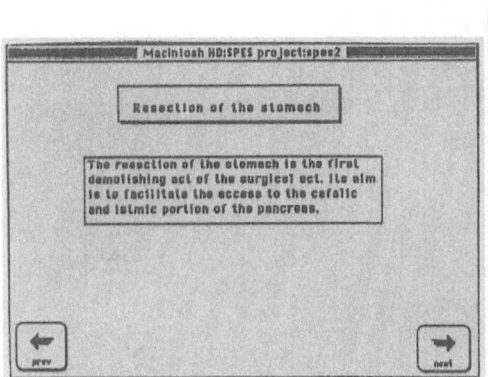
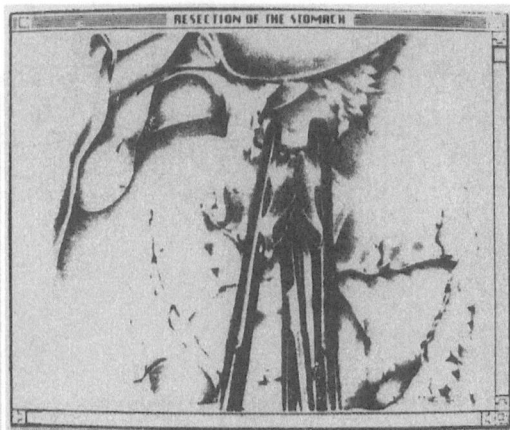

| Fig.2 | Fig. 3 |

5. The post-operative phase
In this phase, temporally identified from the exit out of the operating room to the hospital discharge, the expert system elaborates the previous informations in order to suggest the post operative management and the follow-up. The Medical Record is upgrated and a report for the family doctor is prepared.

6. The Databases
A Medical Record oriented to the pancreatic disease has been defined the SPES (Surgical Pancreatic Expert Systems) project. In Spes-1 information regarding personal data, clinical findings and diagnostic procedures data, and final diagnosis are stored in this medical record of the Spes database. In Spes-2 such a medical record is increased by information regarding the points listed in the previous section 1. Such a database is linked to the knowledge base of the expert system, as well as the other two (visual and textual) databases. A supervisor program manages such links and the interface towards the user. The system architecture of Spes-2 is shown in Fig. 4.

7. Discussion
Different expert systems could be fruitfully implemented for surgical applications [MO84], [MI84], [FA85], but at present *there is no system known designed to be used in the operating room*. The expert system Spes-2, implemented using commercial tools (running on Macintosh, PC-IBM, Vax-station, etc.), at present has a knowledge base which consists of about 1,000 rules. The static knowledge is implemented by classes, objects and the relative properties, but they, as well as the rules, are transparent to the user, generally a surgeon. He interfaces with the system by an hypertextual user friendly interface. The

implemented prototype is running on Macintosh. At present the prototype is not yet completed (it considers only two surgical procedures), but all the implementation problems have been solved and all the expertise elicited and written.

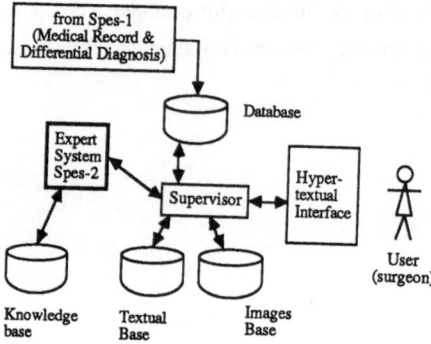

Fig. 4

8. Conclusions and future developments

In this paper the Authors propose a prototype of an expert system, in which the knowledge base was implemented by objects, classes and relative properties (static knowledge) and by rules (inferences). Three different phases of the surgical procedure have been discussed, and some examples have been shown. In particular, ; and of the different databases linked to it are shown. The number of rules of the knowledge base are, at present, about 1,000. The pictures of the visual database are "black and white"; the POMR is structured in an hypertextual way on the screen. The implementation is still in progress and at the end will consider the main surgical procedures regarding the pancreatic diseases (in particular, the pancreas cancer).

References

[FA85]   Fagan L., Differding J., Langlotz C., Tu S. *"Knowledge acquisition and strategic therapy planning for cancer clinical trials"* Proceed. of the International Confer. on Artificial Intelligence in Medicine, Pavia, 13-14 September 1985

[MI84]   Miller P.L. *"Critiquing approach to expert computer advice: ATTENDING"*, Research Notes in Artificial Intelligence, Vol.1, London, 1984

[MO84]   Molokva O.S., Chernyakovskaja M.J. *"Results of implementation of the first version of medical expert systems CONSULTANT"*, Artificial Intelligence and Information-control Systems of Robots, North Holland, 1984, 7-10 Nov. 1986

[RA89]   Rafanelli M., Maceratini R., Crollari S., Maggi M., S.Mascolini S. :"Pancreatic cancer: an object oriented based system for the pre-operative differential diagnosis" Proceed. of the 6th World Confer. on Medical Informatics, Singapore, 11-15 Dec. 1989

[RA90]   Rafanelli M., Maceratini R. "Proposal of an expert system in surgical domain" Proceed. of the 9th Int. Confer. on Medical Informatics Europe, Glasgow, GB, 20-23 Aug. 1989

COMPUTER-AIDED EXPERT SYSTEM OF DIAGNOSTICS AND TACTICS IN ACUTE URGENT NEUROLOGIC PATHOLOGY

E.N. Krupin, M.Ya. Charnis, T.Yu. Telesheva, T.N. Gribanova,
S.L. Leontiev, S.I. Goldberg
Sverdlovsk Regional Medical Information Computer Center
Volgogradskaya St. 187, 620102, Sverdlovsk, USSR

ABSTRACT

The expert system is developed for differential diagnostics of some acute neurologic diseases. The "diagnostic games" and "complex antisyndrome" methods are utilized. The system is based on a considerable number of clinical observations in reliable verification. The diagnostic accuracy amounts to 92%.

INTRODUCTION

The computer-aided (consultative) expert system of diagnostics and tactics in acute urgent neurologic pathology (CCS-"AUNP") has been worked out by collective of authors mentioned above. It is aimed at medical workers lacking practical experience in neurology. The system can be useful in serving any organized contingents, specifically, ship lines whose vessels are on autonomous cruises or in remote areas and, having no physicians on board, do not offer any possibility of consulting a specialist.

The medical technology provides for either organizing a remote diagnostics center on the basis of a medical institution with computer technology and a special staff of neuroreanimatologists/consultants, as it is organized in Sverdlovsk, or a network of personal computers at the disposal of users instructed for working with such a system. The computer's conclusions should be considered as additional consultative ones, but any ultimate decision should be taken by a doctor. Channels of optimal communication with a remote diagnostics center are clearly defined according to conditions and possibilities of the region.

METHOD

The expert system is a product of the long-standing joint work of honored scientists: Prof. D.G. Schefer, M.D., Urals branch of the USSR Academy of Sciences, academician; N.N. Krasovsky, the RSFSR Chief neuropathologist; Prof. L.G. Erokhina, M.D.; and the collective of the computing diagnostics department of the Sverdlovsk Regional Medical Information Computer Center under the supervision of, and in collaboration with, Prof. E.N. Krupin, M.D., Head of the Neurology and Neurosurgery Chair (Sverdlovsk Medical Institute).

The "AUNP" expert system was drawn up according to the special purpose Republican Program P.02, supervised by Prof. S.A. Gasparyan, M.D., Head of the Medical and Biological Cybernetics Chair at the 2nd Moscow Medical Institute. It is intended for emergency recognition of 73 urgent states followed by acute disorders of conscience, mobility, sensitivity, and attacks of pain. It runs along generally accepted symptoms known to a physicians. The coding list for information entering into the computer contains 180 signs characterizing complaints, anamnesis data, data from objective examination, including a neurological status.

The anamnesis data contain characteristics of the patient's past diseases, the development of the acute episode, details of the clinical picture from the intitial stage of the disease. Objective data characterize peculiarities of the respiratory and cardiovascular systems taking into account the arterial pressure level. Neurologic symptoms are put in order of the generally accepted scheme of description with emphasis on dynamics of the development of the disease.

After examination of a patient, the clinician enters available symptoms of the disease into the computer while omitting absent symptoms (indicated in the list).

Actually, the description of a disease or a case can be put within the limits of 12–15 symptoms and requires no special efforts or a lot of time. The computer program works both in a "dialog mode" and in the usual coding variant. The mode can be selected by the user. Work time, from the moment of entering the information until the answer is obtained, is 2 minutes.

There is a logic control of input information and its accumulation in the data bank with subsequent mathematical statistical processing demands. Some of the algorithms used for the solution of the task were worked out in the Mathematics and Mechanics Institute of Urals branch of the USSR Academy of Sciences for the Sverdlovsk Regional Medical Information Computer Center. Every algorithm worked with a certain high accuracy although having some shortcomings. Taking into account the latter circumstance, we paid particular attention to the method of modelling real situations (diagnostic games), developed in the laboratory of mathematical methods of Moscow State University under the supervision of academician L.M. Gelfand [2].

The informative signs and combinations of signs obtained in this way are being used at a procedure of decision-making similar to algorithms entering the expert system (ES) "Internist" [3]. But as opposed to "Internist", the "AUNP" algorithm is based on an analysis of informative combinations of signs (syndromes) but not on separate signs.

The knowledge base consists of 580 syndromes for differentiation, some of which may be given as an example here:

(15)_____
118. Consciousness is clear.
147. Asymmetry of face.
    160. Disturbance of pain sensitivity in limbs of one side. I 35 I 1

(65)_____
118. Consciousness is clear.
55. There was a speech disturbance before development of
 the episode.
155. Difference in power of muscles and capacity of
    movements of the limbs, left and right.   I 40 I 1

(405)_____
120. Sopor, coma.
139. Vomiting.
38. Development of the acute episode in sleep, immediately
 after sleep.
    97. Arterial pressure is normal.   I 13 I 1

(213)_____
118. Consciousness is clear.
149. Vertigo (dizziness).
    152. Disorder of phonation, swallowing.   I 25 I 7

Giving the differential diagnosis is being realized on the basis of "pattern recognition" method "complex antisyndrome" [4]. There are two working modes of the program:

(1) Data communications in the dialog process from the ES. 7–10 questions are usually assigned in this case for diagnosing a pathological finding, or "candidates" are picked for the differential diagnosis. Settling for the final diagnosis requires 5–15 additional questions.

(2) Data communications in the form of a list of a patient's signs from the formalized history of the disease.

For the production of the decision rules, a sufficiently representative sample from the formalized case histories of Sverdlovsk neurological hospitals was used. At present, a data bank of casuistic cases is being prepared to be used in searching for precedents according to the degree of similarity [5].

Besides the diagnostics, the ES offers tactical recommendations aimed at physicians of ambulance and emergency services of Sverdlovsk and at physicians of district medical institutions of the region.

The program for PDP-11 and IBM PC/XT computers is written in FORTRAN-4, FoxBASE+ with the operating systems RAFOS and MS-DOS, respectively.

For a diagnostic game, the list of most valuable (i.e. informative) signs obtained as a result of statistic processing of 1500 histories from Sverdlovsk neurological hospitals was offered to highly qualified specialists. In the final run, models of real situations were obtained that covered all the 73 variants of diagnostic solutions and tactical recommendations concerning medical aid, hospitalization, and special emergency consultations.

Tactical recommendations are aimed at physicians of first-aid stations in the city of Sverdlovsk and at district medical institutions of the region.

In direct tests under field conditions at first-aid stations of Sverdlovsk and the region, the "AUNP" expert system made more precise diagnoses according to subsequently finalized diagnoses based on the data from clinical examination. During the testing stage of the system (remote variant), necessary corrections in the medical data and the software were made. There was a total of 1400 computer-aided consultations. Catamnesis was known in 896 cases. The principal diagnosis was verified with autopsy, computer tomography, and cerebral angiography. The accuracy of the system's diagnostics among patient groups with reliable verification amounts to 92%, which corresponds to the accuracy of a highly qualified specialist.

DISCUSSION

In Sverdlovsk, the "AUNP" expert system has found its application in conditions of the consultative diagnostics center serving hospitals and prophylactic institutions of the city and the region. Here, the computer-aided expert system really shortens the time of ad- minstering specialized urgent aid, it solves diagnostic and tactical problems with sufficient reliability, and it may also be useful for young physicians in acquiring and mastiern the basics of urgent aid for neurologic patients.

REFERENCES

[1] E.N.Krupin, M.Ya.Charnis, M.A.Khinko, T.Yu.Telesheva, V.Ya.Kunis, S.I.Goldberg. Use of Computers for the Improvement of Quality in Neurological Service. Problems of Quality in Psychiatric and Neurological Service. Col. of papers. Moscow, 1988, p. 142

[2] I.M.Gelfand, B.I.Rosenfeld, M.A.Shifrin. Structural Organization of Data in Medical Diagnostic and Prognostic Problems. Medical Diagnostic and Prognostic Problems from the Mathematician's Viewpoint. Moscow, 1985, p. 5-65

[3] R.A.Miller, H.E.Pople, Jr., J.D.Myers. "Internist-1": An Experimental Computer- Based Diagnostic Consultant for General Internal Medicine. N.Eng.J.Med., 1982, 301, p.468-476

[4] S.I.Goldberg. Diagnostics on the Basis of the Informative Space of Antisyndroms. Problems of Control and Information Theory. 1984, Vol.13(6), p. 401-411

[5] S.I.Goldberg, O.A.Scripotchenko. Nearness Estimations for Objects with Complex Structure. Problems of Control and Information Theory. 1986,

Differential Diagnosis in Breast Histopathology

DK Bose[1], HA Heathfield[2] and N Kirkham[2]

IT Research Institute, Brighton Polytechnic[1], IBM UK Scientific Centre, Winchester[2]
and Royal Sussex County Hospital, Brighton, UK[3].

Abstract

The problem of accuracy and consistency in the histological typing of breast disease has been addressed by the development of a decision support system, which assists the pathologist through the identification of important differential tests and ranking of competing diagnoses. The inference model embodied within the system is based upon the notion of a vertex covering of a hypergraph and the Kemeny social choice function. The hypergraph model is in sense 'dual' to that of the set covering model developed by Reggia and has several advantages over the set covering approach. Initial trials with the system have demonstrated the potential of the hypergraph model.

1 Introduction

Histological typing of breast tumours provides important prognostic information. However, the technique is problematic for several reasons, including:

1. There are many histological types of breast disease, some of which are rare and not often seen in routine practice.

2. There are benign and malignant counterparts which can exhibit similar appearances.

3. There are numerous features which have to be taken into consideration when making a diagnosis.

4. There is inherent uncertainty and incompleteness associated with the manifestations exhibited by a histological type.

2 Design Philosophy

A characteristic of pathologists involved in the histological typing of breast disease, is the highly skilled manner in which they can quickly identify a differential set of diagnoses[1]. For example a lesion exhibiting central sclerosis and varying degrees of epithelial proliferation, may lead the pathologist to explore the differential set consisting of tubular carcinoma, radial scar and complex sclerosing lesion. Once a differential problem has been defined, the ability of pathologists to differentiate between the diagnostic alternatives may be less well-developed than their skill in recognising the differential problem. It was observed that pathologists often found it difficult to recall detailed criteria of differential diagnosis, or failed to apply these criteria consistently. It is also apparent that pathologists may inadvertently omit a potential diagnosis due to its rarity or unfamiliarity.

Given the particular characteristics of the diagnostic process, we wish to design our system to take account of the strengths and weaknesses' of pathologist problem-solving ability. Thus our main objectives are:

1. Appending to a user supplied differential diagnostic set, those relevant rare or unusual histological types that have been overlooked, i.e. ensuring completeness of the differential problem.

2. Generating significant tests in an efficient and natural manner.

3. If, as a result of incomplete or uncertain knowledge it is not possible to reach a unique diagnosis, we wish to be able to rank the alternatives in a 'sensible' and systematic manner.

3 Knowledge Representation

The diagnostic definitions used in the knowledge base have been taken from the 'Draft Guidelines for Pathologists' document produced by the Department of Health. Diagnostic knowledge is organised in a frame structure:

```
ENTITY papilloma BEGIN
  CLASS benign lesions;
  OCCURRENCE a rare lesion occurring primarily in middle age;
  ASSOCIATES multiple papilloma, papillary carcinoma insitu;
  FOUND-WITH sclerosing adenosis, epitheliosis;
   SET clinical features BEGIN
     tumour location = subareolar(H);
     age group = middle age (H);
     nipple discharge = blood stained(L); END
   SET microscopic features BEGIN
     epithelial proliferation = yes(A), no(N);
     stromal proliferation = yes(N), no(A);
     growth type = infiltrating(N), non infiltrating(A);
     lesion type = benign(A), malignant(N);
     papillary growth = yes(A),no(N);
     double cell layer = present(A);
     cytological atypia = yes(N), no(A);
     mitosis = absent(H), infrequent(H), frequent(N);
     abnormal forms = absent(M), infrequent(N), frequent(N);
     foci of papillary growth = single(A), multiple(N);
     apocrine metaplasia = absent(H);
     lesion features = necrosis(M), haemorrhage(M); END
  END
```

The symbolic certainty factors shown in angular brackets are subjective, non-numeric estimates of how frequently an event occurs. Given a disease d_i and manifestation m_k these translate as; A = m_k always occurs with d_i, H = m_k has a high likelihood of occurring with d_i, M = m_k has a medium likelihood of occurring with d_i, L = m_k has a low likelihood of occurring with d_i and N = m_k never occurs with d_i.

4 The Inference Model

The inference model is an extension of that described in [2]. Consider a set of diseases **D**, a set of manifestations **M** and an incomplete relation $C = (c_{k,j})$, such that:

$$c_{k,j} = \begin{cases} 1 \text{ if } m_k \text{ is always present in } d_j \\ 0 \text{ if } m_k \text{ is never present in } d_j \\ ? \text{ if } m_k \text{ is sometimes present in } d_j \text{ or if it is unknown} \end{cases}$$

For each pair of diseases d_i and d_j, a manifestation m_k distinguishes between them if it occurs with certainty in one disease and never in the other, or vice versa.

For all pairs of diseases d_i and d_j then $e_{i,j} = \{m_k \; : \; m_k \text{ distinguishes between } d_i \text{ and } d_j \}$. Note, for n diseases d_i there are $\frac{n(n-1)}{2}$ sets $e_{i,j}$, some of which may be empty.

If
$$E = \{e_{i,j} \; : \; \forall_{i,j}\}$$

and
$$S = \bigcup_{i,j} e_{i,j} \subset M$$

then $H = (S, E)$ is a hypergraph. Here the vertices correspond to manifestations and the edges correspond to the sets of manifestations that distinguish between pairs of diseases.

In the dual hypergraph $H^* = (S^*, E^*)$ a vertex $e_{i,j}$ corresponds to a pair of diseases d_i and d_j and the set of all manifestations that can distinguish between them, while an edge e_j^*, corresponds to the set of all disease pairs that a particular manifestation m_j can distinguish between. A minimum cover of H^* corresponds to the minimum set of manifestations that will distinguish between all pairs of diseases. This problem can be solved heuristically or more precisely through integer programming, which also enables the cost of tests to be taken into account.

Uncertain information (i.e. certainty factors H,M and L) may incorporated into the questioning strategy in an incremental manner, beginning with the H certainty factors and progressing to M and L. This is achieved by setting $c_{k,i} = 1$ and reformulating the minimum cover of H^*.

The notion of minimal covering is also been used by Reggia in the set covering model[3]. The relation $C = (c_{i,j})$ captures the notion of causal association between disorders and manifestations in a Boolean matrix where:

$$c_{i,j} = \begin{cases} 1 & \text{if } d_i \in D \quad can \quad cause \quad m_j \in M, \\ 0 & otherwise. \end{cases}$$

If the set of specific case manifestations is known as $\mathbf{M^+}$, where $M^+ \subset M$, the set covering model searches for a set of diseases $A \subset D$ (such that A has the smallest cardinality) which can 'explain' the presence of the manifestations in $\mathbf{M^+}$ i.e $M^+ \subset \bigcup_{d_i \in A} man(d_i)$.

The search for the set A can also be formulated in the following manner.

$$e_i = man(d_i) \cap M^+, \quad provided \quad e_i \neq \varnothing \quad (1)$$

and

$$E = \{e_i \quad : \quad \forall d_i \in D\}$$

then

$$\bigcup_{e_i \in E} e_i = M^+ \quad (2)$$

The search for the smallest subset of $\mathbf{D}$ which explains $\mathbf{M^+}$ is equivalent to finding the smallest $A \subset E$ such that

$$\bigcup_{e_i \in A} e_i = M^+ \quad (3)$$

The diseases that explain $\mathbf{M^+}$ are then given by $\{d_i \quad : \quad e_i \in A\}$. Equations (1) and (2) define the concept of a hypergraph, and (3) corresponds to the minimum cover of the vertices of a hypergraph. Thus, central to the set covering model is the problem of finding a minimum cover of the vertices of a hypergraph.

In Reggia's model, the vertices of the hypergraph $H = (M^+, E)$ correspond to the manifestations M^+, while the edges e_i correspond to the disease d_i and the set of all manifestations that d_i can cause. In the dual hypergraph H^*, the vertices correspond to the diseases d_i, while the edges e_i^* correspond to the diseases that can cause manifestation m_i. In the hypergraph model, the vertices of H^* correspond to disease pairs (d_i, d_j), while the edges e_i^* correspond to all disease pairs that a manifestation m_i can distinguish between. Hence, the Hypergraph model can be viewed as 'dual' to Reggia's set covering model, in that it seeks to find a minimum cover of manifestations capable of differentiating a set of diseases, rather than a minimum set of diseases capable of covering (i.e. explaining) a set of known manifestations. The hypergraph model utilises the differentiation property of a manifestation rather than just the causal connection between diseases and manifestations.

5 Ranking Diagnostic Hypotheses

As a consequence of the inherent incompleteness and uncertainty of histological knowledge, it may not be possible to accomplish a unique diagnosis after testing. In this situation, we treat each manifestation as a 'voter', generating a preference list based upon it's symbolic likelihood in each remaining disease. The objective is now to produce a consensus preference list from the lists of all voters. The theory of social choice addresses this objective. In particular, the Kemeny social choice function achieves a consensus, whilst exhibiting certain advantages over the usual scoring techniques, e.g. it is Condorcet while conventional scoring method are not.

6 Results

The histology system was tested using two sets of samples; the first comprising 14 retrospective cases of breast disease in the form of slide preparations, the second consisting of 5 hypothetical cases. From a total of 19 possible correct diagnoses, the system's recommendation was judged 'correct' by the evaluating pathologist in 15 cases, 'acceptable' in 3 cases and 'incorrect' in the 1 remaining case. The three results classed as acceptable were due to incomplete disease descriptions in the knowledge base and can be easily remedied. The incorrect result was caused by a relatively new disease not yet included in the knowledge base. Note that when this case was presented to a group of pathologists, they too gave the same incorrect diagnosis as the system due to the fact they were unaware of the existence of the new disease.

7 Discussion

The hypergraph model embodies two fundamental concepts. Firstly, the principle of 'minimum effort' (i.e. avoid questions that are not directly relevant to the problem) and secondly the concept that definite information is preferable to doubtful information.

This work has illustrated the implicit assumptions made in the set covering model and demonstrated that improved performance can be achieved using the hypergraph model and Kemeny function. It has also demonstrated the feasibility of providing decision support in the problem of breast histopathology. This investigatory study will be followed by the incorporation of more extensive domain knowledge and systematic evaluation of the system.

8 Bibliography

[1]. Heathfield HA. *Differential diagnosis and decision support in histopathology*. Ph.D. Thesis 1990, Brighton Polytechic.

[2]. Gondrian M and Minoux M. *Graphs and algorithms*. John Wiley and Sons 1979.

[3]. Reggia JA, Nau DS and Wang PY. Diagnostic expert systems based on a set covering model. *Int J Man-Machine Studies* 1983; 19: 437-60.

FUMIDS (Fever of Unknown origin in MIscellaneous diseases Diagnosis System) : DEVELOPMENT AND ASSESSMENT

Katsuhiko Takabayashi*, Sinji Ogaki**,
Yoichi Satomura*** and Sho Yoshida*
Department of Internal Medicine II* and Devision for Medical
Informatics***, Chiba University, School of Medicine
and Mitsui System Engineering Research Co. Ltd**, Japan

ABSTRACT

FUMIDS (Fever of Unknown origin in MIscellaneous diseases Diagnosis System) has been developed for the practical use in the hospitals to assist doctors in making a differential diagnosis among febrile diseases, or fever of unknown origin (FUO). The diagnostic approach is devided into two main steps with a hypothetico-deductive method, in which FUMIDS selects the probable diseases from essential data and deals with more specific data to compare a case with diagnostic criteria. The level of intelligence of FUMIDS was considered as the same or better than that of interns and whole working time for one case was in twenty minutes on the average. More than 95% of simulation cases it selected a correct diagnosis and offered proper procedures to make a more precise diagnosis.

INTRODUCTION

Most of the expert systems in medicine have been built with the goal of diagnosis selection whereas only a few provide assistance in therapy selection. Examples for the varying domains are : cancer therapy (1), infectious diseases (2), connective tissue diseases (3) and the wide area of general internal medicine (4). We have chosen the Fever of Unknown Origin as the application area of our expert system.

Fever of Unknown Origin (FUO) has been one of the main subjects in internal medicine especially in the diagnostic area. FUO is defined by a body temperature of 38.3 °C or greater appearing on multiple occasions lasting three weeks or longer and remaining undiagnosed after one week of in-hospital evaluation (5). A physician must find the basic disease which causes fever. The causes of the fever are scattered in many fields in internal medicine, so that a lot of medical knowledge is necessary to solve this problem. FUMIDS was intended to assist general physicians to solve them instead of the specialists of each field.

CONCEPTS OF DIAGNOSTIC APPROACH IN FUMIDS

The idea of the diagnostic strategy used in FUMIDS is to imitate the specialist's diagnostic process as far as possible. There is no statistical approach in FUMIDS since most of the diseases in FUO are rare diseases and prior probabilities and prevalences are quite different between facilities or doctors. Instead FUMIDS makes a diagnosis using a hypothetico-deductive method which is thought to be a common way that doctors take. They select probable diseases by collecting some essential information in the first step by forward reasoning and verify them by checking specific diagnostic criteria in the second step by backward reasoning.

A cross diagnostic table of diseases, signs, symptoms and laboratoty tests forms the fundamental basis (figure 1). The scores of each symptom in relation to the diseases were decided in each category by considering all the relation between the diseases and signs, symptoms and laboratory data.

The scores range from -10 to +10 and some items have also negative scores to some diseases when they are absent (or negative).

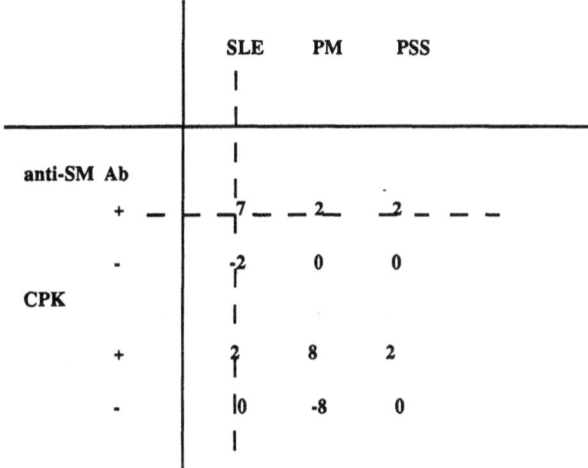

(fig 1)   Cross diagnostic table

       SLE: systemic lupus erythematosus, PM: polymyositis
       PSS: progressive systemic sclerosis (collagen diseases)
       anti-Sm Ab : anti-Sm antibody, CPK : creatinine phosphokinase

During the diagnostic process these scores are added and total scores for each disease are compared. Diseases which obtain higher scores are thought to be more probable. Many combination rules between more than two symptoms or data were also prepared to avoid simple summation of the scores and to imitate expert's complicated diagnostic logics. Thus, in FUMIDS the total score for one disease does not mean the absolute value for the probability of that disease, but the relative value of that disease compared with the other diseases in the same category.

In a second step diagnosis, FUMIDS asks more specific questions for probable diseaes and checks whether a case matches to the diagnostic criteria or not. Many diseases have each authorized diagnostic criteria at the present time however some criteria were newly created for those which do not have one.

DIAGNOSTIC PROCESS OF FUMIDS

The whole diagnostic process consists of four parts.

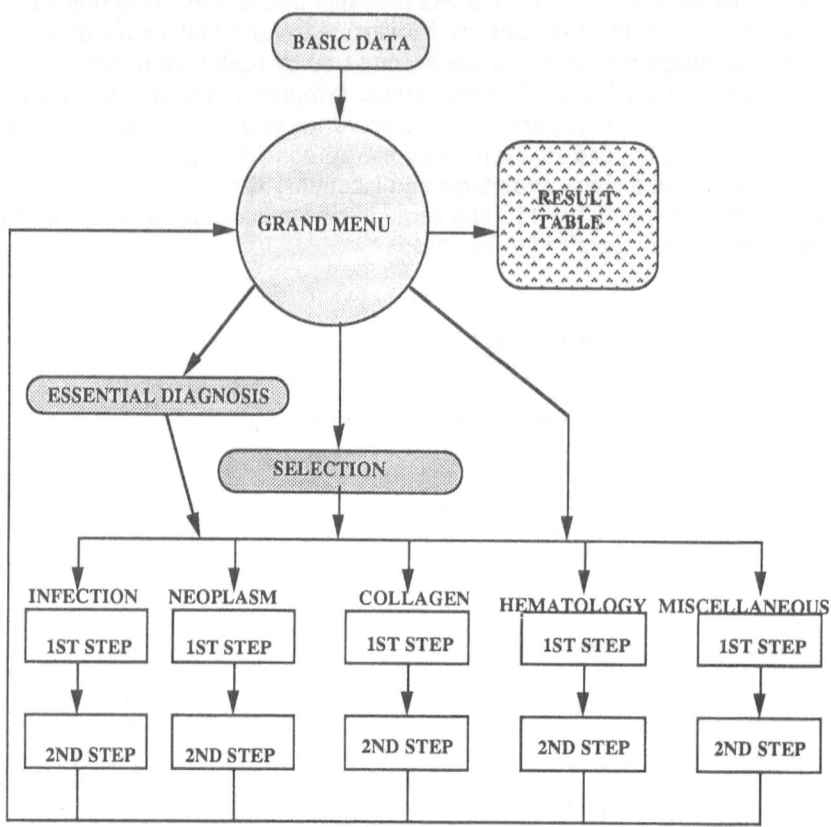

(fig 2)   Overview of the diagnostic process in FUMIDS

The first part is to rule out of the primary or common diseases which should be essentially diagnosed (essential diagnosis).

The next two parts are equal to the first step of the hypothetico- deductive method described above.   Generally, FUO can be classified into five categories depending its origin (infection, collagen diseases, neoplasmas, hematological diseases and other miscellaneous diseases).   At first FUMIDS selects more probable categories from those five by counting the scores for each category (selection).

The third part is a first step of a diagnosis in each category.   Questions are already prepared for each category (less than 100 questions at most).   By answering these questions, the scores of each disease are counted.   All the diseases are shown in order of high scores on the screen with the scores as well as their contents of positive and negative factors .

The fourth is a second step of a diagnosis in each category, or final confirmation of a diagnosis by comparing a case with the diagnostic criteria. Users can select some diseases to compare them with their cases by taking into account the results of the third part. Each disease has a criteria to make a diagnosis "definite", "probable" or "possible" and FUMIDS shows the results of diagnosis for the disease with its criteria and further procedures to make a diagnosis.

A user can start from any of above four parts.

IMPLEMENTATION

FUMIDS is written in OPS5 and FORTRAN and runs on a MICROVAX. The diagnostic process is written in OPS5, while the part of the man-machine interface and calculation is performed by FORTRAN. The size of the executive file is approximately 3MB and occupies 15 MB in use. Windows are used for the information and detailed questions.

The number of target diseases is 108, using approximately 720 items and 1500 rules. The medical knowledge was obtained from three experts. One of the two knowlege engineers is an expert himself.

RESULTS

FUMIDS was tested by experts, young doctors and medical students using more than 80 typical simulated cases and also 30 real cases.

In 95 % of the simulation cases, a correct diagnosis was included among the top five probable diseases that FUMIDS selected in a first step diagnosis of each category. In real or complicated cases it could provide proper suggestions to users. One diagnostic process took about twenty minutes on the average.

FUMIDS worked better with the person who is acquainted with that field, and the best results were obtained when the expert used it.

Users´ impression after using this system was summarized as follows,

1) Sometimes they can not put in data correctly because they can not evaluate the data well.
2) As for time-oriented data they can not easily select suitable one from them for FUMIDS .
3) FUMIDS is useful to summarize the data and avoid from overlooking diseases.

DISCUSSION

FUMIDS was initially designed for attempting to imitate an expert´s diagnostic process and to be a practical system in a hospital. In that sense it achieved the object because FUMIDS almost satisfied the level of intelligence and speed for the users.

Although this system can not surpass the level of the expert theoretically, it sometimes worked better than the experts in summarizing the patient´s data and arranging the probable diagnosis in order and it was useful for users to prevent from overlooking diseases and laboratory tests.

This expert system can solve only simple cases, while practically many cases of FUO are complicated such as overlapping of diseases or modified with drugs or treatment. However these complicated cases are also difficult for the experts to solve and to analyze or simplify the complicated cases is a basic method to work out a problem.

In this system we prepare a set of "ready made" questions for the users in each category. By using these question sets, we can avoid redundant questions and answers and we can store cases in the same quality. From that point of view, we can say that FUMIDS is a case database system which can make a diagnosis.

FUMIDS worked better when the user was a person who knew well in that field. This fact suggests that a diagnosis by FUMIDS depends on the quality of the data input. To minimize the difference between the user´s level of knowledge, we tried to make windows for the information but we should provide further information system as a huge text file or graphics to users.

We must always consider the user´s need if we attempt to make a real feasible expert system. We thought that doctors´ need in making a diagnosis of FUO is knowing which disease should be suspected and which procedure is necessary to make a final diagnosis rather than knowing precise probability for each diagnosis. From this point of view FUMIDS was focused on not making a complete diagnosis by calculating the accurate certainty factors, but providing proper suggestions to users.

REFERENCES

1) Shortliffe, E.H., Scott, A.C., Bischoff, M.B., Campbell, A.B., Melle, W. van, Jacobs, C.D. : ONCOCIN: An Expert System for Oncology. Protocol Management. Proceedings of the Int. Joint Conference on Artificial Intelligence (UCAI), pp.876-881, 1981.
2) Davis, R., Buchanan, B, Shortliffe, E. : Production Rules as a Representation for a Knowledge-based Consultation Program. Artif. Intel. 8:15-45, 1977.
3) Lindberg, D.A.B., Sharp, G.C., Kingsland, L.C., Weiss, S.M., Hayes, S.P., Ueno, H., Hazelwood, S.E. : Computer Based Rheumatology Consultant. In Lindberg, D.A.B., Kaihara, S. (Eds) : Medinfo 80, pp.1311-1315 (Amsterdam : North-Holland 1980).
4) Pople, H.E. : Heuristic Methods for Imposing Structure on Ill-structured Problems : The Structuring of Medical Diagnostics. In Szolovits, P. (Edit.): Artificial Intelligence in Medicine, p.p.119-190 (Boulder, CO : Westview Press,1982).
5) Petersdorf RG, Beeson PB : Fever of unexplained origin : Report on 100 cases. Medicine 40:1, 1961

A Bayesian Approach to the Detection of Acute Disorders in a Respiratory Intensive Care Unit

Robert B. Fraser, Ph.D., Northwest Research Associate, Inc., 300 120th Ave. N.E., Bldg. 7, Suite 220, Bellevue, WA 98005, U.S.A.
Stephen Z. Turney, M.D., Maryland Institute for Emergency Medical Services Systems, 22 South Green Street, Baltimore, MD 21201, U.S.A.

Abstract

Acute pulmonary and systemic disorders occur in mechanically ventilated intensive care patients frequently enough to be of concern. We selected twelve routinely monitored parameters in order to detect certain of these acute disorders (specifically, pneumothorax, pulmonary embolism, ARDS, and sepsis) before they lead to obvious clinical distress. A systematic approach to early detection utilizing changes in the twelve parameters was developed using the sequential Bayesian method. Fifty patients were monitored over a period of one to several days. Six of these patients developed one of the four disorders under study as determined by conventional diagnostic means, such as by x-ray. An examination of the records of these six patients over the time period prior to the actual diagnosis showed that the disorders of three of these six would have been predicted by our Bayesian approach.

Introduction

A number of biomedical monitors have been developed to provide alarms (e.g., for apnea) in intensive care unit (ICU) environments; however, there is a need for a system to alert ICU personnel before emergencies occur by responding to more subtle physiological indicators. Specifically, the means for providing the early detection of certain acute pulmonary and systemic disorders would prove to be a valuable asset. Examples of such acute disorders include pneumothorax and atelectasis, pulmonary embolism, adult respiratory distress syndrome (ARDS), and sepsis. The occurrence of these disorders in ventilated ICU patients is relatively frequent (ranging from a few percent for ARDS and pulmonary embolism to as high as 25% for sepsis) and patient survival rate is usually improved with early treatment.

Since the early days of routine respiratory monitoring there have been several efforts to improve patient care in the ICU by observing parameters which could uncover the early signs of disease. These efforts include the work of Gardner et al (1982), Osborn (1977), Riker and Haberman (1976), Siegel and Coleman (1986), Sittig (1987), Turney et al (1972), and Turney (1988). What their approaches have in common is the use of central monitors to observe the current status and long-term trends of several patients as well as the use of alarms keyed to a single respiratory variable such as end-tidal CO_2, respiratory rate, or arterial O_2. However, there is a need for more research into the use of patterns of monitored physiological parameters to alert ICU staff to the presence of acute pulmonary or systemic disorders.

Methods

The data for this program were collected at the Maryland Institute for Emergency Medical Services Systems (MIEMSS) under the direction of the second author. Each patient admitted to the MIEMSS ICU requiring ventilatory support is routinely monitored for a number of respiratory and cardiovascular parameters (Turney et al, 1972; Turney, 1988). The system used for gathering the real-time respiratory data, the respiratory assessment system (RAS), has been described by Fraser and Turney (1985). Approximately 40 parameters are taken directly or derived from these respiratory waveforms, including respiratory gas concentration and lung volume measurements, and lung mechanics and gas exchange calculations. Other data collected manually and calculations from these data include blood gases, blood chemistry, hematological parameters, cardiovascular parameters, ventilation/perfusion calculations, and ventilator status.

The four acute disorders with which we will be concerned in this study are acute atelectasis and/or pneumothorax (AA/PT), pulmonary embolism (PE), adult respiratory distress syndrome (ARDS), and sepsis. From the routinely collected patient data, twelve parameters, $P_i(i=1$ to 12), and/or changes in these parameters were selected from clinical experience as being most indicative of these disorders and include: total lung compliance (C in ml/cm H_2O), change in total lung compliance (ΔC), change in total non-elastic airway resistance (ΔR in cm H_2O/ml/min), change in partial pressure of alveolar CO_2 ($\Delta PACO_2$ in torr), change in CO_2 production (ΔVCO_2 in ml/min), change in heart rate (ΔHR in beats/min), body temperature (TEMP in ^oC), change in the ratio of arterial to inspired O_2 partial pressure ($\Delta PaO_2/PIO_2$), change in venous O_2 saturation (ΔS_vO_2), change in the fraction of intrapulmonary blood flow effectively shunted away from ventilation ($\Delta Q_s/Q_t$), change in the ratio of alveolar dead space to alveolar volume ($\Delta V_D/V_T$), and change in the white blood cell count (ΔWBC in number per mm^3).

Our initial approach to this problem was to examine the possible development of a rule-based expert system built on physiological modeling and heuristic reasoning. However, we eventually sought a more systematic approach to reflect the fact that as the number of diagnostic indicators of a disorder increases, there should be a corresponding increase in the probability of that disorder being present. This suggested the use of the sequential Bayesian method to calculate the probability, $p(D_j|E_i)$, of a patient having disorder D_j given some evidence, E_i (see, for example, Sox et al, 1988). E_i, in our case, is some clinical evidence of the patient's condition as determined by a measurement or an observation made on that patient.

To calculate the probability, $p(D_j|E_i)$, we must first know the probability of E_i given D_j, or $p(E_i|D_j)$, which is the probability that certain evidence, E_i, is present given the disease, D_j. The $p(E_i|D_j)$ are generally the probabilities most accessible in a clinical setting and were estimated for each E_i and D_j by the co-author from clinical experience. A piece of evidence, E_i, is determined by the value of P_i (listed above) relative to some predetermined threshold. The probability, $p(E_i|D_j)$, was considered to have a constant, non-zero value if P_i exceeded this threshold. D_j is one of the four disorders listed above or a fifth category which includes other disorders or normals.

Finally, the probability that the disorder, D_j, is present after obtaining the ith piece of evidence is given by:

$$p(D_j|E_i) = \frac{p(E_i|D_j) * p(D_j|E_{i-1})}{\sum\limits_{j=1}^{5} p(E_i|D_j) * p(D_j|E_{i-1})} \qquad (1)$$

The calculation of $p(D_j|E_i)$ for a particular disease, D_j, is a sequential one in which $p(D_j|E_1)$ is calculated first and then is used in calculating $p(D_j|E_2)$, which is in turn used to calculate $p(D_j|E_3)$, and so on to $p(D_j|E_{12})$. If there is no value for the probability, $p(E_i|D_j)$, then the calculation for $p(D_j|E_i)$ is skipped. When i=1 we note that $p(D_j|E_0) = p(D_j)$, which is the prior probability that the disorder, D_j, is present in the population under consideration. In our case $p(D_j)$ is the probability that the disorder, D_j, will appear in an ICU patient during a 24-hour period. Finally, we define:

$$p(D_5) = 1 - \sum\limits_{j=1}^{4} p(D_j). \qquad (2)$$

An assumption implicit in Equation (1) is that all $p(E_i \mid D_j)$ are independent. This may not be true in our case, but since the number of E_i per D_j is not too large, the performance of our system may not suffer greatly (Fryback, 1978).

Data were collected prospectively from 50 patients at the MIEMSS ICU over a six month period. Each patient was monitored continuously for at least 24 hours. The measured data, as well as bedside notes, clinical interventions, and any diagnoses made by the staff were collected for each patient. This allowed us to compare a diagnosis suggested by the Bayesian calculations in Equation (1) with the actual diagnosis made by the staff.

Results and Conclusions

Of the fifty monitored patients, six were diagnosed by the staff at some point in time as having one of the four pulmonary or systemic disorders under study. (This is about the average rate at which these disorders appear in ICU patients at MIEMSS.) Of these six, three patients showed effects which could be said to be other than artifact. A summary of the evidence suggesting the Bayesian diagnoses and the probabilities calculated from Equation (1) are shown in the Table for each of the three patients. One of the cases for which no Bayesian diagnosis could be found is also listed in the Table. The calculated probabilities for the first three cases are at least a factor of ten greater than the prior probabilities. These preliminary results suggest that the automatic calculation of Bayesian probabilities from Equation (1) at frequent intervals could serve as a means for the early detection of certain pulmonary and systemic disorders.

Case No.	Actual Diagnosis	Bayesian** Diagnosis	Probability from Eq(1)	t_B (hrs)	t_E (hrs)	Evidence in order of importance				
1	PT	AA/PT	0.32	-8	-1	$\Delta C=-5.4$	$\Delta R=+11.7$	$\Delta PACO_2=+7.6$	*$\Delta VCO_2=+41$	*C=12 to 17
2	Sepsis	Sepsis	0.92	-10	-3	$\Delta WBC=+2200$	$\Delta VCO_2=+50$	TEMP=38.6	*$\Delta C=-15$	*$\Delta PACO_2=-40$
3	ARDS	ARDS	0.12	-15	-3	$\Delta PaO_2/PIO_2=-.13$		C=22.3 at t=0 (respiratory monitor started at t=0)		
4	PT (by x-ray)	None		-24	0	C, R, $PACO_2$, V_D/V_T all showed no significant change; $\Delta Q_s/Q_T = .06$				

* evidence suggesting other disorders

**when the minimum probability for detection is set at 0.1

t_B = beginning of monitoring period over which change was calculated (t=0 at time of actual diagnosis)

t_E = end of monitoring period over which change was calculated

Table. Comparison of actual and Bayesian diagnosis

In this preliminary study only the six cases with diagnosed disorders could be examined in detail. In the next phase of this study a much larger patient group will be studied. This should lead to more refined probabilities, $p(E_i | D_j)$, establish a better understanding of the difference between artifact and changes actually associated with a disorder, and allow us to determine a more rigorous measure of performance, i.e., sensitivity and selectivity.

Acknowledgments

This project was supported by a Department of Health and Human Services grant (1R43GM42306-01). We would like to thank James Clark (Capt., U.S. Army Nurse Corps) for his assistance with the arduous task of data collection.

REFERENCES

Fraser, R.B. and S.Z. Turney (1985), "New Method of Respiratory Gas Analysis: Light Spectrometer," J. Appl. Physiol., 59, (3), 1001-1007.

Fryback, D.G. (1978), "Bayes' Theorem and Conditional Nonindependence of Data in Medical Diagnosis," Computers and Biomedical Research, 11, 423-434.

Gardner, R.M., B.J. West, T.A. Pryor, K.G. Larsen, H.R. Warner, T.P. Clemmer, and J.F. Orme (1982), "Computer-based ICU Data Acquisition as an Aid to Clinical Decision-making," Critical Care Medicine, 10 (12), 823-830.

Osborn, J.J. (1977), "Cardiopulmonary Monitoring in the Respiratory Intensive Care Unit," Medical Instrumentation, 11 (5), 278-282.

Riker, J.B. and B. Haberman (1976), "Expired Gas Monitoring by Mass Spectrometry in a Respiratory Intensive Care Unit," Critical Care Medicine, 4 (5), 223-229.

Siegel, J.H. and B. Coleman (1986), "Computers in the Care of the Critically Ill Patient," Urology Clinics of North America, 13 (1), 101-117.

Sittig, D.F. (1987), "Computerized Management of Patient Care in Complex, Controlled Clinical Trial in the Intensive Care Unit," Proc. Symp. Computer Appl. Med. Care, IEEE Computer Society, Los Angeles, 225-232.

Sox, H.C., Jr., M.A. Blatt, M.C. Higgins, and K.I. Martin (1988), Medical Decision Making, Butterworths, Boston, MA.

Turney, S.Z. (1988), "Monitoring Considerations," Chapter 6 in Acute Respiratory Care, Eds., S.E. Linberg and J.J. Applefeld, Blackwell Scientific, Boston.

Turney, S.Z., C. McCluggage, W. Blumenfeld, T.C. McAslan and R.A. Cowley (1972), "Automatic Respiratory Gas Monitoring," Ann. Thor. Surg., 14 (2), 159-172.

EXPERT SYSTEM "DINAR-2". METHODOLOGICAL BASIS FOR THE PEDIATRIC EMERGENCY AID ORGANIZATION IN A LARGE REGION

S.I. Goldberg, V.E. Lomovskikh, A.O. Makhanek , M.S. Sklyar
Biophysics Department, Physiology Institute USSR Acad.Sci
Popov str., 30, 620014, Sverdlovsk, USSR

ABSTRACT

The Expert System is presented for assessing the severity of a child's organism in critical states and deciding tactical problems of its treatment. The mathematical apparatus of the Expert System realizes an unstatistical approach to the analysis of the possible intentional distortion of information. This approach is based on the verification of stability of the decisions taken in relation to the distortion of the information.

THE ROLE OF THE EXPERT SYSTEM IN PEDIATRIC EMERGENCY AID ORGANIZATION

Considering the problem of providing the emergency aid for children in a large region (with the territory radius up to several hundreds kilometers) it is necessary to take into account the possibility of life-threatening situations occuring in very different as to their treatment and diagnostic facilities medical institutions and with the not always highly experienced or specialized personnel in charge of them. With this in mind it is vital to have a system making it possible for doctors in charge of such cases to consult the specialists,a system allowing to transfer the patients to the Intensive Therapy Centre and the prompt specialists-reanimatologists arrival to the patient. To some extent these problems could be solved with the help of a Reanimation Consultative Centre (RCC) connected through a communication network with all the medical institutions in various localities of the region and thus receiving the necessary information on all critical cases and working out the optimal treatment tactics. The RCC controller would then be able to provide consultation and make decisions on the priority of reanimation aid. However in real life such a controller-consultant will have to cope with lots of problems:

- the necessity to provide "blind-consultations" from the local
doctor's description;
- providing consultations for children of all the ages with the
problems of a very different nature;
- making a great number of vital decisions in a limited time;
- the necessity to coordinate the different controller's actions
in what concerns one and the same patient;
- the possibility of acquiring inaccurate or completely false
information on a case;
- the need to have current information on the reanimation
facilities in hospitals nearest to the patient.

Besides such a Centre must apart from providing emergency aid to the patients take the responsibility for all the regional emergency aid network operation in what concerns the doctor's qualification upgrading, working out the unified estimates of the gravity of the patient's conditions, unification of medical definitions and concepts.

The expert system with the functions listed below may prove very effective in the work of such a centre and provide a solid support for the controller-consultant's decisions.

1.Dynamic observation of the seriously ill children of the region.

2.Clarifying-dialogue function to obtain exhaustive information on a child's condition and to give the corresponding treatment recommendations.

3.Determination of a complete syndrome diagnosis.

4.Elimination of errors in the information transmitted.

5.The patient's condition dynamic evaluation.

6.Help in specific treatment prescription.

7.Actions coordination in a particular case treatment.

8.Tactical aid in central resourses distribution.

9.Display of analitic information on RCC operation, general picture of children health condition in the region, defects in the hospitals operation, the reasons for the impossibility of providing thenecessary aid.

10.Reports on RCC operation.

11.Reference materials on concepts and terminology employed in the system.

12.Reference information on the hospital's aid facilities, treatment methodics, pharmacology, special treatment methodics, diagnostics etc.

13.Building-up of a comfortable informational environment for the RCC controller-consultant.

All these functions are realized in ES "DINAR-2". "DINAR-2" is the further development of the ES "DINAR-1" which is based on the ideas of Gubler and Tsibulkin [1].

DINAR-2 consists of an information-reference subsystem organized as a connected graph, subsystem for the RCC operation and the condition of the pediatric emergency aid service in the region analysis, and the expert system "inquiry" itself for the diagnostics and treatment of the critical conditions of the children.

The very first problem being solved by the expert system is the evaluation of the degree of urgency for making a decision. If the patient's condition is critical the expert system carries out a dialogue over the a-priori given question-and-derivation tree. In case there is no immediate danger for the patient's life within the nearest 20-30 min the controller-consultant is expected to take an active part in the expert system operation. He is able then to choose his questions independently, correct the intermediate derivations and suggestions, exclude the unnecessary local derivation chains. A block diagram of the expert subsystem operation is given in Fig.1.

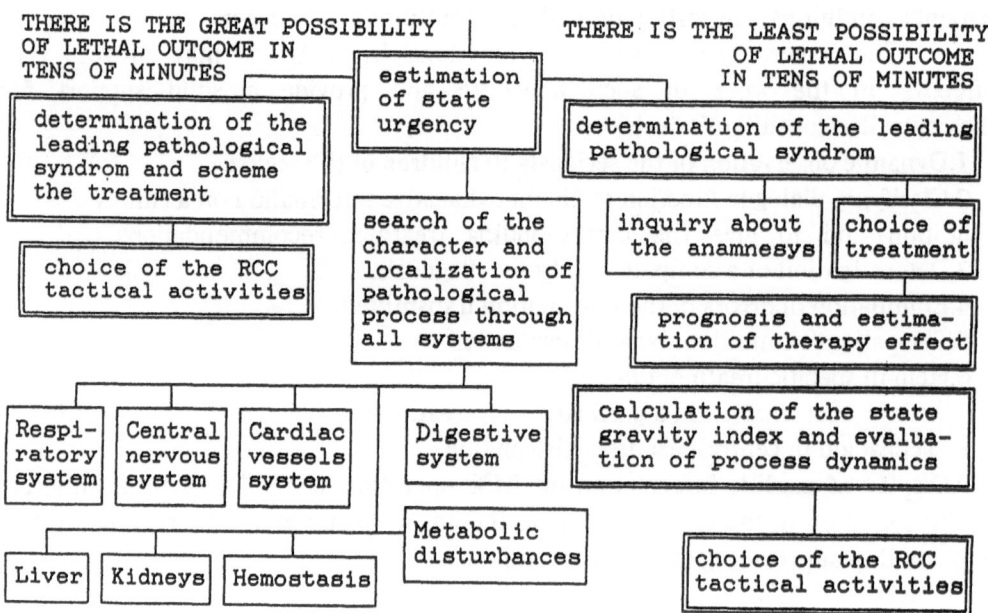

Fig.1 Flowchart of the expert subsystem operation.
Double lined blocks are due to execute.

MATHEMATICAL AND MEDICAL CHARACTERISTICS OF THE EXPERT SYSTEM

Mathematics. The suggested decision making model's peculiarity is the partial divergence between the local doctor's and the RCC controller-consultant's interests. As a result apart from misunderstandings because of the lack of qualification or concept discrepancies etc., a deliberate purposeful misrepresentation of information is also possible. Traditional statistic approaches to this kind of problems can't be applied here because of the difficulties in the necessary distribution functions determination. In the given original mathematic method employed in this expert system a true picture of the case is presented as a fuzzy set. Membership function of this set is determined by the information transmitted. The system of derivations on a fuzzy set is assumed to be proved if stable with regard to the purposeful distortions of information transmitted. Membership function values, and information shift's values and directions, are being changed in the dialogue process and are dependent upon transmitted information coordinateness, the extent to which the doctor in charge can be trusted, and the additional discussion of dubious responces. Algorithm strategy consists in offering a hypothesis, additional information collection with the aim of its confirmation and stability verification. If the hypothesis is unstable additional data are collected until a stable derivation is acquired. The software is based on "Turbo-PROLOG 2.0" language for IBM-PC/AT personal computers.

Medicine. The medical basis for this kind of systems is the methodics of the degree of gravity of the patient's condition evaluation and providing an adequate emergency aid. Traditional methods of the adequate emergency aid. Tra evaluation in the form of the "threat to life" scales fails to give a clear understanding of the pathological process character, the necessary treatment, and the therapy adequacy.

We have elaborated an original method for the degree of gravity of a critical state evaluation, determined by the degree of urgency of the intensive therapy measures, the degree of the affected function compensation, the degree to which the patient's condition is under control, the previous treatment adequacy evaluation and the advisability of the treatment intensivity alteration.

Thus evaluating the patient's condition over the above listed criteria it is possible to determine the gravity vector component evaluation. In the process of this patient's condition evaluation the expert system calculates the case gravity index. Such a description of the patient's condition gravity predetermined the necessity of gravity-dependent syndroms, treatment methodics, and tactical decisions classification. The necessary medical component of the expert system is the computer conclusions verification by man. In this system verification is based on the degree of correspondence between the prognosis and the real condition of the patient. The algorythm for the degree of the therapy adequacy is also prognosis oriented.

We suppouse that this approach can be used at the organizing of emergency aid service.

ES EFFICIENCY

ES "DINAR-1" and "DINAR-2" are in operation from January 1989. Expert systems became an indispensable element in the RCC routine. The level of the diagnosis accuracy and the choice of the tactical decisions of ES "DINAR-2" is quite compatible with the level of a qualified reanimatologist. From the moment the expert systems were introduced into operation the number of lethal outcomes among the children of the region became significantly less than in other similar localities. The authors have at their disposal convincing statistical data that it was achieved not in the least becouse of the described division efficiency, though it is of course very difficult to estimate the expert system contribution to the process. Now the expert system has already been introduced in a number of regions in Russia.

REFERENCES

1.Цыбулькин Э.К., Кукулевич М.А., Гублер Е.В. Вычислительное прогнозирование исходов угрожающих состояний при острых респираторно-вирусных заболеваниях у детей раннего возраста. Вопросы охраны материнства и детства. 1977, N12, с.45-50.

An Expert System for the Diagnosis, Treatment, and Triage of Head Injuries in Remote Environments

Robert B. Fraser, Ph.D., *Northwest Research Associates, Inc., 300 120th Ave. NE, Bldg. 7, Ste. 220, Bellevue, WA 98009, U.S.A.*

Aizik Wolf, M.D., C. Michael Dunham, M.D., Stephen Z. Turney, M.D., Brad M. Cushing, M.D., Ameen I. Ramzy, M.D., and James N. Eastham, Ph.D., *Maryland Institute for Emergency Medical Services Systems, 22 So. Greene St., Baltimore, MD 21201, U.S.A.*

Abstract

We describe the development of an expert system, TRAUMA ADVISOR, to aid clinical staff in remote locations in the diagnosis, treatment, and triage of trauma victims with head injuries. The expertise was derived from the current literature, an experienced trauma neurosurgeon, a committee of trauma physicians, and a large trauma database. The emphasis was placed on variables obtainable in the field by emergency medical personnel. The program, developed on an expert system shell, runs on a laptop or desktop IBM-compatible 80286 (or better) personal computer.

Introduction

In remote environments or small communities the diagnosis and treatment of severe injuries with minimal staff and simple diagnostic equipment can be a major challenge. In response to this, we are developing a rule-based expert system for trauma care (TRAUMA ADVISOR) which incorporates the expertise of several trauma physicians practicing at the Maryland Institute for Emergency Medical Services Systems (MIEMSS), one of the major level-one trauma centers in the United States. Although expert systems for abdominal pain (de Dombal *et al*, 1972) and chest injuries (Clarke *et al*, 1988) have been described in the literature, we are not aware of similar developments for head injuries. In this paper we describe the development of the portion of TRAUMA ADVISOR which specifically addresses the diagnosis, treatment, and triage of head injuries with the assumption of limited diagnostic facilities and medical supplies. We also assume that the clinical staff has a knowledge of basic life support techniques but that the more serious injuries will be treated only to the extent necessary to stabilize the patient for transportation to the appropriate treatment center. The specific emergency interventions and drugs recommended by this expert system are those available to

U.S. Navy medical corpsmen; additions and deletions are easily made for other applications because of the modular nature of the expert system.

Methods

We identify four stages in the development of this expert system: a review of the literature, interview with a single expert, consensus with a group of experts, and refinements with the use of a trauma database.

A review of the literature uncovered a variety of emergency treatment and triage schemes for head trauma (e.g., American College of Surgeons, 1989; Boyd *et al*, 1987; McSwain and Kerstein, 1987; Ornato *et al*, 1985; and West *et al*, 1988). However, there were such differences in approach that only the major diagnostic indicators, such as the systolic blood pressure or the Glasgow Coma Scale (GCS), were found to be useful in the development of our expert system. (GCS is a broad numerical indicator of the level of consciousness and varies from 3 to 15, with 15 being normal.)

In the second stage, these diagnostic indicators were used as a focal point for knowledge acquisition via interview. The expert in our interview was an experienced trauma neurosurgeon at MIEMSS. From this interview we developed a preliminary approach to the diagnosis, treatment, and triage of head injuries. As our discussions broadened to include other members of the MIEMSS staff, it became apparent that other than strictly neurologic indicators would have to be considered in making the proper decisions for treatment and triage. This led to the third stage in which the preliminary approach was presented to a committee of trauma physicians at MIEMSS representing all aspects of trauma care. The logical scheme was then modified to incorporate a broader patient assessment and treatment. In the final stage of this expert system development, some of the more subtle logical distinctions were made with the help of a trauma database comprised of over 10,000 cases collected over a ten-year period at MIEMSS (Dunham *et al*, 1989).

The programming of TRAUMA ADVISOR was carried out in the expert system development shell, Personal Consultant Plus (PC Plus, Texas Instruments, Inc., Houston, TX). We customized portions of the user interface by employing both PC Plus and external graphics software. Once a program is fully developed and tested it may be converted into "C" object code, which requires less memory (usually running under the conventional 640K of RAM).

Results and Discussion

We do not have the space here to show a flow chart of the logic for TRAUMA ADVISOR's head-injury module; however, we will describe its most salient features. The major logical branch points occur at GCS = 11 and systolic blood pressure (SBP) = 90 mmHg. For

GCS < 11 (indicating a serious deficit in neurologic function) the program will recommend immediate evacuation to a level-one trauma center unless one of the recommended interventions (such as the administration of naloxone) results in a new GCS $\geq$ 11.

For SBP < 90 mmHg a series of interventions will be recommended starting with the administration of one liter of Ringer's lactate intravenously. If the successive interventions to increase SBP above 90 mmHg all fail then immediate evacuation will be recommended.

All logical branches eventually lead to a series of questions about various signs and symptoms of head injury. Some signs or symptoms, such as uncontrolled seizures, will lead to a recommendation of an immediate evacuation. Some signs, such as unequally dilated pupils or leaking cerebral spinal fluid, also lead to a recommendation of evacuation, but the level of urgency is dependent upon the patient's GCS. The level of GCS at which the evacuation priority should change was determined from the MIEMSS trauma database by examining the relationship between GCS at admission and the requirement for serious interventions (e.g. craniotomy) or the appearance of central nervous system disabilities. One result of this review, for example, showed that if the patient has unequal pupils and the GCS $\leq$ 13, then it would be appropriate to recommend *immediate evacuation*, but when the GCS > 13 the recommendation could be relaxed to *evacuation when possible*.

If GCS $\geq$ 11 and SBP $\geq$ 90 mmHg, some relatively minor signs or symptoms, such as head lacerations or severe headache, will lead the program to suggest specific treatments and continued observation, but not evacuation.

When run on an IBM-type 80386 computer, the program responded to the user within one or two seconds. After all the prompts are answered and the responses to suggested interventions are given, the program displays in order: the evacuation priority, the suggested diagnoses, and the suggested treatments. After a consultation, the program is designed to explain its conclusions (each major conclusion is assigned an explanation during development). The output file (evacuation, diagnoses, and treatments) can be saved by a keystroke. Finally, the user can change any one of the inputs and rerun the program to see what effect it will have on the output. A conclusion screen for a head injury serious enough to warrant evacuation is shown in the Figure.

TRAUMA ADVISOR has been evaluated by the co-authors and is currently being evaluated by the U.S. Navy. Preliminary results indicate that the program is appropriate as written for U.S. Navy medical corpsman. Modifications in treatment and evacuation priorities would be made for other emergency treatment centers depending upon the tests and drugs available and the proximity of a fully equipped trauma center.

IMMEDIATE EVACUATION RECOMMENDED

DIAGNOSIS OF HEAD INJURIES:

A GCS of 10 or less suggests a head injury serious enough to warrant evacuation.
Possible neurogenic shock.
Possible intracranial hematoma suggested by lateralizing signs.

TREATMENT OF HEAD INJURIES:

Insure a proper airway and administer oxygen as needed. Control bleeding.

Unequal pupils or lateralized motor responses suggest an intracranial hematoma. To reduce intracranial pressure give mannitol, 0.25 to 1 gm/kg intravenously. A 0.25 gm/kg bolus may be repeated every 6 to 12 hr. Insert a Foley catheter if the patient is immobile.

Increase in blood pressure in response to dopamine suggests neurogenic shock. To control any associated bradycardia (heart rate < 60) give atropine, 0.5 to 1 mg IV. Repeat once or twice at 5 to 10 min. intervals as needed to bring the heart rate above 60 bpm. Patient should be kept well covered to prevent hypothermia.

SUMMARY OF PATIENT ASSESSMENT

Initial systolic blood pressure *(at start of consultation)*: 50-70 mmHg
Final systolic blood pressure *(after administration of dopamine)*: >90 mmHg
1st Glasgow Coma Scale *(at start of consultation)*: 9
2nd Glasgow Coma Scale *(after dopamine and improved GCS)*: 10
Trauma Score *(at end of consultation)*: 10

Figure. Abbreviated summary of a sample consultation with TRAUMA ADVISOR for a hypothetical patient with a serious head injury.

Acknowledgment

This project is being supported by a contract from the Office of Naval Research (N00014-89-C-0136). We are grateful for the technical assistance of Mahnaz Namini at MIEMSS.

References

American College of Surgeons (1989), "Advanced Trauma Life Support Course," American College of Surgeons, Chicago.

Boyd, C.R., M.A. Tolson, and W.S. Copes (1987), "Evaluating Trauma Care: The TRISS Method," *J of Trauma*, 27. 370-378.

Clarke, J.R., D.P. Cebula, and B.L. Webber (1988), "Artificial Intelligence: A Computerized Decision Aid for Trauma," *J of Trauma*, 28, 8, 1250-1254.

de Dombal, F.T., D.J. Leaper, J.R. Staniland, A.P. McCann, and J.C. Horrocks (1972), "Computer-Aided Diagnosis of Acute Abdominal Pain," *Brit. Med. J.*,2, 9-13.

Dunham, C.M., R.A. Cowley, D.R. Gens, *et al* (1989), "Methodological Approach for a Large Functional Trauma Registry," Maryland State Medical Journal, 38:227-233.

McSwain, N.E. and M.D. Kerstein, eds., (1987), *Evaluation and Management of Trauma*, Appleton-Century-Crofts, Norwalk, CT.

Ornato, J., E.J. Mlinek, E.J. Craren, and N. Nelson (1985), "Ineffectiveness of the Trauma Score and CRAMS Scale for Accurately Triaging Patients to Trauma Centers," *Ann. Emerg. Med. 14*, 11, 51-54.

West, J.G. and A.B. Eastman (1988), "Field Triage," in *Trauma*, Mattox, K.L., E.E. Moore, and D.V. Feliciano, eds., 76-90.

EXPERT SYSTEMS—KNOWLEDGE REPRESENTATION

A MODEL FOR THE SYSTEMATIC APPLICATION OF ARTIFICIAL INTELLIGENCE IN THE DIAGNOSIS OF PATHOLOGIC CONDITIONS IN A SYSTEM OR APPARATUS

P. Ferrer-Salvans *, L. Alonso-Vallès *, R. Rubio-García **,
O. Juan-Babot *, E. Vidal-Casas *
* Unitat de Farmacologia Clínica, Ciutat Sanitària de Bellvitge
Hospital Duran i Reynals. Autovia de Castelldefels, Km 2.7,
08907 Hospitalet de Llobregat, Barcelona, Spain
** Andersen Consulting, Madrid, Spain

Abstract

A model of structure for a complementary expert system to the AEDMI project (An Epidemiological Approach to Computerized Medical Diagnosis) is proposed. Starting from a diagnosis of abnormality in a system or apparatus, the model identifies the organ affected, and determines which of the possible illnesses is the one we are faced with in a particular case. The resoning is based on a tree-like structure divided into a set of three levels, assuming that greater sensitivity and less specificity of the questions, clinical variables, and the signs and symptoms to be taken into consideration is found at level I than at level III. Each time that the system is consulted for a real patient, the system offers the possibility to register all the parameters in a data base. The modules, rules, and diagnoses are registered and compared with physicians' judgment. The study of conflicting patterns helps to analyze clinical judgment and rule-based reasoning techniques in greater depth. The system is being implemented for more than one year and the data from 825 patients introduced are being currently assessed.

Introduction

The AEDMI general diagnostic system (Epidemiological Approach to Computerized Medical Diagnosis), designed at Hospital de Bellvitge and presented in another paper at this meeting (1), is based on the assessment of sensitivities, specificities, and predictivities of different symptom patterns associated with each diagnosis. The first 1-year experience of the program and the development of an expert system for the detection of adverse drug reactions (2) are current lines of research.

The AEDMI diagnostic system provides a context of the general complaints of the patient which are grouped by systems or apparatus. In order to continue the diagnostic process it is necessary to limit the knowledge domain and to build a clinical record with some defined objectives. The expert system described below is an example of this methodology.

Method

To maintain the proposed AEDMI epidemiological approach it would appear not operational to use different methodologies or to fall in the diversity of the existent expert systems (3). On the other hand, it is difficult to define a precise diagnosis if a broad spectrum scanning of signs and symptoms is used as in the AEDMI program (4). Moreover, any particular expert system requires to be applied in a previously defined context. The background epidemiological approach of the AEDMI general system is a prevalence study design. To continue the diagnostic procedure in the different systems, the use of a case-control design is foreseen (5-7). The knowledge systematization is adapted to the structure 'system - organ - disease'. In the current state of development of the project, the main syndromes or multisystem pathologies are analyzed without considering the connections among the different organs or systems involved.

Expert system model

The expert system model has been developed for the diagnosis of gastrointestinal disorders which are one of the most common pathologic conditions. The same model will be later progressively applied to remaining systems and apparatus included in the AEDMI program. The Aion Development System (8) is used as a tool to build the model due to its possibilities of forward and backward running, and the modular and tree-like knowledge representaton.

The model can be adapted to different levels of depth in the diagnostic procedure, such as:

```
I/    System or apparatus
II/   Organ or location
III/  Disease
```

The questions in the present program distinguish between normal and abnormal conditions. According to their location in the general sequence of the program, it is possible to determine which apparatus or system they belong to (level I). Once the system or apparatus to which the possible pathological data has been identified, the questions necessary to locate the organ affected are then included, i.e. esophagus, stomach, etc. (level II). The delimitation of the affected organ only by the information provided by symptoms is

difficult, especially in disorders of boundary areas sharing clinical
expressivity (i.e. gastroesophageal junction). In these cases,
results of complementary examinations are requested. The model asks
interactively for the necessary questions to open each organ module
program. Those modules whose answers fulfill a set of predifined
criteria are read by the expert system and proceeds to the next level
of questions.

Once the organ has been identified, the parameters necessary to
deduce which of the possible illnesses is the one we are faced with,
should be determined (level III). At this level the characteristics
of the disease contributes to the diagnosis as much as anatomical and
physiopathological correlation that permitted to achieve this third
level. A series of rules are being developed horizontally to
establish the differential diagnosis (9).

DIAGNOSIS

It is foreseen to compare and contrast patterns, so that different
patterns established by vertical structuring can be compared with
other possible patterns within the same level. The hypothesis may be
ventured that sensitivity and specificity of the questions, clinical
variables, and the signs and symptoms to be taken into consideration
are stratified according to their level within the diagnostic
process, so that greater sensitivity and less specificity is found at
level I than at level III (10,11).

It should be noted that the progression to a higher level at level II requires the incorporation of additional data, such as results of laboratory tests, imaging techniques, etc. These may be obtained using an integrated system of clinical data which at present are introduced by the user. All data obtained from real clinical interviews are stored in a clinical data base.

The process ends with the establishment of a diagnosis of the illness or a list of the most likely diagnostic possibilities. A summary of the abnormalities observed is also provided (Figure 1). The system has been already developed up to level I.

Once the system has provide a diagnosis, the doctor in charge of the patient is asked whether he/she agrees with the diagnosis or not. If both diagnosis coincide, the case in then included in the epidemiological data base. If not, the data or rules which were interpreted differently are recorded, and the case in included in a files for 'special cases' and 'critical reasoning'. The list of cases in which discrepancy in the diagnosis was observed may help to define the diagnosis more clearly. On the other hand, the study of conflicting patterns can help to add case based reasoning techniques to rule-based reasoning techniques usually used.

Using the proposed methods, medical knowledge may be updated and revised, epidemiological data assessed, and clinical judgment (12) analyzed in greater depth.

Current experience

Since February 1989, data from 825 patients have been collected and data from 466 of them have been statistically analyzed. In addition to the staff physicians involved in the design of the project, the data collection team is formed by four interviewing nurses and three postgraduate students. It has to be emphasized that the major investment of the project is the time spent with the patient with the aim of collecting a complete medical record. Interviews are carried out using five lap-top computers and despite our initial uncertainty, patients have not shown any kind of surprise; on the contrary, most of them have repeatedly expressed their appreciation for being submitted to such a complete interview. When patients are interviewed in such a way, a general perspective of the patient's condition is obtained without being influenced by the previous diagnostic orientation. Our experience confirms the importance of medical interview in medical diagnosis, as has been pointed out by different authors (13,14).

Preliminary results of the population sample reveal a high proportion of illiterates and low-income groups which impedes the use of a self-administered questionnaire (45.4% of them having incomplete primary education). It has to be mentioned that people referred to our hospital are not representative of the total population.

Subsampling techniques (15) by hours have been developed due to differences in the daily number of patients appointed over the morning and evening hours. The sampling coefficient of each patient during the process of the analysis of data, as recommended by Cochran et al. has been taken into account.

At the same time, physicians' diagnostic reasoning are being collected. A study on the acceptance of the AEDMI project by personnel, doctors, and patients is being prepared as well as the impact of the project on health care provided by the hospital (16).

Acknowledgments

The authors would like to thank the management authorities of Bellvitge Health Complex, Dr Eng F Moreu, Dr C Serra, Dr F Ramos, and Mr JM Deparés for the use of Hospital facilities for our research work, and Dr Marta Pulido for editorial assistance and copy editing.

References:

[1] Ferrer-Salvans P, Alonso-Vallès L, Rubio-García R, Juan-Babot O, Vidal-Casas E. Epidemiological approach to computerized medical diagnosis. The AEDMI project as a multicentric design for implementing artificial intelligence. Porceedings of Medical Informatics Europe '91. Lecture Notes in Medical Informatics. Springer-Verlag, Berlin 1991.

[2] Juan-Babot O, Ferrer-Salvans P, Alonso-Vallès L, Ferrer-Salvans I, Castells-Nat C, Rubio-García R. Foundations to build an expert system to control adverse drug reactions. Proceedings of Medical Informatics Europe '91. Lecture Notes in Medical Informatics. Springer-Verlag. Berlin 1991.

[3] Barr A, Feigenbaum EA. The handbook of Artificial Intelligence (Vol. 2). 1986 Addison-Wesley.

[4] Ferrer-Salvans P, Alonso-Vallès L. An epidemiological approach to computerized medical diagnosis: the AEDMI program. Comput Biol Med 1990; 20: 433-43.

[5] Kleinbaum DG., Kupper LL., Morgenstern H. Epidemiologic Research. Principles and quantitative methods. Lifetime Learning Pub. 1982.

[6]   Bulpitt C.J.   Randomised controlled clinical trials.   Martinus
      Nijhoff. The Hague. 1983; 28-34.
[7]   Spiegelhalter DJ.   A statistical view of uncertainty in expert
      systems.   In Artificial Intelligence and Statistics.   William A.
      Gale Ed. Addison-Wesley 1986; 17-55.
[8]   Aion   Development   System.   ADS/PC   guidebook.   1988   Aion
      Corporation. Palo Alto CA, USA.
[9]   Barahona P., Veloso M., Amador R. and Menezes F.   Some issues in
      the control of interactive differential diagnosis.   In AIME 89
      Lecture Notes in Medical Informatics.   (Hunter J., Cookson J.
      and Wyatt J. eds.) Berlin. Springer-Verlag. 1989; 72-76.
[10] Bernardo J.M.   Bayesian linear probabilistic classification; in
      Statistical Decision Theory and Related Topics 4. (S.S. Gupta
      and J.O. Berger, eds.) New York. Springer. 1988; 151-162.
[11] Lopez de Mántaras R., Sanz F., Sierra C., Verdaguer A.   MILORD +
      PNEUMON-IA: Un outil et une application en medicine. in AAVV:
      Colloque Intelligence Artificiel et Santé.   Toulousse. 1987; 45-
      54.
[12] Chaput de Saintonge DM.   and Cookson M.J. The role of clinical
      judgment analysis in the development of medical expert systems.
      In AIME 89 Lecture Notes in Medical Informatics. (Hunter J.,
      Cookson J. and Wyatt J. eds.) Berlin. Springer-Verlag. 1989; 3-
      13.
[13] Hampton JR, Harrison MJG, Mitchell JRA   et al.   Relative
      contributions of history taking, physical examination, and
      laboratory investigation to diagnosis and management of medical
      outpatients. Br Med J 1975; 2: 486-9.
[14] De Dombal FT.   Medical diagnosis from a clinician's point of
      view. Methods Inf Med 1978; 17: 28-35.
[15] Cochran   WG.   Técnicas   de   muestreo.   Compañía   Editorial
      Continental, S.A., México 1971.
[16] Jessen K.   How does a hospital information system add value to
      health in Denmark. In O'Moore R, Bengtsson S, Bryant JR, Bryden
      JS.   Proceedings of Medical Informatics Europe '90.   Lecture
      Notes in Medical Informatics n. 40.   Springer-Verlag, Berlin
      1990. pp 118-22.

UnPatient: A KNOWLEDGE BASE FOR MEDICAL DIAGNOSTIC EXPERT SYSTEMS

Christian Stary[1] and Karl Fasching [2]

[1] School of Computer Science, Florida International University, University Park, Miami, Florida 33199, USA

[2] Department of Applied Computer Science, Technical University of Vienna, Paniglgasse 16, 1040 Vienna, Austria

Abstract

Medical diagnosis is based on a variety of tasks: accumulation of patient data, application of patient-independent knowledge, generation and evaluation of diagnostic hypotheses, and the integration of patient-dependent and -independent findings. *UnPatient* supports the application and the integration of patient-independent findings. It provides a knowledge representation mechanism which can be applied to any medical problem domain used for diagnosis. The medical knowledge can be accessed by symptoms as well as by diseases. Finally, it supports the integration of static knowledge and procedural heuristics for effective diagnostic support.

1. Introduction

Medical decision making starts with an initial set of patient-related findings, which are tested against hypothetical diagnoses. The knowledge required for medical decision making is constituted by the acquired medical knowledge in the course of studying the field of medicine as well as by the practical experiences of the diagnostician, regardless of the case at hand [Ben-Bassat, 1984]. Diagnostic support tools have been mainly oriented towards a dedicated set of diseases, such as rheumatological diagnoses [Kingsland, 1985]. As a consequence, medical practicioners refused to use such kind of tools because of the lack of comprehensive knowledge for diagnostics. According to their opinion effective support can only be achieved, if more than the original diagnostic domain is covered by support tools [Singer et al., 1983]. In particular, if diagnostic hypotheses of different problem domains have to be triggered, comprehensive medical knowledge (extending the original problem domain) is required. In such cases, certain diagnostic goals have to be set to proceed in decision making. According to these goals, several problem domains (e.g., internal medicine, physical examination) have to be scanned to evaluate hypotheses [Horak et al., 1988]. In order to meet these requirements for effective support, a patient-independent knowledge base for diagnostic expert systems has been developed. It corresponds not only to a complete medical source-book accessable by factors (e.g., etiology), findings, and diseases, it also provides procedural guidelines for active diagnostic support (e.g., finding differential diagnoses).

In the course of evaluating existing diagnostic support tools, we found out that there is still a lack of comprehensive frameworks for the representation of medical knowledge [Fasching, 1990]. Most of the approaches which have been investigated pursued the goal to assist physicians or medical specialists in finding a diagnosis within a limited area of medicine. Different techniques for knowledge representation, such as rules [Buchanan et al., 1985], objects [Ben-Bassat, 1984] or combination of methods [Miller and Fisher, 1987] have been applied. Tools, such as CASNET [Patil et al., 1987] or RX [Miller and Fisher, 1987] address consultation and therapy in particular medical disciplines (internal medicine, rheumatology, etc.). Few of the tools focus on general principles of knowledge-based diagnosis, e.g., Patrec, MDX [Chandrasekaran et al., 1984]. In general, hierarchical structuring of diagnoses have been provided. In some approaches findings have also been hierarchically structured.

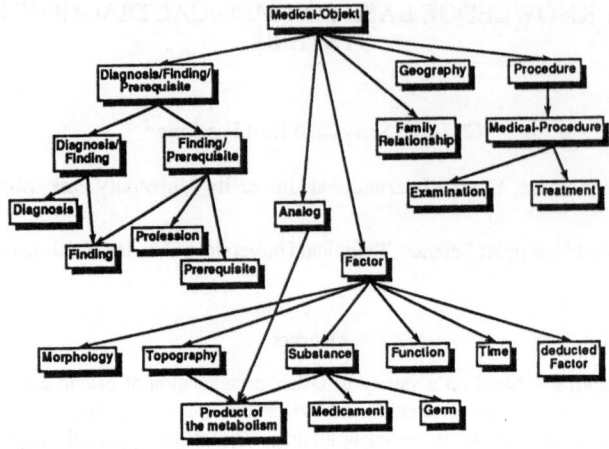

Figure 1: Knowledge Categorization in UnPatient

However, we derived some general principles to provide effective diagnostic decision support: For instance, it turned out to be extremely useful to represent medical procedures, such as therapy or treatment, in addition to symptoms and findings. Moreover, categories of diseases, such as 'syndrome' and 'common' have been attached to diseases. In addition to conventionally identified properties of diseases (such as observable symptoms) the a-priori-probability, the degree of threatening, and the prognosis are required for effective diagnostic support. Finally, relationships between diseases, such as succeeding and causal diseases, are helpful to identify a final diagnosis.

In the following we discuss the development of *UnPatient*, a medical knowledge base which

1. represent patient-unspecific medical knowledge

2. is applicable to all medical disciplines

3. provides static objects as well as

4. supports actively the process of medical diagnosis.

2. Knowledge Base Design

The problem to define suitable structures for medical knowledge in general is complex because essential parts cannot be formalized appropriately. Moreover, inaccurate knowledge often renders diagnosis difficult. Thus, we had to apply a representation mechanism which enables accurate mapping from medical reality to computable structures. Object-oriented modeling (see e.g., [Kim and Lochovsky, 1989]) allows direct mapping of medical entities, such as *diseases*, to computable structures. Properties and methods are associated with each object. Classes are sets of similar objects. In a class hierarchy, objects of superior classes inherit properties and methods to objects of classes below. Dynamic behaviour is supported by message exchange between objects to activate methods. However, in order to support diagnostics we had enhance the mutual activation of methods by a rule-based control flow model.

Figure 1 shows the defined classes for *UnPatient*. On one hand, a medical object can be a diagnosis, a *finding* or a *prerequisite*. On the other hand, *medical factors*, such as etiology, have been considered in accordance to additional aspects, such as geographical issues (if relevant, like e.g., for malignant melanoma).

Class Level

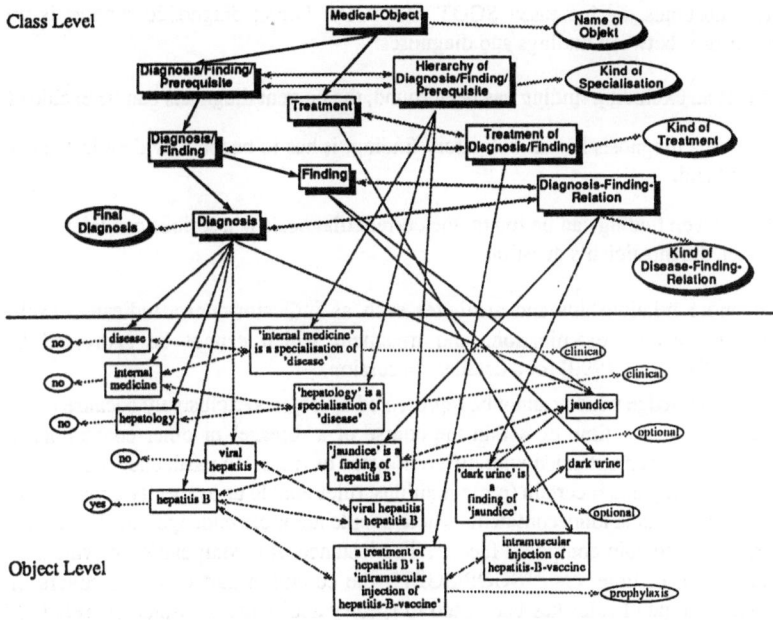

Figure 2: UnPatient Classes and Objects

For diagnostic support medical objects also comprise activities concerning *examination procedures*, and the evaluation of hypotheses. In Figure 2 we exemplify some objects and their relationships. Attributes and their values are illustrated by ellipses, whereas classes and objects are denoted as rectangles. The dotted lines represent relationships. For instance, the class 'Diagnosis' contains the following diagnostic attributes in addition to conventional description items, such as endemic information or SNOMED-Codes for factor classification:

- *Phase.* The course of diseases can be described by certain phases. According to each phase different symptoms may be required for testing diagnostic hypotheses - which means, different relationships may be activated.

- *Early Diagnosis Indicator.* Sometimes it is necessary to find out very early that a patient has a certain disease, e.g., when suffering cancer. If this indicator is 'on', special prevention methods can be suggested (if available).

- *Final Diagnosis Indicator.* This indicator tells the user of the knowledge base, if the current diagnosis is a final one (e.g., Hepatitis B) or the user has to proceed to a subclass.

Findings are structured according to several aspects: topography or product of metabolism, their cause, alterations being caused by them, the function being concerned, temporal aspects, etc., i.e. factors. Factors are primarily attached to findings which are actually results from a variety of examinations. *Procedures* comprise both medical measures (examination, dose of a medicament, operation, injection) and activities of the patient (going, standing, sports, breathing, intake of food or poison).

In order to provide appropriate relationships between symptoms and diseases we developed the *disease-finding-graph*. Its nodes correspond to diagnoses and findings, which can be related by clinical, etiological, topographical, phase and morphological relationships. Moreover, findings, prerequisites, and diagnoses can be combined by "and", "or" and "extra" – where "extra" is used for identifying a valuation. For example, "Transaminases raised" is a combination of "SGOT raised" and "SGPT raised" - thus, "Transaminases raised strongly" subsumes the increased SGOT and SGPT. Direct diagnostic support is provided by particular relationships between findings and diagnoses:

- *Exclusion.* If an excluding finding has been found, the current diagnosis can be excluded.

- *Obligation.* If a diagnosis has an obligatory finding, it has to become evident in the course of the diagnosis at hand.

- *Proof.* If a proven finding can be found, the current diagnosis is a serious candidate to be a correct answer to the diagnostician's question.

There are a lot more relationships and attributes such as indicator-contra indicator, exclusive finding, probability, succeeding examination, and treatment which cannot be addressed here. See [Horak et al., 1988, Fasching, 1990] for a detailed discussion.

In order to handle knowledge which cannot be represented by objects exclusively because of its dynamics (e.g., changes of values over time or within the course of a disease) or other constraints, the object-oriented framework has been extended with different types of *rules*. In particular, if some properties or relationships are valid only under certain (pre)conditions, rules enable us to specify additional constraints, e.g., in case of malignant melanoma continents where people are more endangered. We also had to apply rules for objects which contain composed factors. For instance, if a computation of values makes only sense at a certain point of time, e.g., "SGOP/SGPT", the condition part of a rule covers the relevant information. Another type of rules has been used to specify additional, non-medical relationships, e.g., 'mother' between persons. This type of rules are primarily used for relationships which have not to be built-in into the class hierarchy because of their particular application domain, e.g., for a small group of diseases.

3. Implementation and Use

To enable the storage of a large amount of knowledge we had to find appropriate technical means. Prolog-DB is a pre-compiler which combines all pro's of logic programming and data base management systems [Fleischanderl, 1987]. *UnPatient* is based on Prolog-DB which consists of a relational data base (db++), Prolog, and an interface between Prolog and db++. In order to store the medical knowledge we had to map our object-oriented framework to relations as well as to Horn clauses. For instance, the relation '*class* (Object-name, Class-name, Final-diagnosis, Early-diagnosis-necessary, Excluding-diagnosis)' identifies an object not only by its class but also by its relationships. The relation '*diagnosis-finding-graph* (Diagnosis/finding, Subordered-diagnosis/finding, Type-of-subordering)' maps the diagnosis-finding-graph to relations. It contains the name of the medical term, one or more reference to sub-terms, and the type of relationship to the referred medical term, e.g., its succeeding element in the object hierarchy (if available) according to clinical criteria. Finally, diagnostic knowledge concerning the application of a medical procedure is defined by the relation '*risk* (Procedure, Topography, Substance, Valuation-Interval, Time, Result-Type, Frequency)'.

The rules of our framework are defined within the Prolog part of Prolog-DB. In addition, information from the objects (relations) can be activated to generate conditions or hypotheses dynamically. Hence, it becomes possible to embed static knowledge (represented by relations) into clauses to represent diagnostic procedures, and support diagnostics directly. By introducing meta-levels, the diagnostician can map strategic knowledge concerning additional constraints and restrictions to control the application of the derived knowledge.

Advanced diagnostic expert systems are largely based on knowledge bases, such as *UnPatient*, which support diagnostics effectively. They do not only provide comprehensive patient-independent knowledge but also specialized diagnostic procedures to solve complex tasks. In our approach we have made a step further to more comprehensive modeling medical knowledge without respect to a specific application domain. Based on previous systems we derived an object-oriented schema which can be embedded into Prolog-clauses for effective diagnosis support.

UnPatient provides a direct manipulation interface which supports the retrieval, acquisition, and updates of the entire medical knowledge. The diagnostician is able to browse the class hierarchy as well as its instances. In particular, the disease-finding-graph supports the explanation of correlations which have to be explicit for the evaluation of hypotheses. Moreover, the diagnostician is able to execute rules which process attributes of values retrieved from the stored objects. To accumulate and test diagnostic strategies he/she may formulate heuristics. Thus, he/she may contribute to a steady improvement of the quality of the acquired knowledge.

References

[Ben-Bassat, 1984] Ben-Bassat, M.: The Role of Expert Systems in Clinical Diagnosis: A Conceptual Model; in Proc. of the 4th Jerusalem Conference in Information Technology, IEEE, pp. 632-644; 1984.

[Buchanan et al., 1985] Buchanan B.G., Shortliffe E.H. (eds.); The MYCIN Experiments of the Stanford Heuristic Programming Project; Addison-Wesley; 1985.

[Chandrasekaran et al., 1984] B. Chandrasekaran, Jon Sticklen; Patrec: A Knowledge-Directed Database for a Diagnostic Expert System; in Computer, Vol. 17, No. 8, 1984.

[Fasching, 1990] K. Fasching; Knowledge Acquisition and Representation for a Medical Knowledge Base; Thesis, Department of Applied Computer Science, Technical University of Vienna, 1990.

[Fleischanderl, 1987] G. Fleischanderl; PROLOG-DB - Pre-Compiler, User Manual, Version 1.0; Technical University of Vienna, Department for Applied Computer Science; 1987.

[Horak et al., 1988] W. Horak, E. Neuhold, Ch. Stary; Implementing A Medical Knowledge Base, A Feasible Study; Technical Report TR 25.148, IBM-Laboratory Vienna, Austria, 1988.

[Kim and Lochovsky, 1989] W. Kim, F. H. Lochovsky (Editors); Object-Oriented Concepts, Databases and Applications; Department of Computer Science, University of Toronto; 1989.

[Kingsland, 1985] L. C. Kingsland III; The Evaluation of Medical Expert Systems: Experience with the AI/RHEUM Knowledge-based Consultant System in Rheumatology; in Proceedings of the 9th International Joint Conference on Artificial Intelligence, pp. 292-295; 1985.

[Miller and Fisher, 1987] P. L. Miller, P. R. Fisher; Causal Models in Medical Artificial Intelligence; in Proceedings of the 11th Annual Symposium on Computer Applications in Medical Care, IEEE, Washington D. C., pp. 17-22; 1987.

[Patil et al., 1987] R.S. Patil, O. Senyk; Efficient Structuring of Composite Causal Hypotheses in Medical Diagnosis; in Proceedings of the 11th Annual Symposium on Computer Applications in Medical Care, IEEE, Washington D. C., pp. 23- 29; 1987.

[Singer et al., 1983] Singer, J.; Sacks, H.S.; Lucente, F.; Chalmers, T.C.: Physician Attitudes towards Applications of Computer Data Base Systems, in: JAMA, Vol. 259, pp. 1610-1614, 1983.

INTERPRETATION OF CLINICAL BIOCHEMISTRY TEST PROFILES BY A METHOD ALLOWING COMMUNICATION BETWEEN LINKED ORGAN-RELATED KNOWLEDGE BASES.

G Boran (1), D Alexander (2), J Grimson (2) and R O'Moore(3)

Department of Clinical Biochemistry, Lewisham Hospital, London (1). Department of Computer Science, Trinity College, Dublin (2). Central Pathology Laboratory, St. James's Hospital, Dublin (3).

Abstract

We have studied how the conclusions from one knowledge-based system can be transferred into another so that interpretative tasks can be divided among several smaller communicating knowledge bases without impairing the quality of the final interpretation. The ability of one knowledge-based system to consult another is becoming more important as the number of domain-specific systems increases. Accordingly, methods are required to allow cooperativity between domain-specific programs. This paper describes one such method where individual knowledge-based systems are allowed to communicate by means of a top-level integrating knowledge-based system.

Introduction

There are increasing demands for effective decision support systems in clinical biochemistry laboratorie [1,2], not least because the use of organ-related test profiles introduces several opportunities for interpretative error. First, profiles are more difficult to interpret than individual tests and there is a risk of overlooking significant findings as the number of available results increases. Second, assumptions may be made by the inexperienced that tests are only used to diagnose conditions pertinent to the allocated profile. Third, pre-analytical factors, analytical and biological variation and the predictive value of laboratory tests are not widely appreciated outside of the laboratory but have dramatic effects on interpretation [3].

An interpretative report is an analysis of clinical and laboratory data whose purpose is to elucidate the full significance of laboratory results for the requesting physician. Decision support systems have been developed to provide interpretative reports for laboratory tests, including multiple tests and profiles [4,5]. We have recently described a method for interpretative reporting using automatic knowledge acquisition by computer [6] and this has now been applied to produce interpretative reports for several organ-related profiles of clinical biochemistry tests. We have also explored how the conclusions from one knowledge-based system can be transferred into another so that the interpretative task can be divided among several smaller communicating knowledge bases without impairing the quality of the final interpretation.

Principle

The program classifies quantitative laboratory tests into mutually exclusive decision ranges. All decision ranges are user-defined, revisable, and age-specific. Qualitative and semi-quantitative results are entered by selecting the appropriate finding from user-defined expandable lists of options. The patient's age and sex are also included.

The program generates a rule from any available data. It then solicits an interpretation from the observer and links it to the rule so that the interpretation can be provided automatically whenever similar data are encountered.

One of the features of this approach is that the main knowledge base can be constructed from several smaller knowledge bases, called primer knowledge bases. These ASCII files contain lists of interpretations and associated typical cases from which rules are derived.

When primer knowledge bases are used for commonly encountered cases or sub-domains, the main knowledge-based system rapidly achieves high performance while retaining the ability to enter or modify interpretations on a case-by-case basis.

Individual tests from the total repertoire were allocated to organ-related profiles (renal, bone, cardiac, liver profiles) as shown in Table 1.

Primer knowledge bases were then written for each of the four organ-related profiles. When used separately in the main knowledge-based system, these primer knowledge bases provide interpretations for their own profile only.

Table 1 . Allocation of tests to profiles. Note that certain tests appear in more than one profile.

RENAL PROFILE

- Sodium
- Potassium
- Urea
- Creatinine

BONE PROFILE

- Calcium
- Albumin
- Corrected calcium
- Phosphate
- Alkaline phosphatase (ALP)

LIVER PROFILE

- Bilirubin
- Albumin
- Total protein
- Aspartate aminotransferase
- Alkaline phosphatase (ALP)
- γ-glutamyltransferase

CARDIAC PROFILE

- Cholesterol
- Triglyceride
- Creatine kinase
- Lactate dehydrogenase

Table 2 shows examples of interpretations for a renal and a bone profile performed on a patient with renal disease and a secondary bone disorder where the results for each profile are considered separately. In order to allow communication between the individual knowledge bases, a set of diagnostic outcomes was defined for each of the four profiles studied (see Table 3).

Table 2. Example of non-communicating interpretations for renal and bone profiles: the results for each profile are considered separately. Each test name is followed by the result, its units of measurement and the reference range. Diagnostic outcomes for the profiles are shown in square brackets below the interpretations.

RENAL PROFILE

Sodium	133 mmol/l	(135-145)
Potassium	5.8 mmol/l	(3.3-4.8)
Urea	30.5 mmol/l	(3.0-7.0)
Creatinine	400 umol/l	(60-120)

Renal failure with hyperkalaemia and mild hyponatraemia.

[Diagnostic outcome: renal failure]

BONE PROFILE

Calcium	1.94 mmol/l	(2.10-2.55)
Albumin	35 g/l	(35-45)
Corrected Calcium	2.04 mmol/l	(2.10-2.55)
Phosphate	1.88 mmol/l	(0.80-1.20)
ALP	450 u/l	(100-285)

Hypocalcaemia, raised phosphate and ALP: osteomalacia pattern.

[Diagnostic outcome: osteomalacia pattern]

For the renal profile interpretation shown in Table 2, the diagnostic outcome was 'renal failure' and the outcome for the bone profile was 'osteomalacia pattern'. When data for multiple profiles are available for a single patient, each of the four profile systems is called in turn. Diagnostic outcomes for each sub-system are determined and these are transferred into a fifth top-level knowledge-based system which integrates the conclusions of the individual four sub-systems. Other factors such as the patient's age and sex are also taken into account by the top-level system. Using typical cases drawn from the routine laboratory workload, integrating comments were entered into the top-level knowledge base in the same way as the individual sub-systems were constructed.

The interpretation shown in Table 4 shows how the separate renal and bone profile interpretations given in Table 2 are reconciled by the integrating comment, which explains the connection between the two sets of findings.

Table 3. Selected diagnostic outcomes for the renal, bone, liver and cardiac profiles.

RENAL PROFILE

- Prerenal impairment
- Renal failure
- Hyponatraemia
- Hypokalaemia
- Hypernatraemia

BONE PROFILE

- Osteomalacia
- Renal osteomalacia
- Primary hyperparathyroidism
- Ectopic PTH production
- Hypoparathyroidism

LIVER PROFILE

- Isolated hyperbilirubinaemia
- Hepatocellular damage
- Cholestasis
- Focal hepatic lesion
- Alcoholic hepatitis

CARDIAC PROFILE

- Myocardial infarct
- Hypercholesterolaemia
- Hypertriglyceridaemia
- Mixed hyperlipidaemia
- Skeletal muscle damage

Table 4. The report where two profiles have been requested, showing how the conclusions (diagnostic outcome) of the renal and bone profiles are used to produce an integrating comment from the top-level knowledge-based system.

RENAL PROFILE COMMENT

Renal failure with hyperkalaemia and mild hyponatraemia.

[Diagnostic outcome: renal failure]

BONE PROFILE COMMENT

Hypocalcaemia, raised phosphate and ALP.

[Diagnostic outcome: osteomalacia pattern]

INTEGRATING COMMENT

These results are consistent with renal failure and associated renal osteodystrophy.

Conclusion

The ability of one knowledge-based system to consult another is becoming more important as the number of domain-specific systems increases. Although knowledge-based programs for general medicine have been developed, it is unlikely that their performance for individual disciplines will be superior to domain-specific systems. Accordingly, methods are required to allow better communication between domain-specific programs. The present program implements a communication protocol which is effective for the application of interpretative reporting and results in an integrated conclusion. At the same time, the detailed findings from each participating system are included in the final report.

References

1. Killingsworth LM. Editorial: What do the numbers say? Clin Chem 1988;34:996.
2. Pringle M. The new agenda for general practice computing. Br Med J 1990;301:827-828.
3. Fraser CG. Interpretation of clinical chemistry laboratory data. Oxford (UK): Blackwell Scientific Publications, 1986.
4. McConnell TH, Ashworth CT, Ashworth RD, Nielsen CR. Algorithm-derived, computer-generated interpretive comments in the reporting of laboratory tests. Am J Clin Pathol 1979;72:32-41.
5. Dito WR. An octal algorithm for pattern coding and computer-assisted interpretative reporting. Am J Clin Pathol 1977;68:575- 583.
6. Boran G, Eldridge P, Nolan J, Brosnan P, O'Moore R. A decision support tool for laboratory medicine based on automatic knowledge acquisition. In: O'Moore R, Bengtsson S, Bryant JR, Bryden JS, editors. Lecture Notes in Medical Informatics, Berlin: Springer-Verlag, 1990;40:329-333.

Declarative and operational in knowledge based systems

M. Popper, M. Hauskrecht
Medical Bionics Research Institute
Jedľová 6, 83308 Bratislava, Czechoslovakia

Abstract: The contribution deals with some aspects of complementing declarative and procedural knowledge representation in knowledge based systems from the object-oriented perspective.

Introduction

The inspiring review article [2] by Buchanan et al. on knowledge based systems (KBS for short) is for the concerned community not only informative but motivating, too. Many of our notions based on experiences with KBS, particularly with expert systems aspiring to be attentive for solving realistic medical problems, are in concordance with the ones we are referring to. In this regard, as the heading suggests, some conceptual aspects of the nonprocedural and procedural components of knowledge representation is to be discussed in this contribution. Another closely related paper in this proceedings [4] based on some illustrations elaborates the given views. In both contributions the paradigm of object-oriented approach is getting into foreground.

Complementing the declarative and operational

In evolvement of KBS and of expert systems particularly, one may observe a changing attitude to their nonprocedural and procedural components. While in early systems significantly higher stress was put on the first one, nowadays it is realized that their operational complement is alike vital knowledge counterpart: not only concepts of the domain but dependencies resulting from them as well as many of the related reasoning processes need to be explicitly represented [2]. As a matter of fact, the operational component was and yet is mostly understood as a more-or-less given method or technique of a general inference strategy to be simply accepted by a knowledge base (KB for short) designer. The same concerns the furnished means for approximate reasoning. The result, regardless the attained performance, is not only the KB designer's discomfort but, more importantly, he is frequently forced to surpass the given constraints by inventing obscure tricks when nontrivial representation problems occur. The affairs with nontrivial real problems, without any doubt, let us conclude that simplified approaches to the knowledge-able operational components, chiefly regarding the inference control, in very many applications are far for being sufficient and satisfying.

For KBS, as artifacts aiming to mimic some of the man's cognitive capabilities, the knowledgeable inference (reasoning) control is of great relevance. Its audit is actually a subject of its own. If we would constrain ourselves in conceiving the inference control as an issue of me-chanistic logic or logic of machines only, we may miss the main objective of KBS. Consequently, we would prevent ourselves in our attempts to understand

* the occurrence of various elementary control processes, their 'semantics' particularly, frequently exploited in diverse adaptable sequences,

* the man's conscious goal-oriented behavior, his reflection of changing situations and conditions, giving him the chance to adapt himself by proper selection of subgoals and their sequences,

* his many-faced capabilities to form and exploit various schemes for event driven control strategies, from the most simple to more complex ones, including reasoning from first principles, shifting attention, changing abstraction levels, reasoning about and with a variety of constrains, performing reasoned backtracking, conflict resolution, problem decomposition, global perception of fractional problems and integration of partial results, qualitative, imprecise, default, and analogical reasoning, etc.

From these aspects, clearly, any simplified approach to a nontrivial KBS design yields its very constrained performance regarding the aims to comply with. Applications with demanding knowledge representation schemes and demanding structured inference control are evidencing it. For that robust and efficient KBS are needed. In their design, stress must be put on discover-ing and designing suitable symbol and control structures using high performance operational soft-ware. They should exhibit logical and modular architecture: clearly defined units that carry out system's functions and ways of their activation, transparently specified connections that show the routes of transmitting, sharing, and hiding information. They should allow also isolation of in-dividual design decisions from each other.

Frame and object-oriented representation

Between the domain of KBS and the software technologies there is a drawbridge between the aims and the means to attain them. One end of this bridge is anchored into the soil of know-ledge representation schemes while the other one is lowered into the field of software tools and software design. Without tracing down all the possible implicit or explicit influences stemming from this bridge crossovers, let us touch at least one - the object-oriented programming and knowledge representation.

Each from the well known knowledge representation formalisms - from formulas of logic to frame structures - encompass various knowledge representation schemes with differing expressiveness and computational power. Each of them posses some specific inherent advantages and limitations. In more complex applications, requiring structured knowledge representation and structured inference control, the frame constructs are rather generally accepted as the most advantageous. This is propped also by convinction that the regarding representational schemes in many respects provide a kind of resemblance to both, the ways people structure (organize) knowledge in their memory and the ways they think.

Object-oriented design uses classes of objects (concepts) as building blocs (units) of software architecture. Classes are specified in terms of their structure and behavior. In their hierarchies inheritance relationships can be specified: a sub-class acquires the structure and behavior of a super-class either in a strict hierarchy from a single parent or in a lattice with multiple parents. A class or object combines both data and operations on data. Operations - also called procedures, methods, messages, or services - can be provided for both, classes and objects. A class and its operations is defined as a single unit. The operations can be exploited for selection and specification of general functions provided by the program interpreter (a virtual machine) as well as for setting up designer own operational infrastructures enabling to intervene with the interpreter functions giving thus in both cases possibilities for specifying methods and strategies. This is important from the perspective of a KBS knowledgeable operational component.

One can clearly see the considerable overlap among the ideas of frame and object-oriented knowledge representation. However, while the frame schemes provide rather comfortable aptitude for declarative kind of knowledge representation, it is not so for the operational (procedural) one. Let us elaborate somewhat on advantages and disadvantages of both techniques, namely with respect to their capability to represent operational knowledge.

Operational knowledge in frames and objects

It gives sense to discern two different types of procedural knowledge apparently embodied in a KBS: The type (1), regardless whether represented by instruction sequences, subroutines, or functions, is for the KB designer a given complementing counterpart of his representation schemes. This procedural knowledge is actually incorporated into the KB interpreter (a virtual machine) providing general operational semantics to any specific KB content. The type (2), again regardless of its various forms, unlike of the previous one, is provided by the KB designer. By him set up and placed software pieces represent various operational knowledge on top of furnished ones. They enable him to specify new or modify the given methods and strategies - hence directly influence the inference process.

301

The program constructs and control data structures, comprising the KB interpreter, its infrastructure actually, represents in fact the type (1) operational knowledge. This infrastructure is, however, not directly accessible to the KB designer: he has no legitimate way to examine purposefully its internal data structures or modify them. With the type (2) operational knowledge it is different: in spite it has to follow the governing principles of the chosen representation formalism, it is represented by own consrtucts and thus by own infrastructure also. As it together with declarative knowledge comprise the KB, it is fully under KB designer control and thus easily modifiable. From this aspect the main difference between frame and object-oriented repre- sentations results from the way the constraints of imposed representation limits the designer in defining his own methods and strategies (general or domain specific). This is also closely related to the way the responsibilities in the control are shared among the interpreter and the designer, i.e. what is provided - the procedural knowledge of type (1) - and what is allowed - procedural knowledge of type (2) - by the system's interpreter.

Frames are evaluated in rather fixed manner: filling in their slots. The same holds for carrying out system's functions, for transmitting or sharing information, and connections that show explicitly how the various functions are activated. The control flow can be somehow directed by procedures attached to some of their slots. The respective slot specific procedures are activated when some operation or action within the slot is to be performed, e.g. when the slot value is needed, added, or changed. This type of procedural knowledge attachments, providing the user with clear and easy understandable tool for directing inference process, can be utilized efficiently in many applications. However, they lack power and flexibility especially regarding situations that require more sophisticated reasoning control. The two following cases, for example, are evidencing it:

* Many decisions can't be adequately reached without global evaluation perspective, without notion of the status of various frames concurrently, i.e. whether and in which active control data structure are they referenced. A frame-slot action - a local view - hardly can provide the needed information.

* Many efficient operations require changes in existing control data structures, alterations of their significance, creating new or destroying existing ones. Unlike the former case, when for a situation overview poring over the infrastructure is needed only, this one; for example when major revision or suspension of the current reasoning line might be efficient, besides more global panorama may require vital changes in the infrastructure for what again a frame-slot action hardly yields the needed effect.

Accommodation of the frame based system to deal properly with such and similar situations can be resolved either by enabling access to the KB interpreter infrastructure, by modification and/or extension of the representational formalism enabling to build new procedural constructs, or by making the type (1) procedural knowledge modifiable by the user, meaning its partial transformation to the type (2) knowledge. The last case means leaving for the type (1) procedural knowledge only basic elementary interpretation routines that hardly mirror any knowledge representation schemes (no semantic concerned knowledge processing is present), giving however sufficient freedom for defining any type of procedural constructs in it. If such an approach enables the procedural component to be modularly structured while capturing both general and specific problem solving methods, then it can be defined incrementally in the remaining interpreter. Intermediate levels of defining the needed operational constructs in course of design stages can be thus viewed as a stepwise definition and implementation of a virtual inference mechanism.

Conclusion

The underlaying principles of object-oriented approach, besides flexibility it grants for representing declarative knowledge, seems to be an appropriate tool for defining procedural constructs of various types. They fulfill not only the criteria of modular structuring but provide many more advanced musters to satisfy the discussed requirements for operational knowledge. The paradigms of object-oriented approach renders the KB designer with transparent system organization and the possibility to define easily new pieces of procedural knowledge. In similar fashion they allow him also to change and adjust representational formalism by modifying its interpretative counterpart.

In evolvement of means for KBS design the object-oriented approach seems to be very promising. It provides both, the support for transparent and expressive declarative knowledge representation and the possibility to maintain modular and lucid system interpreter components by the same resources.

References

[1]   Anderson B.: Object-oriented programming. Microprocessors and Microsystems. 12, 8, 433-442, 1990.

[2]   Buchanan B.G., Bobrow D., Davis R., McDermott J., Shortliffe E.H.: Knowledge-based systems. Annu. Rev. Comput. Sci., 4, 395-416, 1990.

[3]   Cox B.: Object-oriented programming: an evolutionary approach. Addison-Wesley, Reading, Mass., 1986.

[4]   Stanek J., Popper M., Hauskrecht M.: The operational aspects of object-oriented approach in medical expert system design. In this proceedings.

[5]   Wasserman A.I., Pircher P.A., Muller R.J.: The object-oriented structured design notation for software design representation. Computer, 50-62, March 1990.

The operational aspects of object-oriented approach in medical expert systems design

J. Stanek, M. Popper, M. Hauskrecht

Medical Bionics Research Institute

Jedlová 6, 833 08 Bratislava, Czechoslovakia

Abstract: In the contribution some of the issues of object-oriented paradigm in the knowledge based systems (KBS) design technology are considered, particularly with regards to expert systems in medical domain. Some illustrating examples are provided.

Introduction

As it is reasoned in the closely related paper in the current proceedings [3], the demanding inference control requires explicit operational constructs in hands of the knowledge base (KB) designer. They enable setting up event specific interventions and modifications of the standard course of inference performed by the furnished KB interpreter. In concordance with the AI paradigms, the expert level problem solving is confined to knowledge-based and strategy-directed exploration of problem spaces [1]. However, it does not exclude exploitation of classical domain-specific solution algorithms whenever possible and of advantage. Nevertheless, in the respective KBS processes the problem-space exploratory techniques, especially those ones inspired by man's intelligence - his efficient cognitive capabilities, play the dominant role. In consonance with these assertions some of the related issues are discussed in the following.

When the procedural is to be preferred

As the KB design rests predominantly or exclusively on declarative knowledge representation, the designer is most frequently forced to express even typical procedural knowledge by declarative schemes. This yields undesirable representation, as well as, procedural complexity. The following trivial example illustrates it.

Let us consider classification of acid-base disorder according to increased, decreased, or normal pH, pCO_2, and HCO_3 values, respectively. When for this purpose a decision tree is constructed, it consist of 40 nodes: a root, then 3, 9, and 27 nodes on next levels. Regardless the form of the tree representation (e.g. production rules, frame system, etc.) and its exploitation a considerable amount of overhead control activities are required compared with a procedure (even for qualitative computation) using the listed variables as input and returning the name of the resulting acid-base disorder as output.

This illustration stands for many situations in which the classical algorithmic solving processes are to be preferred.

Declarative-procedural representation in hierarchies

A classification task frequently rests on hierarchical taxonomies of the considered concepts (e.g. diagnoses, findings, constrains, etc.). Such a hierarchy lends itself to declarative representation. However, it does not mean that each possible process representing a cognitive activity related to a hierarchy yields automatically from the respective data structures.

Taxonomy evaluations most typically correspond with the (Aristotelian) intensional concept definitions giving possibility for sorts of truth value inheritance, or more broadly, their propagation in the hierarchy. Nevertheless, this kind of taxonomy is not the only way to perceive a hierarchy. Many other semantically different hierarchical dependencies can be defined, e.g. diagnose refinement, constraint propagation, context relations, ordering patient examinations according to their specifity, sensitivity, or severity (invasiveness), etc.

A hierarchy in general is a relation defined on a set of elements enabling their ordering according to chosen reliance. The declarative representation formalisms themselves, regardless of the form, provide only basic hierarchy interpretation. For instance, in frame-based representation a hierarchy is most frequently a means for inheritance of specified slot values. In case of a class hierarchy represented in object-oriented environment it is most frequently a relation enabling to inherit a class structure and its operations. Then implementation of differently perceived hierarchy meanings grounded only on its basic interpretation may be rather opaque. Therefore semantic clarity in design of such functions can be very useful in attaining problem solving efficacy.

For instance in a hierarchy reflecting intensional logic, the operational knowledge for transitive propagation of specific truth value should be explicitly determined: the **false** value should be propagated from more general to more special entity, while the **true** value in the opposite direction. This corresponds to a general task (operation) representing a method [1] which might be further specified: its employment can be conditioned by real needs, i.e. only when essential and in a desired spread.

Such tasks exercising the hierarchies can be written ranging from trivial and general ones to more sophisticated and specific - representing complex propagation schemes for whatever entries incorporated in respective symbolic constructs. The latter ones are frequently more or less domain or even case-specific and therefore their implementation as user-defined operation is of more advantage than as they would be a part of the general inference engine. Propagation of fuzzy qualified truth values and their (qualitative) combination, accomplishment of the propose-and-refine strategy, situation and context dependent selection of patient investigations hierarchized according their invasivity and relevance of attainable results are only some examples of that.

The objected-oriented environment provides for the KB designer rather straightforward possibilities for method design. He has the means for setting up his own semantically clearly defined operational components, say in form of generic tasks. These can be implemented as a couple of procedures with eventual restrictive conditions enabling control of any propagation process (e.g. for expressing exceptions from a general property or for optimising the system's performance).

Searching layers of the problem space

As our concern is the knowledge-based and strategy-directed exploration of problem spaces, it is clear that the problem space needs to be defined before any search can take place. But, in general, a problem-solving does not have a unique problem space. It even can be perceived as a complex multilayer space reflecting that a solving process exploration can be performed on several intertwined strata. When dealing with complex problems, it is useful to distinguish among various layers of a problem space - different kinds of problem spaces can be visualized, each appropriate for some kinds of domain knowledge and not others. This evidently holds for the medical domain, as the reality it is concerned with can be represented and perceived at several levels of detail and from various perspectives. For instance anaemia can be perceived either as a complication of a gastrointestinal bleeding, or as a nosographic entity which is to be evaluated. In the first case anaemia is in direct relation to the causative disease (e.g. gastric ulcer) and besides assessing its severity, anaemia is not a separate diagnostic problem. In the latter case anaemia is such a problem, and is to be appreciated as a whole, including ethiopathogenetic diagnosis and therapy. For this purpose specific knowledge is to be exercised - even a separate embedded KB on anaemia, including eventual specific inference strategies. Clearly, at least two alternative problem space layers depending on the role of anaemia can be placed into the foreground.

To make search in a problem space to be operationally definable, as it is discussed in [1], there have to be problem states and related operators which transform one problem state into a set of successors. Also some ordering knowledge is needed that helps to choose between alternatives. The directly available domain knowledge should be applied to generate successors and choose among them. In the case of above illustration, operational tasks reflecting the problem state can be designed with parameters determining e.g. the needed reasoning detailedness, shift of attention, clinical or etiopathogenetic (causal) reasoning, etc. In fact, several anaemia specific and still independent inference strategies may run upon different but in a way intertwined declarative pieces of knowledge.

Using both, the generic task philosophy [1] and object oriented tools, such behavior can be achieved when proper knowledge representation approach is adopted in KB design.

Complex entities representation and its employment

Many concepts in medicine are complex in their nature - from diagnoses, through pathophysiologic states, even to symptoms (e.g. pain, with its time dependencies, localization, radiation, character, contexts, etc.). Such items can be at least in some extent represented using nested classes.

A good illustration might be the interstitial lung involvement caused by mixed connective tissue disease. This compound diagnostic unit has been specified as a concurrent occurrence of three diseases belonging to the class of collagenoses: progressive systemic sclerosis, systemic lupus erythematodes, and polymyositis-dermatomyositis, all with lung involvement. Depending on the employed formalism various more-or-less efficient and transparent (for operations, as well as, for understanding) representation schemes may stand for this compound diagnostic unit. However, in the object-oriented environment the representation in form of a nested class is of advantage. The following might be the case

```
class interstitial_lung_involvements
     with mixed_connective_tissue disease
.....
        class progressive_systemic_sclerosis
             inherits collagenoses
        .....
        class systemic_lupus_erythematodes
             inherits collagenoses
        .....
        class polymyositis_dermatomyositis
             inherits collagenoses
        .....
.....
```

Such a scheme enables transparent specification of manifold   relations to other associated pieces of knowledge, as well as, embodiment of various clearly defined operational attachments. The operational semantics of a relation can be defined either in more general units, or when its particular interpretation is of advantage, then as a part of the corresponding structure. The use of such a compound representation unit depends upon the specific tasks corresponding to methods applicable in various problem-solving situations.

Using classes (as templates) it is possible to generate objects as instances of a class - in case of a nested class a nested object. Generating multiple objects in this way is also feasible. This can be efficiently employed in a causal reasoning process: the system takes the current object and applies tasks corresponding to the concerned parameters to generate a new object, eventually to be further examined. Hence the complex object can represent a state of a patient and operations can be used to define paths of transition from his considered state to another one. For instance in processing the situation when the pH of the patient changes its value from 7.3 to 7.2 the following equations [2] can be of use

$$\Delta pH = -0.056 * \Delta pCO_2 \pm 0.02$$
$$\Delta K^+ = 4 * \Delta pH$$

Several similar quantitative and qualitative relations can be included. The resulting object represents the status of a patient at pH equal 7.2 and it can be further exercised. Given a complex class including objects and relations among them (as e.g. relation among kalemia and ECG, heart function etc.), first the interstate operations are used to create a new instance of this class, then the internal procedures are applied to make this instance complete and consistent.

Conclusion

The object-oriented approach seems to be very advantageous in KBS design and a challenge in this respect. We have attempted to display some of the arguments for this approach which in our opinion provides rather transparent and flexible medium for representing several types of knowledge - both, procedural and declarative in its nature - in a comprehensive way. Although these tools already proved their relevance, several questions still remain to be answered (e.g. problems with navigation through a complex object network, conflict detection and resolving when multiple inheritance schemes are adopted, etc.) especially in creating large systems.

References
[1]   Brown D.C., Chandrasekaran B.: Design problem solving (Knowledge structures and control strategies). Morgan Kaufmann Publ., California, 1989.
[2]   Dzúrik R. et al.: Disturbances of the Acid-Base Status. Diagnostics and Therapy [in Slovak]. Osveta, Martin 1984.
[3]   Popper M., Hauskrecht M.: Declarative and operational in knowledge based systems. In this proceedings.

Design of a Well-Protected Patient Record Unit for Multi-centre Knowledge-Based System CLINAID

Viswanathan KALIAPPAN and *Ladislav J. KOHOUT*
The Center for Expert Systems and Robotics, Department of Computer Science
Florida State University, Tallahassee, Florida 32306, USA.
and
John ANDERSON
King's College School of Medicine and Dentistry, University of London, U.K.

Abstract

In this paper, we describe the high level design of a general, modular and comprehensive Patient record unit (PRU) that can interface with two distinct environments simultaneously and provide for their mutual secure local or remote interaction. One environment is formed by a community of distributed interacting expert systems, or a multicentre concurrent Knowledge-Based System (KBS). The other environment consists of a community of data bases distributed locally or connected via a remote communication network. The paper is concluded with the description of the way in which the PRU is integrated within a multi-centre, multi-context and multi-environment KBS CLINAID. Further relevant references to this approach are provided.

1 Introduction

Problems of several kinds are created when one attempts to integrate a network of various data bases (DB) with the expert systems (ES) technology. It is well known that these problems are caused by incompatibility of the underlying computational models [1] of the ES and DB parts of the integrated system. The mismatch of the models in conventionally resolved by changing the means of DB or ES realization. For example, choosing PROLOG for the DB, to match it better with ES [1], or choosing the Relational Representation Language (RPL) to implement the ES in relational DB "idiom" [2]. Such an approach imposes computational and performance constraints on some parts of the integrated distributed intelligent system, depending on the choice of the implementation technology. For obvious reasons, this is not apropriate when dealing with health care information systems. A typical scenario in the context of health care informatics consists in having a diverse network of DBs storing patient records that supply ESs with the patient information. Imagine a clinical KBS at a specialised clinic that has to connect to a network of data bases defined by the catchment area of the clinic, each DB belonging to one of the hospitals that may refer their patients to that clinic. Re-implementation of parts of such a complex medical informatics systems is impossible and may not even be desirable. Indeed, the DBs may be used at the same time by other information processing systems, wich may be based on different underlying computational models.

An adequate way of dealing with this rather typical scenario is to use the Multi-Environment approach [3], in which the high level abstract data type (ADT) models are superimposed over the local computational models of the DB, ES, or whatever the local computing system might be. The ADT provides for the reinterpretation of the chosen model of medical activities within the computational models that are underlying the local computing systems supporting the DBs, KBS, patient administration etc. This provides for flexibility, extendability, maintainability. It also increases the computational performance and makes it possible to deal with dynamic protection and security of these systems without performance degradation of unduly increased cost of computational facilities.

In this paper, we describe the high level design of a general, modular and comprehensive Patient record unit that can interface with two distinct environments simultaneously and provide for their mutual secure local or remote interaction. One environment is formed by a community of distributed interacting expert systems, or a multicentre concurrent Knowledge-Based System (KBS). The other environment consists of a community of data bases distributed locally or connected via a remote communication network.

The most significant feature of our design is its reconfigurability and extendibility. The generic shell of the Patient record unit alows the user to reconfigure a specific system *from the general structure*, depending upon the user's requirements, hospital environment, type of other technology available etc. This generic structure also provides protection structures [4], [5] that are imposed on the transactions of information between the KBS and the data-bases with which the KBS communicates. This is a important advance, since the security of patient records against illegal access by the unauthorized human users or on-line computing systems and expert systems has not been dealt with adequately in the Knowledge Engineering literature. The relevant overview of the protection problems in other branches of computing, including databases, the pros and cons of the individual protection schemes and the history of the subject together with a number of references appears in our recent book [4], hence it will not be discussed here. Formal specification of the *protection* and *retrieval* structures, consequently applied in this design can be found in [4] and [9] respectively, and in the references quoted therein. Both conceptual schemes are represented by means of fuzzy triangle relational products [6], [7], which have considerable computational advantages.

The Patient record described here was designed to cooperate with any community of expert systems that have adequate functional competency, which can be provided by the knowledge elicitation and acquisition methods [3] based on Activity Structures methodology [4]. We shall conclude the paper with a specific instance of such an environment that is provided a multi-centre KBS CLINAID. The Activity Structures methodology [4] has been used not only in the design of the main centres of CLINAID [8], but also for representing the structures and functional features of the design of Patient record unit presented here.

2 Specification and Design of Patient Record Unit

The Patient record unit serves as a agent between users (which can include not only expert systems of KBS but also human users) and databases. To deal with all the requirement in a general and unified manner, we have defined a *generalised knowledge user* and a *knowledge source* [9]. These conceptual objects form the base for relational definition and realization of both, the schemes for the retrival of relevant information and for protection. The relational structures based on this scheme that are used in the design are discussed further in Sec. 4 below. The grouping of *knowledge users* in a distributed system might consist of both, *human users* such as clinicians, hospital management etc. and of the *units of a KBS* such as Diagnostic unit, Treatment recomendation unit etc. The main requirement is that *not all users* should have access to *all information* about the patient. A strategy that the user's access should be limited only to the relevant parts of a patient record is strictly adapted in the design of Patient record unit. Control of the interaction as well as of all the information exchange is also realized exclusively via fuzzy triangle relational products.

3 Developing the design

The substratum structure of the Patient record unit consists of several substructures listed below. Each of these is providing for substratum relization of some specific functions:

1) Satisfaction Structures (SS).
2) Protection Structures (PS).
3) Structure for data types error checking.
4) Structure for data abnormality checking.
5) Structure for time checking and date stamping.
6) Implementation Constraints Structures (ICS).

The process of building a general model for Patient record unit based on the Activity structures methodology of Kohout [4] applies the following sequence of design transformations:
$EAS \rightarrow Activity\ graph \Rightarrow SUB \Rightarrow IPM - AS$
From the medical activities mapping the Environment Activity Structure (EAS) of both environments is formed. Then the activity graph capturing the dynamics of the Patient record unit is constructed from the specification of its major activities. This provides the input and output details of the activity flow at various activity nodes of the Patient record unit. The purpose of the activity graph is to capture the dynamics of the broad categories of the functions of the information processing machine. The activity graph therefore a refinement of the dynamics of the EAS structure of the Patient record unit. The graph defines the interaction of the hyper-processes that form the activity structure, capturing the interactions between the users and the Patient record unit. Finaly, the substratum structure (SUB) which represents the "anatomy" of the Patient record unit is formed (Fig. 1).

The design of the substratum structure satisfies the following requirements:
a) Each structure will form a part of the overall system of Patient record unit and database; it cannot have the overall authority over the other structures.
b) No direct communication is allowed between users and database during retrieval or update of information.
c) Not all the users are permitted access all the available fields in the database; the access is permitted only in accordance with the individual permission profiles.

4 Use of Fuzzy Triangle Relational Products in the Design

The overall coordination of the retrieval of patient data as well as its dynamic protection is achieved by means of two structures: it satisfaction structure and *protection* structure.

Satisfaction structure (SS) evaluates request from the users and also ascertains their relevance. The participant satisfaction is measured by means of fuzy set inclusion. The function of the satisfaction structure is to monitor the users' satisfaction during the process of their interaction with the Patient record unit. For each participant of multi-centre interaction (that can be either a Knowledge User (KU) or a Knowledge source (KS)) appearing in either environment, the permitted information relevant to the interest of each participant is retrieved, providing that the degree of satisfaction with the source exceeds a particular predetermined, fixed or variable, treshold.

The following specific fuzzy satisfaction relations are used in the design [9]:
$(U \Rightarrow F)@(F \Rightarrow R);$ $(U \Rightarrow R)@(R \Rightarrow F)$ FILE DEMAND SATISFACTION
$(U \Rightarrow R)@(R \Rightarrow DB);$ $(U \Rightarrow F)@(F \Rightarrow DB)$ PARTICIPANT SATISFACTION
where @ is either $\Box$ or $\triangleleft$ product [6], [7]. The meaning of the sets in the above satisfaction relations is as follows: KB represents the Knowledge base, DB a Data base, U Users, F Fields and R files of a patient record. The relations over these sets are of two types: *demand* and *availability* relations.

Fuzzy relational products [6], [7] are defined by the following formulas:
$\pi[a(R \triangleleft S)b] = \pi(aR \subseteq Sb)$ $\pi[a(R \Box S)b] = \pi(aR = Sb)$
where $\subseteq$ and $=$ represent fuzzy set inclusion and equality, respectively. The type of fuzzy power set theory

determining the properties of set inclusion and equivalence is given by the choice of many-valued logic (MVL) implication operators. Readers not familiar with this matter are refered to [10] which provides a comparative study of mathematical properties of several distinct fuzzy power set theories and has become a standard reference. Mathematically equivalent direct relational formulas are summarized by the generic formula: $(R@S)_{ik} ::= \#(R_{ij} * S_{jk})$ where * represents either MVL implication or equivalence operator and # is either an MVL *and* operator or the normalized arithmetic sum. Definitions of ten different implications, further mathematical details on the products and the description of applications appear in [6], [7].

The *Protection structure* of the system also employs fuzzy relational products. For details of precise relational specification and further references see [5]. This protection scheme is capability based [4]. It should be noted that the choice of the MVL operators is strongly application dependent. In the protection mechanism we have used *standard strict* operators, while in data base retrieval *Lukasiewicz* and *Klene-Dienes* operators. For the mathematical definitions see [7], [10].

5 Integrating the Patient record unit into CLINAID

The unit has been integrated into the generic architecture of the multi-centre medical knowledge based system CLINAID [8]. The basic architecture of CLINAID consists of the co-operating units [11] of the Basic Shell Substratum (see Fig. 2). The development of a PRU based on the new design techniques adumbrated here was neccessary, as CLINAID dealt with a very complex dynamic scenario. The design covers several medical specialties (with more than ten body systems); this leads to the need to handle problems of multiple context and of coordination of multiple knowledge users. The multiplicity of DBs leads to the necessity of dealing with multiple environments.

In integrating the PRU into CLINAID, the medical activity mapping has provided the information on how all the current activities work and how the medical processing fits together. Identification of medical activities and the functions corresponding to it played the primary role in defining the scope of the Patient record unit of CLINAID. Functions of the Patient record unit include dealing with the requests from users – human users as well as the units of CLINAID, such as the Treatment recommendation unit and the Diagnostic unit, etc. Other functions include interacting with the databases and giving feedback to the users. Considerable attention had to be paid to the operating environment of CLINAID since it operates in a multi-environmental situation [3]. To enhance the security, the information from the databases linked to CLINAID is not to be directly accessible by the human users of the knowledge-based system. It can be accessed by the human users only through the front end-unit of CLINAID. Furthermore, as this information has to be also accessible by the programs and various subsystems of CLINAID. This access is done exclusively through the protected structures of the Patient record unit.

References

1. Brodie, M.L. and Myopulos, J. (eds.). *On Knowledge Base Management Systems*. Springer, Berlin, New York, 1986.

2. Delacambre, L.M.L. and Etheredge, J.N. The relational production language: A production language for relational databases. In Kerschberg, L., editor, *Expert Database Systems*, pages 333–351, Benjamin Cummings, Redwood City, Calif., 1989.

3. Kohout, L.J., Anderson, J., and Bandler, W. *Knowledge-Based Systems for Multiple Environments*. Gower, Aldershot, U.K., 1991.

4. Kohout, L.J. *A Perspective on Intelligent Systems: A Framework for Analysis and Design.* Chapman and Hall & Van Nostrand, London & New York, 1990.

5. Kohout, L.J. and Bandler, W. Computer Security Systems: Fuzzy Logics. In Singh, M.G., editor, *Systems and Control Encyclopedia*, Pergamon Press, Oxford, 1987.

6. Bandler, W. and Kohout, L.J. Mathematical relations. Ibid. pages 4000 – 4008.

7. Bandler, W. and Kohout, L.J. A survey of fuzzy relational products in their applicability to medicine and clinical psychology. In Kohout, L.J. and Bandler, W., editors, *Knowledge Representation in Medicine and Clinical Behavioural Science*, pages 107–118, an Abacus Book, Gordon and Breach Publ., London and New York, 1986.

8. Kohout, L.J., Anderson, J., Bandler, W., Gao, S., and Trayner, C. CLINAID: A knowledge-based system for support of decisions in the conditions of risk and uncertainty. In [3], chapter 10.

9. Kohout, L.J. and Bandler, W. The use of fuzzy information retrieval techniques in construction of multi-centre knowledge-based systems. In Bouchon, B. and Yager, R.R., editors, *Uncertainty in Knowledge-Based Systems (Lecture Notes in Computer Science vol. 286)*, pages 257–264, Springer Verlag, Berlin, 1987.

10. Bandler, W. and Kohout, L.J. Fuzzy power sets and fuzzy implication operators. *Fuzzy Sets and Systems*, 4:13–30, 1980.

11. Kohout, L.J., Bandler, W., Anderson, J., and Trayner, C. Knowledge-based decision support system for use in medicine. In Mitra, G., editor, *Computer Models for Decision Making*, pages 133–146, North-Holland, Amsterdam, 1985.

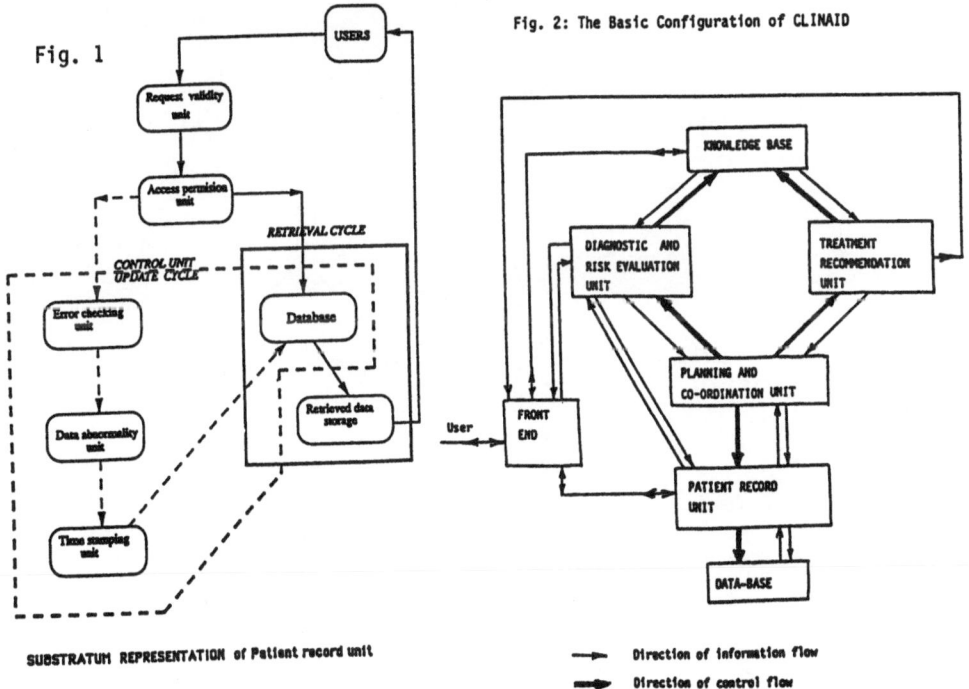

Fig. 1

Fig. 2: The Basic Configuration of CLINAID

SUBSTRATUM REPRESENTATION of Patient record unit

→ Direction of information flow
⇒ Direction of control flow

313

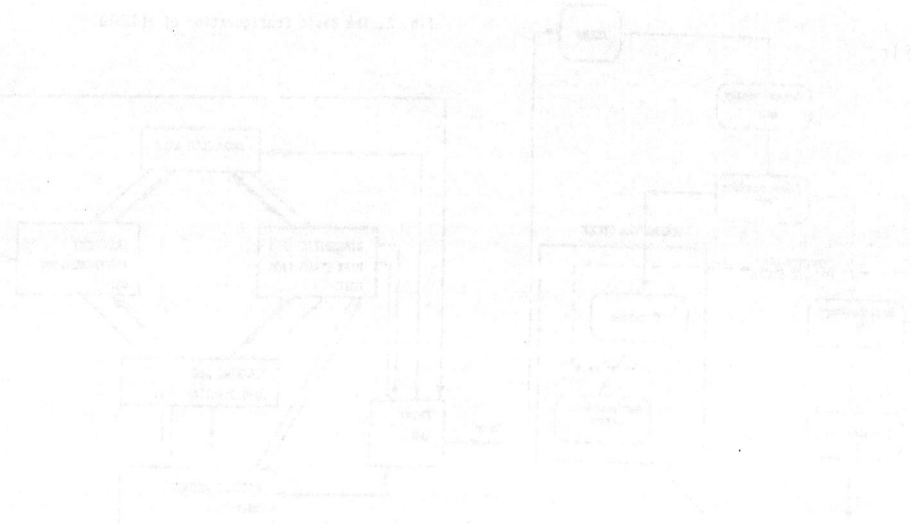

EXPERT SYSTEMS—KNOWLEDGE ACQUISITION AND LEARNING

Better Justifiability and Less Rules by Using Deep Knowledge

Kindler H.*,**, Densow D.*, Fliedner T. M.*

*) Institute of Occupational and Social Medicine of the University of Ulm,
**) Institute of Applied Knowledge Processing at the University of Ulm

Abstract

An expert system in medicine has for legal and ethical reasons special charges, i. e., justifiability and intelligibility. It will be shown that justifiability and intelligibility of knowledge can be achieved. This is obtained by modeling medical knowledge as deep knowledge. Another advantage of this is a substantial reduction of the number of rules which have to be represented to achieve the same problem-solving capacity compared to surface knowledge. The medical domain is the acute radiation syndrome.

Keywords

acute radiation syndrome, deep knowledge, expert system, justification

1. Introduction

As far as the result is concerned, expert systems that were previously constructed almost match the problem-solving capacities of human experts [15]. They were thought to be of use in domains in which physicians have a lack of expertise. This is especially true concerning the management of radiation accidents. There is often a clearly recognized pattern and consistency in the symptoms and signs, particularily the time sequence of events following acute radiation exposure and resulting in some form of the acute radiation syndrome. Early indicators exist to perform a grading of the acute radiation syndrome according to its severity. This classification could be done by defining all possible cases with surface knowledge. A low number of rules would be sufficient to classify the most common cases. For the more special cases a large amount of additional rules would

be necessary. The following advantages can be obtained by using deep knowledge, i. e., about pathophysiological mechanisms:

- significant reduction of the number of rules, thus, improved maintenance,
- equal quality of classification of ordinary cases compared to the use of surface knowledge,
- better classification of exceptional cases,
- better intelligibility, and
- justifiability of rules in an epistemological sense.

Intelligibility and justifiability are crucial for the application of expert systems in a medical domain. In medicine the personal responsability has to remain with the physician and cannot be handed over to a machine. Thus, medical expert systems lacking the ability to explain their reasoning in an intelligible way and to justify the validity of the applied knowledge cannot be employed.

2. Acute Radiation Syndrome

The acute radiation syndrome manifests itself as a characteristic set of clinical pictures when either most of the body or large segments of the body are exposed in a relatively uniform way to ionizing radiation. Radiation doses sufficient to initiate the acute radiation syndrome come from external sources and consist of the more penetrating gamma rays, X-rays, neutrons, or combinations thereof.

The differential diagnosis is limited to the question how intensely the patient has been exposed. The strain is the reaction of an organism to external stress, which in our case means radiation exposure. The strain can be estimated by hematological signs and symptoms of the central nervous system. The early indicators are presented below in accordance to their time of onset:

- Indicator 1: Early vomiting can be caused by irradiation of the central nervous system which results in alterations of membrane permeability. The stronger the irradiation, the earlier the vomiting occurs. This symptom is not as specific as the hematological signs, but a very sensitive and the earliest indicator for radiation lesions.
- Indicator 2: The lymphocytes are the most radiosensitive cells in the peripheral blood. Therefore, there is an immediate sharp drop in their number even at relatively low radiation doses. Thus, higher doses cannot result in a further decrease of their concentration. Nevertheless, the death of the lymphocytes is a specific and early parameter for radiation injuries.

- Indicator 3: After the irradiation the granulocyte concentration increases initially. This mobilisation and intravasation of granulocytes is a reaction to the radiation strain. This reaction, although it is not specific, is a good indicator of the radiation strain.
- Indicator 4: If this initial rise is due to radiation effects then it will be followed by a characteristic pattern of a more or less marked decrease. This decline depends on the limited life expectancy of the mature cells and the disturbed supply. The radiation affects the more radiosensitive immature cells ment to replace the short-lived but relatively insensitive adult granulocytes. This decline is the more significant the more intense the strain is.

3. Grading with Surface Knowledge

Important for the initiation of the therapy is the grading of the acute radiation syndrome. A five grade classification has been generally agreed upon ([1], [7], [11]). These classes are defined by the clinical outcome. Therefore, the definition cannot be utilized to grade during the initial phase of the acute radiation syndrome. Nevertheless, a grading is required for an optimized therapy. By combination of the above mentioned early indicators the grading can be estimated properly. The rule in first order predicate calculus for the estimation of degree III is depicted in fig. 1.

fig. 1:

If
a patient has been vomiting between half an hour and two hours after the end of the radiation exposure,
the patient's concentration of lymphocytes has been at least one time between 40% and 60% of his normal value until day 2,
the patient's concentration of granulocytes has been at least one time higher than 120% of his normal value until day 4, and
the patient's concentration of granulocytes has been at least one time between 50% and 80% of his normal value between day 4 and 7,
then
it will be certain that he has an acute radiation syndrome of degree III.

Every of the indicators 1 - 4 is a premise of the rule. The indicator 4 for the degree III will exist if the time of a time-value-pair of the concentration of granulocytes is in the interval [4d, 7d] and the value of the time-value-pair is in the interval [50%, 80%].

For each of the degrees a comparable rule for the early estimation exists. An overlapping of the intervals of the value of a single indicator may occur, e. g., the concentrations of lymphocytes of higher degrees of the acute radiation syndrome are similar. With five rules similar to the rule in fig. 1 most of the cases of the acute radiation syndrome are covered. Nevertheless, inconsistency may occur due to, e. g., multiple injuries and marked inhomogeneity. Therefore, combinations of the early indicators may occur which are not covered by the five rules. In order to cover all cases at least 625 rules would be needed.
Every chunk of knowledge used in a medical expert system should be justifiable by reason of the physician's personal responsability. A justification of a chunk of knowledge is an argumentation about its correctness in an epistemological sense. A justification of the rule in fig. 1

would be a long essay containing chapter two of this publication.

4. Grading with Deep Knowledge

Regarding the rule in fig. 1 shows that it is composed out of four premises. Each of the premises is a condition for the time-value-pair of one indicator. The justification of each of the premises can be given based on the pathophysiological knowledge of chapter two. The rule depicted in fig. 1 can be decomposed in five rules. Four of the rules are of the same type: The premise is one of the premises of the rule in fig. 1 and the conclusion is that an indicator for degree III is found. An example for this type of rule and its pathophysiological justification is given in fig. 2:

fig. 2:

If
the patient's concentration of granulocytes has been at least one time higher than 120% of his normal value until day 4
then
indicator 3 for an acute radiation syndrome of degree III will exist.

The granulocytes are highly radiosensitive and are most critical to the immediate prognosis because of their role in coping with bacterial infections. After the irradiation the granulocyte concentration increases initially. This mobilisation and intravasation of granulocytes is a reaction due to the radiation strain. Nevertheless, this effect is not specific. Other health impairments may also lead to a granulocytosis.

A rule and its pathophysiological justification.

Each of the three other similar rules can be justified. A scoring table is provided for every patient as shown in fig. 3. If an indicator for a certain degree is deduced with a rule as depicted in fig. 2, this will be marked in the patient's scoring table.

fig. 3

	Ind.1	Ind.2	Ind.3	Ind.4
degree I				
degree II				
degree III	x	x	x	x
degree IV				
degree V				

In the patient's scoring table the four indicators for the degree III of the acute radiation syndrome are already marked. The patient's scoring table is a property which is attached to every patient's object in the fact base.

Using the scoring table another set of rules permits the patient's scoring. The combination of the indicators pointing to one degree is a measure for the evidence of this degree. The rule in fig. 4 means that four out of four indicators pointing to one of the patient's possible degrees of his radiation syndrome certify this degree. This rule will deduce from the scoring table in fig. 3 that the patient's acute radiation syndrome is certainly of degree III. Even for this type of rule a plausible justification (compare fig. 4) can be given. The rule in fig. 1 expresses the same knowledge as the four rules of the type shown in fig. 2 and the rule in fig.4, although, it is not explicitly represented and justified.

fig.4:

If
all out of four early indicators indicate an acute radiation syndrome of the same degree
then
it will be certain that it is an acute radiation syndrome of this degree.

* Four indicators are choosen because of their early occurence as cardinal signs and symptoms of the acute radiation syndrome. Standing alone each single parameter is not specific enough to obtain a valid grading of the radiation syndrome. Nevertheless, the combination of the four indicators is specific. By higher redundancy a higher reliability of the decision is achieved.*

Rule to determine the evidence of a degree of the acute radiation syndrome and its justification.

In case that there is evidence for diverging degrees of the acute radiation syndrome, always the higher degree is considered. Generally in medicine the upper border of risk has to be taken into account. Even in special cases of the acute radiation syndrome decision-making is alleviated by this conservative approach. The number of rules (25) used for this reasoning model is dramatically lower compared to the use of surface knowledge (more than 625). The numerical treatment of uncertain reasoning which cannot be justified epistemologically is avoided, also.

5. Conclusion

A demonstrator for this reasoning with deep knowledge is implemented on KEE™. Apart from the justifiability described in the publication this implementation uses a truth maintenance system [6] to provide "How"-explanations of all deductions. The justification network can be represented as a hypertext approach [4]. For every rule which has been applied, both, its textual representation and its justification can be provided by this. The work presented above has been carried through for the development of a full-scale second generation expert system for the medical management of radiation accidents.

6. Literature

[1] Bundesgesundheitsamt der Bundesrepublik Deutschland (ed.): "Grundsätze und allgemeine Verfahren bei Strahlenexpositionen in beruflichen Notfall- und Unfallsituationen", Veröffentlichungen der Internationalen Strahlenschutzkommission ICRP, vol. 28, Gustav Fischer Verlag, Stuttgart, 1980

[2] Chandrasekaran B., Smith J. W., Sticklen J.: " 'Deep' models and their relation to diagnosis", in Sadegh-Zadeh K. (ed.): "Artificial Intelligence in Medicine", vol. 1, no. 1, Burgverlag, Tecklenburg, 1989

[3] Clancey W. J.: "Viewing Knowledge Bases as Qualitative Models", IEEE-Expert, vol. 4, no. 2, IEEE Computer Society Press, 1989

[4] Conklin J.: "Hypertext: An Introduction and Survey", IEEE-Computer 20, 9, IEEE Computer Society Press, 1987

[5] Densow D., Kindler H., Fliedner T. M.: "RADES - Radiation Accident Decision Support System", in "Proceedings of the 10th International Symposium of the Electricity Section of the ISSA 1990", Vienna, to appear

[6] Doyle : "A Truth Maintenance System", Artificial Intelligence Journal 12, North Holland, Amsterdam, 1979

[7] Fliedner T. M.: "Strategien zur strahlenschutzmedizinischen, ambulanten Versorgung von "Betroffenen" bei kerntechnischen Unfällen", in Messerschmidt O., Betz B., Fliedner T. M.: "Medizinische Erstmaßnahmen bei kerntechnischen Unfällen", Thieme, Stuttgart, 1981

[8] Kernavou E. T., Washbrook J.: "Deep and shallow models in medical expert systems", in Sadegh-Zadeh K. (ed): "Artificial Intelligence in Medicine", vol. 1, no. 1, Burgverlag, Tecklenburg, 1989

[9] Kindler H.: "Wissensmodellierung als Grundlage eines intelligenten Tutors in der Elektromyographie", in Reuter A.: "20. GI-Jahrestagung", vol. 2, Springer, 1990

[10] Kuipers B., Kassirer J. P.: "Knowledge Acquisition by Analysis of Verbatim Protocols", in Kidd A. L.: "Knowledge Acquisition for Expert Systems", Plenum Press, London, 1987

[11] Mettler jr. F. A., Kelsey C. A., Ricks R. C.: "Medical Management of Radiation Accidents", CRC Press, Fort Lauterdale, 1990

[12] Patil R., Szolovits P., Schwartz W.: "Modeling Knowledge of the Patient in Acid-Base and Electrolyte Disorders", in Szolovits P. (ed.): "Artificial Intelligence in Medicine", AAAS Selected Symposium 51, Westview Press, Boulder, 1982

[13] Szepesi T., Naudé J., Schneider B.: "Blood Cell Changes as Indicators of Reversible and Irreversible Hemopoietic Damage to the Stem Cell Pool", in Seidel H. J.: "The Hemopoietic Stem Cell", Universitätsverlag Ulm, Ulm, 1990

[14] WHO: "Acute Radiation Effects in Victims of the Accident at the Chernobyl Nuclear Power Plant: Report from the USSR", in WHO Regional Office for Europe: "Nuclear Accidents and Epidemiology", Copenhagen, 1987, (Environmental Health Series No. 25)

[15] Yu. V., Buchanan B., Shortliffe E., Wraith E., Davis S., Scott R., Dohen A.: "Evaluating the Performance of a Computer-Based Consultant", Computer Programs in Biomedicine 9, 1979

Learning Specialized Disease Descriptions in a Rheumatological Expert System[1]

Werner Horn[†‡], Gerhard Widmer[†‡], Bernhard Nagele[†]

[†]Department of Medical Cybernetics and Artificial Intelligence,
University of Vienna, Freyung 6, A-1010 Vienna, and
[‡]Austrian Research Institute for Artificial Intelligence, Vienna
Email: werner@ai-vie.uucp

Abstract. MESICAR is a second generation expert system which contains very general disease descriptions about rheumatological disorders in the primary medical care field. With the help of a detailed hierarchical description of the human anatomy the system is able to support diagnostic decisions. The current paper describes how Machine Learning techniques are used to automatically build more specific disease descriptions for common, frequently occurring cases. Integrating learned concepts into the hierarchy of disease descriptions supports efficient and fast reasoning on common cases in addition to the general diagnostic support for rheumatological problems of anatomical structures.

1. Introduction

Second generation expert systems are characterized by their capability of a more principled form of reasoning (Steels 1985, 1990). This is done using some basic knowledge about the structure, the function, and the behavior of components of the domain – often called "deep" knowledge. The problem–solving methods used tend to be robust but also very expensive. MESICAR is such an example of a decision support system (Horn 1989). It demonstrates the usage of detailed anatomical knowledge when diagnosing rheumatological problems in the primary medical care field.

MESICAR incorporates extensive anatomical knowledge which provides the basis for the reasoning methods. During a consultation disease concepts are instantiated to form hypotheses describing the patient's problem. The disease concepts point to expected manifestations with conditions for associated attributes. The concepts are very general in the sense that these conditions are given for classes of anatomical structures. The inference process supplies elementary values for these attributes, which now gives the detailed picture of the patient's situation. Complex "bindings" (Horn, 1991) allow to maintain consistency with respect to anatomical constraints, both during hypothesis generation and hypothesis testing. Checking the bindings makes the inference process expensive.

The advantage of (first generation) expert systems based on surface knowledge is their ability to diagnose common cases (covered by the surface knowledge) very fast. This ability is required for second generation expert systems, too. But instead of manually acquiring surface rules from the domain expert we can apply machine learning techniques to build such surface rules. This is done using a combination of Explanation–Based Learning (EBL) and empirical learning techniques (Widmer

---

[1] We are grateful to Dr.Kurt Ammer for providing the rheumatological knowledge and to Prof.Robert Trappl for his continuous support of the project. The project was funded in part by the Austrian "Fonds zur Foerderung der wissenschaftlichen Forschung". The Austrian Research Institute for Artificial Intelligence is supported by the Federal Ministry for Science and Research, Vienna.

1989). Successfully solved problems are generalized with the use of the deep knowledge which forms the domain theory. We have built MESICAR-LEARN which is a learning apprentice (Wilkins et al.1986) for MESICAR. Incrementally it constructs specific disease descriptions by generalizing disease instances, which represent patients' problems correctly diagnosed. The generic disease descriptions of MESICAR (section 2) serve as the domain theory for the learning methods described in section 3.

2. MESICAR's generic disease descriptions

MESICAR's original knowledge base consists mainly of generic disease concepts and knowledge about the human anatomy. A generic disease concept is a high–level description of a prototypical disease. It is abstracted from the anatomical localization of the disease. Figure 1 shows part of the disease concept *Tendinosis*, which is a shorthand for non–inflammatory disease of a muscle and tendon insertion point.

The description of a generic disease concept (D) consists of several parts:
- the "D–attributes" section, specifying the attribute slots each instance will have. The CHARACTERISTIC-ATTRIBUTE identifies the instance, i.e., it allows to distinguish between several instances of the same disease concept.
- the "D–binding" section defines places where the disease instance gets its attribute values from;
- the "Manifestations" section contains several *D–M–expressions*. Each D–M–expression points to one manifestation (M) which supports or opposes the disease hypothesis D. It contains several *matching conditions*. Each one defines expected

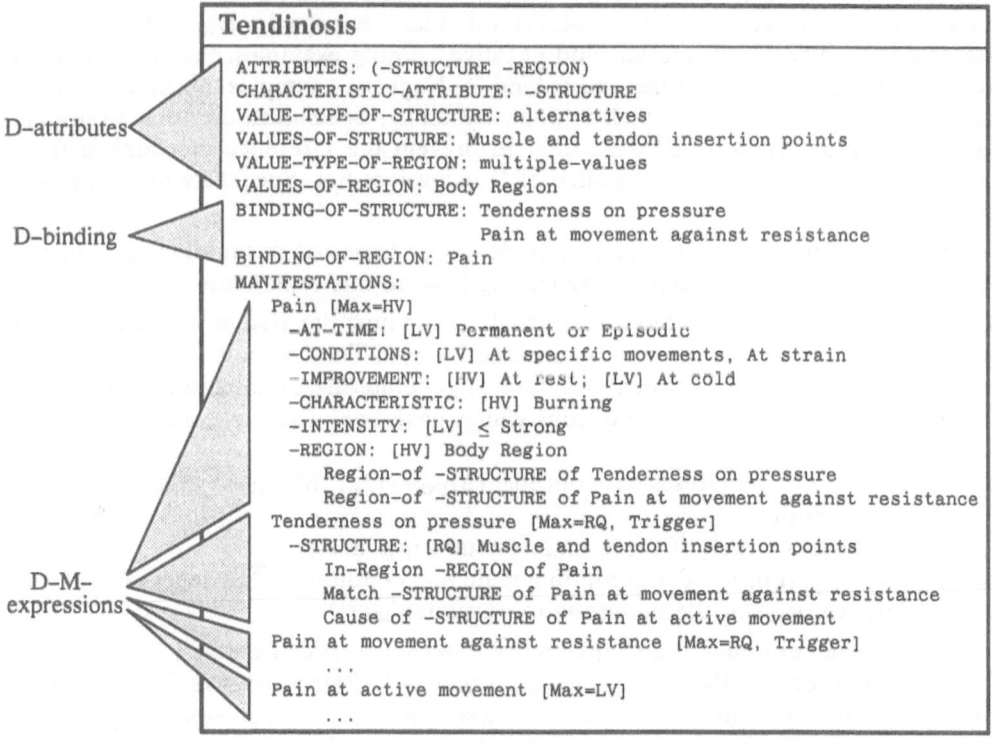

Figure 1: Description of the generic disease concept *Tendinosis*.

values for one attribute of the manifestation together with the support it gives (*ReQuired, High–Valued, Low–Valued, UnSpecific*). In addition, each matching condition may contain a *D–M–binding* part. This part gives consistency conditions between attributes of manifestations which are to be satisfied by the attribute values. For example (see Fig.1), the structure showing *tenderness on pressure* must be in that region of the body, where the patient complains about *pain*.

This description is generic. It supports the creation of specific instances in the presence of patient data. When confronted with a patient showing manifestations of a "tennis elbow" on the left arm, the inference mechanism of MESICAR creates the disease instance *Tendinosis–1 (Epicondylus radialis humeri)*. In this case the two attribute slots of *Tendinosis–1*, –STRUCTURE and –REGION, are filled with *Epicondylus radialis humeri*, and *Elbow front left*, respectively.

Each generic disease concept together with the hierarchical description of the anatomy and the attributes defines the background knowledge for MESICAR–LEARN. It is used as the *domain theory* (Mitchell et al. 1986) when building the explanation for a disease instance.

3. Building explanations and learning new disease descriptions

MESICAR–LEARN creates and extends specialized disease concepts ($\bar{D}$) with the guidance of an expert rheumatologist. In principle the system is able to create a $\bar{D}$ after completion of the inferencing about one case of the disease D (resulting in instance D_{INST}). But such a $\bar{D}$ will be meaningful only after the system has seen several (slightly different) cases of the same problem, which allows the generalization process to create a $\bar{D}$ more general. MESICAR–LEARN divides the instances $D_{INST}-1,...,D_{INST}-n$ into positive (correctly diagnosed) and negative training examples. Positive examples are used to automatically create and extend $\bar{D}$. Negative examples are used to guide the expert at specialization, which is done manually. Specialization adds additional clauses to the description of $\bar{D}$, in order to prevent the inference mechanism from diagnosing a case as being an instance of $\bar{D}$ when it is not. Specialization is not described in this paper.

Learning from the positive training example $D_{INST}-i$ consists in building an explanation for $D_{INST}-i$ and in creating or extending $\bar{D}$ from this explanation.

An explanation is a tree of depth five which shows how the system was able to conclude positively about the presence of disease $D_{INST}-i$. The contents of the levels are:

0: the disease concept D which was used to generate the explanation;
1: pointers to those D–M–expressions which have been used in concluding about $D_{INST}-i$.
2: the instantiated manifestation concepts ($M_{INST}-1$, ..., $M_{INST}-k$) that contributed to the conclusion;
3: the attributes of each of those manifestation instances;
4: the atomic part of the corresponding matching condition ▨▨▨ together with the attribute value(s) of the manifestation instance ⸢*values*⸥ .

Figure 2 gives an example of an explanation tree for one specific case which resulted in confirmation of the disease instance *Tendinosis–1 (Epicondylus radialis humeri)*. Comparing the explanation tree with the description of the corresponding disease concept given in Figure 1 we can see several characteristics:
· the structure of the tree resembles the structure of the disease description;

- only those D–M–expressions are used here which have their corresponding manifestation concepts instantiated and used. For instance, in the example there is no pointer to the D–M–expression for *pain at active movement*, since it was not found in this case;
- there may be several manifestation instances for one D–M–expression – see, e.g., the two *pain at movement against resistance*–instances representing pain at two different movements;
- at levels 3 and 4 only those attributes and atomic matching conditions are present, which deal with attribute values present in the specific case.

Several cases of the same specialized disease concept (e.g., *Tendinosis-1, ..., Tendinosis-5*, all with the same characteristic attribute –STRUCTURE: *Epicondylus radialis humeri*) produce several explanation trees with the same root D (*Tendinosis*). The learning algorithm uses generalization when creating the new specialized disease concept D̄ (*Tendinosis (Epicondylus radialis humeri)*). The basic principle is to generalize over corresponding attribute values given at level 4 of the explanation trees. This generalization is dependent on the type of the attribute (integer, real, yes/no, ordered alternatives, alternatives, or multiple values) and of the operators used in the matching conditions. It uses heuristics for performing generalization steps in the attribute hierarchy. The generalization process is constrained by the values given in the atomic matching conditions. In this way (and in other ways, too) the explanations provide guidance to the generalization algorithm (see also Widmer 1991). The learning process can be applied incrementally, too: MESICAR-LEARN may later on modify the description of D̄ after having seen more cases.

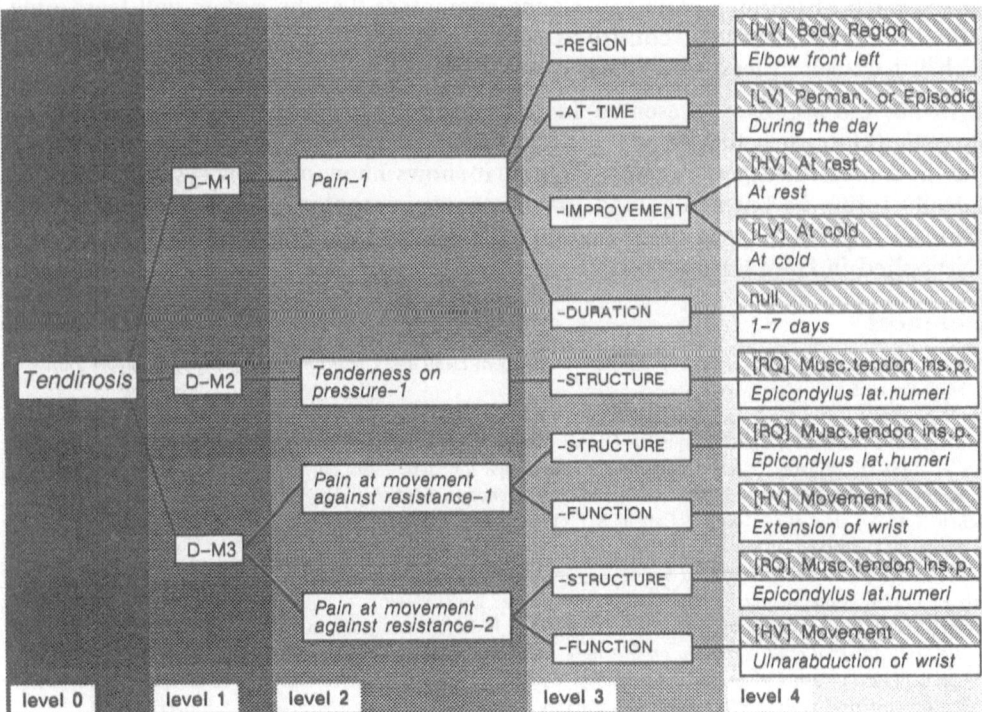

Figure 2: Explanation for disease instance *Tendinosis-1*.

The newly created specialized disease concept $\overline{D}$ becomes a sub–concept of D. $\overline{D}$ has a formal structure which is identical to the formal structure of D. The D–M–expressions of $\overline{D}$ are constructed from the result of the generalization process. D–bindings and D–M–bindings are established only if non–elementary attribute values are related. Compared to the generic disease concept D the specialized concept $\overline{D}$ will not contain bindings for leaves in the attribute hierarchy, since the inference process has already checked these elementary relations to be ok. Due to this integration of learned (specific) disease concepts and generic disease concepts it is possible to use the same inference methods for both knowledge types.

4. Conclusion

With the help of MESICAR–LEARN it is possible to integrate general and specific disease concepts into the knowledge base of MESICAR – thus integrating deep and surface knowledge. This contrasts the usual separation (e.g. KARDIO: Bratko et al. 1989) and allows the use of the same reasoning methods for both types of knowledge. By applying focusing techniques the inference engine preserves the efficiency when confronted with a common case. Only when focusing on specific disease hypotheses is not possible are the general disease concepts used; they provide the full anatomical background for the reasoning process. Efficient reasoning for common cases is achieved since MESICAR–LEARN has eliminated the complex binding conditions in the description of a learned disease concept.

Moreover, this construction and integration of specialized knowledge into the knowledge base is performed *automatically*, through *learning*. It should also be noted that this approach of learning from experience guarantees that the system will learn only useful concepts, because it constructs specialized descriptions only for diseases of which it has seen at least one actual case.

All in all, the approach presented in this paper is not meant to be a method for automatically constructing knowledge bases from scratch (which would be rather dubious in a medical expert system). Rather, it shows how an expert system can automatically refine its knowledge and make its own reasoning process more efficient. This is an important capability if second generation expert systems are to be successfully applied in complex domains.

References

Bratko I., Mozetic I., Lavrac N. (1989): *Kardio – A Study in Deep and Qualitative Knowledge for Expert Systems*, MIT Press, Cambridge, MA.

Horn W. (1989): MESICAR – A Medical Expert System Integrating Causal and Associative Reasoning, *Applied Artificial Intelligence*, Special Issue on Causal Modeling, 3(2–3)305–336.

Horn W. (1991): Utilizing Detailed Anatomical Knowledge for Hypothesis Formation and Hypothesis Testing in Rheumatological Decision Support, *Artificial Intelligence in Medicine*, 3(1)21–39.

Mitchell T.M., Keller R.M., Kedar-Cabelli S.T.(1986): Explanation–Based Generalization: A Unifying View, *Machine Learning*, 1(1)47–80.

Steels L. (1985): Second Generation Expert Systems, *Future Generations Computer Systems*, 1(4)213–221.

Steels L. (1990): Components of Expertise, *AI–Magazine*, 11(2)28–49.

Widmer G. (1989): A Tight Integration of Deductive and Inductive Learning, in A.M.Segre (ed.), *Proceedings of the Sixth International Workshop on Machine Learning*, Morgan Kaufmann, Los Altos, CA.

Widmer G. (1991): Using Plausible Explanations to Bias Empirical Generalization in Weak Theory Domains, in Y.Kodratoff (ed.): *Proc.Fifth European Working Session on Learning (EWSL–91)*, Springer, Berlin.

Wilkins D., Clancey W., Buchanan B. (1986): Overview of the ODYSSEUS Learning Apprentice, in T.Mitchell et al.(eds.): *Machine Learning: A Guide to Current Research*, Kluwer, Boston, Mass.

INDUCTIVE LEARNING AS A METHOD FOR MEDICAL DECISION MAKING

Gjuro Deželić and Josipa Kern

Andrija Štampar School of Public Health, Medical School,University of Zagreb, Zagreb, Yugoslavia

SUMMARY.- A system for inductive learning is used in automatic construction of decision trees. The results and experience in its use in the field of rheumatology are presented. The decision trees have been obtained under different conditions, i. e. without and with pruning. Variability of results has been noted and discussed. It is concluded that such decision trees could be a useful guide in clinical decisions.

INTRODUCTION

Each human being possesses a knowledge base which contains knowledge acquired during the whole life by different ways of learning. Among them learning from experience - the inductive learning - is a continuous process in which existing knowledge is checked against reality for validity and efficiency. If there are some discrepancies or opportunities for improvement, the knowledge base is revised (1). Such approach can also be applied in automatic methods of learning. One of them is the so-called method of structured learning introduced by Quinlan (2) and thoroughly investigated by Bratko and collaborators (3). Quinlan's method is based on an algorithm which constructs a decision tree from examples used for learning.

All examples are specified by the values of all attributes and by the class to which the example belongs. The decision tree is constructed by choosing attributes according to its informativity. The leafs of the tree are assigned a class containing all the corresponding examples. The procedure continues until the tree classifies correctly all the examples used for learning (4). In such a way the rules for problem solving are established and can be applied to the classification of new examples.

As a result of research performed by Bratko and his group a software tool for inductive learning of decision trees, named ASSISTANT Professional, has been developed (5). ASSISTANT has been applied in many fields, among them also in solving various medical diagnostics problems. In one of our recent papers (6) the problems in the fields of perinatology and rheumatology have been studied. Initial experience with decision trees obtained by the ASSISTANT system has been presented and a variation of results of inductive learning has been noted. In continuation of this work a thorough examination of this phenomenon seemed to be of interest in view of the possible use of decision trees in practical clinical work.

MAIN FEATURES OF THE INDUCTIVE LEARNING TOOL

ASSISTANT, the system for inductive learning, belongs to the TDIDT class (Top Down Induction of Decision Trees). The system presumes existence of an appropriate number of learning examples described by a set of attributes and by classes representing conditions (diagnoses, anatomical stages, courses of disease etc.).

The algorithm for decision tree construction searches for the most informative attribute as follows.

The information amount necessary to classify an example, E, equals to

$$E = - \Sigma_i p_i \log_2(p_i),$$

where p_i is the a priori probability that the observed example belongs to class i. If the root of the tree is attribute A with V different values, the new amount of information necessary to classify an example appears to be

$$I(A) = - \Sigma_v p_v \, i(p_{vi}/p_v) \log_2(p_{vi}/p_v),$$

where p_v is the a priori probability that the observed example has the v-th value of attribute A, and p_{vi} the probability that the observed example has the v-th value of attribute A and belongs to class i. The best attribute is the one minimizing the function $I(A)$ as it renders the maximum of information. The informativity of attribute A is defined as

$$\text{Inf}(A) = E - I(A).$$

The system includes, among others, the possibility to work with continuous attributes, incompletely specified learning examples, automatic choosing of good learning examples, tree pruning, etc. A detailed description of the algorithm is given in the paper by Kononenko et al.(7).

MATERIALS AND METHODS

The data used for experimenting with the inductive learning of decision rules are from a study on clinical evaluation of serologic tests for rheumatoid factors in patients with rheumatoid arthritis (8). Data of 377 patients, shown in Table 1, include the course of disease and present diagnostic criteria of the American Rheumatism Association (ARA): morning stiffness (ARA-1), pain in at least one joint (ARA-2), joint swelling (persisting for at least six weeks, ARA-3), swelling of an additional joint (during three months, ARA-4), symmetrical swelling of joints (ARA-5), subcutaneous nodules (ARA-6), typical x-ray changes (ARA-7), and positive test for rheumatoid factors (ARA-8). As the data have been collected in mid-seventies, these are the 1958 ARA diagnostic criteria (9).

Table 1

Number of rheumatoid arthritis patients with ARA criteria in dependence of the course of disease

Class			Attributes							
Course of disease:	No. of cases:	ARA criterion:	ARA-1	ARA-2	ARA-3	ARA-4	ARA-5	ARA-6	ARA-7	ARA-8
episodic/ intermittent	175	present	174	175	165	125	171	1	169	80
		absent	1	0	10	50	4	174	6	95
contin. progredient	202	present	199	199	193	185	201	38	202	149
		absent	3	3	9	17	1	164	0	53

The programming system ASSISTANT has been applied in the version ASSISTANT PROFESSIONAL (Ver. 3.31), installed in a personal computer IBM AT compatible equipped by a Hercules graphic card and matrix printer.

RESULTS

In the experiments of automatic decision tree construction 70% of instances have been used as learning examples, and the 30% of remaining instances served for testing of decision rules. The decision trees and their prognostic characteristics depend on the degree of pruning the tree. The tree is pruned if the classification errors computed on the basis of the existence of a subtree under a node are greater than the error in the node itself. The degree of pruning is determined by the prune factor which is greater with stronger pruning.

The learning examples are chosen at random, so each new tree construction can be expected to produce a different result. Experiments have been made both without and with pruning. The experiments have been repeated a number of times (ten or more). Differences have been observed in several factors: the prognostic accuracy, the root of the decision tree, the arrangement of nodes under the root and in the total number of nodes in the tree. Table 2 presents a summary of results on automatic tree construction obtained in our experiments. The most frequent tree obtained with pruning is shown in Fig. 1.

Table 2

Summary of experiments in construction of decision trees for classification of rheumatoid arthritis patients regarding the course of disease

Condition of construction	Number of experiments	Root attribute	Number of resulting trees	Maximal freq. of identical trees	Range of prognostic accuracy (%)	Average prognostic accuracy (%)
without pruning	16	ARA-8	9	2	63.7-77.9	71.4
		ARA-6	7	3	68.1-79.7	74.6
with pruning	10	ARA-8	9	7	70.8-76.1	73.3
		ARA-6	1	1	70.8	-

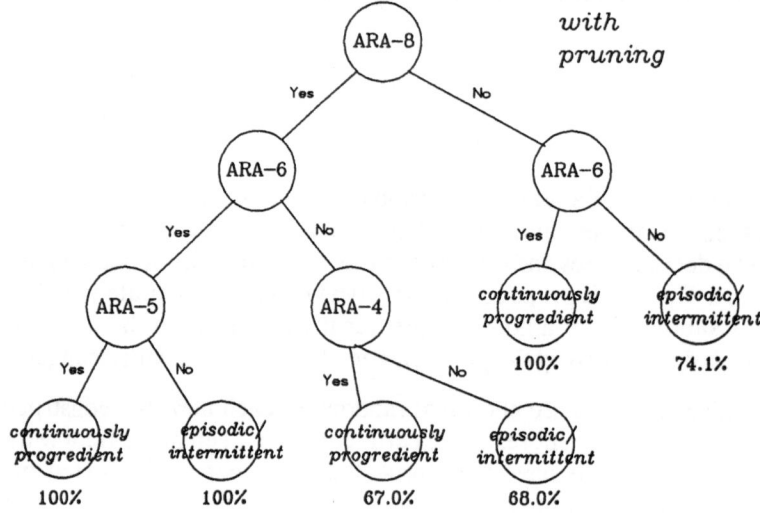

Fig. 1. Course of disease in patients with rheumatoid arthritis; the tree is constructed with pruning and the probabilities of outcome in leafs are indicated in percentages

DISCUSSION

The prognostic accuracy in our decision trees differs in a rather great range indicating the sensitivity of tree construction on the sample used for learning. This is more pronounced if the trees are not pruned. Trees obtained under this condition are more different either in content and shape with less identical trees and broader range of prognostic accuracy. Pruning leads to more uniformity reflected in the increase of the number of identical trees and in a narrower range of prognostic accuracy.

A possible explanation for the variability could arise from a rather small number instances used for learning and testing. Hojker et al. (10) recommend numbers over 1000 if better and more reliable classification results are wanted. This is, of course, not easily met in clinical investigation. The results obtained, however, are reasonable from the medical point of view, thus leading to a general conclusion that if there are sets of patient data with well defined attributes, such decision trees could be a useful guide in clinical decisions.

REFERENCES

1. W.R. Arnold and J.S. Bowie, Artificial Intelligence: A Personal, Commonsense Journey. London: Prentice-Hall,Inc., 1986.

2. J.R. Quinlan, Iterative Dichotomizer 3 (ID3). Stanford University, Artificial Intelligence Laboratory, California, June 1979.

3. B. Cestnik, I. Kononenko and I. Bratko, ASSISTANT 86: A Knowledge Elicitation Tool for Sophisticated Users. EWSL, Bled 1987.

4. I. Bratko and P. Mulec, An Experiment in Automatic Learning of Diagnostic Rules, Informatica 4:18-25,1980.

5. Cestnik B. ASSISTANT PROFESSIONAL a Software Tool for Inductive Learning of Decision Rules. System User Manual, Ver. 3.30. Ljubljana: Edvard Kardelj University 1987.

6. J. Kern, Gj. Deželić, M. Težak-Benčić and Th. Duerrigl, Medical Decision Making by Using a Program for Inductive Learning (original in Croatian), Proceedings 1st Yugoslav Congress for Medical Informatics, Belgrade, December 6-8, 1990, 221-228.

7. I. Kononenko, I. Bratko and E. Roškar, A System for Inductive Learning ASSISTANT (original in Slovenian), Informatika 10:43-52, 1986.

8. Gj. Deželić, Th. Duerrigl, N. Deželić, V. Zergollern, H. Jurak, M. Vitauš and S. Androić, The Photometric Latex Test for Rheumatoid Factors in Patients with Rheumatoid Arthritis. II. Clinical Evaluation, Z. Rheumatol. 37:112-122, 1978.

9. M.W. Ropes, G.A. Bennett, S. Cobb, R. Jacox and R.A. Jessar, 1958 Revision of Diagnostic Criteria for Rheumatoid Arthritis, Bull. Rheum. Dis. 9:175-176, 1958.

10. S. Hojker, I. Kononenko and A. Karalič, Experiments with Automatic Learning of the Thyroid Gland Illnesses (original in Slovenian), in: Proceedings 8th International Symposium CAD/CAM, Zagreb, 1986.

KNOWLEDGE ACQUISITION STUDY AND ACCURACY RATE EVALUATION FOR CADIAG-2/RHEUMA WITH 308 CLINICAL CASES

Harald Leitich[1], Klaus-Peter Adlassnig[1], Gernot Kolarz[2]

[1]Department of Medical Computer Sciences
(Director: Univ.Prof. Dr. G. Grabner)
University of Vienna, Garnisongasse 13, A - 1090 Vienna, Austria
and
[2]Ludwig Boltzmann Institute for Rheumatology and Focal Diseases
(Director: Univ.Prof. Dr. N. Thumb)
Kaiser-Franz-Ring 8, A - 2500 Baden, Austria

Abstract

CADIAG-2/RHEUMA is a medical expert system assisting in the differential diagnosis of rheumatic diseases. The aim of this study was to establish a set of criteria for diagnosing definite rheumatoid arthritis (RA) that provides optimal accuracy and to implement this set of criteria as an IF-THEN rule for application in CADIAG-2/RHEUMA. First, two different sets of criteria for the classification of definite RA described in medical literature were implemented and their respective diagnostic accuracies were evaluated with 154 patients suffering from RA and 154 control subjects. Second, that set of criteria which had performed best became the starting point for establishing an improved set of diagnostic criteria that eventually reached an accuracy of 88.7% (81.8% sensitivity and 95.5% specificity). This improvement was possible by combining literature definition of RA with specific clinical experience of a rheumatology expert.

1. Introduction

CADIAG-2/RHEUMA is a medical expert system designed to assist in establishing differential diagnoses of rheumatic diseases. Its theoretical background and integration into a medical information system were described in [1,2,3,5]. The expert system's accuracy has been evaluated before, reaching 93.7% sensitivity by evaluating 426 patients with rheumatoid arthritis, gout, ankylosing spondylitis, psoriatic arthritis, Sjögren's disease, systemic lupus erythematosus, Reiter's disease, and systemic sclerosis [2].

This study is focused on the diagnosis of rheumatoid arthritis (RA). Three different sets of RA diagnostic criteria were used and applied to RA patients and a control group with non-RA rheumatic diseases. All three sets were based on RA classification criteria edited by The American Rheumatism Association (ARA, now The American College of Rheumatology) [4,5]. In CADIAG-2/RHEUMA, each set of diagnostic criteria was implemented as one IF-THEN rule. The three established rules are:

- rule 1 was implemented according to the revised 1958 ARA criteria for the classification of definite RA [6];

- rule 2 was implemented according to the revised 1987 ARA criteria for the classification of (definite) RA [4];

- rule 3 combined both literature definition and specific clinical experience of a rheumatology expert: As rule 1, it was implemented according to the revised 1958 ARA criteria for the classification of definite RA; however, several criteria were changed and redefined by the rheumatology expert.

The aims of the study were: (a) which of the two initial sets of RA diagnostic criteria performed best; (b) whether the best performing set of criteria could still be improved; and (c) whether splitting both RA patients and control subjects into subsets (according to disease stages, disease characteristics, and concomitant diseases) would give a more detailed picture of the expert system's performance.

2. Patient data

All 154 RA patients and 154 control subjects of this study underwent treatment in a 140-bed hospital for rheumatic diseases in Baden/Austria. Only adults with disease onset after age 16 were included. The mean ages of RA and non-RA patients were similar, whereas sex percentages differed because of a larger number of male control patients.

RA patients: 150 of the 154 RA patients had a confirmed clinical diagnosis of RA. The remaining 4 patients were diagnosed as suspected RA cases. (At time of data collection, a more specific diagnosis was not possible; they were, however, confirmed as definite RA cases later.) The confirmed RA patients were additionally subdivided into the following groups:

- disease stage (The disease staging used in this study is based on radiographic findings and was introduced by Steinbrocker et al. [7]);
- presence or absence of rheumatoid factor (seropositivity/seronegativity); and
- concomitant rheumatic diseases with no relation to RA according to the following categorization: (1) concomitant diseases of the vertebral column; and (2) concomitant osteoporosis.

Control subjects: Any patient with a rheumatic disease other than RA was designated a control subject. The clinical diagnoses represent a cross-section of patients that were treated in the hospital mentioned above.

3. Method

The results shown in Tables 1–5 were obtained by comparing CADIAG-2/RHEUMA's diagnostic results with the available confirmed clinical diagnoses. In addition, it has to be mentioned that a CADIAG-2/RHEUMA diagnosis was taken as established if it was either a confirmed diagnosis or a diagnostic hypothesis with a degree of confirmation of at least 0.5 (cf., [1,3]).

4. Results

4.1. Results obtained with rules 1 and 2 (based on literature definition)

True positive results (sensitivity) with RA patients: As shown in Table 1, rule 1 performed best reaching a sensitivity of 75.3%. Tables 2–4 show the different diagnostic results obtained in the RA subgroups. Cases with early disease stage (stage 1), cases with seronegative RA, and cases with concomitant diseases of the vertebral column tended to cause a lower sensitivity.

False positive results (100%−specificity rate) with control subjects: As shown in Table 5, rule 1 performed best reaching a specificity of 87.7%. A substantial number of patients with psoriatic arthritis and systemic lupus erythematosus yield incorrect results, a fact which lead to further developments, as is described in Section 4.2.

Table 1: True positive results (sensitivity) obtained by the literature-based rules 1 and 2 in patients with rheumatoid arthritis (RA).

diagnosis	total number of patients	rule 1 (ARA 1958 definite)	rule 2 (ARA 1987 definite)
suspected RA	4	1	1
seropositive RA, stage 1	9	7	6
seronegative RA, stage 1	19	10	10
seropositive RA, stage 2	25	22	21
seronegative RA, stage 2	26	17	16
seropositive RA, stage 3	28	23	25
seronegative RA, stage 3	20	18	15
seropositive RA, stage 4	17	13	12
seronegative RA, stage 4	6	5	5
total number of diagnoses	154	116	111
sensitivity rates		75.3%	72.1%

Table 2: True positive results (sensitivity) obtained by the literature-based rules 1 and 2 in RA patients, disease stages 1–4.

diagnosis	total number of patients	rule 1 (ARA 1958 definite)	rule 2 (ARA 1987 definite)
RA, stage 1	28	17 (61%)	16 (57%)
RA, stage 2	51	39 (76%)	37 (72%)
RA, stage 3	48	41 (85%)	40 (83%)
RA, stage 4	23	18 (78%)	17 (74%)

Table 3: True positive results (sensitivity) obtained by the literature-based rules 1 and 2 in seropositive and seronegative RA patients.

diagnosis	total number of patients	rule 1 (ARA 1958 definite)	rule 2 (ARA 1987 definite)
seropositive RA	79	65 (82%)	64 (81%)
seronegative RA	71	50 (70%)	46 (64%)

Table 4: True positive results (sensitivity) obtained by the literature-based rules 1 and 2 in RA patients with and without concomitant spinal diseases.

diagnosis	total number of patients	rule 1 (ARA 1958 definite)	rule 2 (ARA 1987 definite)
no concomitant diseases	74	59 (80%)	54 (73%)
diseases of the vertebral column	50	36 (72%)	34 (68%)
osteoporosis	26	20 (77%)	22 (85%)

Table 5: False positive results (100%−specificity rate) obtained by rules 1 and 2 in control subjects.

diagnosis	total number of patients	rule 1 (ARA 1958 definite)	rule 2 (ARA 1987 definite)
osteoarthrosis	44	2	0
gouty arthritis	32	0	4
ankylosing spondylitis	30	2	0
psoriatic arthritis	20	10	10
joint tuberculosis	4	1	1
other joint infections	4	1	1
Reiter's disease	4	0	0
systemic lupus erythematosus	4	2	3
systemic sclerosis	4	0	0
polymyositis	3	0	1
chondrocalcinosis	3	1	0
polymyalgia rheumatica	2	0	0
total number of diagnoses	154	19	20
specificity rates		87.7%	87.0%

4.2. Development of an improved rule 3 (based on literature definition and clinical experience)

To improve CADIAG-2/RHEUMA's performance, clinical experience of a rheumatology expert was needed to modify the established rules. Rule 1 was selected for further improvement because of its obtained high sensitivity and specificity. Its criteria were consecutively changed to reach higher rates of sensitivity and specificity. Finally, the problem was successfully approached in two different ways:

(a) redefinition of some diagnostic criteria

The symptom "morning stiffness" was redefined in a more restrictive way, but had to last for only 30 minutes instead of 60 minutes.

The sign "symmetrical joint swelling", which had to be observed by a physician, was re-modelled to "symmetrical joint involvement", with the additional inclusion of patient history data.

(b) addition of some further exclusion criteria

To avoid false positive results in cases of psoriatic arthritis, an exclusion in case of present psoriasis was added to rule 1. This exclusion prevents the diagnosis of definite RA if there is sufficient evidence that a patient might actually suffer from psoriatic arthritis.

4.3. Diagnostic results obtained with the improved rule 3 (based on literature definition and clinical experience)

All improvements lead to a definite rule for RA which showed a sensitivity of 81.8% and a specificity of 95.5%, thus reaching a total accuracy of 88.7% (means of sensitivity and specificity rates) as is shown in Table 6.

Table 6: Sensitivity, specificity, and accuracy rates obtained by
rules 1 and 2 and improved rule 3

	rule 1 (ARA 1958 definite)	rule 2 (ARA 1987 definite)	rule 3 (improved rule 1)
sensitivity	75.3%	72.1%	81.8%
specificity	87.7%	87.0%	95.5%
accuracy	81.5%	79.6%	88.7%

5. Discussion

It could be shown that an expert system using diagnostic criteria published in the medical literature can perform successfully. As the ARA criteria were developed for classification purposes to get more uniform cohorts of RA patients for various clinical studies, an improvement might still be reached adding subjective clinical experience of a medical specialist for diagnostic purposes.

Acknowledgements. We thank I. Gröger for secretarial assistance and C. Schuh and F. Fischler for extended programming work. This research was partly supported by IBM Österreich.

References

[1] Adlassnig, K.-P. (1986) Fuzzy Set Theory in Medical Diagnosis. *IEEE Transactions on Systems, Man, and Cybernetics* SMC-16, 260–265.

[2] Adlassnig, K.-P., Kolarz, G., Scheithauer, W., Effenberger, H. & Grabner, G. (1985) CADIAG: Approaches to Computer-Assisted Medical Diagnosis. *Computers in Biology and Medicine* 15, 315–335.

[3] Adlassnig, K.-P., Kolarz, G., Scheithauer, W. & Grabner, H. (1986) Approach to a Hospital-Based Application of the Medical Expert System CADIAG-2. *Medical Informatics* 11, 205–223.

[4] Arnett, F. C., Edworthy, St. M., Bloch, D. A., McShane, D. J., Fries, J. F., Cooper, N. S., Healey, L. A., Kaplan, St. R., Liang, M. H., Luthra, H. S., Medsger, Jr., Th. A., Mitchell, D. A., Neustadt, D. A., Pinals, R. S., Schaller, J. G., Sharp, J. T., Wilder, R. L. & Hunder, G. G. (1988) The American Rheumatism Association 1987 Revised Criteria for the Classification of Rheumatoid Arthritis. *Arthritis and Rheumatism* 33, 315–324.

[5] Kolarz, G. & Adlassnig, K.-P. (1986) Problems in Establishing the Medical Expert Systems CADIAG-1 and CADIAG-2 in Rheumatology. *Journal of Medical Systems* 10, 395–405.

[6] Ropes, M. W., Bennett, G. A., Cobb, S., Jacox, R. & Jassar, R. A. (1958) Revision of Diagnostic Criteria for Rheumatoid Arthritis. *Bulletin on Rheumatic Diseases* 9, 175–177.

[7] Steinbrocker, O., Traeger, C.H., & Batterman, R.C. (1949) Therapeutic Criteria in Rheumatoid Arthritis. *The Journal of the American Medical Association* 140, 659–662.

Knowledge Acquisition in Medicine: Enforcing Consistency

Dario A. Giuse[1,2], Nunzia Bettinsoli Giuse[1], Randolph A. Miller[1]

1 Section of Medical Informatics, Department of Medicine, University of Pittsburgh
2 Robotics Institute, Carnegie Mellon University
Pittsburgh, PA 15213 - U.S.A.

Abstract: Some aspects of knowledge base creation can be partially or completely automated, resulting in higher quality and smaller effort. Computer assistance is particularly valuable in ensuring the internal consistency of a knowledge base. The paper describes several techniques for consistency enforcement in QMR-KAT, an interactive knowledge base editor for the INTERNIST-I/QMR medical knowledge base. Two strategies which improve consistency are applicable to a wide range of situations. The first strategy prevents simple (but common) inconsistencies. The second strategy reveals facts that are potentially (but not necessarily) inconsistent with known data, and may require further evaluation. Both strategies use the contents of an existing knowledge base in the evaluation of new facts.

1. Introduction

Medical knowledge bases are computer-readable collections of medical facts. Knowledge bases are an integral component of most medical decision-support systems [5]. Major medical knowledge bases represent the contributions of several individuals, and are produced with significant investments of time and effort.

The information used in constructing a medical knowledge base ranges from the clinical expertise of individuals to peer-reviewed medical publications. An important issue connected with knowledge base creation and maintenance is that of consistency. Computer assistance can be quite valuable for this purpose, since a program can check large amounts of data in a short time. This paper describes some of the techniques used in QMR-KAT [1], an interactive knowledge editor program for the QMR knowledge base.

QMR [3] [4] [6] is a medical decision support system for internal medicine. The QMR knowledge base contains the detailed descriptions of more than 600 diseases. A *disease profile*

---

[1]The research described in this document was supported in part by the National Library of Medicine, Research Grant no. R01 LM04622.

is the description of a disease in terms of its manifestations (called *findings*) and its relations to other diseases (*links*). The structure of the INTERNIST-I/QMR KB has been described in detail elsewhere [2].

While the original INTERNIST-I profiles were created manually, in the last couple of years all disease profiles have been created via QMR-KAT, an interactive knowledge acquisition program. QMR-KAT uses a combination of menus, dialog boxes, and direct editing techniques. It allows physicians to create new disease profiles interactively.

In addition to its role for knowledge acquisition, QMR-KAT ensures the consistency of the knowledge base. This is done incrementally, as individual facts are added, rather than *post facto*. This strategy is not difficult to implement efficiently, and is most helpful to the user because it detects (or prevents!) errors at a very early stage, when they are easiest to handle.

2. Consistency Enforcement in QMR-KAT

An important technique for enforcing consistency is to prevent users from entering inconsistent information. QMR-KAT uses this technique as much as possible. It does so by relying on knowledge about the structure of the knowledge base, and by using the existing knowledge base as a guideline for consistency checking.

Static Knowledge Base Constraints

The user interface of the program enforces the built-in constraints imposed by the QMR knowledge base. This kind of consistency enforcement is static, in the sense that its behavior depends purely on the structure of the knowledge base, rather than on its actual contents.

QMR frequency numbers, for example, describe how often a finding is seen in patients with a certain disease (i.e., they indicate the sensitivity of the finding for the diagnosis). A frequency number must be an integer between 1 and 5, inclusive. The QMR-KAT interface enforces this constraint by presenting a dialog box where only legal values can be selected. Similarly, only values between 0 and 5 are allowed for evoking strength. This interaction style, which is based on dialog boxes and only shows permissible values, is used extensively in the program interface.

Dynamic Knowledge Base Constraints

The second type of consistency enforcement, which uses the current contents of the knowledge base, is dynamic. This feature addresses a frequent cause of errors by profile creators who are less familiar with the rules of the QMR knowledge base. One rule says, for example, that once a finding is marked as *non-specific*, it must always be marked as such (non-specific findings are those which give no indication about a possible diagnosis).

When a finding is added to a new disease profile, the program consults the current knowledge base. The user is not allowed to mark as specific a finding which the knowledge base indicates as non-specific, and vice versa. Since non-specific findings are indicated by an evoking strength of zero, the program uses a dialog box which only contains the appropriate values for the evoking strength.

Heuristic Consistency Determination

A different category of consistency problems arises from failure to consider certain interactions between findings and links in a profile. It is not uncommon for more than one QMR disease to occur simultaneously in a patient. Different patterns are possible: For example, one disease may cause another disease. Such situations are handled in the QMR knowledge base via *links*. A link expresses the relationship between one disease and another.

Whenever links are created, one must carefully distinguish between findings that properly belong to the disease being profiled and other findings which might occur through a linked disease. If a finding is caused by a linked disease, but not by the disease being profiled, it should not be added to the profile. Doing so would cause "double counting" of the finding by the QMR diagnostic algorithm, possibly leading to incorrect diagnostic behavior.

A recently developed feature of QMR-KAT is aimed at preventing this type of error. This feature is heuristic, since in general it is impossible to determine exactly whether a true link/finding conflict exists. Rather than making a definite statement, this heuristic simply suggests to the user that a potential conflict might exist.

When a finding is added to a new disease profile, the heuristic checks whether the finding might also occur as part of a linked disease. If the conditions are appropriate, the program issues a warning. Note that the heuristic also works for the opposite situation: When a link is added to a new disease profile, the program checks whether some of the findings might cause a conflict.

Figure 2-1 shows an example of the behavior of this heuristic. The user, who was not aware of the potential problem, found the warning extremely useful and modified the profile accordingly. The figure shows a snapshot of the QMR-KAT display. The user has retrieved a list of QMR findings in the left-hand window, and has just attempted to add the finding "FECES FAT OTR THAN 7 GRAM <S> PER DAY" to the disease profile being constructed in the window on the right.

The pop-up window at the top shows the effect of the heuristic. The heuristic determines that a potential conflict would arise by adding the finding, since the QMR disease "MALABSORPTION" was already linked to the disease being profiled. The user is then given the option to accept or reject the suggestion. The suggestion from the heuristic is very relevant in this particular example, since the QMR entity "MALABSORPTION" is often used in the knowledge base as a marker for a condition of steatorrhea, which is what the profile creator intended to indicate.

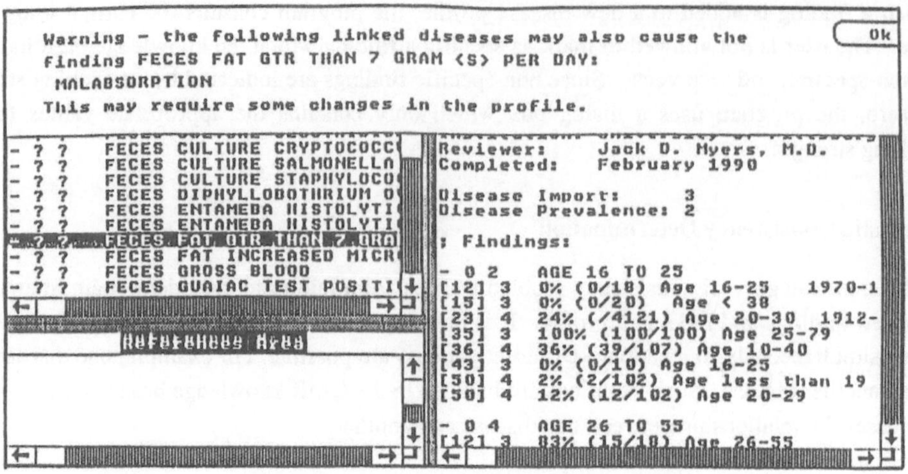

```
Warning - the following linked diseases may also cause the        ( Ok )
finding FECES FAT GTR THAN 7 GRAM <S> PER DAY:
  MALABSORPTION
This may require some changes in the profile.

- ? ?    FECES CULTURE CRYPTOCOCC(    Reviewer:      Jack D. Myers, M.D.
- ? ?    FECES CULTURE SALMONELLA     Completed:     February 1990
- ? ?    FECES CULTURE STAPHYLOCO(
- ? ?    FECES DIPHYLLOBOTHRIUM O(    Disease Import:     3
- ? ?    FECES ENTAMEBA HISTOLYTI(    Disease Prevalence: 2
- ? ?    FECES ENTAMEBA HISTOLYTI(
- ? ? .. FECES FAT GTR THAN 7 GRA     : Findings:
- ? ?    FECES FAT INCREASED MICR(
- ? ?    FECES GROSS BLOOD            - 0 2       AGE 16 TO 25
- ? ?    FECES GUAIAC TEST POSITI(+   [12] 3    0% (0/18) Age 16-25      1970-1
←                                →    [15] 3    0% (0/20)  Age < 38
                                      [23] 4    24% (/4121) Age 20-30  1912-
           References Area            [35] 3    100% (100/100) Age 25-79
                                   ↑  [36] 4    36% (39/107) Age 10-40
                                      [43] 3    0% (0/10) Age 16-25
                                      [50] 4    2% (2/102) Age less than 19
                                      [50] 4    12% (12/102) Age 20-29

                                   ↓  - 0 4       AGE 26 TO 55
←                                →    [121] 3   83% (15/18) Age 26-55    →
```

Figure 2-1: Warning the user about possible conflicts between findings and links.

This heuristic attempts to be selective. Demographic conditions are never flagged as potential problems. All QMR diseases, for example, contain findings which describe age and sex of the patient population. The heuristic immediately discards such findings. A scoring algorithm is also used to eliminate findings that are very unlikely to cause potential conflicts. The algorithm uses a combination of the import of the finding and its evoking strength. This algorithm tends to concentrate on "important" findings and discard those which happen infrequently enough that a warning would not be justified. Whenever a reasonable doubt exists, however, the heuristic will issue a warning, under the assumption that it is better for the disease profile creator to be alerted of these situations as early as possible.

3. Future Directions

In addition to the consistency enforcement techniques described above, many other approaches are possible. We have recently begun to experiment with new ideas, with the goal of developing techniques that can simplify the users' task even further.

One technique which is planned for implementation is also based on a heuristic. This heuristic can suggest possible frequency numbers for a finding or a link, based on numerical data entered as supporting evidence. Based on a study of the fifteen most recent disease profiles, we have developed different heuristics which attempt to approximate the ''correct'' frequency number. The best heuristics in this class suggest the correct frequency in 90% of the cases where enough evidence is available. It is evident that this technique could be valuable in improving the inter-subject consistency of frequency numbers.

Another idea is enforcement of consistent terminology in the naming of new findings. When new disease profiles are created, it is sometimes necessary to create new findings (i.e., findings that are not yet present in the QMR knowledge base). A well established set of conventions is used when naming new findings, and it might be possible to have the program enforce these conventions and suggest the appropriate wording to the user.

Finally, we are evaluating new techniques to detect inconsistencies by using QMR properties, which express logical relations among findings. A property, for example, might specify that a finding is logically implied by the presence of others. It seems that building the transitive closures of certain properties might enable the program to detect inconsistencies and missing connections. More work is needed to determine whether this technique would provide valuable information.

Bibliography

[1]   Giuse, D.A.; Giuse, N.B.; Miller, R.A.
        Towards Computer Assisted Maintenance of Medical Knowledge Bases.
        Artificial Intelligence in Medicine 2(1):21-33, March, 1990.

[2]   Masarie, F.E.; Miller, R.A.; Myers, J.D.
        INTERNIST-1 Properties: Representing Common Sense and Good Medical Practice in a
           Computerized Medical Knowledge Base.
        Computers and Biomedical Research 18:458-479, 1985.

[3]   Miller, R.A.; and Masarie, F.E.
        The Demise of the "Greek Oracle" Model for Medical Diagnostic Systems.
        Methods of Information in Medicine 29(1), 1990.

[4]   Miller R.A. and Masarie, Jr. F.E.
        Quick Medical Reference (QMR): A Microcomputer-Based Diagnostic Decision-Support
           System for General Internal Medicine.
        In *Proceedings of the Fourteenth Annual Symposium on Computer Applications in
           Medical Care (SCAMC)*, pages 986-988. IEEE Press, Washington, D.C., 1990.

[5]   Miller, R.A. and Giuse, N.B.
        Medical Knowledge Bases.
        Academic Medicine , January, 1991.

[6]   Miller, R.A.; McNeil, M.A.; Challinor, S.M.; Masarie, F.E., Myers, J.D.
        The INTERNIST-1/Quick Medical Reference Project - Status Report.
        The Western Journal of Medicine 145:816-822, December, 1986.

Medical Knowledge Base Consistency Checking and Its Application to CADIAG-1/BIN

Wolfgang Moser[†], Klaus-Peter Adlassnig[‡]

[†]GSF-Forschungszentrum für Umwelt und Gesundheit GmbH
Institut für Medizinische Informatik und Systemforschung
Ingolstädter Landstrasse 1, D-8042 Neuherberg, Germany
and
[‡]Universität Wien
Institut für Medizinische Computerwissenschaften
Garnisongasse 13, A-1090 Wien, Austria

Abstract

Knowledge bases of medical expert systems have grown to such an extent that formal methods to verify their consistency seem highly desirable; otherwise, decision results of such expert systems are not reliable and contradictory entries in the knowledge base may even cause totally erroneous conclusions.

This paper presents a new formalization of the finding/finding, finding/disease, and disease/disease relationships of the medical expert system CADIAG-1. This formalization also helps to clarify the differences between the application of propositional logic and of quantificational logic to capture the meaning of some fundamental categorical relationships in the area of medical diagnostics. Moreover, this formalization leads to a very simple yet provable correct and complete algorithm to check the consistency of a medical knowledge base containing a set of these relationships.

1 Introduction

CADIAG-1's knowledge base [1] consists largely of binary finding/finding, finding/disease, and disease/disease relationships. This part of the system, hereafter called CADIAG-1/BIN, contains at present more than 50.000 relationships of this type. Because of this enormous quantity of medical relationships provided by several medical experts, a formal algorithm to check their logical consistency seems highly desirable.

Although such an algorithm has already been presented in [3], a reworking of the underlying formalization seems to be necessary because this algorithm turned out to be incomplete for the detection of *all* possible inconsistencies [5].

After providing an informal account of CADIAG-1/BIN's relationships, some differences between the interpretation of these relationships in terms of propositional and quantificational logic are highlighted. This discussion helps to motivate a new formalization of these relationships which leads directly to a remarkably simple and efficient algorithm for correct and complete consistency checking.

2 Relationships in CADIAG-1/BIN

In CADIAG-1/BIN, two aspects of the relationship between two medical entities E_i and E_j (e.g., symptoms, signs, test results, and diseases) occurring at the same time in a patient are taken into account: (a) the necessity of occurrence of E_i with E_j and (b) the sufficiency of occurrence of E_i to conclude E_j. These two aspects are combined, yielding the following five types of relationships as was proposed in [7]:

1. E_i oc E_j (*obligatory occurrence* and *confirmation*):
   the occurrence of E_i is *necessary* and *sufficient* for the occurrence of E_j in a patient.

2. E_i on E_j (*obligatory occurrence* and *non-confirmation*):
   the occurrence of E_i is *necessary*, but *not sufficient* for the occurrence of E_j in a patient.

3. E_i fc E_j (*facultative occurrence* and *confirmation*):
   the occurrence of E_i is *not necessary*, yet *sufficient* for the occurrence of E_j in a patient.

4. E_i ex E_j (*exclusion*):
   the occurrence of E_i is *not necessary* and *not sufficient* for the occurrence of E_j, yet *sufficient* for the absence of E_j in a patient.

5. E_i fn E_j (*facultative occurrence* and *non-confirmation*):
   the occurrence of E_i is neither *necessary*, nor *sufficient* for the occurrence of E_j, nor *sufficient* for the absence of E_j in a patient.

3 Meaning of the Relationships

By giving informal meaning to the five types of relationships in terms of necessity of occurrence and sufficiency of occurrence, one is tempted to translate these relationships directly into propositional logic. In formalizing (a) "E_i is necessary for E_j" by the implication $\neg e_i \rightarrow \neg e_j$, which is logically equivalent to $e_j \rightarrow e_i$; and (b) "E_i is sufficient for E_j" by $e_i \rightarrow e_j$, the following formal characterization of the relationships is obtained:

1. E_i oc E_j: $e_i \rightarrow e_j \wedge e_j \rightarrow e_i$.
2. E_i on E_j: $e_j \rightarrow e_i$.
3. E_i fc E_j: $e_i \rightarrow e_j$.
4. E_i ex E_j: $e_i \rightarrow \neg e_j$.
5. E_i fn E_j: no formula.

This formalization seems intuitively appealing. It captures what might be concluded from these types of relationships for a single patient.

Consider a knowledge base consisting of the single, validated entry E_i fc E_j. If E_i is present in a patient, e_i is added to the working memory. From e_i and $e_i \rightarrow e_j$, a single application of the modus ponens inference rule derives e_j; thus E_j must occur in this patient, too. However, if E_i is absent in a patient, $\neg e_i$ is added to the working memory, from which neither e_j nor $\neg e_j$ can be derived. Therefore, neither the occurrence nor the absence of E_j in this patient can be concluded in this situation.

Although this formalization leads to intuitively correct conclusions in cases of a single patient, it is too weak to grasp the full meaning of the above-mentioned medical relationships. It is not clear at all, how one should deal with the fn relationships during consistency checking. Another consequence of this formalization for example is that E_i fc E_j is logically entailed by E_i oc E_j.

However, these relationships intuitively contradict each other, because facultative occurrence is supposed to be complementary to obligatory occurrence. These examples indicate that a procedure to test the consistency of CADIAG-1/BIN's knowledge base cannot be built upon this formalization.

Nor are these limitations overcome by adding the corresponding formulas for "not necessary" and "not sufficient" to the above formalization. In fact, this extension results in an inconsistent set of formulas. The formalization of E_i fn E_j yields $\neg(e_i \to e_j) \wedge \neg(e_j \to e_i) \wedge \neg(e_i \to \neg e_j)$. The first two implications of this conjunction already constitute a contradiction. An inconsistent set of formulas is obviously no sensible candidate to attach formal meaning to the relationships.

The failure to give a formal account of these relationships in propositional logic can be traced back to two closely related misconceptions: (a) the actual domain of interpretation of these relationships; and (b) the role of the implication sign in modelling empirical knowledge.

The propositional formalization allows to draw reasonable conclusions for a single patient, while assuming, however, that the respective relationships can be applied to any patient. In this respect the propositional implication $e_i \to e_j$ is an instantiation for an individual patient of an actually universally quantified implication $\forall X (e_i(X) \to e_j(X))$, where the variable X ranges over all patients.

The merits of changing to a formalization in quantificational logic, and thus from interpretations about a single patient to interpretations about a set of patients, become apparent in the analysis of the relationship E_i fc E_j. This relationship does not refer to a single patient at all. If the occurrence of E_i is not necessary but sufficient for the occurrence of E_j in a patient, at least two different groups of patients must exist: (a) a first group of patients having E_j, but not E_i; and (b) a second group consisting of patients all having E_i. Moreover, all patients in the second group must exhibit E_j as well. It is impossible to claim E_i fc E_j to be true when considering only one single patient.

To ensure that these groups of patients really exist, the corresponding sets of patients have to be non-empty. If one group is allowed to be the empty set, these interpretations refer to situations where the corresponding combination of entities is not present in any patient and therefore unobservable. Obviously the relationships express empirical knowledge that is not justified by non-existing patients but based on observable evidence. To protect against such possible misinterpretations, the formalization must be extended by appropriate existentially quantified formulas. Because the implication $\forall X (e_i(X) \to e_j(X))$ is true even in the case where its premise is false for every X and e_i therefore denotes the empty set, the addition of the existentially quantified formulas is absolutely necessary to ensure the correct meaning of these relationships.

Putting things together, E_i fc E_j can be characterized by the formula $\forall X (e_i(X) \to e_j(X)) \wedge \exists Y \, e_i(Y) \wedge \exists Z \, (\neg e_i(Z) \wedge e_j(Z))$. With this formalization at hand it becomes clear why interpreting the fc relationship as the propositional implication $e_i \to e_j$ was so appealing. By instantiating the quantificational formula for a single patient, only this part of the instantiated formula is able to actually provide additional information for a patient, namely the occurrence of E_j simultaneously to E_i. Nevertheless, the relationship itself is not a statement about a single patient but about a set of patients.

Instead of presenting the formulas for the other relationships as well, the above discussion is graphically summarized by Venn diagrams [6] in Figure 1. A cross indicates that the corresponding subset should not be empty and a hatched region marks a definitely empty subset. As can be seen from the fc relationship, it is easy to translate a Venn diagram directly into quantificational logic using the one-place (monadic) predicate symbol e_i for the corresponding entity E_i. If CADIAG-1/BIN's knowledge base is formalized in this way, we will end up with a set of formulas denoted by F_m.

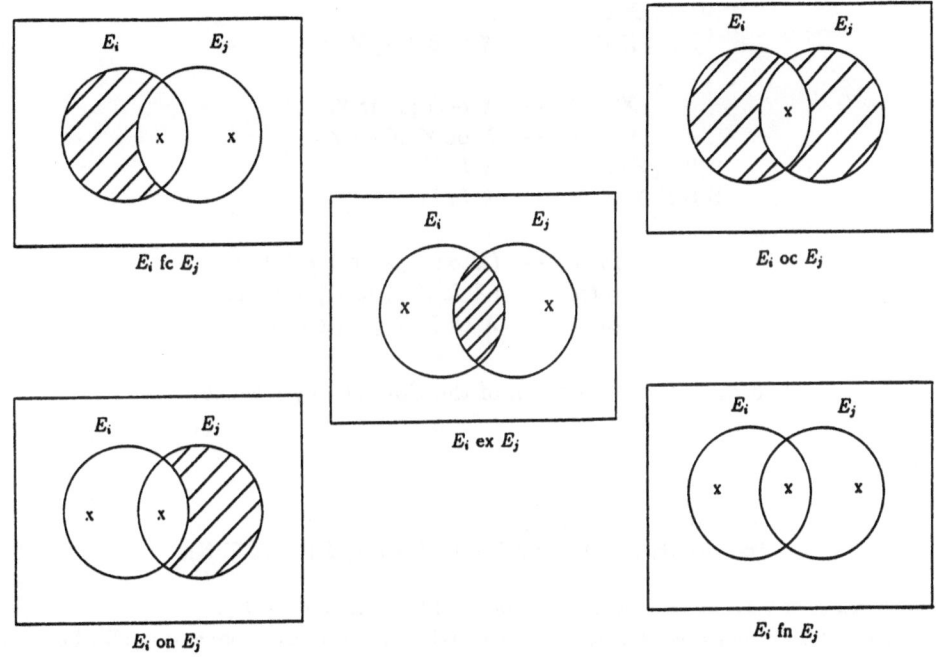

Figure 1: CADIAG-1/BIN's Relationships as Venn Diagrams.

4 A simple formalization

In formalizing the relationships between medical entities in terms of logical relationships between predicate symbols we provide—from a logical point of view—definitions of the five types of relationships in terms of second-order predicate logic.

The question may arise whether it is possible to give an equivalent formalization of these relationships directly in first-order logic, where (a) the relationships are represented themselves by predicate symbols; and (b) the entities are denoted by constant symbols rather than predicate symbols. Such a formalization would have the great advantage to be directly applicable to CADIAG-1/BIN's knowledge base without all relationships having to be translated into a set of logical formulas first.

For the formalization in first-order logic, we introduce the new two-place predicate symbol $\sqsubseteq$. The intended interpretation of $e_i \sqsubseteq e_j$ is that E_i is a subset of E_j.

Bearing this intended interpretation in mind, the following equivalences should be self-evident:

$$\forall X \forall Y \, (X \text{ oc } Y \equiv \ X \sqsubseteq Y \wedge Y \sqsubseteq X).$$
$$\forall X \forall Y \, (X \text{ on } Y \equiv \ \neg X \sqsubseteq Y \wedge Y \sqsubseteq X).$$
$$\forall X \forall Y \, (X \text{ fc } Y \equiv \ X \sqsubseteq Y \wedge \neg Y \sqsubseteq X).$$
$$\forall X \forall Y (X \text{ ex } Y \equiv \ \neg \exists Z \, (Z \sqsubseteq X \wedge Z \sqsubseteq Y)).$$
$$\forall X \forall Y \, (X \text{ fn } Y \equiv \ \neg X \sqsubseteq Y \wedge \neg Y \sqsubseteq X \wedge \exists Z \, (Z \sqsubseteq X \wedge Z \sqsubseteq Y)).$$

Formally however, $\sqsubseteq$ is not different from any other predicate symbol in that it can be interpreted in arbitrary ways. By providing the following two axioms, we limit its possible

$$X \sqsubseteq X \quad \leftarrow \quad .$$
$$X \sqsubseteq Y \quad \leftarrow \quad X \sqsubseteq Z, Z \sqsubseteq Y.$$

$$X \sqsubseteq Y \quad \leftarrow \quad X \text{ oc } Y; X \text{ fc } Y.$$
$$Y \sqsubseteq X \quad \leftarrow \quad X \text{ oc } Y; X \text{ on } Y.$$
$$@f(X,Y) \sqsubseteq X \quad \leftarrow \quad X \text{ fn } Y.$$
$$@f(X,Y) \sqsubseteq Y \quad \leftarrow \quad X \text{ fn } Y.$$

$$false \quad \leftarrow \quad (X \text{ on } Y; X \text{ fn } Y), X \sqsubseteq Y.$$
$$false \quad \leftarrow \quad (X \text{ fc } Y; X \text{ fn } Y), Y \sqsubseteq X.$$
$$false \quad \leftarrow \quad X \text{ ex } Y, Z \sqsubseteq X, Z \sqsubseteq Y.$$

Figure 2: Specification of the Consistency Checker.

interpretations:

Reflexivity : $\forall X (X \sqsubseteq X)$.
Transitivity : $\forall X \forall Y \forall Z ((X \sqsubseteq Y \wedge Y \sqsubseteq Z) \rightarrow X \sqsubseteq Z)$.

A formalization of CADIAG-1/BIN in terms of $\sqsubseteq$ will be denoted by $F_\sqsubseteq$.

Although this formalization seems to be intuitively correct, it is not obvious at all whether $F_\sqsubseteq$ is inconsistent if and only if CADIAG-1/BIN's corresponding formalization in monadic predicate logic F_m is inconsistent. But fortunately the following theorem can be established [5]:

Theorem 1 F_m *has a model if and only if $F_\sqsubseteq$ has a model.*

As a set of formulas has then no model if and only if the set of formulas is inconsistent, $F_\sqsubseteq$ and F_m are proved to be equivalent with respect to consistency.

5 Consistency Checking

For consistency checking, the relationships between the medical entities in the knowledge base are given in advance. Therefore we are only interested in the left to right direction of the above equivalences of our medical relationships. Transforming these formulas into a set of clauses, where skolemization introduces the new two-place function symbol $@f$, yields a set of horn clauses. Replacing each goal $\leftarrow G$ in this set by a new rule $false \leftarrow G$ results in a set of definite horn clauses equivalent to the PROLOG program depicted in Figure 2 [8].

CADIAG-1/BIN's knowledge base is inconsistent if and only if $false \leftarrow$ is entailed by this set of clauses [5]. The first rule for $false$ should therefore be read in the following way: The underlying knowledge base is inconsistent if Xon$Y$ or Xfn$Y$ is an entry in the knowledge base and if $X \sqsubseteq Y$ is a logical consequence of the other entries. This captures precisely what intuitively constitutes a contradiction for these types of relationships.

From this set of clauses it becomes obvious that consistency checking of CADIAG-1/BIN's knowledge base is reduced to the computation of the reflexive and transitive closure of the $\sqsubseteq$ relation and the lookup of the corresponding $\sqsubseteq$ entries for the $false$ rules. If the entities are stored in a matrix, this computation takes at most time in $O(|E|^3)$, where $|E|$ denotes the number of entities in the knowledge base [4, pp. 550ff].

It should be noted that the clauses in Figure 2 have to be modified for the use with a standard PROLOG system in order to detect all possible inconsistencies. Due to PROLOG's incomplete depth-first, left to right strategy, the system will encounter an infinite loop for every cycle in the $\sqsubseteq$ relation, e.g. for every oc relationship.

6 Conclusions

The paper on hand presents a new formalization of the five types of relationships in CADIAG-1/BIN which leads to a remarkable simple algorithm for consistency checking.

This formalization was only possible by realizing that any knowledge base generally claims statements about different sets of patients to be true. What is true of a single patient is a logical consequence of the placement of this patient within these sets. Hence, only a formalization in quantificational logic as opposed to propositional logic suffices to capture this situation.

Based on this formalization, a program was developed to check the consistency of CADIAG-1/BIN's knowledge base. On the first run, it detected 17 inconsistencies which could be corrected subsequently.

Furthermore, a suitable mapping of binary relationships of some medical expert systems (such as QMR [2]) into the relationship categories of CADIAG-1 makes the developed consistency checking algorithm a broadly applicable one.

References

[1] K.-P. Adlassnig, G. Kolarz, G. Scheithauer, W. Effenberger, and G. Grabner. CADIAG: Approaches to Computer-Assisted Medical Diagnosis. *Comp. Biol. Med.*, 15: 315–335, 1985.

[2] R.A. Bankowitz, M.A. McNeil, S.M. Challinor, R.C Parker, W.N. Kapoor, and R.A. Miller. A Computer-Assisted Medical Diagnostic Consultation Service. *Annals of Internal Medicine*, 110: 824–832, 1989.

[3] F. Barachini and K.-P. Adlassnig. CONSDED: Medical Knowledge Base Consistency Checking. In *Proc. Medical Informatics Europe 87*, Rome, 974–980, 1987.

[4] T.H. Cormen, C.E. Leiserson, and R.L. Rivest. *Introduction to Algorithms*. The MIT Press, Cambridge, Massachusetts, 1990.

[5] W. Moser. *Konsistenzprüfung einer medizinischen Wissensbasis*. Diplomarbeit, Studiengang Medizinische Informatik, Universität Heidelberg und Fachhochschule Heilbronn, Heilbronn, 1990.

[6] W.V.O. Quine. *Methods of Logic*. Holt, Rinehart and Wilson, New York, 1964.

[7] W. Spindelberger and G. Grabner. Ein Computer-Verfahren zur diagnostischen Hilfestellung. In K. Fellinger (Hrsg.) *Computer in der Medizin — Probleme, Erfahrungen, Projekte*. Brüder Hollinek, Wien, 189–221, 1968.

[8] L. Sterling and E. Shapiro. *The Art of Prolog*. The MIT Press, Cambridge, Massachusetts, 1986.

ASSOCIATIVE MEMORIES IN MEDICAL DIAGNOSTIC

J. M. Barreto*, F. de Azevedo**§, C. I. Zanchin**, L. R. Epprecht***§§
*Lab. of Neurophysiology. & Lab. of Control Systems,
Université Catholique de Louvain (UCL), Belgium
**Dept. Eng. Elétrica, Universidade Federal de Santa Catarina (UFSC), Brazil
***Dept. de Medicina Geral, Universidade do Rio de Janeiro (UNIRIO), Brazil

ABSTRACT

Neural networks are used as associative memories to build an expert system for diagnostic. Similarly to expert systems implemented using symbolic manipulation, here the knowledge is introduced by a knowledge engineer using a collection of known cases. Fuzzy sets are used as interpretation for connection values and/or excitation state of units. The main result is that the proposed neural network allows not only to find a solution in some cases, but also to suggest to obtain more clinical data if the data available is insufficient to conclude. To illustrate the approach the case of two diseases with similar symptoms (difficult diagnostic) are presented.

INTRODUCTION

Traditional expert systems are sometimes not very well suited to deal with real world problems, due to its inconsistencies, exceptions to the rules and incomplete specifications. Medical diagnosis involves these difficulties and more: a good diagnostic is often achieved by similarity with previous studied cases, where imprecision is pervasive.

It is possible to identify two types of domains where an expert system can actuate: man made (artificial) domains and natural domains. Examples are respectively computer aided design and medical diagnosis. In the first case the functioning of the system is known because it is man made. In the other the functioning is known only partially, as result of research and most knowledge derives from particular cases observed. If in the first case, rules of type IF...THEN...ELSE are natural, in the other, they are not: it is necessary to extract the structure of the causal reasoning from examples and to arrive at conclusions by analogy. Neural networks can be considered as a good programming paradigm in these ill defined cases [1], where the knowledge is available by examples and inferences taken by analogy. Some previous neural networks were used in the medical diagnostic field. Without being exhaustive, it is possible to mention the work of

§ Presently in "Institut d'Informatique, FUNDP, Namur, Belgium, sponsored by CNPq (Conselho Nacional de Desenvolvimento Científico e Tecnológico"), Brazil.

§§ Presently in "Clinique Universitaire Mont Godinne" - UCL, Belgium, sponsored by UNIRIO in Brazil.

Gallant (1988) that considered 6 symptoms and two diseases and using a feedforward network showed how explanations can be obtained. He trained the network to learn associations between symptoms and diagnostic. After presenting a set of symptoms it is possible to get the corresponding diagnostic. This approach was followed by some other researchers, for example [4,7].

Here a different approach is followed. The paradigm of associative memories in medical diagnosis is considered. The available cases are represented directly by weights of connections between units representing symptoms, diseases and names of the corresponding patients. The intensity of connections is a number in the interval [-1 1] representing the fuzzy value of importance of symptom or degree of illness, [-1 0] standing for inhibition and [0 1] for excitation. A consultation is done by exciting a particular element and corresponding symptoms. To test the approach a difficult case was chosen: a case where it is difficult to arrive easily to a conclusion.

STRUCTURE OF THE NEURAL NETWORK

The network (Fig.1) has neurones grouped in three pools. They represent respectively the diseases, the symptoms and particular patients (localized knowledge representation). This knowledge and the convenient values of connections constitutes the knowledge base with which inferences about a different patient will be done. All units are supposed visible. The connections are all bi-directional, as the network considered by Kosho [4].

No connection internal to the disease pool is completely inhibitory. A patient can present two diseases. Diseases that can occur simultaneously have low inhibitory connection between them. Between the units representing the patients there is maximum inhibition - each patient is an isolated case. This leads to a competition and the system is driven to find a similar case to the case whose diagnostic is desired. In the pool of symptoms, (not mutually exclusive), the connections are set to 0 representing ignorance.

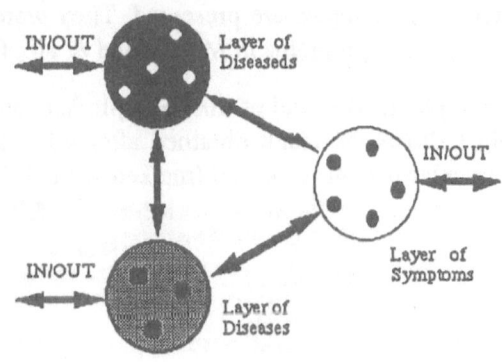

Fig.1 Structure of the Neural Network used

The particular case used in this work to exemplify and study the approach considers 2 diseases, 14 symptoms and 12 patients forming 12 known cases.

• The diseases are: Rheumatoid Arthritis - Adult Form (RA) and Systemic Lupus Erythematosus (SLE). RA is a chronic inflammatory disease of unknown etiology. It is a common disease affecting about 1.5% of the population in North America. It may occur at any age, but most often strikes between the ages of 20 and 60, with a peak incidence in women from 40 to 60. Women are affected more frequently than men, the ratio being about 3:1. SLE is a chronic, inflammatory disease of unknown cause affecting skin, joints, kidneys, nervous system and often other organs of the body.

This one, if less frequent than RA, affects essentially the same population. As they have similar symptomatology in the initial phase of disease development, a correct diagnosis is difficult if based exclusively in clinical data, except if specific symptoms of each disease are present. However these specific symptoms appear generally in a latter phase. However the use of laboratory examinations generally give sufficient data for a diagnosis.

- The following symptoms were considered: Fever, Arthralgia, Arthritis, Morning Stiffness, Myalgia, Subcutaneous Nodules, Butterfly Rash, Raynaud's Phenomenon, Photosensitivity, Alopecia, Renal Manifestations, Central Nervous System Manifestations, Pulmonary Manifestations and Rheumatoid Hand. No speculation about possible relation between symptoms is made.
- The cases considered were in number of 12 (real patients), 6 of them with a RA diagnostic and the 6 others with a SLE diagnostic.

The data described was used to build a synaptic matrix representing the relations between units of a pool and between two different pools. In these synaptic matrix, the membership values representing the several fuzzy membership were considered, expressing a clinical classification. All connections are symmetric and no unit is connected to itself. This implies a symmetric matrix with null main diagonal. This choice implies that the equilibrium points of the neural network are stable [2].

RESULTS

Here two examples are presented. They were programmed taking as starting point the collection of programs in McClelland & all., (1988) [6].

Example 1: The goal of this example is to show the structure of the data.
Fig.2 shows the result obtained after 40 cycles when the neurone corresponding to a particular patient is excited (marked with: **).

```
0 Rheumatoid_Arthritis      68    cycle  40
0 Lupus_Erythematosus       77

0 Fever                     23    0 Anne          70
0 Arthralgia                57    0 Helen         68
0 Arthritis                 32    0 Mary          68
0 Morning_Stiffness         46    0 Susan         68
0 Myalgia                   30    0 Lucy          65
0 Subcutaneous_Nodules      10    0 Carol         65
0 Butterfly_Rash            62    ** Pat          82
0 Raynaud's_Phenomenon      48    0 Jackie         5
0 Photosensitivity          23    0 Sue          33
0 Alopecia                  47    0 Beth          5
0 Renals_Manifestations     15    0 Linda        31
0 CNS_Manifestations        15    0 Mag          31
0 Pulmonary_Manifestations   3
0 Rheumatoid_Hand           46    0 Patient       68
```

Fig.2 Final screen for a particular case of the data base

It is possible to remark:

- In the data base "Pat" is associated with Arthralgia, Raynaud's Phenomenon, Alopecia e Butterfly Rash. However, the result indicated by the stable point found by the neural

350

network indicate other symptoms of the universe of considered symptoms that are not related with this disease (negative excitation-reverse video).

- In the pool of the known cases three other cases are excited: Sue, Mag & Beth. This indicate a similar symptomatology, and the degree of excitation is the fuzzy membership value of this degree of similarity.
- The diagnosis given by the network is really an stable point. This was verified by observation of the transient of excitation levels of neurons.

Example 2: A consultation

Let us consider a patient with two symptoms: Arthralgia and Arthritis. These two symptoms are not sufficient to a diagnostic, as shown in Fig.3, where the equilibrium point of the network is attained with both diseases excited. Fig.4 shows the transient of the values of excitation of the units representing the two diseases and it is possible to see that really the steady state was attained. So it is necessary some supplementary information. However as the symptomatology is very similar in these two cases, a choice must be done, because a new symptom can not be sufficient to make the selection between the two diseases.

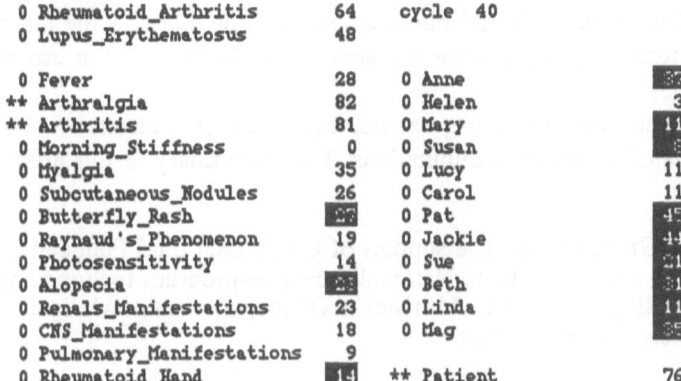

0 Rheumatoid_Arthritis	64	cycle	40		
0 Lupus_Erythematosus	48				
0 Fever	28	0 Anne		80	
** Arthralgia	82	0 Helen		3	
** Arthritis	81	0 Mary		11	
0 Morning_Stiffness	0	0 Susan		8	
0 Myalgia	35	0 Lucy		11	
0 Subcutaneous_Nodules	26	0 Carol		11	
0 Butterfly_Rash	27	0 Pat		45	
0 Raynaud's_Phenomenon	19	0 Jackie		44	
0 Photosensitivity	14	0 Sue		21	
0 Alopecia	22	0 Beth		31	
0 Renals_Manifestations	23	0 Linda		11	
0 CNS_Manifestations	18	0 Mag		35	
0 Pulmonary_Manifestations	9				
0 Rheumatoid_Hand	14	** Patient		76	

Fig.3 Patient with two symptoms after 40 cycles.

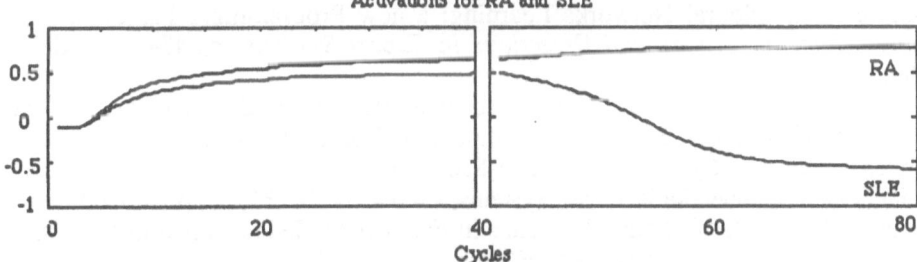

Fig.4 Transient of the activation level

Considering the universe of discussion, only three symptoms are capable of making the distinction: exactly the three presented in reverse video (Fig.3) (negative excitation!), or in a worst case a low excitation level: Butterfly Rash, Alopecia & Rheumatoid Hand. Clearly the symptoms with higher excitation are common to the two diseases and so have low discriminatory power. This is exactly the reasoning followed by a physician. After introduction of a new symptom (reumatoid hand) a new stable state is achieved in more 40 cycles indicating clearly the diagnostic.

CONCLUSIONS

The examples show the viability of the approach . However we are yet very far from real possibility of clinical use of the approach. For example, it must be remarked that the cases presented, if dealing with a difficult diagnostic, are very limited: they consider only two diseases. There are however other possibilities of diseases since Arthralgia and Arthritis are also symptoms of Arthrose, for example, and it is not considered here.

It is claimed that a neural network expert system is not capable of explaining why it arrived at a conclusion. On the contrary, traditional expert systems, generally are able to do so, by tracing the rules that were activated to produce the answer. The answer to this claim can be a higher interaction between the physician and the computer. If the physician is able to follow the transient of the neural network and interpret it the explanation of the "reasoning" becomes clear. It is natural that some training will be necessary. Will it be too difficult? For example any one that saw the interpretation of a computerized tomography or even an ecography, knows that a strong training is necessary...

Presently the system is being extended to consider 4 diseases, 17 symptoms, 24 cases and results of laboratory examinations. The preliminary results are promising.

ACKNOWLEDGEMENTS: The support of CNPq (National Foundation of Scientific Research), Brazil, and the Belgian National incentive-program for fundamental research in Artificial Intelligence, Prime Minister's Office, are acknowledge. The scientific responsibility rests with its authors.

REFERENCES

[1]–Barreto, J., "Neural Networks Learning: a new Programming Paradigm?" *ACM Inter. Conf. on Trends and Directions in Expert Systems*, pp.434-446, Orlando, Oct.31-Nov.2,.1990.

[2]–Cohen, M. A. & Grossberg, S. G., "Absolute Stability of Global Pattern Formation and Parallel Memory Storage by Competitive Neural Networks", *IEEE Trans. on Systems, Man and Cybernetics* 13: 815-826, 1983.

[3]–Gallant,S., "Connectionist expert systems, Comm. ACM, 31, 2, pp.152-169.

[4]–Kosho, B., 1987, "Adaptive Inference in Fuzzy Knowledge Networks", *Proc. First Inter. Conf. on Neural Networks*, IEEE, pp.II-261-268.

[5]–Kosko, B., 1988, "Bidirectional Associative Memories", *IEEE Trans. on Systems, Man and Cybernetics*, vol.18, 1, pp.49-60, 1988.

[6]–McClelland, J. & Rumelhart, D., *"Explorations in Parallel Distributed Processing"*, The MIT Press, 1988.

[7]–Peng, Y. & J. Reggia, "A Connectionist Model for Diagnostic Problem Solving", *IEEE Trans. on Systems, Man and Cybernetics*, vol.19, 2, pp.285-298, 1989.

USING CONNECTIONIST APPROACH FOR FINDING IDEAL CUT-OFF VALUES FOR QUANTITATIVE LABORATORY TESTS

Jari Forsström[1] and Mårten Fogström[2]

1. University of Turku, Department of Medicine, SF-20520 Turku, FINLAND
2. Åbo Akademi University, Department of Computer Science, SF-20520 Turku, FINLAND

ABSTRACT

A connectionist method is used in order to produce decision making limits for clinician from example patent data. A clinical patient material with symptoms and signs typical for Nephropathia epidemica (NE) is used as an example material. A single layer neural net was built using Minsky-Papert's perceptron algorithm. Half of the material was used for learning and half for testing. The performance of the net was measured as a correctness rate for the classification of test material. A clear improvement was detected in the performance after the optimal cut-off points were searched using the connectionist method. We conclude that with connectionist algorithm we can imitate the learning process of a clinician and produce from example cases decision making limits which correlate more or less to those learned by clinician in their work.

1. INTRODUCTION

In diagnostic tasks laboratory tests are an essential source of information. The correct interpretation of the results needs much experience and knowledge about the test used as well as about the disease which is suspected. For clinicians laboratories produce normal values which are based on a distribution from the results of healthy volunteers. This information is not very helpful in diagnostic reasoning. Many patients may have laboratory tests within the normal range but values near the end of the normal range may be significant. Also in many laboratory tests the values which are little above or below the normal range may not have any clinical significance. Clinicians learn in their work to do judgements which are more or less based on disease specific decision making limits. Because the interpretation is very much based on the whole clinical picture of the patient it has been difficult to estimate the decision making limits mathematically. The clinical diagnosis is like listening to a symphony. None of the instruments itself is enough for recognizing the music but many instruments are plaid together the music can be identified. In this study we use a connectionist method based on Minsky - Papert's perceptrons [1] for searching the decision making limits for Nephropathia epidemica (NE) which is a common viral infection in Scandinavia and in parts of Central Europe.

2. MATERIAL

The clinical picture of NE varies a lot and the disease has many signs and symptoms customary in infections and usually also symptoms of renal diseases [2-5]. The diagnosis can be confirmed with a very specific viral antibody test [6]. We collected 425 cases retrospectively from those patients where the viral antibody test had been taken. 140 of these patients had antibodies against the disease and they were classified to NE group. Other 285 cases had negative result in the antibody test and they formed the non-NE group. The definite diagnoses in the non-NE group were mainly some infections or an acute renal failure of some other reason. NE is a very suitable disease for our purpose. The viral antibody test is very sensitive and it can be used as the "golden standard method" for the diagnosis of NE. The neural net is based on clinical signs and symptoms and the antibody test is used only for classifying the patients in NE and non-NE groups. Thus, no circular reasoning occurred. We chose 27 signs and symptoms which are helpful in the clinical diagnosis of the NE (see Table 2). Sixteen of these attributes were qualitative and 11 were quantitative. For the qualitative attributes the most abnormal value obtained during the hospitalization was selected. The missing data was replaced with random values based on the distribution of values in the two groups.

3. METHODS

We programmed a single layer neural net based on Minsky-Papert's perceptrons. Each attribute constituted one input neuron. Our net did not support quantitative data and the numerical values were changed to qualitative attributes using predefined cut-off values which were based on experience of a clinician. The material was divided in two subsets: the learning set and the testing set. A more detailed description of the net is presented elsewhere [7]. The learning set was used for learning of the net. After 10 iterations the learning result was tested and success rate of 88% for NE and 88% for non-NE group was detected. After this basic result we started to search the ideal cut-off point for each quantitative attribute. We started with fever. The net was learned with the same learning set using 10 different cut-off values for the fever. After every learning phase the performance of the resulting net was tested with the testing set. From the different cut-off values we selected the one where the test gave the best results. The cut-off points were selected in the same manner for the 16 numerical attributes. Each time we used the original cut-off values for other attributes - not the tuned ones. After this searching process we replaced the original cut-off values with the ones found by the searching algorithm and the net was learned using these new cut-off values. This tuning can be iterated several times. It is supposed that the cut-off values will convergence towards the optimal decision making limit which can be used in clinical decision making.

4. RESULTS

The original cut-off values and the tuned cut-off values are shown in Table 1. The weights for the attributes in NE and non-NE net are shown in Table 2. When tested with the testing set the net using the tuned cut-off values diagnosed the NE better: correctness rate 90% for NE and 93% for non-NE group. The weights for the attributes changed remarkably after the tuning. The weights using original cut-off values are not directly comparable to those weight obtained using tuned cut-off values because the thresholds are differs between the nets. However, it can be seen although the threshold for NE net was lower in the latter nets most of the weights for the numerical attributes increased. Thus, they had much more influence on the diagnosis. The weights decreased notably after tuning only for serum proteins, thrombocytes, creatinine and fever. For creatinine the cut-off value (1660 μmol/l) was so high that none of the patients had such values. However, this cut-off level gave the best result and thus it is seen that the diagnosis can be more accurately without using the creatinine value at all.

TABLE 1. Original and tuned cut-off values for numerical attributes.

Attribute	original cut-off	tuned cut-off
Fever (°C)	38.0	39.0
CRP (mg/l)	40.0	60.5
ERS (mm/h)	30.0	78.3
Leukocytes (E9/l)	10.0	4.4
S-Creatinine (µmol/l)	100.0	1670
dU-Proteins (g/d)	0.5	5.2
Maximum DUO (ml/d)	2000	6322
Minimum DUO (ml/d)	400	50
Max DUO / Min DUO	4.0	50.7
S-Ca (mmol/l)	2.0	1.6
S-Pi (mmol/l)	2.0	3.8
S-Proteins (g/l)	60.0	60.0
Thrombocytes (E9/l)	100.0	26
Hematuria (Scale 0-3)	1.0	0.5
Heart rate (1/min)	60.0	84.0
Systolic BP (mmHg)	100.0	60.0

Abbreviations: ESR = Erythrocyte sedimentation rate, CRP = C-reactive protein, DUO = daily urinary output, BP = blood pressure.

5. DISCUSSION AND CONCLUSIONS

In clinical diagnosis experience of a clinician has an important role. The knowledge of an expert is derived from theoretical domain knowledge as well as learning from example patient cases. The background knowledge can systematically be described but the knowledge learned by the clinician is hard to formulate. However, the differences in the clinical skills of physicians is very much related to the learning from example cases. Interpretation of laboratory results is one of the clinical skills scrutinized in this study. The decision making limits for laboratory tests for different diagnoses is mainly acquired through learning from a large mount of example cases. Because there is a considerable need for such information we tried to build an "artificial clinician" using a learning algorithm based on neural computing. The aim was to find optimal decision making limit for numerical attributes. In the results it was clearly seen that the signs and symptoms were interdependent. When the net was learned using the tuned values there were considerable

TABLE 2. Weights for the attributes after learning with 10 iterations. ORIGINAL: weights when original cut-off values were used and TUNED: weights when tuned cut-off values were used. In the attributes T = the cut-off value used.

Attribute	ORIGINAL NE	not-NE	TUNED NE	not-NE
Fever (°C) ≥ T	36.4	-7.0	5.3	-11.1
Headache	12.8	-1.3	17.2	-9.9
Nausea	-23.7	19.6	24.0	-26.4
Vomitus	-37.2	17.8	-4.6	9.4
Cough or flu	-34.8	29.9	-9.3	-2.8
CRP (mg/l) < T	42.0	-35.5	32.1	-29.4
ESR (mm/h) < T	-10.1	-8.7	-18.1	34.9
Leukocytes (E9/l) < T	-18.9	4.3	-27.9	21.4
Thorax abnormal	2.9	-5.3	0.7	7.8
S-Creatinine (μmol/l) ≥ T	32.1	-20.2	0.0	0.0
dU-Proteins (g/d) ≥ T	-9.6	6.7	-17.2	29.5
Maximum DUO (ml/d) ≥ T	52.8	-51.8	-6.4	13.9
Minimum DUO (ml/d) < T	-25.9	18.5	-31.8	43.2
Max DUO / Min DUO ≥ T	-5.2	12.3	-43.6	56.1
Edema of the extremities	-35.4	40.5	-53.5	40.9
S-Ca (mmol/l) < T	22.2	-25.2	18.1	-15.4
S-Pi (mmol/l) ≥ T	2.3	-15.6	-43.0	63.7
S-Proteins (g/l) ≥ T	-42.1	46.1	-14.5	28.9
Thrombocytes (E9/l) < T	91.3	-90.9	-0.9	11.4
Hematuria (Scale 0-3) ≥ T	-19.1	13.0	0.4	-5.4
Diarrhea	-16.6	27.2	23.5	-21.7
Heart rate (1/min) < T	22.7	-30.5	3.9	-10.2
Systolic BP (mmHg) < T	-27.7	30.7	-20.1	13.1
Backache	-8.3	-0.9	-8.3	-14.0
Abdominal pain	33.5	-23.2	21.2	-19.2
Myopia for 1-5 days	79.3	-44.6	35.7	-42.8
Typical sonography	-3.6	15.6	-1.0	-2.3
Threshold	49.9	-58.4	10.3	-28.9

changes in the weights for non-numerical attributes as well. We have shown that weights obtained using the connectionist approach for this material had a good correlation to the sensitivity of each attribute for diagnosing the NE [8]. In this study the cut-off values were most often changed to a more abnormal direction. This leads to better specificity and poorer sensitivity for each test. As a result the net performed the diagnosis by finding a decision making limit with a good specificity and then combining these tests in order to get the overall conclusion. Low level of thrombocytes (below 100) in the original net showed a high diagnostic significance. After tuning the cut-off level was adjusted to 26. The weight in the NE net was negative suggesting that values below 26 is evidence against the NE. This can be interpreted so that a typical level of thrombocytes for NE patients is between about 25 and 100. Values below 25 are more typical to other diseases. In order to find this typical range of values (if there is any) for a numerical attribute we should increase the number of input nodes. Each numerical attribute should have two input nodes. The other node could be adjusted to find upper limits and the other node lower limits of the diagnostic range.

The increase in the performance of our net in diagnosing the test group suggests that this approach can be of great value in finding the optimal decision making limits. This method is also very suitable for clinical practice: The decision making limits found are easy to understand for clinicians and they can be used also in expert systems based on other methods, for example probabilistic systems based on Bayes' formula.

REFERENCES

1. Minsky ML and Papert S. Perceptrons: An Essay in Computational Geometry, (The MIT Press 1969).
2. Lähdevirta J. Nephropathia epidemica in Finland: A clinical, histological and epidemiological study. Ann Clin Res 3 (Suppl 8) 1971. pp. 1-154.
3. Lähdevirta J. Clinical features of HFRS in Scandinavia as compared with East Asia. Scand J Infect Dis Suppl 36 1982, 93-95.
4. Settergren B, Juto P, Trollfors B, Wadell G and Norrby SR. Clinical characteristics of Nephropathia Epidemica In Sweden: prospective study of 74 cases, Rev Infect Dis 1989;11:921-927.
5. Cosgriff T. Hemorrhagic fever with renal syndrome: four decades of research. Annals od Internal Medicine 1989;110:313-316.
6. Lähdevirta J, Savola J, Brummer-Korvenkontio M, Berndt R, Illikainer, R and Vaheri A. Clinical and serological diagnosis of Nephropathia epidemica, the mild type of hemorrhagic fever with renal syndrome. J Infect 1984;9:230-238.
7. Eklund P, Forsström J. Diagnosis of Nephropathia Epidemica by Adaptation through Lukasiewicz inference. Computational Intelligence 90, Milano, September 24-28, 1990, in press.
8. Forsström J, Eklund P, Virtanen H, Waxlax J, Lähdevirta J. DIAGAID: A connectionist approach to determine the information value of clinical data. Artificial Intelligence in Medicine. 1991;3:XXX-XXX (in press).

EXPERT SYSTEMS—
EVALUATION

A METHODOLOGY FOR EVALUATION OF KNOWLEDGE-BASED SYSTEMS

Kevin Clarke[1], Rory O'Moore[1], Raymond Smeets[2], Jan Talmon[2], Jytte Brender[3], Peter McNair[4], Pirkko Nykanen[5], Jane Grimson[1], Barry Barber[6].

1.Dept. Computer Science and Laboratory Medicine, Trinity College, Dublin.
2.University of Limburg., Dept. of Med. Informatics and Statistics, Maastricht.
3.Computer Resources International a/s, Copenhagen.
4.Hvidovre Hospital, Dept. Clinical Chemistry, Copenhagen
5.Technical Research Centre of Finland, Med. Engineering Lab, Tampere.
6.National Health Service, Information Management Centre, Birmingham.

INTRODUCTION

Knowledge based systems (KBS) are of great potential use in medicine. However, the progress in development and actual day to day use of KBSs in medicine has been disappointing. Shortliffe (1989) believes that this is because medical decision aids are not user friendly, they do not explain their reasoning adequately, they are too time consuming to use in the actual work environment, and particularly because of physician fears of e.g. legal liability and intrusion of the systems into their practice. We believe that lack of rigorous scientific evaluation studies on KBSs is an additional factor which hinders their acceptance by the medical community (O'Moore et al, 1990 a). Evaluation should confront these and other issues, and so should contribute substantially to the diffusion of KBS technology into the clinical environment. This paper is a summary of a rigorous evaluation methodology as outlined in O'Moore et al. 1990a and 1990b, developed and experimented with (Nolan et al 1990) in the KAVAS (A1021) AIM project.

AN APPROACH TO CONTINUOUS DEVELOPMENT AND EVALUATION

Following a comprehensive review of the literature (O'Moore et al, 1990 a) and some experimentation on the transferability of KBSs (Nolan et al, 1990), we are of the opinion that both development and evaluation of KBS should be iterative with continuous cycles of development and evaluation taking place. Feedback should be sought throughout from expert collaborators and potential end-users. This feedback serves to define the major problem areas in the system's development and guides the next iteration of development/evaluation. The cycles are also guided by Wyatt's (1987) principle that the most likely reasons for failure of each phase should be anticipated and included in the evaluation methodology at each phase. In this way, if a phase of an evaluation indicates failure, the reason for the failure, the type of failure, and the consequence of the failure will be known. This should allow a focussed backtrack to the appropriate point for modification of the system. Anticipation or prediction of the reasons for failure (of any given phase in any particular system) is also useful in the selection of the relevant metrics for the evaluation of the phase.

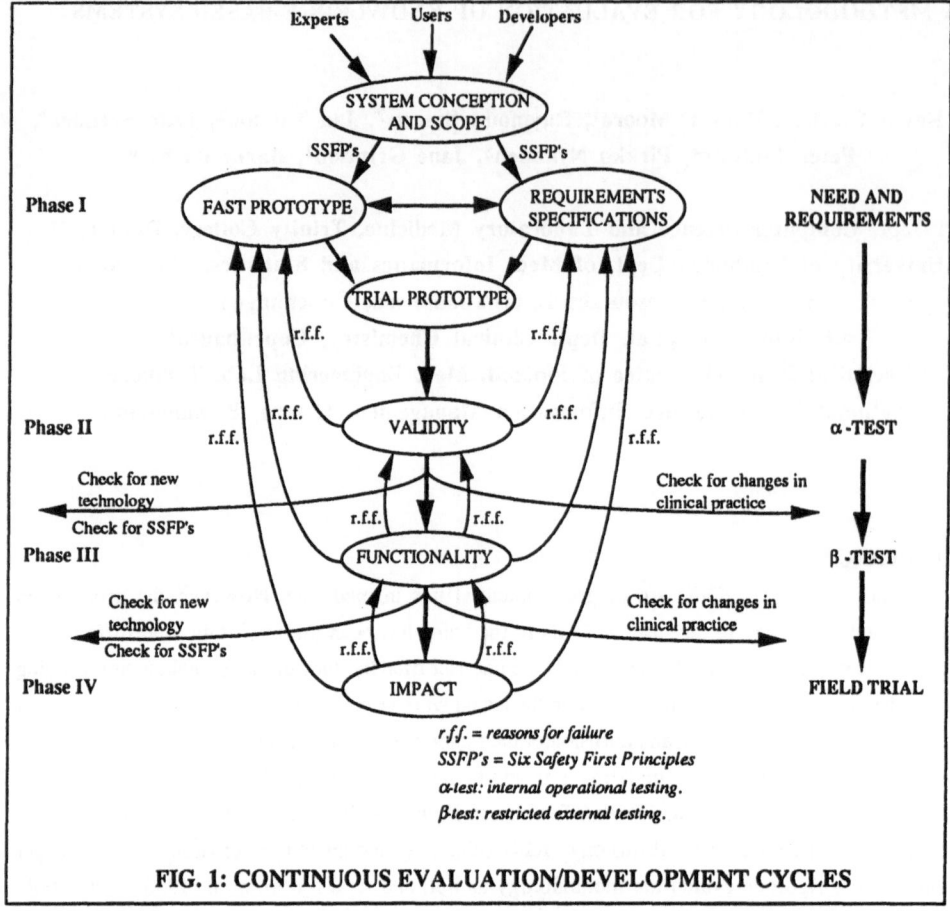

r.f.f. = reasons for failure
SSFP's = Six Safety First Principles
α-test: internal operational testing.
β-test: restricted external testing.

FIG. 1: CONTINUOUS EVALUATION/DEVELOPMENT CYCLES

Figure 1 outlines a four phased methodology for evaluating KBSs. Progress through each of these phases is guided by:

a) The results of the evaluation of the phase using the relevant metrics which have been chosen by the anticipation or prediction of the reasons for failure of the phase in question.

b) A check to determine whether changing technology may render the results invalid.

c) A check to determine whether changes in medical practice have an impact on the relevance of the evaluation results.

d) The conformation of the system to the Six Safety First Principles of Data Protection / Integrity (Barber et al, 1990).

Not all items in this formal evaluation methodology should be measured in every trial: the methodology should be tailored to the developers' own requirements. It is important to note that throughout system development, the legal aspects should be considered. Important legal questions are: who should bear the responsibility for compiling knowledge within the knowledge base, who should be responsible for applying it in prescriptive situations, and who is responsible for keeping the knowledge base up to date? We believe, because of the recent legislative initiatives throughout Europe in Data Protection / confidentiality, that the Six

Safety First Principles developed by the AIM Requirements Board (Barber et al, 1990) should be included at each appropriate stage of the evaluation of a KBS.

The First and Second Safety First Principles call for a safe and secure environment for patients and users. The Third Principle requires that the system makes few demands in terms of training effort for individuals to become effective in using it. The Fourth and Fifth Principles place demands on the modification of the legal systems within the European Community in order that the responsibility for all aspects of the development and use is unambiguously clarified, and that there is adequate legal protection of software to encourage development and marketing of systems. The Sixth Principle establishes a system requirement for multi-lingual capability so that it can be deployed effectively throughout the European Community.

PHASE I : The Early Development/Evaluation Process

Some fundamental questions should be asked before embarking on major efforts in developing a system: 1) Is there a need for the system? 2) what role is the system to play in the intended environment? 3) what kind of user is the system aimed at?

After having a systems conception (see figure 1) two approaches for further system definition may be taken, i.e. fast prototyping or specifications of detailed requirements, or a combination of the two. These two approaches have built in evaluation/development cycles (Smeets et al 1990).

Having built a prototype (from either of these methods) which is performing well on most examples, it is appropriate to progress to a more structured formal evaluation. The actual evaluation may take very different forms depending on, for example: the role the system is asked to play, the goals of the project, and the character of the domain, (Miller 1986). During formal evaluation of the suggested iterative development cycles, the major focus will be seen to shift in emphasis from the validity in the early prototype phases, through functionality of the system in its intended environment, and finally to impact as the KBS matures.

PHASE II: Validity of System.

Phase II validity of system evaluation may be seen as having two sub-phases, the first aiming at the detection of errors, the second aiming at "proving" the validity of the system (O'Moore et al 1990 b, Smeets et al 1990). The first subphase is much more aimed at **development**, the next at **application** of the system. Two issues of validity evaluation are relevant: 1) Structural validity of the knowledge base, and 2) Semantic validity of the knowledge when applied.

Structural validity: Validation of a knowledge base involves testing of the knowledge base to decide if it satisfies reliability and consistency requirements. This may be done by running many sample cases or by using tools designed for the validation of knowledge based systems. The appropriateness of the inference mechanism to the particular problem domain should also be evaluated.

Semantic Validity: In the measurement of reliability of a KBS its intended role must be considered: will it be used as a decision support system (DSS) or as an expert system. In measuring the accuracy one has to define a Gold Standard against which to compare the performance of the system. Difficulties often arise when there is no single best answer and it must be decided what is the acceptable rate of error. It is important to exclude system builders from the panel assessing the results and also to avoid testing with data used in the development of the system, in order to eliminate bias.

PHASE III: Functionality of the System

This phase is concerned with the evaluation of the DSS in the user's environment.

User Interaction: Aspects of man-machine interaction are of crucial importance when validating a DSS: it has to be established whether or not the user is able to operate the DSS correctly and with confidence. To facilitate the acceptance of the system, it is necessary that it is easy to use and does not require much special learning. The amount of required human interaction should be minimised and the work environment should be disturbed as little as possible on introduction of the system. The user should be made aware of the limits of the system's expertise. Also, the performance of the system should degrade gracefully at the edge of its application.

Broad Evaluation of the System: Transferability is the degree to which the system retains its reliability and confidence when applied in another location of the same domain (Nolan et al 1990, Schioler et al 1991). Domain features which may cause difficulties in transferability are terminological, epidemilogical, and methodological differences. Features which have an impact on the transferability of a KBS are: the knowledge representation, the theoretical framework for inferencing, and the knowledge acquisition technique.

PHASE IV: Impact of the System

The expert system may lead to permanent changes in the user's attitudes and in the whole organisation of the work environment. The long range effect may be positive, i.e. a sort of permanent educational update; or negative, i.e. a form of "acritic agreement" or perhaps boredom with the routine of a normally correct device. In order to determine the impact on patient care the population morbidity and mortality may be measured as well as looking for fewer misdiagnoses/management errors. Rossi-Mori and Ricci (1989) believe that the impact of the KBS on the health field may depend on its effects on such things as the routine management of a health service, the awareness and timeliness of the health planning, and the advancement of the medical research. A Cost benefit analysis should include the cost of purchasing the hardware and software, of educating the staff on using it, and of updating and maintaining it. This should then be weighed against the benefits from the system such as resources saved, and increase in efficiency and patient health. However, the problem in cost benefit analysis is that of attaching monetary value to ethical and legal issues. Decision aids may have side-effects which should be taken into account as part of the evaluation. Wyatt & Spiegelhalter (1990) have recommended monitoring:-

- feedback of performance and educational effects on health care personnel.
- improvement in performance of decision makers when under study.
- improvement in quality of decisions because of more complete data collection.
- the placebo effect on patients because they are getting more attention.

These should be measured in order to prove *how* the system had its effect: for example if the effect is entirely due to a more complete data collection, then a KBS was not necessary (De Dombal 1983).

CONCLUSION

It is important to note that the four phases of the methodology presented here, should not be employed in isolation from one another. The major focus of the evaluation merely shifts in emphasis from one phase to another. While carrying out an evaluation in one phase, it may be advisable / necessary to refer to issues in other phases. Broadly, the evaluation of KBSs has two purposes:

1) to guide the design of the system

2) to quantify various performance aspects of the system and to verify the acceptability of the system.
Frequently evaluation is employed in isolation, rather than as an integral part of system development. Evaluation should start at system conception to ensure a more rigorous evaluation, and also to forewarn of possible reasons for failure, thus saving time and wasted effort.

REFERENCES

Barber, B., Jensen, O.A., Lamberts, H., Roger, F.H., de Schouwer, P., Zollner, H. "The Six Safety First Principles of Health Information Systems, Computer Perspectives in Health Care - CP90, UK National Conference of Medical Informatics 2-4 April (1990), Brighton, pub. British Journal of Health Care Computing.

De Dombal, F.T. "Towards a more objective evaluation of computer aided decision support systems". In MEDINFO '83. Ed, Van Bemmel J., Ball M.J., Wigertz O. 436-439 (1983).

Miller, P.L. "Evaluation of artificial intelligence systems in medicine." Comp. Prog. Method Biomed, 22 5-11 (1986 a).

Nolan, J., McNair, P., Brender, J. "Factors Influencing the Transferability of Medical Decision Support Systems". Int J Biomed Comput, 27, 7 - 26. (1990).

O'Moore R., Clarke K., Smeets R., Brender J., Nykanen P., McNair P., Grimson J., Barber B. "Items of Relevance for the Evaluation of Knowledge Based / Expert Systems and Influence from Domain Characteristics". KAVAS (A1021) Report EM 1.1. EEC AIM Office, 62 Rue de Treves, Brussels. (1990 a).

O'Moore, R., Clarke, K., Brender. J., McNair. P., Nykanen. P., Smeets, R., Talmon, J., Grimson, J., Barber, B. "Methodology for Evaluation of Knowledge Based Systems". Technical report EM 1.2, KAVAS (A1021) Project, CEC AIM Programme, (1990 b).

Rossi-Mori, A., Ricci, F.L. "Comprehensive criteria for evaluation and design of knowledge based systems in Medicine." In System Engineering in Medicine. Ed. Talmon, J. & Fox, J. Springer Verlag (1989).

Schioler, T., Nolan, J., McNair, P. "Transferability of Knowledge Based Systems, Information Technology Factors", MIE '91.

Shortliffe, E.H. "Testing reality - the introduction of decision support technologies for physicians. Meth. Inform. Med., 28, 1 - 5 (1989).

Smeets, R.P.A.M., Talmon, J.L., O'Moore, R. "General Methodology and Problems in Assessment of Decision Support Systems". In Lecture Notes in Medical Informatics, MIE '90, Vol 40, 225-230. (1990).

Wyatt, J. "The evaluation of clinical decision support systems: a discussion of the methodology used in the ACORN project. AIME '87. Ed. Fox, J., Fieschi, M., Engelbrecht, R. Lecture notes in medical informatics 33, Springer Verlag, 229-238 (1987).

Wyatt, J., Spiegelhalter, D. "Evaluating medical decision aids: What to test, and how." In System In Medicine Eds. Talmon, J. and Fox, J. Springer Verlag 1-13 (1990).

Outcomes Assessment, Quality Assurance and Evaluation of Expert Diagnostic Systems

Christian Nøhr,
Aalborg University, Department of Development and Planning,
Fibigerstræde 2, 9220 Aalborg Ø, Denmark.

Improvement of the quality in health care and the assessment of health outcomes of medical technologies have attracted an increasing attention in the implementation phases. In this paper 12 recent evaluation studies are reviewed to investigate to what extend they reflect the structure, process, outcome conceptual framework. It is found that all the evaluation studies focus on structure measures. But if computer programs to support medical decision making are to be considered in the planning process of the health care system, the evaluation studies must strive to evaluate process and outcomes measures as well.

Introduction

During the last couple of years there has been an increasing attention to the assessment of the end result of medical care. Arnold S. Relman [17], who is the editor-in-chief of the New England Journal of Medicine, has even termed it as the third revolution in medical care. Arnold Epstein [8] has referred to it as the "outcomes movement", which describes the growth in activity directed at the assessment of outcomes, the analysis of effectiveness and quality assurance. These discussions raise a number of issues in relation to evaluation of computer programs to support medical decision making. Will the use of medical expert systems improve the effectiveness of health care? Will they improve the health status in a population? Can the quality of care be improved etc.

As with the development of any new technology, expert systems have always been evaluated in different ways and on different stages throughout the development process. The medical field has a long tradition of clinical trials and a heritage of experimental design and analysis. The literature holds a wealth of relevant experience in the theories underlying the practical accomplishment of evaluations. Although the medical computer science have been criticized for an informal approach to evaluation, often based on anecdotal accolades alone [5] there is a considerable methodological literature on the topic [5,10,11,12,18,21,22,23]. However, most of the specific methodological guidance is on the evaluation of system performance, but all the papers would probably agree, that the most fundamental issue is the impact on patients health, and it is probably also the most difficult to measure.

In order to assess emerging systems from an outcomes assessment or health care quality point of view it can be fruitful to turn to the structure, process, outcome conceptual framework.

General conceptual framework

In the wake of the development of systems theory in the 1940's it was also found applicable in health services research. The idea can be illustrated in a simple diagram showing three aspects of the delivery of health care.

STRUCTURE ----------> PROCESS ----------------> OUTCOME

Quantity	Variations in use	Effectiveness
Efficacy	- Quantity-	health status
	- Quality-	mortality
	- others	

The diagram indicates, that any health care system requires structure a certain *quantity* of resources such as hospitals, equipment, sufficiently trained personnel etc. *Efficacy* is generally referred to as a measure of the effect under optimal conditions: "the probability of benefit to individuals in a defined population from medical technology applied for a given medical problem under ideal conditions of use" [14] (P. VIII). Therefore efficacy can be regarded as that which in our present state of knowledge and skill we consider to be achievable and is consequently a structural entity [6] (P.175). Efficacy is determined by randomized clinical trials.

Within this structure the *process* of health care takes place. Certain procedures are carried out, patients are diagnosed, treated, cared for and rehabilitated etc. *Variations in use* is an entity characterizing the process of care and can be defined as: "Different observed levels of per capita consumption of a service, especially hospital care, office visits, drugs, and specific procedures" [4]. It can be *quantified* by utilization rates and the frequency of different procedures as for instance: visits, medications, referrals, tests ordered, hospitalization etc.

There is no shortage of definitions of the *quality* of the health care process, and it is beyond the scope here to discuss all the attempts. Avedis Donabedian has put In more than two decades of work in this area and states in general terms that "Quality consists in the ability to achieve desirable objectives using legitimate means" [7] (P. 173). Since quality is described under process of health care it can only be judged "direct by examining the attributes of care itself or ... indirectly by examining the characteristics of the settings in which care is provided (structure) and the effects of care on the health and welfare of individuals or populations (outcome)" [7] (P. 177).

Finally the process has *outcomes*, which include the desired results as well as undesired results. The outcome of a medical procedure can be characterized by the term *effectiveness* which reflects the performance under ordinary conditions by the average practitioner for the typical patient [4]. Effectiveness is estimated by methods similar to those used to define the efficacy, but it is far more difficult because of the absence of rigorously controlled settings.

There is of course a fundamental relationship between the three issues. The structural characteristics of the settings in which care takes places, will influence the process of care and thereby diminish or enhance the quality of the care process. Further the chances in the process of care will influence the effect on the health status [6] (P.84).

Review of Evaluation Studies

To investigate to what extend the most recently evaluations of expert systems reflects structure, process or outcomes estimates, 12 recent evaluation studies were reviewed. MEDLINE, the computerized bibliographic data base of the National Library of Medicine (USA) was used to identify articles published in the period 1985-90. The references in those articles were scrutinized and in addition proceedings from relevant congresses in the same period were scanned for evaluation studies. A total of more than 50 studies were identified, but as the primary goal of this investigation is expert systems for clinical decision aid in diagnostic procedures, and in addition only those systems that are beyond the proposal stage of development, only 12 qualified for review.

The method of annotation is based on the framework discussed and the evaluation criteria derived above.

Results

The results of the review are shown in the table below. The twelve studies have been reviewed to determine to what extend the research questions reflect structure, process or outcome variables.

SYSTEM	DOMAIN	STRUCTURE (research question)	PROCESS	OUTCOME
Nelson (1985) RECONSIDER	Differential diagnosis	Does the system include the correct diagnosis? Rank of the correct diagnosis	-	-
Barnett (1987) DXplain	Differential diagnosis	Does the system include the correct diagnosis?	Does the system change the phycisians diff. diagnosis	-
Bankowitz (1989) QMR	Differential diagnosis	Does the system include the correct diagnosis?	Does the system influence phycisians diff. diagnosis	-
Waxman (1990) MEDITEL	Differential diagnosis	Does the system include the correct diagnosis? Rank of the correct diagnosis	-	-
Plugge (1990) EVINCE-I	Psychiatry	Determine false/neg and false/pos rate Agreement between domain expert and system	-	-
Reggia (1985) TIA	Neurology	Agreement between domain expert and system	-	-
Kingsland (1985) AI/RHEUM	Rheumatology	Determine diagnostic accuracy	-	-
Adlassnig (1989) CADIAG-2	Rheumatology Gastroentero.	Determine false/neg and false/pos rate Use of ROC curves	-	-
Shamsolmaali (1989) ICU MACPEE		Comparing system with a junior clinician	-	-

368

As seen in the table all the evaluation studies are mainly focused on determining the efficacy of the system.

The four systems that provide help in making differential diagnosis are not designed to come out with *the* correct diagnosis. The goal of these systems is to provide the physician user with a list of possible diagnosis that match a set of input findings, so failure to provide an efficacious intervention, when it is needed, can be omitted. This is the reason for the research question: "Does the system *include* the correct diagnosis".

The rest of the systems works within a specific medical domain, and they are designed to come up with a correct diagnosis. The output of the system is compared to various "gold standards", and thereby evaluates the correctness of the output by determining the diagnostic accuracy.

Only two of the studies evaluate issues that are related to the care process. The DXplain study evaluates whether the advice from the system changes the physicians differential diagnosis. The QMR evaluation studied the impact of the system on the differential diagnosis of a ward team, as a measure of change in the diagnostic strategy of clinicians caring for patients.

None of the evaluations studies consider any outcomes measures.

Discussion

Because only a very limited number of expert systems have reached the level of routine use it is of course difficult to perform process evaluations and impossible to perform outcomes evaluations on any great scale. If, however, computer programs to support medical decision making are to be considered seriously in the planning process of the health care system, it will be necessary to perform objective assessments of the impact of the system on patients outcome and the quality of care. Medical expert systems have the potential of becoming widely diffused, if they show beneficial reductions in crucial outcomes measures as for instance length and cost of hospitalization. The quality of care can only be judged directly by examining the attribute of the care process itself. In the context of medical expert diagnostic systems the specific systems ability to influence the frequency of for example patients visits, referrals or tests ordered.

For systems not used on a routine basis, it can be very difficult to assess the effectiveness of the system. But if a functional relationship between process measures and outcomes measures can be established, indicators of patient outcomes can be estimated from process measures obtained on a smaller scale, and the system will have better chance to become widely used.

List of references

1. Adlassnig K.P., Scheithauer W.: *"Performance evaluation of medical expert systems using ROC curves"*. Computers and biomedical research: 1989 22(4) P. 297-313.

2. Bankowitz R.A., McNeil A.M., Challinor S.M., Parker R.C., Kapoor W.N., Miller R.A.: *"A Computer-Assisted Medical Diagnostic Consultation Service. Implementation and Prospective Evaluation of A Prototype"*. Annals of Internal Medicine: 1989 110 P. 824-32.

3. Barnett G.O., Cimino J.J., Hupp J.A., Hoffer E.P.: *"DXplain: Experience with Knowledge Acquisition and Program Evaluation"*. Proceedings 11th Symposium on Comp. Appl. in Med. Care: 1987 P. 150-4.

4. Brook R.H., Lohr K.N.: *"Efficacy, Effectiveness, Variations and Quality. Boundary Crossing Research"*. Medical Care: 1985, 23(5), P. 710-22.

5. Buchanan B.G., Shortliffe E.H. (Eds.): *"Rule-Based Expert Systems. The MYCIN Experiments of the Stanford Heuristic Programming Project"*. Addison-Wesley Publishing Company: 1984.

6. Donabedian A: *"Explorations in Quality Assessing and Monitoring. Vol. 1. The Definition of Quality and Approaches to its Assessment"*. Health Administration Press. Ann Arbor, MI: 1980.

7. Donabedian A.: *"Quality Assessment and Assurance: Unity of Purpose, Diversity of Means"*. Inquiry (Blue Cross and Blue Shield Association): 1988 25(spring) P.173-192.

8. Epstein A.M.: *"The Outcomes Movement - Will It Get Us Where We Want to Go"*. The New England Journal of Medicine: 1990 323(4) P. 266-70.

9. Kingsland L.C. III: *"Evaluation of Medical Expert Systems: Experience with the AI/RHEUM Knowledge-Based Consultant System in Rheumatology"*. US Government work: .

10. Lundsgaarde H.P.: *"Evaluating Medical Expert System"*. Social Science and Medicine: 1987, 24, P.805-19.

11. Miller P.L.: *"The Evaluation of Artificial Intelligence Systems in Medicine"*. Computer methods and programs in biomedicine: 1986 22 P 5-11..

12. Miller P.L., Sittig D.F.: *"The Evaluation of Clinical Decision Support Systems: What is Necessary versus what is interesting"*. Medical Informatics: 1990, 15(3), P. 185-90.

13. Nelson S.J., Blois M.S., Tuttle M.S., Erlbaum M., Harrison P., Kim H., Winkelmann B., Yamashita D.: *"Evaluating Reconsider. A Computer Program for Diagnostic Prompting"*. Journal of Medical Systems: 1985 9(5/6) P. 379-88.

14. Office of Technology Assessment: *"The Quality of Medical Care. Information for Consumers"*. OTA-H-386 Washington D.C. U.S. Government Printing Office: 1988.

15. Plugge L.A., Verhey F.R.J., Jolles J.: *"A Desktop Expert System for the Differential Diagnosis of Dementia. An Evaluation Study"*. International Journal of Technology Assessment in Health Care: 1990 6(1) P. 147-56.

16. Reggia J.A.: *"Evaluation of Medical Expert Systems: Case Study in Performance Assessment"*. Proceedings of the 9th Annual Symposium on Computer Applications in Medical Care: 1985 P.287-91.

17. Relman A.S.: *"Assessment and Accountability. The Third Revolution in Medical Care"*. The New England Journal of Medicine: 1988 319(18) P. 1220-1222.

18. Rossi-Mori A., Pisanelli D.M., Ricci F.L.: *"Evaluation Stages and Design Steps for Knowledge-Based Systems in Medicine"*. Medical Informatics: 1990, 15(3), P. 191-204.

19. Shamsolmaali A., Collinson P.O., Gray T.G., Carson E.R., Cramp D.G.: *"Implementation and Evaluation of a Knowledge-Based System for the Interpretation of Laboratory Data"*. Hunter J. et al. (Eds.): AIME 89. Springer Verlag: 1989 P. 167-76.

20. Waxman H.S., Worley W.E.: *"Computer-Assisted Adult Medical Diagnosis: Subject Review and Evaluation of a New Microcomputer-Based System"*. Medicine: 1990 69(3) P. 125-36.

21. Whitbeck C., Brooks R.: *"Criteria for Evaluating a Computer Aid to Clinical Reasoning"*. The Journal of Medicine and Philosophy: 1983 8. P. 51-65.

22. Wyatt J.: *"The Evaluation of Clinical Decision Support Systems: A Discussion of the Methodology Used in the ACORN Project"*. Fox J. et al. (Eds.): AIME 87. Springer Verlag: 1987 P. 15-24.

23. Wyatt J., Spiegelhalter D.: *"Evaluating Medical Expert Systems: What to Test and How?"*. Medical Informatics: 1990, 15(3), P. 205-17.

Software Tools for the Development and Validation of HEPAR, an Expert System for the Diagnosis of Hepatobiliary Disease

Peter Lucas
University of Amsterdam
Department of Medical Physics and Informatics
Meibergdreef 15, 1105 AZ Amsterdam

Abstract

HEPAR is an expert system which can be used as a supportive tool for the clinical management of patients with hepatobiliary disease. For the purpose of the construction of this expert system, we have developed a collection of simple software tools as extensions to a rule-based expert system shell. These tools provide valuable information about the effects of modification of the HEPAR knowledge base, and indicate places in the knowledge base for refinement. This set of tools has also been applied in two successive performance validation studies of HEPAR. It is believed that similar software tools may prove helpful in the development of other medical expert systems as well.

Keywords & Phrases: medical expert systems, medical knowledge engineering, medical decision-making.

1   Introduction

HEPAR is an expert system that offers support in the diagnosis of disorders of the liver and biliary tract [1]. It is widely recognized that the diagnosis of disorders of the liver and biliary tract on purely clinical grounds is a difficult task, requiring much experience [2]. Several studies indicate that experienced clinicians are able to differentiate between biliary obstructive and hepatocellular disease in 80 - 90% of their patients [3-5]. Clinicians with limited hepatological experience seem to be able to make a correct specific diagnosis in jaundiced patients in less than 45% of cases [6]. The latter group of clinicians may therefore benefit from using the HEPAR system.

The development of the HEPAR system, which started in 1984, provides a typical instance of how a medical expert system may evolve. During its development, the need for the development of several software tools, which were not provided in the expert system shell applied, arose. In this paper, several of these tools will be described and related to the basic problem of representing medical knowledge.

2 Development of the HEPAR system

It is now well-recognized that the acquisition of domain knowledge in the process of building an expert system is a difficult task [7]. In recent years, many methodologies have therefore been developed, suggesting systematic methods to be followed in building an expert system. Some of these methodologies include a set of software tools which help the knowledge engineer in building a specific application, mainly by assisting in the analysis of the problem domain [8].

2.1 Structured development

The knowledge concerning diagnosis in liver and biliary disease incorporated into the HEPAR system was derived from the experience of a specialist in internal medicine and hepatology and from the medical literature. Expert hepatologists usually follow a clear and unambiguous strategy in diagnosing hepatobiliary disease; this strategy has been taken as the point of departure for the domain structure of the HEPAR system. The development of the system was decomposed into several subtasks, according to this domain structure. After completing a considerable portion of the knowledge base, it was decided to carry out some experiments with the system using data from real patients to investigate whether the system was able to meet our expectations. It appeared that the system was unable to come up with an acceptable advice in many cases. An analysis of the results of this experiment yielded the following reasons for the disappointing performance:

- Many rules were formulated too rigorously, such that these rules almost never applied to a patient with the given disease.

- Many rules were defined without explicitly mentioning the medical context in which they should hold. These rules frequently succeeded in patients for which they had not been designed.

These problems may actually be taken as an indication of the way in which clinicians operate in medical practice. Firstly, the knowledge of the clinician is partly based on the descriptions given in medical textbooks, in which there is little place for the description of atypical disease patterns, and partly on experience in the management of specific disorders. Clinicians often have to base their early decisions on incomplete clinical evidence; likewise, expert systems must be able to deal with incomplete evidence as well. Rules which have been formulated too rigorously tend to describe the typical picture of the disease, and may in addition assume the availability of an unrealistic amount of data for the patient. Secondly, the clinician has considerable experience with disorders frequently observed in clinical practice. However, these disorders carry a clinical context which the clinician may not be able to make explicit. Formalizing such knowledge may yield rules with a wider application than intended. In designing a medical expert system, the availability of information obtained at certain stages of the diagnostic process should explicitly be taken into account. Therefore, rules were drafted covering only the symptoms and signs of a disorder, whereas other rules were drafted only covering the results of laboratory tests. In this way a more or less layered structure of the knowledge base was obtained.

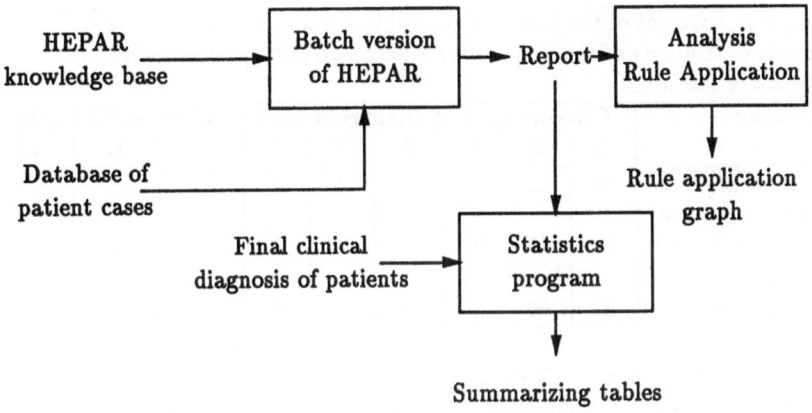

Figure 1: Environment for incremental development.

2.2 Knowledge refinement

For the purpose of the refinement (and later also the validation) of the HEPAR system, a special testing environment was implemented under the Unix operating system consisting of a set of interacting software tools. The environment consists of a non-interactive batch version of the expert system shell which is able to use a database of patient cases as its input. This system produces a report containing the results for each individual patient. The report together with a file containing the final clinical diagnosis of the patient is then processed by a program producing a table summarizing the results. Figure 1 shows the overall structure of the testing environment. An example of such a table, produced after refinement of the HEPAR system using the software tools, is reproduced in Table 1, which shows the results of the HEPAR expert system for 82 patient cases from the Leiden University Hospital. An additional method adopted for the refinement of the HEPAR knowledge base, supported by the same environment, had the aim of studying the effects of incompleteness of information on the conclusions of the HEPAR system. An example of a table produced using the environment is shown in Table 2. The same database of patient cases from the University Hospital Leiden has been used here. As can be seen in Table 2, the number of correct final diagnoses decreased considerably when the patient data entered into the system was more incomplete. However, the system was still capable of producing a correct final diagnosis in about one fourth of the cases. More important

Table 1: Diagnostic results for a population of 82 patients with hepatobiliary disease.				
Conclusion	Correct n (%)	Incorrect n (%)	Unclassified n (%)	Total n (%)
Type of hepato-biliary disorde	74 (90)	4 (5)	4 (5)	82 (100)
Benign/malignant nature of disorder	78 (95)	4 (5)	0 (0)	82 (100)
Final diagnosis	71 (86)	8 (10)	3 (4)	82 (100)

Table 2: Assessment of the effects of incompleteness of information on the diagnostic conclusions of the system, for a database of 82 patients with hepatobiliary disease.									
Conclusion	Correct (%)			Incorrect (%)			Unclassified (%)		
	A	B	C	A	B	C	A	B	C
Type of hepato- biliary derangement	90	90	50	5	5	0	5	5	50
Benign or malignant nature of disorder	95	95	94	5	5	6	0	0	0
Final diagnosis	86	49	24	10	9	10	4	43	66

A: All available data presented to system.
B: Only data concerning symptoms, signs, haematology and bloodchemistry
    (no data from ultrasound or serology presented).
C: Only data from medical interview and physical examination.

was that the percentage of incorrectly classified cases did not increase significantly, only the percentage of unclassified cases did increase in most cases.

3   A profile of the HEPAR knowledge base

In the previous section, we have discussed how the study of the results of the HEPAR system for individual patient cases, has been employed for refining the diagnostic quality of HEPAR. A second source of information that can be used for the refinement of the system, is the contents of the HEPAR system itself, by studying the behaviour of the system when provided with patient data. In order to obtain information concerning the frequency of rule application over certain patient populations, the testing environment discussed in Section 2.2 was extended by a collection of tools which again used the report produced by the batch version of the expert system for a database of patient cases. The following results are produced by these programs:

- An enumeration of all production rules used, with for each rule information about how often it has been used for a given database;

- An overview of the frequency distribution of the rule application, both in textual and in graphical form.

Figure 2 which was automatically produced by the environment, contains the results after refinement of the HEPAR knowledge base for the 82 patient cases from Leiden University Hospital. Most production rules (72 of about 500 rules contained in HEPAR) were applied only once. The accompanying textual form, which is not reproduced here, showed that from the rules that were applied several times, those with highest frequency were applied to conclude about the intermediate hypotheses. Only few, one to three, production rules were applied several times to reach a final conclusion.

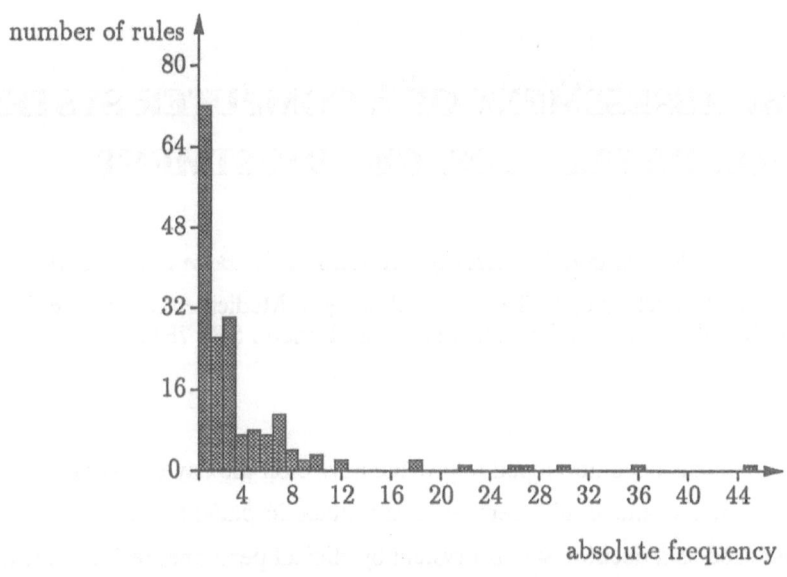

Figure 2: Rule-application bar graph for 82 patients.

References

[1] Lucas PJF, Segaar RW, Janssens AR. HEPAR: an expert system for the diagnosis of disorders of the liver and biliary tract. *Liver* 1989: **9**: 266-275.

[2] McIntyre N. Computer-aided diagnosis in jaundice and liver disease. *Journal of Hepatology* 1986: **3**: 269-272.

[3] Berkowitz, D. Pitfalls in the differential diagnosis of jaundice. *American Journal of Gastroenterology* 1964: **41**: 488-498.

[4] Haubek A, Pedersen JH, Burcharth F, *et al.* Dynamic sonography in the evaluation of jaundice. *American Journal of Radiology* 1981: **136**: 1071-1074.

[5] Theodossi A, Spiegelhalter D, Portmann B, *et al.* The value of clinical, biochemical, ultrasound and liver biopsy data in assessing patients with liver disease. *Liver* 1983: **3**: 315-326.

[6] Theodossi A. *An assessment of the value of diagnostic techniques in hepatobiliary disease.* M.D. Thesis, London: University of London, 1986.

[7] Guida G, Tasso C. Building expert systems: from life cycle to development methodology, in: Guida G, Tasso C (eds.), *Topics in expert systems design: methodologies and tools,* North-Holland, Amsterdam, 1989.

[8] Breuker J, Wielinga B. Models of expertise in knowledge acquisition, in: Guida G, Tasso C, *Topics in expert systems design,* Amsterdam: North-Holland, 1989.

CLINICAL ASSESSMENT OF A COMPUTER SYSTEM FOR INSULIN DOSAGE ADJUSTMENT

E.D. Lehmann, A.V. Roudsari, T. Deutsch, E.R. Carson, J.J. Benn & P.H. Sönksen

Departments of Endocrinology, Chemical Pathology & Medicine, United Medical and Dental Schools, St. Thomas's Hospital, London SE1 7EH, U.K.

Abstract

A computer system has been developed to provide advice on the day-to-day adjustment of carbohydrate intake and insulin regime in the diabetic patient. The prototype is intended to be used as a decision support system by clinical personnel in the context of day-to-day management of insulin-treated diabetic patients. It is designed for use during consultations, as a simulator of patient response following changed insulin and dietary regime and as a system to provide education on planning insulin therapy. Advice is generated by a qualitative knowledge based system which suggests what the next step in improving glycaemic control might be for a given patient, e.g. 'decrease evening medium-acting insulin'. A clinical model is being developed to allow predictions of the patient's blood glucose profile to be generated based on these adjustments. Clinical scenarios taken from postgraduate teaching cases have been used to compare the advice given by the computer with that of four independent diabetologists. The results of seven case studies are presented.

Introduction

Diabetes mellitus is a major chronic disease in industrialised countries. It affects 3% of the population of Europe and approximately one hundred million people worldwide[1]. While the incidence of the disease is currently on the increase in Western society, the incidence and severity of the later life complications which accompany it can be considerably reduced if the diabetic patient receives effective treatment leading to good glycaemic control[2]. In general such treatment attempts to achieve normoglycaemia by maintaining a careful balance between diet, physical activity and insulin therapy. However, education of the diabetic patient to achieve this balance requires a level of clinical expertise which, although present in specialised diabetes units and some general practices with an interest in diabetes, is not always to be found in other sectors of the health service. A prototype computer system has been developed to assist in making this clinical expertise more widely available.

A number of computer based approaches to aid in the treatment or long-term management of diabetic patients have been previously reported in the literature. These include knowledge based systems to advise on patient management in out-patient clinics[3], computer algorithms for insulin dosage adjustment[4] and mathematical models as a means of predicting or simulating patient blood glucose levels[5]. Deutsch *et al*[6] have used 'period orientated' knowledge based reasoning to analyse blood glucose profiles and hypoglycaemic episodes in insulin-treated diabetic patients. They have incorporated the dynamics of glucose and insulin interactions in a manner which reflects their clinical importance, as a way of providing advice to the referring clinician. The clinical assessment of this approach, which is presented here, draws on work which also introduced qualitative insulin algebra to predict changes in the blood glucose profile brought about by alterations in the insulin regime[7].

Overview of the system

The prototype is an integrated PC based computer system which consists of three main components: a data processing (DP) module, a simulator module and a knowledge based system (KBS). The DP module serves as the control module for the whole system. It combines clinical data such as blood glucose measurements, insulin injection doses and special event markers such as hypoglycaemic episodes with nutritional data including the carbohydrate content of meals to produce a 'modal day' current patient profile which represents a 'snapshot' of the patient's current metabolic status with respect to insulin-treated diabetes. The clinical model which is still under development allows a 24 hour simulation of the patient's blood glucose profile to be produced on the basis of the carbohydrate intake and insulin regime data contained in the current patient profile. It consists of a one compartment glucose model linked to a model with free and bound insulin compartments. This part of the system represents a simplified version of a three compartment model which has already been validated against short-term data[5].

The KBS provides qualitative advice on how to improve the patient's blood glucose profile on the basis of information contained in the current patient profile. This advice is useful in indicating the *direction* of changes which need to be made to either the patient's diet or insulin regime. The only types of insulin catered for in the version of the system evaluated are short and medium acting preparations such as soluble insulin and NPH. The KBS is described in greater detail elsewhere[7]. The linked system allows the effects of advice from the KBS to be simulated using the model. This is done by modifying the current patient profile on the basis of advice from the KBS. As the advice generated by the KBS is only qualitative (i.e. 'increase morning short-acting insulin') this link provides the facility to quantify the advice by using the simulator module. Furthermore as the KBS can provide a number of different pieces of advice for any one given current patient profile, the link with the simulator provides an opportunity to identify the 'optimal' suggestion for an individual patient. The integrated system is described in greater detail elsewhere[8].

Clinical assessment

As a first step towards a full scale clinical evaluation of the whole integrated prototype work is in progress to separately validate the individual components of the system. The simulator module is still undergoing testing so the first part of the system to be formally evaluated has been the KBS. Previous validation work has focused on the collection of patient test cases which have been used to generate advice from the KBS for comparison with a clinician[8]. However, for a comprehensive validation of the KBS it is necessary to subject the system to as wide a range of clinical situations as is likely to be encountered in clinical practice. Since the test cases previously collected[9] only covered a portion of the spectrum of diabetic management, a range of clinical scenarios which exhibited a greater breadth of clinical problems were used[10]. Fig. 1 shows these clinical scenarios which contain information about insulin doses and blood glucose measurements for seven hypothetical patients.

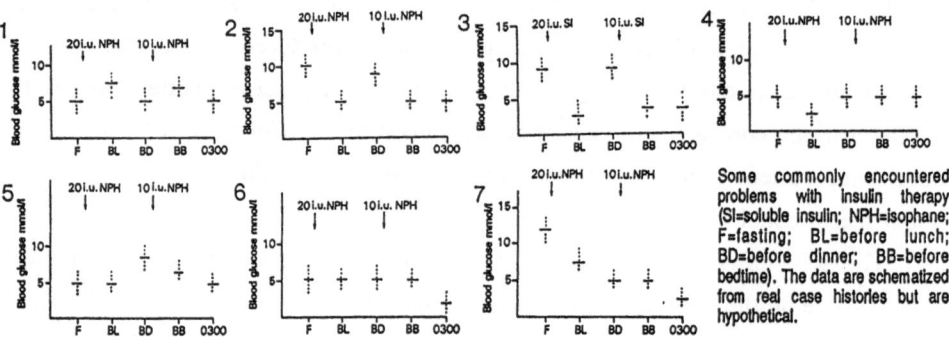

Fig. 1. Seven clinical scenarios (modified from Sönksen[10]).

Dietary information in terms of the carbohydrate content of the various meals was provided separately by a diabetologist. This data was fed into the KBS which generated advice on the basis of it. The same data was made available to four clinicians who independently provided their suggestions as to how the blood glucose profiles could be improved. The clinicians' suggestions are shown in Fig. 2. As can be seen changes were suggested for the insulin regime, injection times as well as the insulin dose. The version of the KBS evaluated, however, was limited to only making insulin dosage adjustments. The qualitative advice generated by the KBS is shown in Fig. 3.

Case	Clinician (1)	Clinician (2)	Clinician (3)	Clinician (4)
1	needs BD mixed soluble & NPH	add soluble am & pm	add 2-5u soluble am	needs soluble added to NPH
2	needs BD mixed soluble & NPH	try monotard	split evening dose 4u soluble BD & 6u NPH BB	change to lente, increase dose
3	change to NPH	change to NPH & add soluble if required	change to BD NPH	change to NPH or lente
4	decrease am NPH to 16u or take am snack	try decreasing am NPH	add lunchtime injection or try monotard	needs (?bigger) mid-morning snack
5	mixed am regimen & adjust	top up soluble BL	reduce am NPH; take 15u NPH am & 5u soluble BL	needs extra lunchtime injection or try lente
6	decrease pm NPH to 8u initially	give soluble BD & NPH BB	reduce pm NPH; if it fails give soluble BD & NPH BB	split pm dose with 5u soluble BD & 5u NPH BB
7	split pm dose with injection of NPH BB	try decreasing NPH at night first	reduce pm NPH, split pm dose; if BD glucose normal reduce am NPH	split pm dose with extra injection BB or try lente

Fig. 2. Clinical advice provided by four diabetologists for managing the clinical scenarios.

Case	Computer
1	KBS suggested no change
2	increase BD NPH dose
3	decrease soluble dose & increase carbohydrate content of breakfast and dinner
4	decrease am NPH dose - c.f. clinicians (1) & (2)
5	decrease am NPH dose - c.f. clinician (3)
6	decrease BD NPH dose - c.f. clinicians (1), (3) & (4)
7	decrease BD NPH dose - c.f. clinicians (2) & (3)

Fig. 3. Suggestions provided by the KBS for the clinical scenarios.

Discussion

In this preliminary clinical assessment the KBS was able to provide advice which matched that of at least one of the diabetologists in over half of the cases studied. Those cases for which the KBS could *not* give comparable advice were the ones which required changes to be made to the insulin regime. Knowledge about such regime changes has not, as yet, been coded for in the KBS. Without the option of altering the type of insulin preparation prescribed the computer's suggestions for cases (1-3) appear quite reasonable. For example the suggestion for case (2) to 'increase the before dinner NPH dose' seems valid given that the early morning blood glucose reading was raised; although a clinician might be concerned that this could lead to hypos in the night. It would appear, however, from this preliminary clinical assessment that another layer of knowledge needs to be incorporated into the system to cater for situations where more complex control actions are required.

A number of problems posed by the medical validation and clinical evaluation of medical decision support systems have been identified. For example, on occasions the diabetologists gave quite different advice from each other. In previous studies we have collected data from 12 insulin-treated diabetic patients over a 5 day period and employed a single diabetologist to provide expert advice which we have compared with the computer's suggestions for each day of the study[8]. Even with a relatively small number of patients this is quite a time consuming exercise. Furthermore, as we have shown here the view of one diabetologist may not necessarily be representative of his colleagues' and a *panel* of clinical experts may be needed to obtain a more acceptable 'standard' against which to compare the computer's advice. The difficulty of achieving a consensus is clearly another problem which would need to be overcome as part of a full scale validation. It is interesting to note, however, that clinicians when given *theoretical* scenarios react differently to real life situations. For example if presented with case (1) in a clinic most diabetologists would *not* make any changes to the insulin regime.

Another problem which needs to be addressed is making the computer system as flexible as possible in its suggestions. As we have shown a whole host of difficulties arise if the computer is not able to match the variety or flexibility of advice given by a clinician. In particular constraining the system to particular types of suggestions will raise questions about the clinical validity of the advice. However, despite this it is vital to be able to assess the individual components of the system as they are developed. Attempting to validate the *whole* integrated system in one go could lead to major problems in terms of software integrity and validity, and could potentially cause concern about future patient safety.

The overall goal of our work is to improve the patient's glycaemic control. We aim to do this by using currently accepted clinical practice. However, accepted medical practice varies among different groups of doctors in different countries and changes with time as medical science develops. Thus whatever approaches are adopted for the validation process must be easily repeatable as the *re*-validation of any medical decision support system will become an integral part of its on-going maintenance. One way round this problem would be to go straight to the clinical endpoint in diabetes care and see whether the computer system, when used by patients either directly or indirectly, improved glycaemic control. Such an approach is appealing but relies on total confidence in the safety of the system developed. We have decided on a slightly different approach whereby we are formally verifying the knowledge base of our 'expert' system. This is being done by translating the PROLOG clauses from the KBS into English sentences which have been given to expert diabetologists at St. Thomas's Hospital for checking. It is hoped that in this way it will be possible to identify omissions from the knowledge base as well as expose the reasoning process of the KBS to as wide an audience of diabetologists for clinical debate.

In conclusion, a prototype computer system has been developed to provide advice on the day-to-day adjustment of carbohydrate intake and insulin regimen in the insulin-treated diabetic patient. This fulfils an important part of the total information management and decision support requirement for the management of the diabetic patient. A preliminary medical validation of one component of the system has been performed. Work is currently in progress to formally verify the knowledge base of this. Future work will undertake a major clinical evaluation of the whole system based on a scheme defined with a much higher degree of methodological rigour. Advice other than insulin dosage adjustments will be dealt with, a panel of diabetologists will be employed, and a further 'judgemental' panel established in order to assess the relative merit of the prototype's advice. A larger representative set of patient test cases and clinical scenarios will be used.

Acknowledgements: *This work was supported by the EEC AIM Exploratory Action [EURODIABETA Project No. A1019], the Wellcome Trust and IBM (UK) Ltd.*

References
1. EURODIABETA (1990) *Diabetic Medicine* **7**:639-650.
2. Engerman *et al.* (1977) *Diabetes* **26**:760-769.
3. Carson *et al.* (1990) *Comput. Meth. Prog. Biomed.* **32**:179-188.
4. Skyler *et al.* (1981) *Diabetes Care* **4**:311-318.
5. Boroujerdi *et al.* (1987) in: *International Symposium on Advanced Models for Therapy of Insulin-dependent Diabetes* (Raven Press, New York) 41-46.
6. Deutsch *et al.* (1989) *Comput. Meth. Prog. Biomed.* **29**:75-88.
7. Deutsch *et al.* (1990) *Comput. Meth. Prog. Biomed.* **32**:195-214.
8. Lehmann *et al.* (1991) *Diab. Nutr. Metab.* **Suppl 2**: in press.
9. Roudsari *et al.* (1990) in: *Whither Computers in Diabetes Care?*, Köge, Denmark. 28.
10. Sönksen (1985) *Update Postgraduate Centre Series* **5**:30-38.

A Validation Methodology for Testing Decision-Support Systems for Insulin Dosage Adjustment

A.V. Roudsari [1], H.J. Leicester [1], E.D. Lehmann [2], R. Hovorka [1],
S. Andreassen [3], T. Deutsch [1,4], E.R. Carson [1,2] P.H. Sönksen [2,1]

1. Centre for Measurement and Information in Medicine,
Department of Systems Science, City University, London.
2. Department of Endocrinology and Chemical Pathology,
St. Thomas's Hospital, London.
3. Department of Medical Informatics and Image Analysis,
Aalborg University, Denmark
4. Computer Centre, Semmmelweis University, Budapest.

Abstract

A medical validation protocol has been developed to test three decision-support systems in the management of insulin-dependent diabetic patients. The systems have been chosen as representative of the range of computational strategies recently reported and the protocol is designed to compare their relative merits directly using retrospective data, before planning full, clinical evaluations.

In particular, the protocol allows computer advice on insulin therapy adjustments to be compared with that provided by the individual clinician acting in the clinic, or acting independently on recorded data alone, as well as comparing computer advice with a consensus view of a group of clinicians. It is sufficiently flexible to match available clinical resources, incorporating statistical and domain-specific checks to ensure that staff and time are used appropriately. The new validation protocol is considered a fairer and more informative test for decision-support systems in a domain that has as yet few rigid standards for information technology and is characterised. By performing a strictly controlled clinical trial to test the efficacy of a new proposed treatment. It is, therefore, considered appropriate for use in other areas of chronic health care.

Introduction

In recent years, many decision-support systems have been developed to assist in the treatment of diabetic patients. They have ranged from the rule-based to the adaptive system [1-3]. Though they share patient management objectives, they differ in their computational techniques. There is a need, therefore, to evaluate the efficacy of such techniques in the overall management of chronic health care and in the management of diabetes in particular. Evaluation must be an important and integral part of a system's development [4-6]. It is a wide-ranging process, considering features such as ease of use, clinical acceptability and costing, which are more realistically studied in prospective hospital and primary care trials [7]. Medical validation is that part of the process which concentrates on the more fundamental issues of medical accuracy, acceptability and scope. Systems are usually tested with retrospective patient data, against pre-defined clinical criteria or expert consensus [8].

The results of medical validation should determine which systems require modification and which can proceed to more substantial evaluation. It is important, therefore, that the validation is both fair and informative. In this case, three decision-support systems have been selected for validation. They use similar, and commonly measured, data (eg. blood glucose, insulin injection and carbohydrate intake) to generate insulin dosage advice for the daily management of diabetic patients. Each uses a different computational strategy; they have been selected, in addition, to be representative of the range of strategies reported in the literature.

The Decision-Support Systems

Metabolic Prototype (KBS Module) [MP]

This is written in MicroPROLOG using an APES expert system shell. The aim of the system is to provide advice on how to improve the patient's blood glucose profile on the basis of clinical and nutritional data. However, the system is not a day to day controller, instead it is based on the concept of the 'modal day': the patient's response to unaltered therapy assessed over a minimum of two days. The advice generated by the system is qualitative and is expressed as an increase or decrease in the insulin dosage regimen. Explanations of the advice are also provided [9].

Consultation System [CS]

This is written in Turbo Pascal and consists of three main sub-systems; first, a mathematical model of insulin pharmacodynamics which can establish the effects of an insulin therapy; second, an adaptive/learning module which can use blood glucose measurements to estimate patient-specific parameters; and third, a proposal module which is used to generate insulin therapy advice based on predicted blood glucose levels [10].

Causal Probabilistic Network [CPN]

A differential equation model of carbohydrate metabolism was implemented in the form of a causal probabilistic network. This permitted explicit representations of the uncertainties associated with model-based predictions of 24 hour blood glucose profiles. In addition the implementation gave automatic learning and adjustment of model parameters based on measured blood glucose profiles. Insulin therapy was adjusted using a decision theoretical approach. Penalties were assigned to blood glucose values that deviated from normal, and the insulin therapy was adjusted to minimise the expected occurrence of penalties [12].

Preliminary Validations and Summarised Results

The three systems have already been tested with several days' recorded data from 12 patients treated with two common drugs [13]. Figures 1 and 2, respectively, summarise the clinical advice which the patients followed and the advice from an independent diabetologist acting on recorded data alone. The difference between the independent diabetologist's advice and that of the patient's clinician is shown in Figure 3, and the Metabolic Prototype's recommendations are compared with independent diabetologist advice in Figure 4.There are noticeable variations between the clinical advice and that of the independent diabetologist, which are more pronounced for one of the insulin formulations. These may result from real differences in the advice between clinicians who see the particular patients and those who see only records. Similarly they may arise through acceptable variations in individual clinicians' standard practice. The results do not reveal, however, whether some of the variance is due to superficial therapy adjustments, making changes between different insulin formulations.

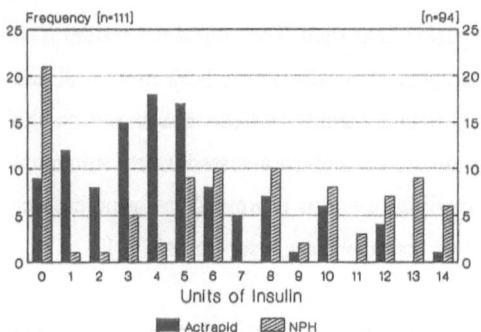

Figure 1. Distribution of injections received by 12 patients for 5 days, advised by their own clinician.

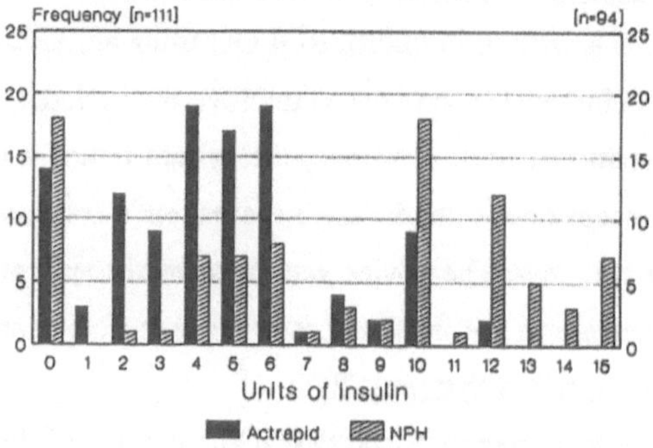

Figure 2. Distribution of injections advise by an independent diabetologist seeing recorded data alone, for patients as given in Fig.1.

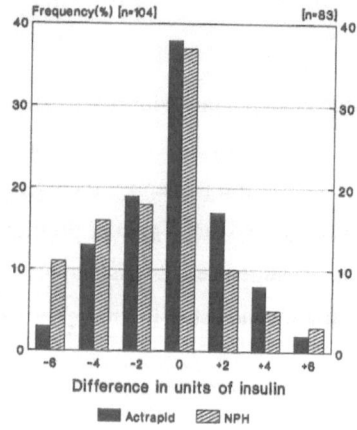

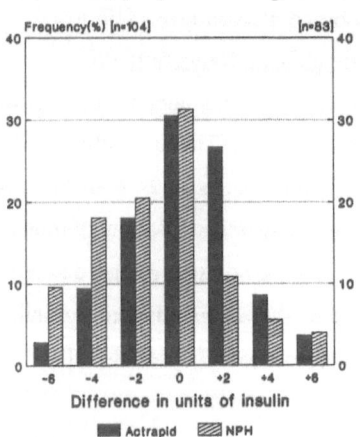

Figure 3. Difference in advice between an independent diabetologist and patients as given in Fig.1.

Figure 4. Difference in advice between an independent diabetologist and the (MP) for the patients as given in Fig.1.

All the systems tested were reported to have acceptable performance levels against a single, independent diabetologist and against the actual therapy [13]. The comparative representations in Figures 3 and 4 do not reveal, however, the degree to which insulin dosages were actually adjusted from day to day. It is generally reported that a majority of diabetics, once tested, can maintain a common daily insulin regime with only mild fluctuations. It is possible, therefore, for computer systems to be highly accurate, in such cases, simply by restating the previous therapy.

The design of the computer systems themselves becomes important in cases which are considered by experts to require immediate or continuous insulin adjustments. The CS, for example, tends to make small changes, particularly when patient data are limited. In contrast, the CPN advises greater adjustments which would be clinically more acceptable if made in smaller steps over longer periods. These behaviours have been termed "conservative" and "aggressive", respectively; their medical accuracy and appropriateness is not clear.

Requirements of a Medical Validation Protocol

The results of the preliminary validations suggest that a more rigorous protocol should accommodate features to:

1. ensure that the patient test cases represent a broad range of diabetic states with a significant number requiring active changes in the therapy;
2. compare therapeutic agents with different periods of activity, but which are equally acceptable in similar patient circumstances;
3. compare advice between clinicians acting independently;
4. compare advice between clinicians who treat the patient and those who see only recorded data;
5. compare the advice between individual computer systems;
6. compare computers' advice with that of doctors acting for their own patients, acting individually on retrospective data and acting collectively on the same data.
7. be accepted by a panel of experts, when 'masked'

To be accepted, the protocol must also have the flexibility to match the availability and endurance of hospital staff.

The Medical Validation Protocol

An extended peer review technique is proposed with three levels of clinical assessment. Statistical filters are incorporated to reduce the amount of data passing to lower levels. Figure 5 summarises the protocol.

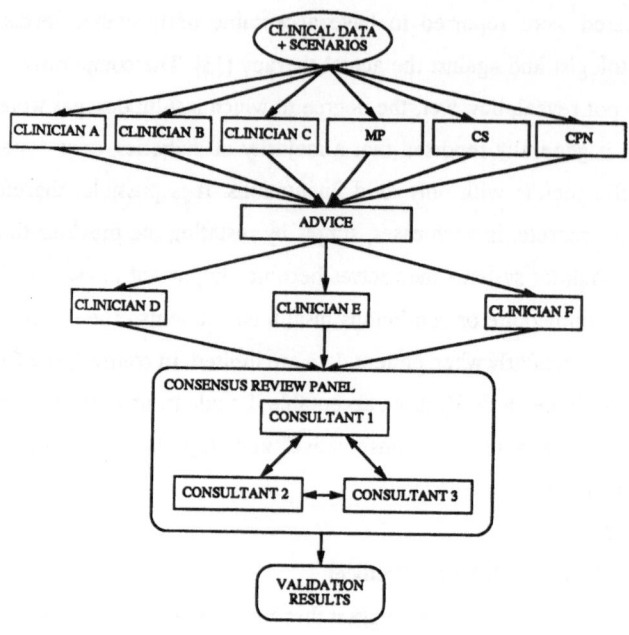

Figure 5. Schema for validation methodology. [MP=Metabolic Prototype; CS=Consultation System; CPN=Causal Probabilistic Network].

Initially fifty patients are selected, each having at least three days' retrospective data and a case history.

The third day's data in each case are withheld, as "clinical" or "actual therapy" for comparison with later results. Data from the other days pass to the first level of clinical assessment. Here, three independent clinicians (A, B and C) and the three computer systems, are instructed to advise on insulin dosage adjustments for the missing days.

The dosage recommendations are then statistically analysed for variations between the computer systems, between the clinicians and between both groups. Any recommendations which are clearly distinguished as computer-generated advice are recorded and eliminated before the second clinical assessment.

The remaining recommendations are then transcribed to preserve the information but to conceal the sources. The transcriptions, together with the original patient data, are presented to a further three clinicians (D,E and F). Acting again independently, D, E and F should rate each recommendation on a series of numeric and verbal scales presented as a questionnaire. The scales are designed to test features such as: safety, effectiveness, ease of patient data interpretation, considered medical accuracy and acceptability.

The results from clinicians D, E and F are again statistically filtered to record and remove computer recommendations which are clearly distinguishable. The remaining cases will be marked by good computer performance or by substantial variation in the clinicians' views. Relevant information from these cases, still with the sources concealed, are passed to the third clinical assessment level.

This final level is composed of three consultant diabetologists who can act collectively to resolve conflicts or anomalies from previous levels. To do so, they must reach a consensus or majority decision. The consensus panel may also be used to interpret any ambiguous therapy recommendations at earlier stages of the validation process and to highlight any patient categories which have not been represented.

Discussion

The medical validation protocol described is currently under test as part of the process of selecting decision-support systems for evaluation in the diabetic clinic. It is rare for such systems to be compared directly, under the same conditions or, indeed, to compare a single system with several experts. Such comparisons are being made through this protocol, with special steps to make efficient use of clinicians.

Modifications could be made to ensure a patient mix that is more representative of the diabetic population or to concentrate the process on the more interesting features of computer performance revealed in earlier validation stages. Such modifications are, however, governed by local patient populations and clinical practices.

Above all, the new medical validation methodology recognises the inherent variation between clinicians in the field of diabetes management. It should provide a more objective test of decision-support systems that is informative to both medical assessors and system designers. With such important features, the protocol may well be applicable in other areas of chronic health care.

Acknowledgements

This work was supported in part by the EEC AIM (Advanced Informatics in Medicine) Exploratory Action [EURODIABETA Project No. A1019].

References

1. Carson, E.R., Carey, S., Harvey, F., Sönksen, P.H., Till, S. and Williams, C.D. (1990) Information technology and computer-based decision support in diabetic management. *Comput. Meth. Prog. Biomed.* 32:179-188.
2. Salzsieder, E., Albrecht, G., Fischer, U., Rutscher, A. and Thierback, U. (1990) Computer-aided systems in the management of type I diabetes: the application of a model-based strategy. *Comput. Meth. Prog. Biomed.* 32:215-224.

3. Sano, A. (1986) Adaptive and optimal schemes for control of blood glucose levels. *Biomed. Meas. Infor. Contr.* 1:16-22.

4. Albisser, A.M., Schiffrin, A., Schulz, M., Tiran, J. and Leibel, B.S. (1986) Insulin dosage adjustment using manual methods and computer algorithms: a comparative study. *Med. & Biol. Eng. & Comput.* 24:577-584.

5. Gaschnig, J., Klahr, Ph., Pople, H., Shortliffe, T., Terry, A. (1983) Evaluation of expert systems: issues and case studies. in: *Building Expert Systems*, Hayes-Roth, F., Waterman, D.A. and Lenat, D.B. (eds.) Addison Wesley, 241-280.

6. Wyatt, J. and Spiegelhalter, D. (1990) Evaluating medical expert systems: what to test and how? *Med. Inform.* 15(3):205-217.

7. Holland, J., EURODIABETA (1990) Modelling and implementation of information systems for chronic health care - example: diabetes. in: *Lecture Notes in Medical Informatics, MIE'90*, O'Moore, R., Bengtsson, S., Bryant, J.R. and Bryden, J.S. (eds.) Springer-Verlag, Berlin, 40:48-53.

8. EURODIABETA. Information technology for diabetes care in Europe: the EURODIABETA initiative. *Diabetic Medicine* 7:639-650.

9. Deutsch, T., Carson, E.R., Harvey, F.E., Lehmann, E.D., Sönksen, P.H., Tamas, G, Whitney, G. and Williams, C.D. (1990) Computer-assisted diabetic management: a complex approach. *Comput. Meth. Prog. Biomed.* 32:195-214.

10. Hovorka, R., Svacina, S., Carson, E.R., Williams, C.D. and Sönksen, P.H. (1990) A consultation system for insulin therapy. *Comp. Meth. Prog. Biomed.* 32:303-310.

11. Boroujerdi, M.A., Williams, C.D., Carson, E.R., Piwernetz, J.K., Hepp, K.D., Sönksen, P.H. (1987) A simulation approach for planning insulin regimes. in: *Int. Symp. on Advanced Models for Therapy of Insulin-dependent Diabetes*, Brunetti, P., Waldhurst, W.K. (eds.) Raven Press, New York, 37:41-47.

12. Andreassen, S., Benn, J.J., Carson, E.R., Hovorka, R., Kjaerulff, U. and Olesen, K.(1990) A causal probabilistic network model of carbohydrate metabolism for insulin therapy adjustment. in: *Proceedings of the Twelfth Annual International Conference of the IEEE Engineering in Medicine and Biology Society*, Pedersen, P.C. and Onaral, B. (eds.) IEEE, New York 12(3):1011.

13. EURODIABETA Deliverable 15, Andreassen, S., Bauersachs, R., Benn, J., Carson, E., Gomez, E., Hovorka, R., Lehmann, E., Nahgang, P., del Pozo, F., Roudsari, A., and Schneider, J. (1990) Report on developed prototypes integrating KBS and other methodologies for insulin therapy advisory systems. *Technical Report to the EEC Advanced Informatics in Medicine (AIM) Exploratory Action*, Brussels.

Clinical Value of a Decision Support System for the Assessment of Thyroid Function

P. Nuutila[1], K. Irjala[2], J. Viikari[1], J. Forsström[1], M. Välimäki[3], P. Nykänen[4], K. Saarinen[4]

[1]Department of Medicine and [2] Central Laboratory, University of Turku, SF-20520 Turku, [3]Third Department of Medicine, University of Helsinki, SF-00290 Helsinki, and [4]Technical Research Centre of Finland, Medical Engineering Laboratory, SF-33100 Tampere, Finland

Abstract

We studied the practical implication of a decision support system for thyroid diagnostics (THYROID) by testing the correctness of reports, the clinicians' attitude toward them and the general level of knowledge about thyroid diagnostics among users. The THYROID-system was tested on 1664 consecutive patients with suspected thyroid disease. The system found 153 patients from 166 patients with clinical disease (sensitivity 92.2%). The diagnostic accuracy was 98.0% and specificity 88.7%. The clinicians read printed the reports of the THYROID-system in 85.6%, and they considered the reports useful in 55.9% of the cases. The general knowledge level about thyroid diagnostics among users was tested on selected cases; it was insufficient in a fifth of the answers. In conclusion, the THYROID -system is valuable for diagnosis of thyroid disorders and it can be coupled easily with routine work.

Introduction

In the past decade several computer programs have been developed as consultants for the diagnosis of thyroid disorders (1-7). The major aims of these systems are to increase the diagnostic accuracy by improving test selection strategies, to reduce the numbers of tests carried out and to train unexperienced clinicians. The decision support system THYROID has been in use in the University Central Hospital of Turku for 28 months for thyroid function diagnostics (8). In this paper the experiences of the use of this system are discussed in terms of effectiveness in the users' environment and the users' attitudes toward it.

Principles of THYROID-system

The THYROID-system is designed to diagnose only thyroid function. The system is integrated with the laboratory information system and with the work flow of the laboratory in order to minimize the users' work flow. The only change to the routine test request practice includes an extra question regarding the clinical suspicion of the thyroid state. The interpretation is based on the initial clinical suspicion of thyroid disease (i.e. hypothyroidism or hyperthyroidism) and on the test results of thyrotropin (TSH) as the first line test and free thyroxine (FT4) and/or total T4 as the second line tests (9,10). The THYROID-system produces a suggestion for the diagnosis or alternative diagnoses of thyroid function and request for further tests, if needed, which is printed automatically for each patient.

Evaluation of diagnostic accuracy

The system has been tested for diagnostic accuracy in 1664 consecutive cases. The correctness of the classifications of the THYROID-system was checked using all the data which was available concerning the patient's clinical features, medication, nonthyroidal illnesses and additional test results. If needed, patients were re-checked later. Finally, only 70 patients were overtly hypothyroid and 96 patients were hyperthyroid. Abnormal hormone results were found in 480 additional cases.

TABLE 1. Patients in the THYROID-system (N = 1664).

Systems' Diagnosis	N	% Overall
Normal and correct	1018	61.2
Normal and incorrect	0	0.0
Abnormal and correct	612	36.8
Abnormal and incorrect	34	2.0

The THYROID-system agreed with the final evaluation in 98.0% of all cases. When patients with normal TSH and thyroid hormones are excluded, the accuracy of the THYROID-system was 94.7%. The reports were misleading in 34 patients. Thirteen of these patients were overtly hypothyroid and two hyperthyroid although laboratory measurements led to the interpretation of subclinical disease. In 21 cases the clinical disease was not yet obvious or non thyroidal illness (not available to the system) influenced the test results.

A broad category of reports was 'euthyroidism or further tests indicated in selected cases to screen rare clinical conditions' (N = 151, Table 2). This category of the reports is difficult to fit into the system as regards the sensitivity and the specificity. If it is assumed that the instructions to select patients for further tests were always followed, the number of euthyroid patients not requiring any further tests, according to the THYROID system, was 1329 and the specificity of identifications was thus 88.7% (1329/1498, Table 2). The THYROID-system found 153 of 166 patients with clinical disease (sensitivity 92.2%).

TABLE 2. Reports in euthyroid and overtly hyperthyroid or hypothyroid cases.

THYROID system's report	Clinically Hyper/Hypothyroid N	Euthyroid N
Hyper/Hypothyroid	150	21[b]
Not definitive[a]	3	148[c]
Euthyroid	13[d]	1329
Total	166	1498

[a] euthyroid or further test indicated in selected cases
[b] clinical disease soon in 7 cases, nonthyroidal illness in 8 cases
[c] clinical disease soon in 7 cases, nonthyroidal illness in 57 cases
[d] interpreted as subclinical disease

Need for THYROID-system

TABLE 3. The clinicians' attitude toward the THYROID-system was asked among users and non-users.

	Reports of the THYROID-system			
	Read regularly	Consider useful	Consider misleading	System interpretation welcomed
USERS				
Internists (N=11)	79.5%	55.9%	1.8%	37.3%
General practitioners (N=9)	99.0%	60.4%	4.2%	52.2%
All (N=20)	88.3%	57.9%	2.9%	44.0%
NONUSERS (N=16)	-	-	-	18.7%

Most of the reports of the interpretation system were read and considered as useful. According to the users the THYROID-system helped to interpret the results of thyroid hormone assays, was generally didactic in diagnostics of thyroid diseases and helped in planning further tests. The clinicians wanted less help in interpretation of thyroid hormone results, if the THYROID-system had not been available for them (18.7% vs. 44%).

The general level of knowledge of thyroid diagnostics was tested in a group of doctors working in a department of internal medicine (n=31), general practitioners (n=38) and medical students (n=49). The test consisted of three patient cases: 1. nodular goiter, 2. subclinical hypothyroidism, and 3. total T4 elevated due to high thyroxin binding globulin. Only 54.8 percent of all answers contained the correct diagnoses and conclusions. Some of the diagnostic alternatives were missing or decisions were misleading in 26.2% of answers, and 18.9% of all the interpretations were incorrect. There was no difference between the test groups.

Discussion

The main purpose of the THYROID-system was to produce a program, which is sensitive in screening thyroid diseases, and guides the clinicians in selecting the tests and helps them to interpret the results. According to the evaluation of the THYROID-system and clinicians' opinions these purposes were reached. Although the diagnoses of overt thyroid diseases are usually easy to establish, general practitioners and even internists had problems in the interpretation of thyroid hormone results.

Unlike many other expert systems (4, 7) our system was made without measures of uncertainty or probability, because the expert system shell that is used (Expertech's Xi+) does not support any certainty factors or use probabilities directly. Any uncertainty in choosing between competing diagnoses was dealt with by producing less conclusive or qualified diagnoses of thyroid function. Because broad diagnostic categories were defined, it is very unlikely that the system produces totally incorrect suggestions. The less conclusive diagnoses or tentative suggestions could have been more precise if more details and clinical information would have been available. On the other hand, the system identifies the cases in which only proposals can be given, and the final decisions are made by clinical grounds. Either in an ambulatory or in a hospitalized patient setting, a normal serum TSH value is strongly suggestive of euthyroidism if the patient has an intact hypothalamic-pituitary function and is not receiving drugs known to suppress pituitary TSH secretion (10, 11). According to this strategy FT4 and T4 are not needed if TSH is normal. This strategy was also very sensitive in this study.

Although several interpretation systems have been developed (1-7), little is known about their effects on the behavior and attitudes of the users. Clinicians wanted more assistance in interpretation of thyroid hormone results, if they were familiar with the THYROID-system. This may indicate that users were more aware about their true knowledge level of thyroid disorders than nonusers.

This study demonstrates that the THYROID-system can be applied successfully on primary thyroid diagnostics in the clinical laboratory. The program proved to be satisfactory for classifying thyroid function. We are currently improving the clarity of the diagnostic comments and the transferability of the knowledge base.

References

1. C. A. Kulikowski. Expert systems for thyroid function testing. Diagnostic Medicine 1981; 2: 99-102.

2. J. M. Fattu, E. A. Patrick, W. Sutton. Thyroid disorders: Automatic diagnosis in CONSULT I. Computer in Biology and Medicine 1982; 12: 285-293.

3. K. A. Horn, P. Compton, L. Lazarus, J. R. Quinlan. An expert system for the interpretation of thyroid assays in a clinical laboratory. Australian Computer Journal 1985; 17: 7-11.

4. J.B. Beck: Laboratory decision science applied to chemometrics. Strategic testing of thyroid function. Clinical Chemistry 1986; 32: 1707-1713.

5. P. Brosnan, G.Boran, J.B. Grimson, R. O'Moore. A decision support system for the assessment of thyroid function. Automedica 1987; 8: 169-178.

6. F. L. Degner, R. Santen. DES: A Domain Independent Expert System Running on a Microcomputer: Diagnostics of Thyroid Disorders. In: P. L. Rechertz and D. A. Lindberg (Eds.), Lecture Notes in Medical Informatics, Springer-Verlag Berlin 1988, pp 334-337.

7. P. J. Compton. Expert systems for the clinical interpretation of laboratory reports. In: den Boer, der Heiden, Leijnse and Souverijn (Eds.). Proc. of the 13th International Congress of Clinical Chemistry, Plenum Press New York 1989, pp. 615-627.

8. K. Saarinen, K. Irjala, P. Nuutila, P. Nykänen. A knowledge based system in a hospital - a discussion of improvements in clinical practice. In: Rienhoff O, Lindberg D A B (Eds), Lecture Notes in Medical Informatics, Springer-Verlag Berlin 1990, pp 343-347.

9. G. Caldwell, H.A.Kellett, S.M. Gow, G.J.Beckett, V.M.Sweeting, J.SEth, A.D.Toft. A new strategy for thyroid function testing. Lancet 1985; ii: 1117-9.

10. P.Nuutila, K.Irjala, J.Viikari, V.-P.Prinssi, H.-L.Kaihola. Comparative evaluation of serum thyroxine-, free thyroxine-and thyrotropin-determinations in screening of thyroid function. Annals of Clinical Research 1988; 20: 158-163.

11. C.A Spencer. Clinical utility and cost-effectiveness of sensitive thyrotropin assays in ambulatory and hospitalized patients. Mayo Clinic Proceedings 1988; 63: 1214-1222.

Transferability of Knowledge Based Systems
Information Technology Factors

Thomas Schioler*, John Nolan** & Peter McNair*

* Dept. of Clinical Chemistry, Hvidovre Hospital, University of Copenhagen, Denmark
** Division of Endocrinology and Metabolism, University of California, San Diego, USA

ABSTRACT

This presentation illucidates the impact information technology factors may have on transferability of knowledge based systems. The paper describes how database content, knowledge acquisition and knowledge representation may hamper or enhance viable transfer of knowledge based systems. Furthermore through experiments we demonstrate that the appropriateness of a chosen technology may be dependent on domain factors such as the epidemiological composition of training databases.

INTRODUCTION

The term "Transferability" (of a Knowledge Based System) can be defined as the degree to which the system retains its credibility and therefore reliability and usefulness when applied in another organisational environment [1]. Transferability is a key issue in the development of viable Knowledge Based Systems (KBS) in medicine. In previous work [1] we have proposed a separation of the many basic factors which influence a systems transferability under two main headings, see table 1. Domain factors belong to the medical problem area. Technology factors are independent of clinical medicine, belonging instead to the discipline of knowledge engineering. However as we shall show the appropriateness of a technology can be dependent on domain factors. We have previously described the impact of Domain factors [1]. In this paper we give experimental examples showing the effect of Technology factors.

Table 1, Transferability Factors.

Domain factors	Technology factors
Epidemiology	Knowledge acquisition
Terminology	Knowledge representation
Methodology	System functionality
Resources	Database content

METHODOLOGY

In order to study transferability factors we follow the structured approach suggested by the KAVAS-AIM project, see figure 1 [1,2]. In setup A, a KBS is exposed to databases from different sources and its ability to produce reasonable/sensible output is studied (i.e. correctness of output compared with clinical verified diagnosis). In setup B, a single database is used as input source to several different KBS's. Sensibility of output is then studied.

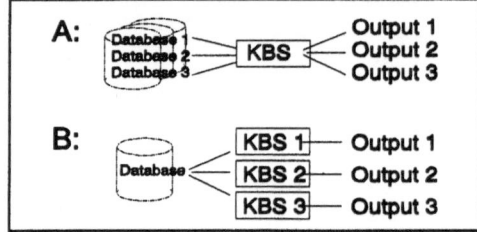

Figure 1, Two approaches to assess transferability.

Databases

We have used 3 different databases on Thyroid disease. One database of 140 thyroid patients from Trinity College, Dublin, Ireland collected from 1988 to 1989 [1]. The Dublin database consists of data on 7 possible thyroid function tests, clinical details and final clinical diagnosis, see table 2. Two consecutive databases on Thyroid diseases, collected at Hvidovre Hospital, University of Copenhagen, Denmark from 1980 to 1982 and from 1983 to 1985. The first database consist of 202 thyroid patients and normal controls and the second database 174 thyroid patients. See table 2.

Source of patients, biochemical analysis, diagnostic criteria, etc. were identical for both database. The first database was originally used for the development of a sequential test selection algorithm, at Hvidovre Hospital, Copenhagen [3]. Hence called the "Training database". The second database, used to evaluate the sequential test selection algorithm. Hence the called "Testing database". Both databases consist of data on 5 Thyroid function tests and final clinical diagnosis.

Table 2, Thyroid DataBases (DB).

Diagnosis Category	Dublin	Copenhagen	
	DB	Training DB	Testing DB
Thyrotoxic	35	50	59
Myxedema	42	20	19
Euthyroid	48	55	96
Controls	15	77	-
All	140	202	174

Knowledge Based Systems

Four different knowledge based systems/ algorithms were used for our experiments. The last 3 were all trained on the same Copenhagen training database as mentioned above:

1) Dublin KBS, a rule-based system designed to interpret any permutation of test results, giving a textual comment in the form of advice regarding diagnosis. Because of the huge number of possible permutations a very extensive decision tree is provided, with forward and backward chaining inference mechanism [4].

2) An inductive machine-learning program for automated construction of binary decision trees through multiple successive divisions. At each division the route offering the greatest reduction in entropy of the data is chosen [5].

3) A naive, manually constructed rule-based algorithm developed for sequential thyroid function test selections and diagnosis support at Hvidovre Hospital, Copenhagen, Denmark [3].

4) A probabilistic system of causal networks using statistical methods to make a causal model relating the data elements. Various models of conditionality or connectedness are tried for goodness of fit to the data. The final conditionality model is used to derive a KBS. The output is expressed as a probability that the case fits a given diagnosis [6].

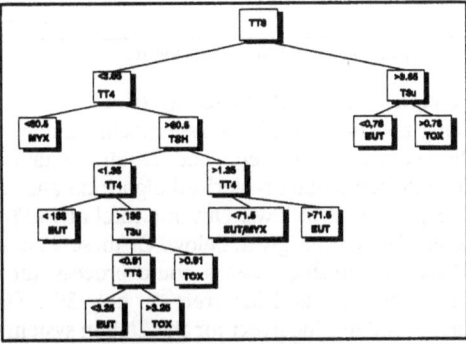

Figure 2, Induction algorithm decision tree.

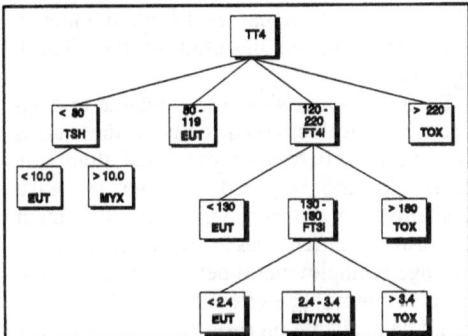

Figure 3, Manual algorithm decision tree

The three different algorithms derived by the three last systems were represented as decision trees. For the manually constructed and the induction algorithms, this is their "natural" mode of representation, see figures 2 and 3. The probabilistic KBS does not represent its derived algorithm as a decision tree or as a set of rules. However by simulating all possible variations it is possible to represent the knowledge as a decision tree see figure 4.

RESULTS

The distinction between the different information technology factors are not as clear as the distinction between domain factors. Our experiments concentrated on elucidating possible information technology factors, focusing on "knowledge acquisition" and "database content".

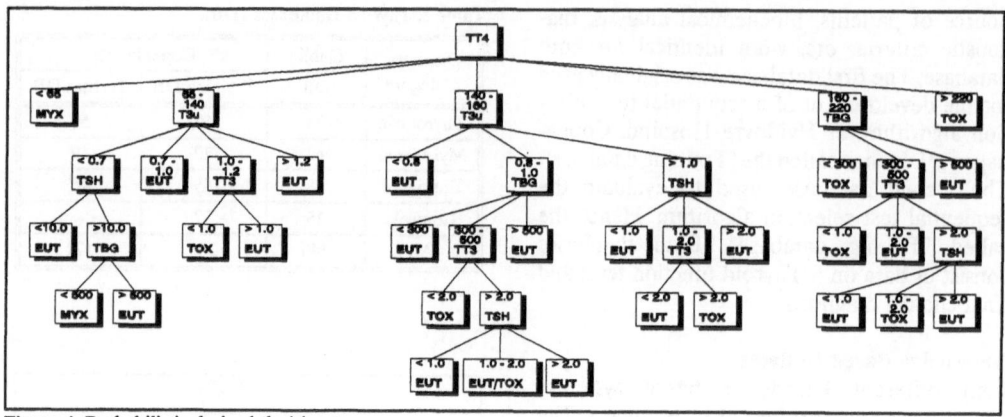

Figure 4, Probabilistic derived decision tree.

Example 1: Two Rule Based Systems

Using approach B of our assessment strategy (see figure 1), two rule-based systems for Thyroid Disease was compared. The Dublin database were processed by the Dublin KBS and the Copenhagen manually derived algorithm and their outputs compared, see table 3. The results may be explained as follows: Out of a total of 140 Irish cases, only 91 could be processed by the Danish system for reasons given below. Of these 91 cases 14 had diagnosis modified by the Danish system. Of the processable cases it could process, the Danish system was fully correct on 79%, partially correct on 18% and incorrect on only 3%. This compares with 81% fully correct, 13% partially correct and 6% incorrect for the Dublin system on the same cases. However the Danish system had the following problems:.

1) Difference in the available laboratory tests on the Dublin cases causes a large number of cases (35%) to be unsuited to the Danish algorithm.

2) The simpler decision tree is unable to diagnose "subclinical" cases correctly. As these cases are borderline between normal and abnormal, more rules are required to cater for each possibility. In conclusion, this experiment demonstrates differences in sensitivity and case-coverage (completeness) between two decision support systems. The effect of the rules was to impose inflexible demands on what laboratory tests should be available on cases from a foreign centre. This is a fundamental obstacle to transferability.

Table 3, Comparison of Dublin KBS output with Copenhagen KBS output.

Correctness	DUB	CPH
Fully Correct	113	72
Partially Correct	19	16
Incorrect	8	3
Unable to Process	-	49
% Fully Correct	81	51

Example 2: Rule Based versus Probabilistic versus Induction Algorithm

Using approach B of our assessment strategy (see figure 1), the 3 different decision trees described previously were compared for the correctness of their output. All 3 decision trees were trained on the same Copenhagen Training database (see table 2). In order to evaluate the Copenhagen testing database was applied according to the "rules", described by the decision trees. The test-cases were then sorted. The end-diagnosis of the terminal branches of the decision trees were compared with the clinical verified diagnosis of the sorted test cases. For results see table 4. The 3 derived trees showed large differences in structure. The manually constructed algorithm and the probabilistic derived algorithm both used the TT4 as the primary test, whereas the induction algorithm used TT3 as the primary test. The probabilistic derived decision tree showed far greater complexity than the two other trees, using more steps and having far more terminal branches (26) in comparison with the manually constructed decision tree and the induction algorithm decision tree (9 terminal branches each). See figures 2, 3 and 4.

It appears that the poorer performance of the probabilistic derived decision tree is due to its performance on the thyrotoxic cases. Even though the tree is applicable to 54 out of 59 thyrotoxic cases, which gives the coverage as for the two other trees, its correctness performance is very poor being only 68% of cases covered, in comparison with the manual tree's 95% and the induction tree's 87%. However the probabilistic and the induction tree's poorer performance on thyrotoxic cases, could indicate that the thyrotoxic cases of the testing database differ from the thyrotoxic cases of the training database. If this is the case, then the probabilistic derived tree is more dependent on the completeness of the data/attributes in its training database than is the rule-based manual approach and the machine-learned induction system. In this sense it is more constrained by local habits and therefore less amenable to transferability.

Table 4, Correctness of decision trees, % applicable cases.

Diagnosis Category	Manual		Probabilistic		Induction	
	Coverage	Correct	Coverage	Correct	Coverage	Correct
Euthyroid (N=96)	98 %	96 %	91 %	94 %	89 %	98 %
Thyrotoxic (N=59)	93 %	95 %	92 %	69 %	92 %	87 %
Myxedema (N=19)	84 %	94 %	90 %	100 %	100 %	90 %
All (N=174)	95 %	95 %	91 %	86 %	91 %	93 %

Example 3: Impact of Epidemiological Change of Training Database

In this experiment we have applied both the A and the B approach of our assessment strategy, see figure 1. By representing each hypothyroid case twice in the database (direct duplication) a new more hypothyroid training database is created, see table 5. The probabilistic and the induction algorithm systems were then trained on the new "myxedema" training database and the process of deducting decision trees was repeated, see figures 5 and 6. Again the Copenhagen testing database was used to evaluate the two "myxedema" trees for the correctness of outputs. The change of training database in a more hypothyroid direction gave large changes in the structure and composition of the new decision trees. Primary thyroid tests were changed from TT4 to TSH on the probabilistic tree and from TT3 to TT4 on the induction algorithm tree. Both these changes seems reasonable from a physiological point of view, if the aim is to "screen off" the hypothyroid cases. Again the probabilistic derived decision tree showed far greater complexity than the other tree having far more terminal branches (37) than the induction algorithm decision tree (10), see figures 5 and 6. Comparison of outputs when changing the epidemiological composition of the training database for the probabilistic derived decision trees showed an overall increase in correctly diagnosed cases when applying the "myxedema" setting (86 % to 92 %) due to an increase in correctly diagnosed thyrotoxic cases (69% to 92%). See tables 4, 6.

Table 5, Thyroid Training Databases.

Diagnosis Category	Epidemiological Setting I	Epidemiological Setting II
Thyrotoxic	50	50
Myxedema	20	40
Euthyroid	55	55
Controls	77	77
All	202	222

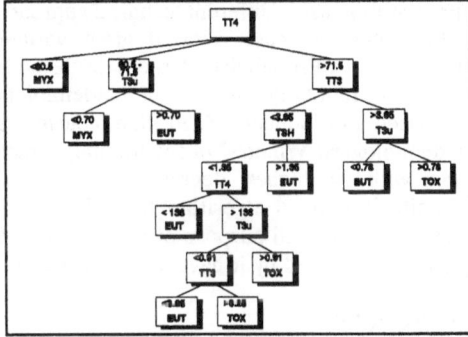

Figure 5, Induction algorithm decision tree, setting 2.

Table 6, Correctness, epidemiological setting 2.

Diagnosis Category	Probabilistic		Induction	
	Coverage	Correct	Coverage	Correct
Euthyroid (N=96)	80 %	90 %	90 %	93 %
Thyrotoxic (N=59)	49 %	92 %	92 %	87 %
Myxedema (N=19)	15 %	100 %	100 %	90 %
All (N=174)	83 %	92 %	91 %	91 %

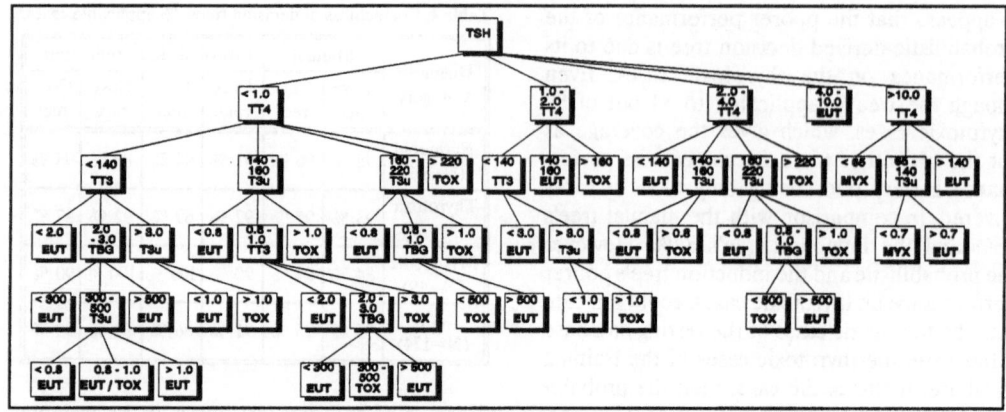

Figure 6, Probabilistic derived decision tree, epidemiological setting 2.

Thus the change of epidemiology of the training database resulted in not only a higher degree of correctness for the probabilistic tree, but also in a more even degree of correctness over disease categories. The induction derived decision tree showed no major change in the number of correct diagnosis. In conclusion, this experiment demonstrates differences in sensitivity to changes in the epidemiology of the training database, which not only causes changes in the structure of the decision trees (by different technological approaches) but also has impact on the correctness of their output.

CONCLUSION

The mode of Knowledge Acquisition and Database Content are key transferability factors in the Information Technological area. In our experiments we have shown how different Rule-based systems, for the same medical problem can vary greatly. Regional differences in data profile (due to local laboratory or medical practice) may hamper transferability, giving a higher number of unprocessable cases. Different technical approaches to knowledge acquisition from databases, trained on the same database, showed great variation in knowledge representation and in output performance. A Probabilistic System displayed less transferability because it was more constrained by domain limitations, such as the epidemiological composition of the training database, than its Rule-based and Induction Algorithm "cousins". However the most robust system to changes in the "Epidemiological Window" of the training database (the induction algorithm), is not necessarily the system with the highest degree of correctness on output performance in a given setting (the Probabilistic derived algorithm trained in a hypothyroid setting). Therefore both the technical approach, design and purpose of a Knowledge Based System as well as the design and content of databases processed by it have a role in the ultimate transferability of a system.

REFERENCES
[1] Nolan, J., McNair, P., Brender, J. "Factors influencing transferability of medical decision support systems". Int. J. Biomed. Comp, 27, 1991, pp 7-26.
[2] McNair, P., Nolan, J., Brender, J. "A pilot study of factors hampering transferability of medical knowledge based systems" In McNair, P., Brender, J. (eds.) Proceedings of AIM Workshop, Bruxelles, October 1990, Trans-4.1, KAVAS (A1021) Project, AIM programme, 1990, pp. 69-80.
[3] McNair, P. et al "Thyroid function test strategy", Eur. J. Clin. Invest., Vol 15, no. 2, pp A57, 1985.
[4] Brosnan, P. et al "A decision support system for the assessment of thyroid function", Automedica, 8, 1987, pp 169-178.
[5] Talmon, J.L. "A multiclass Nonparametric Partitioning Algorithm", Pattern Recognition Letters, 4, 1986, pp 31-38.
[6] Andersen, L.R., Krebs, J.H., Andersen, J.D. "STENO: An expert system for medical diagnosis based on graphical models and model search", J. Applied Stat., 1991 (in press).

THE ROLE OF DIAGNOSTIC UNCERTAINTY IN HEALTH CARE OUTCOMES AND ITS POTENTIAL FOR MODIFICATION WITH DECISION SUPPORT

Richard A. Bankowitz, MD

The Section of Medical Informatics, LB 50A Lothrop Hall, University of Pittsburgh School of Medicine, Pittsburgh, PA 15261 USA.

Abstract: INTERNIST-1 and its successor Quick Medical Reference (QMR), are computer programs which utilize an extensive knowledge base of diseases in internal medicine to assist clinicians in the task of diagnosis. The provision of medical care, in general, and the utilization of the diagnostic laboratory, in particular, are known to exhibit wide variation among physicians. A neglected reason for some of this variation may be the degree of diagnostic uncertainty accompanying each patient case. We propose that computer programs like QMR may decrease some of this variability by providing more information to the physician, and we discuss a methodology for testing this proposal.

Introduction

For over 15 years, a project has been under way at the University of Pittsburgh to develop and maintain a computerized knowledge base of diseases in the domain of general internal medicine. INTERNIST-1, and its successor Quick Medical Reference (QMR), are computer programs which utilize this extensive knowledge base to assist the clinician with the process of medical diagnosis [1,2]. The INTERNIST-1/QMR knowledge base contains detailed information on the frequencies and predictive values of more than 4200 history, physical and laboratory findings occurring in each of more than 600 diseases in internal medicine. Pilot data using QMR on hospital medical wards suggest that the system can be both accurate, and can impact upon the utilization of the diagnostic laboratory [3,4].

To extend this research, we are currently studying the effectiveness of QMR on patients admitted to the general medicine wards of a university hospital when the program is operated by health care personnel familiar with its use. Outcome measures of effectiveness will include information on hospital lengths of stay, diagnostic test utilization, and hospital charges. A goal of this project is to determine the incidence of diagnostic uncertainty among patients admitted to a general medical hospital ward, and to determine how, if at all, cost of diagnosis is related to the diagnostic uncertainty at the time of admission. The purpose of this paper is to discuss the methodology for this aspect of the study and to provide the theoretical background for the work.

Evidence for variation in medical practice

Wide variations have been uncovered in the amount of medical services delivered to patients with identical or similar medical problems. Variation has been described in almost every area of medical practice and can be demonstrated in rates of diagnostic testing [5,6] and rates of medical procedures [7]. Hospitalization rates are highly variable. Wennberg et al. compared hospital bed utilization and hospital expenditures for residents of Boston, Massachusetts and New Haven, Connecticut. By any measure, utilization was significantly higher in Boston. Six medical diagnoses accounted for 25% of the variability. Although this wide disparity in utilization existed, there was no difference in the 30-day Health Care Financing Administration (HCFA) mortality between these two communities [8].

Variation in surgical utilization is well documented [9-13]. In an early study published in Science, Wennberg and Gittlesohn examined the variation in utilization of services between regions of Vermont. They demonstrated a fourfold difference in hysterectomy rate, sixfold variation in tonsillectomy rate and a fourfold variation in prostetectomy rate [9]. A similar study by Roos, revealed a fivefold variation in hysterectomy rates in Monitoba Canada [10]. Other studies have disclosed similar variation [11-13].

Variability in the use of the diagnostic laboratory

The utilization of the diagnostic laboratory exhibits wide variation among practitioners; not all of this variation is appropriate [5]. Many factors affect this variability. Physician characteristics such as specialty, age, and type of training have been shown to influence the practitioners' practice style. General Practitioners (not necessarily family practitioners) order fewer diagnostic tests then internists. [6]. Subspecialists order more tests than do general internists [14]. Older physicians use fewer laboratory tests and order fewer x-ray studies [15]. Whether this reflects increased utilization by younger physicians, or underutilization by older physicians is not clear, but younger physicians tend to have shorter lengths of stay for their patients [16].

The role of diagnostic uncertainty in practice variation

One largely neglected component of the high rate of variability encountered in diagnostic laboratory utilization is the physician's initial level of diagnostic uncertainty. Relatively few studies have explored physicians' attitudes concerning diagnostic uncertainty. There is some general evidence that physicians are not skilled at handling expressions of probability. In a study which evaluated physicians' expressions of probability, Bryant and Norman found a striking inconsistency in the way these expressions were applied. For example, when asked to assign a numerical probability to the word "sometimes," the estimates ranged from 5% to 75%. The range exceeded 50% for more than half of the expression [17]. Though Pauker and Kassirer have proposed the threshold approach to the use of the diagnostic laboratory, [18], there is evidence that this approach is consistently violated in actual clinical practice.

The role for computerized medical decision support

Potential roles of computer-based systems in modifying physicians' use of the diagnostic laboratory follow a continuum of invasiveness from educational software to decision support to managed care [See Figure 1]. Although some have proposed managed care, and other more "invasive" solutions to decreasing the variability in laboratory utilization, we are proposing utilizing the QMR program and its knowledge base as a guide to more rational laboratory use.

Figure 1: Possible Roles of Computer Assisted Medical Decision Making in Decreasing
Variation in Medical Practice.

```
I
N        Education
V               Cost-Effective use of Laboratory
A        Process of Care
S               Efficient /Effective Diagnosis
I               Efficient/ Effective Therapy
V               Practice "Reminders'
E               Optimal Scenarios
N        Managed Care
E               Practice Guidelines
S               Quality Assurance
S               Pre-admission Certification
```

We have devised and are currently implementing a randomized controlled trial of the impact of a computer-based decision support system, the University of Pittsburgh version of Quick Medical Reference (QMR), on patient care outcomes. In the context of this evaluation, we are seeking to determine the incidence of diagnostic uncertainty with regard to admissions to a general medical hospital ward, and to determine how, if at all, cost of diagnosis relates to diagnostic uncertainty at the time of admission. We further wish to explore the level of diagnostic uncertainty at which use of computer-based decision support software becomes optimal or even desirable.

Patients are recruited prospectively. Those that meet eligibility criteria are further grouped by the level of house staff diagnostic uncertainty at the time of admission. This uncertainty will be quantified by means of a modification of the standard reference gamble technique. The study protocol calls for the evaluation of patients by a diagnostic consultation team which utilizes the QMR program. A physician's assistant will enter the preliminary clinical data into the QMR program and a study investigator will review the procedure. After the protocol intervention, patients are randomly assigned to a study group, in which the results of the QMR diagnostic intervention are revealed to the house staff caring for the patient, or to a control group, in which the results of the intervention are concealed. Primary outcome measures of the effectiveness of the system will include: patient length of hospital stay, accuracy of house staff diagnoses, time required for diagnosis, number of diagnostic services utilized by medical personnel, and total as well as categorical charges incurred.

This data will allow an examination of the relationship of diagnostic uncertainty to patient outcome. In addition, the analysis will allow us to determine the relationship between diagnostic uncertainty and cost of diagnosis. The methodology utilized in this study confronts several problem areas which should be of interest to others developing or evaluating decision support systems.

References

1. Miller RA, Pople HE, Myers JD: INTERNIST-1, An experimental computer-based diagnostic consultant for general internal medicine, N Engl J Med, 1982, 307:468-476.
2. Miller RA, McNeil MA, Challinor, SM, et al., The INTERNIST-1/Quick Medical Reference Project - Status Report, West J Med, 1986, 145:816-822.
3. Bankowitz RA, McNeil MA, Challinor, SM et al., A Computer-Assisted Medical Diagnostic Consultation Service: Implementation and prospective evaluation of a prototype, Ann Intern Med, 1989, 110:824-832.
4. Bankowitz RA, McNeil MA, Challinor, SM, Miller RA, Effect of a computer-assisted general medicine diagnostic consultation service on house staff diagnostic strategy, Meth Inform Med, 1989, 28:352-356.
5. Schroeder SA, Myers LP, McPhee SJ, Use of Laboratory tests and pharmaceuticals: variation among physicians and effect of cost audit on subsequent care, JAMA 1984; 252:225-30.
6. Noren J, Frazier T, Altman I and DeLozier J. Ambulatory medical care: A comparison on internists and family-general practitioners. N Engl J Med 1980;302:11-16.
7. Chassin MR, Kosecoff J, et al. Does inappropriate use explain geographic variations in the use of health care services? N Engl J Med 1986;314:285-90.
8. Wennberg JE, Freeman JL and Culp WJ. Are hospital services rationed in New Haven or over-utilized in Boston?. Lancet May 23, 1987; 1185-1189.
9. Wennberg JE, Gittleshon A, Small area variations in health care delivery. Science 1973;18:1102-1108.
10. Roos NP, Flowerdew G, Wajda A, et al., Variations in physicians' hospitalization practices: A population-based study in Manitoba, Canada. American Journal of Public Health 1986:;76(1):45-51.
11. Lewis CE. Variation in the incidence of surgery. N Engl J Med 1969;281:880-884.
12. McPherson K, Wennberg JE, Hovind OB, et al. Small-area variation in the use of common surgical procedures: an international comparison of New England, England and Norway. N Engl J Med 1982; 307: 1310-1314.
13. Wennberg JE, Mulley AG, Hanley D, et al. An assessment of prostatectomy for benign urinary tract obstruction. JAMA 1988;259:3027-3030.
14. Manu P, and Schwartz SE, Patterns of diagnostic testing in the academic setting: The influence of medical attending ; subspecialty training. Soc Sci Med 1983; 17:1339-42.
15. Eisenberg JM, Nicklin D, Use of diagnostic services by physicians in community practice. Med Care 1981; 19:297-309.
16. Goldfarb MG, Hornbrook MC, Higgins CS, Determinants of hospital use: A cross-diagnostic analysis. Med Care 1983; 21:48-66.
17. Bryant GD and Norman GR. Expressions of probability: Words and numbers. N Engl J Med 1980;302:411.
18. Pauker SG, Kassirer JP. Decision Analysis. N Engl J Med 1987;316:250-258.

FUZZY SET THEORY
IN MEDICINE

DECISION-AID UNDER UNCERTAINTY BASED ON
SEPARATING POWER AND FUZZY MEASURES
Christiane DUJET - Hamza SI-KADDOUR
Laboratoire Modélisation des Systèmes et Reconnaissance des Formes
Centre de Mathématiques - INSA - Bâtiment 403
F - 69621 Villeurbanne Cedex

ABSTRACT: Facing the problem of mecical diagnosis assistance under uncertainty, whatever should be the adopted methodology, if based on fuzzy sets, the final step is to take a non-fuzzy decision, which means to assign some diagnosis to the patient. To tell it briefly, after some "fuzzyfication" of the problem comes the "defuzzification". This defuzzification may be achieved by means of the separating power (of a fuzzy set). The separating power was first introduced by Dujet in 1980 [3], to solve the problem of finding the "best (crisp) partition" of a referential set, elements of which may satisfy a given property to some imprecise degree and was first applied to help for diagnosis in Inflammatory Syndroms by E. Sanchez and R. Bartolin in 1987.
Here is proposed a review of the methodology based on fuzzy sets which may be worked up, involving fuzzy measures and separating power. A rapid view about new mathematical results will follow, in order to show how to answer some specific problems encountered in the "continuum" case.

KEYWORDS: knowledge base, data representation, matching, fuzzy sets, separating power, fuzzy measures.

INTRODUCTION: What is proposed is a methodology based on fuzzy sets, when the data are vague, imprecise, uncertain, which methodology consists mainly of three steps:
- representation of knowledege and data by means of fuzzy sets,
- matching of pattern with the patient's condition by means of fuzzy measures,
- decision making (assignement of diagnosis to the patient) by means of the separating power.
As an example of medical application, we shall refer to the use of protein profile to help for diagnosis in Inflammatory syndroms (I.S.). [8].
Let us recall that I.S. are characterized by specific protein variations: what matters in the protein I.S. model is the relative variations of serum protein levels, thus uncertainty is not of a probabilistic nature; moreover, thresholds cannot be defined precisely to allow classification of patients; on the opposite, variations of serum protein levels may be easily interpretated in linguistic terms by internists, and thus are well adpated to a fuzzy representation (see [1]).

407

I - REPRESENTATION OF KNOWLEDGE AND DATA

The medical knowledge pattern takes the form of tableau with linguistic entries [6, 10], which are fuzzy propositions of standard form: " S is P". S is the label of an attribute (symtom, sign ...) taking values in universe of discourse E, P is a fuzzy set of E.

Example: interpretation of fuzzy concept *Increased biliburin*.

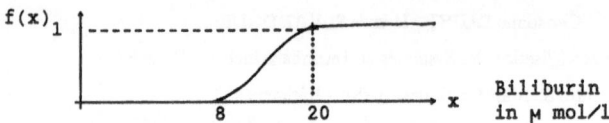

Biliburin
in μ mol/l

Example of a typical serum protein pattern

Diagnoses \ Symptoms	Total Protein	Albumin	α Globulin	β Globulin	γ Globulin
Hepatitis	Usually Normal	Decreased	Slightly Decreased	Slightly Decreased	Increased

Then, diagnosis Δ (hepatitis) is interpretated by conjunctions (and's) of fuzzy propositions: total protein (S_1) are usually normal (P_1) and albumin (S_2) is decreased (P_2) and ... . This conjunction defines a proposition Q, representing diagnosis hepatitis.

The data representation takes the standard form: S_i is D_i, where D_i is a fuzzy set of E_i. It means that, in order to compare the patient's condition with the reference proposition Q in the knowledge base, we assign to each symptom S_i occuring in Q, its value (which is a fuzzy set D_i) for the given patient.

II - MATCHING

For a given patient, we have to compare a reference proposition Q: (S_1 is P_1) and ... and (S_n is P_n), and the corresponding data: (S_1 is D_1) and ... and (S_n is D_n).

The matching is realized by means of fuzzy measures; in the medical illustrations, three indexes were used: Possibility index [2], Necessity Index [2], Truth Qualification Index [11].

Let us recall, for example, the definition: of the possibility index: Pos(P/D) = Sup {P(x) ∧ D(x)}; it is clear from definition that this index expresses the "degree" of intersection of fuzzy sets P and D.

The rule for interpretating the conjunction of propositions was the "min operator", it is not the best choice, but the more simple. The following procedures is then adopted for a given patient:

For every diagnosis $Δ_i$, let us compute, for every sign S_j occuring in $Δ_i$

The possibility index, denoted by P_{ij} (= Pos P_j / D_j)

The necessity index, denoted by N_{ij}

The truth index, denoted by Q_{ij}.

This, for a given patient, let us define the following mappings:

h, ℓ, k, respectively associated to possibility, necessity and truth indexes

$$h(\Delta_i) = \min_j P_{ij}$$

The mapping h may be interpreted as a fuzzy set of the class of optimal diagnoses.

III - DECISION MAKING

Up to this step, every patient is associated to some fuzzy set h (ℓ, k respectively) of the class Δ of all optionnal diagnoses. The final step consists of applying the separating power [4] to fuzzy sets, h, ℓ, k, which leads to find crisp bi-partitions of Δ corresponding respectively to h, ℓ, k. This procedure allows the assignment of one (or a group) of diagnoses to the given patient.

Moreover, the calculus of the separating index allows to get an idea about the degree of concordance between the patient's condition and the suggested diagnoses. We may then compare the obtained results for a given patient with respect to the chosen index.

Let us call A_G, A_H, A_L, respectively, the assigned class of diagnoses for a given patient, with respect to Pos, Nec and Truth indexes respectively. Generally, the classifications respect the following order:

$$A_G \subset A_H \subset A_L$$

which is rather satisfying, because it is well known that

$$\text{Nec Index} \leq \text{Truth Qual. Index} \leq \text{Pos Index}$$

Remark: for the medical studied case, a multiple assignement is not a default of relevance of the method, on the opposite, it reflects evidence that some elements in the protein profile should evoke a pathogenic association.

IV - RESULTS AND DISCUSSION

To work up the described methodology, a software named XFLOU was conceived by V. BONNIOL (Marseille) and implemented on MINI 6 BULL

Sampling: 163 patients

. *56% are well assigned* (in their origin group, or in two groups containing origin group).

. *38% are apparently ill-assigned*, that is: assigned to a group different from the origin group. This missclassification was most of times an apparent error: after analysis, these patients had for example recover a normal profile (by evolution of disease or therapeutical success).

. *6% are assigned* to more than one group, to which their origin group is not belonging. These results were rather satisfying, we point out that our goal in decision-aid for medical diagnoses is to help for evoking diagnoses, not to give a precise diagnosis: Nevertheless, the medical part of the method may be improved by a best choice of proteins for example, by taking in account the evolution of disecase, by a better definition od diagnoses among experts. For the mathematical part, other operators may be used, instead of the min operator; the matching procedure may be achieved by means of a compatibility index, also based on the seprating power in order to ensure more coherence to the method.

V - SEPARATING POWER

A complete axiomatic approach of the separating power is to be found in [5].
This concept was aimed to take into account:

- the average behaviour of a fuzzy set,

- and more specifically, the degree to which a fuzzy set of some referential set E is separating the elements of E, compared to the ideal case (no uncertainty), when f takes only values zero or one (i.g. if f is a boolean characteristic function), in which case, the referential set is "naturally" partitioned into two complementary subsets.

Obviously, the more separation we get, the more fuzziness we get. Therefore, any measure of separation will be tightly linked to and determined a measure of fuzziness.

Let us recall, in the discrete case, a very simple way of getting a separating power. Given a finite referential set E, and given a fuzzy set f of E (f is a mapping from E into interval [0, 1]) an example of separating power of f on E is a mapping denoted by *, from $\mathcal{P}(E)$ into [0,1] , defined as follows:

$$f * B = \frac{1}{Card\ B} \sum_{x \in B} f(x) - \frac{1}{Card\ \overline{B}} \sum_{x \in \overline{B}} f(x) \quad ; \quad \forall B \in \mathcal{P}(E), \quad B \neq E \quad B \neq \emptyset$$

where $\overline{B}$ denotes the complementary set of B with respect to E, and $\mathcal{P}(E)$ denotes the class of all (crisp) subsets of E.

Then, the separating index of f is the positive real number denoted by S(f), and equal to Sup $|f * B|$, $B \neq \emptyset$, $B \neq E$

$$B \in \mathcal{P}(E)$$

In the discrete case, this Sup is always attained for some proper subset A of E, determining by the way a partition (A, $\overline{A}$) of E, which is a non-fuzzy partition and realizes the "best separation of elements of E with respect to fuzzy set f of E.

As examples of separating power of fuzzy set f of E, if E is not a finite set, it was proposed the use of Lebesgue's integral (or Sugeno's integral) as follows:

$$f * B = \frac{1}{\mu(B)} \int_B f\ d\mu - \frac{1}{\mu(\overline{B})} \int_{\overline{B}} f\ d\mu$$

where μ is a Lebesque's measure, and B belongs to the class of μ measurable subsets of E, with $\mu(B) \neq \emptyset$ (For more details, see [5]).

In the continuum case, given an infinite set E of elements, it may happen that this Sup is not reached, even for a continuous fuzzy set f of E.

Moreover, in the case of a continuous fuzzy set f, we have to find a method to compute the separating power.

As it was already proved in [5], if the Sup exists, the corresponding partition of E is an α-cut. This fact inspired us to look at the decreasing rearrangement f* of the given continuous fuzzy set f (see [9]), and we prove in [7] that S(f*) = S(f).

The main consequence is that we can compute the separating index of any continuous fuzzy set by determining the separating index of a decreasing mapping, which is an easy task. Anyway, the problem still remains, that even for a decreasing mapping, the separating index should not be reached at some proper subset A of E; we propose then in [7] another way of defining the "best partition" with respect to the notion of separation, which turns out to solve an equation and which always gives an answer.

CONCLUSION: The use of the separating power was an original approach in the medical case reported here as an example; particularly, it gives rise to a standard method for "defuzzifying" a problem, which can be used in any problem of Decision-aid under uncertainty, in which, a non-fuzzy decision is required at the end.

REFERENCES

[1] K.P. ADLASSNIG - A survey on medical diagnosis and fuzzy subsets. Approximate reasoning in decision analysis - Gupta, Sanchez Eds. - 203-219 - North Holland (1982).

[2] D. DUBOIS - H. PRADE - Fuzzy sets and Systems - Theory and Applications - Academic Press - New York London (1980).

[3] C. DUJET - Valuation et separation dans les ensembles flous - Informations et Questionnaires - Publications CNRS (1980).

[4] C.DUJET - Complementation and information on the separating power of a fuzzy set - Fuzzy Information and Decision Process - Gupta, Sanchez Eds. - North Holland (1982).

[5] C. DUJET - Separation and measure of fuzziness - Fuzzy sets and systems - 28 - 245-262 - North Holland (1988)

[6] C. DUJET, E. SANCHEZ, R. BARTOLIN - Fuzzy sets and partitions - A new approach applied to medical decision assistance: inflammatory syndroms - Technical report, Laboratoire Modélisation des Systèmes et Reconnaissance des Formes - INSA Lyon (1987).

[7] C. DUJET, H. SI KADDOUR - On the separating power of a fuzzy set - Preprint - Submitted for publication.

[8] J.C. FROT, H. HOFMANN, P. MULLER, M.F. BENAZET , P. GIRAUDET - Le concept du profil protéïque - Ann. Bio. Clin. - 42 - 1-8 (1984)

[9] T.V. RYFF - Measure preserving transformations and rearrangments - Journal of Math. Analysis and Applications - 31 - 449-458 (1970).

[10] E. SANCHEZ - Medical applications with fuzzy sets - Fuzzy Sets Theory and Applications - A. Jones and Als eds - D. Reidel - 331-347 (1986).

[11] E. SANCHEZ - On truth qualifications in natural languages - Int. Conf. on Cybernetics and Society - Tokyo Proceedings - 1233-1236 (1978).

HYPERTHYROIDISM DIAGNOSIS SUPPORTING USING IMPRECISE RULES

Joanna Straszecka

IV Department of Internal Medicine of the Silesian Medical Academy

POLAND

Ewa Straszecka[*]

Institute of Electronics, Silesian Technical University

POLAND

ABSTRACT. A method of transforming a diagnostic pattern in hyperthyroidism, into "IF A THEN B" rules is presented. A representation
of imprecision of some medical concepts and a scheme of reasoning
using it are suggested. Examples of testing the model for patients'
data are given. Results of testing are summarized and conclusions
are drawn.

1. Introduction.

Hyperthyroidism is a frequent disease of thyroid gland. The
diagnosis, however is not easy because symptoms are not always typical
and they may also be characteristic for other diseases (e.g. neurosis).
A tool of diagnosis support can be an expert system with a knowledge
base in the form of IF-THEN rules. Unfortunately, though medical books
are full of diagnostic patterns, it is difficult to rewrite them in a
form that is acceptable for knowledge-based systems. We made an effort
to find a method of transforming one of the diagnostic patterns, namely
the Crooks index [3], into IF A THEN B rules. We also suggest a representation of imprecision useful in some medical problems and a scheme of
reasoning which may be very efficient for the kind of rules under
discussion. Thus a very small know ledge based system modelling the
Crooks index using fuzzy sets is proposed.

2. Method of reasoning.

The proposed method of reasoning is based on generalized modus ponens
[5] and on a concept of similarity of fuzzy sets [2]. The conclusion is
determined by firing an $A \rightarrow B$ rule for the fact A' which is similar,

[*] Address for correspondence: Ewa Straszecka, Inst. of Electronics,
Silesian Technical University, Pstrowskiego St. 16, 44-101 Gliwice,
POLAND

(but usually not identical) to the premise of the rule. The premise of the rule is a logical sum of several conditions. Rules are of the form :

$$A \rightarrow B \qquad \text{where } A = A_1 \cup A_2 \cup \ldots \cup A_n$$

The rule is fired given facts $A' = A_1' \cup A_2' \cup \ldots \cup A_n'$ and conclusion B' is drawn. Values of facts A_i' i=1,...,n (generally imprecise, defined by membership functions of fuzzy sets) are from input data or are unknown. The former are represented by previously or currently constructed membership functions, the latter by a constant membership function of 0.5 value. Some membership functions are proposed in [4].

A rule can be fired even when all facts are unknown but obviously, in this case, the conclusion will also be 'I don't know'. In the most rule-based systems a sum of conditions is transformed into the sum of several rules with the same conclusion, i.e into $\bigcup_i A_i \rightarrow B$. However, specific demands of Crooks index modelling make us find a different solution.

The most important problem in summing membership functions A_i i=1,...,n consists in that that they have different supports. This was the reason why we used a sum of similarity functions not the membership functions themselves. The basics for this method are explained in [4]. Here we only give a brief description necessary for further discussion.

The conclusion in the reasoning process, in which generalized modus ponens is involved, is constructed on the basis of a rule and facts similar to its premise. The more similar the facts A_i' to A_i are, the less different conclusion B' from B is. Assuming that similarity functions for all pairs A_i and A_i' i=1,..n are found, the similarity function between B and B' can be calculated and next the conclusion B' can be estimated. The similarity function is defined using t-norms (and ϕ-operators) or s-norms (and β-operators), e.g. as:

$$A_i \equiv A_i' = \gamma_{A_i} = (\mu_{A_i} \phi \mu_{A_i'}) \, t \, (\mu_{A_i'} \phi \mu_{A_i})$$

or

$$A_i \equiv A_i' = \gamma_{A_i} = 1 - (\mu_{A_i} \beta \mu_{A_i'}) \, s \, (\mu_{A_i'} \beta \mu_{A_i})$$

Other useful definitions for γ, which have been tested for a medical case and some t-norms are proposed in [4].

It is worth noticing that supports for all γ_{A_i} can be the same and thus the sum $\bigcup_i \gamma_{A_i}$ expresses available information for facts A_i' and the premise A. The logical sum is interpreted by an s-norm. Defining similarity function enables us to estimate lower $(\mu_B, -)$ and upper $(\mu_B, +)$ boundaries for the membership function of B, given μ_B and γ_B. It should be also noticed that defining γ for every rule from a collection of the form: $A \rightarrow B$, $C \rightarrow B$, can be helpful in eliminating rules, which are weakly supported by facts.

It is possible to add a factor of imprecision of implication to the scheme of reasoning. To this end, a relation R^{CFi} is calculated between γ_{A_i} and γ_{B}. R^{CFi} shows that the diagnosis does not entirely depend on the similarity between A'_i and A_i. Similarity function γ_{B_i} denotes this element of γ_B, which depends on pair A_i and A'_i.

All in all, the reasoning process is described in Diagram 1.

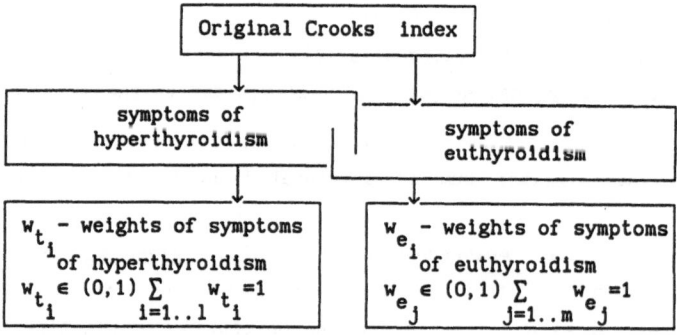

Diagram 1. A scheme of the method of reasoning.

The reasoning method presented above, was used in modelling Crooks index. The results of modelling are considerably better than in case of traditional [1] interpretation of the problem.

3. The Crooks index model.

The Crooks index is a test in which data obtained during an interview and primary physical examination are summed according to some pattern [3]. The pattern consists in assigning integer numbers from [-5,5] interval to symptoms. Numbers are assigned to some symptoms both when they are pre- sent or absent, and these numbers differ in signs and/or in absolute values. Numbers are assigned to other symptoms only when they are present. After gathering all data, an algebraic sum is calculated. If the sum is less or equal to 10, it is assumed that a patient does not suffer from hyperthyroidism. If the result is within

```
          ┌──────────────────────────┐
          │  Original Crooks  index  │
          └──────────────────────────┘
             │                    │
   ┌──────────────────┐    ┌──────────────────┐
   │   symptoms of    │    │   symptoms of    │
   │ hyperthyroidism  │    │  euthyroidism    │
   └──────────────────┘    └──────────────────┘
             │                    │
```

w_{t_i} - weights of symptoms of hyperthyroidism
$w_{t_i} \in (0,1) \sum_{i=1..1} w_{t_i} = 1$

w_{e_j} - weights of symptoms of euthyroidism
$w_{e_j} \in (0,1) \sum_{j=1..m} w_{e_j} = 1$

Diagram 2. The Crooks index modelling.

414

[11,19] interval, further investigation is needed. The result equal to or greater than 20 means that there is 90% chance that patient is ill with hyperthyroidism [3].

The Crooks index is modelled using the reasoning method presented in previous paragraph. Membership functions for symptoms given in an imprecise way are defined. Symptoms are divided into two groups -these which are present in hyperthyroidism and those which indicate euthyroidism (normal function of the thyroid gland). Obviously some of them belong to both groups, but with different significance. The original weights are transformed into (0,1) interval in the model. Diagram 2 illustrates the process of modelling.

Final modelling results in two rules : one for hyperthyroidism, and the other for euthyroidism. E.g. for hyperthyroidism:

IF   <linguistic description> <$symptom_1$>   =>
   OR...   <$weight_1$>

      <linguistic description> <$symptom_n$>   =>   <Hyperthyroidism>(0.9)
                                             <$weight_1$>

Weights w_{t_i} and w_{e_j} are used to calculate R^{CFi}, R^{CFj} relations.

The constructed model of the Crooks index can be used even when some symptoms are not known. The result of reasoning in this case is different from that obtained when the symptoms are absent. For simplification and expecting that the system would be used by doctors who do not know much about membership functions, some membership functions resembling linguistic descriptions commonly used are defined.

Many authors find that one of the most difficult steps in constructing a reasoning algorithm with membership functions is an interpretation of a conclusion. We have decided to simplify the problem and to present the result of reasoning in a figure, in which broken lines represent membership functions of hyperthyroidism and euthyroidism. Broken lines are used to join points equivalent to values of membership functions, calculated as mean values of $\mu_{B'-}$ and $\mu_{B'+}$. Thus the conclusion is presented in the form of an easily understandable figure.

4. Examples *.

The model was tested for data of outpatients of a clinic of the district hospital   for thyroid gland diseases. The Crooks index questions (e.g. 'What is the patient's age?', 'What is his weight?','Is

---

* It is not possible to submit a full example in this short paper. We present a description and diagrams of some results. Original diagrams have been re-drawn to reduce space and avoid unimportant information.

the heart beating present?') were answered by expressions connected with
membership functions (e.g. 'young', 'old'; 'normal','elevated'), "crisp"
concepts ('yes','no') or "I don't know" phrase. Following the scheme of
reasoning presented above, the conclusion is produced in a diagram form.
It is interpreted as follows.

If the broken line representing hyperthyroidism is above the line
representing euthyroidism, it indicates hyperthyroidism. In the opposite
situation the conclusion is: euthyroidism. Crossing membership functions
implies dubious diagnosis - further investigation is needed. Fig.1 shows
examples of conclusions. They are model's conclusions for three patients
for whom doctor's diagnoses were: healthy (a), suffering from
hyperthyroidism (b), needs further examination (c), respectively. As we
can see, in these cases doctor's diagnoses and the model's conclusions
are identical. We have obtained good results for patients with clear
doctor's diagnoses.

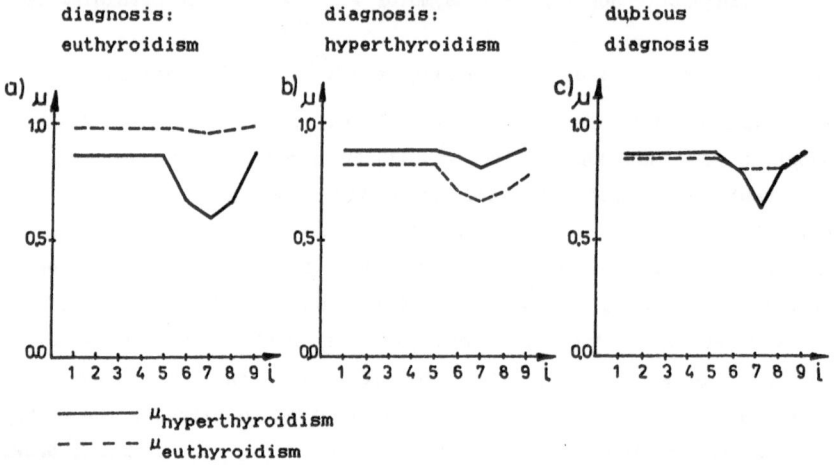

Figure 1. Results of the model of the Crooks index testing.

After testing the system with a number of patients' data we found, that
similar sets of symptoms produce almost identical representation,
creating something which can be called "a picture of a disease". It
means that "typical" hyperthyroidism produces one kind of a picture,
while a different figure is obtained for a healthy person. This property
of the system, which is somehow obvious when carefully considered, can
make the interpretation of results even simpler.

5. Testing results and conclusions.

We hope that the presented method, though not universal can be used
in solving some problems of similar nature. We have obtained promising

results in testing the system for outpatients data from Tychy district hospital clinic for thyroid gland diseases. We have obtained proper results for healthy patients and those who suffered from "typical hyperthyroidism". The system tends to qualify a part of patients with dubious, according to doctors, diagnosis, as ill persons. However, also in this group most of results are proper. We describe the work of the system as "careful" for it does not qualify the latter cases as healthy. We found that our simple interpretation of the model's conclusion is easy to understand and works surprisingly well. Obviously it can not be used in a situation when there are many conclusions. Nevertheless, there are a lot of problems of this kind in medicine, connected with the differentiation, which can be solved in this way.

We have presented a method of building a very small knowledge-based system (which can become a part of a larger one), using information taken from medical books. We feel that this kind of information should be used wider in constructing knowledge bases, because re-writing the whole knowledge, from the very beginning, by a team knowledge-engineer - doctor is too tiring. This leads to a great simplification of rules at the primary stage and thus requires a very long period of supplementing.

We work with the method creating a knowledge base for differentiation between neurosis and hyperthyroidism and we continue testing the Crooks index model.

We hope that the presented method, though not universal, and our experience in using it, can help in solving problems of a similar nature.

6. References.

1. Dubois D., Martin-Clouaire R., Prade H. -"Practical computing in Fuzzy Logic" in Fuzzy Computing, M.M.Gupta, T.Yanakawa Edts, Elsevier Science Publishers BV (North Holland), 1988, pp. 11-34;

2. Gottwald S. Pedrycz W. - "On the Methodology of Solving Fuzzy Relatio- nal Equations and its Impact on Fuzzy Modelling" - in Fuzzy Logic in Knowledge-Based Systems, Decision and Control, M.M.Gupta, T.Yamakawa Edts, Elsevier Science Publishers B.V. (North - Holland), 1988, pp 197-210.

3. Crooks J., Murray J.P.C., Wayne E.J. - "Statistical methods applied to the clinical diagnosis of thyrotoxicosis" - in Quart.J.Med, 1959, 28, 211

4. Straszecka E. - "Modelling imprecision of rules in expert systems for medical decision - making support" - to appear in Modelling Simulation and Control, C, vol 26 1991 p.55-63

5. Zadeh L.A. - "Fuzzy sets as a basis for a theory of Possibility", Fuzzy Sets and Systems No 1, Vol. 3, 1978, pp 3-28.

A Decision Making System in Aviation Medicine

Ludmila Kuncheva[*], Rumen Zlatev[**], Vania Raicheva[**]

[*] Central Laboratory of Bioinstrumentation and Automation, Bulgarian Academy of Sciences, Acad. G. Bonchev Str., Bl. 105, 1113 Sofia, BULGARIA

[**] United Scientific and Research Institute for Aviation Medicine, Georgy Sofiiski Str., 3, 1304 Sofia, BULGARIA

Abstract

A decision support system for assessing of the pilot's resistance to high-G radial accelerations is described. It uses the achievements in the fields of Pattern Recognition, Artificial Intelligence, Fuzzy Set theory, etc. to cope with the specific constraints and requirements in aviation medicine. The structure of the system as well as the classification rules are empirically determined on the basis of a variety of experiments with retrospectively collected data. Although the system is still at a developmental stage, the preliminary results obtained show a sufficiently high classification accuracy.

1. Introduction

The problem to be solved is to distinguish between two groups of pilots - permitted and nonpermitted to fly for a certain period. The decision of the physician is based on the results of an examination subjecting the individual to extreme conditions [1] (e.g. high-G radial accelerations, hypoxia, etc.). The final decision consists of several intermediate ones. One only negative intermediate decision involves a negative final decision.

The most challenging features which the designer of a computer consultation system faces in the field of aviation medicine can be summarized as follows:

(i) Small size of data samples - Due to the specific character of the examination only small sets of reference data are available;

(ii) Impossibility for verification - No physician's

418

decision about the medical ability of a pilot to fly can be directly checked (except in the case of an accident);

(iii) Practical lack of anamnestic data - Usually the pilots try to hide their subjective complaints hoping to obtain a permission to fly from the medical council. Even they make attempts to improve the objective parameters (e.g. to normalize the blood pressure) before the examinations;

(iv) Need of objectively confirmed decision - Usually the pilot does not agree with a negative decision arguing that the physician's decision is too subjectively biased.

Due to the features listed, it may appear that the point of view on Decision Support Technologies of physicians concerned with aviation medicine is slightly different from the negative attitude presented in [5]. A decision support system could help in eliciting more precisely the boundary between a positive and a negative decision and on the other hand to avoid the eventual subjectivity.

Taking into account the constraints it seems reasonable to apply to this kind of problems composite strategies arising from the convergence of pattern recognition and Artificial Intelligence, fuzzy set theory, etc. [2,3,4]. Their combination can cope both with various numerical problems and with the lack of information.

In this paper a decision support system for resistance to high-G radial accelerations is described which uses the achievements from the above mentioned fields.

2. STATEMENT OF THE PROBLEM

Results from annual routine medical examinations of pilots and candidates [6] have been used. The training sample consists of 78 healthy male persons.

The examination for a given individual consists in passing through a profile of high G radial accelerations in a centrifugal cabin. A signal is from time to time transmitted into the cabin, and an immediate answer is required from the pilot. The miss of this answer is an indication for the loss of peripheral vision, and presents an evidence for "bad resistance" decision.

The physician's decision is based generally on cardiac rhythm disorders, loss of peripheral vision, changes in pulse rate, reaction time, etc.

Two groups were formed depending on the physician's decision: "good resistance to high G", and "bad resistance to high G". Furthermore the description of each class is expressed in a more detailed way:

"good resistance": good resistance (code 0); good resistance with nonsignificant cardiac rhythm disorders (code 1); good resistance with nonsignificant loss of peripheral vision (code 2);

"bad resistance": bad resistance with significant loss of peripheral vision (code 3); bad resistance with significant cardiac rhythm disorders (code 4).

3. STRUCTURE OF THE SYSTEM

The purpose of the system is to suggest a decision about the permission of a pilot to fly on the basis of his physiological parameters before, during and after the examination.

Due to the small size of the training data set as well as the lack of anamnesis a parallel structure of the system is chosen as shown in fig 1.

Figure 1: Structure of the system

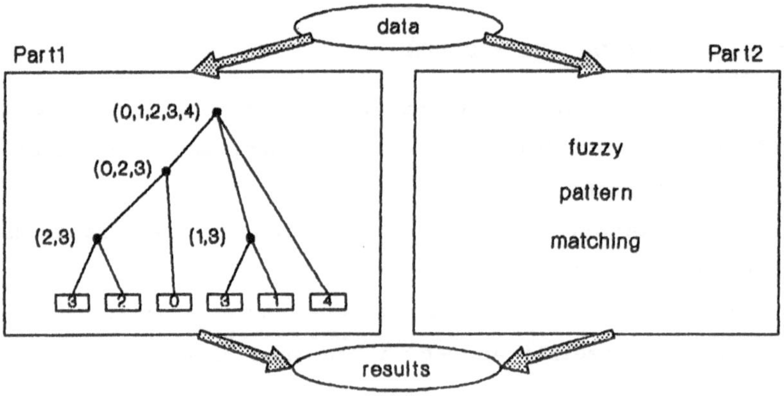

The first decision process is based purely on pattern recognition techniques - treewise scheme using discriminant analysis and k-Nearest Neighbors methods at different nodes of the tree, depending on the results obtained in the training stage. The structure of the decision tree was generated also using the result of testing checking different combinations of groups of classes. The objectivization of this decision making criterion was presented in a previous publication [7]. As a result for an unknown pattern the respective class is pointed at in the form presented in fig. 2.

Figure 2: Output of the parallel results

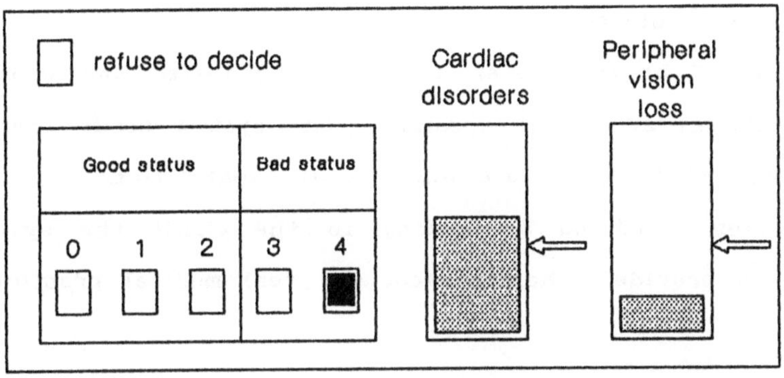

The second decision process is based on expert opinion, described in the form of fuzzy sets. Several prototype patterns were generated and two degrees of membership are attached to each one expressing the degree of cardiac disorders and the degree of loss of peripheral vision of the individual. The description of the information implies that fuzzy pattern recognition method is to be used. The results are two degrees expressing the availability and the strength of the respective characteristics. Form of the decision is shown in fig. 2.

Having this information the physician could draw his own conclusion making use of both results. This competition form enables the user to pay a look to the problem from different points of view.

4. PERFORMANCE EVALUATION AND CONCLUSIONS

The accuracy of the Part 1 of the system was tested on the basis of the training sample complemented with a test sample. As a measure of accuracy an estimate of error rate was used. The results obtained were reported in [7]. Overall classification accuracy calculated on the basis of 154 cases is 96.1 % . The evaluation presented can provide a rough impression about the system performance because the result might be slightly optimistically biased.

Part 2 of the system is now being tested and prototypes for the classes are being specified. The system needs some more improvement of its interface and visual capabilities.

After a period of testing in the clinic the system is supposed to provide a helpful tool for real medical practice.

REFERENCES

1. Burton, R.R. (1986). Simulated Aerial Combat Maneuvering Tolerance and Physical Conditioning: Current Status, Av. Sp. Env. Med., 57 , 712-716.
2. Gelsema, E.S. (1989) (Editorial) Pattern Recognition and Artificial Intelligence in Medical Research and Clinical Practice, Methods of Information in Medicine 28, 63-65.
3. Kissiov, V., Hadjitodorov, S., & Kuncheva,L. (1990). Using Key Features in Pattern Classification. Pattern Recognition Letters, 11, 1-5.
4. Kuncheva, L. (1990) Fuzzy Multi-Level Classifier for Medical Applications, Computers in Biology and Medicine 20, 421-431.
5. Shortliffe, E.H. (1989) (Editorial) Testing Reality: The Introduction of Decision-Support Technologies for Physicians, Methods of Information in Medicine 28, 1-5.
6. Zlatev, R. & Dimitrov, D. (1986). About the Dynamics of Certain Cardiovascular Parameters in +Gz Accelerations with Changing Profiles and Gradient Increase. Proc: XV Workshop of Aviation Physicians from WCA, Sofia.
7. Zlatev, R., L. Kuncheva & V. Raicheva (1990). A Pattern Recognition Criterion for Evaluating of High-G Tolerance of Pilots and Astronauts, I-st Int. Conf. "Modeling and Control of Biotechnological, Ecological and Biomedical Systems, Varna.

MEXYS2: A FUZZY REASONING EXPERT SYSTEM BASED ON THE SUBJECT EMOTIONS CONSIDERATION

Stevo Božinovski[1], Cveta Martinovska[2],

Liljana Božinovska[3], Nada Pop-Jordanova[4]

[1]*Electrical Engineering Faculty,* [2]*Institute of Seismology*
[3]*Institute of Physiology,* [4]*Clinic of Child Deseases*
University of Skopje, Yugoslavia

ABSTRACT: An expert system for personality and emotional profile assessment is developed and here reported. The expert knowledge and the basic computational procedure are based on a standard psychological test. Fuzzy reasoning and uncertainty assessment are also features of this system.

INTRODUCTION

MEXYS2, as a medical diagnosis expert system (3) is designed to give insight into the basic personality features and internal conflicts of a subject. Theoretical background is taken from a personality theory which assumes personality features to be a representation of some emotional structures (7). The basic computational procedure as well as the required expert knowledge are taken from the standard psychological inventory EPI (1).

Some personality analysis measurements, such as the partial ordering of the subject personality features according to the subject preference, and synthesis of the facial emotional expression, are specific to this system and not part of the standard EPI test.

As an expert system, MEXYS2 includes dealing with types of knowledge such as knowledge which is considered with a certain degree of unceirtainty (unceirtainty problem), and knowledge which is not represented precisely enough (fuzziness problem). Uncertainty occurs when one is not absolutely certain about a piece of information. The degree of unceirtainty is usualy represented by a numerical value. Fuzziness occurs when a boundary of a piece of information is not clear-cut, e.g "John is *quite* young".(4,6)

THE SYSTEM ARCHITECTURE

Figure 1 shows the architecture of the system. It consists of 9 modules which could be divided into 4 groups: communication interfaces to the subject and to the user, knowledge base, computational procedure including fuzzy reasoning, and ability of the user to adjust the system parameters according to his experience (5). Ability to adjust the system parameters enables adaptation to the given population.

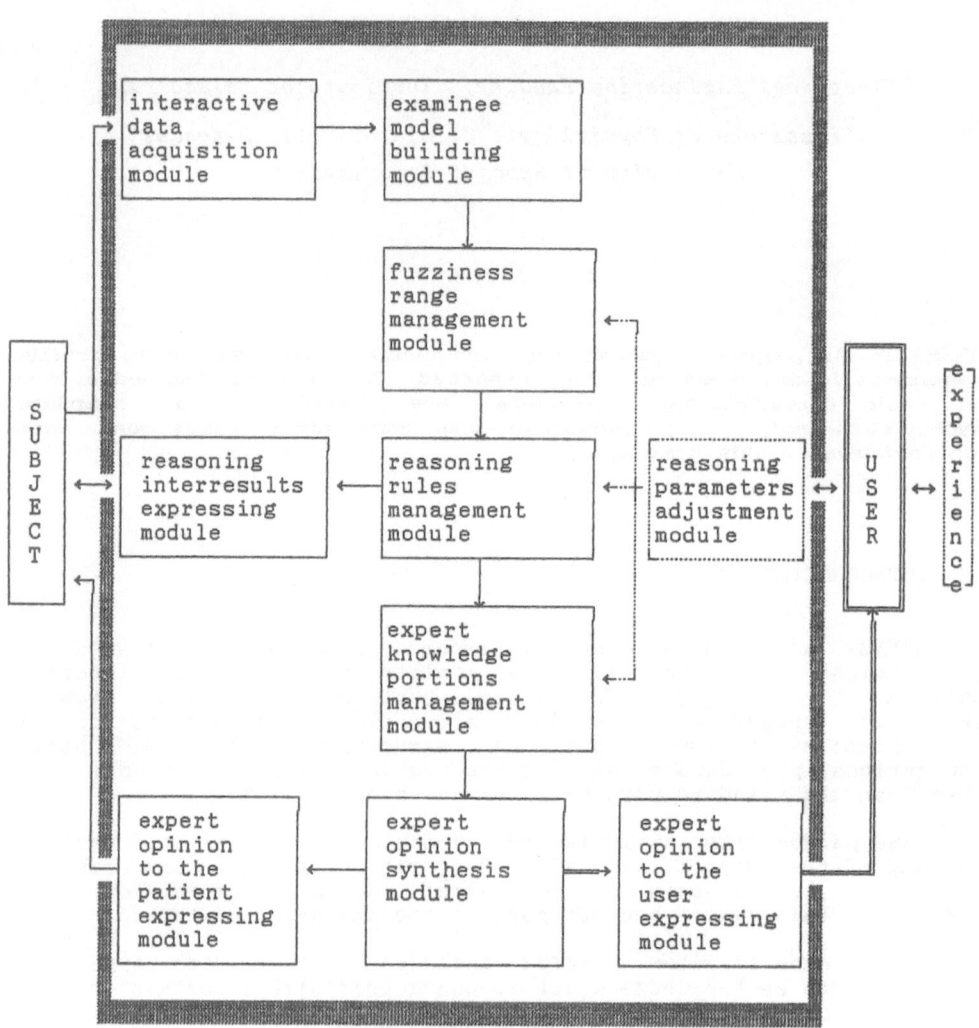

Figure 1. The structure of the MEXYS2 expert system

THE SYSTEM PROCEDURE

The system deals with two predefined sets. The personality features set F is defined as

F = {adveturous, cautious, confused, depressed, disputatious, embittered, hasty, hearty, obedient, sociable, self-biting, self-inconfident }

and the emotional groups set E is defined as

E = { reproduction, incorporation, incontrolability, self-protection, deprivation, oposition, exploration, agression }

The MEXYS2 computational procedure over these sets is described on Figure 2.

---

1. Perform questionaire on the entered subject.

2. Find the subjective preference ordering relation R over F.

3. Compute the subject fuzzy vector V over E.

4. Perform a rule based fuzzy reasoning over V.

5. Synthetise the expert opinion using the appropriate knowledge portions from the expert knowledge base.

6. Synthesize the facial emotion of the recognized emotional state

---

Figure 2. The MEXYS2 computational procedure

The reasoning within the system is performed over the rules of a form

if <antecedent> infer <consequent> with <certainty factor=CF>

where <antecedent> is a relation over fuzzy components computed at stage 3, <consequent> is a portion of the expert knowledge base assigned to the personality feature represented by the <antecedent>, and <certainty factor> indicates the certainty that each rule is believed in. The CF is subject to an empirical assessment. Example: "if rbig and ssmall then display appropriate piece of knowledge with the associated CF" where *rbig* and *ssmall* represent a range of variables reproduction and self-protection obtained in the fuzzufication process.

Each rule that applies for a computed V, produces a paragraph of text which contributes to the description of the subject personality.

THE SYSTEM OUTPUTS

At some stages of the computational procedure the system produces outputs, which are described on Figure 3.

ADV

CON

SBI   CAU

HEA   OBI

SOC

HAS   DIS

EMB

SIN

DEP

Figure 3.1

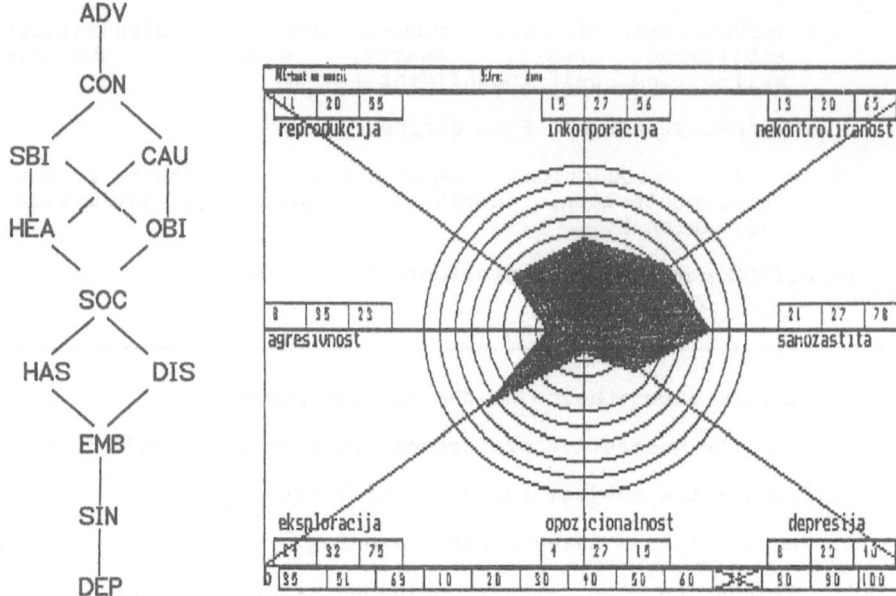

Figure 3.2

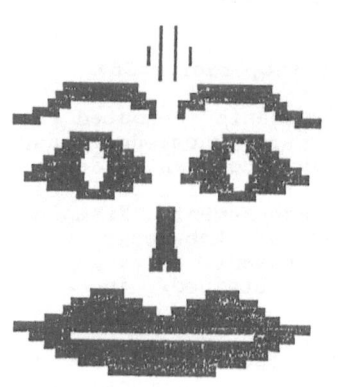

Figure 3.3

The subject is cautious, carefull, and axious. He is constantly worried not to get into troubles which could not deal with. It worries what other people think and talk about him. (FC=.8)

It is a personality which does not tend toward criticism and oposition. It is undecisive, subject to some others influence, non-fighting personality. (FC=.8)

Has tendencies and wishes to understand the environment it lives in, in order to manage it. Has tendency for organized life, and every thing to put on its own place. It wants to work and could express itself as as a well organized personality. Posess a good self-control. The other people consider him as an accurate, organized person, conscious and ambitious. (FC=.7)

The personality is not agressive and do not quarel, seldom is embittered, and even then does not express it out gladly. (FC=.8)

This personality is axious and there is possibility for fobic and opsesive-compulsive behavior. (FC=.7)

Figure 3.4

Figure 3. The MEXYS2 analysis of a subject

At the stage 2, a Hesse diagram of partial ordering of the subject personality features is displayed. Figure 3.1 gives an example of a computed Hesse diagram.

At the stage 3, a fuzzy vector in the emotional space is computed, and displayed in one of the several representation offered by the MEXYS2 system. Figure 3.2 shows a radial polygon representation.

Figure 3.3 shows an example of a facial expression synthesized from the emotional state of the system computed at the stage 6.

Figure 3.4 shows an example of an expert opinion output produced at stage 5. This technique we used in our previous expert systems for psychiatric assesments (2).

CONCLUSION

An expert system is developed which is an useful tool for medical diagnosis of a personality and emotional state of a subject. In includes dealing with knowledge base uncertainty, and fuzzines of the state which is to be recognized, the problems which contemporary expert system research addresses. Being in use for a year now in a medical institution, it showed increasing degree of belief as an instrument to which medical and neuropsychology decisions should rely.

REFERENCES

1. Baskovac-Milinkovic A., Bele-Potocnik §., Hrusevar B., Rojsek J. PIE: Emotions Profile Index, Manual (In Serbocroatian) Zavod za produktivnost dela, Ljubljana 1983
2. Bozinovski S., Jankovski Lj., Naumova M. "MEXYS: An expert system for psychiatric diagnosis based on the MMPI" In A. Luque, A. Figueiras, J. Delgado (Eds.) Bioengineering, Elsevier Publishers, IEEE 1985
3. Bundy A. "An expert system for medical diagnosis" In T.O'Shea, J. Self, G. Thomas (Eds) Intelligent Konwledge-Based Systems, London: Harper and Row, 1987
4. Fox J. "Dealing with unceirtainty" In T. O'Shea, J. Self, G. Thomas (Eds) Intelligent Konwledge-based Systems, London: Harper and Row, 1987
5. Kolonder J., Kolonder R. "Using experience in clinical problem solving: Introduction and framework" IEEE Trans. SMC May/June 1987
6. Leung K.S., Lam W. "Fuzzy concepts in expert systems" IEEE Computer Magazine, Sept. 1988
7. Plutchik R., Kallerman H. "Emotions Profile Index" Western Psychological Services, 1974

KNOWLEDGE-BASED FUZZY CLASSIFICATION OF SIGNAL EVENTS

S. Barro[1], R. Ruiz[2], R. Marín[1], J. Presedo[1], A. Bugarín[1] and J. Mira[3]

1. Dept. Electrónica. Facultad de Física. Universidad de Santiago. SPAIN
2. ETSII de Cartagena. Universidad de Murcia. SPAIN
3. Dept. Informática y Automática. UNED. Madrid. SPAIN

ABSTRACT

This work presents, and exemplifies in the field of electrocardiographic (ECG) signal processing, aspects of the design of Knowledge-based Fuzzy Classifiers of signal events. These classifiers add schemes for the conversion of numerical and symbolic information, and a later knowledge based treatment of this information to the classical processes of numerical feature extraction. This way, a feature space made up of linguistic variables is defined. The classification of an event in this space is approached through a process of comparison with a series of prototypes acquired from the expert.

INTRODUCTION

The detection and later classification of events based on the analysis of the evolution in time of certain physiological variables is of great interest in the context of medical science. The diagnosis/classification of many pathologies or the detection of situations which are dangerous for the patient (ventricular arrhythmias, for example) are founded, in many cases, on the analysis of physiological variables and parameters obtained from diverse sources: electrocardiogram, cardiovascular pressures, temperature, etc. The implementation of computerized systems for the analysis and classification of these events is generally based on the construction of procedures for the exhaustive manipulation of numerical data, such as the statistical classifiers [1]. The design of these classifiers usually starts by determining a set of properties (normally numerical) which will constitute a "definition vector" for the event being classified. After the calculation of this vector, the event will be classified using schemes for the comparison with representative prototypes for the possible categories or discerning classes. These prototypes are derived from a previous analysis (heuristic or statistical) of a large set of preclassified events (training set for the classifier). Despite the good performance of this type of systems, in some cases their design is not possible. This happens, for example, if a sufficiently populated training set is not available, the set of necessary characteristics is not well defined and/or limited, or the available information is of a qualitative nature, not exact, etc. In these cases, the design strategy for the classifier can be based on a process which mimics the one followed by the human experts in the field. This way, the design of the classifier must take into account the adequate representation and manipulation of the knowledge necessary for an efficient classification. Thus we must add to the problems inherent to the operation with signals: inclusion of low level processing steps, need, in most applications, for operating in real time, many artifacts, loss or distortion of the data, ambiguous information, continuous dynamism in the environment, etc., the fact that the knowledge manipulated by the expert is full of descriptive terms, which have a difficult translation into the computational domain, and lack precision in the characterization of multiple situations.

REPRESENTATION OF THE KNOWLEDGE

A general outline of the design process for a knowledge based classifier is shown in fig. 1. A process of knowledge elicitation is needed as a first step, with a frame that includes: a) a representation space with features that carry enough information to describe the patterns or events in the application domain. This point is directly linked to c); b) these features generally impose the need of adequate algorithms for their calculation in representations which are initially of numerical or boolean type; c) a set of linguistic descriptors to match, as nearly as possible, the perceived knowledge of the human expert. These linguistic descriptors will be used to construct classification prototypes in terms of conceptual entities in the format of "if-then" fuzzy rules (Fuzzy Conditional Statements (FCSs)).

After the design stage we enter the operational stage (fig. 2) in which unclassified data is identified in terms of features of the representation space which are translated into linguistic descriptors. On these linguistic descriptors, measurement of analogies with classification prototypes and decision criteria are applied in order to obtain classified data.

Need for fuzzy classification

In the medical environment the problems derived from the imprecision in the frontiers between the different categories to be differentiated, from the sometimes imprecise determination of the parameters on which the classification is based and the non deterministic relationship existing between these parameters and the different categories contemplated are frequent. This situation leads to consider interesting to perform a fuzzy classification (introducing the concept of "assigning degrees" of analyzed events to the categories considered) instead of the traditional deterministic classifications. Formalizing, it is a question of defining an application of the cartesian product of the set of events ($E = \{e_i\}$) to be classified and the set of possible categories ($C = \{c_n\}$), in the real interval $[0,1]$, in the following way:

$$
\begin{aligned}
R: \quad & E \times C \dashrightarrow [0,1] \\
& (e_i, c_n) \dashrightarrow \mu_{c_n}(e_i), \qquad n = 1, \dots, N
\end{aligned}
\tag{1}
$$

being $\mu_{c_n}(e_i)$ the membership degree ("assigning degree") of the event e_i to the fuzzy set indicated by the category c_n.

The events e_i can be defined, for example, using the linguistic variable concept introduced by Zadeh [2]. The values of a linguistic variable are members of a set of

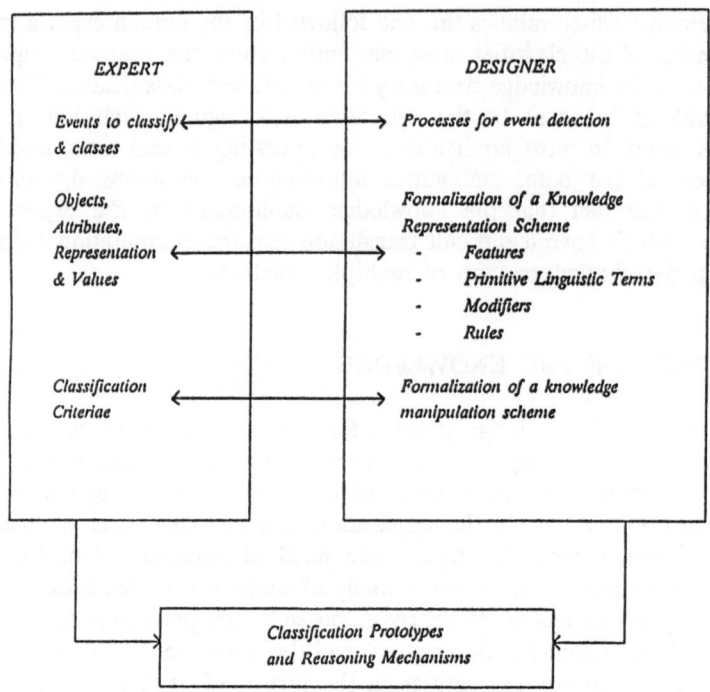

Fig. 1 Interaction Expert-Designer in the design process of a knowledge-based classifier of signal events.

linguistically defined labels. Heart rate, for example, can be interpreted as a linguistic variable with values in the set {very low, low, normal, high, ...}, each of whose member labels L_j is generally constructed from a set of primitives ({low, normal, high, ...}) and a set of modifiers ({not, very, ...}). These linguistic variables are based, in most cases, on numerical variables, whose value is computed using ad-hoc algorithms (heart rate in beats/minute).

For an application involving M linguistic variables P_m, we define the feature space $U = U_1 \times U_2 \times ... \times U_M$, where U_m is the universe of discourse associated with P_m. On the other hand, the knowledge necessary for approaching the classification process takes the form of a set of fuzzy classification rules of the type:

$$R_s = \text{"IF } <p_1 \text{ is } L_{s1}> \text{ and ... and } <p_m \text{ is } L_{sm}> \text{ THEN } <\mu_{c_1}(e_i) = W_{1s}>, ... , ..., <\mu_{c_N}(e_i) = W_{Ns}>\text{"} \quad (2)$$

where the symbols "< >" indicate that its content is optional.

The IF clause of each rule defines a fuzzy subset F_s of U, while the THEN clause defines the vector of membership degrees $\{\mu_{c_n}(e_i)\}$, $n=1,...,N$, of a event e_i belonging to F_s. Membership degrees can also take linguistic values in the set {absolute, ..., medium, ..., null}.

This structure goes well with the way in which medical knowledge is represented. For example, in the definition of ventricular extrasystole [3]: "ventricular extrasystole are premature, wide QRS complexes followed by a T wave with an axis opposite to that of

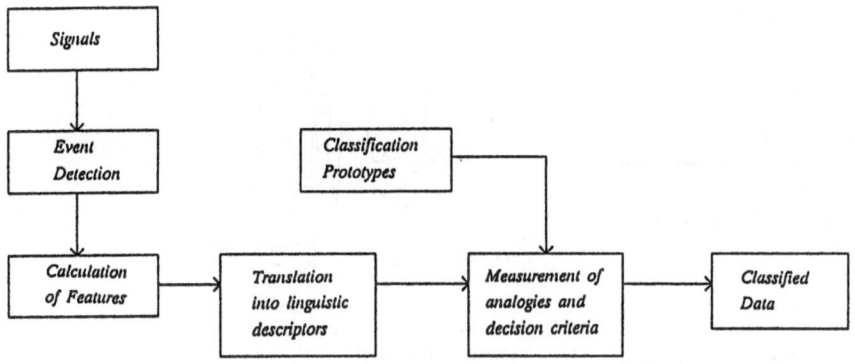

Fig. 2   Data flow in knowledge-based classification of signal events.

the QRS. Characteristically, ventricular extrasystole are not preceded by P waves..."(SIC); the need for the manipulation of linguistic concepts with clinical meaning such as: premature beat or wide QRS complex, is obvious in order to retain the conceptual descriptions of the expert. Thus, the manipulation of symbolic information and the necessary conversion of numerical information into symbolic information is imposed. For example, to use propositions of the type: "QRS width is high", it is necessary to define them according to the numerical parameters on which they are based; in this case QRS width in ms. So, the triplet "object-attribute-value" which is widely used in artificial intelligence [4] can be expanded into a quartet "object-attribute-representation-value" where the representation indicates the way in which the value of the object's attribute is represented.

Fig. 3 illustrates an example of rule extracted from a beat classifier which operates on an ECG signal [5].

KNOWLEDGE MANIPULATION

Apart from establishing the "prototype base" of the classifier (set of rules R_s), it is necessary to define the criteria for the measurement of event-prototype analogies and the final decision or result of the classification. In principle, it could be thought that the knowledge manipulation process for the classification of an event e_i, is reduced to the application of the rule or prototype R_s which defines in its antecedent part a fuzzy subset F_s in which e_i is included with a unity ("absolute") membership degree. However, given the form taken by the definition of events, this is not applicable in most cases. Also, the discourse universe or numerical interval in which an attribute (in its numerical representation) takes values, is divided into a series of fuzzy subsets with linguistic variables associated to them. The definition domains for the fuzzy subsets can overlap, and it is therefore possible for several rules to present non false antecedents for the same event and can thus be considered in the classification process of the event.

The need of having criteria for measuring the event-prototype analogies can be

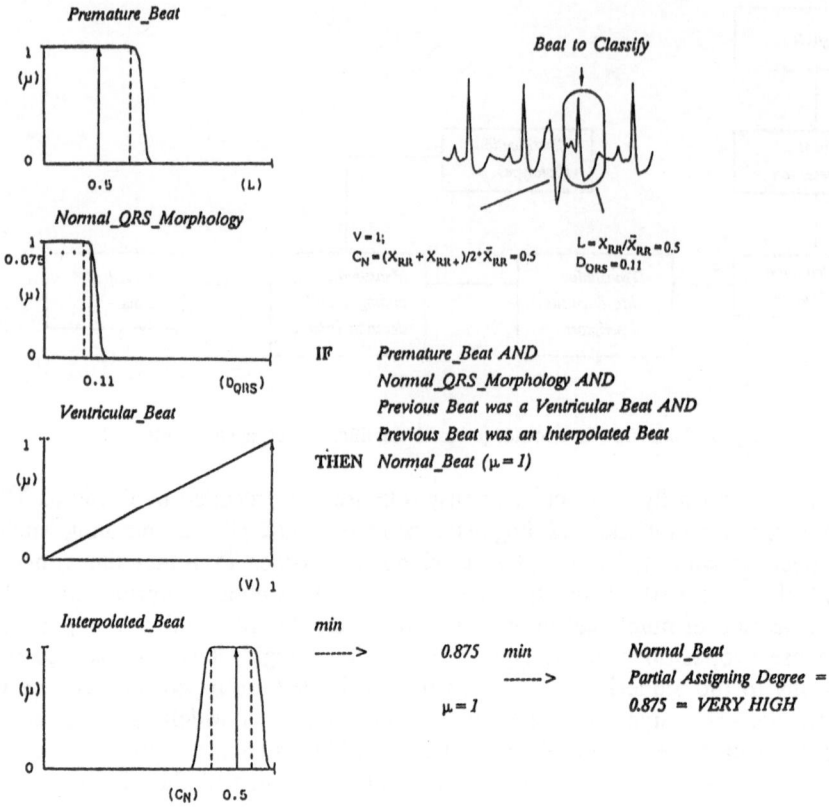

Fig. 3 Graphic illustration of the application of a fuzzy conditional structure in the classification of beats according to their focus of origin. (μ, membership degree of a beat to a category; X_{RR}, RR distance associated with a beat; $\bar{X}_{RR}$, normality average of the values X_{RR}; X_{RR+}, RR interval between a beat and the following one; D_{QRS}, normalized "dissimilarity" index, obtained from the comparison with a QRS template which is representative of normality; V, membership degree of a beat to the category of ventricular origin).

solved with the different techniques for the evaluation of the antecedent part of a FCS in a given situation (event). A classical example [2], would imply the partial classification of an event e_i by comparing it with the prototype R_s according to the following expression:

$$\mu_{c_n}^s (e_i) = \min \{\mu_{c_n} (e_i), \mu_{R_s} (e_i)\}, \qquad \forall \ c_n, \ n=1,...N, \qquad (3)$$

where:

$$\mu_{R_s} (e_i) = \min \{\mu_{L_{sm}} (e_i), \ m=1,...,M\}, \qquad (4)$$

being $\mu_{L_{sm}} (e_i)$ the assigning degree of e_i to the fuzzy subset associated with L_{sm}.

With respect to the final classification criteria, the consideration that each rule "if-then" of the classifier can be understood as a "prototype" permits the use of the same criteria as in conventional classifiers. Thus, in a K-nearest-neighbor classifier, the classification will result from the consideration of the K rules (prototypes) which better match (nearest) event e_i. The final classification can be established as an average of the partial classifications derived from each of these K rules [6].

In any case, the classification of an event can be derived from considering that all the rules in the knowledge base are linked with connectors of the type ALSO (the representation of knowledge is in a single level of rules, not implying chaining inference mechanisms), which permits the use in classical processes of forward data-driven inference through the application of criteria for the composition of the partial results obtained from the evaluation of each rule [5].

DISCUSSION

In this work we present concepts associated with knowledge-based fuzzy classifiers of signal events. This solution for the design of classifiers is specially interesting when the information to be processed is of a qualitative and imprecise nature. The main drawback of this solution is the longer calculation time it imposes, which results specially critical in real time applications. Nevertheless, the enormous advances in the design of VLSI circuits and some realizations in the field [7,8] imply that this will become a less important problem. On the other hand, the exhaustive use of symbolic processing-schemes facilitate not only to mimic human classification processes, but also the manipulation the complexity, uncertainty and contextual information associated with them.

ACKNOWLEDGEMENTS

This work was supported in part by the Spanish CIC_yT under proyect PRONTIC 488/90 and Xunta de Galicia XUGA8040189.

BIBLIOGRAPHY

[1] Cabello D., Barro S., Salceda J.M., Ruiz R. and Mira J. (1990). "Fuzzy K-nearest neighbor classifiers for ventricular arrhythmia detection". Int. J. Biomed. Comput. In Press.

[2] Zadeh L.A. (1973). "Outline of a new approach to the analysis of complex systems and decision processes". IEEE Trans. on Systems, Man and Cybernetics, Vol. 3, No. 1, pp. 28-44.

[3] Pucheu A., Lacroix H., Tonet J.L., Frank R., Fontaine G. and Grosgogeat Y. (1989). "Ventricular Arrhythmias". In "Comprehensive Electrocardiology. Theory and Practice in Health and Disease", Eds. Peter W. MacFarlane and T. D. Veitch Lawrie. Vol. II, Cap. 25, p. 966. Pergamon Press.

[4] Buchanan B.G. and Shortliffe E.H. (1985). "Rule-based expert systems". Addison Wesley.

[5] Barro S., Ruiz R. and Mira J. (1990). "Fuzzy beat labeling for intelligent arrhythmia monitoring", Comput. and Biomed. Research, 23, pp. 240-258.

[6] Marín R. and Mira J. (1990). "On knowledge-based fuzzy classifiers: a medical case study". In Press in a special number of Journal of Fuzzy Sets and Systems.

[7] Togai M. and Watanabe H. (1986). "Expert system on a chip: an engine for real-time aproximate reasoning". IEEE Expert Syst. Mag., Vol. 1, pp. 55-62.

[8] Lim M.H. and Takefuji Y. (1990). "Implementing fuzzy rule-based systems on silicon chips". IEEE EXPERT, February, pp. 31-45.

AntibES/Rabat - A FUZZY COMPUTER-AIDED INSTRUCTION ON THE TREATMENT OF INFECTIOUS DISEASES DESIGNED FOR MOROCCO MEDICAL STUDENTS AND MEDICAL PRACTITIONERS

Joint project of :
- Département d'Informatique Médicale, Université de Bordeaux II,
146 rue Léo Saignat, 33076 Bordeaux Cedex, France (1)
- IRIT , Université de Toulouse III, France (2)
- Département d'Informatique Médicale, Université de Rabat, Maroc (3)
- Clinique des Maladies Infectieuses, CHR de Bordeaux, France (4)
- Institut National d'Hygiène, Rabat, Maroc (5)

Program realized under the aeges of the World Health Organization.

G. Palmer (1)(2), P. Morlat (4),
J.C. Pillet (1), G. Labroille (1), B. Tilly (1), C. Nejjari (5)
J. Luguet (2), J. Aubertin (4), A. Medahoui (3), M. Hassar (5), R. Salamon (1)

ABSTRACT

This paper presents a program designed to help Maroccan students for prescribing antibiotics. The software was realized in the Department of Medical Informatics in Bordeaux, France, while the Knowledge Base was written by French and Moroccan Specialists. This project has been made in the framework of a World Health Organisation project.

I - BACKGROUND

The Medical Informatics Department (MID) of the University of Bordeaux II has realized in 1986 a videotex system to help French General Practitioners (GP) for prescription of antibiotics : ANTIBIOGUIDE [1]. This program had been written especially to answer the GP's requirement (consulted through a needs analysis in a random sample). This study showed that help and permanent training in antibiotherapy was one of their principal requests.

For two years, the system has been freely proposed to two hundred GPs in the context of a Sentinel Health Network [2] created and managed by the MID. This procedure has permitted to observe the reactions of the practitioners when faced with a computer-assisted product, and to evaluate the program both in terms of the satisfaction with use and the medical content.

II - A NEW PROJECT

Following this experience, in 1989 the World Health Organization has called for the DIM to realize a similar program to help Medical Students of Morocco to learn the prescription of antibiotics in ambulatory medecine. According to these objectives, the project had specific and new constraints :
- the program had to run on a simple IBM or compatible micro-computer (640 KO of RAM, monochrom or color screen, CGA, EGA or VGA graphic card, hard drive, no mouse).
- it had to be designed so that it could be used as a training system (for computer-aided instruction) as well as a decision support system (for real prescription practice). This second aim was set in anticipation of a future possible utilization of the program (distribution in some health consulting offices in Morocco).
- the knowledge base had to be adapted specifically to reflect health problems and curative sources of Morocco.
- the knowledge base had to be easily modified by Morocco's specialists. Hence, the program had to be accompanied with specific procedures to analyse and translate "natural written"-like knowledge rules into operational ones.

The decision of carrying out such a program was taken with the consideration of specific problems of developing countries like Morocco (great number of students for example) as well as in front of specific problems of antibiotherapy (evolution of the pharmacopoeia, risks, side-effects, ...).

III - CONSULTING THE PROGRAM

The program, "AntibES/Rabat", is now written. To use it, it is necessary to answer three basic questions :
- what is the diagnosed infection ? This choice is carried out through two menus. The first proposes twelve pathologic areas, and the second, depending on the preceding choice, lists known infectious diseases (the program identifies 53 diseases). Some diseases do not need to be treated in ambulatory medecine. Nevertheless they are proposed as a reminder that an hospitalization is essential, the reasons why this is necessary, and what kind of treatments will be performed.
- what are the etiologic agents ? For most common infections, this question can be skipped (the knowledge base is able to propose a standard

prescription for each of these infections). For other infections, it is imperative to give the isolated or suspected germs. AntibES proposes a list of 153 names of pathologic agents (some of them are synonyms).

- is there one or several clinical or biological particularities ("grounds") : renal insufficiency, pregnancy, ... ?

Once these basic questions are answered, the program is able to compute the list of recommended antibiotics, sorted out in a decreasing order of pertinent prescription. This information is calculated through a numerical weight (between 0 and 1). This number does not consist in a "certainty factor" [3] ; rather it corresponds to the value of the membership function which associates the antibiotic to the final fuzzy-subset [4] of the prescription.

It is clear that the only criterion which is taken into account in the program is the adequacy between antibiotics and the case under study. Other criteria could surely be considered (for example, price) in a second step, but this is not yet possible.

Finally, the program displays three kinds of information for each displayed antibiotic :

- it presents all of the commercial products (the names currently used by the program are only group or pharmalogical names),

- it proposes an explanation on the meaning (in favor, in disfavor) of the weight between 0 and 1 associated to the antibiotic,

- it offers a trace of the evolution of this weight, step by step, after taking in account each information (infectious disease, germs, grounds). This last information shows to the student the relative importance of these data in the final decision. For example, this trace can emphasize that a given germ is the major reason for the decrease of an antibiotic weight in one case, while it can be due to a special ground in another case...

IV - DEVELOPMENT OF THE KNOWLEDGE BASE

The medical content of the system has been written through the collaboration of two organizations : the Medical Clinic of Infectious Diseases of the Hospital of Bordeaux (who already wrote the knowledge Base of ANTIBIOGUIDE), and the National Hygiene Institute of Rabat (to adapt the system to the local particularities and pharmacopeia).

V - THE SYSTEM

AntibES is based on the Fuzzy Expert System Shell "MENTA", which has been developed by the DIM. In fact, the proposed program is using only part of MENTA possibilities : the management of fuzzy subsets. MENTA is also able to work in fuzzy logic instead of the classical boolean one, but it has been decided that the first version of AntibES will not use it.

So, MENTA is using two kinds of knowledge rules : "inference" ones to describe and deduct information, and "set" ones to describe and operate fuzzy subsets. Both of these rules are using logical fact in the hypothesis part (so they are examined and triggered off by an inference engine), but the conclusion of a set-rule is not of a logical nature. It is the expression, in extension form, of a fuzzy subset.

In general, the hypothesis of our set-rules is made up of only one information (a germ, for example). The conclusion of this rule is so constituted by the fuzzy set of the adequate antibiotics. If two germs are isolated, or suspected, the system searches for the antibiotics which are efficacious for both of them (the association of antibiotics has not been considered adapted to ambulatory medecine). This result is obtained by executing a fuzzy intersection between the conclusions of the two adequate rules.

However, these rules are not sufficient to build a correct prescription. It is frequent that a germ can be treated with a whole group of antibiotics, while another one can only be treated with one pharmacological speciality of this family. If the two germs are to be treated, the correct prescription is the second alternative. But the program will not be able to deduct this if the hierarchical relation between the two names is not provided beforehand.

So another important part of the knowledge is the Oriented Acyclic Graph of all the elements that belong to the used fuzzy sets. For example, the following subgraph describes the group of Penicillins :

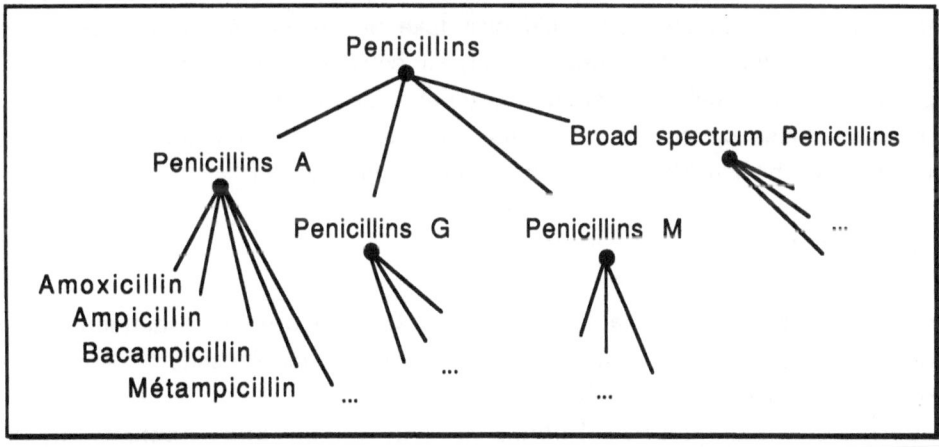

The complete base represents a graph of 342 nodes, describing groups, sub-groups, pharmacological specialities and commercial names.

The complete and final system delivered to the World Health Organization consists in three parts :
- the inference and set engine MENTA v.2,
- a module for tracing and commenting the final prescription,
- a group of programs to enter, analyse and compile the knowledge rules and to manage the graph of antibiotics.

VI - TEST AND ASSESSMENT

Since October 1990, the program has been installed in the Medical Informatics Department of the University of Rabat. The Department's task is to test the program, and then to build an evaluation protocol in collaboration with the World Health Organization. It will also be responsible for the evaluation.

For the World Health Organization, the present evaluation have a dual objective :
- testing the program, its performance and the concistancy of its medical content,
- but also provide data on the feasibility of implementing knowledge-based systems in developing countries.

VII - FUTURE DIRECTIONS

Extensions to the model can now be imagined. First, the system could take into account new kinds of information (allergies, parallel prescription of drugs in other therapeutic classes). It could also take advantage of using fuzzy logical facts instead of pure boolean ones. Lastly, it could consider new criteria in the computation of the antibiotics adequacy (cost, side-effects, ..).

Although these extensions where not the goals of the first program, some of them will surely be included in a new version of the system.

REFERENCES

[1] Palmer G., Morlat P., Prague Y., Corson C., Aubertin J., Salamon R. : A Videotex System to Help the General Practitioner for Prescribing Antibiotics. Proceedings of MEDINFO 1986, 1030-1032.
[2] Maurice S., Salamon R., Dabis F. : Telematics and sentinel health information system with general practitioners in Aquitaine, southwest France. Medical Informatics, 1989, Vol. 14, n° 4, 281-286.
[3] Buchanan B.G., Shortliffe E.H. : Rule-based Expert Systems. Addison-Wesley Publishing Company, USA, 1984.
[4] Zadeh L.A. : Fuzzy Sets. Information and Control, 1965, Vol. 8, 338-353.

EXPERT SYSTEMS—KNOWLEDGE MODELS

Maccord: a metamodel for problem solving competence applied to medicine

D. Kraus, B. Petkoff
RG Expert Systems,
CT Biomed,
Center for Technology Transfer Biomedicine
Brahmsstr. 2,
W-4970 Bad Oeynhausen

H. Mannebach
Heart Centre Northrhine-Westphalia
Department of Cardiology
Georgstr. 11
W-4970 Bad Oeynhausen

Abstract

The problematic aspects of knowledge acquisition, representation and maintenance, the development of modular, extendable, flexible, reflective and explainable knowledge based systems can only be addressed with reasonable hope of success if an appropriate conceptual structure of the system has been gained. The ACCORD-methodology provides an interpretation framework for the mapping of domain facts - constituting the world model of the expert - onto conceptual models, which can be expressed in formal representations. Applying ACCORD to the domain of clinical medicine a framework is yielded - Maccord - which supports a stepwise and inarbitrary reconstruction of the problem solving competence of medical experts as a prerequisite for an appropriate architecture of both medical knowledge bases and the "reasoning device". ACCORD thus shows a way to bridge the large conceptual gap between mental models of human experts and formal representations in programming languages or AI-toolboxes.

Introduction / The Problem

Over the past fifteen years a great deal of research has been directed towards the development of knowledge based systems (kbs) for problem solving in complex domains. Nevertheless, there can be no doubt that a knowledge engineer planning to implement a kbs has little effective guidance in identifying, formalising and represénting the relevant concepts, notions and phenomena of the universe of discourse. This not seldom forces an intuitive approach to the problem, emphasising "rapid prototyping" rather than a formal analysis of the domain. The availability of a "shell" or "tool" system may of course reduce the complications which arise when implementing systems based on experts´ knowledge, but offers no help in the analysis or validation of this knowledge. Despite the vast amount of work dedicated to these problems there is still no means of bridging the large conceptual gap between domain concepts and representational formalisms, a fact which renders knowledge engineering an art rather than a science. As Winograd puts it: "*..designing a knowledge base [...] is the creation of a systematic domain - a new construct that reflects what is important in the situation of interest*" [Davis 89]

Attempts to support the building of kbs have to be viewed with respect to the following problematic aspects

- **modelling of the reasoning and explanation process**

- **knowledge acquisition and representation**

- **modularity and transparency, portability and maintainability of knowledge bases**

Much of the unsatisfactory behaviour exhibited by many existing kbs may be regarded as due to the fact that the models of expertise - upon which problem solving behaviour relies - have been disregarded in favour of forms of knowledge enabling sufficient mimicking of the expert´s behaviour. Models of expertise have to comprise knowledge of various kinds and at different levels of abstraction, according to the cognitively and epistemologically different problem solving activities, in order to enable effective communication between experts and knowledge engineers during the knowledge acquisition process.

Thus what is really needed is a **methodology**, providing an interpretation framework for the building of *conceptual models* of the universe of discourse. "Conceptual model" denotes an abstract description of the problem solving process(es) and the different categories of knowledge employed therein. In the case of a medical domain this modelling requires an **in depth epistemological analysis** of the medical reasoning process. This analysis has to include the identification, formalisation and representation of the relevant concepts, notions and phenomena of the domain and their epistemic roles in medical reasoning. This is what has been done in Maccord.

Our approach

The ACCORD-metamodel has two major sources: the Experiential Learning Model (ELM) - developed by Lewin, Lippitt and White (1939), elaborated by Kolb and Fry (1975)- and the epistemological studies of the structuralist philosophers Sneed, Balzer, Moulines and Stegmüller. By integrating both views a framework is yielded which allows for a **dynamic description of individual or collective learning & problem solving processes.** Assuming that what a human problem solver is doing when confronted with a problematic situation can be interpreted as *learning*, this framework can be used as an **epistemological structure for knowledge based systems.**

The ELM and the epistemological results of the structuralists make similar propositions about the nature of learning and problem solving as worked upon by cognitive scientists, and about theory formation and validation as a subject of epistemology respectively. Essential common ground between these approaches is the **circular nature of the problem solving process,** which is illustrated by the hypothetico-deductive cycle (fig 1).

ACCORD tries to integrate both approaches into what can be called a "methodology of knowledge based systems". Developing a medical knowledge based system using the ACCORD-model means reconstructing the problem solving behaviour of the medical expert in terms of empirical, hypothetical, theoretical or experimental models at various levels of abstraction and the transitions between these. Empirical Models (EM) are phenomena which can be "experienced" and which deserve to be "understood" or "explained". Hypothe-

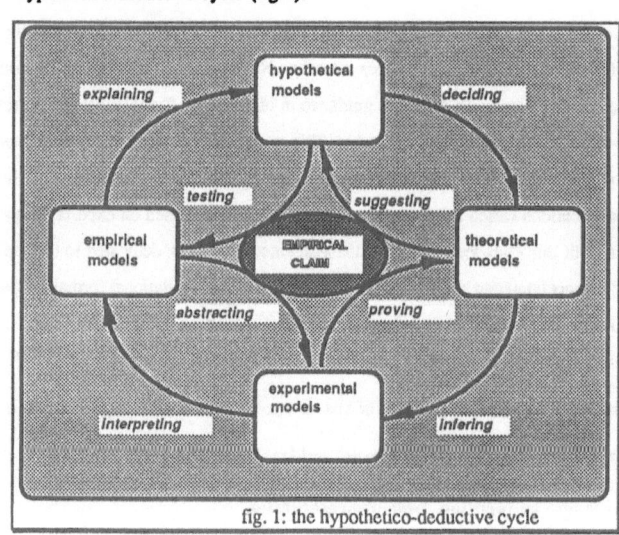

fig. 1: the hypothetico-deductive cycle

tical Models (HM) are entities which can be assumed as being possible explanations for EM. Theoretical Models are HM further enriched with **theoretical terms** which describe new, unobservable concepts. These prescribe the application of Experimental Models (XM) in order to produce new EM.

442

Applying **ACCORD** to Medicine: **Maccord**

When the attempt is made to apply these ACCORD-concepts to a domain as complex as medicine several difficulties arise:

First of all, the very nature of medicine makes it extremely hard merely to *represent* the knowledge categories of medical reasoning appropriately. The following areas of medical knowledge are commonly utilized in daily clinical practice: symptomatological knowledge, nosology, epidemiology, etiology, pathophysiology, anatomy and knowledge about diagnostic and therapeutic procedures (specifity and sensitivity, invasiveness, etc.).[1]

This leads to the introduction of **conceptual levels**. In ACCORD any such level has the form of an hypothetico-deductive cycle, extended by backward leading transitions. The highest, **strategical**, level involves *"global knowledge"* about the environment in which problem solving takes place. With regard to medicine this may be the constitutional or situative factors of the patient (expositions, psychic and social situation), seasonal or epidemiological circumstances and the like, plus the "never changing" anatomical and etiological categories, but may also be the ("meta-") criteria for the evaluation of procedures (specifity, sensitivity, invasiveness, risk...) and the patient's health status (comfort, abilities, development potential). The knowledge provided by medical *specialities* is found mainly at the **tactical** level : pathognomonic constellations of findings and principal signs, specific knowledge concerning the etiological nature of disorders at various anatomical sites, detailed pathophysiological knowledge (...). Knowledge organized at the lowest, the **operative**, level is most concrete: the raw, uninterpreted observations, specific hypotheses as well as diagnoses or particular tests and therapies reside at the operative level. To a certain degree, the operative level amounts to what constitutes expertise in a domain. Whereas the concepts localized on the operative and on the tactical level constitute "possible worlds" which can be freely introduced, altered or disregarded in the reasoning process, the strategic level determines the context in which reasoning takes place. Similar to the intuitive notion of levels, one may circumscribe the meaning of the columns which develop from the "corners of the circle" by juxtaposing several levels: the **empirical column** simply contains everything which is (or has been) observable. Signs, symptoms or values as well as historical facts or epidemiological constellations. The **hypothetical column** is the location of hypotheses which may be *assumed* on the basis of observations. Such assumptions may concern anatomical localisations of varying precision (such as *hepatobiliary system* and *ductus choledochus*) or etiological classes

(such as *infectious disease* and *inborn metabolic disturbance*). Theoretical concepts can be found in the **theoretical column**. What we mean in clinical medicine by theoretical concepts are mainly physiological or patho-physiological notions describing functional properties of the human body.

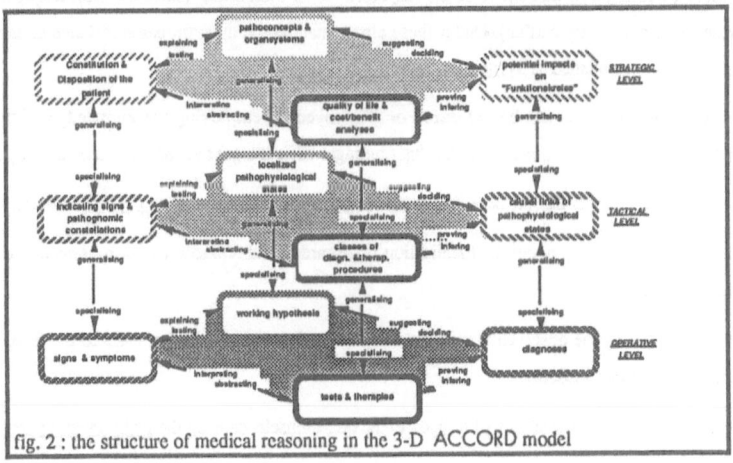

fig. 2 : the structure of medical reasoning in the 3-D ACCORD model

---

[1] Of course, common sense knowledge and ethical principles ("primum nil nocere") are engaged as well

The **experimental column** contains the elements which render medicine an actional science, oriented towards influencing the signs & symptoms of the patient. These are tests & therapies, procedural classes (such as *substitution, provocation, determination*) which are subject to "meta"-criteria such as *sensitivity, specifity, invasiveness* and the like.

The above considerations prepare the way for a **descriptive language for medical reasoning**, which may be the target language for the mapping of the medical domain onto the ACCORD structure. It is essential that this mapping covers the full range of concepts and argumentational modes employed in medicine. Of course, this work seems very difficult, since it is the *construction* of a sound and complete medical methodology. The terms denoting methodological elements of internal medicine are depicted in fig 2.

It also shows a typology of relations between concepts which is very similar to that of the levels and columns.

The following (partial) transcript of a cardiological consultation, formulated in the terminology of the proposed methodical structure[2], may clarify our point:

• the patient exhibits <u>signs</u> of *pain in the chest region,*

• which can be **subsumed** under the <u>principal sign</u> *thoracodynia.*

• for a <u>sign</u> to be *thoracodynia* it has to have a **specific** location, quality and duration.

• the <u>principal sign</u> at hand has to be **evaluated** in the individual (*sex, age, exposition, risk factors*) and situative (*seasonal, epidemiological*) <u>context</u>

• one has to **adopt** for the time being an **hypothesis** about what may have caused the pain. It may be selected from the following classes: *cardial, oesophageal, vertebragene, pleural* (...) causes.

• this selection can only be made with regard to various <u>pathogenetic modes</u> (e.g. *degenerative, inflammatory, neoplastic* ...), one of which in turn has to be provisionally adopted with respect to the <u>context</u> (infants are, for example, unlikely to suffer from degenerative diseases).

• in the current case of a, say, 55 year old woman, who smokes heavily, the <u>pathoconcept</u> *degenerative* is chosen, which induces the location *cardial site* to be the suspected "locus morborum" (since the most frequent degenerative diseases which cause thoracal pain are cardial). Under these circumstances the most probable instance is *degenerative coronary disease,* which is now established as a <u>tentative diagnosis.</u>

• This tentative diagnosis can be **validated** or **disproved** by employing the knowledge of the obligatory and facultative <u>signs</u> it produces. It is in this case likely that (amongst other things) the *pains are triggered by stress.*

• The unexpected answer that the *pain occurs at rest* gives rise to the new <u>principal sign</u> *thoracal rest pain.*

• the previous assumption about the localisation is discarded and replaced by "*oesophageal*"; the new <u>tentative diagnosis</u> is "*sliding hernia*".

• **disproving** this by the observation that the *pain occurs in a sitting position* leads to the reactivation of the old hypothesis *degenerative coronary disease.*

• this disease leads to a low supply of oxygen to the heart muscle, causing the <u>pathophysiological state</u> "*cardial hypoxia*".

• there are several <u>testing procedures</u> for *cardial hypoxia* including *provocative tests* and *image producing procedures.*

---

2 note that medical concepts appear underlined, instances of these in italics and the transitions in bold face

- In order to decide which procedure to apply in the given situation the medical test theory (*sensitivity, specifity* of tests) and other test attributes such as *risk, invasiveness, side effects* have to be engaged.

- In the example an *exercise electrocardiogram* is performed, since it is able to combine well a high specifity of result and low discomfort for the patient.

- ...

The previous section indicates that the entire diversity of medical reasoning can be described adequately in a formal terminology derived from epistemology and cognitive science regardless of the medical application. Even very abstract features, for example the difference in attitude between a practitioner in an emergency case, who tends to remain at the operative level of symptoms, hypotheses and remedies, and the specialist in a complicated situation concerning differential diagnosis, can be expressed easily as "preferences", say, for the operative level or the "theoretical corner". It should then be possible to say that all this *paves the way to a rational and comprehensible restructuring of medical knowledge*. This restructured knowledge, we emphasise, should in no way be regarded as inherently embodying a "technicist" or "reductionist" view, or as being forced to use stipulated disease concepts or pathophysiological models. On the contrary, a "holistic" approach may well fit the proposed structure.

Yet this model of medical reasoning should be *close enough to formalisation to allow for a computer implementation* which could turn out to be a satisfactorily performing "medical expert system".

Conclusion

To summarise, the ACCORD-framework allows for a stepwise and inarbitrary reconstruction of the domain specific problem solving competence, which must be seen as a prerequisite for an appropriate architecture of a planned kbs. It stands as an interpretation framework for the mapping of domain facts onto conceptual models which can be expressed in formal representations, and which are thus a step nearer to implementational constructs. We feel justified in stating that the problematic aspects of knowledge acquisition, representation and maintenance, the development of modular, extendable, flexible, reflective and explainable systems can only be addressed with reasonable hope of success if such an appropriate conceptual structure of the system has been gained.

- **Modelling of the reasoning and explanation process** is a key issue in the building of knowledge based systems in domains which comprise a manifold of argumentational structures, as is the case with medicine. Most "medical expert systems" simply neglect the clinical decision problem,.i.e. the problem of deciding which action (be it diagnostic or therapeutic) is to be carried out next in order to maximise the benefit for the patient. Many medical kbs only attempt to *order* (diagnostic/therapeutic) *alternatives by "plausibility"* based on *given* data. But the question underlying any consultation of a medical xps is not *"what is patient X's illness?"* but *"what should I do next in order to obtain more specific information and to initiate a rational therapy?"*. Obviously any reconstruction of medical knowledge led by the Maccord-methodology is forced to lay emphasis on such genuine problem solving knowledge.

- **Knowledge Acquisition** - widely regarded as a "bottleneck" in the construction of knowledge based systems - is at least *supported* by means of the systematic structure offered by the ACCORD-model. If one adopts the view that knowledge acquisition implies modelling and representing the acquired knowledge, then an epistemological framework is even a *prerequisite* for a reliable and reproducible knowledge *elicitation process*.

• **Modularity and transparency, portability and maintainability** are attributes which strongly determine the utility of knowledge bases. Obviously the goals of modularity and portability can be achieved if, and only if there is a common systematic structure of domain and problem solving concepts and processes imposed on the knowledge bases. Similarly, transparency and maintainability largely depend on the extent to which the architecture of the knowledge base reflects the domain structure.

The application of the ACCORD-methodology even to very complex domains, as, for instance, medicine, seems to be possible and desirable. We attribute the heuristic power and guiding force of ACCORD to the fact that it was not an ad hoc development, but rather a methodology based on results in epistemology and cognitive psychology, developed without regard to medicine.

References:

[Balzer/Moulines/Sneed 87] Balzer W., Moulines C.U. Sneed J.D. (1987) An Architectonic for Science- The Structuralist Program, D.Reidel Publishing Company

[Davis 89] Davis R., Expert Systems: How far can they go?, Part I, AI Magazine, 1, 89

[Kolb/Fry 75] Kolb D. A., Fry R..(1975): Towards an Applied Theory of Experiential Learning, in: Cooper C. (ed): Theories of group processes, New York

[Kraus/Petkoff/Mannebach 91] Kraus D; Petkoff B, Mannebach H: Reconstructing Medical Problem Solving Competence: Maccord, Proc AIME-91, Springer, Heidelberg

[Petkoff 85] Petkoff B. (1985) Artificial Intelligence and Computer Simulation of Scientific Discovery. Artificial Intelligence - Methodology, Systems, Applications, Proc. AIMSA 84 , North-Holland, Amsterdam.

[Petkoff 85] Petkoff B. (1986) Ein Kybernetisches Modell der Wissenschaftsentwicklung. Struktur und Dynamik Wissenschaftlicher Theorien, Verlag Peter Lang, Frankfurt am Main, Bern, New York.

[Petkoff 88] Petkoff B. (1988) ACCORD - a Metamodel for IInd Generation Expert Systems, Artificial Intelligence - Methodology, Systems, Applications, Proc. AIMSA 88, North-Holland, Amsterdam

A CLINICAL KNOWLEDGE MODEL AS BASIS FOR CONSTRUCTING A DECISION SUPPORTING SYSTEM

CICM Buiting-van der Zon, JMJ van den Berg and HM Berger.
Working Party of Medical Decision Making and
Department of Medical Informatics, State University,
and Department of Neonatology, University Hospital,
Leiden, The Netherlands.

ABSTRACT

Only a few of the existing medical expert systems have really found acceptance in the clinic. An important reason for this fact is that most knowledge models of the expert systems have been designed outside the clinic and are not well integrated in the routine procedures and way of thinking of the clinic. We found in the clinic a systematic model already in use for teaching purposes that seems suitable as knowledge model for an expert system. Because of the similarities of the model to object oriented programming we developed an expert system in an objected oriented way. We implemented a part of the teaching model concerning the circulation and respiration of neonates.

INTRODUCTION

In designing a medical expert system one of the major problems is to find the proper knowledge model to reflect the problem domain: the gap between technology and clinical practice is wide. The model in use in an expert system is in general quite different from the way of thinking of the clinic, and therefore the chance that the system will really be accepted by clinicians is not large.

In the Department of Neonatology of the Leiden University Hospital we found the situation that a coherent model was already in use for teaching purposes. This model, called SOOPA MD, had been designed to improve the teaching by using a systematic and consequential approach to the whole range of medical problems [Berger 1986,1990].

Although this model was developed years before the advent of object oriented programming (one of us had been working on it for twenty years), it has some very useful similarities to the way an object oriented system is constructed.

Therefore we started a project to try to develop the model further in an object-oriented way and to implement the model in an expert system that also must be clinical usable for problem solving.

This paper reports about the approach.

SOOPA MD (Structured Object Oriented Problem Analysis for Medical Diagnosis)

The SOOPA MD approach for teaching was developed in the clinic in an attempt to integrate the often very different methods of approaching the diagnosis of similar clinical problems in different specialties, or of approaching the same diagnosis at different ages. The model emphasizes the similarities instead of the differences of clinical problems, and thus provides the medical undergraduate or postgraduate student with a common pathway to reach diagnoses. Thereby it stimulates a more integrated and effective collection, analysis and usage of clinical findings. The model is briefly illustrated below by our model for "FLOW" problems in pulmonology and cardiology.

In for example central cyanosis (i.e. inadequate saturation of haemoglobin) the problem in every age group can be described as being due to oxygen not reaching the red blood cells (disturbed ventilation) or to the red blood cells not reaching the oxygen (disturbed perfusion) (figure 1). Both ventilation and perfusion are then described by the so-called model for "FLOW", which is based on Poisseuille 's law that flow in a tube is positively related to an increasing pressure gradient (dP) and inversely related to the resistance (R) (due mainly to the diameter of the tube (r) and the viscosity of the content (v)). Thus inadequate ventilation can be simply classified as being due to inadequate development of ventilation pressure or obstruction of the path of the air flow. Airway obstruction can be analyzed further by following the normal pathway of air from the nose to the alveoli. At each anatomical site the airway obstruction can potentially be in the lumen, in the wall or due to compression from outside.

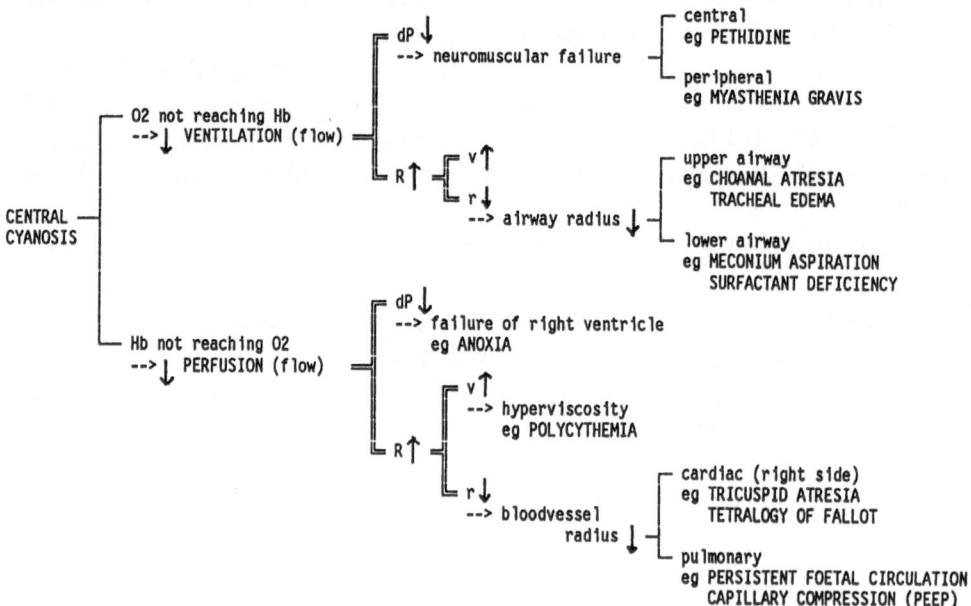

Figure 1. Part of the SOOPA MD model (simplified), showing the repeated occurrence of the "FLOWMODEL" (═══).

Using this approach similarities in pathophysiologic mechanisms, clinical signs, special investigations and therapy in diseases such as meconium aspiration at 8 minutes, bronchiolitis at 8 weeks, cystic fibrosis at 8 months, asthma at 18 years and chronic emphysema at 80 years of age can easily be recognized.

Furthermore, the model for "FLOW" can be used in a similar way to analyze the causes of cyanosis due to inadequate perfusion of the lung, by again following the anatomical pathway to find e.g tricuspid atresia.

THE LINK OF SOOPA MD TO TECHNOLOGY

It was felt that this model might also be useful in the support of clinical activities when properly supported by an adequate information system. So the motivation for designing an expert system based on the SOOPA MD model was to try to reduce the frequency of missed diagnoses, and at the same time to improve the effectiveness of collection, analysis and usage of clinical findings. To realize this the expert system has to integrate medical (expert) knowledge with clinical up-to-the-minute parameters.

Components of the expert system

Standard models

The bare version of the expert system we designed provides the expert-physician with the modules needed to implement parts of the SOOPA MD model. This bare version is filled by the expert-physician with the needed models for an application to describe the analysis of a certain type of problem. For instance the model for "FLOW" in the clinical example is defined by the possible "states" it can be in (normal flow, increased flow and decreased flow), and its analysis factors (pressure gradient and resistance). One other model is the model for "INPUT-OUTPUT" for problems concerning too high or too low concentration of for instance electrolytes. The analysis factors of this model are disturbance of input and disturbance of output.

Instantiated system

Next a network of instantiated models (or "devices" in the more classical reasoning literature [Kuipers, Chandrasekaran]) and their relations is formed. This is done by defining specific pathofysiologic problems as a derivative of one of the standard models e.g. "decreased flow in the circulation" is a derivative of the model "FLOW". By filling in the analysis factors with other devices, the links are created.

Thus an instantiated system consists of a network of devices with pointers, where each device is based on one model. The device has several important properties:

-   One property is the usage of "states" which makes it possible to define the behavior of a device in different situations (e.g. normal flow, increased flow and decreased flow).

At run time the device can evualuate its own state by gathering the parameters needed to do this from the system or from the user.

- The device uses causal analysis factors for causal reasoning on the direction of further analysis (e.g. increased pressure is compatible with increased flow etc).

- Within each device related devices that can give useful information about the analysis factors are listed (e.g. if a pressure problem of the respiration is investigated the list refers to possible causes in the respirator or the respirator-neuro-muscular system).

- The structure of the device makes it extreme simple to change the device or network according to new insights.

Applicability of the system

At run time the system will be fed with clinical parameters of a patient coming from anamnesis, physical examination and special investigations, which are organized in a qualitative or quantitative way. These parameters will be integrated throughout the system to determine the state of relevant devices. Besides they will be used in the causal reasoning to give evidence in favour of or against each further analysis path. If enough data is supplied the system can reason about the likelihood of various diseases. By looking at the missing data and their relative importance for analysis the system can give recommendations about further clinical investigations and order of importance.

DESIGN CONSIDERATIONS

Smalltalk was chosen for the implementation of the expert system. The first reason to use an object oriented system is the close fit of the metaphor to our model. The models, such as "flow", become the objects, and the relations between the models can be represented as pointers. Other reasons are the good reusability of concepts and software, the possibility of fast prototyping and the relatively simple standard Smalltalk classes simplifying the structure of programming.

The disadvantages of object oriented systems such as memory use and lack of speed are known, but we circumvent these by using a fast processor (80386 33 MHz) with a large memory (4 MegaByte).

THE STATE OF THE PROJECT

In our design and implementation of the system we focused on the analysis of problems concerning the circulation and respiration of neonates. We will show how the system gives support in reaching a diagnosis, and how the therapies given have their influences throughout an instantiated model.

Our present investigation concentrates on developing the teaching model with weighted factors so the system can give relative weights for each of the possible diagnoses.

REFERENCES

1. Bylander T and Chandrasekaran B, "Understanding behavior using consolidation", Proc. Ninth International Joint Conference of Artificial Intelligence, IJCAI, Los Angeles, 1985.
2. Berger HM, Van Zoeren D, Kardson J. "Antioxidant capacity of uric acid and adaptation to a terrestrial environment". Spec Sc Technol 1986; 9:83-4.
3. Berger HM and Van den Berg JMJ, "An approach to integrating medicine and increasing competence: 'SOOPA MD'", International Conference on Teaching and Assessing Clinical Competence, Groningen BoekWerk Publications (1990) 55-60.
4. Berger HM, "Clinical examination of the newborn", in: Enkin MW, Keirse MJNC and Chalmers J (eds) Effective Pregnancy and childbirth, Oxford University Press, 1990.
5. Chandrasekaran B, Bylander T and Sembugamoorthy V, "Functional Representations and behavior composition by consolidation: two aspects of reasoning about devices", SIGART Newsletter, nr 93 (July 1985) 21-4.
6. Kuipers B, "Commonsense reasoning about causality: Deriving behavior from structure" Artificial Intelligence, nr 24 (1984) 169-203

Integration of the Causal and Functional Approaches for Robust Medical Diagnosis

Pedro Barahona
Departamento de Informática
Faculdade de Ciências e Tecnologia
Universidade Nova de Lisboa
2825 Monte da Caparica
PORTUGAL

Mário Veloso
Hospital Egas Moniz
Serviço de Neurologia
R. da Junqueira, 126
1300 Lisboa
PORTUGAL

Abstract

In this paper we present a causal-functional approach that we are developing for the representation of medical knowledge which integrates features from both the causal and functional approaches, and may thus take advantage of the kinds of deep knowledge that they exploit, namely temporal transitions between pathophysiological states and function and structure decomposition.

1. Introduction

Early medical knowledge based systems (KBS), were based on associative models aimed at modelling heuristic associations between diagnoses and findings. Experience gathered from the use of these systems, has however shown that surface models are not sufficiently deep [KeWa89] to adequately represent medical knowledge and cope with the complexity of the reasoning process. This fact partly explains the difficulties in making medical KBSs accepted by clinicians.

Some systems have attempted to circumvent the limitations of associative models, by explicitly representing pathophysiological knowledge, usually in the form of a causal network of pathophysiological states. CASNET [WKAS78] is a system that has adopted this causal approach. Its domain was the problem of glaucoma, and the nodes of its causal network represented pathophysiological states of the eye system. Other systems that adopted this approach and integrate heuristic associations with deeper causal knowledge include ABEL [PaSS81], and CHECK [ToCo89]. In these systems, several causal networks are organised in different layers. The more superficial layers basically represent associations and their nodes and arcs are abstractions of (and are mapped onto) causal networks of deeper layers, where pathophysiological knowledge is represented in more detail. These deeper layers can therefore be consulted to validate and place in proper context the associations represented at the more superficial layers.

If this multiple layer approach is adequate to represent deeper pathophysiological knowledge, it by and large ignores anatomical knowledge. In particular, it abstracts away the fact that the domain includes many structures (human organs and functional systems) which perform certain functions and whose interaction has to be considered. In medicine, this knowledge is quite important, namely in focussing the diagnosis towards the right structures and their functioning. This type of knowledge is exploited in systems based on a functional approach [Stee89] and [StCh89], where both structures and their functions may be decomposed into arbitrarily deep levels of detail. However, the issue of time is not addressed in such models, thus they are not able to represent causality adequately.

To summarise, one may conclude that whereas the causal approach is appropriate for modeling causality that develops over time, the functional approach is more adequate to model the structure and functioning of a system and decompose it into deeper and more basic components. In our opinion, both these aspects have to be accommodated in medical knowledge based systems, if they are to be sufficiently robust and be acceptable (and adopted) by the medical community.

In this paper we will therefore present the causal functional approach, that we are developing in order to take advantage of the positive features of both the causal and functional approaches. The structure of the paper is the following. In the next section we present a clinical case and describe the main issues involved in diagnosis. The following sections describe how the different kinds of diagnosis are accommodated in our approach. The last section presents the main conclusions and discusses some issues for a future implementation of our approach.

2. Problem description and solving strategy

The clinical method of diagnosis in neurology, is used to illustrate our framework for causal functional reasoning. The explicit analysis of a brief clinical case, summarised below, will show how the different types of knowledge can be represented and exploited in our approach.

> A 28 years old right handed previously healthy female describes in the day before admission the acute onset of right arm and leg numbness. A few minutes later, there was also a decreased strength of right arm and leg. Her past and family history were irrelevant, and there was no history of substances' abuse but for about two months she is taking oral contraceptives. Blood pressure was 130/75 mmHg, being normal her physical examination. Neurologic examination disclosed a flaccid right side hemiparesis, weaker miotatic reflexes in right limbs, an extensor right plantar response, and decreased sensation in the right arm and leg.

Typically, diagnosis includes four major components a) **anatomical diagnosis**, to obtain anatomic structures whose hypothetical damage could explain the patient's findings, b) **syndromic diagnosis**, using associative knowledge between findings and clinical entities, to produce hypothetical disorders, c) **pathologic diagnosis** where the nature of such disorders is assessed, and finally **etiologic diagnosis** where causes of such disorders are asserted.

3. Anatomical Diagnosis

During the anatomical diagnostic phase, the neurologist attempts to hypothesize plausible anatomic structures whose damage should explain the patient's findings. Given the motor problem of the patient, a representation of the motor pathways which are involved in the genesis of such problems is required. In our approach, the anatomy and physiology of these motor pathways are represented as functional and composition schemata. Since an action must have a plan, a program, and an execution, motor action is a complex function depending on the integrity of these three subfunctions. Subfunction action execution may be further decomposed into the exertion of muscular force and its control. The former of these subfunctions may still be decomposed into the generation of nerve pulses, its propagation to a structure and the execution of the action by this structure. Exertion of muscular force is thus represented by the following composition schemata

```
function:    exert muscular force -
                of structure: S,
                exert force : F
  sub_func:       generate nerve pulses -       % some region of primary motor
                    to structure: S,            % cortex of the brain related to S
                    generation: G
                & propagate nerve pulses -       % corticospinal tract and
                    to structure: S,  .          % second neuron related to S
                    propagation: P
                & execute force -                % muscles of structure S
                    by structure: S,
                    execute    force:    E
  such that    exert muscular force composition (F, G, P, E)
```

In general, schemata make use of auxiliary relations to represent how the state of a function may be affected by those of its subfunctions (e.g. exert muscular force composition (F, G, P, E), where the state F of the force exertion depends on the states G, P and E of its subfunctions). Additional auxiliary relations are used to model anatomo-physiological knowledge, namely to represent topographic relations, such as part_of, adjoins, anterior_to, branch_of (for arteries) and in_territory (to map arteries and the structures they irrigate).

Since arm paresis (presented in the clinical case) is a synonym of 'exert muscular force - of structure: arm, exert force: decreased', and this function is a composition of other more basic functions, the system naturally allows diagnostic refinement. In this case, a decreased generation or propagation of nerve pulses will enforce a decreased exertion of muscular force. In our approach, functional schemata are used not only to map these subfunctions onto specific structures, but also to specify the relationship between pathological states of the structures and the corresponding dysfunctions.

In the example below, the pulse gen correspondence(G,l) relationship specifies that a lesion on the motor cortex (l=lesion) causes the pulse generation to decrease (G=decreased). Similar effect is obtained when a lesion in the corticospinal tract or the second neuron affects the propagation subfunction.

```
function:   generate nerve pulses -
            to structure: S         % e.g. S = arm
            generation: G
structure:  motor cortex -
            to structure: S
            integrity:        |
such that   pulse gen correspondence (G,I)
```

Anatomic diagnostic reasoning provides anatomical arguments to relate affected structures with observed dysfunctions. Our knowledge representation lends itself naturally to this kind of reasoning. However, there are many ways in which this knowledge may be used, hence the system must be flexible enough to specify and use them. In our approach, and following similar ideas that were incorporated in the OSM system [NeGF89], reasoning may be specified by means of explicit argument forms. Arguments produced by these forms may be subsequently handled by an adequate decision making procedure. A useful argument in our present clinical case has the following form

```
If    V is observed                                    % V = arm paresis
and   V is an abnormal value of function F             % F = exert muscular force - decreased
and   structure S is responsible for function F        % S = arm motor cortex
and   V is an abnormal value of function F in state St  % St = integrity : lesion
then  S is possibly in state St                        % a lesion of the arm motor cortex is  proposed
```

The same argument would also propose as possible hypotheses a corticospinal tract or second neuron lesion (and the corresponding decrease of nerve pulses propagation). Because both the generation and the propagation of nerve pulses may be affected, the system should decide which one is actually affected.

For this differential diagnosis purpose, argument forms may implement the Occam's razor principle (also known as the principle of parsimony): given hypotheses A and B, prefer that explaining more findings. Using this argument form, a lesion of the 'second neuron' (or lower motor neuron) should be causally discarded taking into account the function schemata of peripheral nerves and roots (components of the second neuron). Actually, muscle testing (together with motor function and sensation charts) provides a means for the diagnosis of a root, nerve or muscle lesion. A lesion of the second neuron would typically explain paresia of only some muscles of the arm. Since in this case all muscles were affected, one would rather consider a lesion of the upper motor neuron (i.e. arm motor cortex or corticospinal tract).

At this point, the system as well as the clinician, can not be more specific concerning the anatomic diagnosis, because of a lack of available data. Hence, other types of knowledge (namely pathological and etiological) must now be explored, and a refinement of anatomic diagnosis is postponed until further and more precise knowledge is obtained.

4. Syndromic, Pathological and Etiological Diagnosis

Our causal functional framework, is not only able to represent and use functional knowledge, but is also able to accommodate the causal knowledge usually exploited in pure causal approaches. To be more specific, causal pathophysiological knowledge is represented in our approach by means of (pathologic) process schemata. For each process, a sequence of one or more state changes occurring in one or more structures are defined. Each change depends upon a multiplicity of triggers (which can be considered the etiology of the process and eventually of the whole disorder). There may be external or internal agents, and the latter include either dysfunctions of functional systems, pathological states of structures, or even abnormal structures (such as tumours, whose states are by and large pathological). Causal networks can thus be represented in our approach, since once a structure is affected and changes into a (pathological) state, the related dysfunction may trigger other processes, modifying the state of other structures.

In order to simplify the description, it is assumed a vascular nature of the lesion, i.e. a cerebral abnormality derived from a pathologic process affecting the blood vessels. Major pathologies include a) any lesion of the vessel wall, b) occlusion of the lumen, c) rupture of the vessel, d) altered permeability of the vascular wall, e) change in the quality of the blood (i.e. increased viscosity).

For the problem in hand, an hyperfibrinogenaemia process, specified below, is considered due to the known contraceptive pill intake. Note that a few findings (i.e. increasing age, pregnancy) which constitute associative knowledge are represented as "+ factors" (positive associations or risk factors). This is the means through which our model copes with syndromic diagnosis, i.e. by favouring processes that mention observed associations (even when these associations could be derived from known causal knowledge).

```
    process:  hyperfibrinogenaemia
    trigger:  contraceptive pill, malignancy, ...
  structure:  blood - component: plasma
 from  state:  fibrinogen - concentration: normal
 into  state:  fibrinogen - concentration: increased
   + factors:  increasing age, pregnancy,
   - factors:  -----
      delay:  -----
```

Processes may be specified in more detail if structure and function states are also represented with corresponding detail. In this case several grades of fibrinogen concentration could be considered, such as normal, mild increase, medium increase, strongly increase (and similar grades for concentration decrease). Together with a specification of the delays in which these state transitions take place (which is currently under study), this improved detail will be very helpful in the future to model time. In this case, time information (from the acute onset of the illness described by the patient) is very important to propose a vascular nature of the lesion.

The additional refinement of structure and function states will also cause longer chains of process steps to be generated. In particular, the above process step could be decomposed into two finer process steps, changing the fibrinogen concentration from normal to mildly increased, and then to medium increased. The exploitation of causal chains of processes, together with related functional schemata, provide anatomical and physiopathological arguments to explain the observed findings.

In this case, the increase of fibrinogen concentration also increases blood viscosity. This increase in blood viscosity may in turn explain a lack of blood in some parts of the brain by means of the schemas shown below. Firstly, blood flow in some artery is a function of blood pressure and vascular resistance. The latter increases with rigidity (or lack of elasticity of the arteries) and viscosity of the blood. The increase of fibrinogen concentration will therefore justify a lack of blood flowing to several structures, namely some parts of the brain.

Argument forms, similar to that shown above, may then be used together with process specification such as hyperfibrinogenaemia to provide not only possible pathophysiological states (increased concentration of fibrinogen), but also their etiology (e.g. contraceptive pill).

Finally, the lesion of some part of the brain could be explained by means of an infarction process. The decreased blood flow to a structure such as the corticospinal tract (a part of the internal capsule), may cause its state to change from normal to hypoxic, and then to ischaemic and eventually to infarcted, all destructive lesions of increasing severity.

Of course, alternative diagnoses could also be explored. For example, polycythaemia could constitute a competing etiologic diagnosis, since a decrease of blood flow can be caused by an increased concentration of circulating particles, instead of fibrinogen. However, in our case, there is no medical evidence for the trigger of such process (e.g an increased production of erythropotein). Moreover, a refinement of the anatomic diagnosis (infarcted region and vascular territory) may now be made, based on the above stated principle of parsimony and making use of some auxiliary relations (in_territory, is_branch_of, and is_terminal_branch of).

Informally, the motor cortex, which includes the arm motor cortex, is directly supplied by the prerolandic artery, and the lenticulostriate arteries supply the internal capsule and adjacent structures. Both arteries are branches of the middle cerebral artery (the left in the present case), a terminal branch of the internal carotid artery which supplies all the cerebral hemisphere. Therefore, assuming a lesion in the internal capsule, the proposed vascular territory should be the one of the lenticulostriate arteries, which is the closer branch to the affected structure. Therefore, this anatomic refinement constitutes in turn a stronger argument for the suspected vascular nature of the pathologic process.

Eventually, a composite solution to our problem should be proposed: brain infarct in the left cerebral hemisphere, plausibly in the posterior limb of left internal capsule, in the territory supplied by the left middle cerebral artery, more specifically the lenticulostriate arteries, caused by a change in blood quality due to high blood viscosity caused by an intake of oral contraceptive pills.

5. Conclusion

This paper described a causal functional approach to knowledge representation which integrates features from both the functional and the causal approaches, and may thus take advantage of the kinds of deep knowledge that the two different approaches exploit. The clinical case that was used to examplify our approach, has shown that our approach is powerful enough to cope with different types of knowledge and diagnostic reasoning tasks.

At present we are developing a formal specification of our approach, and will soon start its implementation. Apart from minor implemnentation details, we antecipate that the major problems with implementation will occur a) on the representation of the argument forms, and b) the modeling of time. As to the argument forms, we are hoping to apply the methodology proposed in [Fox87], given our separation of domain knowledge and control and other meta-level knowledge. As to the second problem, we will first have to verify the adequacy of representing time as a single argument in a process step, and only after gaining some insight in this matter will we engage into implementation.

Acknowledgements

This work was developed at the AI Centre of UNINOVA and funded by JNICT, INIC (Portuguese Research Agencies), and also by programme AIM of the European Community (project LEMMA, A-1042). We would like to thank our colleagues at UNINOVA, in particular Anabela Ribeiro and Susana Nascimento, and our partners in the LEMMA project - the ICRF and Fondation Bérgonié groups, led by John Fox and Jean Louis Renaud-Salis.

References

[Fox87]   J. Fox, *Architectures for decision making under uncertainty*, Imperial Cancer Research Fund, 1987.

[KeWa89]   E.T. Keravnou and J. Washbrook, *What is a deep expert system? An analysis of the architectural requirements of second-generation expert systems*, The Knowledge Engineering Review, vol. 4, no. 3, pp. 205-233, 1989.

[NeGF89]   M. O'Neil, A. Glowinski and J. Fox, *A Symbolic Theory of Decision Making Applied to Several Medical Tasks*, in Procs. of Second European Conference on Artificial Intelligence in Medicine, London, 62-71, 1989.

[PaSS81]   R.S. Patil, P. Szolovits and W.B. Schwartz, *Causal Understanding of Patient Ilness in Medical Diagnosis*, in Procs. of Seventh International Joint Conference on Artificial Intelligence, 893-899, 1981.

[Stee89]   L. Steels, *Diagnosis With a Function-Fault Model*, Applied Artificial Intelligence, vol. 3, no. 2/3, pp. 129-153, 1989.

[StCh89]   J. Sticklen and B. Chandrasekaran, *Integrating Classification-Based Compiled Level Reasoning With With Function-Based Deep Level Reasoning*, Applied Artificial Intelligence, vol. 3, no. 2/3, pp. 191-219, 1989.

[ToCo89]   P. Torasso and L. Console, *Diagnostic Problem Solving: Combining Heuristic, Approximate and Causal Reasoning*, North Oxford Academic, 1989.

[WKAS78]   S.M. Weiss, C.A. Kulikowski, S. Amarel and A. Safir, *A Model-Based Method for Computer_Aided Medical Decision Making*, Artificial Intelligence, vol. 11, no. pp. 145-172, 1978.

Integrating closed form representations and qualitative reasoning for cancer treatment.

S.Gaglio*, M. Giacomini°, C.Nicolini$ and C.Ruggiero°

*Department of Electrical Engineering of Palermo University, Italy
°Department of Communications, Computer and System Sciences
of Genoa University, Italy
$Institute of Biophysics of Genoa University, 16145 Genoa, Italy

Abstract

The present work describes the last version of a consultation system for the development of cancer therapies, NEWCHEM, in which pharmaco-cell kinetic modeling and molecular knowledge about neoplastic processes allow to propose new protocols for adjutant combination chemotherapy. It focuses on the integration of the two kinds of knowledge involved, that is closed form representation for pharmaco-cell kinetics and declarative representation for the basic principles of molecular knowledge relating to cell growth.

Introduction

Adjutant combination chemotherapy has been used for several years with some encouraging result (1), although the problem of cancer treatment is far from being solved. On one hand the results obtained so far, although limited, encourage further research in the field; on the other hand the limitations of these results suggest reconsidering the problem starting from the basic ideas and using recent results on pharmaco-cell kinetic modeling (2,3,4).

A consultation system for the development of cancer therapies, NEWCHEM, is described in which pharmaco-cell kinetic modeling and molecular knowledge about neoplastic processes allow to propose new protocols for adjutant combination chemotherapy.

The present work describes the last version of the system, outlined in (5,6,7), and focuses on the integration of the two kinds of knowledge involved, that is closed form representation for pharmaco-cell kinetics and declarative representation for the basic principles of molecular knowledge relating to cell growth.

This integration takes place according to two closely, interacting stages: the first singles out groups of antineoplastic drugs according to their cycle specific action; the second uses experimental results on tissues and drugs and pharmaco-cell kinetic findings and gives detailed administration recommendations for each group of antineoplastic drugs.

Description of the data bases of NEWCHEM.

NEWCHEM contains a database of drugs, a data base of assertions on specific combinations of drugs, a data base of tissues and a data base of constraints on the groups of drugs.

Group	Subgroup	Action	Drug
Antimetabolites	Pyrimidine analogues	Stop DNA, RNA and Thymine synthesis	Fluoracil
		Stop DNA synthesis	Ara_C
	Folic acid antagonists	Inibit DNA, RNA and protein synthesis	Methotrexate
		Stop DNA synthesis	Hydroxyurea
Antibiotics	Anthracyclinics	Inibit DNA synthesis (are inserted in DNA)	Adriamycin
			Daunomycin
	Not anthracyclinics	Inibit DNA synthesis (divide DNA)	Bleomycin
Alkylating agents	Nitrogen mustards	Modify DNA structure building up intermolecular and intramolecular bounds with DNA	HN_2
			PAM
			Cyclophosphamide
	Sulfonoxialcans	Modify DNA structure	Busulfan
Vinca-alcaloids		Prevent mitolic fuse formation	VCR
			Vinblastine

Table 1

DRUGS IN NEWCHEM

The data base of drugs contains drugs on which a great deal of experimental results are available. Table 1 shows the drugs present in this version of NEWCHEM. The information stored for them is: name, group, subgroup, phase of the cell cycle in which the drug is active, its main action on the cell, the lethal dose for 10% of the animals on which the drug has been tested.

The data base of assertions contains rules relating to combinations of drugs. Every rule contains a parameter representing the extent of reliability and a comment explaining the reasons for adopting the rule. The parameter ranges from -10 to +10. It is a positive number if the rule recommends the combination of drugs, a negative number if this is not the case. The evaluation of each treatment takes place using these rules and assessing a global extent of reliability to the treatment. NEWCHEM allows the user to insert rules, however the rules deriving from clinical findings by the user are given a lower extent of reliability with respect to the ones deriving from laboratory experiments.

The data base on tissues contains information on the cell kinetics of tissues. Taking into account that chemotherapy is not a local treatment limited to one tissue only but rather a global treatment involving the whole body of the patient, many tissues have to be considered, which will respond to treatment in different ways. Basically the tissue data base contains: name of the tissue, type (tumoral or not) and average and variance for each cell cycle.

The data base of the constraints of the groups is at present limited to compatibility conditions at group level, but will be extended to subgroups.

Closed form representation and qualitative reasoning in NEWCHEM.

A branch of NEWCHEM consists of a mathematical model of cell growth. This closed form representation attempts to provide an integrated and realistic approach to optimal cancer treatment. The model considered acts at a time scale of hours-days. Its inputs are: the duration (in mean value and standard deviation) of each phase of the cell cycle; the rate of resting-growing cells; the percentages of cells killed by the action of three (at least) particular doses of a drug (label indexes). The programs constituting this model and their interactions are outlined in fig.1.

Another branch of NEWCHEM consists of a qualitative model of cell growth (8) developed according to qualitative process theory inside an environment for qualitative modeling called WQMS.

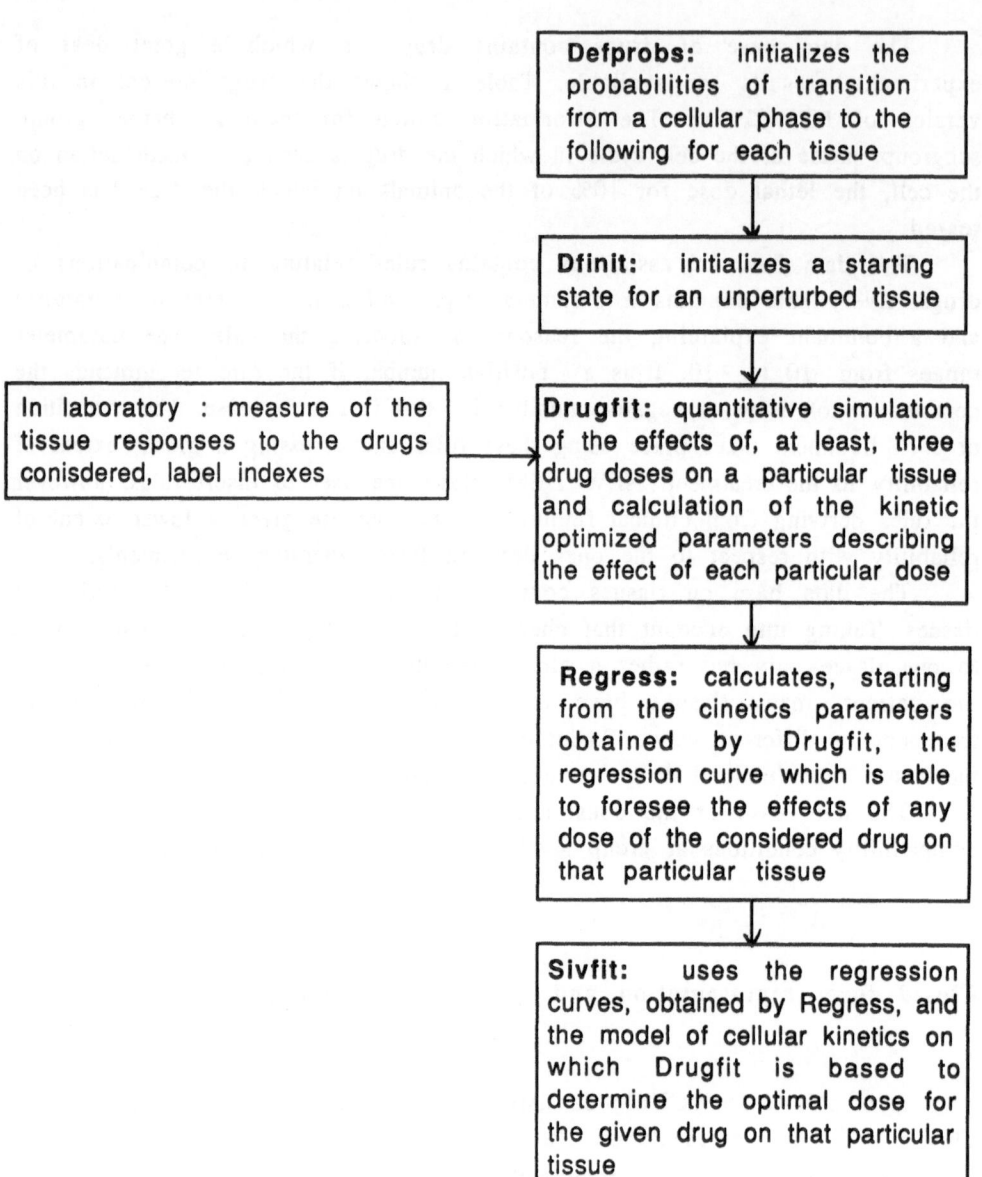

Fig. 1
Closed form representation programs

WQMS (9) has been developed according to the principles of qualitative process theory by Forbus (10), defining the notion of physical process by the property of causing changes in objects over time. The qualitative process theory approach has been integrated by an inference based on the rules of qualitative algebra formulated by Kuipers (11,12). This integration of the process centred approach and of the constraint centred approach has led to an environment that can provide both structural and behavioural answers. Moreover, this approach brought about significant advantages when dealing with particularly complex systems.

The process centred approach is mainly based on two primitives: individual views and processes. Individual views are conditional statements which impose some relations once some conditions are assessed. The relations describe how the features of the objects are related to each other with equality and inequality constraints. Processes are similar to individual views, but they can also influence the features of the objects with proportional and integral differential constraints.

According to this formalism, the classical four phases of the cell cycle have been modelled with four individual views called:
- M, mitosis, the phase in which happens the true cell division;
- G1, the phase just after mitosis, in which both a special protein which triggers the whole growth and the other growth factors are synthesized;
- S, the phase in which the cellular DNA is duplicated;
- G2, the phase just before mitosis, in which the factors that are necessary for mitosis itself are prepared.

Moreover the resting phase G0 is also modelled as an individual view.

The dynamics of the cell cycle is described by several processes reflecting its main features. Some of these processes can be active during the whole cell cycle; others, on the contrary, can be active during a given phase only (phase specific processes).

Problem solving with NEWCHEM

Problem solving with NEWCHEM is organised according to two levels. When all label indexes for all drugs of the combination under examination are available, the closed form representation is used obtaining the recommended protocol. When this is not the case NEWCHEM uses the verbal information contained in the drug data base and builds up rules describing the action of drugs on the cell cycle according to the qualitative process theory. It is then possible to set up a qualitative simulation reproducing the action of the drugs under examination on the particular tissue. In this case the output is a description of the behaviour of a cell population of the tissue. If the action of the combination results into a significant reduction of the tumoral cells, the hypotheses of the effects of the combination are validated and the user is guided in the planning of experiments to determine the label indexes.

So far NEWCHEM has been tested with reference to the qualitative model of cell growth. The behaviour of this model has been tested on several combination of cycle specific antiproliferative drugs, with good agreement with the actual experimental data.

Experiments have been planned to obtain the label index of antiproliferative drugs. When this data is available the mathematical model of cell growth will be tested.

References

(1) G. Bonadonna and P. Valagussa "Adiuvant systemic therapy for resectable breast cancer", *J. Clin. Oncol.* 3R, 1985, p. 259
(2) C. Nicolini "The principles and methods of cell synchronization in cancer chemotherapy", Biochim and Biophys. Acta, Vol. 458, 1976, p. 243
(3) C. Nicolini and R. Baserga "Cell synchrony with lining epitelium of the intestinal tract of mice" in Pulse Cytometry, Amsterdam: European Press, 1976, Vol. II, pp. 46 - 57
(4) C. Nicolini, A. Belmont, M. Grattarola, C. Moor, E. Milgram "Pharmaco-enzym kinetic simulations of experimental intercations among multiple antineoplastic drugs" *Biochem. Pharmacol.*, Vol. 28, 1979, p. 2891
(5) E. Ardizzone, F. Bonadonna, S. Gaglio, R. Marcenò, C. Nicolini, C. Ruggiero and F. Sorbello "Artificial intelligence techniques for cancer treatment planning" *Med. Inform.*, Vol. 13, N. 3, 1988, pp. 199 - 210
(6) E. Ardizzone, F. Bonadonna, S. Gaglio, C. Nicolini, C. Ruggiero and F. Sorbello "Qualitative modeling of cell growth processes" *Appl. Art. Intell.*, Vol. 2, 1988, pp. 251 - 263
(7) C. Nicolini, S. Gaglio and C. Ruggiero "Artificial intelligence techniques for the control of cancer cells" *Cell Biophysics*, Vol. 14, 1989, pp. 117 - 127
(8) S. Gaglio, M. Giacomini, C. Nicolini, and C. Ruggiero "A qualitative approach to cell growth modelling and simulation for cancer chemotherapy", *I E E E Transactions on bimedical engineering*, in press.
(9) S. Gaglio, M. Giacomini, A. Ponassi, and C. Ruggiero "An OPS5 implementation of qualitative reasoning about physical systems" *Applied Artifical intelligence*, Vol.4, pp. 37 - 65, 1990.
(10) K. D. Forbus "Qualitative process theory" *Artificial Intelligence*, Vol. 24, pp. 85-168, 1984
(11) B. J. Kuipers "Commonsense reasoning about causality: deraving behavior from structure", *Artificial intelligence*, Vol 24, pp. 169-204, 1984
(12) B. J. Kuipers "Qualitative Simulation" *Artificial Intelligence*, Vol. 29, pp. 289-338, 1986

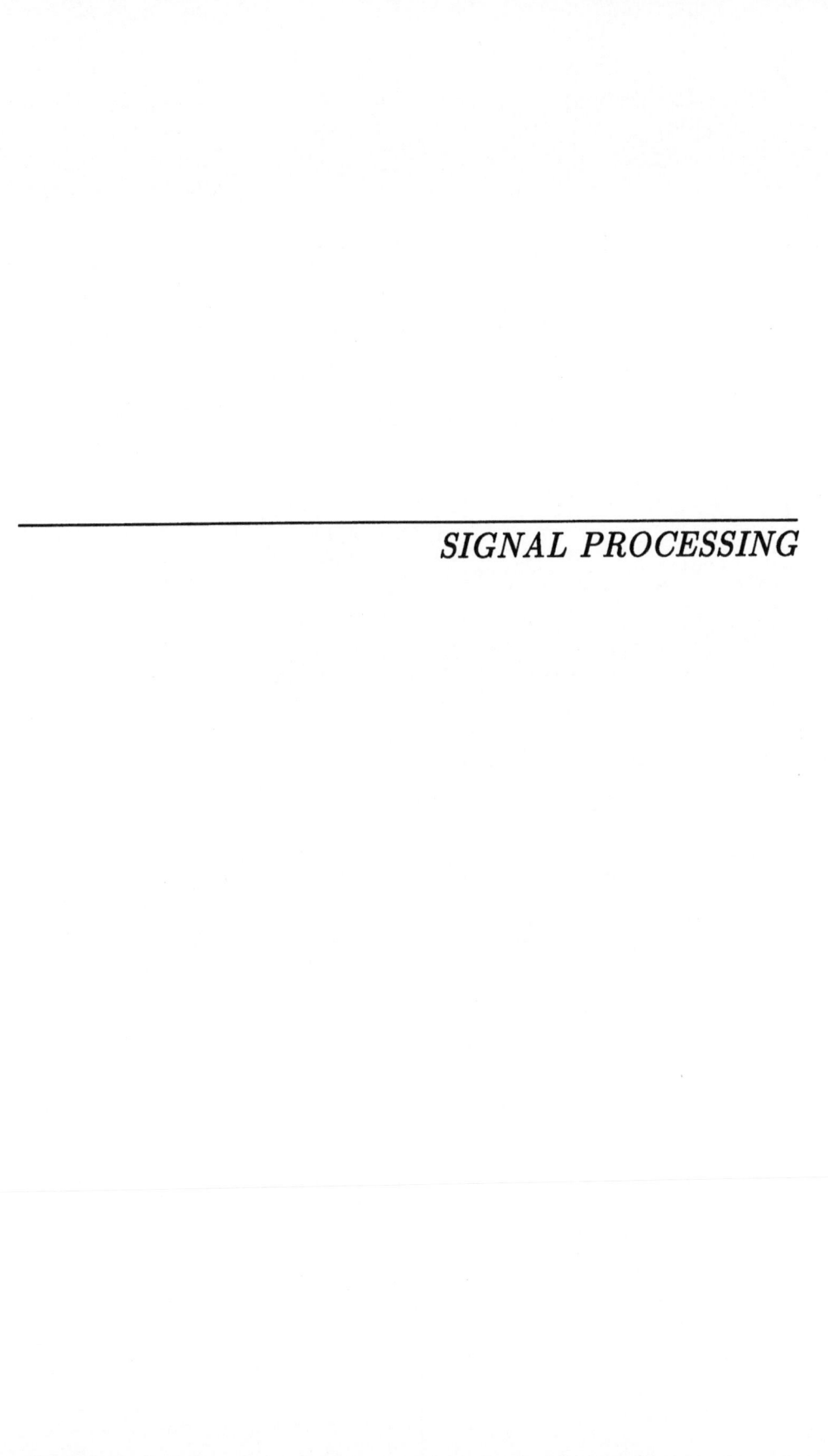

SIGNAL PROCESSING

ECG BEAT CLASSIFICATION USING LINEAR PREDICTION ERROR SIGNAL

Zygmunt Frankiewicz and Anwar Shrouf

Institute of Electronics, Technical University of Silesia,
ul.Pstrowskiego 16, 44-101 Gliwice, Poland.

Summary

This paper proposes a linear prediction method for beat classification in ECG Holter system. We assume that correlation method is used for recognition of up to 40 QRS templates. Since a classifier has to operate in real time mode a computationally efficient algorithm is used. A three state pulse-code train derived from a linear prediction error signal (LPES) is employed for classification instead of a raw signal.

The paper indicates that linear prediction coefficients do not differ significantly from beat to beat and from patient to patient.

This paper also indicates that the sensitivity of the classifier based on the three state linear prediction error signal to shape changes is sufficient for a Holter system. Its noise immunity is sufficient under condition that ECG signal is band-pass filtered and the threshold for LPES is not symmetrical. These conclusions were possible thanks to a special test signal which was generated using the first three Hermite functions.

1. Introduction

24 hour ambulatory ECG analysis is one of the most valuable cardiac tests. It enables early arrhythmias diagnosis.

Modern Holter systems should recognize up to 40 different morphologies according to templates created individually for each patient. When the correlation method is used for classification, what is commonly done, problem with computational load can arise.

An interesting method for ECG signal processing was presented recently by Lin and Chang [3]. They detected premature ventricular contractions (PVCs) using linear prediction error signal. In this paper we propose the same, but slightly improved, method for multitemplate beat classification in Holter systems.

We start with a short presentation of the linear prediction method.

2.Linear prediction method (LPM)

The actual ECG sequence s(i) can be approximated by another sequence $\hat{s}(i)$ which is determined by a unique set of predictor coefficients and the previous P samples s(i). That is

$$\hat{s}(i) = \sum_{k=1}^{P} a(k) * s(i-k)$$

where a(k) is the kth linear predictive coefficient.

The difference between the actual ECG sequence and the predicted sequence is called residual error signal.

$$e(i) = s(i) - \hat{s}(i)$$

There are many different methods available to find the linear predictive coefficients a(i). In this work the most efficient method - Durbin's recursive procedure was applied.

We employed the procedures introduced in [3] to obtain a three state error signal.This signal was used for ECG beat classification instead of the raw signal.

3.Linear predictive coefficients

First of all we checked whether the LPM coefficients had to be individually computed for each ECG beat. We randomly chose 5 records from the AHA arrhythmia database and computed coefficients a(i) for a few normal beats from each record. Durbin's recursive procedure was used to obtain optimal coefficients in lms sense. Values of the coefficients are shown in Table 1 and 2. We present only results for the order P=2 and partly for P=3 but we examined the coefficients for P=2,3 and 4. The fidelity of the reconstructed signal (measured as a rms of a difference between actual and reconstructed signal) was not significantly better for P>2. This was also reported by others [1,3]. So, our further consideration was done for P=2.

One can see from the table 1 that values of a(1) and a(2) are rather similar for different beats and different records.So it is not very important to compute new coefficients for each new beat.

Table 1

Record	N11		N12		N18		V78		V76	
Beat	a(1)	a(2)	a(1)	a(2)	a(1)	a(2)	a(1)	a(2)	a(1)	a(2)
1	−1.88	0.91	−1.82	0.90	−1.60	0.62	−1.88	0.94	−1.87	0.98
2	−1.83	0.86	−1.85	0.94	−1.80	0.85	−1.95	0.96	−1.85	0.94
3	−1.82	0.85	−1.85	0.94	−1.92	0.95	−1.93	0.94	−1.87	0.96
4	−1.84	0.87	−1.86	0.95	−1.91	0.93	−1.95	0.96	−1.75	0.85
5	−1.84	0.87	−1.86	0.93	−1.34	0.37	−1.95	0.96	−1.85	0.95
6	−1.89	0.78	−1.83	0.92	−1.86	0.88	−1.40	0.42	−1.80	0.91
7	−1.74	0.82	−1.85	0.93	−1.85	0.88	−1.46	0.99	−1.85	0.94

First two LPM coefficients for 7 beats from 5 different ECG records.

Table 2

Record	N 11			N12			V78		
Beat	a(1)	a(2)	a(3)	a(1)	a(2)	a(3)	a(1)	a(2)	a(3)
1	−2.670	2.547	−0.873	−1.997	1.265	−0.203	−2.400	1.973	−0.546
2	−2.270	1.698	−0.449	−2.574	2.573	−0.879	−2.561	2.205	−0.640
3	−2.071	1.407	−0.706	−2.580	2.378	−0.784	−2.289	1.673	−0.377
4	−2.235	1.714	−0.459	−2.674	2.548	−0.861	−2.473	2.024	−0.551
5	−2.296	1.839	−0.523	−2.418	2.052	−0.603	−2.648	2.379	−0.728
6	−1.892	1.219	−0.276	−2.290	1.835	−0.500	−1.294	0.070	0.248
7	−2.241	1.880	−0.612	−2.480	2.187	−0.670	−1.323	0.080	0.280

First three LPM coefficients for 7 beats from 3 different ECG records.

4.Sensitivity of the LPES based classifier to shape changes

As a next step we checked the sensitivity of the classifier based on the LPES to changes in the QRS shape. We needed a test signal which could fluently change its morphology.

We employed here an artificial signal modeled with the Hermite functions. The Hermite functions was first proposed for modeling QRS complexes by Sörnmo et al. in [4] and recently as an adaptive process by Laguna et al. [2]. There is an important question whether Hermite functions are adequate for modeling real ECG signal due to a convergence problem but for our purpose they seem to be very useful.

We generated a series of 21 different QRS shapes using a linear combination of the three first Hermite functions: $\Phi_0(i)$, $\Phi_1(i)$ and $\Phi_2(i)$.

$$H_j(i) = \begin{cases} \Phi_0(i)(N - 2j)/N + \Phi_1(i)\dfrac{2j}{N} & \text{for } 0 < j \le N/2 \\[2ex] \Phi_0(i)(2j - N)/N + 2\Phi_1(i)(N - j)/N + \Phi_2(i)(J - N)/N & \\[1ex] & \text{for } 11 \le j < N \end{cases}$$

N was equal to 20.

We obtained templates that could fluently change its morphology from mono phasic to biphasic and from biphasic to three-phasic.

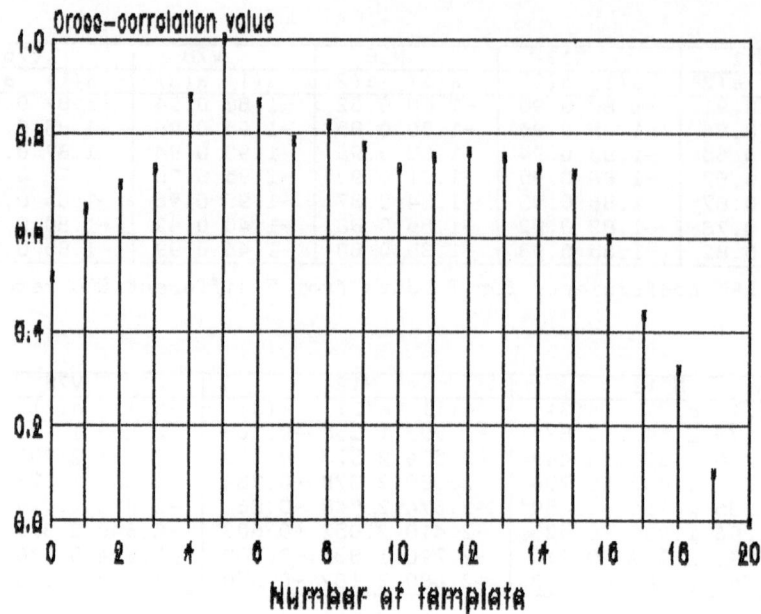

Fig.1. Plot of the cross-correlation values computed for the shape $H(n)$ and for each template from the series $H_i(n)$, $i=0,1,...,20$.

We found that LPES was different for different $H_i(n)$. Even similar shapes ($H_j(n)$ and $H_{j\pm1}(n)$) can be easily distinguished. A cross-correlation is frequently used as a measure of similarity in real Holter systems. Fig.1, for example, depicts a cross-correlation computed for three state error signal of a given signal [$H_5(n)$] and of each one of the series of templates [$H_0(n) \div H_{20}(n)$]. This means that the first point (zero on the horizontal axis) denotes the cross-correlation value computed for the three state error signal of templates H_0 and H_5, the second one H_1 and H_5 etc.

In real world applications where actual ECG signal is often noisy the classifier must still work correctly. In order to test a noise immunity of the classifier we added artificial white Gaussian noise to the generated signal and the pattern recognition procedure was repeated. White Gaussian noise is often used to model muscle artifacts. When the signal to noise ratio was below 20 dB the misclassifications occurred.

We discovered that a band-pass filtering of a current signal is needed. The filtering doesn't have to be compatible with the AHA standards because the filtered signal is used only for classification. We chose cutoff frequencies of 2 Hz and 20 Hz. Digital recursive filters were applied. The templates for the classification was obtained using the filtered signal too. Then the performance of the classifier was satisfactory even when the signal to noise ratio was equal to 5 dB.

We checked that influence of the other disturbances like line interference and baseline wandering was negligible.

Unfortunately, for some shapes misclassifications still occurred when signal was disturbed with a noise. We found out that these happened for QRS complexes with one wave much bigger than the others (for example: QRS with a small Q or S wave).

We came to conclusion that the threshold for the LPES should be separately computed for positive and negative LPES waves.

Upper threshold - for positive LPES waves, was computed as a rms of a signal $e_n(i)$, where :

$$e_n(i) = e(i) \qquad \text{for } e(i) > 0$$

$$e_n(i) = 0 \qquad \text{for } e(i) < 0$$

Lower threshold - for negative waves was computed from the $e_L(i)$ signal respectively,

$$e_L(i) = 0 \qquad \text{for } e(i) > 0$$

$$e_L(i) = e(i) \qquad \text{for } e(i) < 0$$

Then for all shapes from $H_o(n)$ to $H_{20}(n)$ and for SNR=5dB there were no incorrect classifications.

5.Real signal

The classifier was also tested using real data from the AHA arrhythmia database. Five records with the worst signal quality was chosen.

We did not observe any misclassification but this was partly due to a procedure often applied in Holter systems: if the cross-correlation was below a given value (75%) for each existing template a new template was created. No misclassification happened due to an excessive noise.

6.Conclusions

Typical results indicate that the linear prediction coefficients are very similar for different patients and for subsequent, normal QRS complexes. Because of that, these coefficients may by computed only once – at the beginning of the test or taken as constants.

The most important result is that the sensitivity of the classifier based on the pulse code sequence (derived from the linear prediction error signal) is sufficient for multitemplate beat recognition system. The classifier can be realized in real-time mode due to its computational efficiency.

Thanks to special series of artificially generated QRS complexes we found out that some misclassifications could be avoided when the different threshold values were used for positive and negative LPES waves.

We also found that the method introduced by Lin and Chang was very sensitive to noise. When ECG signal was bandpass filtered the classifier readily recognized even similar shapes for signal to noise ratio equal to 5 dB.

It seems that the linear prediction method can be used for comprehensive ECG signal processing including wave detection, noise level measurement, beat classification and data reduction.

In our next step we are setting to work on a data reduction method based on an idea of storage only a difference between actual linear prediction error signal and the same signal obtained for appropriate template.

References

[1] B. Eisenstein, R. Vaccaro, "Feature Extraction by System Identification", IEEE Trans. on Systems, Man, and Cybernetics, vol.SMC-12, no 1, 1982, pp.42-50.
[2] P.Laguna, P.Caminal, N.V.Thakor, R.Jane, "Adaptive QRS Shape Estimation Using Hermite Model",IEEE Eng. in Medicine & Biology Society 11th Annual International Coference, 1989.
[3] K.Lin, W.H.Chang, "QRS Feature Extraction Using Linear Prediction", IEEE Trans. on Biomedical Engineering, vol.36, no 10, 1989, pp. 1050-1055.
[4] L.Sörnmo, P.Börjesson, M.Nygårds, O.Pahlm, "A Method for Evaluation of QRS Shape Features Using a Mathematical Model for the ECG", IEEE Trans on Biomedical Engineering, vol 28, no 10, 1981, pp.713-717.

Averaged Powerspectra of the Electrocardiograms of Patients After Heart Transplantation

Wolfgang Schreiner[1], Guenther Laufer[1], Martin Neumann[2]
Wolfgang Premauer[1], Franz Merksa[3], Rudolf Lahoda[4], and Ernst Wolner[1]

1   2nd Department of Surgery, University of Vienna
    Spitalgasse 23, A-1090 WIEN / AUSTRIA
2   Department of Experimental Physics, University of Vienna
3   Department of Radiology, Krankenhaus Floridsdorf, Vienna
4   Institute of Physiology, Dept. Biotechnology, University of
    Vienna

Data acquisition and beat-by-beat FOURIER analysis is performed on a
PC-based system, aiming at the detection of rejection episodes from
electrocardiograms of heart transplant patients.

1. Introduction

Up to now, endomyocardial biopsy provides the only reliable
diagnostics for rejection of transplanted hearts (3,8). Simple visual
inspection of ECG tracings proved insufficient to diagnose rejection
episodes, at least as long as severe clinical symptoms are not
apparent as well. More refined approaches used the FOURIER analysis of
the ECG (1,6,7,9-11).

Modes of FOURIER Analysis

Two approaches to ECG FOURIER analysis can be envisaged:

(i) Fourier analysis can be performed on the original ECG signal over
     finite intervals, in which case the length of each cardiac
     cycledetermines the discrete set of frequencies for which
     spectral information is obtained. Evidently, this requires an
     accurate software detection of the beginning and end of each
     cardiac cycle and implies variable fundamental frequencies and
     harmonics (due to changes in heart rate). However, windowing (and
     thus distorting) the data prior to analysis is unnecessary.

(ii) Data can be multiplied by a 4-term Blackman-Harris window (4,5)
     and thus smoothly forced to zero outside an arbitrary interval.
     FOURIER analysis then (formally) applies to an infinite interval
     of time. In this case the detection of the length of the cardiac
     cycle is not as critical as in method (i), and the window may
     span part of a cardiac cycle (e.g. QRS-complex, T-wave), the

whole beat, or several beats. However, the multiplication by a window function distorts the data and also changes the spectrum. Moreover, the choices of the window function and the window length are to some degree arbitrary.

We therefore decided to do both types of FOURIER analysis, i.e. based on finite intervals as well as on windowed data.

Triggering on the ECG Vector

Signals from surface leads only yield projections of the 3-dimensional cardiac electrical vector. Depending on the particular lead chosen and on the (individual) orientation of the electrical axis of the heart, the maximum voltage found in each lead occurs in slightly different phases of the cardiac cycle. Generally, the time when the 3-dimensional cardiac vector reaches its maximum length need not coincide with the voltage maximum in any of the leads. Any trigger depending on conventional surface leads would therefore shift within the cardiac cycle if, e.g. between successive follow-ups of a patient, the orientation of the electrical axis should change. We therefore decided to acquire a vector ECG and to trigger on the maximum modulus R of the vector itself ("R-wave of the vector"). The interval (representing a cardiac cycle) obtained in this way was then used as a basis for the analysis of single lead signals.

2. SIGNAL ACQUISITION

Bipolar leads were connected to five electrically independent amplifier channels, featuring large bandwidth (-3dB points: 0.5 and 1100 Hz), low noise (10 μV_{pp} times amplification of channel) and a selectable low pass filter. An IBM-compatible (TANDON) 10-MHz AT computer was equipped with: Two 40 MB hard disks (28 ms), 2.5 MB RAM-disk, EGA graphics screen, numerical coprocessor, streamer tape, 3270 emulation adapter, DASH 16 analog/digital conversion board (METRABYTE), a high-speed hardware scroller board WFS 2000 (DATAQ). The installed software comprised: CODAS high speed data acquisition software (DATAQ), Personal REXX and KEDIT (both MANSFIELD SOFTWARE GROUP), and FORTRAN 77 (MICROSOFT), GRAPHMATIC library (MICROCOMPATIBLES).The CODAS software was used for the simultaneous acquisition of the five 800 Hz data channels and to display them (via the hardware scroller) in real time on the screen (X, Y, Z and the two intracardiac leads A and B). Note that the real-time display utilizes the A/D-converted data. Real-time display proved mandatory to ensure correct setting of electrodes, catheter and amplifier gains prior and during each measurement. If everything was found correct, real-time data logging to hard disk was started with a total throughput of 4000/sec (800 Hz per channel). One minute of logging produces about 0.5 MB data on the hard disk. Also during logging, signals were displayed in real time on the screen.

3. Digital Signal Processing

The evaluation program, written in FORTRAN 77, first extracted the amplifier gains from the calibration signal (for each channel) and rescaled data to millivolts at amplifier input.

Then the time derivatives of the three orthogonal components ($\frac{d}{dt}X$, $\frac{d}{dt}Y$, $\frac{d}{dt}Z$) for each record i were calculated as the slopes of linear regression lines over N_d ($\approx$ 4 ms) points. In the following, numbers of successive sampling points are related to sampling time so as to keep the notation open to different sampling rates. Derivatives were squared, added and summed over a window of $N_E + 1$ successive data points to obtain an "energy collector" for record k:

$$E_k = \frac{1}{N_E + 1} \sum_i \left\{ \left(\frac{d}{dt}X\right)_i^2 + \left(\frac{d}{dt}Y\right)_i^2 + \left(\frac{d}{dt}Z\right)_i^2 \right\} \quad k \le i \le k + N_E \quad (1)$$

where N_E was the nearest integer number of data points spanning a 80 ms window at a given sampling rate. E_k was re-evaluated for successive k and checked against two reference levels $E_{on} = 0.7 \cdot \max\{E_k\}$, $E_{off} = 0.7 \cdot \min\{E_k\}$) defining a hysteresis for the robust detection of QRS complexes. Following each detection of a QRS-complex, the estimates for E_{on} and E_{off} were updated by a running average. Then, in a second pass, the R-waves were accurately located by considering the slopes of two linear regression lines (each extending over $N_{R,pass2}$ data points, $\approx$ 16 ms) fitted to the length of the ECG vector $R = X^2 + Y^2 + Z^2$. Visual inspection following large scale graphic display revealed the algorithm to be stable and accurate to one data point (1/800 sec), even in the presence of local maxima close to the very peak of the R-wave.

The elimination of pacemaker spikes was in fact performed immediately after the detection of amplifier gains, prior to the triggering of R-waves. However, since the algorithm draws on concepts similar to R-wave detection, it is not described in detail.

4. Averaging of Powerspectra

For each cardiac cycle the FOURIER spectra were calculated, based on the the variable fundamental frequency $f_1 = T^{-1}$, where T is the cardiac cycle.

$$A(f_j) = \frac{1}{T} \int_0^T dt\, e^{-2\pi i\, f_j\, t}\, C(t) \tag{2}$$

where C(t) stands for the ECG data (X, Y, Z, R, A or B). Then the power-spectrum $P(f_j)$ was calculated (2) for all harmonics f_j:

$$P(f_j) = \left(Re\left[A(f_j)\right]\right)^2 + \left(Im\left[A(f_j)\right]\right)^2 \qquad 1 \leq j \leq j_{max} \tag{3}$$

where $j_{max} \triangleq 200$ Hz was the maximum frequency component well below the Nyquist frequency (for a sampling rate of $800\ s^{-1}$). According to the heart rate of the respective beat, we then allocated each harmonic frequency, f_j, to a channel number k ($1 \leq k \leq 200$) according to

$$k-1 \leq f_j < k \tag{4}$$

remembering that channel k holds frequencies between k-1 Hz and k Hz. Then the k-th elements of three arrays, $\hat{N}_k$, $\hat{P}_k$ and $\hat{P}_k^2$ were incremented: $\hat{N}_k$ incremented by 1, $\hat{P}_k$ incremented by $P(f_j)$ and $\hat{P}_k^2$ incremented by $P^2(f_j)$. This procedure was carried out for all cardiac cycles within a data file, and finally we calculated the mean and standard error of mean for all channels of each histogram. This procedure ensured a convenient estimate of the statistical spread in the averaged power spectra, which was considered essential in order to assess the statistical significance of intra-individual changes between successive follow-ups of a patient.

We chose data from a patient who was deliberately paced at three different frequencies (59, 89 and 119 bpm) during the same routine follow-up. The QRS complexes were windowed, and beat-by-beat power spectra were averaged as decribed above (see figure 1). The differences between these spectra may be compared with the standard deviation of an averaged spectrum for a fixed pacing frequency, as shown in fig. 2. QRS-power spectra, obtained at different heart rates (and hence at different fundamental frequencies) deviate from each other only by the amount of one standard deviation over the entire frequency range. This is reasonable, since the QRS-complex is almost unaffected if the heart rate changes within physiological limits.

These tests demonstrate the feasibility and consistency (i.e. QRS spectra being independent of heart rate) of results obtained by a beat-by-beat FOURIER analysis with subsequent spectrum averaging according to the method described in this work.

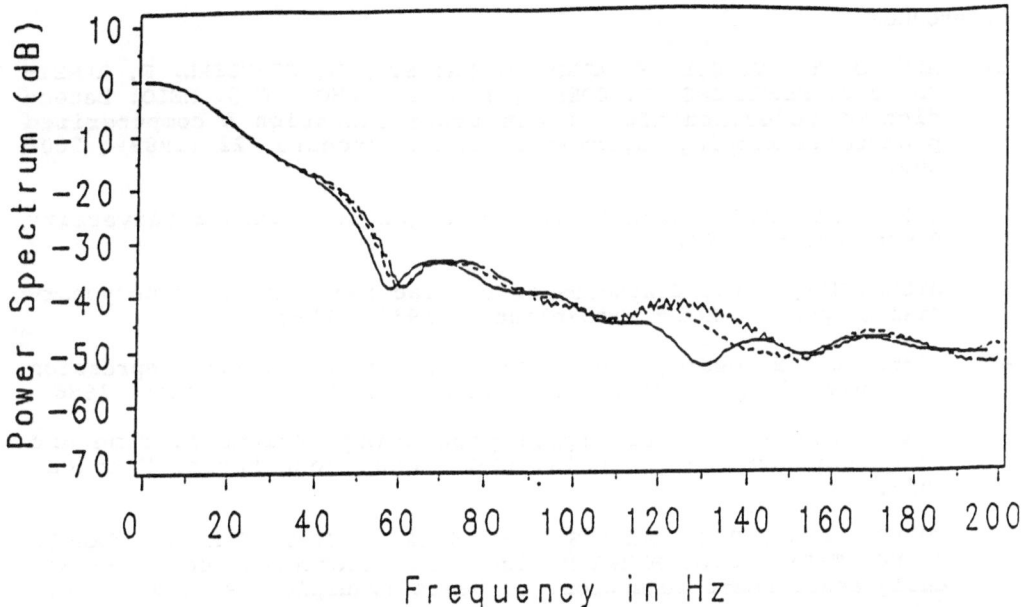

Figure 1: Averaged ECG Power Spectra for Different Pacing Frequencies.
The patient was paced at 59 bpm (solid curve), 89 bpm (short dashes)
and 119 bpm (long dashes). The QRS-complexes were windowed with a
120 ms 4-term Blackman-Harris window centered at the R-peaks.

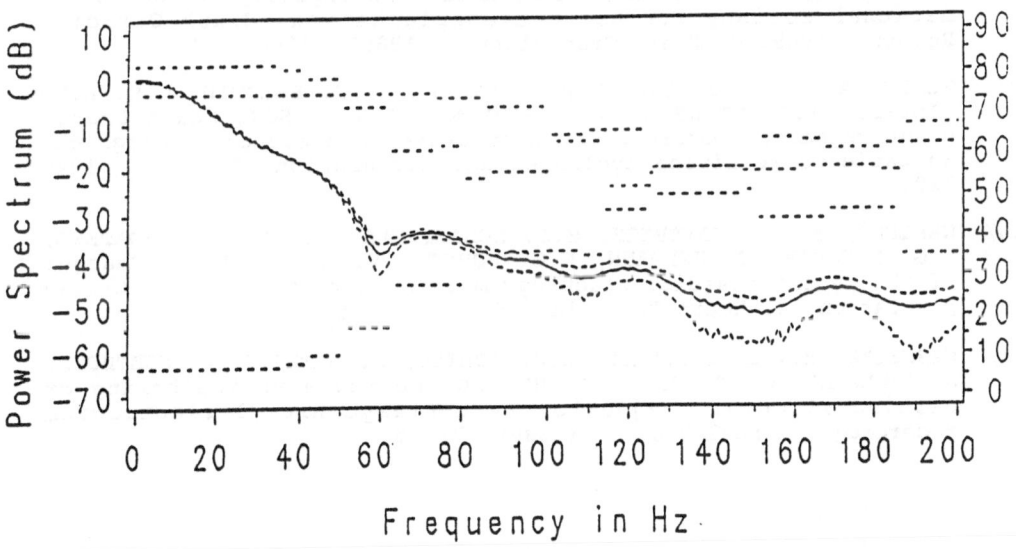

Figure 2: Averaged Power Spectra of Vector Length. Data from 80 QRS
complexes of a patient paced at 89 bpm. Mean values (solid curve) ±
standard deviation (dashed curves) for equidistant frequency bands of
1 Hz width. Right scale: Number of heart beats contributing to each
channel.

References

1/ ALEIXO, A., V. GIL, M. ADAO, J. BATISTA, N. ESPECIAL, F. ALMEI-
   DA, J.C. FERNANDES, R. COELHO, M.J. REBOCHO, J.Q. MELO: Detection of rejection after heart transplantation A computerized
   precordial mapping experience. J. Electrocard. 22 (1989) 200-
   203.

2/ BERUCHAMP, K.G.: Transforms for engineers. Oxford University
   Press Oxford, 1987.

3/ BILLINGHAM, M.E.: Diagnoses of cardiac rejection by endomyocardial biopsy. J. Heart Transplant 1 (1982) 25-30.

4/, COHEN, A.: Biomedical signal processing; Volume II: Compression
   and automatic recognition. CRC Press Boca Raton, Florida, 1986.

5/ COHEN, A.: Biomedical signal processing; Volume I: Time and
   frequency domains analysis. CRC Press Boca Raton, Florida,
   1986.

6/ COOPER, D.K., R.G. CHARLES, A.G. ROSE, R.C. FRASER, S. ISAACS,
   D. NOVITZKY, C.N. BARNARD: Does the electrocardiogram detect
   early acute heart rejection. J. Heart Transplant 4 (1985) 546-
   549.

7/ HABERL, R., M. WEBER, H. REICHENSPURNER, B.M. KEMKES, G. OSTER-
   HOLZER, M. ANTHUBER, G. STEINBECK: Frequency analysis of the
   surface electrocardiogram for recognition of acute rejection
   after orthotopic cardiac transplantation in man. Circulation 76
   (1987) 101-108.

8/ HECK, C.F., S.J. SHUMWAY, M.P. KAYE: The registry of the international society for heart transplantation. Sixth Official
   Report - 1989. J. Heart Transplant 8 (1989) 271.

9/ KEREN, A., A.M. GILLIS, R.A. FREEDMAN, J.C. BALDWIN, M.E. BIL-
   LINGHAM, E.B. STINSON, M.B. SIMSON, J.W. MASON: Heart transplant rejection monitored by signal-averaged electrocardiography
   in patients receiving cyclosporine. Circulation 70 (1984) 124-
   129.

10/ WAHLERS, T., A. HAVERICH, H.J. SCHAEFFERS, K. FRIMPONG-BOATENG,
    H.G. FIEGUTH, G. HERMANN, H.G. BORST, V. ARVANITIDOU: Changes
    of the intramyocardial electrogram after orthotopic heart trans-
    plantation. J. Heart Transplant 5 (1986) 450-454.

11/ WARNECKE, H., S. SCHUELER, H.J. GOETZE, G. MATHEIS, U. SUETHOFF,
    J. MUELLER, U. TIETZE, R. HETZER: Noninvasive monitoring of
    cardiac allograft rejection by intramyocardial electrogram
    recordings. Circulation 74 (1986) 72-76.

EEG MAPPING WHILE LISTENING TO A TEXT: DIFFERENCES BETWEEN CONTROLS AND SCHIZOPHRENICS[1]

Lacroix D., Rappelsberger P., Steinberger K., Thau K., Petsche H.
Institute of Neurophysiology and Psychiatry Unit, Währingerstraße 17, A-1090, Vienna.

ABSTRACT

An EEG mapping study was conducted in controls and schizophrenic males while they were listening to a text. In controls, changes in EEG parameters were observed mainly in brain areas related to language comprehension. These changes were not present in schizophrenics who differed also with a reduction in local and interhemispheric coherences when in a resting state with eyes closed.

INTRODUCTION

Computer assisted EEG analysis can be used to study changes in brain electrical activity during cognitive processes. The changes that occur during the execution of a cognitive task can be characterised by spectral parameters such as power, local coherence and interhemispheric coherence. The topographic distribution of these changes can be represented by different mapping techniques. These type of studies have been conducted in normals (Rappelsberger et al., 1986, 1988) and in psychiatric syndromes such as schizophrenia (Morihisa et al., 1983, Gruzelier et al., 1988, Guenther et al. 1988, Pockberger et al., 1989).

METHODS

19 EEG electrodes were placed on the scalp according to the international 10/20 system. EEG was recorded against averaged signals picked up from both ear lobes (TC 0.3s, Filter 35 Hz). The subjects were sitting comfortably in an arm chair and EEG records were made while they were listening to a text in a resting state with eyes closed. Control EEGs were made whereby the subjects were asked to relax with their eyes closed. Each record lasted at least 1 minute. EEG was recorded from control (n=23) and schizophrenic males (n=8). DSM3-R, ICD9 and Vienna Psychiatric Research criteria were used to establish the diagnostic of schizophrenia in drug-free patients.

EEG was written out on paper and simultaneously digitised at 128/s and stored on hard disc. Artifacts were eliminated from further computation by visual inspection. All artifact free 2 second epoches of one record were Fourier transformed to compute averaged power- and cross-power spectra with a frequency resolution of 0.5 Hz. 19 power spectra and 38 cross-power spectra were obtained for each record. Averaged cross-power spectra were calculated between adjacent electrodes along the transverse and longitudinal electrode rows and also between electrodes on homologous sites of both hemispheres.

For data reduction adjacent spectral lines were averaged to restrict to the frequency bands: theta (4 - 7.5 Hz), alpha (8 - 12.5 Hz), beta1 (13 - 18 Hz), beta2 (18.5 - 24 Hz) and beta3 (24.5 -

---

[1] Supported by the Jubiläumsfonds der Österreichischen Nationalbank, NB 3580

31.5 Hz). Final computations yielded broad band parameters like amplitude and coherence for the different frequency bands (Rappelsberger and Petsche, 1988) which were stored in a data base together with personal data like sex, handedness, age, task relevant data, etc. They served as discrimination criteria for group studies.

Group studies can be performed in two ways. In the first case, for a given task two groups of subjects can be chosen and a Wilcoxon test for independent samples can be applied to show significant differences between the respective parameters (Fig.4). In the second case, two different tasks for one group of subjects can be selected to visualise differences concerning both tasks. The differences can be presented by the mean values of the respective parameters of the chosen group (Fig.1) or by error probabilities according to paired Wilcoxon tests (Fig.2, Fig.3). Absolute EEG parameters were presented in colour coded topographic maps.

RESULTS

1. Effect of listening to a text in a resting state with eyes closed in control males (Fig.1, Fig.2): Amplitude was significantly decreased in left frontal regions of alpha, beta1 and beta3 bands, in left temporo-occipital regions in beta3 band and in right frontal areas of alpha and beta3 bands (Fig.2). Increased amplitudes (Fig. 1) were not shown to be statistically significant (Fig.2). Local coherence (LC) was significantly increased between left temporal, central and parietal electrodes in theta and alpha bands. LC was also increased between right posterior temporal, parietal and occipital electrodes in alpha, beta1 and 2 bands. Interhemispheric coherence was significantly increased in the theta band between posterior temporal and occipital areas and decreased between parasagittal frontal and occipital areas in the alpha band and between central regions in the beta1 band.

2. Differences between control and schizophrenic males when listening to a text in a resting state with eyes closed: Compared to control males, amplitude was not decreased and coherence revealed major differences in schizophrenics (Fig.2, Fig.3). The essential increase of local coherence was no longer present in the left centro-temporo-parietal regions in the theta and alpha bands and in right posterior temporal, parietal and occipital areas in alpha, beta1 and beta2

Fig.1: Spectral parameter maps. The maps show the grand mean of spectral parameter changes while listening to a text as compared with control EEG of 22 male volunteers.

The five rows relate to the five frequency bands examined. The three columns concern: mean amplitude per frequency band, local coherence, i.e. coherence between adjacent electrodes along the transverse and longitudinal rows, and interhemispheric coherence, i.e. coherence between corresponding sites of both hemispheres.

Colour codes for amplitude and coherence differences are given in the figure. Red means increase of the respective parameter during listening to a text.

Fig.2: Probability maps. The maps show the significant spectral parameter changes of 22 control males according to a paired Wilcoxon test. The arrangement of the maps is as in Fig.1.

Significant amplitude differences are indicated by squares at the corresponding electrode positions. A significant transverse or longitudinal coherence change is presented by a square drawn between the two electrodes involved. A significant interhemispheric coherence change is marked by squares at the two electrode locations of homologous sites of both hemispheres connected by a line.

The colour codes of the squares relate to the computed error probabilities. Blue squares indicate amplitude or coherence decrease and red squares amplitude or coherence increase.

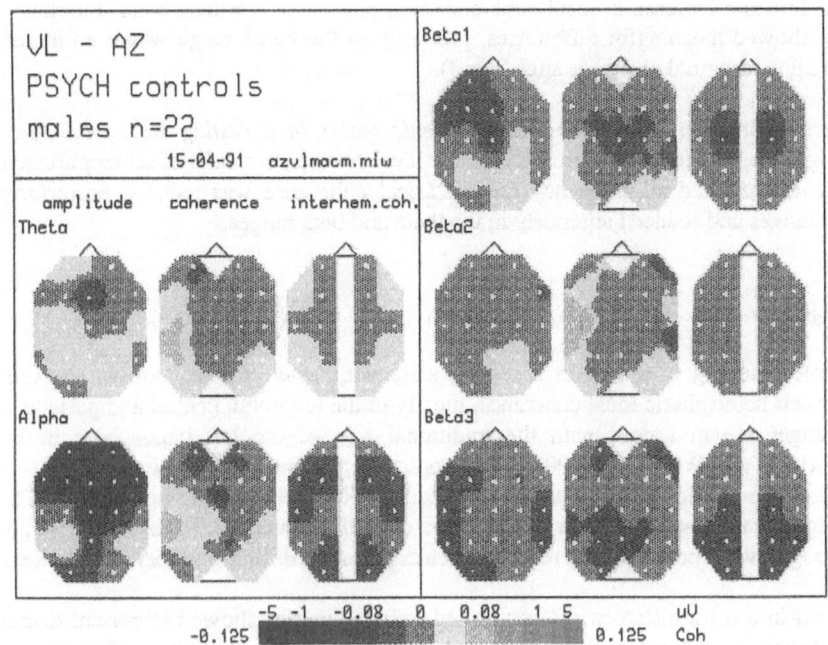

Fig.1: Caption in the text.

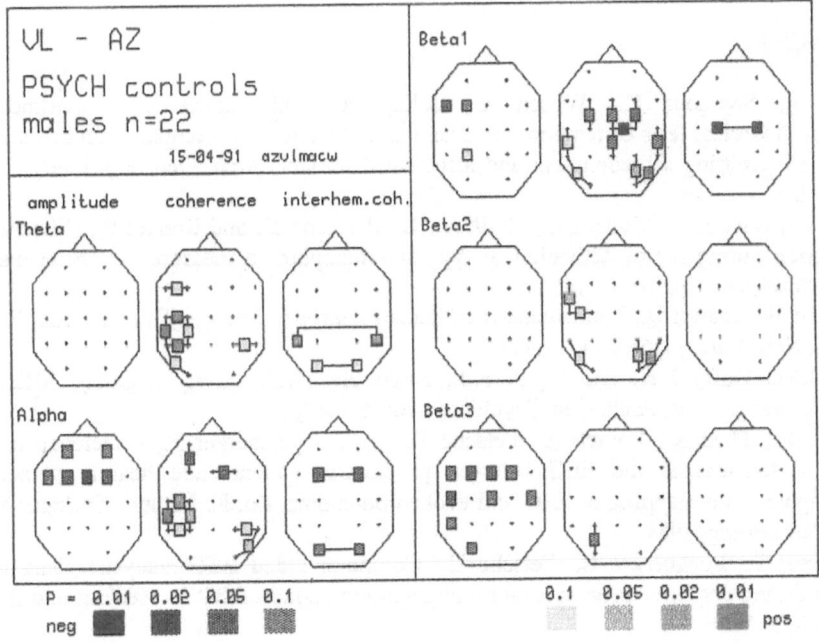

Fig.2: Caption in the text.

bands. An intricate increase in local coherence was present in the theta band. Interhemispheric coherence showed meaningful differences, primarily in the beta1 range where an increase was present in all parasagittal electrode sites (Fig.3).

3. Differences between control and schizophrenic males in a resting state with eyes closed (Fig.4): Significant differences were observed in local coherence results of schizophrenic üs patients which affected all frequency ranges. Local coherence was reduced posteriorly in all frequency ranges and reduced anteriorly in the theta and beta ranges.

DISCUSSION

While listening to a text in a resting state with eyes closed, controls showed major changes in left hemispheric local coherence, mostly in the temporal, central and parietal regions. These changes are in accord with the traditional role of the left hemisphere in language functions. (Kolb and Whishaw, 1990). In schizophrenic patients, changes in the left hemisphere were markedly reduced although the comprehension of the text was not altered. Their left temporal lobe was especially uninvolved in this cognitive function. These results suggest that different cognitive processes are present in schizophrenics during auditory comprehension of language.

When in a resting state with eyes closed, schizophrenics showed important decreases in local coherence in all frequency bands which indicate neurophysiological differences even in such an elementary mental state. Our results also show important differences in interhemispheric coherences in schizophrenic patients suggesting that the cognitive processes relating both hemispheres are altered.

REFERENCES

Gruzelier J., Seymour K., Wilson L., Jolley A. and Hirsch S., Impairments on neuropsychological tests of temporohippocampal and frontohippocampal functions and word fluency in remitting schizophrenia and affective disorders, Arch. Gen. Psychiatry, vol. 45, July 1988.

Guenther W., Davous P., Godet J.L., Guillibert E., Breitling D. and Rondot P., Bilateral brain dysfunction during motor activation in type II schizophrenia measured by EEG mapping, Biological Psychiatry, 21: 295, 1988.

Kolb B. and Whishaw I.Q., Fundamentals of human neuropsychology, Third edition, Freeman and Co., New York, p.568-574, 1990.

Morihisa J.M., Duffy F.H. and Wyatt R.J., Brain electrical activity mapping (BEAM) in schizophrenic patients, Arch. Gen. Psychiatry, vol. 40, July 1983.

Pockberger H., Thau K., Lovrek A., Petsche H. and Rappelsberger P., Coherence mapping reveals differences in the EEG between psychiatric patients and healthy persons, in: Topographic brain mapping of EEG and evoked potentials, Ed. K. Maurer, Springer-Verlag, Berlin, Heidelberg, 1989

Rappelsberger P., Pockberger H., Petsche H.: Computer aided EEG analysis: evaluation of changes during cognitive processes and topographic mapping. EDV in Medizin und Biologie 17(3): 45-53, 1986.

Rappelsberger P., Petsche H.: Probability mapping: power and coherence analyses of cognitive processes. Brain Topography, Vol 1, No 1: 46-54, 1988.

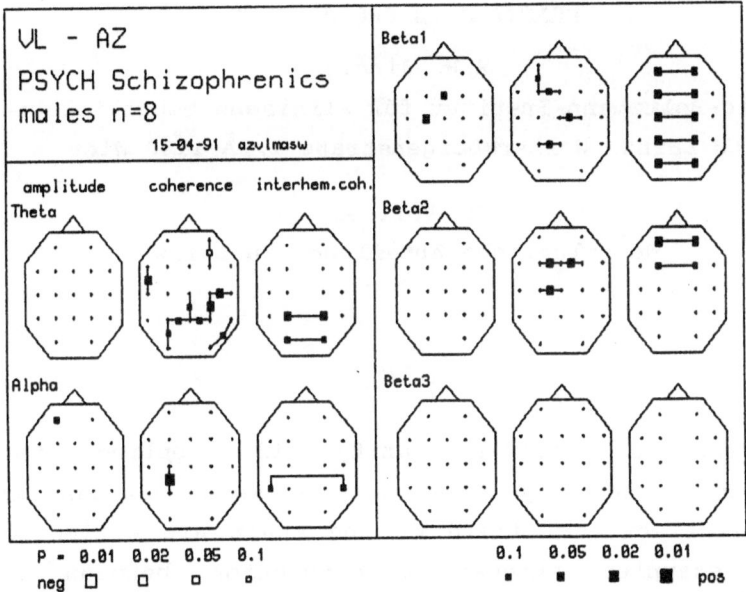

Fig.3: Probability maps. The maps show the significant spectral parameter changes during listening to a text of 8 schizophrenic patients according to a paired Wilcoxon test. The arrangement of the maps is as in Fig.1. Black squares denote significant increase according to the error probabilities shown and empty squares denote significant decrease.

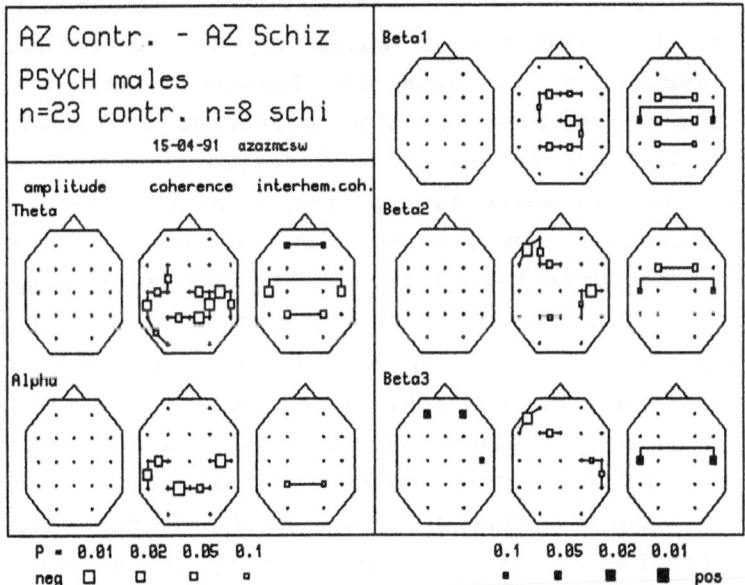

Fig.4: Probability maps. The arrangement of the maps is the same as in Fig.1. The computed error probabilities are due to Wilcoxon tests for independent samples when EEG with eyes closed of 23 healthy males are compared with that of 8 schizophrenic males. Black and empty squares as in Fig.3.

FRACTALS IN EEG MAPPING

R. H. Jindra

Ludwig-Boltzmann-Institut für Klinische Neurobiologie
KH Lainz, Wolkersbergenstraße 1, A-1130 Wien

R. Vollmer

Neurologische Abteilung, KH Lainz

Abstract

The concept of self-similarity is applied to the electroencephalogram. By means of the wave equation fractal maps of the electrical field on the scalp are estimated. The presented examples suggest a connection between fractal dimension and morphological or physical phenomena.

Introduction

During the last years quantification procedures for the electroencephalogram (EEG) were focussed on various algorithms depending on the information which should be pointed out. Currently computation of maps is favoured. Calculation of electrical fields is based on time dependent potential curves available at distinct points only. Consequently field strength or potentials are estimated by application of theorems governing electrical phenomena. In general, from a numerical point of view, these procedures result in certain averaging algorithms. Theorems which are employed for this purpose are most frequently Poisson's equation (for description of an electrostatic field) or wave equation (to consider time dependent properties). Computation, however, lacks of an only small number of electrodes which influences accuracy of numerical evaluation and, moreover, boundary conditions are difficult to determine (a fully comprehensive overview is presented by Gevins and Remond, 1987. For details of error estimation in ill-posed problems Hämmerlin and Hoffmann, 1989, may be consulted). In the following study computation of maps is based on wave equation, representing the potential by multiplication a space varying term with a time dependent function. Results of computation are maps which point out the potential distribution of the electrical phenomena occuring in the brain and projected onto the scalp. There is still another outstanding question: It is possible to obtain information about the structure of the maps? For answer the general concept of self-similarity is used which was first applied for description of the structure of fractals by Mandelbrot (1983) because the authors feel that this concept is a powerful tool to determine self-similarity in the electric field generated on the scalp. If such self-similarity is detected maps may be described by fractal dimension and be related to morphological or functional anomalies. After computing fractal dimension by the box counting method (Mandelbrot, 1983) ideas for future explainings are presented.

Methods

EEG was recorded using 10/20 system (except C2/F2) monopolarily against P2 as reference electrode obtaining 16 channels for this configuration. For further analysis it was analog/digital converted and stored on the system disc of a PDP 11/23. The signals obtained at the location of the electrodes were taken over a time duration of 1 minute divided into samples of 2 seconds succeed one another. Each sample was Fourier transformed and the results were averaged. For use of wave equation the following expression of the potential function was performed (Babister, A.W., 1966):

$$u(x, y, t) = U(x, y) . \exp(ikct) \qquad (1)$$

with x,y as space coordinates and t denotes time, while c represents propagation velocity (it is estimated for each frequency number k by consideration of the phase differences of Fourier transform). Boundary conditions were estimated by spline interpolation. Computation of potential values inside the area bordered by the contour electrodes was performed by use of finite element methods (Zienkiewicz, 1984). To reduce the mesh size additional node points were calculated according the structure function principle (Jindra, 1990), which means that the value at this points, say u_{est}, is obtained by weighted averaging of the actually available values at the electrodes u_i obeying minimum spuare error criterion

$$u_{est} = w_i . u_i \qquad (2)$$

(as usually, the sum is taken over double occuring indices). For each area bordered by the arrangement of four electrodes 25 additional nodes were computed. Subsequently finite element approximation was used to obtain a first solution. By means of this approximation further points were calculated to reduce the mesh size and the proviously described steps were again performed until starting of oscillation of the results (this is a frequently used criterion in computation of inverse problems). Then fractal dimension was estimated by the box counting method. The property of self-similarity is described by a power law. Consider a system of self-similarity determining elements enclosed by a square of length s_0. If the original square is divided into $(s_0/s)^2$ squares of side length s und N(s) is the corresponding number of determining elements and if, moreover, the system under consideration has fractal structure, the following equation holds

$$N(s) = constans. s^{-D} \qquad (3)$$

with D as fractal dimension. If N(s) is plotted against s on a double logarithmic scale the linear graph has slope -D, which means that from the slope the fractal dimension D may be estimated. The properties of the determining elements have finally to be specified (in geophysics, e.g. the number of faults entering a square is often used). Determining the fractal dimension of an arbitrary area requires its representation by a set of discrete points which is obviously fulfilled by the computation procedure. For each point the absolute value of the gradient was computed and all values were averaged. In each box (with decreasing length) those points were counted where the actual absolute value of the gradient exceeds the over all mean value. In the following figures only values of fractal dimension with variance <0.15 are considered.

Results

The results may be observed from two points of view, qualitatively and quantitatively. Primarily it will be pointed out that a fractal structure on the scalp may be detected. Two examples of our investigations are shown in Fig. 1 and Fig. 2, respectively. The small triangle denotes rostral direction (top view). Fractal dimensions from 0.7 to 1.6 are proven in both figures which result implies a self-similarity in the electric field of the brain. Moreover, local changes in the fractal dimension can be seen. Fig. 1 shows such areas of different fractal dimensions on the scalp of a normal proband. Highest values are located parietal. From these two spots fractal dimension decreases with increasing spatial distance. On the other hand, a parieto-occipital located area of high fractal dimension in Fig. 2 corresponds with a meningeom proved by computer tomography below this region.

Discussion

Firstly it may be emphasised that the concept of fractals is able to describe the structure of electrical fields on the scalp. From an energetic point of view the generation of a fractal surface with an high fractal dimension requires more energy than in the case of lower dimension. It may be guessed that barriers in morphology control fractal dimension. In summary, the concept of fractal dimension offers a method for better understanding physical processes generating the electrical activity of the brain.

Literature:

Babister, A. W.: The Mathematical Theory of Fields.
In: Vitkovitch, D.: Field Analysis. Van Nostrand, London. 1966

Gevins, A. S., Remond, A.: Methods of Analysis of Brain
Electrical and Magnetic Signals.
In: Handbook of Electroencephalography and Clinical
Neurophysiology. Elsevier, Amsterdam - New York - Oxford. 1987

Hämmerlin, G., Hoffmann, K. H.: Numerische Mathematik. Springer-
Verlag. Berlin - Heidelberg - New York. 1989

Jindra, R. H.: Topographical EEG mapping by means of the
structure function. Med. & Biol. Eng. & Comput., 28, 286-388,
1990

Mandelbrot, B. B.: The Fractal Geometry of Nature. Freeman.
New York. 1983

Zienkiewicz, O. C.: Methode der finiten Elemente. Hanser Verlag.
München. 1984

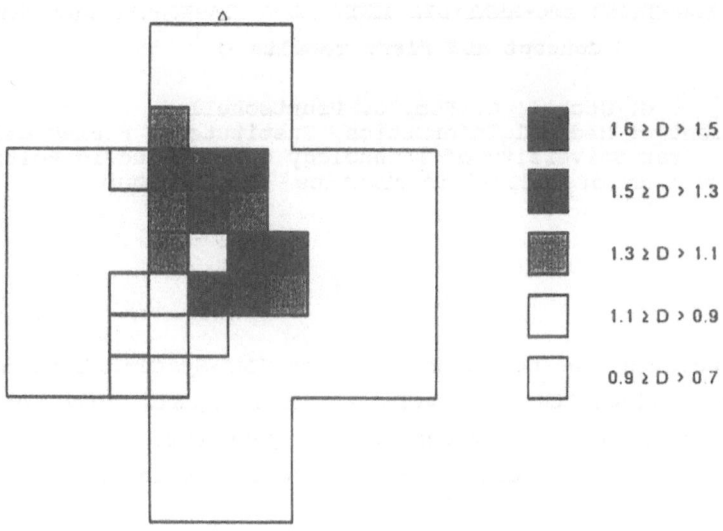

Figure 1: Fractal mapping of a normal proband
(for details see text).

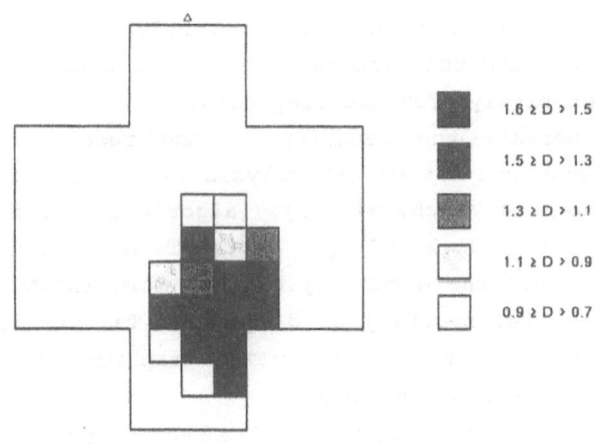

Figure 2: Fractal mapping of a patient suffering of an
occipital leocated meningeom (for details see text).

TRANSPUTER-BASED EMG-ANALYSIS INCLUDING DIAGNOSTIC SUPPORT
Concept and first results [1])

G. Jöchtl, G. Rom, G. Pfurtscheller
Departement of Medical Informatics, Institute of Biomedical
Engeneering, Graz University of Technology and the Ludwig Boltzmann
Institute of Medical Informatics, Graz, Austria.

ABSTRACT

This paper describes the new concept of an EMG-System. A transputer-
based hardware allows the analysis of EMG-signals with different
methods at the same time. Additionally an expert system can run on the
same device, so that a fast diagnosis support is possible.

Key words: EMG; Transputer; Helios; X-Windows

INTRODUCTION

EMG-diagnosis is up to now a time-consuming procedure. Because of
the complex human anatomy and measuring problems, it is easily possible
to get a wrong diagnosis. To reduce the time of EMG analysis and to
increase the security of the diagnosis, we develope a complete EMG
analysis system with diagnosis support. It should also be possible to
control the amplifiers and the stimulator from the central unit and the
expert system, respectively, for the diagnosis.

In order to increase the security of the results, we plan on
implementing more than one method of analysis of the EMG data. Besides
the standard method of Buchthal [1], algorithms similar to the
Automatic Decomposition EMG (ADEMG) [2] or the Turns & Amplitude method
[2] could be added. Thus the expert system has more independent inputs
which should increase the security of diagnosis. The standard features
of common EMG machines, such as fast online graphics and a good user
interface, are of course also included.

Realizing such a system with a PC-based computer will cause
problems. All connections between the hardware components of a PC are
handled by only one bus. This means that if many units are

---

[1] This study is supported by the "Forschungs-Förderungs-Fonds für die gewerbliche Wirtschaft" in Austria and
by the Austrian Ministry of Science and Research

communicating, the speed of every software module, such as graphics or data analysis, will be reduced.

REALISATION OF THE EMG-SYSTEM WITH TRANSPUTERS

To avoid loss of speed when adding software modules, hardware which allows comunication between two processes without slowing down the others is used. This can be done with a transputer network. Transputers are special microprocessors which have four serial connectors called links, so that networks can be built by connecting links between different processors. The optimal topology of the network depends on the software being implemented.

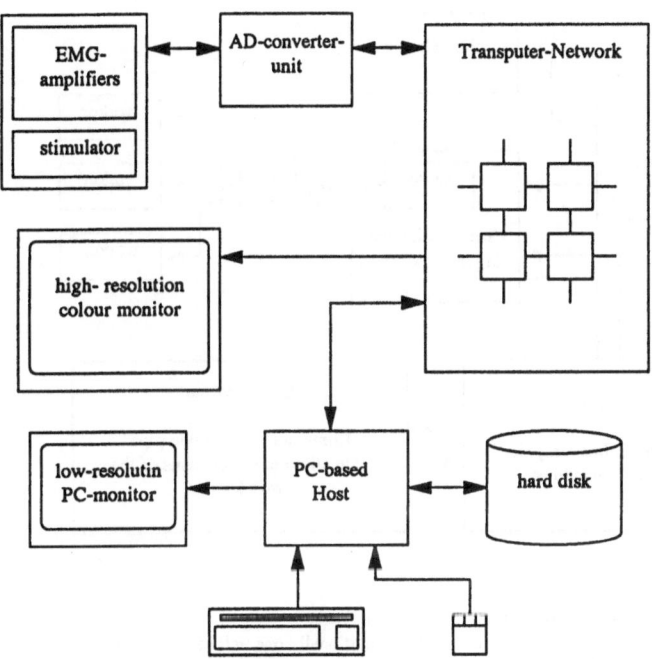

Fig. 1   hardware components of the EMG-System

We decided to use the Helios operating system for transputer networks. This is similar to Unix and also supports the X-Windows software [3]. Therefore there is a standard graphics environment available which simplifies the developement of user interfaces. Under

Helios, we use the programming language C. With the help of a special component distribution language (CDL), it is possible to distribute the software components over the whole transputer network automatically, so that the same software can run on different transputer networks without affecting any task. In Helios, a task is defined as a program which contains one or more concurrent processes and is in the state of execution. A disadvantage of Helios is that communication is slower than under Occam, especially if only a few bytes are transferred. If some kB are being transferred, the difference is no longer relevant.

The hardware concept of the EMG system is shown in Fig.1. In Figure 2, one can see the connection of the software components. One component can run on several transputers. Specifically, classification and analysis can be parallelized on different processors (worker 1..n).

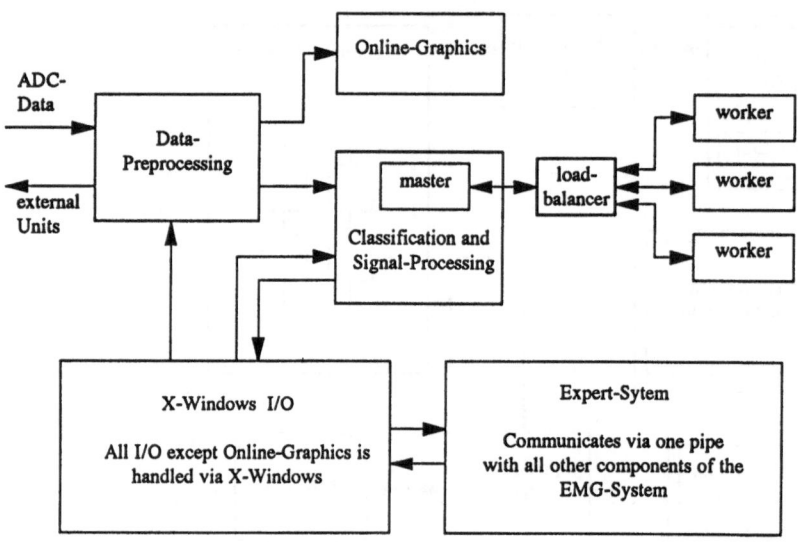

Fig.2: Schematic representation of the software components
The units may run on different transputers, additionally one unit can be divided into more tasks which can also be executed on different transputers. It is possible to use 'farms', where a frequently used worker-task can exist more times and can be distributed over the transputer-network, controlled by a master. The synchronisation is handled via a load balancer. Helios supports a farm constructor, so it is easy to construct farms.

Data acquisition

If continuous data acquisition in the background is desired, one must be sure that the process which receives data is not suspended when a byte is to be read. The transputer has two priorities, but the Helios operating system requires the highest priority for internal purposes. Task switching under Helios is done automatically so the user cannot influence the time when the reading process is ready to accept data.

To solve this problem, we designed our own A/D-Converter with an additional buffer. If the task is not ready to accept data, the data is stored in the buffer which is emptied immediately with maximum link speed when the task is activated again.

A transputer link is a bidirectional asynchronous connector, which means that it is possible to send information to the analog units such as amplifier and stimulator simultaneously during data acquisition using only one link.

Graphics

Online graphics should be very fast and have a very short delay time. Because of the complexity of X-Windows, there is much overhead and so the speed of the transputer graphics card is not fully exploited. Thus the part for online graphics is implemented as a separate task, which does not work under X-Windows, but communicates via streams.

EMG Classification and Analysis

Before analysis, the EMG potentials have to be averaged to increase the signal-to-noise ratio. It is important that only very similar shapes which belong to the same motoric unit are averaged. To obtain similar potentials from a stream of EMG data, these data are triggered and then classified by calculating the mean square error of the deviation between potentials. The similar shapes are placed in one box and then averaged [3].

EMG-analysis for an averaged muscle unit potential (MUP) is performed by extracting amplitude, number of phases, various durations etc.[2]. In addition to the standard method of Buchthal, we plan to implement also a method similar to ADEMG [2].

In a transputer system it is possible to make various calculations from the same raw data on different processors, so the speed of the standard calculation will not go down by adding more analysis software. Even classifications and calculations performed with standard algorithms can be parallized to work more efficiently.

Expert System

The EMG system will also be supported by a rule-based expert system to assist diagnosis. The expert system software runs on the same machine as the data acquisition and analysis software. This allows a fast and efficient communication between these units. The expert system can run on one transputer, on which other tasks are already working. It is also possible to run the expert system on a separate transputer subnet.

The expert system reads the analysed values of the averaged EMG potentials. Depending on the values, it will ask for more measurements or, if some diagnosis suggestion can be made, the measurement will be stopped and the diagnosis displayed. The doctor/physician can decide whether to accept this diagnosis or to disregard this suggestion and start new measurements.

The adjustment of the amplifiers (amplification, filter boundaries), which depend on the type of measurement, can be made directly from the expert system . The user I/O of the expert system has been written under X-Windows in a special window. The communication with other tasks is implemented with stream-oriented I/O.

DISCUSSION

The units shown in Fig. 2 are realized under Helios. In this stage of development it is not certain which combination of analysis methods will be used to get optimal information from the EMG-signal. Till now, only a few rules have been implemented in a first prototype.

Because of the concept it will be quite easy to add or change software and hardware components.

REFERENCES

[1] Buchthal, F.: Einführung in die Elektromyographie. Urban & Schwarzenberg, München, Berlin, (1958)
[2] Desmedt, J. E.: Clinical Neurophysiology Updates, Volume 2: Computer-Aided Electromyography and Expert Systems. Elsevier, Amsterdam, New York, Oxford (1989).
[3] Nye, A.: Xlib Reference Manual for Version 11, Volume 1. O'Reilly & Associates, Inc. (1989)
[4] Stålberg, E., et al: Quantitative Analysis of Individual Motor Unit Potentials: A Proposition for Standardized Terminology and criteria for Measurements. Journal of Clinical Neurophysiologie 3(4), Raven Press, New York, (1986), 313-348.

Computerized cephalometry on orthodontic radiographs: towards flexible and easily customized systems

F. Alte da Veiga and M.J. de Matos Barbosa
Dept. of Biomathematics and Medical Informatics
Faculty of Medicine, University of Coimbra - Portugal

Abstract

Computerized analysis of cephalometric radiographs for Orthodontic purposes has gradually been replacing the classical manual procedure, with outstanding advantages. Unfortunately, this replacement seems to be facing some resistance in several countries such as Portugal. The authors identified the main reasons for this fact and developed a system (AUTOCEF) with the major purpose of overcoming them.

Keywords:　　Orthodontics, Computerized cephalometry, PASCAL-programming, Cephalometric mathematical models and algorithms.

1. Introduction

Although computerized cephalometry is well known to provide considerable gain over the manual procedure, such as a dramatic reduction in execution time (from hours to minutes) and the elimination of drawing errors, among other features, this apparently obvious benefit is being somewhat ignored in a number of countries including Portugal. The main reasons for this fact, as pointed out by our orthodontists and potential end-users of such automated systems, could be described as follows:

- Expensiveness of the available commercial software;

- Submission to the implemented, rigid protocols, leading to the acquisition of systems which are not, most of the time, tailored or adaptable to one's needs as well as to the improvements the protocol models often experience as a result of continuous research;

- The standard values to which the patient's parameters must be compared were, in most of the available commercial systems, obtained for North-american or North-european populations, whose anthropometric characteristics are substantially different from the Portuguese population.

The AUTOCEF (which stands for Automated Cephalometry) system, written in PASCAL for MS-DOS computers, was designed in order to meet the requirements raised by the former topics, and does not intend to provide major advances concerning the kind of the information returned (such as prediction and simulation of treatment and facial-growth joint-effects or three-dimensional cephalometric analysis). Its goals can therefore be summarized as an attempt to build a easily expansible and flexible system, providing an attractive man-machine interface and allowing the introduction of significant changes and/or extensions with a minimum programming effort.

2. Cephalometry protocols

Any cephalometry protocol begins with the identification of a set of points on a side view skull-face radiograph, referring to bone, dental or soft-tissue structures from whose spatial interrelation the orthodontist will be able to extract precious information regarding diagnosis, therapy and follow-up. This two-dimensional spatial relationship is materialized as a set of numerical parameters (distances, angles and proportions between these) which acquire clinical meaning when compared to standard normal values. The first computerized methods were described by Houston [HOUSTON, 1970], Cleall [CLEALL & CHEBIB, 1971] and Ricketts [RICKETTS, 1972] and since then a considerable number of systems has been developed, making use of a digitizer to capture the XY co-ordinates of the X-ray identifiable points which can then be manipulated by appropriate subroutines yielding the wanted cephalometric parameters and their clinical interpretation.

Two protocols were incorporated into the AUTOCEF system, which was itself built according to the above guidelines. The first one is known as the CERVERA's protocol, with the outstanding feature of using standard comparison values obtained for the spanish population, anthropometrically close to the portuguese one. The second one has no particular designation due to the fact of having been developed at Coimbra's Universitary Hospital, as a result of specific research held at the Orthodontics Clinic (we will call it "COIMBRA" for reference).

3. Operation features

Hardware requirements consist on a compatible PC, a digitizing tablet and a printer (a dot-matrix one will do). Special attention was given to man-machine interface, supported by a window and menus system through which the user decides on particular actions to take (such as printing or saving results and executing a specific protocol), controls all the digitization process, visualizes results, enters patient's relevant information and gets messages from the system. With a few exceptions, output information concerning a given cephalometric parameter can be viewed as a record structure of the following type, exemplified for the distance between the points Go (Gonion - vertex of the mandibular angle) and Co (upper extremity of mandibular condyle):

Number and parameter designation		Mean value and acceptable deviation for age and sex	Calculated value	Deviation value	Interpretation
3	Go : Co	53 ± 3	57	+4 (+)	Hypo - meso- (hyper) -plasia ascend. branch

We would then say that, for the present patient, Go:Co exceeds the 3 mm acceptable deviation beyond the mean (the "+"s stand for the number of acceptable deviations that the actual deviation encloses), allowing us to conclude for the presence of a hyperplasia (overdevelopment) of the mandibular ascending branch.

4. Implementation details

AUTOCEF was fully developed in PASCAL, including the digitizer driver routines.

Two versions are available, one of which is database dependent and was designed to be interfaced with any DBMS supporting .DBF files, thus enabling the end-user to store and integrate cephalometry data with other types of information; this implied the development of interfacing routines allowing Pascal code to access .DBF records, for both reading and writing. The second version is database free and is suitable for those users who only wish to visualize and keep printed results.

As was previously pointed out, the main goal was to overcome the problem raised by the wide and growing variety of protocols used, as a result of differences concerning particular needs, concepts of Orthodontics science and anthropometric characteristics of the populations involved. Our primary task was then to distinguish their common and generic features from the specific ones, in order to build a stabilized shell needing no frequent updating or reviewing, to which individual and small modules could be linked.

Procedures such as overall system control, digitization, comparison with standard values, output to screen, printer or database and geometric computation routines were implemented as protocol-independent features, since the data structures they use can be dinamically generated on runtime; consequently, the task of implementing a new protocol or making substancial

modifications in existing ones becomes considerably simplified, involving the following steps:
- Creation of a text file with the designation of the points to be digitized;
- Creation of a text file with standard comparison values, allowed deviations and possible clinical interpretations for all desired cephalometric parameters (this allows the same protocol to be used on anthropometrically different populations); this file may also contain optional configuration information;
- Creation of a PASCAL module containing the computation sequences for distances, angles and proportions; it is our intention to build a parser to allow the user himself to do this in a simple syntax language, with the additional advantage of not having to compile and link the code; however, the PASCAL code involved is straightforward, making use of the following procedures and functions:

Function Distance (Point1,Point2)	returns the distance between two points
Function Angle (Point1,Point2,Point3)	returns the angle corresponding to the vertex Point1
Procedure Straight_Line (Point1,Point2,SL)	assigns to SL the equation of the straight line defined by Point1 and Point2
Procedure Intersection (SL1,SL2,Point)	assigns to Point the co-ordinates of the point where SL1 intersects SL2
Procedure Perpendicular (SL,Point,PSL)	assigns to PSL the equation of the perpendicular to SL passing by Point
Procedure Parallel (SL,Point,PSL)	assigns to PSL the equation of the parallel to SL passing by Point
Function Between (Point,Point1,Point2)	returns TRUE if the orthogonal projection of Point on at least one of the axes (X or Y) is between the projections of Point1 and Point2, otherwise returns FALSE (This is necessary because the values of some parameters are by convention positive or negative depending on the relative situation of the points used on their computation)

The interface language will only need to call the procedures and functions described above, and to manipulate basic arithmetic and logic operators plus a IF-THEN-ELSE control structure.

For example, the Po:V parameter - distance between the Pogonion (most anterior point of chin symphysis) and Cervera's Vertical Axis - which defines the mandible anteroposterior position, could be coded as :

(Remark: for better comprehension we will use meaningful argument names instead of the PASCAL references to pointers, records and arrays; when implemented, the interface simple syntax language could look like the following)

```
{...... assuming Cervera_Vertical has already been determined }
Perpendicular (Cervera_Vertical,Po,Horizontal_Po)
Intersection (Horizontal_Po,Cervera_Vertical,CVHPo)
Intersection (Horizontal_Po,Co_Go,Refl)   { reference point on Co_Go, the
                                             line defined by points Co and Go}
if Between (Po,CVHPo,Refl)
  Po:V =  - Distance (Po,CVHPo)
else Po:V = Distance (Po,CVHPo)
```

The great majority of protocols being used could be easily incorporated into AUTOCEF in this way. However, some of them make use of specific and more or less complex procedures to compute one or more cephalometric parameters, as is the case of CERVERA's protocol whose coding involves simulation of optimized plane rotation to determine Cervera's Vertical Axis (all other parameters can be computed as we have exemplified). Situations such as this one will obviously have to be coded in a language like PASCAL by an experienced programmer, but their reduced frequency fully justifies the existence of generic systems enabling the user to be as independent as possible. Furthermore, by allowing him to explicitly define or redefine the way parameters are obtained, as well as to use the standard comparison values he wishes, we foresee that the system will prove to be helpful in cephalometric methodology research.

References

Begole, E.A. (1980), 'Software development for the management of cephalometric radiographic data', *Comput. Programs Biomed.*, 11: 175-182.

Bernie, D.J. (1983), 'On-line digitizing useful mathematical techniques', *B. J. Orthod*, 10: 78-89.

Cleall, J.F. & Chebib, F.S. (1971), 'Coordinate analysis applied to orthodontic studies', *Angle Orthod.*, 41: 214-218.

Houston, W.J. (1970), 'Automated measurements of photographs and radiographs', *The Dental Practicioner*, 21.

Konchak, P.A. (1985), 'A Pascal program for digitizing lateral cephalometric radiographs', *Am. J. Orthod.*, 87: 197-200.

Ricketts, R.M. (1972), 'An overview of computerized cephalometrics', *Am. J. Orthod.*, 61: 1-28.

EPEXS: AN EXPERT SYSTEM FOR ANALYSIS AND INTERPRETATION OF HUMAN EVOKED POTENTIALS

A. BRAI, R. M. KOUTLIDIS, J.-F. VIBERT

Laboratoire de Physiologie, CHU Saint Antoine
Université Pierre et Marie CURIE, CNRS UA 1162
PARIS FRANCE

Abstract - *EPEXS is an expert system for evoked potentials (a medical examination performed in clinical neurophysiology laboratories), working from available clinical records and numerical data measured from the evoked potential traces. EPEXS integrates two formalisms of knowledge representation: rules and structured objects. The rules represent the elementary concepts (shallow knowledge) and include a model of possibility based on the Dubois and Prade's default reasoning and possibility theory. The structured objects (prototypes) are organized as hierarchical taxinomies (underlying knowledge). They allow the description of both the objects and their relationships. The heuristics used to interpret the knowledge are based on two hypothesis: the unicity of the pathological process leading to several symptoms, and the progression from the general to the specific, leading to decide between the presence or absence of a class of diagnosis. This avoids the problem of the differential diagnosis. These various knowledges are used in a dynamical way that could be described as a four step process: acquisition of clinical data in order to define the nosological frame of the pathology, production of hypothesis about the nature and topography of lesions, interpretation of data in accordance with these hypothesis and finally evaluation of their likelihood.*

Evoked potentials (EP) are the electrical responses recorded from the scalp of a patient few milliseconds after a peripheral sensory stimulus. Three types of EP are commonly used in clinical explorations: somesthetic, visual and auditory. This paper describes an expert system based on classification allowing the analysis and interpretation of EPs. This expert system was primarily thought and tested on brainstem auditory evoked potential (BAEP), and finally generalized and implemented to process any EP type according to the knowledge base used. It is well documented (Chiappa, 1983) that the origin of the accidents (thereafter referred as peaks or waves) on the EP waveform is due to the recordings of electrical fields generated by the synaptic activity in the different anatomical relays on the neural pathways and recorded at the cortex level as far or near fields, according to the considered EP. Their study thus allows to determine the topography and/or nosology of a possible lesion.

EPEXS overview -

The analysis of the way the knowledgeable expert follows to go from the signal recording to the EP interpretation within the clinical context, led us to structure the knowledge into three main categories, each of them corresponding to a step toward the diagnostic. The first step is the signal recording, including the electrode positioning and the recording parameters adjusting. The second step is the pattern recognition, *i.e.* the signal analysis, in order to extract the significant patterns from the EP waveform. The last step is the EP interpretation and the resulting diagnostic. This analysis led us to choose the "blackboard" model (Gomez 1981, Nii 1986) since it allows the different knowledge sources to communicate (Vailly 1986). This model is interesting for several reasons: several types of knowledge can communicate in this model, procedural knowledge as well as declarative one, it is possible to generalize the model of production rules into $condition \rightarrow action$, it is possible to build a solution using stepwise refinements of hypothesis given by the different knowledge sources In our implementation, these different knowledge sources are hierarchically linked. The signal recording knowledge source is at the lower level, the interpretation and diagnostic knowledge source is at the highest level while the pattern recognition knowledge source represents the intermediate level. The recording related knowledge source will not be debated in this paper, since it is always under project at this time, and therefore not yet included in EPEXS.

Knowledge acquisition - The goal of knowledge acquisition is to model the knowledge of one or more experts in a way that allows it to be encoded into an expert system *i.e.* translating implicit knowledge into an explicit form. The expert confrontation led to point out the type of knowledge used during the EP interpretation process. There are the elementary concepts such as the absolute peaks latency and amplitude, the interpeak latencies and the clinical data. On the other hand, there are more reach concepts with a higher level of abstraction such as the hierarchical relationships between concepts of the first group, the clustering of different types of concepts into categories, and the causal relationships corresponding to the physiopathological or anatomo-electrical models used by the expert to conclude to a diagnostic.

These various knowledges are used in a dynamical way and are described as a four steps process:
- acquisition of clinical data in order to define the nosological frame of the pathology,
- production of hypotheses about the nature and topography of lesions,
- interpretation of data in accordance with these hypotheses,
- and finally evaluation of their likelihood.
The heuristics used to interpret the knowledge are based on two hypothesis :
- the unicity of the pathological process leading to several symptoms,
- the progression from the general to the specific, leading to decide between the presence or absence of a class of diagnosis.

Reasoning under uncertainty, whatever its cause, remains a difficult problem. Many alternative methods have been proposed such as bayesian techniques, shafer/dempster approaches, default reasoning, possibility theory, and fuzzy logic. Some of these methods have been successfully implemented. EPEXS uses a model of uncertainty close to those used by Buisson in the Diabeto III system (Buisson, 1985), rooted in the default reasoning and possibility theory by Dubois and Prade (Dubois and Prade, 1988).

EPEXS knowledge representation - Two representational forms have been used to make explicit and to interpret the two types of knowledge:
- *prototypes* (also called structured objects): for the deep knowledge (knowledge of domain facts and their relationships),
- *production rules*: for the shallow knowledge (knowledge about how to apply these facts and

relationships to solve a specific problem).

Prototypes - Prototypes are data structures containing informations about an object. These informations are the name of the object and slots with values to be determined dynamically from the user or from deduction. Values which are not to be derived from rules but asked from the user are called primitive. Each of these slots can be filled with a value according to the type of the slot. There are three types of slots:
- the **interval**: $[Minimum, Maximum]$ characterized by its lower and upper bounds, both bounds could be equals indicating a single value.
- the **set**: $\{X_1, X_2, \cdots, X_n\}$ characterized by a values enumeration.
- the **prototype**: which is a sub-part of this object, itself made of intervals, sets and prototypes. It is recursively defined until there is only intervals and/or set slots.

Prototype trees - The relationship between the prototypes can be described usefully by using the tree representation, where each node represents a prototype. This representation can be drawn graphically and provides an easy way to communicate with the experts, usually not familiar with the knowledge engineers specific language. The root prototype of the main prototype tree represents the main class of the expert system. Classifying an object is finding out which prototype (node) gives the best fit. The finding path goes from the more general (root) to the more specific (nodes) prototypes.

Production rules - A production rule represents knowledge in the form **If** *premisse* **Then** *conclusion*. In EPEXS, rules are used to complete the description of an object during its classification by deducing some values from other slot values, or by transforming numerical values to symbolic ones (*i.e.* transform a given numerical value to the symbolical concepts such as normal, too low or too high.
The EPEXS rules have the following form:
Name: the symbolic rule name.
Class: the class to which the rule is associated.
If   *premisse(s)* (ci) where ci is the coefficient of importance of the premisse and cp
Then   *conclusion(s)* (cp)
the coefficient of possibility given to the conclusion, as described by Dubois and Prade (1988) in their possibility theory. Rules are implicitly grouped according to the prototype they are linked to. Thus during the progression along the tree, EPEXS knows which rules to activate. This is a simple but powerful choice of strategy of rules activation since it eliminates the need of metarules.

Inference type - The methodology of EPEXS inference mechanism is contained in the prototype trees description, and described as follow:
- activate the rules at the level of the current prototype,
- deduce facts,
- complete the object description,
- compare object and prototype,
- if the object fits, the tree exploration goes on, else it stops.
The result is a prototype or a set of prototypes, or is empty if the object does not corresponds to the root.

Production rules and uncertainty - The expert knowledge that must be represented in the expert system knowledge-base is often incomplete or uncertain. Indeed, reasoning in real-world domains is usually pervaded by the need to handle incomplete and uncertain knowledge

(Post 1987) such as missing facts or rules that supply only partial or weak support for their conclusion. The uncertainty concerns mainly the truth or the untruth of propositions representing factual knowledge, or operating rules (production rules), truth and untruth that are not definitively established. The fuzziness is related to the information content expressed using fuzzy predicates ($\approx$, $\succeq$, $\preceq$, near-to, far-from). Consequently, the expert system must be able to take into account this uncertainty and to transfer it correctly from the premisses to the conclusion. The inference engine of EPEXS computes the coefficient of possibility (cp) for each conclusion, according to the faith (ci) credited to the premisses. ci is comprised between 0 (false premisse) and 1 (true premisse). This coefficient becomes then the new cp value for the conclusion. During the rules input, the coefficient of possibility cp defaults to 1, and keeps this value unless the expert explicitly gives a lower value. During the classification phase the computed cp values are compared to the cp values given by the expert. The lowest value is kept.

EP Knowledge modelisation -

This section describes the special organization of the knowledge representation used to specifically process the EPs. The method used by the EP expert to interpret the EP signal and then to establish its diagnostic is rather stereotyped. The EP expert organizes the way the EP examination is done by first examining the available clinical data from the patient record, which may help during both the recording session and the interpretation phase. During this interpretation phase both sides are simultaneously analyzed. The prototypes tree is built by tracing the way the EP expert follows to go from the EPs and clinical raw data to the final interpretation and diagnostic.

The knowledge source of BAEP is constituted by 4 prototypes trees and several prototypes.

The root of the main tree is **EP_exam** which contains 3 slots describing the right ear, the left ear and the clinical context. Right and left ears are described by a prototype called **baep**, and the clinical context is described by a prototype called **clinic**. The **baep** prototype is described by four prototypes called **wave**, auditory threshold and several latency values. The **clinic** prototype is described by several data types such as clinical symptoms and paraclinical exam results (scanner, IRM, etc...).

Evaluation of EPEXS -

The validation of EPEXS was done on a collection of representative and well documented, diagnostic accurate medical records. Two types of clinical records were considered to be eligible: simple and characteristic records, and questionable records, in which the diagnostic was finally well established, but where the available data could lead to hesitations between some diagnostics. The knowledge base was established by one expert, but the validation was performed with the collaboration of three experts, two of them being naive in respect to EPEXS. The evaluation results are summarized on the following table:

Validation of E.P.E.X.S.				
Record types	Records number	Correct diagnosis	Erroneous diagnosis	Supplemental informations
Normals	20	20 (100 %)	0 (0 %)	5 (25 %)
Abnormals	25	23 (92 %)	2 (8 %)	1 (4 %)
Total	45	43 (95.6 %)	2 (4.4 %)	6 (13.3 %)

Forty five clinical records were tested. Among them, 20 records were classified as normal by human experts, and EPEXS gave 100% of correct diagnostic, but find out complementary information (subnormality or liminal pathology) in 25% of these normal instances. These complementary informations were verified and always agreed by the experts. For the pathological records, EPEXS gave 92% of correct diagnostic (topography and nosology), and in 8% of instances, EPEXS gave the correct topography, but a false nosology. EPEXS never considered a pathological record as non pathologic. In 4% of instances, EPEXS find out complementary information, also accepted by the experts.

References

Buisson, J.C., H., Farreny, et H., Prade. Un systeme expert en diabetologie accessible par minitel **5eme Cong. Systèmes Expert Avignon**; (1985)

Chiappa, K.H., Evoked potentials in clinical medicine. **Raven Press, N.Y., 340PP**: (1983)

Dubois, D., et H., Prade. Default reasoning and possibility theory. **Art. Intell.**; 35 : 243-257 (1988)

Gomez , F., et B., Chandraeskaran. Knowledge organization and distribution for medical diagnosis **IEEE Trans. Sys. Man And Cybernetics**; (1987)

Nii, H.P., Blackboard system: The blackboard model of problem solving and the evolution of blackboard architecture. **The Ai Magazine**; 1 & 2 : (1986)

Post, S., Reasoning with incomplete and uncertain knowledge as an integer linear program In: **Avignon 87.EC2 Eds.** 2 : 1361-1377 (1987)

Vailly, A., et M.A., Simon. Des systemes experts cooperants, pourquoi, comment ? **Communication Cognitiva**; (1987)

AN INTEGRATED COMPUTER WORKSTATION FOR EPILEPSY MONITORING: TECHNICAL CONCEPT

T.A.Vuong, M.Dupre', H.Holthausen, A.Sakamoto,
R.C.Burgess [1], T.F.Collura [1],H.Lüders [1]

Epilepsie-Zentrum Bethel, Präoperative Diagnostik,
Maraweg 21, D-4800 Bielefeld 13, Germany
and
[1] The Cleveland Clinic Foundation, 9500 Euclid Avenue,
One Clinic Center, Cleveland, Ohio 44195-5221, USA

Abstract:

Processing of EEG signals recorded from epileptic patients under prolonged video-EEG monitoring can be routinely applied to detect and localize interictal abnormalities, and to analyze ictal EEGs. In our Epilepsy Monitoring Units (EMUs) at the Epilepsy Center Bethel (FRG) and the Cleveland Clinic Foundation (USA), this processing has already been done successfully for years. In the search for useful and cost effective new enhancements to our current hardware and software framework, we are now concentrating efforts on the development of the concept of a workstation at the physicians' hands, which consists of implementation and integration of workstations to this basic system. Desirable features of these integrated workstations are expendability, graphic interface, communication with data acquisition system, communication with patients' data bank, and possibilities of multiple clinical applications. Currently a "prototype" including some of these features has already been implemented (HP 9000/800 and 9000/400 Workstations). In this report we describe the technical concept and the current stand of this development including examples of some clinical applications on EEG filtering, mapping, reformatting, signal measurements, etc.

1. Clinical requirements:

The main indication of video-EEG monitoring is nowadays in the presurgical evaluation of epileptic patients with intractable seizures. For this purpose interictal as well as ictal EEGs have to be extensively examined in order to localize precisely the brain areas to be surgically sessected /1/. The procedure usually consists of 1-4 weeks of continuous "around-the-clock" video and EEG recordings. The number of EEG channels recorded usually ranges from 16 to more than 100 channels for each patient (our current capacity is 256 channels of EEG, and a upgrade to 512 channels is currently under way). At conventional paper speed of 30 mm/sec this represents 8,640 page/24 hours/bank of 16 channels. These figures clearly demonstrate the need of implementation of computer-assisted techniques for the EEG analysis /2/. On the other hand, physicians need a "tool" to handle the recorded EEG-data and collected patient's information. At this point of our development we have defined the features or clinical requirements as a "tools kit" for our integrated computer workstation (see table 1).

2. Technical concept:

We have previously described the structure of the basic system currently in use at the EMUs of Bethel and the Cleveland Clinic. It consists of a HP-1000 computer for the real time EEG acquisition (acquisition subsystem) and a UNIX HP-9000 for the monitoring (monitoring subsystem). The acquisition subsystem is responsible for the digitalization and buffering of the data which are then transferred to a First In First Out (FIFO) buffer. The FIFO is programed for storage on a 570 Mbyte hard disc appropriated to the storage capability of approximately 80 minutes of 256 EEG channels. The monitoring subsystem is responsible for the organization of the data simultaneously recorded from different patients and for the remote control of measure instruments in the units. The EEGer can review the EEG data and print and store selected samples of it.

The "EEG-Workstation " is a postprocessing subsystem (see Fig.1) offers user a "tools kit" for epilepsy monitoring. The inputs of the EEG-Workstation are the EEG-Data stored on the monitoring subsystem and the patient's information. Outputs are selected EEG-samples, iso-potential maps, FFT-spectrum, measurements, special comments, etc. Fig. 2 shows a graphical description of the EEG-Workstation functions. The basic specifications necessary to achieve these goals are listed below:

-     a local area network (LAN) is used to link the workstations with the acquisition-/ monitoring subsystem;
-     the hardware requirements are a minimum of 2 Mbyte RAM for the loading of 256 channels of EEG samples in 20 seconds and a 200

Mbyte hard disc for the data buffering and a SCSI-Bus for future expansion;
-   **high resolution graphic monitor** for the display of EEG data, with capability for 32 channels and a 1000x1000 pixels resolution;
-   **screen speed** capability of 3-4 EEG-page/sec /5/;
-   UNIX and C for software **development environment** (currently most of our software are written in C) and **X-Window for graphic interface** (allows independent development of the graphic presentation /3/).

3. Development:

For this development we have chosen the HP 9000/425t Workstation (performance 20 MIPS and 3.5 MFLOPS) based on the fast MC68040 (25MHz) MOTOROLA microprocessor. An application with an other Workstation is not excluded, because the most part of software is independent from the hardware. While waiting for the HP 9000/425t we developed a package of software based on X-Window on a HP 9000/835 Workstation (the "workstation prototype"). The software has been implemented into the HP 900/425t since Jan. 91.

Network communication with Network File System (NFS) was established /4/. Communication between the Monitoring subsystem and EEG-workstations was also established allowing access to directory of recorded EEG-Data files and transfer them from the monitoring unit to the workstations.

A user-friendly software was then written on language proper for the physicians' use. The layout for the presentation and access of the data was also based on the interaction of the computer and physicians staff. Icons with symbols one can easily understand are applied. For example, we use symbols commonly used on video cassette recorders for the paging or scrolling of EEG-signals, because the EEG-technologist are familiar with them (s. Fig.3).

At this point the following features have been implemented and are currently already used by our physicians:
-   display of any number of channels per patient by any sequence of derivations;
-   display modes: paging, scrolling, zooming, stretching, compressing and zooming of selected channels;
-   cursor for precise amplitude and latency measurements;
-   sensitivity control, reformatting;
-   filtering with FIR-filters, FFT-spectrum;
-   isopotential maps /6/ (in development).

4. Summary:

A project of a workstation at the physicians' hands for post- processing of EEG data is currently being developed, and a "workstation prototype" has already been implemented in our EMUs. The technical specifications and concept which includes modern technology as LAN, NFS, X-WINDOW, SCSI-bus, etc., are described. The main features of the system are presented stressing its wide possibilities of different applications and modes of display.

References:

/1/   Second International Cleveland Clinic Epilepsy Symposium: Epilepsy surgery; June 19-23, 1990, Cleveland, USA.
/2/   R.C.Burgess, E.C. Jacobs; Computer Analysis of Epileptiform EEG Abnormalities. Clev Clin J Med, Vol. 56 (1989), p. 240-247.
/3/   D.A.Young; The X Window System: Programming and Application with Xt, OSF/Motif edition; Prentice Hall, 1990, USA.
/4/   Programming and Protocols for NFS Services/800; Manual Part Number:50970-90010, Hewlett Packard, 1988, USA.
/5/   T.A.Vuong, R.C.Burgess; Video und EEG Darstellung: Technik und Anwenderaspekte; Deutsche EEG-Gesellschaft 35.Jahrestagung; 18-21 Okt, 1990, Bonn, FRG.
/6/   T.A.Vuong, T.F.Collura,R.C.Burgess, E.C.Jacobs; A Versatile Graphic Output Package for Clinical EEG, Journal of Clinical Neurophysiology, Vol. 6, No. 4, Oct. 1989, p. 340.

TOOLS KIT FOR EEG-WORKSTATION

-paperless review (fast review) of EEG data
-reformatting or remontaging capability
-filtering of EMG-artefact
-automatic spike detection
-quantitative measurements of spikes
-averaging
-isopotential maps
-FFT-analysis, correlation calculation
-text edition
-printing of EEG curves (laser printing)
-patient oriented archive of EEG
-Epilepsy data bank access

Table 1: List of clinical applications will be implemented in EEG-Workstation.

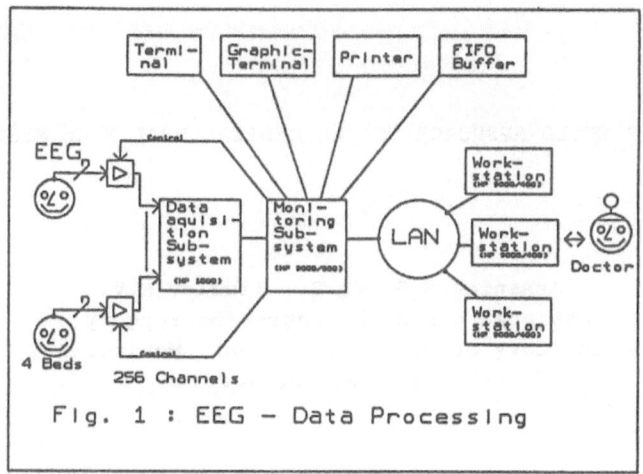

Fig. 1 : EEG - Data Processing

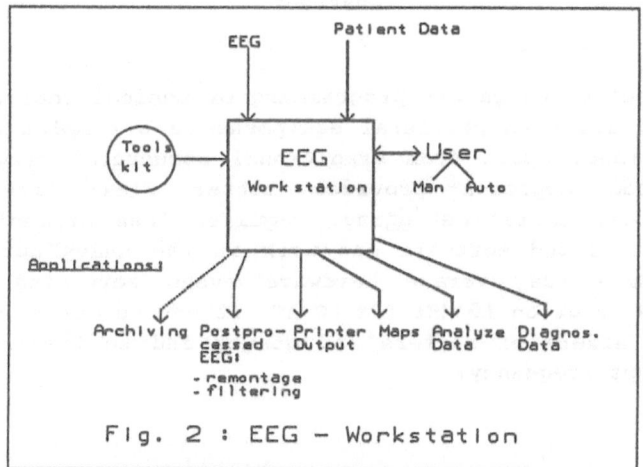

Fig. 2 : EEG - Workstation

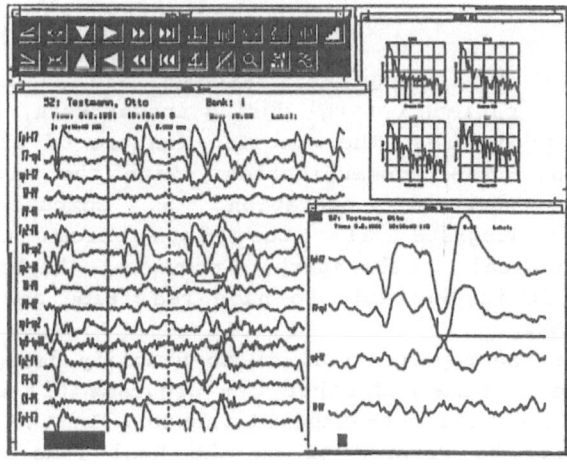

FIG. 3: SCREEN SAMPLE

THE OBJECT-ORIENTED APPROACH TO THE MEDICAL REAL TIME SYSTEM DESIGN

Arseniev S.B.,Ph.D., Kiselev M.V.
National Research Centre for Surgery,
Laboratory of Computer Patient Monitoring,
119874, Moscow, Abrikosovski 2

Abstract

The object oriented C++ programming of medical real time systems which communicate with periferal equipment in a complex non-standard way is described. Apart from traditional structural programming the object-oriented approach provides better flexibility and time characteristics, easier debugging, requires less assembler language usage. The developed software can work in the heavy duty real time systems because its average hardware event servicing time makes approximately 75 μs on 10 MHz IBM PC AT. It can be easily configurated to necessary sizers of buffers and queues and to the most suitable timer interrups frequency.

Introduction

Real time monitoring computer systems are widely used in medicine today for patient control during anaesthesia, intesive care, and diagnostic procedures. The specific feature of such systems is the complexity of the communication with the environment. For example, during surgical operation a computer monitoring station must integrate all the data from the measuring devices, the clinical laboratory, provide keyboard entering etc. Moreover, it is desirable to have real time access to a data base through a LAN.

The purpose of the reported work is to simplify design and support of the real time systems and other C++ programs [2] which interact with the periferals in a non-standard fashion. In the present paper these systems will be refered to as the Real Time / Non-Standard Periferial Interacting systems (RT/NSPI systems).

The drawbacks of the conventional structural programming
the RT/NSPI systems

The following problems seem to be common in programming the RT/NSPI systems:

1) "Traditional" understanding of a program as a linear flow of control or of a set of the time-sharing threads is often inadequate.

2) The immediate control over the hardware requires extensive use of the assembler language.

3) Programs are poorly structured.

4) Debugging a RT/NSPI system is a very difficult task because its object is not only the system itself but also the hardware environment.

5) To transform a RT/NSPI system to its demo or tutorial version the internal structure often has to be rearranged complely (especially the lower level parts).

Probably, the first item in this list needs to be commented. The "old" approach to programming the RT/NSPI systems can be illustrated by the following picture:

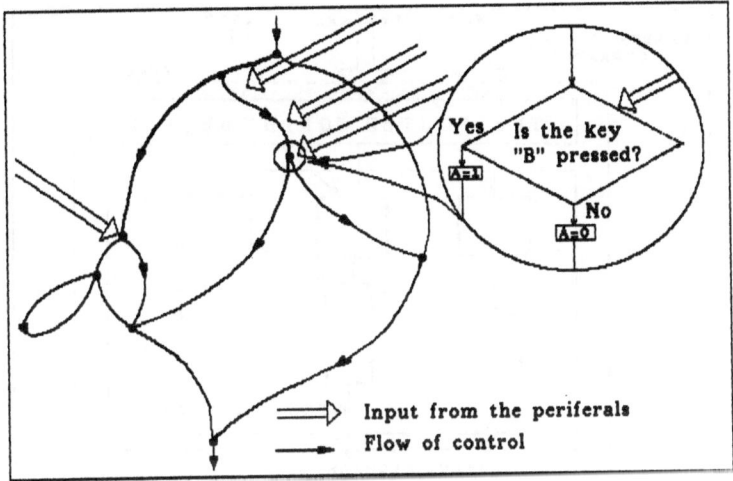

Fig.1 The conventional approach to programming
the RT/NSPI systems

Here a program is represented as the oriented graph on which the "current instruction pointer" runs. Besides, when the "instruction pointer" is at certain points of this graph the program receives some information from the periferals. If this interaction with the periferals fits the schemes provided by the standard I/O procedures, and should not satisfy the strict timing conditions, the clear understandable model of the system can be obtained by the implementation of the conventional structural programming principles [1], namely, a proper choice of the multilevel subroutines hierarchy and data structures. However, in the case of the RT/NSPI systems this representation becomes inadequate because a part of subroutines in this hierarchy has implicit parameters depending on the hardware.

Object-oriented programming the RT/NSPI systems

We propose the following alternative scheme based on the C++ object- oriented programming approach [2] and seems to be more preferable in this case. The whole system is treated as an object which has inputs, outputs and some internal state. This object receives the signals from the outer world, for example, from keyboard, RS232 or network adaptor, which, possibly, change its internal state. The object should respond to them with some output signals in accordance with a specification which can depend on the internal state of the object. These signals may be outputs to screen, sound signals, message sent to the LAN, and so on. The internal structure of such system designed on the basis of our software is shown on Fig.2.

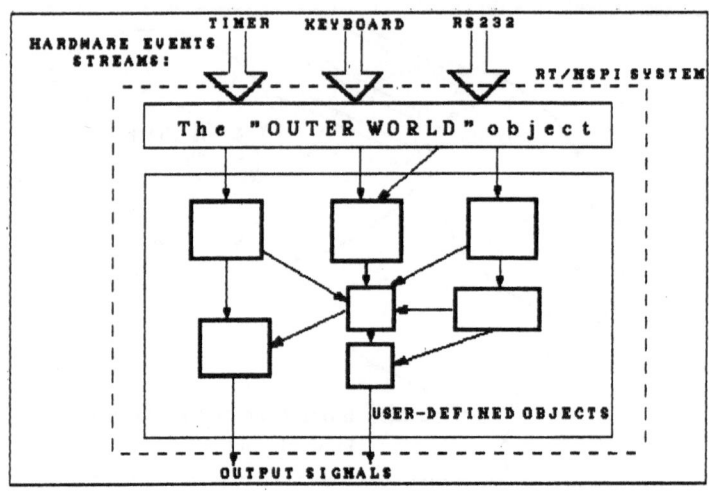

Fig.2 The object oriented programming the RT/NSPI systems.

The fat rectangles denote here the objects constituting the system. They send one to another some messages designated by the thin arrows. Apart from the user-defined objects the system always includes one static object called "the outer world". In fact, this object is nothing more but the universal system of input from the periferals designed by us for use in the C++ RT/NSPI programs.

Let us describe its structure and operation. As it is shown on Fig.2 it receives hardware events. Technically these events are realized as the processor interrupts. It is known that 8 hardware interrupts types can be used in the IBM PC. However, only 4 of them can be interesting for us. These are the timer interrupt IRQ0, the keyboard interrupt IRQ1, and the serial port interrupts IRQ3, IRQ4. Furthermore, it is clear that not all hardware interrupts of these types may concern the user. For example, if the time parameters of the program are not important for the user the timer interrupts are necessary only for the system time support and other operation system purposes. Thus, not all the interrupts should be translated to the "outer world" messages. To select the relevant hardware events the user is to define the three procedures Dt,Dk, and Drs corresponding to the three hardware events streams mentioned above. Besides, these procedures can associate with the generated messages some information in the free format. This information can be accessed by the message addressee by the use of the pointer to it. Only the information associated with the keyboard message always has the fixed format - integer number.

Further, the user is to define three procedures which specify reaction to the "outer world" messages. These procedures can use the message associated information to form messages to be sent to the user-defined objects. Additionally, the user is to specify a procedure which should react to the various malfunction reports from the "outer world" object, for example, about the hardware events queue overflow.

Apart from the periferal devices considered above there is a number of input devices which either do not generate the hardware interrupts, for example, the majority of the analog-to-digital convertors, or generate the interrupts requiring sophisticated servicing performed by the special software as the network adapter does. The data received from these devices could be included in the timer message by the Dt procedure which either reads the A-to-D convertor card or determines if the current input from the computer network has been completed.

Obviously, the ideal realization of such RT/NSPI system would be a network of objects on which the waves of messages triggered by the hardware events travel asynchroneously. However, the implementation of this scheme on the ordinary serial IBM PC requires establishing the event servicing priorities. Therefore the procedures Dt, Dk, and Drs should associate with the hardware messages also their priorities so that a message with lower priority can not interrupt servicing a message with higher priority but is placed into the queue in the order of decreasing priority. Besides, the mechanism allowing to change these priorities is provided.

It should be noted that our system manages only the hardware input because the output is much more diverse and is realized satisfactorily in almost all the cases by the conventional means.

Conclusion

Thus, the described software allows:

1) to represent adequately in the high level language the view on the RT/NSPI system operation as interaction of objects and hardware via the messages exchange;

2) to reduce or even to make unnecessary programming on the assembler language;

3) to simplify debugging the RT/NSPI programs (especially finding hardly detectable real time errors) due to possibility to vary the message priorities easily;

4) to simplify the design of the demo and tutorial versions of the RT/NSPI systems due to possibility of the program emulation of the hardware events.

We can add that the described software can work in the heavy duty real time systems because its average hardware event servicing time makes approximately 75 μs on the 10MHz IBM PC AT. It can be configured easily to necessary sizes of buffers and queues and also to most suitable timer interrupts frequency.

References

1. O.-J.Dahl and C.A.Hoare, Hierarchic Programm Structures, Structured Programming, New York, Academic Press, 1972, pp 174-220.
2. B.Stroustrup, The C++ Programming Language, Massachusetts, Addison-Wesly Reading, 1986.

IMAGE PROCESSING

A Knowledge Base Model for the Interpretation
of Radiographic Densities

Giovanni Braccini [1], Davide Caramella [2] and Ovidio Salvetti [3]

[1] Cattedra di Radiologia, Università di Pisa
Via Roma 67, I-56100 Pisa

[2] Dipartimento di Fisiopatologia Clinica, Università di Firenze
Viale Morgagni 85, I-50100 Firenze

[3] Istituto di Elaborazione della Informazione, CNR
Via S.Maria 46, I-56100 Pisa

Abstract

A knowledge base model suitable for automatic interpretation of densities in digital X-ray images is proposed.

A layered model is defined containing relevant knowledge, processes using this knowledge and results provided by the processes themselves.

In particular, a three-level approach is proposed: identification of images, their projection and relative quality control; extraction of significant characteristics relative to normal or pathological signs; formulation of the diagnostic hypotheses considering also historical, clinical and laboratory data.

Introduction

Image interpretation provides a symbolic description of an input image. The content of a symbolic description may greatly vary due to user requirements and/or application fields.

In our case, a description might contain normal aspects or congenital and pathological abnormalities, in particular if we consider visceral patterns in plain films of the abdomen. Furthermore, with additional knowledge, the description might also contain statements of diagnostic evidence.

Accurate plain film analysis of the abdomen is one of the most difficult challenges of diagnostic radiology and the value of plain film diagnosis in acute abdominal conditions is unquestioned.

Keeping in mind the link with other information relative to the diagnostic and/or therapeutic processes (e.g. different kinds of images, clinical and laboratory data, and so on), we focused our attention on the plain film of the abdomen, having at our disposal a homogeneous ordered series of cases (see Fig. 1).

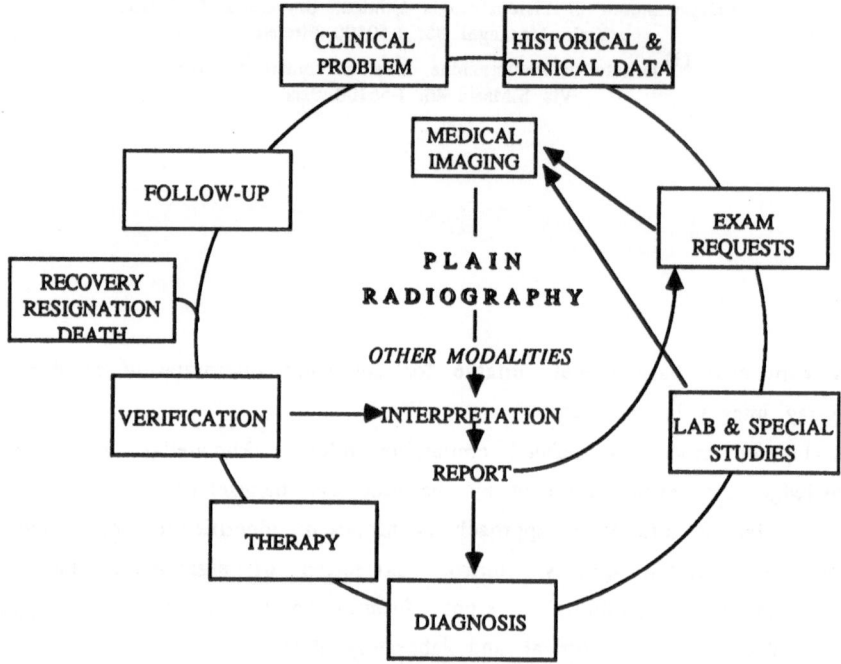

Fig. 1 - General overview of the diagnostic and therapeutic processes

The images and their contents define an optimal and complete base for the design and implementation of an *intelligent system* oriented to automatic diagnosis.

Materials and Methods

For the generation and processing of the images a digital radiological system has been used composed of a standard X-ray device and a computing system equipped with an optical disk mass memory and an image acquisition and handling board.

The data used for the processing phases consist of plain films of the abdomen relating to a series of well known cases.

The X-rays have been digitized with variable spatial sampling steps (from 125 μm to 250 μm), in order to obtain two-dimensional arrays (from 256x256 elements up to a maximum of 1024x1024 elements, each quantized on a byte).

Recognition of visceral patterns and their significant abnormalities is dependent upon three basic factors: visual, physical and anatomic factors.

In particular, we have to consider the perception of the Roengten image and relative quality control, the knowledge about normal anatomic relationships and variants and finally the effect of physical, physiological and pathological processes.

Following the above mentioned concepts, a layered model has been defined which contains relevant knowledge, processes using this knowledge and results provided by the processes themselves.

A three level approach is proposed: a) identification of images, their projections and relative quality control; b) extraction of significant characteristics relative to normal or pathological signs; c) formulation of the diagnostic hypotheses considering also historical, clinical and laboratory data.

Each level is defined by computational models, c_m, composed of sets of algorithms, $\mathcal{A}_k$, and rules, $\mathcal{R}_i$

$$c_m = <\{\mathcal{A}_k\}, \{\mathcal{R}_i\}> \qquad \text{where}$$

$1 \leq m \leq s,$ s = number of basic symbols

$1 \leq k$ k = number of the classes of algorithms

$1 \leq i$ i = number of the classes of rules

Following this approach specific knowledge can be derived from processed images and inserted into the levels a) and b) of the proposed layered model.

At the first level, the knowledge is linked exclusively to the image elements and their attributes. A single image description is carried out on the basis of a computational model for densitometry allowing for the recognition of basic symbols which are present on the examined plain film.

At the second level, elements of knowledge belonging to domains outside the radiographic image, even if strictly correlated, are added. In particular, this knowledge is mainly defined by suitable geometric models of the anatomical structures.

The knowledge derived directly from an input image decreases from the first to the last level while the knowledge based on symbolic elements progressively increase and become the unique information at the level c).

The image is considered a *kernel* in the knowledge structure in levels a) and b). Each digital image is defined as a primary data which is logically and directly linked to its generating scene and it may have its own identity independently from a specific context. An image can be correlated with other images and data belonging to an *external* world through a network of associations which can dynamically evolve. A process applied to an image producing interesting information creates a new element in the network corresponding to a semantic link by which a direct association between processed and produced data is stated.

An example of application

Fig. 2 shows the particular role of an image and its derivative information in the case of the analysis of radiographic densities.

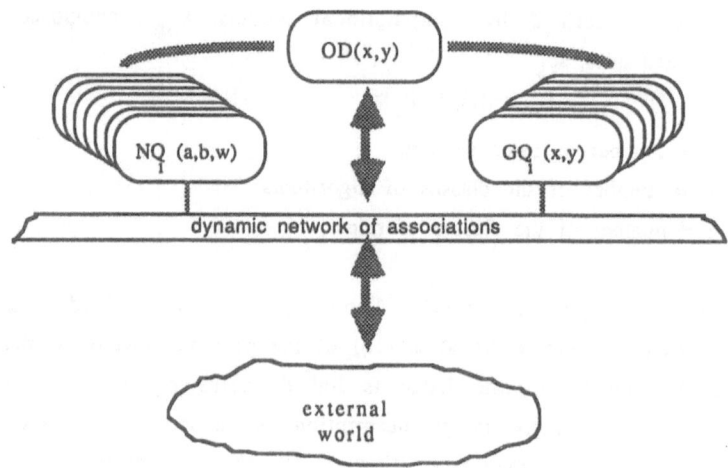

Fig. 2 - Primary and derived data and their relations

The natural radiographic densities can be regrouped into three different categories, i.e. those of air, water and bone.

The digital image OD(x,y) of optical densities, obtained by applying an automatic digitizing procedure to a single film, is first transformed into an image N(a,b,w) where a, b and w are partitions, not necessarily connected, of the *space* S_{xy} which is associated to the processed image. The single pixels are grouped into regions to obtain a map of the prevalent isodensities. An *absorption* operator has been developed to this end, which allows the inclusion of one region into another by operating on parameters such as area, perimeter, form factor, orientation and spatial position.

In parallel, the image $OD(x,y)$ is processed to generate the set of images $\{NQ_i(a,b,w)\}$, $i=1,2,...,k$ and $Q_i < S_{xy}$, for a closer examination of the local characteristics in k regions of interest.

At the same time from the image $OD(x,y)$ is also generated an image $G(x,y)$ of density gradients as well as an image group $\{GQ_i(x,y)\}$, $i=1,2,...,k$, of local gradients in subregions Q_i. Also in this case the image $G(x,y)$ represents a map of prevalent gradients and is obtained by eliminating insignificant information through a comparison with the image $N(a,b,w)$.

The classification of $OD(x,y)$ in $N(a,b,w)$ and $G(x,y)$ has essentially the aim of identifying the type of image under examination.

In fact, according to a predefined model, it is possible to determine the particular plane of projection by making a comparison between the positions of prevalent centres of mass calculated in image $N(a,b,w)$ with the layout and shape of gradient curves in plane $G(x,y)$. On the other hand, the classification of $OD(x,y)$ in $\{NQ_i\}$ and $\{GQ_i\}$ is used to extract the significant characteristics and semeiographic evaluation correctly. The image $OD(x,y)$ is divided into k regions arranged on a regular grid. For each region a corresponding reference anatomic model is defined together with c_m models, if they exist.

Thus a particular pair NQ_s, GQ_s constitutes an *entry* for the model which can be used to provide a response. Usually, the response, based on a comparison of parameters obtained from each single image, provides an overall estimate of morphology and anatomic structures. In some cases it is necessary to provide means of making a comparison between the general analysis (defined by the pair N,G) and the local analysis (defined by the pair $\{NQ_i\},\{GQ_i\}$), when, that is, more detailed information is necessary for the identification of the image type.

However, the analysis of a single image may not be sufficient to discriminate between different densities which are superimposed on the same region.

Indeed the measured density on each point of the image is, in general, dependent on the three primary densities, which are distributed in various ways in the irradiated anatomic volume. In these cases it is necessary to have more images available in order to make evaluation of comparative nature: for example, in order to distinguish an air density superimposed on a water density, two images, complementary orthogonal frontal and latero-lateral, should be processed simultaneously.

In short, additional information may be necessary, deriving from different imaging modalities or clinical or laboratory data.

Acknowledgement

This work has been partially supported by Progetto Finalizzato *Sistemi Informatici e Calcolo Parallelo* of the Italian National Research Council.

Bibliography

[1] O. Salvetti, G. Braccini and A. Frassineti, A Distributed Environment for Quality Control and Diagnosis of Medical Images, Mini & Microcomputers and their Applications, E. Luque Ed., Acta Press, 1988, pages 568-573.

[2] G. Braccini, A. Frassineti and O. Salvetti, , A Database Model for an Intelligent System Oriented to Acute Abdomen Image Understanding, Proc. of the 33rd National Congress SIRMN of Radiology, Monduzzi Ed., 1988, pages 405-409

[3] O. Salvetti, G. Braccini and A. Frassineti, A Knowledge Base for Digital Radiographic Image Understanding in Acute Abdomen, Proc. of the IASTED Int. Symposium "Expert Systems Theory & Applications", M.H. Hamza Ed., Acta Press, 1989, pages 312-314.

[4] L. Azzarelli, M. Chimenti, O. Salvetti, H. Bruenig and H. Niemann, Interactive Processing and Archiving of Images, Image and Vision Computing, Vol.8, No.3, 1990.

[5] G. Braccini, R. Evangelista, A. Frassineti and O. Salvetti, A methodology for automatic understanding of densities in digital images, Proc. IASTED Int. Conf. on Expert Systems and Neural Networks, M.H. Hamza Ed., Acta Press, 1990, pages 174-178.

[6] R. Bozzi, E. Fantini, O. Salvetti, BIS386™: Biomedical Imaging System, Italian Patent No. 10128C/90; 1990.

AUTOMATIC CONSTRUCTIONAL ANALYSIS OF IMAGES
IN VISUOPERCEPTUAL EVALUATION

M.C.Fairhurst and S.L.Smith

Electronic Engineering Laboratories,

University of Kent, Canterbury, Kent CT2 7NT, U.K.

Abstract

Figure copying tasks provide a convenient means of evaluating visuoperceptual functioning which may be related directly or indirectly to neurological factors, but the objective analysis of such tasks can be difficult to achieve in a resource-efficient way. This paper discusses a technique for microcomputer-based automated analysis of figure-copying exercises and, by means of experimental results, shows how a range of factors relating to perceptual functioning can be determined in a convenient and quantitative way.

Introduction

The evaluation of neurological functioning through appropriate cognitive and perceptual tests is very important in the detection and monitoring of neurological disorders such as Alzheimer's disease and other forms of dementing illness [1,2]. For example, dialysis dementia [3], a dementia prevalent in patients undergoing long-term haemodialysis, is particularly difficult to detect early, largely because of the rate at which it advances and the constraints imposed on the applicability of traditional methods of testing, while informal evaluation may be unreliable and inconclusive. In fact, many clinical populations can benefit from an appropriate objective appraisal of cognitive/perceptual function, and of particular interest in this respect are patients who have suffered a cerebral vascular accident (CVA or stroke), for whom some form of monitoring of treatment and therapy can be very important. In particular, such patients can exhibit perceptual and spatial disabilities not dissimilar to those experienced in advanced cases of dementia, and it is precisely this aspect of neurological functioning which is of interest in this paper. Similarly, the monitoring of perceptual functioning in children is clearly important, not only in relation to general developmental studies, but also in the context of the assessment of dysfunction in relation to ability in visuo-motor activity required for participation in communication processes, where perception of signs, signals and symbols can be of primary significance in generating and interpreting dialogue [4].

Conventional methods for this type of evaluation are, however, often either very informal and somewhat subjective, or are highly resource-intensive. This paper describes an approach to the investigation of spatial perceptual functioning which utilises automatic image analysis techniques to overcome many of these difficulties. In particular, figure copying tests suggest an approach to the evaluation of spatial perceptual ability which is potentially very suitable for computer-assisted implementation and which, with appropriate analysis, is potentially susceptible open to interpretation on a widely accepted basis. It is exactly this type of test which provides the basis for the approach to neurological testing which is described in this paper.

An approach to perceptual evaluation

A prototype system for evaluation of spatial perceptual ability uses a task domain which requires a subject to generate line drawings of specified geometric shapes (although clearly other tasks are possible and may be introduced to suit individual requirements) which are analysed interactively by a microcomputer-based system, a schematic view of which is shown in Figure 1.

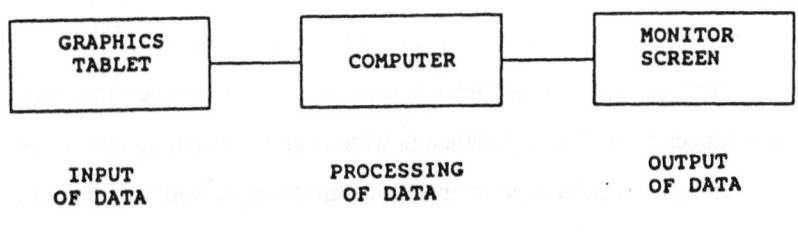

Figure 1

A target shape is copied by the subject on a graphics tablet which is interfaced to the microcomputer to allow the acquisition of the drawing data in terms of a stream of coordinate mappings, and the analysis of the data in real time. The advantage of the interactive capability is that both static and dynamic features of the subject's attempt to generate the target shape can be measured and utilised in the processing. Subsequent analysis seeks to characterise the performance of the subject through a controlled evaluation of the features measured. Although the task domain can be chosen so as to emphasise perceptual characteristics of interest, one task which has been found to be particularly effective is the free-hand drawing of a 3-dimensional regular cube. This task imposes a requirement on the subject of a reasonably high level of visual-motor coordination, and also requires considerable cognitive skills in the spatial visualisation and conceptualisation of the target drawing.

The principal aim of the method adopted is to measure features of the subject-generated drawing which can be used to assess and characterise the "performance" of the subject. A particularly valuable aspect of the approach adopted is that features to be measured can be added to or removed from the system in a modular way so as to match the fine detail of the test to the nature of the behavioural characteristics of interest in any given operational environment. Clearly, many features, both static and dynamic, can be invoked as indices of performance, their value being related also to the target shapes defined, but the studies carried out in an initial investigation have been restricted to a consideration of features related to task execution time {T}, velocity {V} and acceleration {A} of the pen, hesitation in task execution {H}, motor tremor {R}, two measures of drawing accuracy {E,M}, line segment distortion {L} and corner formation distortion {C}. This produces a set of nine parameters which can be used together or in combination in seeking an analysis of subject performance within the specified task domain.

Performance can then be related to values of the measured parameters with respect to defined populations of interest. For example, a "control" population of subjects with no known perceptual or coordination irregularities, with a mix of sexes and covering an age range from 20 to 60 years has been tested, and provides an important reference for other populations.

Experimental results

It is interesting, for example, to compare the performance in the defined task of the reference population with a population consisting of a mixed group of first-year primary (7-year old) children, with no known developmental irregularities, in whom spatial perceptual ability would not be expected to be fully developed [5]. These results are illustrated in Figure 2 where the measured values for two arbitrarily chosen parameters, in this case H and M, define a feature space within which individual performances may be localised according to the values obtained experimentally in the test. These results strongly suggest that the proposed method of evaluation has the degree of sensitivity required to reflect the development of spatial perceptual ability.

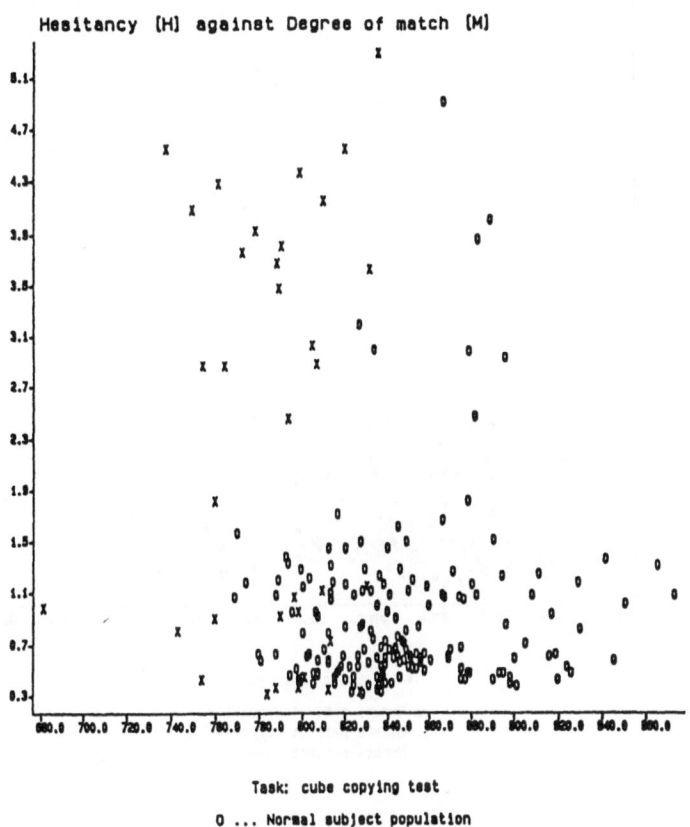

Task: cube copying test

O ... Normal subject population
X ... Child 7 years population

Figure 2

A further useful illustration of the applicability of the test can be observed with reference to a set of measurements carried out with patients who had suffered a right-hemisphere CVA (stroke). These patients were known to have spatial perceptual impairment, and yet in some cases were found to be capable of executing the defined task in a way which, when subjected only to direct visual inspection, showed no apparent difference from the reference population. The proposed test is, however, capable of generating a clear distinction in this respect, as Figure 3 shows.

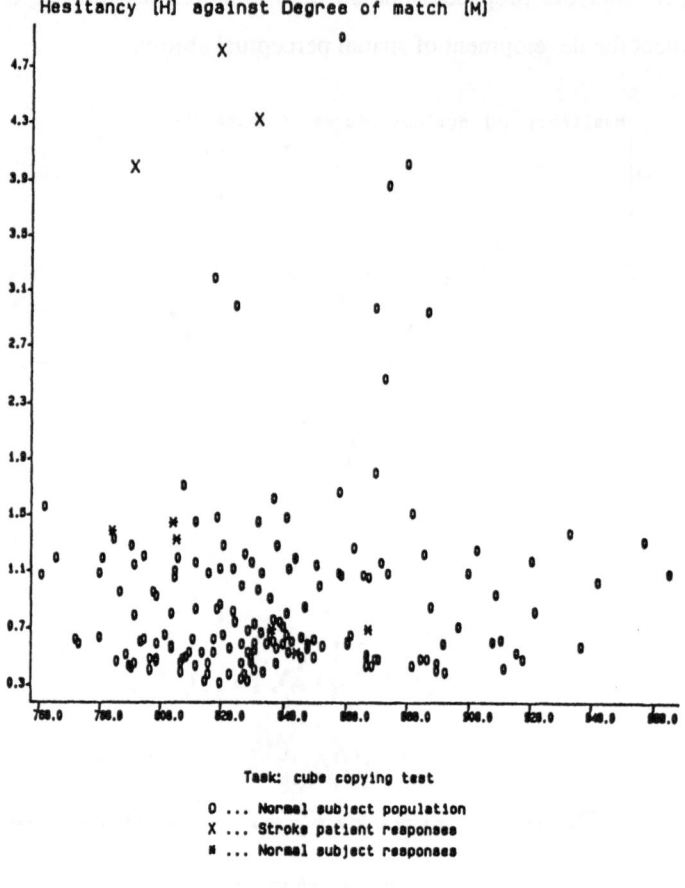

Figure 3

Finally, a consideration of the nature of the proposed application area for the test suggests that any correlation between the age of the subject tested and the response be
quantified so that, if appropriate, compensation can be made in the interpretation of the
responses. The age-related correlation values for each of the nine features of interest were
obtained and are shown in Table 1. Using the established t-test [6], the experimental conditions prevailing here would require correlation values of greater than 0.36 to establish
significance (with a confidence value of 90% (α=0.05)). On the basis of the values
obtained it can therefore be concluded that the age of the subject has little bearing on the

interpretation of performance as measured by this test.

CUBE TASK

Feature	Correlation
Time [T]	0.349
Corner F.D. [C]	0.437
Line S.D. [L]	0.245
Error [E]	0.035
Acceleration [A]	0.150
Hesitation [H]	0.159
Velocity [V]	-0.013
Tremor [T]	0.186
D. of Match [M]	-0.217

Table 1

Conclusions

It is suggested that a novel approach to the evaluation of perceptual functioning based on image analysis techniques may provide the basis of a convenient, very flexible and cost-effective tool for clinical use. Preliminary results have established the viability of the technique and its underlying principles. In fact, exactly this general approach has been very successfully applied in screening and monitoring certain types of dementing conditions [7].

From these observations it is proposed that the same basic principles may prove very effective in the evaluation of spatial perceptual function which impinges directly on the detection and monitoring of a range neurological conditions including dementias and localised stroke damage. It is also relevant to consider the applicability of the technique to the evaluation of individual ability in expressive/receptive communicative processes and in the monitoring of developmental factors. Current work is proceeding to refine, enhance and validate clinically the approach described here, and to extend the analysis to include a more subtle assessment of constructional strategies invoked in task execution.

References

1. Pearce,J. & Millar,E.: Clinical aspects of dementia, Balliere Tindall, London, 197 2

2. Morris, R.G. et al: Computer aided assessment of dementia. In Cognitive Neurochemistry, O.U.P, Oxford, 1987

3. Alfrey, A.C. Dialysis encephalopathy syndrome, Ann.Rev.Med., 29, 93-98, 1978

4. Kiernan,C.: Alternatives to speech, Brit. J. Mental Subnormality, 23, 6-28, 1977

5. Aitken, L.R.: Psychological testing and assessment, Allyn & Bacon, Boston, 1979

6. Chao,L.L.: Statistics - methods and analysis, McGraw-Hill, London, 1974

7. Fairhurst,M.C. & Smith,S.L.: An investigation of dysgraphia using image analysis techniques, Proc.BES 29th Ann. Conf., Bristol, UK, September, 1989

THREE DIMENSIONAL RECONSTRUCTION OF A SMALL FETAL PHANTOM USING REAL-TIME LINEAR ARRAY ULTRASONIC IMAGES

Kenneth L. Watkin, Ph.D.
Samir Khalife, M.D.
Bahij Nuwayhid, M.D.,Ph.D.
Department of Obstetrics and Gynecology
McGill University
Montreal, Quebec CANADA

ABSTRACT

Earlier investigations have demonstrated that 3D computer assisted estimates of volume and weight of only the fetal head and trunk correlated highly with actual fetal volume and weight. Although the estimates of fetal volume were highly correlated with true volume, volumes less than 1000 ml resulted in larger error estimates due to the inability to image the arms and legs as well as errors introduced by the computer assisted volume estimation methods. The present investigation was conducted to determine if the volume and weight of a small (100 cc.) fetal phantom (head, trunk, arms, legs) could be estimated accurately and rapidly using a limited number of ultrasonic phased array images and a computer assisted 3D mesh generation-rendering system. Ultrasonic ultrasonic images were gathered and the digitized contours used to reconstruct the entire phantom surface as a wire mesh, determine the volume of the phantom and render it for color visualization. Results indicated that the computer estimated volume and weight were within 8% of the actural volume and weight using a limited number of ultrasonic scan images.

INTRODUCTION

One of the major diagnostic problems facing the obstetrician is the quantification of changes in the developing fetus and the early identification of abnormalities in fetal growth and development. Our knowledge of intrauterine growth has not developed rapidly since ultrasonic 3D imaging techniques have not permitted the visualization and reconstruction of the entire fetus; the available techniques have been time consuming; and have not been utilized with small volume intrauterine structures. Early reports on the 3D reconstruction of fetuses utilizing 2D ultrasonic images (Brinkley, et al., 1982;1984) revealed that 3D reconstruction of 2D ultrasonic images and associated volume estimates were possible using commercial ultrasound equipment, a transducer localization device and a mini-computer. These studies reported high correlations between measured and estimated volumes. The major difficulties with these studies were (1) the error in volume estimation increased exponentially below 1000 ml, (2) only the head and trunk were reconstructed due to the inability of the reconstruction algorithms to join independent objects across imaging planes, and (3) the reconstruction process was time consuming.

The present investigation was conducted to determine if the volume and weight of a small (100 ml) fetal phantom (including the head, trunk, arms, and legs) could be estimated more accurately using a limited number of ultrasonic phased array images and a computer assisted 3D mesh generation-rendering system.

METHODS

Using commerically available convex phased array ultrasonic images captured via a Matrox MVP/AT video data acquisition board and an IBM PC/AT twelve longitudinal images of a fetal phantom (Figure 1) were gathered. A specially constructed moulding with

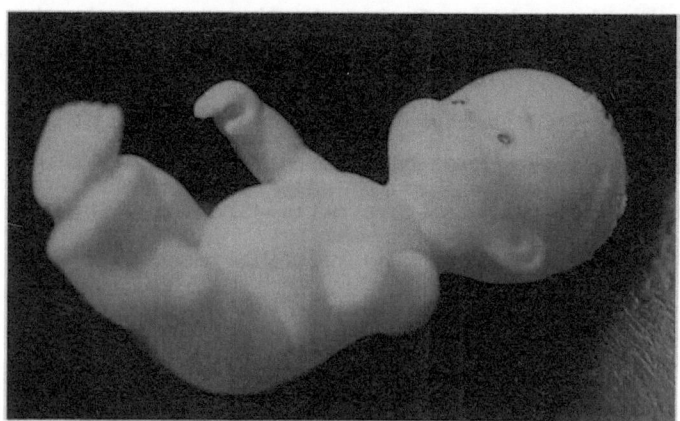

Figure 1. Fetal Phantom

an attached six (6) degrees of freedom position sensing system (3SPACE Tracker, Polhemus, Inc.) was used to determine the real time position of the ultrasonic transducer. The image planes were digitized and stored on the IBM PC/AT. The edges of the fetal phantom were identified using a mouse drive tracing system. The identified x and y values of 2D ultrasonic slices were stored and then converted into X , Y, and Z values based on transducer localization data (Rogers and Adams,1976). Computation of image cross-sectional areas and total volume were accomplished using a DEC VAX3500 computer. Using a specially developed triangulation program with cost effective control criterion, triangular polygons were calculated between each slice.

RESULTS

Identification of phantom edges using the mouse system took approximately 60 sec. per image. Triangulation time between slice pairs was 2 sec. which included determination of the total cross-sectional area of each slice and the volume between the adjacent slices. Solid reconstruction of the image utilized a second program which required the input of the projection direction, any lighting requirements and the choice of wireframe or solid projection. These specially developed programs, calculate the rotation of the object as well as the shading necessary for projection. Projection time was less than 2 minutes. The rendered fetal phantom is present from an anterior oblique and posterior oblique perspective in Figures 2 and 3, respectively.

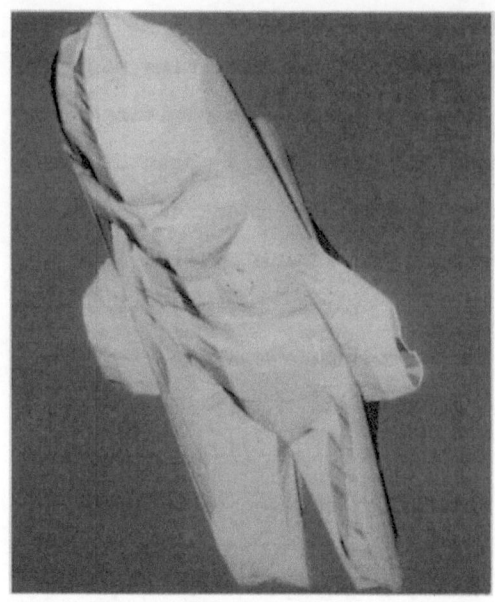

Figure 2. Anterior oblique view of the reconstructed and rendered
fetal phantom

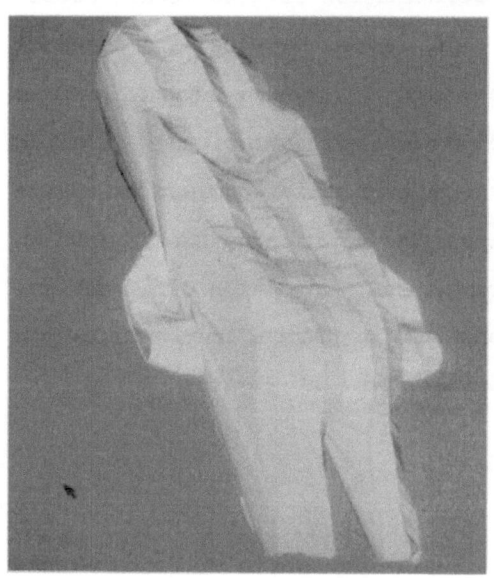

Figure 3. Posterior oblique view of the reconstructed and rendered
fetal phantom

Comparison of the estimated and actual volume and weight of the fetal phantom are presented in Table 1 below.

Table 1 The actual and estimated weights
and volumes of the fetal phantom

	Actual	Estimated
weight	79.9 gms	74.9 gms
volume	100 ml	92.0 ml

DISCUSSION

Results of this investigation revealed that commercially available graphics hardware provided fast processing time for image capture and analysis, advance numerical algorithms can reduce volume/weight calculation times when a limited number of ultrasonic slices through a small fetal phantom are employed, and solid rendering techniques can provide some surface information on small fetal-like objects. Although volume/weight estimation calculation have been reduced, advances in processing ultrasonic images are needed to provide 1) computer assisted extraction of edge contours, 2) algorithms for joining image sections, and 3) 3D databases for visualization.

REFERENCES

Brinkley, JF, et al., Fetal weight estimations from ultrasonic 3D head and trunk reconstructions -evaluation in vitro, Am J Obstet Gynecol, 1982, 144(6):715-721.

Brinkley, JF, et al., Fetal weight estimations from lengths and volumes found by 3-D ultrasonic measurements, J Ultrasound Med., 1984, 3(4):163-168.

Rogers, DF, Adams JA, Mathematical Elements for Computer Graphics, 1976, New York:McGraw-Hill Book Co.

CLUSTERING ALGORITHMS FOR MRI

Vito Di Gesù[+], Robert De La Paz[^], Wiliams A.Hanson[*], Ralph Bernstein[*]
+ *Dipartimento di Matematica e Applicazioni,University of Palermo, ITALY*
^ *Department of Radiology, Stanford University, USA*
* *I.B.M. PASC, Palo Alto, USA*

ABSTRACT.

Magnetic Resonance Imaging (MRI) plays a relevant role in the design of systems for computer assisted diagnosis. MR-images are multi-dimensional in nature; physicians have to combine several perceptual information images to perform the tissue classification needed for diagnosis. Automatic clustering methods help to discriminate relevant features and to perform a preliminary segmentation of the image; it can guide the final manual classification of body-tissues. Three clustering techniques and their integration in a MRI-system are described. Their performance and accuracy was evaluated on synthetic and real image-data. A comparison of our approach with the tissue-classification done by a radiologist was performed.

Key-words: *MRI, clustering, classification, data-analysis.*

1. INTRODUCTION.

Nuclear Magnetic Resonance (NMR) has been discovered in the late 1940's independently by Edwin Purcell and Felix Bloch [1,2]. Owing to the intrinsic spin angular momentum, certain nuclei such as protons, when placed in a magnetic field, develop a net magnetization aligned with the field. By applying pulses of radio frequency power the magnetization may be tilted away from the field. After termination of the pulse, the magnetization tends to realign with the field with two time constants, T1 and T2, which are related to the relaxation spin-lattice and spin-spin respectively. The frequency of the pulse depends on the nature of the nucleus under study. In early 1970's the initial research was done to extend magnetic resonance to imaging (MRI) [3].

Four features vector can be associated with each pixel of an MR-image: T1, T2 (spin and echo image), TI (inversion recovery image) and GRASS (Gradient-recalled acquisition in the steady state image). These measurements are also named the four bands of an MR-image and are computationally treated as multi-spectral images. Figures 1a,b,c,d show GRASS, TI, T1, and T2 respectively; as detected by the a 1.5 Tesla imaging system (GE Sigma) at the Department of Radiology of the Stanford University Hospital. Therefore an MR-image, M, of dimension nxn is a set of pixels, x, in a 6-D space: $x \equiv (i(x), j(x), \eta_1(x), \eta_2(x), \eta_3(x),$

$\eta_4(x)$). The first two coordinates determine the spatial position of x in M, the last four represent the measurements.

The number and kind of tissue classes depends on the anatomical target. For example in the case of MRI of the human skull nine classes may be considered as relevant: background, bone, cerebrospinal fluid, fat, gray matter hemorrhage, tumor and white matter. Manual classification allows experts to discriminate quite easily soft tissues to support the diagnosis of diseases inherent to cerebral matter (cancer, hemorrhage). Other classes of diseases (neoplastic, ischemic,...) are less evident and need the integration of visual information coming from all the four bands.

Full manual classification is difficult for several reasons: the limits of the human perception to synthesize multispectral information and the morphological complexity of MRI-images. Moreover the process is tedious, time consuming and error prone. An incorrect "training set", to estimate statistical indicators, may be generated by the "tired" radiologist, if automatic classification is performed. It follows also that the training process is largely not-reproducible [4,5,6].

The main aim of the paper is to describe a pre-analysis technique, based on unsupervised clustering algorithms, which reduces to one the dimensionality of the parameters space and allows to perform a preliminary rough partition of the pixels in the image. The extracted information is then used to drive the physician to perform the tissue-classification. In particular three integrated "clustering" techniques are described: Hierarchical Single Link Clustering (HSLC), Hierarchical Histogramming Partition Clustering (HHPC) and Histogram Partition Clustering (HPC) [7,8]. Section 2 describes the four clustering algorithms. The integration of the four algorithms is described in Section 3. Section 4 shows preliminary results. Final remarks are given in Section 5.

2. CLUSTERING ALGORITHMS.

Given an universe, X, of samples defined in a d-dimension feature space then clustering algorithms determine a partition of X in the class: $C = \{C_1, C_2,...,C_r\}$, such that: $\forall\, i \neq j\;\; C_i \cap C_j = \phi$ and $\bigcup_i C_i = X$ [9,10]. In the following three techniques, suitable for MRI, are reviewed. Then they will be integrated to achieve the final clustering partition.

Hierarchical Single Link Clustering. This algorithm needs a suitable definition of distance, ρ, between the pixels of an image. In our case it is a function of both the Euclidean distance, ρ_E, and the similarity, ρ_η, in the feature space [11].

The HSLC-algorithm acts in two levels: a) Link each pixel, x, to the nearest-neighbor, y, iff $\rho \leq \alpha$, where α is a positive threshold, which is a not-decreasing function of the mean path in the 6-D space (after this phase the image is segmented in N_α clusters); b) merge the N_α clusters, by using an intercluster similarity function based on a variant of the Mahalanobis distance and function of the feature components of the MRI.

Hierarchical Histogram Partition Clustering. It performs the recursive dichotomy of the image, until the required number of clusters are obtained. Let it be A a cluster obtained at a given level of the hierarchy. The split of A in the sons clusters A_1 and A_2 is performed by assuming an "a priori" distribution of the pixels intensities in the four bands. For example two sons clusters can be generated by assigning each pixel, x, of A as follows: *if* $\eta(x) \le \beta$ *then* $x \in A_1$ *else* $x \in A_2$, where $\eta = f(\eta_1, \eta_2, \eta_3, \eta_4)$ is a global feature (for example: $\eta = \sum a_i \times \eta_i$); β is a cut value, which is computed from the local probability distribution of the feature-space in A.

Histogram Partition Clustering. It is one step unsupervised and non-parametric algorithm. The number of clusters, L, is guessed and for each band, k, the total energy, F_k, is computed. The partition of M is determined by assigning a label λ to each pixel of the image M as follows: $\forall x \in M$ and k=1,2,3,4 $\lambda_k(x) = j \Leftrightarrow \eta_k \in [j \times \Delta F_k, (j+1) \times \Delta F_k]$, where $\Delta F_k = F_k/L$. This procedure induces a natural partition of the 4-D discrete Λ-space. Each element of Λ is a 4-tuple (j_1, j_2, j_3, j_4), with j_k=1,2,...,L. The final labeling is determined by the rule $\lambda(x) = \sum a_i \times j_i$. The coefficients a_i are determined by a principal components analysis algorithm.

3. INTEGRATED CLUSTERING.

The three algorithms have been combined in order to perform an Integrated Clustering (IC). IC is recommended whenever the used methods show complementary properties. In our case HSLC is very sensitive to both spatial and intensity information; HHPC is able to detect relevant differences in the feature space; HPC gives coarse information, but it is very fast ($T_{CPU} \le .8$sec to label an image of size 256x256, on the vector machine IBM3090). Therefore it is useful to perform quick exploratory analysis.

Let it be Cl_1, Cl_2,..., Cl_s the clustering methods used, then the IC algorithm can be sketched as follows: *step 1* set the number of aspected clusters; *step 2* call the algorithms Cl_i and perform a validity test (i=1,...,s); *step 3* perform a cross_validation test; *step 4* output the relevant clusters.

The validation routine tests the *consistency* of each cluster respect to some statistical indicators (for example the size and the internal variance). The *cross_validation* routine tests the agreements between the clustering methods. Given two clustering algorithms Cl_1 and Cl_2 the confusion matrics, $C_{1,2} = \|c_{1,2}(i,j)\|$, represents the number of pixels labeled "i" by the algorithm Cl_1 and "j" by the algorithm Cl_2. The cross-validation algorithm returns the labeling of those pixels for which there is a perfect agreement (diagonal elements).

For more then two clustering methods the procedure could be computationally expensive. In our case we choose to perform the *cross_validation* by considering sequentially two methods Cl_i and Cl_{i+1} for $1 \le i < n$ and returning those clusters that have pass the test at the end of that sequence. This methodology is fast, however must be point out that it may depend upon the order of the tests.

4. EXPERIMENTAL RESULTS.

The clustering algorithms have been implemented in FORTRAN77 under VM/CMS operating system, on a vectorized IBM3090. Their performance and accuracy have been analyzed by using both simulated and real images. The last ones are 8-bits pixel intensity values (224 x 256 pixels per image), and represent a cranial MRI scan, with a hemorrhage localized on the top right corner of the image (see Figure 1a,b,c,d). Simulated images have been generated with 32 classes by using both the uniform (SURAND) and normal (SNRAND) random generator, provided by the IBM Engineering and Scientific Library (ESSL). The accuracy has been evaluated by using two indicators: the clustering tendency (CT) and the merging tendency (MT). These indicators are derived from the confusion matrix, $\|c_{ij}\|$:

$$CT = \sum_{j=0}^{L} T_c(j) \times P_j \qquad MT = \sum_{i=0}^{L} T_m(i) \times P_i$$

where

$$T_c(j) = \frac{\max\{c_{ij} \mid i=1,2,\ldots,L\}}{\sum_{i=0}^{L} c_{ij}} \quad j=1,2,\ldots,L \qquad T_m(i) = \frac{\max\{c_{ij} \mid j=1,2,\ldots,L\}}{\sum_{j=0}^{L} c_{ij}} \quad i=1,2,\ldots,L$$

Here P_i denotes the percentage of the class i in the sample. Table 1 shows TC, MT and T_{CPU} (in seconds) for the proposed algorithms:

Table 1

	CT	MT	T_CPU	P_c %
HSLC	.7	.276	43.7	55
HHPC	.72	.254	22.02	90
HPC	.647	.318	.738	70

Figures 1e,f,g represents the results of the labeling of the MR-image in Figure 1a,b,c,d with the HSLC, HHPC and HPC algorithms respectively. In this case the number of classes was set to 9. An experiment was performed on a set of 20x4 MRI-images to compare the automatic clustering with the tissue classification made by the radiologist. The confusion matrix was used for this purpose. The results are summarized in column four of Table 1, where Pc represents the total percentage of pixels correctly clusterized. The experiment has shown that the main source of mistakes derives by the fact that cerebrospinal fluid and adjacent cortical gray matter may produce mixed clusters.

5. FINAL REMARKS.

MRI has became one of the more powerful tool for medical diagnosis. Full automated procedures are not satisfactory because of the complexity of the data and the dimensions of the feature space (4D). Computer aided analysis can improve the performance of the human decision process. Here three clustering techniques have been described, their performance and accuracy studied. Their integration hallows robust labeling, in order to support the human classification. The system is still under development and the integration of the clustering methods still needs more investigation. The whole performance of the integration of the clustering methods still needs more investigation. The whole performance of the man/machine classification procedure is not yet completed. However the preliminary results are promising and encourage further investigations. A first version of an MR-Image Analysis System is under implementation on the IBM RISC/6000-234.

REFERENCES.

[1]   M.Purcell, H.C.Torrey and R.V.Pound, "Resonance absorption by nuclear magnetic moments in a solid", Phys.Rev., N.69, pp.37-38, 1946.

[2]   F.Bloch, "Nuclear Induction", Phys.Rev., N.70, pp.460-473, 1946.

[3]   P.C.Lauterbur, "Image Formation by Induced Local Interactions: Examples Employing Nuclear Magnetic Resonance", Nature, N.242, pp.190-191, 1973.

[4]   E.Herskovits, M.Walker, "Computer-Aided Classification of Magnetic-Resonance Images", Tech.Rep. N.KSL-89-47, Medical Computer Science, Stanford University, 1989.

[5]   R.Dann, J.Hoford, et al., "Preliminary Clinical Evaluation of Multi-Resolution Elastic Matching Software", Tech.Report, MS-CIS-85-35, Department of Computer Science and Information Science, University of Pennsylvania, 1988.

[6]   W.A.Hanson, E.Herskovits, R.De La Paz and R.Bernstein, "A Maximum-Likelihood Classifier for Automated Radiologic Diagnosis", 1988.

[7]   V.Di Gesu', R.L.De La Paz, W.A.Hanson, R.Bernstein, "A comparison of Clustering Algorithms for MRI", PASC-Tech.Rep., N., 1989.

[8]   V.Di Gesu', et all., "Hierarchical Clustering Algorithms: a comparative analysis", in preparation.

[9]   R.O.Duda and P.E.Hart, "Pattern Classification and Scene Analysis", John Willey and Sons, 1973.

[10] J.C.Bezdek, "Pattern Recognition with Fuzzy Objective Function Algorithms", Plenum Press, NY, 1987.

[11] V.Di Gesù, "A Clustering Approach to Texture Classification", in Real Time Object and Environment Measurement and Classification, A.K.Anil Jain ed., NATO ASI Series F, Vol.42, Springer Verlag, 1988.

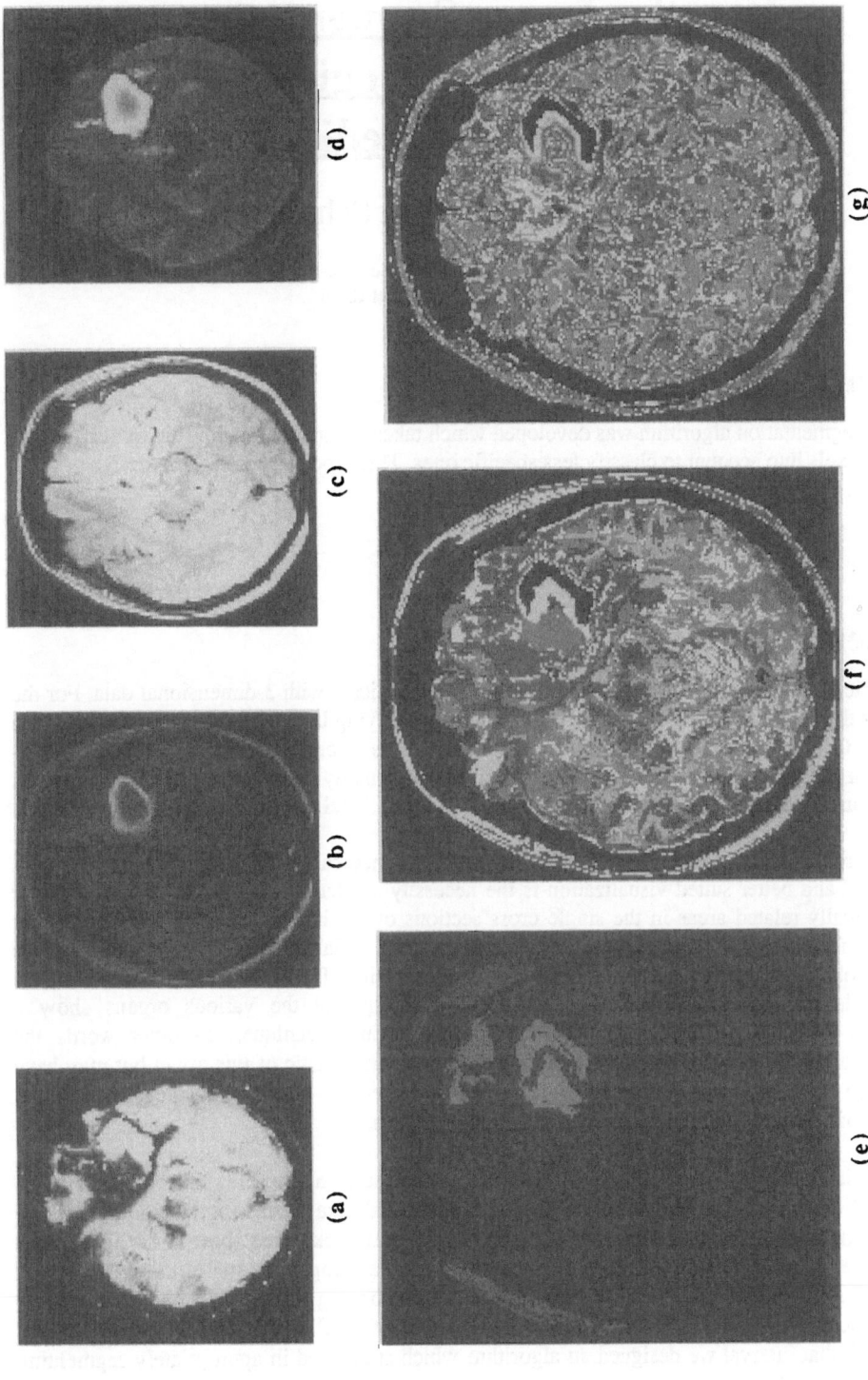

Figure 1 MRI-image of a human skull: (a) GRAS component; (b) TI component;(c) T_1 component; (d) T_2 component. MRI-labeling: (e) HSLC-labeling; (f) HHPC-labeling; (g) HPC-labeling.

Iterative Image Segmentation via 3-valued Logic for 3-D Display of Medical Data

Manfred Gengler, Ernst Schuster

Institute of Medical Computer Science
A-1090 Vienna, Währinger Gürtel 18-20

Abstract

An image segmentation algorithm was developed which takes the spatial relationship of already classified pixels into account to classify less specific ones. This procedure is used in the 3-dimensional display of medical data.

3-dimensional display

Many medical imaging modalities potentially supply the physician with 3-dimensional data. For the time being the visualization of these images is rather dissatisfying because of the way how they are displayed. Generally speaking, the 3-dimensional data is represented as a sequence of 2-dimensional images out of which the physician must mentally reconstruct the 3-dimensional objects. Thus the demand for, and the necessity of, a 3-dimensional display is quite obvious [5, 6].

The main problem in computer-assisted reconstruction of a medical 3-dimensional scene aiming at an improved and better suited visualization is the necessity to identify and extract functionally or morphologically related areas in the single cross sections of the images supplied by the imaging devices. Unfortunately the image data hardly allows for a reliable image segmention into the interesting objects merely on the basis of their numerical values [1, 2]. The main reason for this deficiency is that the various numerical ranges which specify the various organs show a considerable overlap even with the most advanced imaging techniques. In other words the numerical values derived from a specific organ are often characteristic of this organ but may have quite a large range of values in common with other organs because of the wide-spread distribution of the numerical values obtained from the same type of organs.

Since a reliable segmentation into the object(s) of interest is a crucial prerequirement in 3-dimensional display of medical data with the aid of graphical data processing techniques [4], we developed and implemented an algorithm to overcome the drawback stated above. For this purpose we capitalize on the fact that medical objects generally form a compact cluster in the image plane. Taking into account the spatial compactness of the data belonging to the same object as well as their numerical range and considering its decreasing degree of reliability when the data approaches either end of that interval we designed an algorithm which succeeded in appropriately segmenting medical images without any user intervention.

Segmentation Algorithm

Assumption

At present, the input images are assumed to be matrices with values ranging between 0 and 255 (8-bit quantizsation). Apart from limited storage capacities, however, this constraint is not caused by the principle or structure of the algorithm and can easily be altered to any fidelity of quantization. Matrix size and thus the spatial resolution is arbitrary. The most common sizes however are 256x256 (DSA, CT) and 512x512 (MRI, CT). Furthermore the numerical values of the objects to be detected should be contained within a known interval of gray-scale values. This interval should be characteristic of the object inasmuch as the more central the value of a pixel is to that interval the more likely it belongs to that specific object, and the further off the centre it is the less probable is its membership to that object.

Initialization

In an ancillary step we generate from the original matrix of gray-scale values (fig. 1) a 3-valued matrix of classifications:

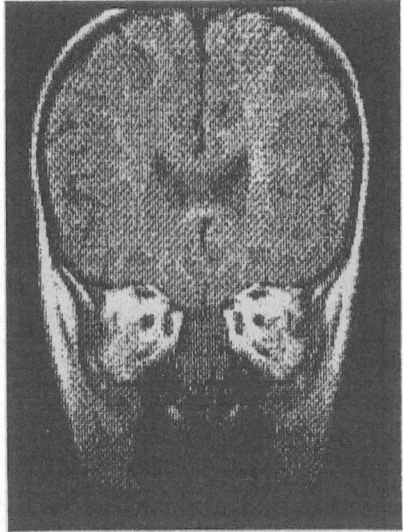

Fig.1: original MR-image (head of a 15 years old volunteer)

- All pixels with values that are within that interval of gray-scale values pathognomonic of the object under consideration with an acceptably high level of reliability are mapped to 1.

- All pixels the values of which are within a range of gray-scale values which indicates on an equally high but optionally different level of certainty that they do not belong to the object are mapped to -1.

- The rest which does not belong to either of these two classes is mapped to 0.

To illustrate this principle, ct: the data given in table 1.

10	16	48	35	11	12
76	74	66	83	92	81
84	79	102	108	86	75
76	83	95	132	154	259
157	206	111	94	78	34
212	178	133	99	75	32

Table 1: original data

Assuming that the typical range of the object is [50,150] and that the reliable range of being no element of the object is [0,25] and [180, 300], respectively, then the initial classification becomes

-1	-1	0	0	-1	-1
1	1	1	1	1	1
1	1	1	1	1	1
1	1	1	1	0	-1
0	-1	1	1	1	0
-1	0	1	1	1	0

Table 2: classified data

Iteration

To assign each point of the image matrix either to the object or to the remaining area in an increasingly reliable way, we analyze both its numerical value and a neighbourhood of certain extent centered around the corresponding element in the previously generated 3-valued classification matrix. From the pixel-related neighbourhood, the proportions of the pixels are calculated which are currently assigned to one of the two classes (i.e. <object>,<non-object>). The more favourable this value is for one of the two classes, the more the gray-scale value of the associated pixel is allowed to differ from the highly reliable range for this class to be still classified as belonging to that class. This is based on a user-specified confidence function reflecting the likelihood of a pixel value of belonging to a particular class [1, 3]. The interval of numerical values for assigning a pixel to the opposite class is in turn narrowed by another user-specified function based upon the ratio of the two membership functions. For example, if 60% of the neighbourhood of the pixel under consideration are assigned to class 1 (e.g. <object>) and 10% of the pixels are assigned to class 2 (e.g. <non-object>) (thus leaving 30% as unclassified) then the interval of the feasible gray-scale values for class 1 is extended by a certain degree (depending n a user-specified function of the computed percentage [= 60%]). Similarily, the interval of feasible gray-scale values for the second class (e.g. <non-object>) is narrowed according to another user-specified function of the computed percentage (10%). On the grounds of these modified intervals, the pixel is (re-)-classified (fig. 2).

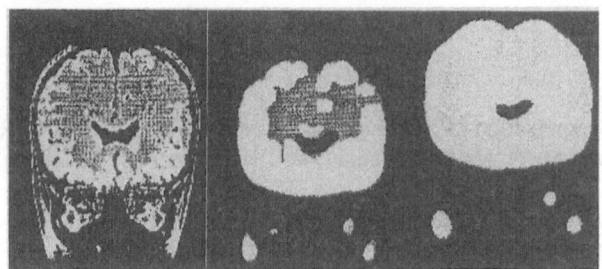

Fig.2: Iterative classification (neighborhood:9x9)

The results are stored in a further 3-valued matrix so as not to interfere with the results of the previous classification, which are still required for calculating the membership functions of adjacent pixels.

Simultaneously the number of pixels which were re-classified is computed. If the number of reclassifications exceeds a certain limit, the classification process continues swapping between the two 3-valued matrices (that is the input matrix of step n becomes the output matrix of step (n+1) and vice versa).

Results

This algorithm was applied to MR data taken from the human head in order to display the brain in a 3-dimensional way (fig. 3). By this algorithm all 64 slices were automatically classified into the two classes *<brain>* and *<non-brain>*. The classification results were used to label those picture elements which were used in the 3-dimensional display of the MR data later on. Both the 3-dimensional view of the brain and the visual classification of the single slices proved the superiority of this approach in comparison with unconstrained classification.

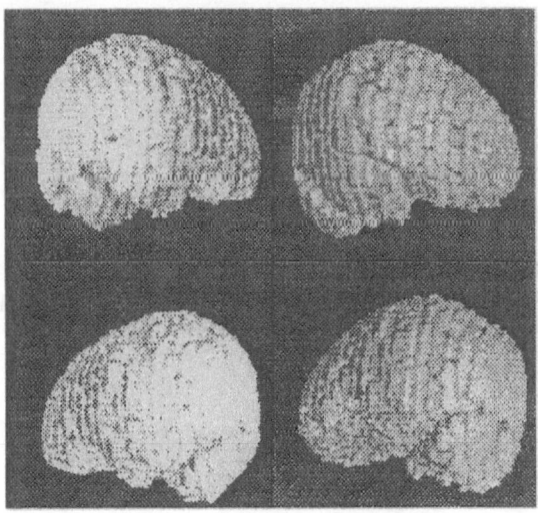

Fig.3: 3-dimensional views of the brain

Literature

1. Sai Prasad Raya:
    Low-level Segmentation of 3-D Magnetic Resonance Brain Images - a Rule-Based System
    IEEE Transactions on Medical Imaging, Vol. 9, No.3, pp 327-337, June 1990.

2. Bomans M., Höhne K., Tiede U., Riemer M.:
    3-D Segmentation of MR Images of the Head for 3-D Display
    IEEE Transactions on Medical Imaging, Vol. 9, No.2, pp 177-183, June 1990.

3. Pedrycz W.:
    Fuzzy Sets in Pattern Recognition: Methodology and Methods
    Pattern recognition, Vol. 23, No.1/2, pp 121-146, 1990.

4. Kapouleas I.:
    Automatic Detection of White Matter Lesions in Magnetic Resonance Brain Imaging
    Computer Methods and Programs in Biomedicine, Vol. 32, pp 17-35, 1990.

5. Dhawan A. P.:
    A Review on Biomedical Image Processing and Future Trends
    Computer Methods and Programs in Biomedicine, Vol. 31, pp 141-183, 1990.

6. Ney D. R, Fishman E.K, Magid D.:
    Volometric Rendering of Computed Tomography Data: Principles and Techniques
    IEEE Computer Graphics and Applications, pp 24-32, 1990.

7. Herman G.T., Liu H.K.:
    Three-dimensional Display of Human Organs from Computed Tomograms
    Comput. Graph. Image Process. 9, 1, 1979.

8. Höhne, K.h:, Riemer M., Tiede U.:
    Viewing Operations for 3D-Tomographic Gray Level Data
    IMDM-Bericht Nr. 87/1

9. Levoy M.:
    Display of Sufaces from Volume Data
    IEEE Computer Graphics & Applications, May 1988, pp 29-37.

10. Vannier M.W., Marsh J.L., Warren J.:
    Three-dimensional CT reconstruction images for craniofacial surgical planning
    Radiology 150, 1984, pp 179-184.

QUALITY ASSURANCE OF READER'S RESPONSE IN MEDICAL IMAGING

Walter R. Steinbach and K. Richter
Institut für Herz-Kreislauf-Forschung Berlin-Buch
Wiltbergstraße 50, D-O-1115 Berlin

Abstract

Among the methodologic criteria which describe the quality of an entire diagnostic imaging system - equipment plus diagnostician - accuracy in form of the observer performance belongs to the most important To consider not only common types of findings but also differential diagnostic problems ROC analysis was modified and applied to a multiple-alternative decision task. It could be shown that the probability of correct classification derived from an allocation-confusion-matrix corresponds to the area under an appropriately constructed ROC curve. Degrees of confidence in the reader's judgement of $0, 1, \ldots, 10$ were used for both classification and ROC rating. The validity of the method had been demonstrated examining a sample of 1.190 chest radiographs to classify cardiovascular conditions. The ROC curves are symmetric, with their points located around the off-diagonal. Differences between the overall probability of correct classification and the ROC curve index calculated from the same evaluator's data were very small, 0,004 to 0,011.

Introduction

In medical imaging the observer is confronted with various types of diagnostic questions. He may have to detect, to recognize, to identify, to discriminate, or to localize findings. Rarely he will be asked to solve a differential diagnostic problem using a multiple classification procedure. The goodness of the reader's response depends on different factors determining the quality of the entire system "Imaging Equipment plus Diagnostician". Among the methodologic criteria fidelity, reliability, validity, utility, and accuracy characterizing the system only the latter can be treated in this lecture. Accuracy should be understood as degree of reduced uncertainty with observer performance as a measurand for it.

Material and Method

Unlike the common measures of diagnostic performance overall accuracy or sensitivity plus specificity ROC analysis is uninfluenced by decision biases and prior probabilities. However, ROC couldn't be applied to multiple classification without modification. Therefore a combination was used between a simple matrix classification and an ROC rating. The diagnosticians were asked to give their responses as degrees of confidence in their own judgement using scores 0,1,...,10. For each classification task the reader had to divide a total 10 (probability 1,0) into no more than two appropriately weighted parts, assigning them to the classifications of conditions considered the most likely and next most likely to be present. The observer responses are arranged into a m-by-m matrix (m = number of classes) which contains the numbers of correct and incorrect classifications. From the classification matrix the matrix of the classification probability is derived. As could be shown the overall probability of correct classification is equivalent to the area under a ROC curve derived from a rearranged matrix outcome. The decision on the modified rating scale now is "correct classification" and "incorrect classification", without prejudice to any class.

Results

To demonstrate the correlation between the overall probability of correct classification and ROC curve index, a large sample of 1190 chest radiographs was evaluated according to the system developed by Richter et al. (1) for classifying cardiovascular conditions detectable by imaging techniques. The reference standard for the five-class system was established by skilled staff radiologists, all of whom had been involved in the developement of Richter's system. Differences between the probability of correct classification and the ROC curve index calculated from the probability matrices for all five readers were small, 0,004 to 0,011. The ROC curves derived from the same data are shown in figure 1 for reader H who had high performance rating, reader M (medium performance), and reader L (low performance). Figure 2 presents these curves in double probability coordinates.

Figure 1: ROC curves constructed from the classification matrix outcomes of five-class task to classify cardiovascular conditions from thorax x-ray films. Reader H made most accurate , reader M had medium and reader L a low rating compared with the others

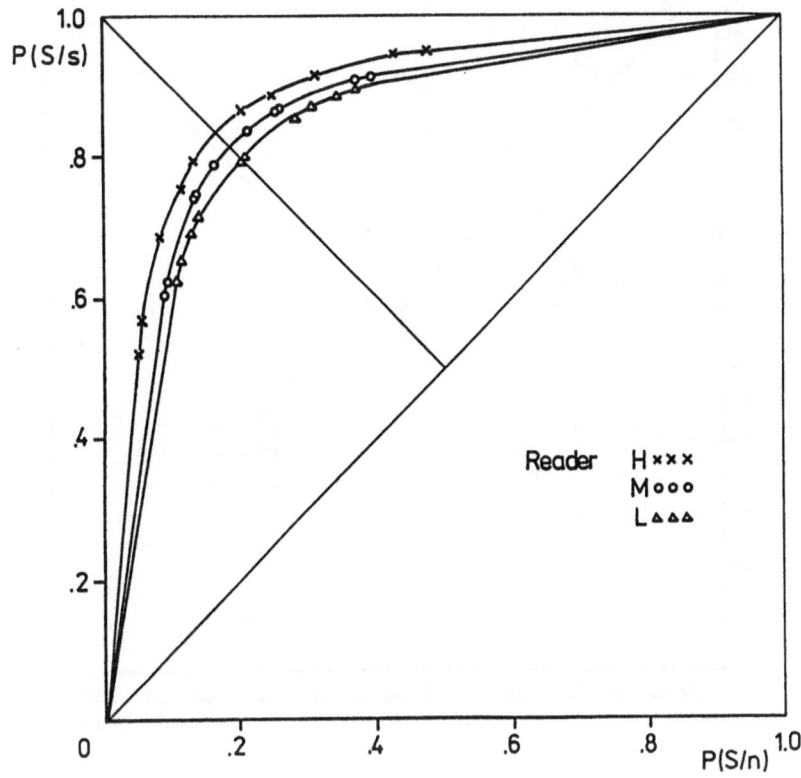

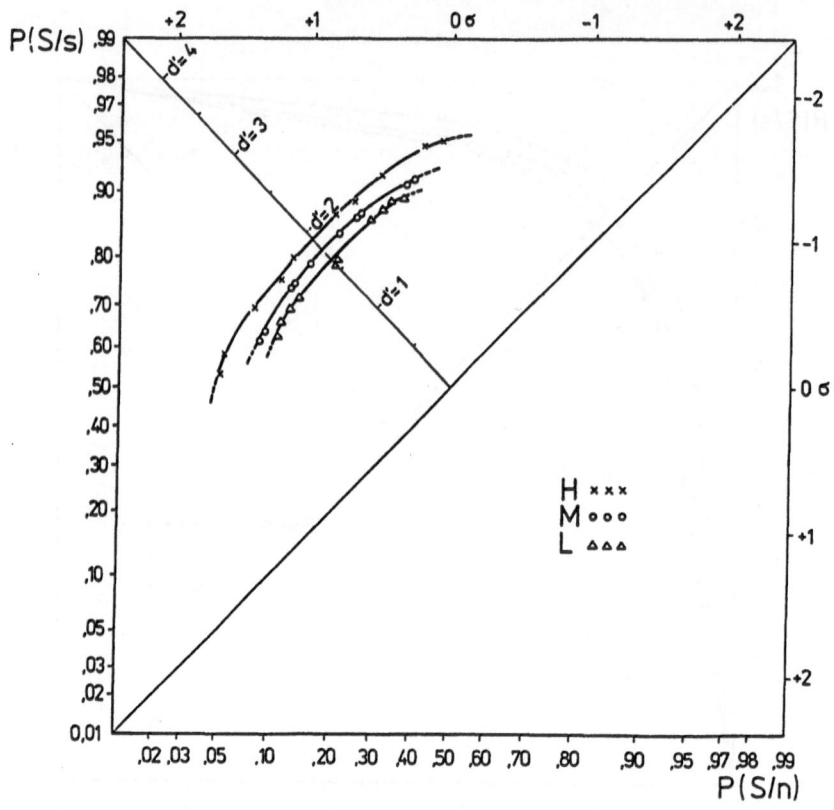

Discussion

Accuracy is an important quality criterion in medical imaging described by an index of observer performance. ROC procedures can be applied to all types of findings with high gain. However, differential diagnostic tasks require a modification of the ROC. Multiple classification with matrix outcomes which shows observer performances in identifying correct choices and yields the probabilities of confusing an identifiable condition with others can be represented graphically. This is shown for the overall probability of correct classification which is equivalent to the area under a ROC curve. An 11-point scale of reader response is useful for both the multiple-classification procedure and construction of the ROC curves. The curves are symmetric around the off-diagonal in the distribution of their points. The smoothness of the curves is explained by the forced symmetry and by large sample size. Double coordinate representation shows a slightly curved ROC which likes more a model category after Luce (4).

References

1. Richter, K. G. Anders et al.: Das Röntgenschirmbild als Herz-Kreislauf-SCREENING: Ztschr. f. Ärztl. Fortbild. 23(1974), 1233
2. Steinbach, W.R., K. Richter: Multiple Classification and Receiver Operating Characteristic (ROC) Analysis. Med. Decis. Making 7(1987), 234
3. To be published
4. Swets, J.A.: Form of empirical ROCs in discrimination and diagnostic tasks: Implication for theory and measurement of performance. Psychol. Bull. 99(1986), 181

USE OF FRACTAL DIMENSION IN SIGNAL ADAPTIVE FILTERS FOR SPECKLE REDUCTION IN ULTRASOUND B-MODE IMAGES

X. Magnisalis   C. Kotropoulos   I. Pitas   M.G. Strintzis

Department of Electrical Engineering, University
of Thessaloniki, Thessaloniki 540 06, GREECE

Abstract

Two novel signal-adaptive nonlinear filters are proposed for speckle reduction in ultrasound B-mode images. The first is a modification of the Signal-Adaptive Median, which uses the Fractal Dimension (FD) as a measure of the local signal activity. The second one is based on the L_2 mean filter which is the maximum likelihood (ML) estimator of a constant signal corrupted by multiplicative Rayleigh noise and uses the above-mentioned measure of local signal activity. The proposed signal adaptive nonlinear filters suppress the speckle noise while preserving the image texture.

1 Introduction

In many object identification problems in Image Processing, the noise corruption includes additive as well as multiplicative and/or signal dependent components. In the ultrasound tissue characterization class of problems the general signal x-observation y relationship is as follows [1] :

$$y = x + x^a n_1 + n_2 \tag{1}$$

where the value of the parameter a, $0 < a \leq 1$, depends on the specific ultrasound sensor used and the preprocessing done, and n_1 , n_2 are independent noise processes. In such cases, the use of signal adaptive algorithms has been seen to be very helpful in general [1,2,3]. This paper developes two signal adaptive algorithms for speckle reduction and texture characterization in ultrasound B-mode images. The first relies on a median filtering formulation similar to that in [3] but with the Fractal Dimension (FD) rather than the Signal to Noise Ratio (SNR) used to effect the needed adaptation. The second, also replaces median filtering by the optimum Maximum Likelihood signal estimate assuming Rayleigh-distributed multiplicative B-mode ultrasound noise. The two above novel algorithms are compared to known ones (such as the SAM algorithm [3]) and to each other as to their computational efficiency and relative effectiveness in texture preservation and speckle removal.

2 Signal Adaptive Median filter based on Fractal Dimension

The Signal-Adaptive Median (SAM) filter [3] is a variable window size nonlinear filter whose output is given by:

$$\hat{x}(k,m) = y_M(k,m) + b(k,m)[y(k,m) - y_M(k,m)] \tag{2}$$

where $\hat{x}(k,m)$ is the signal estimate, $y(k,m)$ is the noisy observation at pixel (k,m), $y_M(k,m)$ is the median of the observations in an $N \times M$ window W centered on pixel (k,m) and $b(k,m)$ is a coefficient which must satisfy the following requirements:

1. it must approach 0 offering maximum noise reduction in uniform regions

2. it must approach 1 preserving and possibly enhancing the boundaries between regions of different texture in textured regions

It can be easily recognized that $b(k,m) = 0$ implies $\hat{x}(k,m) = y_M(k,m)$, while $b(k,m) = 1$ implies $\hat{x}(k,m) = y(k,m)$. An appropriate expression for such a coefficient is given by the following equation:

$$b(k,m) = \frac{1}{1 + \tilde{\sigma}_q^2} \; [1 - \frac{\bar{y}^2(k,m)\tilde{\sigma}_q^2}{\sigma_y^2(k,m)}] \tag{3}$$

where $\bar{y}(k,m)$ is an estimate of $E[y(k,m)]$ over the running window W, $\tilde{\sigma}_q^2$ is the normalized variance of the multiplicative noise and σ_y^2 is the sample variance of $y(k,m)$ over the window W. The value of the factor $b(k,m)$ is used to adjust the window size W pointwize, i.e., to control how many pixels in the neighborhood of $y(k,m)$ will be median filtered, based on the local SNR, where:

$$SNR = 1 - \frac{\bar{y}^2(k,m)\tilde{\sigma}_q^2}{\sigma_y^2(k,m)} \tag{4}$$

This is done in order to avoid abrupt changes in noise suppression and to achieve a better adaptation. In flat regions, it becomes small. Near edges it approaches one. Therefore $b(k,m)$ may be considered as an edge detector, appropriate to the noise model (1).

It is known that the Fractal Dimension (FD) may be used for the representation and classification of texture, and for edge detection and enhancement [4,8]. In the novel method proposed here, we replace SNR in (2) by an estimate of the FD. A space domain estimation of the FD is being used which is based on the fractional Brownian motion model [5,6]. According to this model a fractional Brownian motion surface must satisfy the following relationship:

$$E[|y(k_2, m_2) - y(k_1, m_1)|] \propto (\sqrt{(k_2 - k_1)^2 + (m_2 - m_1)^2})^H \tag{5}$$

where H is the Hausdorf dimension. The FD D_s of the surface is defined by:

$$D_s = 3 - H \tag{6}$$

and, in this paper, is being calculated by the algorithm proposed in [4].

3   Signal Adaptive L_2 mean filter

In this section the following simplification of the model (1) is used:

$$y = xn \tag{7}$$

where n is assumed to be Rayleigh-distributed noise independent of x, with probability density:

$$f_n(\mathcal{N}) = \frac{\pi \mathcal{N}}{2} \exp[-\frac{\pi \mathcal{N}^2}{4}] \; \mathcal{N} > 0 \tag{8}$$

Let us assume that we have N observations. Then the joint conditional probability density function of the observations is given by:

$$f_{y|x}(\mathbf{Y}|X) = \frac{\pi^N}{2^N X^{2N}} \prod_{i=1}^{N} Y_i \exp[-\frac{\pi Y_i^2}{4X^2}] \tag{9}$$

The maximum-likelihood(ML) estimate $\hat{x}_{ML}$ is the value of x maximizing (9). Easily:

$$\hat{x}_{ML} = \frac{\sqrt{\pi}}{2} \sqrt{\frac{1}{N} \sum_{i=1}^{N} Y_i^2} \tag{10}$$

It is seen that the ML estimate (10) is simply the output of an L_2 mean filter defined in [7] multiplied by the constant $\sqrt{\pi}/2$. Therefore instead of the median estimate used in (2) , the ML estimate (10) can be used.

4   Results and Conclusions

Figure 1 illustrates the original ultrasonic image of liver that is used. Figures 2 and 3 illustrate the results of applying a Signal Adaptive ML filter using SNR and FD respectively to calculate the $b(k,m)$ factor that effects the adaptation. It can be easily seen that the FD method does a better speckle reduction than the SNR method. The Fractal Dimension of each pixel has been calculated based on a 7×7 or 5×5 window centered on that pixel.

From the computational point of view, the FD calculation is very time consuming. It takes a full 12 hours to filter a 512x512 image using 5x5 running window on an 68020 based workstation. A parallel version of the program has also been implemented on a 16 Transputer parallel computer, reducing the processing time to under 1 hour. For comparison purposes it is noted that the SNR version of SAM only requires about 35 minutes on the above-mentioned workstation.

The overall effect of such an adaptive filtering is the reduction of speckle in such a way that information inherent in the image is not affected. The better performance of the FD as a local signal activity estimator may be attributed to its texture representation and edge detection properties [8].

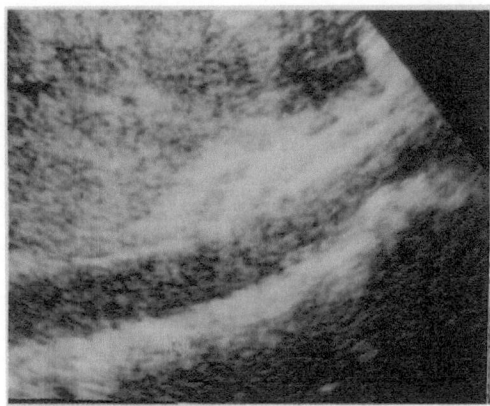

Figure 1: Original ultrasound B-mode liver scan image

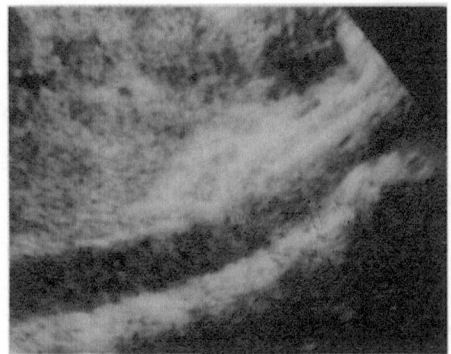

Figure 2: Signal Adaptive ML filter using SNR

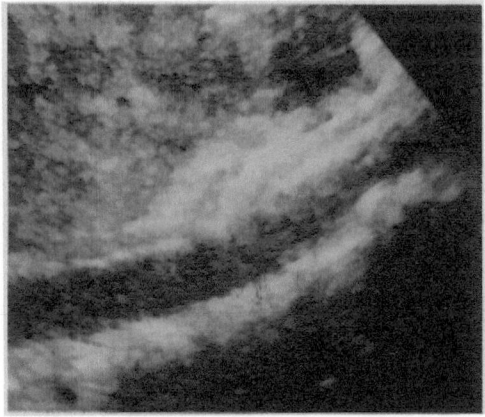

Figure 3: Signal Adaptive ML filter using FD

References

[1] T. Loupas, W.N. McDicken and P.L. Allan, "An adaptive weighted median filter for speckle suppresion in medical ultrasonic images", *Trans. on Circuits ans Systems*, vol. CAS-36, no. 1, January 1989 pp. – .

[2] H.E. Knutsson, R. Wilson and G.H. Granlund, "Anisotropic Nonstationary Image Estimation and its Applications: Part I-Restoration of Noisy Images", *IEEE Transactions on Communications*, Vol. COM-31, No.3, March 1983, .pp. 386–406.

[3] R. Bernstein: "Adaptive Nonlinear Filters for Simultaneous Removal of Different Kinds of Noise in Images", *IEEE Trans. Circuits and Systems*, Vol. CAS-34, No.11, Nov. 1987, pp. 1275–1291.

[4] Chi-Chang Chen, J.S. Daponte and M.D. Fox, "Fractal Feature Analysis and Classification in Medical Imaging", *IEEE Trans. Medical Imaging*, Vol. 8, No. 2, June 1989, pp. 133–142.

[5] Heinz-Otto Peitgen, Dietmar Saupe, Editors, *The Science of Fractal Images*, Springer-Verlag, 1988.

[6] Michael Barnsley: *Fractals Everywhere*, Academic Press, Inc., 1988.

[7] I. Pitas, A.N. Venetsanopoulos, "Edge detectors based on nonlinear filters",*IEEE Trans. on Pattern Anal. and Machine Intelligence*, vol. PAMI-8, no. pp. 538-550, July 1986.

[8] T. Lundahl, W.J. Ohley, S.M. Kay and R. Siffert: "Fractional Brownian Motion: A Maximum Likelihood Estimator and its Application to Image Texture", *IEEE Trans. Medical Imaging*, Vol. 5, No. 3, Sept. 1986, pp. 152-161.

BIOMETRY AND
BIOMATHEMATICS

A Computer Methodology for reducing the volume of the oxytocin used in labour

B RICHARDS, J CADMAN, J LEVITT, B LIEBERMANN

Department of Computation, UMIST, Manchester, England.
St. Mary's Hospital, Manchester, England.

Abstract

This paper describes a regime for controlling the administration of oxytocin during labour. Use of the regime permits much lower volumes of oxytocin to be administered without lengthening labour and with subsequent benefit to the fetus.

Introduction

Many workers in the field of obstetrics and neonatology have been concerned about the damage which can be done to the fetuses born to mothers who have received oxytocin during labour. What follows is a description of the methodology whereby this damage can be reduced.

Oxytocin is produced naturally within the mother's body when the growing fetus reaches Term (40 weeks). However, in some cases the amount available is insufficient to do the job required. In such cases it becomes necessary to introduce synthetic oxytocin into the mother's blood stream either to induce labour or to accelerate labour already in progress. Some 30% of mothers delivered in hospital will receive oxytocin although figures will vary from one hospital to another. Oxytocin infusion brings with it side effects in the mother and causes damage to baby's blood cells. There is a need for a regime which can reduce these risks.

The effect of oxytocin on the fetus

A previous study [1] obtained results from a cohort of 169 patients. The Table 1 below shows that there is a significant reduction in the level of haemoglobin in those babies whose mothers have been induced. This is the result of the breakdown of the red blood cell caused by the uterine contractions working on the uterus like a pneumatic drill. The break-down products of this degradation of the red blood cells include the pigment bilirubin which produces jaundice in the newborn baby. The Table shows that there is a significant increase in bilirubin levels of those babies subjected to oxytocin. The same study [1] shows a significant positive correlation between the bilirubin level in the umbilical cord at birth and the total amount of oxytocin administered to the mother. The equation is:

Cord Bilirubin (mmol/L) = 0.000873 x oxytocin (mu) + 32.2

There is therefore clearly a need to reduce the total volume of oxytocin administered to the mother.

	SPONTANEOUS	INDUCED
Numbers	86	83
Birth Weight (gm)	3372	3388
Hg (g/dl)	17.1	16.1 *
Haematocrit	0.522	0.484 *
RBC ($x10^{12}/1$)	4.88	4.55 *
Bilirubin ($\mu mol/1$)	30	37 **

TABLE 1: The effect of OXYTOCIN on the newborn

A Controlled Study

In order to verify the premise that the volume of oxytocin used during labour could be reduced, a controlled study was devised.

Mothers who were required to have oxytocin were randomly divided into four groups (A,B,C,D). Those mothers in Group A were treated according to the usual Delivery Unit Regime (DUR); which means that the details of the treatment were based on the skill of the midwife. Those mothers in Groups B, C, D, were commenced on an intravenous oxytocin drip. An intrauterine catheter with a pressure transducer at its tip was inserted and continuous monitoring of the fetal heartrate and intrauterine pressure was carried out. Oxytocin (10 units) in 5% dextrose solution (500 ml) was used, the infusion rate being started at 2mu/minute increasing every 30 minutes to 4,8, 16 mu/min until the uterine pressure reached a level of over 1000 K Pascal secs in a 15 minute period. At that stage the protocol was invoked. For those mothers in Group B, the level of oxytocin was halved when the critical pressure was reached. In Group C the oxytocin was quartered, whilst in Group D the oxytocin was switched off when the required pressure was achieved.

Details of the duration of labour, the amount of oxytocin infused and the volume
of dextrose administered, were all recorded. Venous blood was taken from the mothers
on admission to the Labour Ward and again at delivery. Cord venous blood was
collected from a segment of the umbilical cord at birth of the baby. Additionally
a fetus scalp electrode was placed on the baby's head at the commencement of labour
and measurements of foetal pH were thereby made.

Results of the Study

Table 2 below shows that, for those mothers requiring oxytocin, the process of
randomly allocating them to the four Groups A to D, has been successful. These
four goups are evenly matched in all respects. They are also evenly matched with
the Control group, Group E, in every parameter except mother's weight. Here the
"Spontaneous" mothers are somewhat lighter.

			GROUPS			
Numbers	**A** 36	**B** 45	**C** 43	**D** 40	**E** 29	Signif- icance
AGE	27.1	27.6	27.2	25.7	25.8	N.S.
GRAVIDITY	1.14	1.44	1.40	1.25	1.28	N.S.
PARITY	0.89	1.02	0.88	0.65	0.90	N.S.
HEIGHT(CM)	164	164	163	164	160	N.S.
WEIGHT(KG)	72.3	78.7	72.3	73.9	67.0	SIG
CIGS/DAY	4.6	7.2	6.3	5.0	6.7	N.S.
Hg(gm/dl)	11.8	12.1	12.0	11.9	12.0	N.S.

TABLE 2:   Pre-labour Statistics of Mothers

Table 3 shows the details of labour and it will be seen that the spontaneous group,
not surprisingly, have a significantly longer labour. Conversely, oxytocin does
reduce the length of labour. There is no significant difference in the length
of labour between the four groups who had oxytocin. This shows that the methodology
whereby the oxytocin is switched off, does not increase the length of labour in
those same mothers. It is noticeable too that fewer mothers opt for epidurals
when undergoing a spontaneous delivery. It is also noticeable that the mothers
in Group A were subjected to a higher rate of infusion whilst under the control
of the midwife than those mothers in Groups B,C,D, under the control of the
algorithm.

	GROUPS					
Means	A	B	C	D	E	
Numbers	36	45	43	40	29	Signif- icance
1st STAGE (hrs)	7.04	7.35	6.71	6.62	9.14	SIG
2nd STAGE (mins)	38	39	45	46	36	N.S.
Total Oxytocin	4976	5034	2886	2310	0	SIG
Highest rate of Oxytocin (drops/min)	16.17	15.78	12.14	9.55	0	SIG

TABLE 3: Details of Labour

	GROUPS					
Means	A	B	C	D	E	
Numbers	36	45	43	40	29	Signif- icance
Sodium	135	136	136	135	139	SIG
Potassium	3.46*	3.69	3.60	3.70	3.79*	SIG
Urea	3.06	3.24*	3.54*	3.27	2.99*	SIG
Alkaline Phosphatase	144	134*	126*	148	170*	SIG
Total Protein	65	65	65	65	69	SIG

TABLE 4: Maternal Biochemistry prior to delivery

Table 4 shows the results of the analyses of maternal-blood samples taken moments prior to the delivery. The overall message is that the oxytocin groups are suffering from a serum dilution due to the high volumes (as much as 5 litres) of dextrose used as a vehicle for the oxytocin infusion. The maternal serum potassium, alkaline phosphatase, and total protein are all diluted. The urea is considerably raised initially due to breakdown of muscle protein, but then even when it is diluted by the dextrose, it still remains at a signifcantly high level in the oxytocin Groups.

Table 5 shows that the modified APGAR SCORE, cord venous pH, and Cord Venous PO2 are no different between the five groups. However, the table shows that the Bilirubin levels in the oxytocin Groups are significangly raised.

What the tables collectively show is that reducing the oxytocin does not lengthen the duration of labour but does produce healthier babies.

	GROUPS					
	A	B	C	D	E	Signif- icance
Mean "APGAR" Score at 1 min	5.22	5.31	5.19	5.30	5.41	N.S.
Cord Venous pH	7.33	7.34	7.33	7.34	7.32	N.S.
Cord Venous PO2	31.3	32.5	31.0	31.6	30.8	N.S.
Cord Venous PCO2	35.9	33.5	36.4	35.1	40.2	SIG
Hg(gm/dl)	16.9	16.5	17.0	16.6	17.5	N.S.
Serum Sodium	137	135	137	135	140*	SIG
% with clinical jaundice	22%	20%	16%	10%	6%	SIG
% Bilirubin >100μmol/L	8%	5%	7%	2%	3%	SIG
% Bilirubin >200μmol/L	12%	7%	5%	5%	3%	SIG

TABLE 5: Clinical Parameters on the new babies

The Methodology

In those mothers scheduled for oxytocin the membranes are ruptured and an intra-uterine catheter, with a pressure transducer at its tip, was inserted into the uterus. The patient was then wired for continuous fetal heart-rate and uterine pressure measurements. The level of uterine pressure, integrated over each 15 minute period, was determined. The infusion was commenced at 2mU/Min and successively doubled every 30 minutes until an integrated presure (Kilopascals seconds) greater than 1000 is obtained. The methodology then determines that the oxytocin be reduced. As long as the integrated pressure remains above the base-line the current level of oxytocin will be maintained. If the uterine pressure drops, the oxytocin can be restored to its previous level. This control cycle can be maintained throughout pregnancy.

The other benefit from passing the output of the maternal/foetal monitoring system to a computer is that the computer can analyse the foetal heart rate and detect the onset of foetal distress some 20-30 minutes before being detected by the humans[2].

Conclusion

By the application of the methodology described above it is possible to reduce the volume of oxytocin infused into the mother. This does not reduce the length of labour and produces no disadvantages for the mother. However it does produce advantages for the babies in that it reduces the amount of jaundice observed, thereby producing a healthier baby. Finally, if the fetus is being monitored, it makes good sense to use the computer to monitor the foetal heart-rate to search for early onset of foetal distress. This system is highly recommended.

References

1. Richards et al. The effect of oxytocin in labour on neonatal jaundice Br. J. Ob and Gyn. Vol 86, Pg 133, 1979.

2. Jenkins, H "A study of the Intrapartum Fetal Electrogram using a real time computer". MD Thesis 1984.

Non-parametric regression techniques for biometric problems: Concepts and software

Michael G. Schimek
Medical Biometrics Group, Department of Paediatrics
University of Graz, A-8036 Graz, Austria

The biometric application of non-parametric regression models as an alternative to the standard parametric approach is motivated. Some basic concepts of non-parametric regression, uni- (kernel and spline smoothing) as well as multivariate (ACE and GAM), are described. The most important statistical packages for the non-parametric smoothing methodology (BATHSPLINE, XploRe and S-PLUS) are discussed with respect to their features and the types of models they offer.

1 Introduction

Regression techniques play an important role in the analysis of biometric data sets. In classical regression it is required to presume a certain parametric form for the regression curve (e.g. a polynomial). Hence we call this approach parametric. Most recently there is an increasing interest to apply more flexible non-parametric techniques. Numerous reasons can be named for this new trend, often discussed in the context of exploratory data analysis. The main point is to overcome the problem of forcing the regression model into a rigidly defined class, a direct result of the adoption of a single criterion for the estimation, the goodness of fit. For many data sets we do not have a prior knowledge of the functional relationships between the variables. There are also instances where simple parametric regression curves cannot account for the complexity of the parameter dependencies. What we need is a data-driven regression approach which is flexible enough to respond to local data variation while preventing abnormal behaviour, and is controllable in terms of the smoothness of the regression functions.

The basic idea of all univariate non-parametric regression models is the adoption of a goodness of fit and in addition a smoothness criterion in a way, that we can compromise between the effects of these two regarding the regression curve. This makes possible to account for two conflicting aims in curve estimation. The one is to produce a good fit and the other is to avoid too much local variation. Regression smoothing techniques differ basically in their weight functions and in their measures of local variation. What they have in common is a means of tuning the degree of smoothness which is usually called the bandwidth (for kernels) or the smoothing parameter (for splines). Such a parameter controls the rate of exchange between residual error and local variation. The benefit is that trend (regression) functions can be estimated from any given set of noisy observations.

Several different methodological concepts and multivariate generalisations are available by now. Many biometric problems require such regression techniques. Missing is the access to relevant software. As for many recently developed statistical concepts, sufficient computer power (computer intensive methods), graphical representation (exploratory techniques) and suitable environments for individual programming are required. Hardware (AT-compatibles or workstations) is no problem any more. Lacking is alternative software to the standard statistical packages (e.g. BMDP or SAS) not providing the necessary routines or not meeting the above demands.

2 Concepts of non-parametric regression

We confine ourselves to the discussion of non-parametric regression techniques using scatterplot smoothers. These smoothers are tools for summarising the trend of a response variable Y as a function of one or more predictor variables X_1, X_2,..., X_p. What they produce are estimates of the trends, non-parametric in their nature, which are less variable (smooth) than the observations on Y itselve. Scatterplot smoothers are applied in univariate (one predictor) as well as in multivariate (two or more predictors) estimation problems. In this paper we deal with some uni- and multivariate concepts which are of general interest from a biometric point of view. Smoothers for multiple predictors (e.g. thin-plate splines) are not considered because of computational and interpretational difficulties.

The two most frequently applied scatterplot smoothers for a single predictor are kernel, respectively cubic spline based. A kernel smoother uses an explicitly defined set of local weights defined by the kernel. In general weights are applied that decrease in a smooth fashion as one moves away from the target point.

$$ w_{0j} = \frac{c_0}{\lambda} \, d\left[\, \left| \frac{x_0 - x_j}{\lambda} \right| \, \right] $$

defines the weight assigned to the jth point in producing the estimate at x_0, where $d(t)$ is an even function decreasing in $|t|$. The parameter λ denotes the bandwidth and c_0 is a normalising constant. A number of different kernels (e.g. Gaussian) can be adopted (for details see [3]). They contrast in the shape of their weight functions and in their asymptotic behaviour. Of computational relevance is the fashion in which the kernel smooth is obtained. Discretizing the data into bins (WARPing technique, i.e. weighted averaging using rounded points; [3]) can reduce the computational burden almost to linearity.

The cubic spline smoother differs from the kernel concept as it can be introduced via an optimisation problem. Let us have a penalised sum of squares equation

$$SS = \sum_{i=1}^{n} (y_i - g(x_i))^2 + \lambda \int_{a}^{b} (g''(t))^2 dt$$

where $g(x_i)$ is the regression function, λ the smoothing parameter ($\lambda > 0$ and fixed) and $a \leq x_1 \leq x_2 \leq \ldots \leq x_n \leq b$. The cubic smoothing spline is that function $\hat{g}(x_i)$ with two continuous derivatives that minimises SS. The above optimisation problem has an explicit, unique minimal solution. The minimiser is a natural cubic spline with knots at the unique values of x_i (for details see [8]). There are numerous approaches to the estimation problem with different numerical and interpretational consequences. Computationally convenient is an evaluation by B-splines [8]. Only linear time algorithms are involved. Another consequence are straight forward Bayesian interpretations.

For several predictor variables we discuss two additive regression models, the alternating conditional expectation model (ACE; [1]) and the generalized additive model (GAM; [4]). The idea of the ACE model is to find non-linear transformations $\theta(y)$, $\phi_1(x_1)$, $\phi_2(x_2), \ldots, \phi_p(x_p)$ of the response y and the predictors x_1, $x_2, \ldots, x_p$, respectively, such that the additive model

$$\theta(y) = \sum_{j=1}^{p} \phi_j(x_j) + \varepsilon$$

is an adequate approximation for the data, where the error ε is independent of the x_js. In the iterative backfitting procedure the conditional expectations are evaluated by scatterplot smoothers. The convergence criterion is based on a goodness-of-fit measure.

Having a response and predictors as introduced above a GAM is defined by

$$y = g_0 + \sum_{j=1}^{p} g_j(x_j) + \varepsilon$$

where the g_j are regression functions and the error ε is independent of the x_js. The predictor effects are additive and can be examined separately in the absence of interactions. The estimation is based on the backfitting algorithm in an iterative manner until some convergence criterion, usually the residual sum of squares, is fulfilled. Again the conditional expectations are evaluated by scatterplot smoothers. For a model with a logit link (binomial response) the local scoring algorithm [4] is applied in which backfitting is the core.

3 Software for non-parametric regression techniques

3.1 BATHSPLINE

Univariate non-parametric regression with cubic smoothing splines can be carried out in BATHSPLINE [7]. BATHSPLINE is an interactive spline smoothing package in which all aspects of Silverman's approach [8] are realised. This includes the handling of weighted observations, the cross-validatory choice of the smoothing parameter, inference regions, and regression diagnostics. The B-spline approach is used throughout the package. Other scatterplot smoothers are not implemented.

Data editing facilities are available in BATHSPLINE. It is operated by control words in an easy-to-use manner. The package is written in FORTRAN and supports external systems for interactive high resolution graphics. It runs on mainframes and workstations. For a discussion and examples see [5].

3.2 XploRe

All discussed non-parametric regression techniques, uni- as well as multivariate, are implemented in XploRe [2], a graphically oriented computing environment for exploratory regression and data analysis. Kernel approximations using WARPing are extensively used. The standard kernel functions are of uniform, triangle, Epanechnikov, quartic or triweight shape. Cross-validation and several other methods for bandwidth (smoothing parameter) selection are at one's disposal. Bias corrected and robust techniques are available. Confidence bands can be calculated. Kernel-evaluated cubic spline smoothing is offered as well. In the ACE model a special scatterplot smoother, called supersmoother, is used. For GAM there are both kernel (i.e. WARPing) and k-nearest-neighbors smoothing at one's choice, the latter not very valuable from our experience. Cubic splines are missing in the two models.

XploRe is a menu-operated, object oriented, open system, implemented in TURBO PASCAL, which can be programmed. Associated problems including examples are described in [6]. XploRe does not comprise an editor but offers vector manipulations. XploRe runs on AT-compatible personal computers.

3.3 S-PLUS

Several of the described non-parametric regression techniques are or will be available in S-PLUS [9]. S-PLUS is an interactive computing environment which consists of a powerful graphics system, a data analysis system and an advanced statistical programming language called New S. Standard kernel smoothing is implemented, comprising box, triangle, Parzen and normal kernel functions. Cross-validation is available for bandwidth selection. S-PLUS does not offer spline smoothing. The ACE model and a variance stabilising variant of it are also implemented. As in XploRe the supersmoother is used. Specific transformation types (e.g. monotone) are an option. GAMs will be availabel in the next release of S-PLUS including all the features described in [4]. Different from the XploRe realisation, numerous scatterplot smoothers will be provided and a more sophisticated convergence criterion considering also the single regression functions will be used.

S-PLUS is a command operated, object oriented system, implemented in FORTRAN and C with an interface to these languages. External editors can be activated by S-PLUS functions. S-PLUS runs on workstations and AT-compatible personal computers.

4 Conclusions

The available software allows biometricians to analyse variousregression problems in a non-parametric fashion. The most versatile package in terms of implemented techniques is XploRe. When being exclusively interested in univariate cubic spline smoothing, BATHSPLINE is the best choice. S-PLUS can be recommended for statistical programming and in the near future also because of its sophisticated implementation of GAMs.

[1] BREIMAN, L. & FRIEDMAN, J.H. (1985): Estimating optimal transformations for multiple regression and correlation (with discussion). JASA 80, 580-619.
[2] BROICH, T., HÄRDLE, W. & KRAUSE, A. (1991): XploRe. A computing environment for eXploratory Regression and data analysis. Springer, New York.
[3] HÄRDLE, W. (1990): Applied nonparametric regression. Cambridge University Press, Cambridge.
[4] HASTIE, T. J. & TIBSHIRANI, R. J.(1990): Generalized additive models. Chapman and Hall, London.
[5] SCHIMEK, M. G., (1990): Non-parametric spline regression by BATHSPLINE: Foundations and application. In FAULBAUM, F., HAUX, R. & JÖCKEL (eds.). SoftStat '89. G. Fischer, Stuttgart, 224-234.
[6] SCHIMEK, M. G., KUBIK, W. & SCHMARANZ, K.: The programming of XploRe (in preparation for Statistics and Computing).
[7] SILVERMAN, B. W. & WATTERS, G. W. (1984): BATHSPLINE. An interactive spline smoothing package. University of Bath.
[8] SILVERMAN, B. W. (1985). Some aspects of the spline smoothing approach to non-parametric regression curve fitting (with discussion). JRSS B, 47, 1-52.
[9] STATISTICAL SCIENCES, INC. (1990): S-PLUS for DOS. Seattle, Wa.

Confidence Regions on Optimal Drug or Treatment Combination

M.J. de Matos Barbosa and Rosa O. Reis

Department of Biomathematics and Medical Informatics

Faculty of Medicine, University of Coimbra - PORTUGAL

Abstract

With Toxic drugs, to find the optimal dosage levels, when two or more drugs are combined in the treatment, is a rather complex problem. The best way to analyse this kind of problem is to apply Response Surface Methodologies (RSM) which can be presented through Contours of Continuous Response. In theses contours , the darker shade or the higher digits represent the optimal treatment region and whithin its bondaries will lie the best dosage levels for each drug in the combination. However, some constrains must be set in order to avoid significant toxicity. And a confident region of $100(1-\alpha)\%$, which includes the optimal treament level, is indeed the best solution to help the analysis of the problem. In this paper, we are concerned mainly how to calculate such confidence regions. But a brief explanation about the whole process will be given.

Keywords: Response surface methodologies, Optimization methods, Multi Logistic Regression, Asymptotic properties, Maximum-likelihood estimation.

1 - Introduction

With the toxic drugs, the traditional way of doing the pre-clinical or clinical analysis, is applying the various dosages of the drugs in the combination, simultaneously or at different times, to several groups of animals or patients and comparing the results of the treatments with a group used as control, to which no medication is given. Of course, experimentation on patients has very severe ethical problems and toxicity has to be avoided at all costs. However, the simplest way to do this kind of the analysis is through a traditional two-dimention graphic. This process is effective if a single drug is used. But adding more drugs to the treatment, all the process becomes a rather complicated and cannot be done efficiently through the above type of graphic, because with two drugs it would need a three dimension one and with three a fourth dimension and so forth... Things can get yet more complicated if the drugs are given at different dosage and time combinations. To deal with this kind of problem, the best way, so far, is applying the Response Surface Methodologies (RSM), which involves statistical inference, mathematical optimization and multi-regression analysis techniques. With this method, the optimal area of response dosage levels used in the treatment, can be observed visually as it is indicated by the most dark shade area or by the area which enclose the highest digits used in the contour plots, as represented in figure 1.

2 - The Logistic Model

The best type of Multi-Regression applied to solve this kind of problems is Cox's Multi-linear Logistic Regression if does not envolve the variable time. But if it does, then the Porportional or the Non-Proportional Hazard Function, according to the situation, is more adequate. The main reason which makes this type of model more proper, is due to the fact that it envolves the identification of risk factors and the perdiction of the probability of developing, for exemple, certain type of cancer or the probability of response to risk factors, such toxicity, on an individual. The variable is of dichotomous type, that means that: either $y=1$ if there is success or $y=0$ if there is insuccess. Besides, the independent variables can be of quantitative or qualitative types. The probability of success may be expressed by

$$P_i = \frac{\exp\left(\alpha + \sum \beta x\right)}{1 + \exp\left(\alpha + \sum \beta x\right)} = \frac{1}{1 + \exp\left(-\left(\alpha + \sum \beta x\right)\right)} \tag{2.1}$$

And we know that $\lambda_i = \ln\left(\dfrac{P_i}{1 - P_i}\right) = \alpha + \sum \beta x$ is a linear function of $\underline{x}$

One of the most efficient way to estimate the coefficients $\underline{\beta}$ is through the Maximum-likelihood method which is done on the following lines. Let $y_1, y_2, \dots y_n$ be the dichotomous observation on the n individuals. The Likelihood of $P_i / (1-P_i)$ is given by :

$$L(\alpha, \hat{\beta}_1, \hat{\beta}_2, \dots \hat{\beta}_r) = \frac{\prod\limits_{i=1}^{n} \exp\left(\alpha + y_i \sum \hat{\beta} x\right)}{\prod\limits_{i=1}^{n} \left[1 + \exp\left(\alpha + \sum \hat{\beta} x\right)\right]} \tag{2.2}$$

If we put $T_j = \sum\limits_{i=1}^{n} x_{ij} y_i$ the Log–Likelihood function will be:

$$LL(\alpha, \hat{\beta}_1, \hat{\beta}_2, \dots \hat{\beta}_r) = \sum\limits_{j=1}^{r} \hat{\beta}_j t_j - \sum \ln\left[1 + \exp\left(\alpha + \sum\limits_{j=1}^{r} \hat{\beta} x_{ij}\right)\right] \tag{2.3}$$

So that the Maximum-likelihood estimates of $\underline{\beta}$ that maximize LL can be obtained by solving the following r equations:

$$T_j = -\sum_{i=1}^{n} \frac{x_{ij} \exp\left(\alpha + \sum_{j=1}^{r} \hat{\beta}_j x_{ij}\right)}{1 + \exp\left(\alpha + \sum_{j=1}^{r} \hat{\beta}_j x_{ij}\right)} \qquad (2.4)$$

3 - The application of the model to N groups

If we are analysing N groups, with n_j animals or patients in the jth group, and if k_j represents the number of individuals in the which the jth group had a favorable result with the probability p_i, the function 2.2 can be expressed as :

$$L(\alpha,\hat{\beta}_1,\hat{\beta}_2, \dots \hat{\beta}_r) = \alpha \prod_{i=1}^{N} P_i^{k_i} (1 - P_i)^{n_i - k_i} \qquad (3.1)$$

And if the equation system is solved by an iterative process, such as the Newton-Raphson, we need a second derivative of the Log-likelihood function, and our model will result in a system of linear equations. The solution of this system of equations gives us the possibility of analysing the surface indicating, in general terms, the most adequate dosages. And through the significance of the parameters β estimated, we can also observe the significance of the effects of the drugs used, its toxicity and interaction between them. However, before we utilizing the model to make any prediction we should do a Goodness-of-fit χ^2 test. The significance of the χ^2 can be tested by comparing its value to the $\chi^2_{n-r \, df}$ where r is the number of parameters estimated. Then if $\chi^2 < \chi^2_{n-r \, df}$ the model is adequated. The optimal treatment can be obtained by maximizing $\Sigma \beta x$ in relation to x_{ij}. This optimization can be done either employing a Ridge analysis or by obtaining the minimization of the function $\Sigma \beta x$ by a Simplex method, imposing upon it some determined constraints. To avoid toxic levels we may come to obtain a rather limited space and from the referred optimization, we may get treatment levels which fall outside of the region imposed by our constraints. And as such, we may get areas of toxicity associated within an optimal treatment. Therefore it is very convenient to estimate a region of confidence for the optimal drug combination.

4 - Confidence Region for the optimal drug combination

Taking in consideration the asymptotic properties of the Maximum-likelihood estimators, we can estimate a $100(1-\alpha)\%$ confidence region for the optimal drug combination. If the favorable outcome is the survival behond a certain point in time, such as: days, weeks, months or years, it is adequate to apply the Logistic Regression for finding the probabibity of a favorable outcome. If, for example, we consider the case of applying two drugs, d_1 and d_2, in a treatment, the probability of a favorable outcome is then given by the expression 2.1. Where : d_1 represents the dosage of drug 1; d_2 represents the dosage of drug 2; d_{11} represents the squared dosage of drug 1; d_{22} represents the squared dosage of drug 2; d_{12} represents the interaction of drugs 1 and 2; α is the parameter associated with no treatment or level 0; β_1 is the parameter associated with drug 1; β_2 is the parameter associated with drug 2; β_{11} is the parameter associated with the toxicity of drug 1; β_{22} is the parameter associated with the toxicity of drug 2; β_{12} is the parameter associated with the interaction of drugs 1 and 2. So,the probability of a favorable outcome is related to treatment levels through the expression $\Sigma\beta d$ in such a way that it should be quadratic and the following function should fit:

$$\frac{\partial \sum \beta d}{\partial d} = \beta_j + 2\beta_{jj}d_j + \sum_{i=1}^{m} \beta_{ij} d_i \qquad j = 1,2,....,m \qquad j \neq i \tag{4.1}$$

where m is the number of drugs in the combination used in the treatment. Assuming that the model is correct, the optimal dosage levels $(l_1, l_2, ..., l_m)$ will satisfy the expression:

$$\beta_j + 2\beta_{jj}l_j + \sum_{i=1}^{m} \beta_{ij} l_i = 0 \qquad j = 1,2,....,m \qquad j \neq i \tag{4.2}$$

If the L_j represents the Maximum-likelihood estimator of the equation 4.2 we get:

$$L_j = \hat{\beta} + 2\hat{\beta}_{jj}l_j + \sum_{i=1}^{m} \beta_{ij} l_i \qquad j = 1,2,....,m \qquad j \neq i \tag{4.3}$$

Let $\underline{L}$ represent a vector of m elements of L_j, so that from the asymptotic properties of the Maximum-likelihood estimators we may get $\underline{L} \underset{Asymp}{\cap} N(\mu, V)$ where $\mu = \underline{0}$ and the elements of V are the variances and co-variances of the elements of $\underline{L}$. From this asymptotic distribution we get $\underline{L}^1 V^{-1} \underline{L} \underset{Asymp}{\cap} \chi_m^2$ where all values of $l_j(j=1,2....m)$ satisfy this expression. χ_m^2 df will be in the confidence region of $100(1-\alpha)\%$. So, for the case of two drugs, m=2, and the optimal treatment levels $(l_1$ and $l_2)$ satisfy:

$$\begin{aligned} \beta_1 + \beta_{12}l_2 + 2\beta_{11}l_1 &= 0 \\ \beta_2 + \beta_{12}l_1 + 2\beta_{22}l_2 &= 0 \end{aligned} \tag{4.4} \qquad \begin{aligned} L_1 &= \hat{\beta}_1 + \hat{\beta}_{12}l_2 + 2\hat{\beta}_{11}l_1 \\ L_2 &= \hat{\beta}_2 + \hat{\beta}_{12}l_1 + 2\hat{\beta}_{22}l_2 \end{aligned} \tag{4.5}$$

The variances of $\underline{L}_i$ and $\underline{\beta}_i$ are respectively :

$$V = \begin{bmatrix} \text{Var } L_1 & \text{Cov } (L_1 L_2) \\ \\ \text{Cov } (L_1 L_2) & \text{Var } L_2 \end{bmatrix}$$

(4.6)

$$\text{Var } \hat{\beta}_i = \begin{bmatrix} a_{11} & & & & \\ a_{12} & a_{22} & & & \\ a_{13} & a_{23} & a_{33} & & \\ a_{14} & a_{24} & a_{34} & a_{44} & \\ a_{15} & a_{25} & a_{35} & a_{45} & a_{55} \end{bmatrix}$$

(4.7)

The variance of β is simetrical. All values of (l_1 and l_2) which satisfy $L' V^{-1} L < \chi^2_{2 \text{ d.f}}$ will be in the confidence region of $100(1-\alpha)\%$ for the optimal values of l_1 and l_2, as in figure 2.

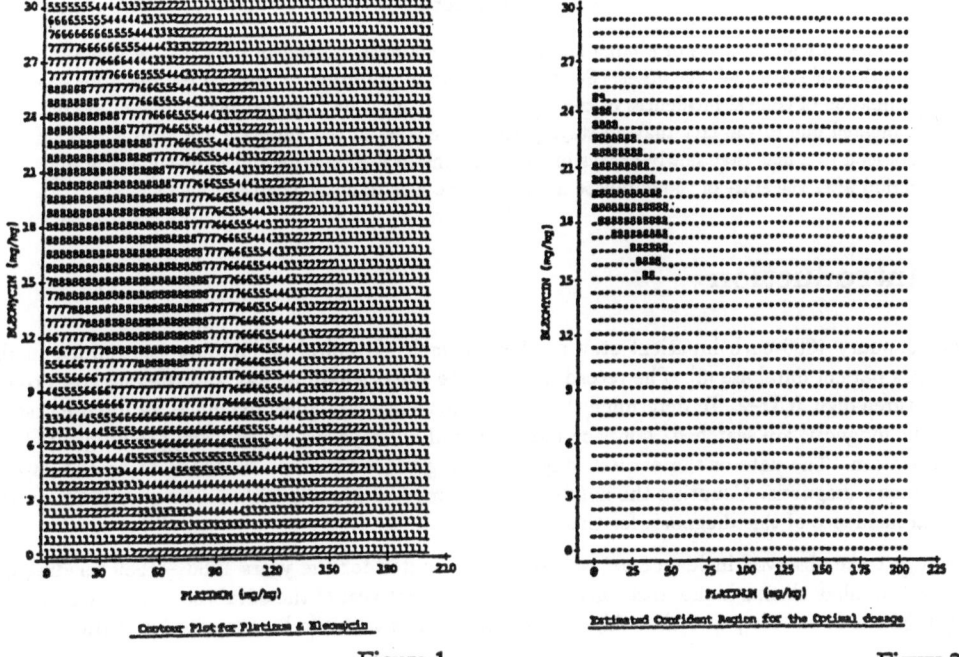

Figure 1   Figure 2

References

Barbosa M.J. (1990)-The use of contour plots for the interpretation of multi-drug combinations. Lecture Notes in Medical Informatics Nº 40 pp 45-47

Box G.E. and Hunter J.S. (1954)-A confidence region for the solution of a set of simultaneous equations with applications to experimental desiign. Biometrika Nº 41, pp 190-199.

Cox D.R. (1972) Regression models and life tables. J.Royal Stas. Society Nº 34, pp 187-220.

Hoerl A.E.(1959) Optimum solution of many variable equations.Chem.Eng.Prog.Nº55,69-82.

Wampler G.L., Carter W.H. and Williams V.R. (1978)-Combination chemotherapy arriiiving at optimal treatment levels by incorporating side effects constrains. Cancer Treat. Rep. Nº62,pp 333-340.

Errors in Estimating the Incidence due to Left-Truncated Data when Using the Hospital's Patient Database — A Modelling Approach —

U. Schrader   A. W. Zaiß   R. Klar

Department of Medical Informatics at the Albert–Ludwigs–University

Freiburg i. Br.

Federal Republic of Germany

Abstract

The patient database of a large hospital contains a huge amount of data that describe the duration of stays and diagnoses. So it is a promising approach to use the database for the estimation of clinical incidences of certain diseases. It must be observed that the data are left truncated due to the fact that no stays prior to the start of the database are recorded. This can lead to a bias that slowly decays in time. A numerical estimation of the bias and the time period after the start of the database needed for the bias to decay is given.

1 Introduction

Since January 1986 each inpatient stay at the University Hospital of Freiburg is recorded in the hospitals patient database [3]. The record includes the start, length of stay and the diagnoses coded in the three-digit ICD–9. To determine the clinical incidence of a given diagnosis all inpatient stays with the diagnosis are searched. For each patient found all stays are linked using the unique patient identification. The date of the earliest stay with the given diagnosis is assumed to be the date of the primary diagnosis. Counting the number of all primary diagnoses within a time period gives the clinical incidence of this diagnosis for this period.

In figure 1 the observed incidence per one year is computed for the years 1986 – 1989 for different diseases. In all of them a higher incidence in 1986 — the first year of the database — can be observed. It will be shown in this paper that this is a systematic bias that can be estimated numerically.

The clinical incidence of a disease is biased by all patients having acquired the disease before the start of the database but returning to the hospital for a further treatment or checkup after the start of the database. Thus there are some patients in the database with only a left truncated history recorded in the database. The date of the first follow–up is then erroneously assumed to be the date of the primary diagnosis. The number of these cases has to be estimated to determine the bias.

2 Deriving the model

To determine the clinical incidence at a given time t_1 the size of the observation period Δt — the time window — must be known. All patients having their primary diagnosis in the time interval $[t_1, t_1 + \Delta t]$ will be counted for the incidence $I(t_1)$ at time t_1. According to figure 2 the patients can be divided into five types:

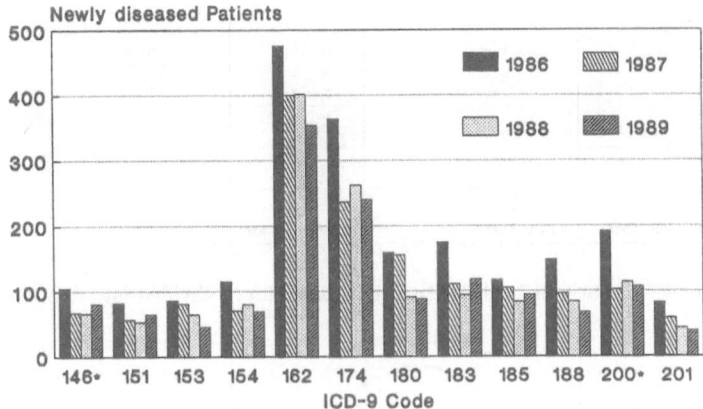

Figure 1: Observed clinical incidence for different carcinoma

1. Patients having their primary diagnosis t_p in the period since the start of the database at t_0 and the start of the window at t_1. These patients are correctly not counted for the incidence. $t_0 \leq t_p < t_1$.

2. Patients having their primary diagnosis t_p after the end of the window at $t_1 + \Delta t$. They are correctly not counted.
$t_p > t_1 + \Delta t$.

3. Patients having their primary diagnosis t_p within the window $[t_1, t_1 + \Delta t]$. They are correctly counted and contribute to the observed incidence.
$t_1 \leq t_p \leq t_1 + \Delta t$.

4. Patients having their primary diagnosis t_p before the start of the database at t_0 but having their first recorded follow-up t_f within the window $t_1, t_1 + \Delta t$. They are *erroneously* counted and so causing the bias in the observed incidence.
$t_p < t_0$ and $t_1 \leq t_f \leq t_1 + \Delta t$.

5. Patients having their primary diagnosis t_p before the start of the database at t_0 but having their first recorded follow-up t_f before the start of the window at t_1. They are correctly not counted.
$t_p < t_0$ and $t_0 \leq t_f < t_1$.

Thus the problem in determining the incidence from the patient database can be stated as follows:

If it was only possible to record all patients after a time t_0, then the incidence is biased by patients having acquired the disease before t_0 and returning after t_0 for a follow-up. This date is assumed to be the date of the primary diagnosis.

So it is possible to start with the approach that the observed incidence I_{obs} at time t_1 consists of a correct I_{corr} and an erroneous part I_{error} adding up:

$$I_{obs}(t_1) = I_{corr}(t_1) + I_{error}(t_1) \quad \text{with} \quad I_{corr}(t_1) = \int_{t_1}^{t_1+\Delta t} i(t)dt. \tag{1}$$

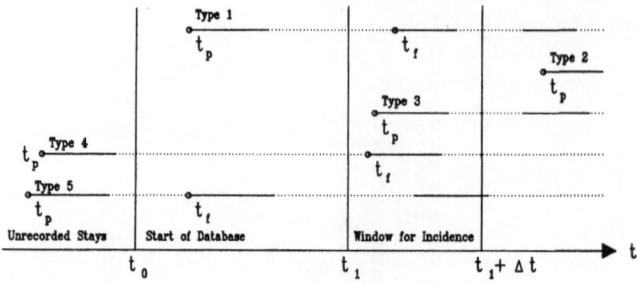

Figure 2: All patients in the patient database can be divided into five types

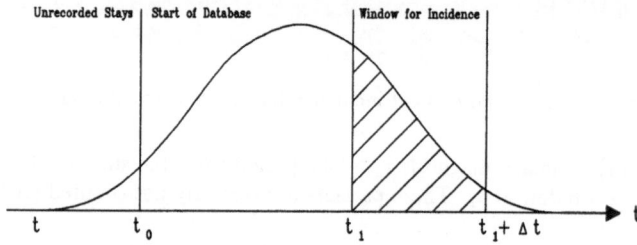

Figure 3: Distribution of the treatment's duration for patients with primary diagnosis at $t < t_0$.

Here $i(t)$ is the number of newly diseased per unit time. To estimate the erroneous part I_{error} the distribution of the duration of the treatment (including follow–ups) must be known. It is assumed that the distributions follows a function $N(\mu, \sigma)$, i. e. a normal or log–normal distribution, that does not change in time. This assumption could be violated by dramatic changes in the treatment itself like the introduction of new procedures. The contribution $\Delta I_{error}(t)$ of all patients diseased at time t before the start of the database t_0 to I_{error} can be discribed as

$$\Delta I_{error}(t_1) = i(t) \int_{t_1}^{\infty} N(\mu + t, \sigma) P(t, t_1 \leq t_f \leq t_1 + \Delta t) d\tau \Delta t. \tag{2}$$

Hereby is $P(t, t_1 \leq t_f \leq t_1 + \Delta t)$ the probability that the first in the database observed follow-up of the patient is within the window $[t_1, t_1 + \Delta t]$ used to determine the incidence. This context is illustrated in figure 3. The complete erroneous contribution to the observed incidence can then be determined by integration over all times t prior to the start of the database at t_0.

$$I_{error}(t_1) = \int_{-\infty}^{t_0} i(t) \int_{t_1}^{\infty} N(\mu + t, \sigma) P(\tau, t_1 \leq t_f \leq t_1 + \Delta t) d\tau \, dt. \tag{3}$$

The only remaining problem is the determination of the probability to observe a follow-up in the window $[t_1, t_1 + \Delta t]$. To estimate this the patient's pattern of recurrence for the specified disease must be known. So a a generalized patient model is contructed. To do this a function $r_i(\tau)$ describing the recurrence of the i–th patient with his primary diagnosis at t_p^i is defined as:

$$r_i(\tau = t - t_p^i) = \begin{cases} 0 & : \quad \text{no begin of a follow–up at t} \\ 1 & : \quad \text{begin of a follow-up at t} \end{cases} \tag{4}$$

If there are n different patients with the specified disease in the database the recurrence of an averaged patient is discribed by:

574

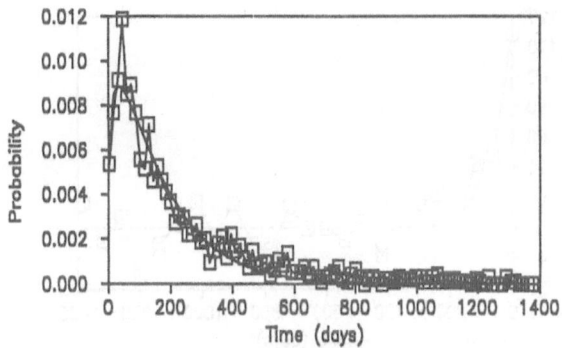

Figure 4: Averaged recurrence of a patient and analytical approximation

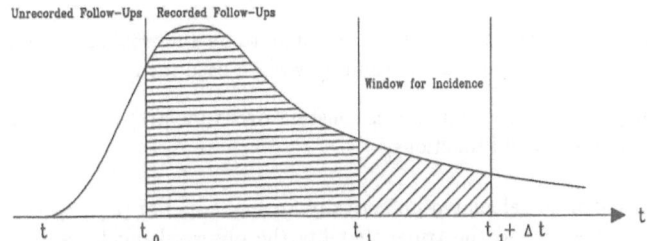

Figure 5: Recurrence of the patients with primary diagnosis at t

$$r_{ave}(\tau) = \frac{1}{n} * \sum_{i=1}^{n} r_i(\tau) \approx a * \tau^b * e^{c\tau} = r(\tau). \tag{5}$$

The value of r_{ave} at time τ is equal to the probability that a patient will return for a follow-up at τ units of time after his primary diagnosis. The area under r_{ave} is equal to the average number of recurrences. The function r_{ave} is further approximated by an analytical function $r(\tau) = a * \tau^b * e^{c\tau}$ for ease of computation. The parameters a, b and c have to be determined for each disease. In figure 4 the averaged recurrences and the analytical function are shown for ICD–174 (breast cancer). Using function $r(\tau)$ the probability $P(t_1 \leq t_f \leq t_1 + \Delta t)$ that a patient diseased at time t will have a first observed follow-up at t_f within the window $[t_1, t_1 + \Delta t]$ can be calculated (see figure 5) as the probability $\neg P_r(t_0 \leq t_f < t_1)$ that he will not come during $[t_0, t_1]$ times the probability $P_r(t_1 \leq t_f \leq t_1 + \Delta t)$ that he will come during $[t_1, t_1 + \Delta t]$.

$$P(t_1 \leq t_f \leq t_1 + \Delta t) = \begin{cases} 0 & \text{if } 1 - P_r(t_0 \leq t_f < t_1) < 0 \\ (1 - P_r(t_0 \leq t_f < t_1)) * P_r(t_1 \leq t_f \leq t_1 + \Delta t) \end{cases} \tag{6}$$

$$\text{with} \quad P_r(t_0 \leq t_f < t_1) = \int_{t_0}^{t_1} r(\tau - t)d\tau.$$

With the help of equation 6 the erroneous part of the incidence as determined by equation 3 can be computed if the distribution $N(\mu, \sigma)$ of the therapy's duration and the rate $i(t)$ of newly diseased per unit time is known. An important conclusion of equation 6 is that the erroneous incidence is reduced to zero at time τ_0 after the start of the database where τ_0 is defined by: $\int_0^{\tau_0} r(\tau)d\tau = 1$.

Under the two assumptions:

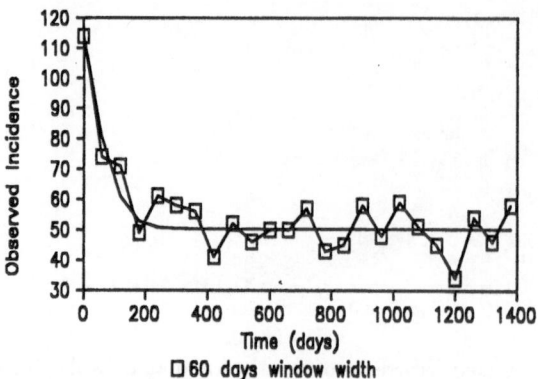

Figure 6: Observed and modeled incidence of ICD–174

- the shape of the distribution is known, for example, to be a normal or log–normal distribution. In the following example a normal distribution will be used for illustration,

- the rate of newly diseased per unit time is constant over time $[i(t) = i]$. This concept can easily extended to time–dependend functions,

the observed incidence can be calculated numerically for any tripel of (i, μ, σ) using equation 3 and 1. This makes it possible to find the tripel that fits the observed incidence best. Generally this is a straight forward minimization problem that can be solved by the Davidon–Fletcher–Powell [1] or Broyden–Fletcher–Goldfarb–Shanno methods [2]. It is helpful that starting values for the mean duration of the therapies and its standard deviation can be calculated directly using the patient database. In figure 6 the observed incidence for the breast cancer (ICD–174) in relation to a two–month wide window since the start of the database is shown. A least square fit using the Davidon–Fletcher–Powell method found the constant incidence to be 306 patients per year. Clearly the bias of the incidence at the start of the database can be seen.

3 Conclusion

In principle it is possible to use the large amount of data in the hospitals patient database for the estimation of incidences. It must be considered that the data may be left truncated and might bias the observed incidences early after the start of the database. An estimate to determine the start of the unbiased data has been given. Under the assumption of constant incidence the effect of bias can be calculated. This assumption can be extended to over known time dependend functions. The above method may be important for early estimation of incidences and early detection of changes in areas like clinical epidemiology, quality assurance, hospital planning, health economy.

References

[1] *Cohen, A.M.:* Numerical analysis. Halstead Press, Wiley, New York 1973.

[2] *Dennis, J.E. and Schnabel, R.B.:* Numerical methods for unconstrained optimization and non-linear equations. Prentice Hall, Englewood Cliffs, N.J. 1983.

[3] *Klar, R. et. al.:* The information system of the Freiburg University Hospital (see these proceedings)

Case Study: Estimation of Drug Effectiveness– Inverse Interpolation of Noisy Data by Nonlinear Least-Squares

Brian R. Stonebridge,* Teresa Lai,† Michael O. Symes†

*Department of Computer Science, Bristol University, University Walk, Bristol, U.K.
†Department of Surgery, Bristol University, Bristol Royal Infirmary, Bristol, U.K.

Abstract

This paper describes a method of using in vitro measurements of drug effectiveness to predict drug performance in vivo. The inhibitions obtained for different drug concentrations in vitro were fitted using a family of non-linear functions, the best of the family being found using a least-squares criterion. In this way, the drug concentration in vitro which would give the same inhibition as observed in vivo was estimated.

The choice of the mathematical model for the general inhibition function, the number of parameters and the asymptotic conditions are considered. The program, which is written in standard Fortran77, forms a package suitable for other applications involving more than one independent parameter.

Here the package is used to give the "best" approximation to the underlying shape of the data and thus allows predictions at intermediate values either of inhibition or concentration. In particular, it allows the prediction of the drug concentration at which the inhibition of protein formation rises to the 50% level.

The results of applying this nonlinear least-squares method to the problem are sufficient to indicate that it gives satisfactory values in the sense that they agree with the in vivo results of drug administration.

A diagram illustrating the method and a table of typical results are included.

Introduction

The ability to predict the effects of an anti-cancer drug before its administration to a patient is of considerable value. However, attempts to do this are dogged by innumerable problems, both in the experimental design and in the processing of the resulting observations.

The aim of this paper is to overcome the problem of noise in the observations when estimating the effects of drugs.

The experimental method

The in vitro inhibition of protein synthesis by cancer cells from 4 mouse mammary tumours following their exposure to 3 increasing concentrations of either Adriamycin (Adr), Cisplatin (Cis-P) or 5-Fluorouracil (5-FU) was measured. It was on the assumption that this would give a good indication of performance in vivo that a comparison was made with the anti-tumour effect (measured as inhibition of pulmonary tumour nodule formation following intravenous infection of isogenic tumour cells) of a single dose of each drug injected into tumour-bearing mice (Table 1).

These sparse sets of data were sufficient for a pilot study. The computer package developed for this investigation will work as well or better for large data sets. It is also applicable to sets of data with non-uniform error expectations, provided these can be quantified and input with the observations.

The choice of the general form of the formula for inhibition

Let the general form of the formula for inhibition be

$$I = f(c, \mathbf{x}) \text{ where } I \text{ is inhibition (\%)}$$

$$c \text{ is the concentration } (\mu g/ml)$$

and $\mathbf{x}$ is the set of unknown parameters.

The formula, $f(c, \mathbf{x})$, must satisfy the end conditions, namely:

when c=0, I=0,

when c is large, I=100.

It is also desirable that the formula shall have as few parameters, the components of $\mathbf{x}$, as possible, whilst still conforming to the characteristic shape predicted by experience of the response obtained when different concentrations of drug are administered in vitro. This ensures that the general *trend* of the observations is fitted rather than the specific readings, which, due to factors outside the control of the observer may be in error compared with accurate readings obtained under ideal conditions.

Any constraints which are known necessarily to prevail are best incorporated into the mathematical formulation, so allowing unconstrained techniques, which are easier to implement and which give identical results, to be employed. Much more is known about the behaviour, the convergence and stability of unconstrained methods than constrained systems and there are thus benefits to be gained by casting the problem in this form.

For the experiments under consideration it was anticipated that the observed response would have a rate of increase which decayed exponentially with increasing concentration. This is most simply expressed as

$$I = 100(1 - e^{-cx^2}) \tag{1}$$

where the value of x (and hence x^2) is to be determined for each set of observations. The x is squared to ensure the desired negativity constraint on the exponent, $-cx^2$, since c is always nonnegative. This means that for all c, I lies in the range 0 to 100.

This choice has restricted the shape of the I to a family of functions, $f(c, \mathbf{x})$, whilst allowing the scale along the c-axis to be determined from the observations.

The least-squares criterion

The choice of the least-squares criterion in fitting noisy data of the type obtained in biological experiments needs some justification. It assumes that the errors of the ordinate, here I, are normally distributed (or are weighted to make them so) and then that the sum of their squares is minimized. This is a statistically sound way of generating the best fit to such data. For further details of the method a numerical methods text, such as Whittaker *et al.* [1], or Stonebridge [2], Section 1, and [3] should be consulted.

Inversion of the formula for inhibition

By straightforward algebraic manipulation we obtain the following formula for the concentration of the drug which would give the same inhibition as the **in vivo** observation, I_v :

$$c_v = -ln(1 - 0.01I_v)/x^2 \qquad (2)$$

The value of x which allows the formula (1) to fit closest to the data was calculated. Then the required concentration, c_v, to give a particular inhibition I_v is determined using the expression on the right-hand-side of equation (2).

At this stage a valuable statistic, denoted IC_{50}, may be calculated. This is the estimated concentration of drug for which 50% inhibition of protein synthesis is obtained:

$$IC_{50} = -ln(1 - 0.01 * 50)/x^2 = -ln(0.5)/x^2 = 0.6931/x^2.$$

Figure 1 shows the fitted curve and sample values for I_v, c_v and IC_{50}.

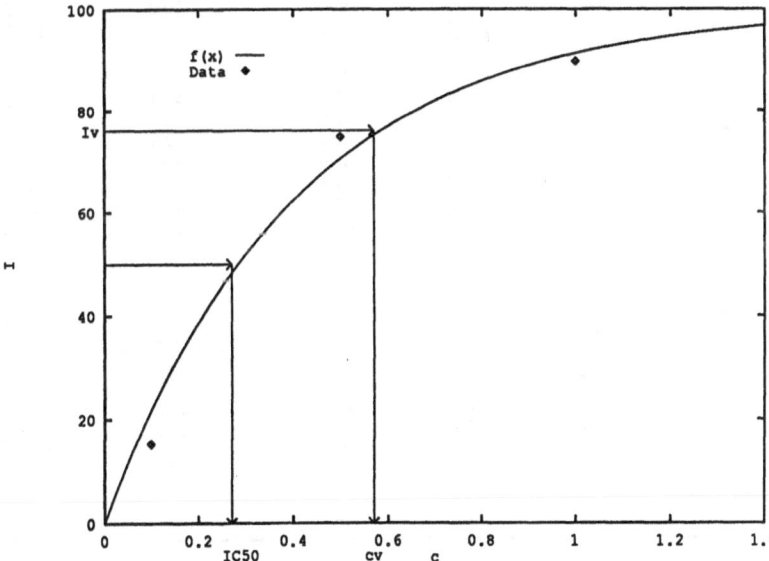

Figure 1: Fitting of Observations and Deduction of the Concentration for 50% Inhibition

Results

The results in Table 1 show the in vitro concentrations of the drugs necessary to produce a degree of inhibition corresponding to the degree of the tumour inhibition observed in vivo.

Comparing the drugs, the most effective, Adr (Adriamycin), was required at a mean concentration of 4.52μg/ml, Cis-P (Cisplatin) at concentration 8.23μg/ml, and 5-FU (5-Fluorouracil) at 75.03 μg/ml in order to produce similar degrees of tumour inhibition in vitro to those seen in vivo. The variances of these 3 figures were in rough proportion to their magnitudes.

Other references to the use of the method are given in the bibliography.

The following table from Lai *et al* [4], p432, contains observations with their corresponding results, c_v, in the final column:

Table 1. Series 1 (8 experiments): a comparison of the percentage inhibition of protein synthesis by mouse mammary carcinoma cells exposed *in vitro*[a] to increasing concentrations of drugs, and the ability of these drugs given *in vivo*[b] to inhibit pulmonary tumour formation following intravenous injection of the tumour cells[c] into isogenic hosts.

Drug	Tumour	Inhibition of protein synthesis (per cent)			Inhibition[d] of pulmonary tumour formation (per cent)	Drug conc in vitro to produce tumour inhibition equal to in vivo effect
ADR (μg/ml)		0·1	1·0	10·0		
	F_1	44·4	82·6	98·0	84·2	0.32
		38·2	98·2	98·6	76·7	0.30
		Nil	Nil	96·7	85·1	9.67
	A_1	17·3	70·1	83·7	95·1	2.35
		0·1	31·8	83·6	88·3	8.30
	A_2	Nil	67·6	93·1	88·8	2.08
		20·2	76·3	91·6	95·3	1.98
	A_3	Nil	15·8	91·5	91·2	11.17
Cis-P (μg/ml)		0·1	1·0	10·0		
	F_1	6·1	16·8	95·3	53·6	3.14
		4·4	4·4	83·4	92·1	16.10
	A_1	22·1	49·2	80·3	92·8	3.60
		15·4	47·7	81·6	96·5	4.99
	A_2	Nil	23·9	77·5	97·5	20.20
		4·2	62·6	92·8	86·4	2.76
	A_3	5·3	35·1	86·7	92·8	6.83
5-FU (μg/ml)		1·0	10·0	100·0		
		0·7	15·9	18·1	24·0	124.53
	F_1	43·3	48·9	54·1	29·2	32.54
		47·8	70·6	73·9	6·8	0.20
		14·7	21·5	35·8	Nil	NIL
	A_1	9·7	Nil	10·3	27·2	292.42
		28·8	58·3	60·0	63·5	65.50
	A_2	3·8	23·4	47·1	39·7	72.38
	A_3	17·5	19·6	1·7	0·5	12.70
Rank difference coefficient		0·28	0·22	0·46		
Significance		NS	NS	<0·025		

[a] Cultured with drug for 2 days and then in the presence of ^{75}SeM for 2 days.
[b] ADR 7·5 mg/kg, Cis-P 5 mg/kg, 5-FU 20 mg/kg i.p. on day 7.
[c] 10^5 cells on day 0.
[d] Inhibition was calculated from the means ($\pm$ S.E.) for lung tumour numbers of treated/untreated mice: E.g. ADR (inhibition) 84·2% = 15·3/97·0 × 100. 5-FU (inhibition) 29·2% = 68·6/97·0 × 100.

Conclusions

The apparent lack of consistency amongst the values obtained is probably an indication of the inherent imprecision which accompanies measurement of response to drugs. Nevertheless, the orders of magnitude of most of the results are consistent, and if more experiments were conducted, the Central Limit Theorem leads us to expect the mean values to be good estimates of the required concentrations. Thus, even with these sparse data sets, valuable results predicting in vivo performance from in vitro observations can be obtained using this technique. This is substantiated by the significant concordance between in vitro observations and in vivo predictions of inhibition at the highest levels of drug concentration tested, Lai *et al* [4]. From this it may be inferred that the effective in vivo concentration of drug obtained is near to the highest tested in vitro. "Better" results would be achieved if one were prepared to eliminate "rogue" readings. However, at this stage, we are loth to discard any information, especially if this is justified only by such slender arguments as a desire for consistency.

This case study was a most satisfactory application of the method described. The data gave well-conditioned equations to solve, which were not susceptible to small changes in the data. Neither weighting of the observations to ensure a "satisfactory" shape of the function, nor damping, to force convergence for an unstable problem, was necessary.

Further work which is envisaged

Several new directions are suggested by these results. To obtain more reliable values, a greater number of observations should be made for each drug at concentrations which are more closely spaced, particularly in the region effective for inverse interpolation from I_v to c_v. If more data were collected, it would be interesting to average those sets of values which are expected to be the same, and so to obtain data for which conform much more closely to one of the family of curves represented by equation (1).

References

[1] E.T. Whittaker and G. Robinson, *The Calculus of Observations*, Blackie and Sons, London, 1937, 214-259.

[2] B.R.Stonebridge, "A Modification of the Levenberg/Marquardt Algorithm for Damped Nonlinear Least-Squares Using a Line Search with Equal-Interval Quadratic Interpolation", Department of Computer Science Technical Report, CS-77-00, University of Bristol, 1977.

[3] B.R.Stonebridge, "Ill-conditioned Least-Squares – Case Study; Trend Surfaces", Department of Computer Science Technical Report, CS-88-01, University of Bristol, 1988.

[4] Teresa Lai, B.R. Stonebridge, Jane Black and M.O. Symes, "Inhibition of protein synthesis, pulmonary tumour formation by drug treated tumour cells, as a means of predicting their chemosensitivity", *Clinical & Experimental Metastasis*, 7, 4, 1989, 427-436.

A CELLULAR GRAMMAR

TO MODEL

METABOLIC PROCESSES

Ralf Hofestädt
Department for Computer Science, University of Koblenz-Landau
Rheinau 3-4, D-5400 Koblenz

Abstract:
A cell is the basic unit of life and can be interpreted as a chemical machine. To study metabolic processes, modelling and simulation are necessary. In this paper a new metabolic model will be presented. We define a grammatical formalism which represents the specification for a simulation program. The advantage of the grammatical formalism is that this formalism allows the definition of metabolic terms to discuss metabolic processes and metabolic phenomena in an easy way. The power of formal languages and automata is a great advantage. So it will be shown that every cellular grammar can be simulated by a chomsky type-3 grammar. This means that metabolism is computable.

1 INTRODUCTION

Every human being consists of approximately 10^{12} cells [1]. With exception of neurons each cell carries a complete set of genetic information which regulates the metabolism. For any medical influence it is necessary to understand the metabolism. To get information about the behaviour of complex metabolic processes, modelling and simulation is an accepted method.

Modelling of chemical processes and biosynthesis is done by theoretical graph approach [2], [3]. The disadvantage of this approach is that it is not possible to handle complex graphs. An algorithm which simulates the metabolism of a whole cell (E. coli) is presented by Weinberg [4]. In this paper we develop a new model which will use a special grammar.

2 CELLULAR GRAMMAR

We base our theory on a simple cell model. This model regards the cell as a compartmented structure, which consists of four components: genetic storage ($\underline{D}$NA), substance concentration, enzyme concentration and substance concentration of the environment ($\underline{u}$). Each component can take on various of states and each cell can be characterized by a 4-tuple of such states. By this way it is possible to give each cell a well defined state in every discrete time interval. Special relations between these sets describe metabolic and genetic processes.

Let Σ_E, Σ_S, Σ_D and Σ_U be finite and not empty sets, then the set
$\qquad \Sigma = \Sigma_E \times \Sigma_S \times \Sigma_D \times \Sigma_U$ is called the $\underline{alphabet}$.

If Σ denotes any alphabet and $e \, \varepsilon \, \Sigma_E$, $s \, \varepsilon \, \Sigma_S$, $d \, \varepsilon \, \Sigma_D$ and $u \, \varepsilon \, \Sigma_U$, than any 4-tuple $z = (e, s, d, u)$ is called $\underline{state}$ of G.

The relations $P_E \subseteq ((\Sigma_E \times \Sigma_D \times \Sigma_U) \times \Sigma_E)$, $P_S \subseteq ((\Sigma_S \times \Sigma_E \times \Sigma_U) \times \Sigma_S)$,
$$P_D \subseteq ((\Sigma_D \times \Sigma_E \times \Sigma_S) \times \Sigma_D) \text{ and } P_U \subseteq ((\Sigma_U \times \Sigma_E \times \Sigma_S) \times \Sigma_U)$$
are defined by $((e, d, u), e') \varepsilon P_E, ((s, e, u), s') \varepsilon P_S, ((d, e, s), d') \varepsilon P_D$ and $((u, e, s), u') \varepsilon P_U$.

Each relation will define a <u>product class</u> and the set $P = P_E \cup P_S \cup P_D \cup P_U$ is called <u>product set</u>. $p \varepsilon P$ is called <u>p-rule</u>.

<u>Def.</u>: *non-deterministic cellular grammar* (ZG)
$G = (\Sigma, P, A)$ with Σ a finite and not empty alphabet, P a finite and not empty product set and the axiom A will be called cellular grammar.

$G = (\Sigma, P, A)$ will be called deterministic cellular grammar, iff P_E, P_S, P_D and P_U are functions.

Moreover, we have to define the derivation of a cellular grammar. This will be done stepwise. First we define the term of applicable rules, after that the action of a p-rule. The derivation will be defined by the parallel action of applicable p-rules.

Any rule $p \varepsilon P$ is called <u>applicable</u> on z, iff

$$\exists e' \varepsilon \Sigma_E \quad p = ((e, d, u), e') \varepsilon P_E \text{ or } \exists s' \varepsilon \Sigma_S \quad p = ((s, e, u), s') \varepsilon P_S \text{ or }$$
$$\exists d' \varepsilon \Sigma_D \quad p = ((d, e, s), d') \varepsilon P_D \text{ or } \exists u' \varepsilon \Sigma_U \quad p = ((u, e, s), u') \varepsilon P_U.$$

For any state z the set $P_E^Z, P_S^Z, P_D^Z, P_U^Z$ and P^Z will be defined by:

$$
\begin{aligned}
P_E^Z &:= \{ p \varepsilon P_E \mid p \text{ is appl. on } z \}, & P_S^Z &:= \{ p \varepsilon P_S \mid p \text{ is appl. on } z \}, \\
P_D^Z &:= \{ p \varepsilon P_D \mid p \text{ is appl. on } z \}, & P_U^Z &:= \{ p \varepsilon P_U \mid p \text{ is appl. on } z \} \text{ and} \\
P^Z &:= P_E^Z \cup P_S^Z \cup P_D^Z \cup P_U^Z.
\end{aligned}
$$

The application of any p-rule $p \varepsilon P^Z$ on z is called the <u>action</u> on z. Every action will produce a state z', which will be constructed as follows:

$$
z' = \begin{cases}
(e', s, d, u) & \text{if } p = ((e, d, u), e') \varepsilon P_E^Z \\
(e, s', d, u) & \text{if } p = ((s, e, u), s') \varepsilon P_S^Z \\
\\
(e, s, d', u) & \text{if } p = ((d, e, s), d') \varepsilon P_D^Z \qquad \text{For the application } p \\
(e, s, d, u') & \text{if } p = ((u, e, s), u') \varepsilon P_U^Z \qquad \text{on } z \text{ we write } z \xrightarrow{p} z'.
\end{cases}
$$

All catalysis, regulation and communication processes in the metabolism are concurrent processes. This is a characteristic of the cellular grammar and can be implemented by simultaneous application of the appropriate p-rules.

Let $G = (\Sigma, P, A)$ be any ZG and $z \varepsilon \Sigma$. A non empty set, $X \subset P^Z$ is called <u>simultaneous applicable</u>, iff for all $y \varepsilon \{E, S, D, U\}$:

$$
|X \cap P_y| = \begin{cases} 0 \text{ if } P_y^Z = \emptyset \\ 1 \text{ if } P_y^Z \neq \emptyset \end{cases}
$$

The set MS^z is given by $MS^z := \{ X \subset P^Z \mid X \text{ is simultaneously applicable on } z \}$.

The concurrent application of the appropriate p-rules on z is called <u>action</u> from X on z. Any action will produce a state $z' = (e', s', d', u')$, which is given by:

- if $X \cap P_E^Z = \emptyset$ than $e' = e$ — if $X \cap P_S^Z = \emptyset$ than $s' = s$
  otherwise $((e, d, u), e') \varepsilon X$ otherwise $((s, e, u), s') \varepsilon X$
- if $X \cap P_D^Z = \emptyset$ than $d' = d$ — if $X \cap P_U^Z = \emptyset$ than $u' = u$
  otherwise $((d, e, u), d') \varepsilon X$ otherwise $((u, e, s), u') \varepsilon X$.

z is called a <u>one-step derivation</u> to z' in G (notation $z => z'$), iff $\exists\, X \,\epsilon\, MS^z$ and the simultaneous action of X on z will procduce z'.

For $n\,\epsilon\, N$ and $n > 1$ z *will be called* <u>*n-step derivation*</u> to z' in G (notation $z \overset{n}{=>} z'$), iff

$$- z = z' \text{ iff } n = 0$$
$$- \exists\, z'' \,\epsilon\, \Sigma \; z \;\; => \; z'' \text{ and } z'' \overset{n-1}{=>} z' \text{ iff } n > 0.$$

z is called <u>derivative</u> into z' (notation $z \overset{*}{\Rightarrow} z'$), iff $\exists\, n\,\epsilon\, N \; z \overset{n}{\Rightarrow} z'$.

The derivation is defined inductively. Any word $x \,\epsilon\, \Sigma^+$ is called <u>derivation</u>, iff

$$|x| = 1 \text{ or}$$
$$|x| > 1 \text{ and } \exists\, y' \,\epsilon\, \Sigma^* \, \exists\, z', z'' \,\epsilon\, \Sigma \text{ with } (x = yz'z'' \text{ and } yz' \text{ is a}$$
$$\text{derivation and } z' => z'').$$

This formalism represents the specification of a simulation program. Advantages of the presented grammatical formalism can be thus summarized:

- theory of automata and languages is powerful (see section 3),
- we can define basic metabolic terms (living-grammar, finite-state),
- we can discuss metabolic phenomena by theory and simulation.

Any state $z \,\epsilon\, \Sigma$ is called <u>attainable</u> in G, iff $A^* => z$.

Σ is called <u>cell-space</u> and attainable states of any cellular grammar can be summarized in a set which will be called <u>metabolic-space</u> R(G).

$AR(G) = \{Ax \mid x \,\epsilon\, \Sigma^* \text{ and } Ax \text{ is a derivation in G }\}$ is called <u>derivation-space</u> of the cellular grammar G.

$z_0 \cdots z_n$ is called <u>cyclic-derivation</u>, iff $\exists\, i\,\epsilon\, \{1, \cdots, n\}\, z_0 = z_i$. Any cyclic-derivation $z_0 \cdots z_n$ is called <u>reproduct</u>, iff $\forall\, i\,\epsilon\, \{0, \ldots, n-1\}\, z_i = z_{i+1}$.

$z \,\epsilon\, \Sigma$ is called <u>finite-state</u>, iff $P^z = \emptyset$.

A cellular grammar $G = (\Sigma, P, A)$ is called <u>living-grammar</u>, iff
$\forall\, n\,\epsilon\, N^+ \, \exists\, v \,\epsilon\, AR(G)\, v = A \cdots z_n$.

As any cell-space is a finite set, the following result is consistent.

<u>Result</u>
Any grammar G is a living-grammar, iff the derivation is cyclic or reproductive.

It is well known that molecular counters regulate metabolic processes. Currently, we do not know a lot about these structures and their function. We will show that a molecular counter can implemented easily using cellular grammar. Fundamental is the reciprocal action between cell components.

Let $G = (\Sigma, P, A)$ be a cellular grammar with the axiom $A = (a, \alpha, k, \beta)$,
$\Sigma_E = \{a, b, c, d, \sigma\},\ \Sigma_S = \{\alpha\},\ \Sigma_U = \{\beta\}$,
$\Sigma_D = \{k, l, m, o\},\ I = \{a, b, c, d\} \subseteq \Sigma_E,\ i\,\epsilon\, I$ and P:

$P_D =$	$P_E =$	$P_S =$	$P_U =$
$\{\,[k_{\overrightarrow{i,\alpha}}\, l],$	$\{\,(a_{\overrightarrow{m,\beta}}\, b),$	$\{\,(\alpha_{\overrightarrow{i,\beta}}\, \alpha)\,\}$	$\{\,(\beta_{\overrightarrow{i,\alpha}}\, \beta)\,\}$
$[l_{\overrightarrow{i,\alpha}}\, m],$	$(b_{\overrightarrow{m,\beta}}\, c),$	Notation : rules in braces	
$[m_{\overrightarrow{i,\alpha}}\, k]\,\}$	$(c_{\overrightarrow{m,\beta}}\, \sigma)\,\}$	denote product classes.	

$(a, \alpha, k, \beta) \overset{*}{\Rightarrow} (\sigma, \alpha, k, \beta)$ is a derivation of G which can be characterized by one-step derivations as follows:

$t_0 = (a, \alpha, k, \beta)$, $\quad t_1 = (a, \alpha, l, \beta)$, $\quad t_2 = (a, \alpha, m, \beta)$, $\quad t_3 = (b, \alpha, k, \beta)$, $\quad t_4 = (b, \alpha, l, \beta)$
$t_5 = (b, \alpha, m, \beta)$, $\quad t_6 = (c, \alpha, k, \beta)$, $\quad t_7 = (c, \alpha, l, \beta)$, $\quad t_8 = (c, \alpha, m, \beta)$, $\quad t_9 = (\sigma, \alpha, k, \beta)$

Component D represents a local cycle which will be count by component E. Moreover, the external regulation can be realized by a specific element $u \, \varepsilon \, U$ which will break the cycle: We have to expand P_E by $[i_{\overrightarrow{j,u}} \, \sigma]$ with $\sigma \, \varepsilon \, \Sigma_E - I$, $i \, \varepsilon \, I$ and $j \, \varepsilon \, J = \{k, l, m\} \subseteq \Sigma_D$.

The cycle will break, if the environment enters the state u (specific hormone) and the derivation of G is in the described cycle.

3   CELLULAR GRAMMAR - FORMAL LANGUAGES

It is not necessary to discuss the metabolic-space of any ZG, because this is always a finite language. In the case of finite languages it is known:

Proposition 1   ([5] proposition 1.3.1)

Every finite language $L \subseteq \Sigma^*$ is a chomsky type-3 grammar.

Just as R(G) is a regular set ([5] proposition 1.3.19), which will be recognized by the finite automata ([5] proposition 2.2.11).

Moreover, AR(G) is regular:

Proposition 2

For every cellular grammar G = (Σ, P, A) there exists a finite automata M= $(Q, \Sigma, \delta, q_0, F)$, with T(M) = AR(G).

Proof:
The finite automata M = $(Q, \Sigma, q_0, F, \delta)$ will be defined by:
   R(G) = $\{z_0, \cdots, z_{n-1}\}$ and $\mid$ R(G) $\mid = n$.
The set of states Q = $\{q_0, q_1, \cdots, q_n\}$ of M will be defined by
   Q = R(G) $\cup \{q_n\}$ with
   f: R(G) $\rightarrow$ Q - $\{q_n\}$ is bijective and $\forall i = 0 \cdots n - 1$ $f(z_i) = q_i$
   $q_0 = f(A)$ is the start-state of M and F = Q - $\{q_n\}$ is the set of the finite-states.

Σ is the input tape and δ be defined as:
   $\delta \subseteq (Q \times \Sigma) \times Q$ is a relation with
            $((q_0, \varepsilon), q_0) \, \varepsilon \, \delta$, because the axiom belongs to AR(G),
            $((q_i, z_j) \, q_j) \, \varepsilon \, \delta$ $\Leftrightarrow$ in G there exists a derivation
                        $f^{-1}(q_i) \Rightarrow z_j$ and $f(z_j) = q_j$,
            $((q_i, z_j), q_n) \, \varepsilon \, \delta$ $\Leftrightarrow$ no one-step derivation
                        $f^{-1}(q_i) \Rightarrow z_j$ and
            $\forall z \, \varepsilon \, \Sigma \, ((q_n, z), q_n) \, \varepsilon \, \delta$ $(i, j = 0 \cdots n - 1)$.

It is easy to see that the finite automata M will simulate the derivation of G so that T(M) = AR(G).

Proposition 3 ([6])

If M is any finite automata, than there will exist a chomsky type-3 grammar G with
L(G) = T(M).

From proposition 1,2, and 3 we can follow that for any ZG G there exists a chomsky
type-3 grammar which will produce AR(G).

4 DISCUSSION

The cellular grammar represents the first grammatical formalism of metabolism. This formalism makes it easy to define and discuss metabolic phenomena and metabolic processes.
The advantage is that formal languages and automata are well-known and powerful. So it
is easy to show that any cellular grammar can be simulated by finite automata or chomsky type-3 grammar (see section 3). This result means that the metabolism of any cell is
computable because any cell component is a finite set. In comparison with mathematical
modelling and quantitative modelling the grammatical formalism is easy to handle, the
abstraction level can be chosen by user.

The developed formalism models the metabolic processes which form the basis of genetic
processes. Moreover, there exist phenomena, which don't respect any legal behaviour.
Such phenomena will rately occur, but they must be taken into account for any simulation. The effects of these phenomena can not be realized in any formalism, but it is easy
to include them in a simulation program. In our simulation program [7] the well-known
phenomena recombination and mutation are described in a special algorithm specification
language. The developed formalism and the simulation program permit the definition,
simulation and discussion of metabolic processes [7].

References

[1] Lewin, B. (1985): Genes, John Wiley & Sons, New York

[2] Kaufmann, S.A. (1969): Metabolic Stability and Epigenesis in Randomly Constructed Genetic Nets, in: Journal of Theoretical Biology, 22, 437-467

[3] Kohn, M. and W. Letzkus (1983): A Graph-theoretical Analysis of Metabolic Regulation, in: Journal of Theoretical Biology, 100, 293-304

[4] Weinberg, R. (1970): Computer Simulation of a living Cell, University of Michigan,
Phd., Department for Computer Science

[5] Maurer, H. (1977): Theoretische Grundlagen der Programmiersprachen, B.I., Mannheim

[6] Aho, A. and J. Hopcroft and J. Ullmann (1975): The design and analysis of Computer Algorithms, Addsison-Wesley Publishing Company, London

[7] Hofestädt, R. (1990): Vom Metabolismus zur genetischen Sprache, University of
Bonn, Phd., Department for Computer Science

A THEORETICAL STUDY OF THE STABILITY OF RESPIRATION

Bruno VIELLE, Gilbert CHAUVET
Institut de Biologie Théorique
10 rue André Boquel, 49100 Angers, France

Abstract : A mathematical model of the human respiratory system is developed for studying the stability of respiration from a theoretical point of view. This model is based on simple assumptions (CO_2 exchanger system and linear controller system), and leads to a nonlinear differential system with delays. By using further mathematical tools such as the Lyapounov-Krasovskii functional techniques, it is demonstrated there exist stationary states which are stable for any values of the delays involved in the respiratory system, i.e., circulatory delays and controller delay. Numerical simulations show the influence of controller parameters on the behaviour of the respiratory system in case of high disturbance.

INTRODUCTION

The stability of respiration is a basic problem in respiratory physiology from both a clinical (Cheyne-Stokes breathing) and a theoretical (respiration control mechanisms) point of view, and has been investigated extensively (e.g., Cherniack [3], Longobardo [8], and Milhorn [9]). However, only few strict mathematical studies of the stability of respiration has been conducted, particularly by Khoo [6].

For the last twenty years, further mathematical tools for the study of delay differential systems have been developed. In this work, they are used in order to study further properties of the stability of the respiratory system, i.e., how the system returns to its steady state after having been disturbed.

MODEL OF THE RESPIRATORY SYSTEM

The respiratory system can be schematically described by two subsystems (Fig.1) :

- *the exchanger system*, made of three components : lungs, tissues, and cardiovascular loop ; only CO_2 is considered ; lungs are represented by a single compartment (monoalveolar representation) which is ventilated by a unidirectional air flow, and where CO_2 is eliminated ; tissues are represented by a single compartment where CO_2 is produced ; CO_2 is carried by circulating blood through the cardiovascular loop which connects lungs and tissues ;

- the controller system : CO2 partial pressures are sensed by chemoreceptors and provided to bulbar centers which adjust lung ventilation in order to maintain CO2 tissue concentrations within physiological range.

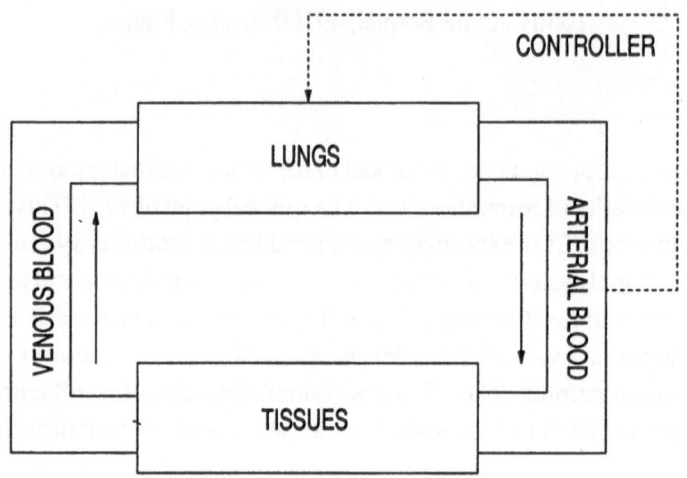

Figure 1 : The two subsystems of the respiratory system : exchanger and controller systems.

The assumptions for this model are : 1) alveolar air and arterial blood leaving the lungs are in equilibrium, i.e., the respective CO2 partial pressures are equal ; 2) tissues and venous blood leaving the tissues are in equilibrium ; 3) CO2 partial pressures and CO2 concentrations in blood and tissues are related by the same linear function ; 4) diffusion and mixing of CO2 have negligible effects in blood along the cardiovascular loop ; and 5) the controller system is a CO2 linear controller, i.e., lung ventilation is a linear function of the CO2 partial pressures.

By using law of mass conservation for lung and tissue exchange areas, the respiratory system is described by the following system (S) :

$$
\begin{cases}
\dfrac{dP_T}{dt}(t) = -\dfrac{Q_B}{V_T}P_T(t) + \dfrac{Q_B}{V_T}P_L(t - r_A) + \dfrac{M}{\alpha V_T} \\[2ex]
\dfrac{dP_L}{dt}(t) = \dfrac{\alpha\gamma Q_B}{V_L}P_T(t - r_V) - \dfrac{\alpha\gamma Q_B + \mu}{V_L}P_L(t) + \dfrac{\lambda P_I}{V_L}P_L(t - r_N) - \dfrac{\lambda}{V_L}P_L(t)P_L(t - r_N) + \dfrac{\mu P_I}{V_L}
\end{cases}
$$

The CO2 partial pressures in tissues P_T and in lungs P_L are state variables. The following parameters are assumed to be constant : volume of tissues V_T , volume of lungs V_L , blood flow in the cardiovascular loop Q_B , CO2 production in tissues M , external CO2 partial pressure P_I , arterial transport delay r_A , venous transport delay r_V , action delay of the controller r_N, factor of conversion between CO2 partial pressures and CO2 concentrations in blood and tissues α, total pressure in air γ, slope of the controller curve λ, and intercept of the controller curve μ.

RESULTS

System (S) is an autonomous differential system with bounded delays, which first is studied analytically and then simulated numerically. Concerning the first part, a straightforward calculus shows the existence and uniqueness of a constant solution Y:

$$Y = \begin{pmatrix} \dfrac{\lambda P_I - \mu + \sqrt{(\lambda P_I + \mu)^2 + 4\lambda\gamma M}}{2\lambda} + \dfrac{M}{\alpha Q_B} \\ \dfrac{\lambda P_I - \mu + \sqrt{(\lambda P_I + \mu)^2 + 4\lambda\gamma M}}{2\lambda} \end{pmatrix}$$

By choosing an appropriate Lyapounov-Krasovskii functional [7] and using a theorem on autonomous differential systems with bounded delays [5], it is demonstrated that solution Y is uniformly asymptotically stable under the following condition (C)

$$(\lambda P_I + \mu)\sqrt{(\lambda P_I + \mu)^2 + 4\lambda\gamma M} - (\alpha\gamma Q_B)^2 > 0$$

for any value of the controller action delay, r_N.

Concerning the simulation, a numerical study of the system (S) is conducted in order to analyze the behavior of solutions that are distant from solution Y. A fourth-order Runge-Kutta method is adapted for solving the differential system with bounded delays. It is shown that the solutions of the system (S) are oscillating time functions (Figs.1 and 2). The controller slope acts on the magnitude of oscillations (Fig.1), and the controller action delay has a substantial effect on both the period and the magnitude of oscillations (Fig.2). By increasing the value of these parameters, solutions of the system (S) do not return to solution Y, as t tends to infinity.

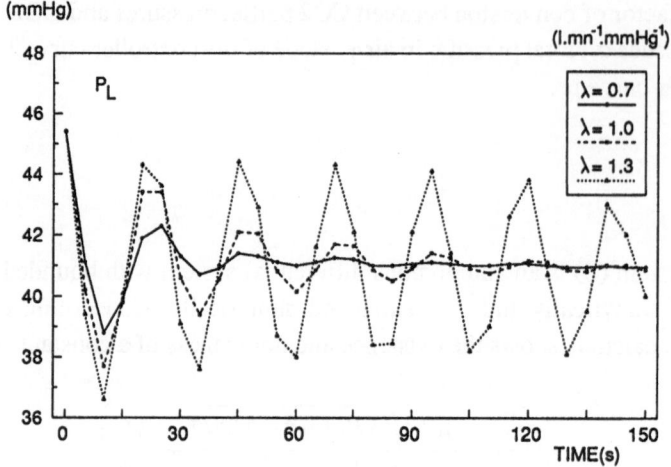

Figure 2 : Influence of controller slope λ on the behavior of solutions of system (S).

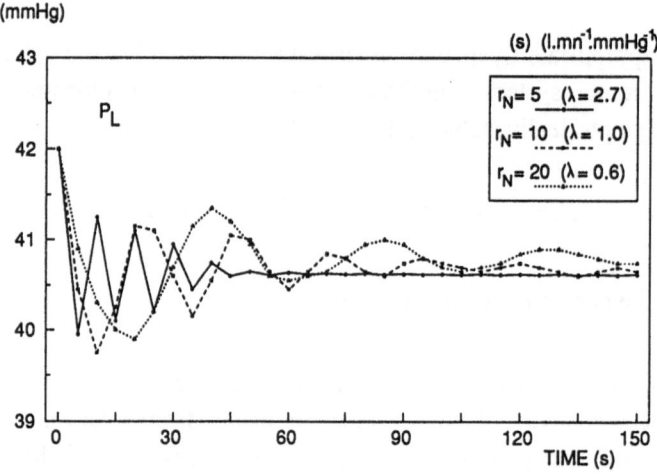

Figure 3 : Influence of controller action delay r_N on the behavior of solutions of system (S).

DISCUSSION

The present model of the respiratory system is similar to that of Milhorn [9] and much simpler than those of Grödins [4] and Saunders [11]. However, this model leads to a differential system whose mathematical properties of stability can be studied analytically. The Lyapounov-Krasovskii functional method seems to be more powerful than the Laplace transform method [6] for the mathematical analysis of stability. Indeed, the results obtained with the former method are independent of the value of the delays included in the differential system.

For any value of the controller action delay, the respiratory system is demonstrated to be stable in the vicinity of the stationary states defined by condition (C). For these stationary states, periodic breathing cannot be induced by small disturbances. It should be noted that condition (C) is sufficient but not necessary. Therefore, the stability of the respiratory system can be enhanced if condition (C) is restricted [12]. Under conditions of high disturbances, controller action delay plays a significant role : for increased values of this parameter, the respiratory system can become unstable. This outcome agrees well with clinical data in humans with brain stem lesions [1] or congestive heart failure [10]. Moreover, preliminary results with such a model in a multialveolar representation [13] lead to do a numerical analysis of stability for cases of ventilatory inequalities [2], which will be applied to obstructive pathology.

REFERENCES

1. BROWN H., PLUM F. - The neurologic basis of Cheyne-Stokes respiration, *Am. J. Med.*, 30, 849-860 (1961).
2. CHAUVET G. - Mathematical study of flow in a non-symmetrical bronchial tree : application to asynchronous ventilation, *Math. Biosc.*, 42, 73-91 (1978).
3. CHERNIACK N.S., LONGOBARDO G.S. - Mathematical model of periodic breathing during sleep, in *Modelling and control of breathing*, Whipp B.J. and Wiberg D.M. Eds., Elsevier Science Publishing Co., 361-368 (1983).
4. GRÖDINS F.S., BUELL J., BART A.J. - Mathematical analysis and digital simulation of the respiratory control system, *J. Appl. Physiol.*, 22, 260-276 (1967).
5. HALE J.K. - *Theory of functional differential equations*, Springer Verlag (1977).
6. KHOO M.C., KRONAUER R.E., STROHL K.P., SLUTSKY A.S. - Factors inducing periodic breathing in humans : a general model, *J. Appl. Physiol.*, 53, 644-659 (1982).
7. KRASOVSKII N.N. - *Stability of motion*, Stanford University Press (1963).
8. LONGOBARDO G.S., CHERNIACK N.S., FISHMAN A.P. - Cheyne-Stokes breathing produced by a model of the human respiratory system, *J. Appl. Physiol.*, 21, 1839-1846 (1966).
9. MILHORN H.T., GUYTON A.C. - An analog computer analysis of Cheyne-Stokes breathing, *J. Appl. Physiol.*, 20, 328-333 (1965).
10. PRYOR W.W. - Cheyne-Stokes respiration in patients with cardiac enlargement and prolonged circulation time, *Circulation*, 4, 233-238 (1951).
11. SAUNDERS K.B., BALI H.N., CARSON E.R. - A breathing model of the respiratory system : the controlled system, *J. Theor. Biol.*, 84, 135-161 (1980).
12. VIELLE B., CHAUVET G. - A mathematical study of stability in the respiratory system (submitted) (1991).
13. VIELLE B., CHAUVET G. - A multialveolar model of lungs : application to ventilatory inequalities (submitted) (1991).

TSOBM: A Tool for the Simulation and Optimization of Biorhythmical Models

T. Sykora, R. Richter
Institut für Angewandte Informatik und Formale Beschreibungsverfahren
Universität Karlsruhe (TH), D-7500 Karlsruhe, Germany

Abstract

TSOBM is a tool designed for users with little skills in computer programming which want to use a personal computer for the development and utilization of simulation models. With TSOBM simulation models can be quickly defined using a comprehensive graphical language. If desired a model can be specified with "open" parameter values. TSOBM will then determine these values by comparing simulation results of the model with data gathered in experiments, thereby tailoring the model to experimentally measured phenomena.

1. Introduction

Computer simulation is attracting increasing interest in medical informatics since it provides a possibility to investigate the behaviour of a biological system under various conditions, without the need of practical experiments. The quality of a simulation depends on the used simulation model. On the basis of experimental data and theoretical research such a simulation model has to be developed. It should fulfil the following requirements:

— Computed data of the model should coincide with experimental data.

— A model should be usable to make predictions (for situations where no experimental data is available).

In this paper we concentrate on the simulation and optimization of biorhythmical simulation models and introduce a tool that was developed in cooperation with the department of psychology at Flinders University in Adelaide, Australia. A first version of the tool was implemented and applied for simulations with small amount of data. Experiences have shown that the system´s execution time is too long for large amount of data. Therefore the tool is presently being tuned. Although it was originally designed for modelling circadian rhythms in sleep research it is also suitable for modelling various other biological rhythms.

Most of the models quoted in the literature consider the biological system of man as a dynamical system. They describe it by using an equation system where all equations depend on time and where the results are also time dependend. Some of the models try to maintain the analogy between biological objects and the structure of the model, whereas others merely describe the external behaviour by giving a mathematical equation system or a biocybernetical description that leads to similar results but regard biological analogies to the model structure as of lower interest.

These dynamical models are suitable for numerical simulation on computers. However, there are a number of difficulties that have to be taken into account:
— The translation of mathematical or biocybernetical models into computer programs is not always trivial.
— The optimization problem of finding the best set of model parameters is very time consuming because it usually goes along with a permanent dialogue between the simulating system and the programmer.
— There are no standardized functions that evaluate the similarity between the model and reality. This decision has to be made by the programmer.
In order to overcome these difficulties, TSOBM was developed.

2. Basic Idea of TSOBM

The basic idea was to develop a tool that would be convenient for building simulation models by providing the following advantages:
— Users not skilled in computer programming should be able to define simulation models.

- Simulation models are presented graphically in a way that is related to the presentation of biocybernetical models.
- The evaluation of the model, based on the comparison between computed and experimental data, is already part of the functionality of the tool.
- The tool is able to find an optimal set of parameter values in order to show whether a simulation model is able to explain experimentally measured phenomena.

A simulation model is defined by a collection of objects, i.e. logical units representing concrete or abstract biological entities (e.g."body temperature"), a collection of dependencies between objects (e.g."body temperature is decreased by sleep"), and a collection of numerical parameters (e.g. "1", giving the decrease of the body temperature). An object is described by characteristic attributes and is graphically represented by an appropriate symbol. The values of the attributes reflect the state of an object. A dependency is described by a function and is graphically represented by a "wire" connecting the associated objects. Parameters are used to complete functions, thereby tailoring a simulation model to specific purposes. Connected objects influence each other: At a time the state of an object depends on its input parameters and its "predecessor objects", which in turn may depend on the object itself (feed-back loop).

Not all values of the parameters need to be known at the time when the simulation model is defined. The tool is able to determine these values by using an appropriate optimization algorithm.

Using integral and differentiation operators as functions the analogy to differential equations is given. Yet, the approach proposed in this paper is far more comprehensive.

3. Developing Simulation Models with TSOBM

TSOBM is based on LabVIEW, a graphical programming language produced by National Instruments for Apple personal computers.

The definition and evaluation of a simulation model has the following phases:

1.) Model specification using the graphical interface of TSOBM.

In order to specify a simulation model, a user sets up a graphical structure of block elements representing objects and parameters by placing the elements on a spreadsheet and connecting them via "function wires". All graphical elements are predefined and provided by TSOBM. For more complex structures the user may aggregate several elements into a module which then can be used as a simple element at a higher level. In essence, a simulation model is represented as a network of object and parameter symbols and wires (see fig. below).

An example for a very simple model structure:

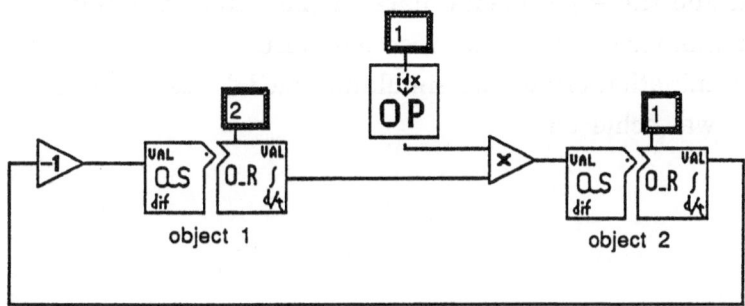

The elements of the structure are
— "objects": dynamical parts of the model which change their value with time (the integral and first differential is stored with them as well)
— "functions": here: a multiplication (x-symbol) and a negation (-1 symbol)
— "wires": connections between all other elements passing their values as inputs into other elements
— "open parameter": represented with the OP-symbol is a numerical value which stays constant during a simulation but is not defined. Its exact value must be found during the optimization.

Two objects in the model influence each other in a feedback-loop:
— object 1 is the negative of object 2
— object 2 is the integral of object 1 multiplied by an unknown value (OP-symbol).
The result is a sinusoide.

2.) Simulation.

After the objects have been initialized, subsequent states are computed for discrete time steps by interpreting the simulation model. The length of a time step can be set by the user.

3.) Optimization of parameters and evaluation of a simulation model.

It often occurs that a simulation model is based on an idea of a certain structure, while the values of some parameters still have to be determined. TSOBM allows to define such "open" parameters, i.e. parameters that have no predefined fixed values. Instead, the user may define estimated (most probable) values and probabilistic distributions. Using these informations and experimental data, TSOBM tries to find optimal values in the sense that the obtained simulation model closely mirrors the desired part of the real world.

In order to find out the quality of a simulation model the user defines an appropriate criteria. Usually, this is done by specifying a bound for the difference between the computed and the experimental data. If the criterion is fulfiled, the optimization algorithm terminates, otherwise new values for the parameters are tried. After termination either the simulation model has to be redefined or a "good" model was achieved.

4. Conclusion

With TSOBM even users not skilled in computer programming are able to develop simulation models for biological systems. Simulation models can be easily defined and executed. If "open" parameters are used, the system will determine suitable values for them.

References

[1]   R.W. Danielis: An Introduction to Numerical Methods and Optimization Techniques, 1978
[2]   Emshoff and Sisson: Design and Use of Computer Simulation Models, New York, 1970
[3]   G. Gordon: System Simulation, Prentice-Hall, 1969
[4]   Moor-Ede and Czeisler: Mathematical Models of the Circadian Sleep-Wake Cycle, Springer-Verlag, 1986
[5]   National Instruments: LabVIEW - Scientific Software for the Macintosh, National Instruments Corporation, Austin, Texas, 1988
[6]   Seaty and Alexander: Thinking with Models, Oxford, 1981
[7]   Strogatz: The Mathematical Structure of the Human Sleep-Wake-Cycle, Springer-Verlag, 1986
[8]   Trappl: Cybernetics - Theory and Applications, Springer-Verlag, 1976

A NON-LINEAR MODEL OF INSULIN KINETICS

R. Hovorka[1,2,3], J.K. Powrie[2], G.D. Smith[4],
E.R. Carson[1,2], P.H. Sonksen[2,1] and R.H. Jones[2]

[1] City University, London, U.K., [2] St. Thomas's Hospital, London, U.K.
[3] Charles University, Prague, Czechoslovakia, [4] MRC Clinical Research Centre, Harrow, U.K.

Abstract. A five compartment model including receptor-mediated insulin degradation is proposed to simulate insulin processing during hyperinsulinaemic euglycaemic clamps. Several physiological constraints were employed to limit the number of parameters which remained to be resolved from the experimental data. The model gave estimates of otherwise inaccessible parameters and also predicted the time course of insulin concentration in various physiological compartments. The model was validated by comparing the summarised variables, i.e. receptor association, receptor affinity, basal degradation in kidney, liver and periphery, to corresponding values from the medical literature.

INTRODUCTION.

Various compartmental models have been proposed to mimic the processing and disposal of insulin [1,3,7]. The majority of these models are linear although there is strong evidence that the insulin degradation pathway in the liver is saturable [5] and that metabolic clearance rate of insulin decreases as insulin concentration increases [17,19]. Insulin is degraded in the liver and in the peripheral tissues via a receptor mediated pathway [4]. The saturation of insulin degradation is due to the finite number of insulin receptors. The process of insulin binding can be modelled by Langmuir dynamics [2]. We have employed two such receptor systems, one to represent the periphery and one to represent the liver, as there is a significant difference in their access to insulin. In addition, linear degradation was included in the plasma compartment, modelling non-receptor mediated degradation, e.g. renal excretion. Prior to modelling, we calculated prehepatic insulin secretion from C-peptide data and directed this input into the liver compartment thus distinguishing between endogenous production (directed into the liver) and exogenous infusion (directed into the systemic circulation). This allowed us to estimate model parameters which correspond to both basal and experimental conditions.

MODEL DESCRIPTION.

A five compartment model is proposed to mimic insulin kinetics in man during hyperinsulinaemic euglycaemic clamp studies, see Fig. 1. This model is an extension of previous work published by Jones et al [15]. The three compartments (plasma insulin, hepatic insulin and interstitial insulin) are linearly connected, the remaining two compartments (insulin bound to hepatic receptors and insulin bound to peripheral receptors) are connected to hepatic and interstitial insulin via a receptor-mediated link. Insulin degradation appears in the two receptor compartments (endocytosis) and in the plasma compartment (linear degradation, e.g. renal excretion). The differential equations which uniquely define the model are given in the Appendix.

The model has two inputs: endogenous insulin secretion and exogenous insulin infusion. Endogenous secretion is calculated from individual C-peptide levels using the deconvolution technique [6] and is directed into the hepatic compartment. The exogenous insulin infusion is directed into the plasma compartment.

The following constraints have been adopted in the model:
i) hepatic plasma volume V_3 is 4.95 ml kg^{-1} [14], plasma volume V_1 is 45.05 ml kg^{-1} and interstitial volume V_2 is 150 ml kg^{-1} [13]

ii) net flow between plasma and interstitial compartments is given by the concentration gradient thus

$$k_{12} = k_{21} \frac{V_1}{V_2} \tag{1}$$

iii) plasma hepatic flow is 30% of cardiac output [9,13] and thus

$$k_{31} = \frac{0.3 \; CO}{V_1} \tag{2}$$

$$k_{13} = \frac{0.3 \; CO}{V_3} \tag{3}$$

where cardiac plasma output CO is a product of body surface area S and cardiac index CI [13]

$$CI = 1760 \; ml \; m^{-2} \tag{4}$$

$$S = 0.007184 \; W^{0.425} H^{0.725} \tag{5}$$

$$CO = CI \; S \tag{6}$$

where W is weight [kg] and H is height [cm].

iv) the association, dissociation and endocytotic rate constants of liver receptors are equal to those of peripheral receptors

Figure 1. The five compartment model of insulin kinetics. Several constraints (see text) have been employed to limit the number of parameters to be estimated from the experimental data. The free parameters are indicated by ‡ (7 parameters out of 16).

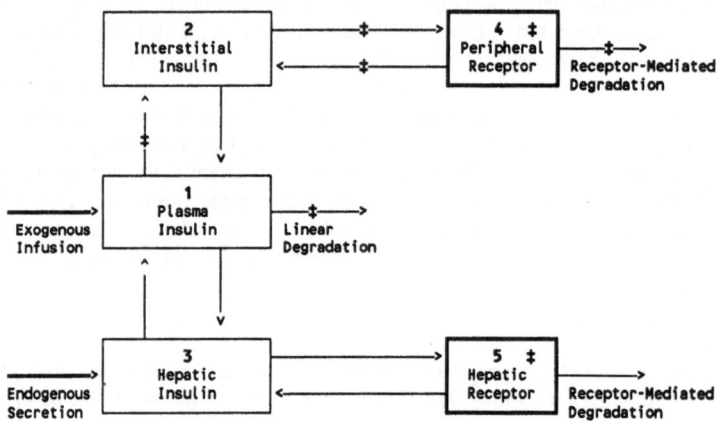

EXPERIMENTAL PROTOCOL.

Ten patients with non-insulin dependent diabetes mellitus underwent two stage, hyperinsulinaemic euglycaemic clamps. A primed continuous infusion of human soluble insulin was introduced at a rate 1 mU kg^{-1} min^{-1} and continued for 2 hours. It was immediately followed by a primed continuous 8 mU kg^{-1} min^{-1} infusion for a further 2 hours. The exogenous insulin infusion was then stopped but the glucose clamp continued for a further 90 min. More details about the protocol and assay procedures are given in [18].

MODEL IDENTIFICATION.

In each subject, seven model parameters (k_{01}, k_{21}, k_{42}, k_{24}, k_{04}, R_4 and R_5) remained to be estimated. The model can be shown to be theoretically identifiable although not uniquely [2]. Parameter estimation was carried out using a non-linear least-square regression of Marquardt [16] with in-house implementation. The sum of weighted squares of differences between predicted and observed plasma insulin concentrations was minimized. The error in plasma insulin measurement was assumed to have a Poisson distribution, i.e. weights were defined as reciprocals of each datum. The precision of estimation of an individual parameter for one experiment was calculated from the inverse of the Fisher information matrix [2] and expressed as the coefficient of variation (CV) of the parameter estimate.

RESULTS.

A typical experiment is shown in Fig. 2. The mean values of 7 parameters estimated from 10 experiments are shown in Table 1 together with the CV of parameter estimates. In one subject, the CV of two parameter estimates are over 100 % indicating that these parameters are resolved from the experimental data with decreased precision.

Figure 2. *Typical experiment showing measured plasma insulin, computer fit of plasma insulin and simulated concentrations of hepatic and extracelluar insulin.*

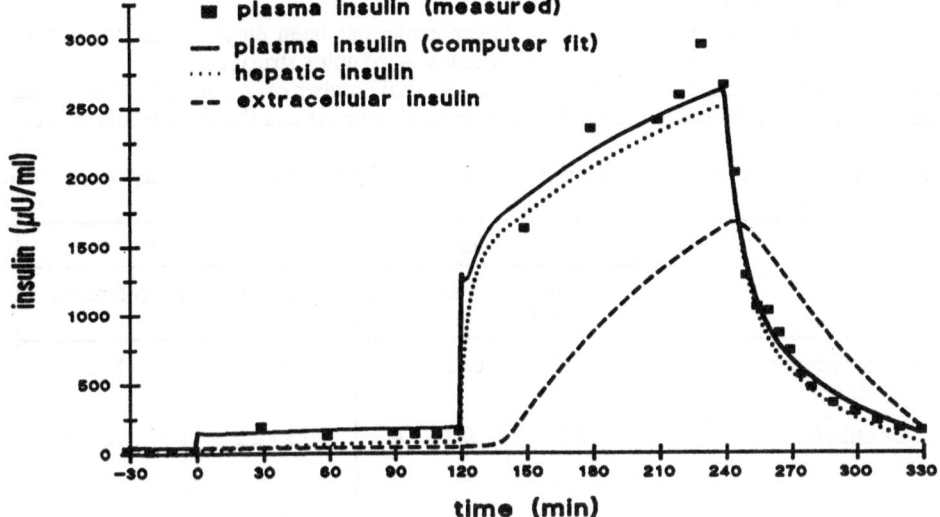

Table 1. *Estimated parameters and the CV of parameter estimates for 10 patients.*

	parameter estimates N = 10		coefficient of variation of parameter estimates (%)	
	mean	range	mean	range
k_{01} (min^{-1})	0.041	0.018 - 0.068	31	11 - 130*
k_{21} (min^{-1})	0.050	0.011 - 0.090	29	4 - 150*
k_{42} (min^{-1})	.84	0.11 - 2.92	17	2 - 43
k_{24} (min^{-1})	0.080	0.018 - 0.163	47	4 - 93
k_{04} (min^{-1})	0.015	0.005 - 0.023	21	4 - 52
R_4 (μU kg^{-1} 10^3)	134	65 - 229	36	7 - 93
R_5 (μU kg^{-1} 10^3)	208	83 - 461	21	5 - 49

* The CV of parameter estimate is greater than 100 % in subject 10 (CV of k_{01} = 130 %, CV of k_{21} = 150%)

DISCUSSION.

A non-linear model including receptor-mediated insulin degradation has been employed to model insulin kinetics in man during hyperinsulinaemic euglycaemic clamp studies. The need for a non-linear model is illustrated by the observation that the metabolic clearance rate of insulin falls from 11.9 to 5.1 ml kg^{-1} min^{-1} when plasma insulin concentration increases from 124 to 2114 mU ml^{-1}.

A complex model structure has been selected. The model was built to represent basic physiological structure rather than to mimic the observed plasma insulin profile using a minimal approach. Physiological constraints are used to limit the number of free parameters to be resolved from the experimental data. However, these constraints may limit the validity of the results obtained for individual patients. The model distinguishes between two insulin inputs. The endogenous insulin secretion is directed into the hepatic pool, the exogenous infusion into systemic plasma, and therefore the processing of these two inputs differs.

Several other parameters can be derived from the model parameters and can be employed to validate the model. Table 2 contains some derived parameters and compares them to values reported in the literature.

In summary, a five compartment non-linear model has been employed to mimic insulin kinetics during hyperinsulinaemic euglycaemic clamps. A complex structure enables estimates of otherwise inaccessible parameters to be obtained, e.g. total number of insulin receptors, and also, the time course of insulin concentration in the hepatic circulation and the extracelluar space.

Table 2. *Some other parameters as derived from the model parameters and corresponding values reported in the literature.*

	derived		reported	
	mean (N=10)	range	range	reference
receptor association (l nmol^{-1} min^{-1})	0.12	0.02 - 0.34	0.025 - 0.23[*]	[11,12]
receptor affinity (l nmol^{-1})	2.1	0.3 - 7.4	0.3 - 2.5[*]	[10,12]
linear degradation at basal state (% of total degradation)	9	4 - 13	10[+]	[8]
peripheral degradation at basal state (% of total degradation)	9	3 - 18	9	[8]
liver degradation at basal state (% of total degradation)	82	72 - 92	80	[8]

[*] Association and affinity as assessed in *vitro* studies
[+] The value reported is the kidney degradation

ACKNOWLEDGEMENT.

The study was supported by grants from the Wellcome Trust, the British Diabetes Association, the Hordern Fund and the Robert Graves research fund.

APPENDIX.

The model is described uniquely by a set of differential equations:

$$\frac{dx_1}{dt} = - (k_{01} + k_{21} + k_{31})x_1 + k_{12}x_2 + k_{13}x_3 + u_1 \tag{7}$$

$$\frac{dx_2}{dt} = + k_{21}x_1 - k_{12}x_2 - k_{42}(1 - \frac{x_4}{R_4})x_2 + k_{24}x_4 \tag{8}$$

$$\frac{dx_3}{dt} = + k_{31}x_1 - k_{13}x_3 - k_{53}(1 - \frac{x_5}{R_5})x_3 + k_{35}x_5 + u_2 \tag{9}$$

$$\frac{dx_4}{dt} = + k_{42}(1 - \frac{x_4}{R_4})x_2 - (k_{04} + k_{24})x_4 \tag{10}$$

$$\frac{dx_5}{dt} = + k_{53}(1 - \frac{x_5}{R_5})x_3 - (k_{05} + k_{35})x_5 \tag{11}$$

$$y = \frac{x_1}{V_1} \tag{12}$$

where x_i is the mass of insulin in compartment i [μU], $R_{4(5)}$ is the mass of peripheral (hepatic) receptors sites [μU], k_{ji} is the fractional turnover constant from compartment i to compartment j [min^{-1}], V_i ($i = 1,2,3$) is the volume of compartment i [ml], u_2 is endogenous insulin secretion [μU min^{-1}], u_1 is exogenous insulin infusion [μU min^{-1}] and y is plasma insulin concentration [μU ml^{-1}].

REFERENCES

1. BERMAN, M., E.A. MCGUIRE, J. ROTH, and A.J. ZELEZNIK. Kinetic modeling of insulin binding to receptors and degradation in vivo in the rabbit. *Diabetes* 29:50-59, 1980.
2. CARSON, E.R., C. COBELLI, and L. FINKELSTEIN. *The mathematical modeling of metabolic and endocrine systems*. New York:John Wiley & Sons, 1983,
3. COBELLI, C., and G. PACINI. Insulin secretion and hepatic extraction in humans by minimal modeling of C-peptide and insulin kinetics. *Diabetes* 37:223-231, 1988.
4. DUCKWORTH, W.C. Insulin degradation: mechanism, products, and significance. *Endocr. Rev.* 9:319-345, 1988.
5. EATON, R.P., R.C. ALLEN, and D.S. SCHADE. Hepatic removal of insulin in normal man: dose response to endogenous insulin secretion. *J. Clin. Endocrinol. Metab.* 56:1294-1300, 1983.
6. EATON, R.P., R.C. ALLEN, D.S. SCHADE, K.M. ERICKSON, and J. STANDEFER. Prehepatic insulin production in man: kinetic analysis using peripheral connecting peptide behaviour. *J. Clin. Endocrinol. Metab.* 51:520-528, 1980.
7. FERRANNINI, E., and C. COBELLI. The kinetics of insulin in man. I. General aspects. *Diabetes/Metabolism Rev.* 3:335-363, 1987.
8. FERRANNINI, E., and C. COBELLI. The kinetics of insulin in man. II. Role of the liver. *Diabetes/Metabolism Rev.* 3:365-397, 1987.
9. FERRANNINI, E., J. WAHREN, O.K. FABER, P. FELIG, C. BINDER, and R.A. DEFRONZO. Splanchnic and renal metabolism of insulin in human subjects: A dose-response study. *Am. J. Physiol.* 244:E517-E527, 1983.
10. FOLEY, J.E., A.L. LAURSEN, O. SONNE, and J. GLIEMANN. Insulin binding and hexose transport in rat adipocytes. Relation to cell size. *Diabetologia* 19:234-241, 1981.
11. GAMMELTOFT, S., and J. GLIEMANN. Binding and degradation of ^{125}I-insulin by isolated fat cells. *Biochem. Biophys. Acta* 320:16-32, 1973.
12. GAMMELTOFT, S., L.O. KRISTENSEN, and L. SESTOFT. Insulin receptors in isolated rat hepatocytes. Reassessment of binding properties and observations of the inactivation of insulin at 37 C. *J. Biol. Chem.* 253:8406-8413, 1978.
13. GANONG, W.F. *Review of medical physiology*. Norwalk:Appleton & Lange, 1989,
14. GREENWAY, C.V., and R.D. STARK. Hepatic vascular bed. *Physiol. Rev.* 51:23-65, 1971.
15. JONES, R.H., P.H. SöNKSEN, M.A. BOROUJERDI, and E.R. CARSON. Number and affinity of insulin receptors in intact human subjects. *Diabetologia* 27:207-211, 1984.
16. MARQUARDT, D.W. An algorithm for least squares estimation of nonlinear parameters. *J. Soc. Ind. Appl. Math.* 2:431-441, 1963.
17. MORISHIMA, T., C. BRADSHAW, and J. RADZIUK. Measurement using tracers of steady-state turnover and metabolic clearance of insulin in dogs. *Am. J. Physiol.* 248:E203-E208, 1985.
18. POWRIE, J.K., G.D. SMITH, F. SHOJAEE-MORADIE, P.H. SöNKSEN, and R.H. JONES. Mode of action of chloroquine in patients with non-insulin dependent diabetes mellitus. *Am. J. Physiol.* 1991.(in press)
19. RADZIUK, J. On linearity of insulin kinetics. Reply. *Am. J. Physiol.* 251:E249-E250, 1986.

The model is described (uniquely) by a set of differential equations.

$$\frac{dC_1}{dt} = k_{21}C_2 - k_{12}C_1 - A_p \qquad (1)$$

$$\frac{dC_2}{dt} = \frac{V_1}{V_2}k_{12}C_1 - \left(k_{21} + \frac{k_{32}}{V_2}\right)C_2 + \frac{k_{23}}{V_2}C_3 \qquad (2)$$

$$\frac{dC_3}{dt} = k_{23}C_2 - k_{32}C_3 + \frac{k_{43}}{V_3}C_4 - k_{34}C_3 \qquad (3)$$

$$\frac{dC_4}{dt} = k_{34}C_3 - k_{43}C_4 \qquad (4)$$

$$\frac{dA}{dt} = k_{45}C_4 - k_{54}A_p \qquad (5)$$

$$\qquad (6)$$

where c_i is the number of identity in cell (per unit volume); A_p is the mass of peripheral (hepatic) release into blood; k_{ij} is the distribution between compartments; the compartment i (or j); V_i is the volume of compartment i (ml); r_i is endogenous insulin secretion (ju) and r_i is peripheral insulin infusion (μU/ml); and r is plasma insulin concentration (μU/ml).

REFERENCES

1. CERASI, E. and LUFT, R., ...

(references largely illegible)

CURRICULA AND
COMPUTER-ASSISTED EDUCATION

THIRTEEN YEARS OF A NATION-WIDE CURRICULUM IN MEDICAL INFORMATICS: DOES IT STILL MEET THE REQUIREMENTS?

Reinhard Busse, Otto Rienhoff

Institute of Medical Informatics, Philipps University Marburg
Bunsenstr.3, W-3550 Marburg, Germany

In 1978, the Federal Republic of Germany was the first country in the world to include medical informatics (MI) in its nation-wide medical curriculum. A survey among medical students at Marburg University today shows that the teaching does not meet their wishes concerning contents, timing within the curriculum, and the amount of practical training. These results as well as proposals from professoral expert groups and experiences with model curricula in the Netherlands and the USA demand changes: Necessary are computer-literacy prior to university, mandatory teaching of data privacy and security, optional practical courses, and an integration of MI teaching into traditional disciplines. If such a reform does not occur, MI will be in danger of being neglected or even abolished by students as well as politicians.

1. Background

In the Federal Republic of Germany, medical informatics (MI) has been included in the nation-wide curriculum for medical students since 1978. According to the ordinance regulating the medical education (Approbationsordnung fuer Aerzte), statistics and MI have to be taught in the so-called "ecological course" in the second or third clinical year together with forensic medicine, hygiene, social and occupational medicine.

The catalogue for the nation-wide multiple-choice exams after the third clinical year lists the following contents within "statistics and MI" for which the students have to be prepared:
* Controlled clinical trials,
* Retrospective case-control and prospective cohort studies,
* Methods for diagnostic support,
* Basic definitions: signal, data, information, algorithm, hardware, software, information systems,
* Medical documentation,
* Application systems (patient records, medical information systems, biosignal analysis),
* Data privacy and security, and
* Health system analysis (1).

In the exam, between 5 and 10 of a total 580 questions are asked about these items.

The inclusion of MI into the curriculum had the advantage of promoting the foundation of institutes of MI and Biometrics at almost all 27 faculties in the western part of Germany. All but one of these faculties are public and all are comparable in size and quality. This institutionalization of MI was necessary to meet the requirement of teaching MI to all medical students. Teaching has to take place according to 13-year old requirements and was mainly theoretical until very recently. Around 1985, institutes started to equip teaching facilities with personal computers funded to 50% by the federal government. At our own university in Marburg, we installed a computer laboratory with 13 PCs in 1986.

2. Surveys

In view of the mainly theoretical instruction in MI at a rather late time within the medical curriculum, 93 fifth-year medical students were interviewed at the Philipps University in Marburg. This sample represents more than 50% of the participants of the "ecological course" and was taken during a break in the teaching of hygiene. The MI instruction within that course at our university was made up of an introductory lecture, 20 hours of teaching with 2 students working with one PC and the possibility to use the computers individually under the supervision of tutors.

The students were asked to fill in a questionnaire about their experiences with computers, their opinion about the use of computer technology in health care, their evaluation of various areas in MI in respect to their future career, their opinion about the need to include these areas in the curriculum and their ideas concerning teaching in MI.

As far as their experience with computers is concerned, 15% of the students interviewed had never used a computer before, while 22% had only tried it. 25% have been using a computer infrequently and 38% regularly. 72% of the regular and 35% of the infrequent users have access to a computer in their own flat; the average figure for all students is 40%. Since the majority of students having been using a computer gained the basic knowledge to do so outside university (59% privately, 14% at high school) and only 28% through our instruction, we assume that the results are not very influenced by our MI courses.

In the evaluation of the importance for their career, the students ranked "data privacy and security" as most important out of nine areas. On a scale from 0 to 6, the items were rated in the following order. In each case, the answers were distributed roughly normally:

data privacy and security	4,9
general knowledge about computers	4,3
text processing	4,3
search for literature by computer	4,0
usage of data bases	3,9
application systems in hospitals	3,6
statistical analysis	3,4
systems for management of physician's practice	2,9
independent programming	1,7

As far as the inclusion of these areas into the curriculum is concerned, the majority of students think mandatory teaching is necessary only in the case of data privacy and security while they favour voluntary instruction for all other areas:

	mandatory	voluntary	no teaching necessary
data privacy and security	53%	42%	4%
general knowledge about computers	26%	72%	2%
application systems in hospitals	22%	68%	10%
search for literature by computer	21%	75%	5%
usage of data bases	18%	70%	12%
text processing	15%	80%	4%
statistical analysis	13%	79%	8%
systems for management of physician's practice	9%	69%	22%
independent programming	3%	65%	32%

44% of all students want the instruction in MI to begin within the pre-clinical years and an additional 42% within the first clinical year, i.e. 86% think it should be taught earlier. Also 86% want practically oriented instruction, 11% a half-and-half mixture of theory and practice while only 2% favour theoretical teaching.

Since this spring semester, the MI course in Marburg was re-designed according to these results as far as possible e.g. by introducing data privacy and security into each course. But major changes, e.g. concerning placement within the entire medical curriculum, would violate nation-wide regulations.

In a similar survey, the 25 professors responsible for MI instruction at the German medical faculties (18 of whom returned the questionnaire) were asked about contents and extent of their teaching as well as their opinion of MI areas in respect to the career of today's medical students: While they ranked "data privacy and security" only in fifth place, "general knowledge about computers" was considered most important. The professors offering more than 13 hours of instruction (i.e. more than 1h weekly) put the first three items in the same order as the students.

3. Proposals for a revision of informatics teaching

As in other countries, structure and contents of medical education has been widely discussed in Germany during the last couple of years and a number of proposals for changes were published. Best known is the report "physician of the future" from 1989 which analyzed the requirements of future physicians and their consequences for medical education (2). As far as MI is concerned, teaching of medical information systems and technology was recommended for first year students.

In 1990, a group of professors of biometrics, epidemiology, and MI were selected by the professional society GMDS. They formulated a revision of the contents of MI instruction within the nation-wide medical curriculum (3). Without changing the general frame, they propose adjustments due to technological progress, i.e. hospital information systems instead of systems for storage of patients' records.

In a report on the role of information and communication technologies to the enquete commission "education 2000" of the German parliament in 1990 (4), Rolff et al. proposed mandatory teaching in information and communication systems for all pupils at secondary school. If their proposals are actualized, teaching in MI at university level could be restricted to the medical aspects instead of teaching basic aspects, as well.

4. International Comparison

The latest developments in curricular design were discussed at the IMIA·(International Medical Informatics Association) working conferences in Victoria and Prague. Out of many examples, the two most prominent curricula presented during these conferences are at the Erasmus University in Rotterdam and at Harvard in Boston.

In the Netherlands, the curriculum designed by van Bemmel et al. (5) has constantly been adapted to changes. It now provides 72 hours of mandatory instruction during the pre-clinical years. Two thirds of these are practicals. The areas covered are basic skills training (operating system, text processing, data bases), aspects of information, analysis of biomedical signals, computer-assisted diagnoses and literature searches. During the clinical training, a further course about hospital information systems is mandatory while other fields (programming, expert systems) are optional. This design of teaching in MI does fulfill many of the demands of the participants of our survey and is well worth to be partly implemented in Germany.

In the US and Canada, teaching of MI is entirely dependent on persons convinced of its importance. This has led to the existence of teaching at some medical schools but virtually no teaching at many others. Harvard was one of the first medical schools to include information science in medical instruction as part of the "new pathway program" which encourages student-directed problem-solving study. The students are expected to make intensive use of computer simulations, text processing and on-line search of the literature.

The initial approach to informatics as an entirely voluntary offer proved to have weaknesses which according to Barnett (6) were:
1. The tight curriculum leaves no time for optional resources.
2. The lack of integration makes computer applications less valuable.
3. The faculty invests in computers only if they are essential to the curriculum.
Therefore, he proposed to replace part of the classical curricular activities by computer applications. Teaching of MI in a classroom environment like in Europe is hardly known in North America. Barnett believed it to be "less than effective" (6) and Haynes et al. stated: "We are unconvinced that computer-aided learning in centralized computer labs constitutes an adequate introduction to informatics to medical students." (7)

5. Conclusion

Considering the results of our surveys, the proposals for a revision of teaching and experiences with curricula in other countries, we conclude that in order to prepare today's medical students for being physicians in the next century, basic knowledge in certain areas of MI should be known by all medical students. This includes system support for patient care, education, and clinical research. These objectives require a reform of the 13 year-old MI curriculum in the Federal Republic of Germany:

Inclusion of MI in the nation-wide curriculum is necessary to ensure that every faculty provides an institut of MI which is necessary to keep teaching on a high level. The diverse backgrounds of German medical students as far as experiences and needs are concerned as well as new developments in this area require flexible and innovative teaching in the framework of federal regulations.

All students should be computer-literate at the time they enter medical school. An introductory course is needed during the pre-clinical years for those who did not acquire the necessary skills at school which apparently will still be the majority for quite some time.

The mandatory MI teaching in a classroom setting should be restricted to some introductory lessons about general principles and very important areas like data privacy and security.

The use of computer applications in the medical environment should be taught in conjunction with the disciplines involved. Teaching of clinical applications should take place in a hospital setting.

In Marburg, various institutions try to follow these conclusions f.e. by integrating informatics into the teaching of radiology and theoretical surgery. If such an integration fails, MI will continue to be considered a "minor subject" and secondary to most other medical disciplines.

Literature

1. Institut für medizinische und pharmazeutische Prüfungsfragen (IMPP): Gegenstandskatalog für den Zweiten Abschnitt der Ärztlichen Prüfung. 2. Auflage. Mainz, 1979
2. Arbeitskreis Medizinerausbildung der Robert Bosch Stiftung (Murrhardter Kreis): Das Arztbild der Zukunft - Analysen künftiger Anforderungen an den Arzt; Konsequenzen für die Ausbildung und Wege zu ihrer Reform. Gerlingen: Bleicher, 1989
3. Konferenz der Fachvertreter für Medizinische Biometrie und Medizinische Informatik: Überarbeitungs-Vorschlag für den Gegenstandskatalog in Medizinischer Statistik und Informatik. Mannheim, 1990
4. Rolff HG, Pfeiffer H, de Witt C, Zimmermann P: Die Bedeutung der Informations- und Kommunikationstechnologien/ Neue Medien für die zukünftige Bildungspolitik des Bundes. In:Zukünftige Bildungspolitik - Bildung 2000. Schlußbericht der Enquete-Kommission des Deutschen Bundestages. Bonn, 1990: 444-454
5. van Bemmel JH, Sollet PCGM, Grashuis JL: Education in Medical Informatics in The Netherlands: A Nationwide Policy and Erasmus Curriculum. Meth Inf Med 1989; 28(4): 227-233
6. Barnett O: Information Technology and Undergraduate Medical Education. Acad Med 1989; 64(4): 187-190
7. Haynes RB, Ramsden M, McKibbon KA, Walker CJ, Ryan NC: A Review of Medical Education and Medical Informatics. Acad Med 1989; 64(4): 207-212

INTRODUCING MEDICAL INFORMATICS AS A HORIZONTAL THEME INTO A MEDICAL SCHOOL CURRICULUM

P.A. Jennett, Ph.D.; S.M. Edworthy, M.D.; T. W. Rosenal, M.D.
Faculty of Medicine, University of Calgary
3330 Hospital Drive N.W., Calgary, Alberta, Canada T2N 4N1

ABSTRACT

Recent reports and publications strongly recommend that medical school curricula should introduce medical informatics (MI) instruction, and promote information science and computer technology applications. In addition, academic centres have been encouraged to foster leadership and research in the MI field. This paper describes how the discipline of MI was adopted into a medical school curriculum as a <u>repeated theme</u> throughout the three-year M.D. program. First year learning opportunities consisted of ten formal learning contact hours, including orientation, lecture/ demonstrations, applications, and projects. This was supplemented by both optional student-led tutorials and special interest group activities. Reference to planned second and third year activities are addressed. Preparing our physicians for tomorrow to cultivate life long and self-directed learning habits by introducing information management tools into medical education programs merits the attention of deans, associate deans, practitioners, and medical educators across the medical education continuum.

INTRODUCTION

The University of Calgary (U of C) Faculty of Medicine, in 1989, began exploring the feasibility of introducing Medical Informatics into its undergraduate curriculum. This step was taken in response to: 1) recent AAMC recommendations[1,2] indicating that learning objectives for specific instruction and applications in the fundamentals of medical informatics for patient care, education, and research should be introduced into medical school programs, and 2) the philosophy of the University of Calgary Faculty of Medicine, which emphasizes the development of skills and habits useful for self-directed, independent, and life long learning.

METHOD

The Curriculum Committee at the Faculty of Medicine formed an ad hoc committee of five members to advise them regarding the need for providing the medical students with learning opportunities to acquire information skills. The committee's mandate was to provide recommendations specific to four areas: 1) content, 2) content organization, 3) management, and 4) evaluation. Committee membership included three faculty members [two clinicians (both graduates of the U of C M.D. program), one P.D. educator] currently working in medical informatics, one medical student, and one research assistant.

The ad hoc committee based its final recommendations on a pertinent literature review, a review of international and national conference proceedings on medical informatics, personal contact with international, North American, national, and local experts in both health informatics and computer sciences, and on the local experiences of medical, nursing, and student environments. Recommendations were placed into a core document and presented to the Curriculum Committee. All recommendations as described below were accepted by the Curriculum Committee and implemented in the Fall of 1990.

RESULTS

Content and Content Organization: The ad hoc committee recommended that the learning opportunities not be packaged as a course or series of courses, but be spread throughout the curriculum as a horizontal theme. A horizontal theme is defined as a body of knowledge or discipline which has consistency or continuity within the curriculum, i.e., it is common to years 1, 2, and 3, and is interwoven and repeated throughout each year. Horizontal themes already established in the curriculum include pathology, biochemistry, infectious diseases, gross anatomy, physiology, and pharmacology. Six areas of medical informatics were recommended for the undergraduate curriculum: 1) computer-assisted learning (CAL)--i.e., (CAI and expert systems); 2) searching information from computerized bibliographic data bases (off-line and on-line); 3) medical informatics applications to biostatistics and critical appraisal of the literature; 4) patient information system (hospital-based); 5) physician office-based information systems; and 6) communication systems, i.e., electronic mail, bulletin boards, and conferencing systems. The rationale, competencies (knowledge, skills, and attitudes), and place in the curriculum was outlined for each of these areas.

Management: It was recommended that the horizontal theme be managed by three faculty members who would act as horizontal theme managers. This triumvirate would provide guidance to course, clerkship, and elective committees regarding: 1) the faculty, student, and staff resources who possess the required expertise and skills in the field; 2) appropriate hardware and software requirements; and 3) how elements of medical informatics might optimally be introduced into units within courses or within mandatory clerkship rotations.

Resources and Equipment: A central core of expertise and support were identified in the student, faculty, and administrative arenas to facilitate the adoption of this theme. These key players were instrumental in the organization and teaching of the discipline.

It was suggested that computer and programming staff as well as key hardware resources currently scattered among educational divisions be housed in one location to provide leadership and the availability of on-site assistance for student and faculty development and needs. A start-up budget for a coordinator and basic hardware/software network equipment was prepared and submitted.

The current technical environment consists of a Sunsparc Station Server along with 11 microcomputer work stations which are connected to the server by twisted pair wiring systems. The Server can be accessed by two modes: 1) microcomputers using the Server drive as the source of programs which run under DOS. These microcomputers can run computer assisted learning programs, word processing programs, spreadsheets, or data base programs, and 2) terminals which permit mail systems such as BITNET and INTERNET and permits access to a conferencing system called COSY.

Learning Opportunities: First year learning opportunities consisted of ten formal learning contact hours, including orientations, lectures/ demonstrations, applications, and projects. These activities were supplemented by both optional student-led tutorials and special interest group activities. Initially second year experiences were incorporated into electives and third year experiences delegated to family medicine clerkship.

Evaluation:

Program Evaluation: The introduction of the medical informatics program into the undergraduate curriculum is being evaluated by a Stuffelbeam model of program evaluation. This approach permits appropriate adjustments to be made on an ongoing basis.

Student Evaluation: This consisted of both informal and formal methods of evaluation. The informal feedback sessions took place during demonstration and practice settings. Summative evaluation took place at the end of the ten hours of formal instruction during the first year of medical school. Seventy-one of the 72 medical students being formally evaluated met the required criteria for our pass/fail system.

DISCUSSION

Physicians in training must be provided with the tools and habits which can assist them to manage information and therefore optimally practice educational, patient, and research activities in their chosen profession.[3,4,5] As information management continues to impact on all aspects of medical practice, introducing developments in medical informatics into curricula has major implications for all levels of medical education program.[6] As medical schools begin to systematically integrate the discipline of medical informatics into their curriculum, guidelines from other medical schools will be of value. It is in this context that this paper is presented.

In general, the introduction of medical informatics has been well received by all stakeholders, that is medical students, faculty, and administration. The biggest obstacle to the implementation of the theme was difficulty in obtaining funding to hire a full-time coordinator. Responses to external requests for support for this position now have been positive, and it is anticipated that the theme will continue to grow and evolve in a positive manner due to this recent advancement.

REFERENCES:

1. *Panel on the General Professional Education of the physician and College Preparation for Medicine. Physicians for the Twenty-First Century: The GPEP Report.* Association of American Medical Colleges, 1984.
2. Executive Council of the Association of American Medical Colleges. Evaluation of Medical Information Science in Medical Education. *Journal of Medical Education*, 61(6):487-543, 1986.
3. Haynes RB, Ramsden M, McGibbin KA, Walker CJ, Ryan NC. A review of medical education and medical informatics. *Academic Medicine*, 64(4):207-12, 1989.
4. Weed LL and Miller MC. Physicians of the future. *NEJM*, 304(15):903-907, 1981.
5. Shockley J. Health education for the twenty-first century. *Medical Informatics*, 9(3&4):313, 1984.
6. Barnett O. Information technology and medical education at Harvard Medical School. *Proceedings of the International Symposium of Medical Informatics and Education*. R. Soloman, D. Protti, J. Moehr (eds.), pp. 3-5, May 1989.

A NEW APPROACH TO COMPUTERIZED MEDICAL KNOWLEDGE ASSESSMENT

Joan M. Carbó, Joan J Sancho, M. José Miravitlles,
Joan C. González, Ferran Sanz.
Departament d'Informàtica Biomèdica. Institut Municipal d'Investigació Mèdica
Universitat Autónoma de Barcelona. P. Marítim 25. 08003. Barcelona. Spain.

ABSTRACT

The development of "smart" test programs to assess the knowledge acquisition during the learning process and to identify areas in which to concentrate the effort, is a potential area of development in Computer Assisted Medical Instruction. We developed a "smart" interactive system, SuperTest, to train students to pass the test to have access to Residency Training Programs. We used object oriented techniques all over the project, from design up to the implementation phase, and developed it under a graphical interface. The program developed is able to assess the student initial knowledge in each area and produces a study plan balancing knowledge extension needs in each area with student proficiency. The plan is surveyed by small, one-area, tests, and continuously adapted to student progress. Eventually, a real test emulation is offered. The students acceptance has been encouraging. Similar techniques could be applied to a variety of tests.

INTRODUCTION

Computer Assisted Medical Instruction (CAMI) is rapidly evolving in two main areas: clinical cases simulation[1] and electronic books[2]. The development of "smart" test programs to assess the knowledge acquisition during the learning process and to identify areas in which to concentrate the effort, is a potential third area of development in CAMI.

Many kinds of tests have been devised to evaluate student's erudition. Multiple choice test (MCT) are widely used as a main form of exam in Medical Sciences both at undergraduate and graduate levels. As far as we know, all previous computerized aids for a MCT were not different from reading a MCQ book and checking correct responses. In Spain, to enter the official Residency Training Program (RTP) graduate medical students must pass a National Exam (called MIR Exam; Medical Internship and Residency Exam) which is a MCT. RTP vacancies in each hospital are strictly allocated by MIR score.

Between fifteen and twenty thousand graduates take the exam yearly. Only two to three thousand pass it and can therefore embark a medical or surgical specialty. Reputation of medical schools are strongly dependent from the number of its graduates able to enter a RTP. Professors are faced with the dilemma of focusing the instruction of medical students for the MIR Exam or instead prepare them as general practitioners, approaches with limited overlapping.

Those considerations lead us to develop a "smart" interactive system, SuperTest, to train students to pass the MIR exam. This system would allow the faculty to prepare physicians according with the WHO guidelines without wasting efforts in exam-oriented teaching.

OBJECTIVES

The objectives were to offer a program able to: 1) assess the student's initial knowledge in each area of the curriculum; 2) determine the areas in which the student needs to concentrate the effort in order to pass the exam and suggest a work strategy; 3) reassess the progress in those weak areas and update the work strategy and 4) offer the opportunity of eventually taking a MIR-like exam as a global evaluation.

For such a program to succeed had to fulfil the requirements of accuracy in the scoring of students knowledge, good emulation of MIR Exam and high adictivity to catch the student attention.

MATERIAL and METHODS

We have chosen a widely spread user interface to implement Super Test (Fig.1). This interface is called Microsoft Windows 3.0 (Microsoft Co., Seattle, USA) to run under most IBM PCs and compatibles. The minimum hardware requirements are: 80286 based PC with 1Mb RAM and a 10Mb hard disk. For development phase we used a Intel 386-based compatible PC with 8Mb of RAM (Random Access Memory) with a colour VGA (Video Graphics Array) graphics card and a 200Mb SCSI (Small Computer Systems Interface) hard disk. Super Test has been written in C++ language (Zortech Ltd., London, UK) and Microsoft Windows Software Development Kit. At the time of this writing, the data bank includes more than 15000 MCT questions.

DESIGN

We used object oriented techniques all over the project, from design up to the implementation phase (4). Now, we will present the system in the same way. Our design focuses upon three main objects: Users, Tests and Inference Engine. Each of them has its own properties and abilities to react to specific messages. To put it plainly, an object should be regarded as an entity with a certain number of private characteristics. The only way for an object to communicate with the outer world is through messages. The User object takes care of everything related to administering users. The Test object main task is choosing a random set of questions from the question data base given a couple of constraints (ie: subject, difficulty, etc). The heart of the system lies upon the Inference Engine object. This object acts like a daemon, always checking system consistency. Its main propose is to issue recommendations to students and assessing their degree of proficiency, while trying to early detect possible lacking. Another important task of the Inference Engine is to dynamically update the difficulty level of each question in the database. This level is assigned taking into account how many correct responses has the question got so far.

DESCRIPTION

When a student first faces SuperTest he/she is asked for personal data along with a password to identify him or herself in future sessions. The student is next prompted to take an initial exam of 250 MCT questions to asses his/her current knowledge in every area of medical science. Once finished, the inference engine compares the scores in each area with the specific requirements for the MIR exam, identifying the areas with insufficient achievement. From this comparison, SuperTest builds a list of suggested areas of study. Those areas include the specialty and the basic science involved (i.e.: cardiovascular anatomy). In successive SuperTest sessions, the student is allowed to take short sets of 25 questions covering specifically each area, to reassess his/her knowledge. Those short tests are build according to the previous score of each particular student in each specialty, and progress in complexity until the score achieved is considered by SuperTest good enough to pass that particular part of the MIR exam. The list of suggested areas to study is updated after each passing each set. Although the student is free to choose those short test in any order, he/she would ideally follow the order suggested by SuperTest to attain maximum effectivity.

The program lets the user check answer's accuracy once a test is finished. Checking means reviewing correct responses against student's responses and viewing help screens with explanations related to each question and arranged with hypertext links.

Eventually, the user is allowed to take a full MIR Exam simulation with 250 randomly chosen questions, with time limitation and penalty score for wrong answers identical to the real test. SuperTest maintains a log of the activity of each student, reflecting date of each session and time spent, suggestions provided, tests taken and the scores achieved in each area.

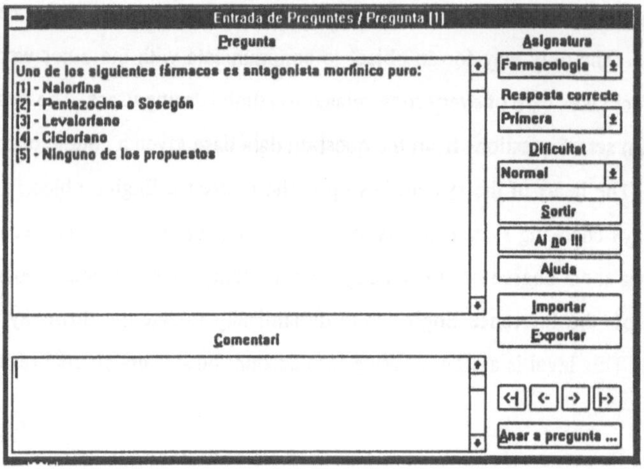

Fig 1. *Supertest main screen under MS Windows 3.0*

PRACTICAL RESULTS

We are very encouraged by SuperTest first practical results. It has smoothly caught students interest and they have quickly got used to it. Its weakest points are the relative time consuming task of creating and validating the questions database and hardware required to run effectively the program.

The process of entering and validating the data bank is carried out by a selected group of 6th year medical students supervised by the authors. Although an inexpensive Intel 80286-based computer can run MS Windows 3.0, an acceptable performance with good interactivity requires an Intel 386-based computer with 2 Mb of RAM and a mouse. The key points in SuperTest are the student's interactive evaluation and the ability to compile recommendations. Both were stressed as of utmost importance in a review about the subject (4).

BIBLIOGRAPHY

1. Pinckell GC, Medal D, Mann WS, Staebler RJ. Computerizing clinical patients problems: an evolving tool for medical education. Med Educ 1986; 20:201-203.

2. Corvetta A, Pomponio G, Salvi A, Luchetti MM, Leven FJ. Hypertext application and clinical simulation: Innovative approaches in computer aided teaching of medicine. In: O'Moore R, Bengtsson, Byrant JR, Bryden JS, eds. Medical Informatics Europe '90. Glasgow: Springer-Verlag, 1990; 402-405. (Rienhoff O, Lindberg DAB, eds. Lecture Notes in Medical Informatics; vol 40).

3. Sanchez J, Canton MP. Systems Application Architecture. Common User Access Advanced Interface Design Guide. In: IBM Microcomputers. A Programmer Handbook. New York, McGraw Hill, 1990.

4. Piemme TE. Computer-assisted learning and evaluation in Medicine. JAMA 1988; 260:367-372.

THE USE OF THE COMPUTER IN GASTROENTEROLOGY
FOR DOCTOR-TRAINING AND PATIENT-DIAGNOSIS

B. RICHARDS [+], T. LUGOVKINA [*], A. OBUKHOV [Ø]

\+ Department of Computation, UMIST, Manchester, UK
* Medical Institute, Clinical Hospital N40, Sverdlovsk, USSR
Ø Institute of Mathematics and Mechanics, Ural Branch of the
Academy of Sciences of the USSR, Sverdlovsk, USSR.

ABSTRACT

This paper introduces the various types of clinical problems which present to the Gastroenterologist and goes on to describe how an Expert System can help in the diagnosis and thence indicate the appropriate remedial action. The package can be used for the training of students and house-men and can also be used by the most senior clinicians as a decision-support tool.

INTRODUCTION

One must recognize that the early work in the field of gastroenterology and computers was done by Card [1]. This was then taken up by de Dombal [2] and subsequently on a much wider scale by additions to the database through the efforts of de Dombal and his colleagues [3].

The Therapeutic Chair at the Medical Institute in Sverdlovsk and the Operations Research Department of the Institute of Mathematics and Mechanics (Ural Branch of Academy of Sciences of the USSR) together with the Computation Department of The University of Manchester Institute of Science and Technology are also carrying out researches on Artifical Intelligence systems in gastroenterology with the aim of diagnosis and education.

The value of a careful interview and physical examination of the patient is still of great importance in the diagnostic process in gastroenterology. Information Technology can assist doctors (especially beginners) in their training and in improving the diagnosis.

Such a package would enable the recruits to gain experience via the computer, whilst for their more experienced colleagues it would serve as a second, or even a third, opinion when they were performing in the absence of their consultant.

GASTROENTEROLOGY

Very often the doctor in General Practice cannot carry out the detailed examination procedures necessary to diagnose correctly the cause of abdominal pain. However, such examination procedures are of extreme importance in Gastroenterology. Most of the typical gastroenterological diseases may be recognised using traditional methods when used by a skilled specialist [4].

Usually when the General Practitioner has found signs of gastroenterological disease he refers the patient to the Consultant Gastroenterologist for an expert opinion (diagnosis) and a recommendation as to a course of action (treatment). Such a two stage procedure makes the wait for a diagnosis somewhat lengthy. Such problems are exacerbated in District Hospitals who do not have a resident Consultant in Gastroenterology. It is felt that these problems may be solved by the use of a computer programme for decision support.

THE AIMS OF THE INVESTIGATION

The main aims governing the production of this computer package have been three in number viz:

(i) To create a model for the training of the recruits in the technique of interviewing patients and obtaining their medical history, and in the techniques of examination procedures.

(ii) To have a computer system which can be used to assess the clinician's performance, ie to carry-out a medical audit.

(iii) To produce an Expert System capable of performing as good as the Consultant, or a team of Consultants.

Therefore such a computer package must prompt the doctor during the patient interview and examination, and take in the answers to the questions; it must make decisions based on pre-determined rules; and it must explain why it has arrived at those conclusions. In this way the junior doctors can learn from the package and can thereby advance in knowledge and skill as a result of the logic built into the programme. Also, the use of a structured history-taking questionaire has previously been shown to be of enormous value.

THE PATIENT INTERVIEW AND EXAMINATION

As was stated above, the computer must first of all ensure that all the information it requires is obtained, therefore it must prompt the doctor to obtain the answers.

The information required is patient's name, sex, date of birth (to give age), height, weight (now) and previous/normal weight, current smoking and drinking (alcoholic) habits. Previous history of gastro-intestinal problems, eg Ulcerative colitis, Appendicitis; previous surgery (eg Cholecystectomy, Appendectomy).

The patient's pulse-rate (heart-rate), blood-pressure and temperature will be recorded. The site of any pain will be identified (as to upper/lower, right/left quadrants) and the patient will be questioned as to both relieving and aggravating factors. Bowel action must be ascertained.

At this stage on initial assessment might be made as to the immediate subsequent course of action. An accurate diagnosis requires special tests, eg X-ray, Barium meal, Ultrasound scan, Sigmodoscopy, Endoscopy, etc. The physician may use the computer programme to avoid unnecessary and sometimes dangerous and rather expensive diagnostic procedures.

EXPERT SYSTEM STRUCTURE

The strategy used in this programme differs somewhat from that used by de Dombal [2] and others as it follows initially the ideas used by Richards [7]. The main part of the expert system is the knowledge base that includes formalized experience of highly qualified doctors and is organized as a system of frames. Every disease is described by qualitative parameters with quantitative characteristics.

The first subsystem of data input is intended for a dialog to enable the entering of the interview and examination results. This initial information may be read from the standard patient's data record.

The subsystem of making the decision rule consists of two functional blocks: logical rules and a pattern recognition block. The last is one based on the committee methods [5,6] and is used in the complicated cases.

The explanation sub-system allows the user to access the logical path used by the computer to arrive at its diagnosis: dislaying of this route is optional. Trainee doctors often find this the most helpful part of the package.

THE RESULTS OF THE USE OF THE EXPERT SYSTEM

The results from using the Expert System on a patient are:

(a) Recommendations as to the appropriate diagnostic procedures to be carried out.

(b) A list of Differential Diagnoses with assigned probabilities.

(c) The ability to check the diagnosis of the learners against the computer.

CONCLUSION

The work with the prototype of the Expert System showed a high percentage of correct diagnostic results especially in typical cases. Further development of The Expert System to a Mark II version will provide the ability for recognition of non-typical forms of diseases. We consider that the key to the future for improving the gastroenterological service is in the cooperation between clinicians and computer scientists. The results so far have proved very encouraging with the emphasis being handled within the training model. The diagnostic sector needs refining in the light of the cases being accumulated in the USSR. It is hoped to be able to build on the vast experience now having been built-up within Europe due to the fine work of de Dombal and his co-workers [3].

REFERENCES

1. Card W.I. et al. A comparison of doctor and computer interrogation of patients. Int Jour. of Biomedical Computing 5, 175-187, 1974.

2. Dombal F.T. de et al. Computer-aided diagnosis of acute abdominal pain. Br. Med. J. 2, 9-13, 1972.

3. De Dombal F.T. The European Community concerted action objective medical decisionmaking in patients with acute abdominal pain. Theo Surg 5, 112-117, 1990.

4. Lugovkina T. Expert system in gastroenterology. Abst. of International Conference "Medical informatics and medical education", Prague, 1990, p. 94.

5. Mazurov V.D. Dual problems of treatment choice. Mathematical modelling of medical and biological systems. Sverdlovosk, Ub AS USSR, 1988.

6. Mazurov V.D., Krivonogov A.I., Kazantsev V.S. Solving of optimization problems by committee methods. Pattern Recognition, vol 20, No 4 pp. 371-378, 1987.

7. Richards B., Jeffrey C. The Computer Diagnosis of Congenital Malformations. MEDINFO 80, p 779-783, North Holland, Amsterdam, 1980.

LINKING EXPERT-SYSTEMS AND INTERACTIVE VIDEO FOR MEDICAL EDUCATION

Michael Hobsley, Dept of Surgery, University College & Middlesex School of Medicine, The Rayne Institute, University Street, London WC1E 6JJ.
Gordon Jameson, Audio-Visual Dept, University College London, Windeyer Building, Cleveland St, London W1P 6DB.
Matthew Wallis & Tim Webb, Multi-Media Lab, University College London, Windeyer Building, Cleveland Street, London W1P 6DB

Abstract

Expert systems are potentially valuable tools in teaching medical decision making. Their potential in this field was identified early in the history of the technology (Clancey & Letsinger 1981). In areas where decisions depend on visual clues, the addition of a store of illustrative video sequences greatly enhances the educational potential of an expert system. A system is described which combines an expert system on surgical management of lumps in the head and neck, with a videodisc containing patient examinations, and illustrative animations. The current system is aimed at students in their first year of clinical studies. Further developments required to make the system useful to more advanced students are identified.

Introduction

University College and Middlesex School of Medicine (UCMSM) faces the same problem as many other centres of medical education; namely, how the academic staff are to meet their clinical commitments and still cover the increasing demands of the curriculum. Students face similar problems as the ever growing curriculum reduces their opportunities for 'hands on' experience with real patients. In response to these problems UCMSM has funded a pair of projects in collaboration with the Multi-Media Lab at University College London, developing multi-media systems to supplement the school's regular teaching.

One of these projects is the development of expert-system based interactive video to help teach surgical management to students in their first year of clinical studies. The first phase of this project has produced a shell capable of presenting knowledge from a knowledge base in a number of ways, including by recourse to illustrative material stored on an accompanying videodisc. The domain of the prototype system is the surgical management of lumps in the head and neck.

The approach to management adopted in developing the expert system is one of 'working' diagnosis (Hobsley 1986). In contrast to the traditional approach of 'differential' diagnosis, the emphasis in working diagnosis is not on finding a 'correct' diagnostic label for the patient's presentation, but on ensuring that the doctor can take the appropriate action to benefit the patient. Thus, while it is possible at times to attach labels to some specific diseases, the most important decision in working diagnosis is whether the doctor is faced with a lump which should be left, or biopsied, and if it should be biopsied which form of biopsy is likely to be best for this patient.

The Prototype System

The prototype system developed provides access to information in two main modes. The student can either look at case studies or use the system as a 'medical dictionary' in which to find descriptions of lumps, explanations of expert terms, or demonstrations of important clinical signs. Both modes employ the same knowledge base, applying slightly different inference rules to provide information in different forms (fig 1.)

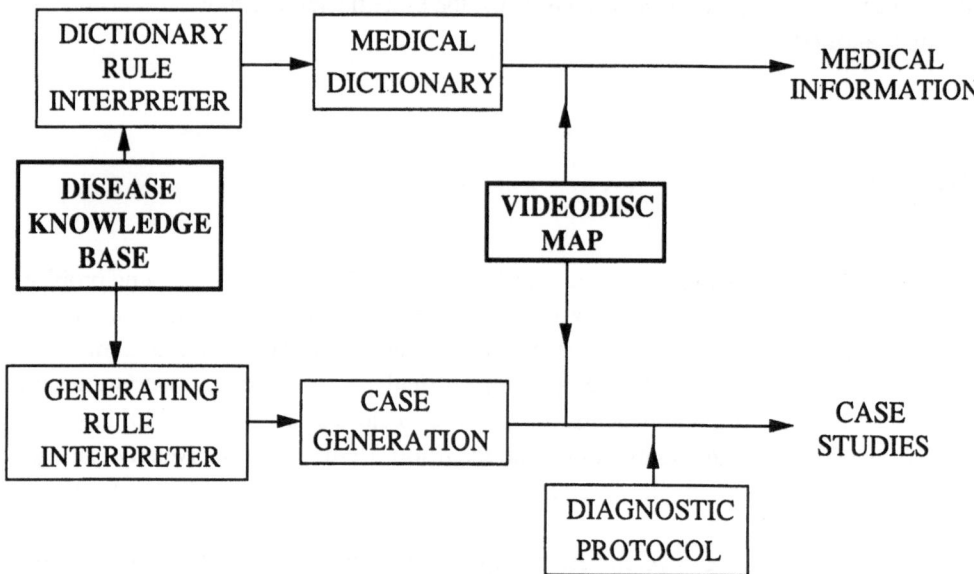

Fig. 1 Domain knowledge and knowledge about videodisc contents are shared by the two main application modes.

Case Studies:-

Having generated a case, the system proceeds to conduct the learner through the process of management. The student is shown a series of video clips of patient examinations. After each clip (s)he is asked a question designed to refine the current working diagnosis. The learner may ask 'why?' the question was asked, and 'how?' to answer it. The response to a student's 'why' states the system's current aim (e.g. clinical diagnosis or treatment decision), and how the current question will further this aim, (e.g. how the answer will affect the current working diagnosis). In responding to 'how?' the system will produce some exemplary video to illustrate the sign being asked about (this may be video of a patient or an animated sequence).

Since the aim of the system is to help to bring students' knowledge up to the level of an expert, the rules the expert system uses by default during its management process are expert-level. However, it has long been recognised that for such rules to be useful to non experts, they must be explained in non-expert terms (Swartout 1981). Accordingly the user may respond 'unknown' to many questions. The system has a set of 'condition' rules which describe when some expert requirement is fulfilled - e.g. lump is fluctuant if lump is deformable without loss of volume - and which are used to produce supplementary questions in lay terms so as to establish an answer to the expert-level question. The system's explanations of 'why?' such supplementary questions have been asked includes an explanation of why the question to which the student responded 'unknown' has been asked.

system:- 'Is the lump inflamed?'
student:- Unknown
system:- 'Does the lump blanch under pressure?'
student:- 'Why?'
system:- 'I am trying to establish a clinical diagnosis for the lump,
I know that the swelling of the parotid gland is an ascending infection if the lump is inflamed, and I know that the lump is inflamed if the lump does blanch under pressure'

The system also provides a facility for the learner to 'retrace' its steps through the lump classification process, asking what evidence was used to make each step, and where the evidence came from.

The 'Medical Dictionary':-
The dictionary provides descriptions of lumps, explanations of expert terms and illustrations of clinical signs. Descriptions of lumps take the form of a list of 'minimal diagnostic criteria', to which a list of signs and symptoms commonly associated with that lump, but not necessary for its diagnosis, may be added. Having seen this list, the learner is offered the chance to see video demonstrations of the signs appearing on it. Expert terms are explained by reference to their associated 'condition' rules, and where relevant, a video demonstration of the appropriate sign(s) is offered. Clinical signs not judged to require any explanation are simply demonstrated using appropriate clips of patient examinations or illustrative animations.

Initial Assessment

The system is currently undergoing assessment under student use (Hilton et al 1990). Initial reactions have been very positive. Students value the opportunity to see diseases, and signs and symptoms they would be unlikely to encounter during their six weeks on general surgical firms. Observation of the first students to use the system also indicates that they do pick up on the distinguishing features of the different lumps described in the system, and do successfully assimilate the meaning of expert terms.

Further Developments

Early indications are that the current prototype is useful to, and will be popular with novice students. In order to extend the use of the system to students at a later stage in their careers, it will be necessary to add a facility which allows students to practise their own diagnostic skills on the system's cases. An initial design for such a facility has been put forward (Hobsley et al 1991).

References

Clancey, W.J. and Letsinger, R. 1981. NEOMYCIN: Reconfiguring a Rule-Based Expert System for Application to Teaching. In 'Proceedings of the Seventh International Joint Conference on Artificial Intelligence', Vol 2, pp 829-836, Los Altos, CA,: William Kaufmann Inc.

Hilton, C., Hobsley, M., Jameson, G., Wallis M., & Webb, T.W., 1990, Expert-System based Interactive Video for Medical Education- Testing and further Development. To appear in Proceedings of CTICM Cruise into the '90's.

Hobsley, M. 1986, 'Pathways in Surgical Management', London, Edward Arnold Ltd.

Hobsley M., Jameson G, Wallis M, & Webb T, 1991, Design of a diagnostic tutor Linking Expert-Systems and Interactive Video, to appear in 'Proceedings of the 8th International Conference on Technology in Education', Toronto 1991.

Swartout, W.R. 1981, Explaining and Justifying Expert Consulting Programs. In Proceedings; of the Seventh International Joint Conference on Artificial Intelligence, Vol 2, pp 815-823, Los Altos CA, William Kauffmann Inc.

ILIAD : AN EXPERT SYSTEM FOR DIAGNOSTIC ASSISTANCE AND TEACHING: IMPLEMENTATION IN FRANCE

Eric Lepage (1, 2), Omar Bouhaddou (2, 3), Jean Tredaniel (1), Olivier Chassany (1), Homer Warner (3), Homer R. Warner (2).

(1) Département de Biostatistique et Informatique Médicale, CHU Lariboisière Saint-Louis, 1, Avenue Cl. Vellefaux, 75010 Paris, France.
(2) Medical Informatics Department, University of Utah, Salt Lake City, USA
(3) Applied Informatics Inc, Salt Lake City, Utah, USA.

Abstract

Iliad is an expert system written in C for the Macintosh computer. The system operates in two modes : as an expert consultant to teach differential diagnosis and as knowledge-based patient case simulator to teach and test medical problem solving. An approach was proposed to create and maintain, in a syncronized fashion, a French version of the Iliad system. The French version is now being evaluated at the Faculté Lariboisière Saint-Louis school of medicine and its evolution follows faithfully that of the master English version.

1. Introduction

Iliad is a microcomputer-based expert diagnostic system intended for use in general internal medicine. It was developped by Applied Informatics, Inc and the Medical Informatics Department of the University of Utah. A French version was jointly developed with the Département de Biostatistique et d'Informatique médicale, Faculté Lariboisière Saint-Louis. Iliad objective is to provide to students and all health care professionals with immediate expert consultation and advice that will facilitate learning the problem solving skills required of a good physician. Iliad is able to recognize each of the diseases we expect a medical student to become familiar with but also different situations occuring more infrequently and then less known to physicians. It allows entry of observations obtained by the student during his workup of the patient, provides consultation to the student at any stage of the process regarding the differential diagnosis. At any stage of the workup, Iliad can help the student in the choice of the optimal information to seek and give the different references according to the diagnosis selected by the user. Also, Iliad uses its knowledge base to generate realistic patient cases to train and test clinical problem-solving skills. The program evaluates the user's workup strategy by comparing it to its own under the same clinical situation.

A French version was developed in early 1990 and is now implemented at Lariboisière Saint-Louis, School of medicine on 12 Macintosh workstations made accessible to students and faculties. The greatly modular structure of the Iliad system and the hierarchical coding scheme of its vocabulary component have facilitated the translation of the entire system operation into French. In fact, a translation table is now automatically generated by the Iliad authoring tools to help support the synchronization between the English and French version (or any other translation) [1].

2. Structure of the Iliad system.

Iliad is structured according to a frame-based version of the Bayes model which formulates the diagnostic problem in term of deciding whether a patient does or does not have each disease [2]. Since each disease is considered separately, this allows for more than one disease to be present in a patient. From observations about a case, inferences regarding diagnoses likelihood are carried out through a sequential Bayesian decision model which requires that the disease manifestations be independent of each other in patients with disease. To avoid the limitations imposed by this contrainst, clusters of manifestations are defined which are not independent and are usually caused by some common underlying process most often recognized as "syndrome" by the physician. Boolean expressions were introduced in the model to represent expert physician logic used to describe relationships among items in these clusters in a form that can be learned by medical students.

3. Components of the system

The Iliad program is written in C and run on the Macintosh personel computer. As others expert systems [3, 4], Iliad includes three components: the knowledge base, the data dictionary and the user interface.

3.1 The Knowledge Base

The Iliad knowledge base component represents the subject-specific knowledge. It associates the data dictionary used to describe the subject and a set of frames (tables) written in a loosely-structured text frame format that describes explicitly diagnostic medical logic. This knowledge base represents a four year of effort spent in comprehensive medical information and weekly meeting associating medical experts in each field and cogniticians. Information sources used include litterature review, patient data base derived from different Hospital Information Systems (more than 500,000 patients) and expert subjective judgement. Knowledge is obtained after different cycles of refinement and validation including experimentation on real patients cases before a satisfactory representation evolves. This medical knowledge base contains diagnostic information about 1000 internal medicine diseases and 5600 patients findings and covers the main diseases corresponding to the level of knowledge required of a student [5] .
The building block of the knowledge base is represented by the Iliad frame : a comprehensive list of the different clinical and biological findings reliably reported to

occur in patients with the disease. Diseases frames in Iliad are designed using probabilistic model whenever possible. This facilitates the ranking and comparison of multiple hypotheses. A typical disease frame would include the following slots : 1) an apriori probability, 2) the list of findings, 3) the frequency of these findings in patients with and without this disease. Each disease is modelized by grouping its manifestations into subsets named "intermediate decisions" and corresponding to the syndrome used by physicians in medical practice. This approach is considered to closely emulate the logical analysis used by domain expert in making medical decisions in practice. In many instances, such a subset of manifestations represents a physiopathological process that may be shared by different diseases.

3.2 The data dictionnary

The data dictionnary is organized according to a hierarchical structure. Each item in the dictionnary has a text string describing it and a unique corresponding code. The code identifies uniquely the finding in the hierarchy and is used for internal processing while the text (in English or French) is used to interact with the users. Each finding has also two numbers associated with it:
- the cost of acquiring the piece of information,
- the probability of the symptome that represents the frequency estimate with which the feature or attribute occurs in the subject population based on the combined population of three hospitals located in Salt Lake City. To each term is also linked a set of synonyms that permits to better recognize the considered term.
In addition, the dictionary files include information about words relationships and findings relationships independently of a disease context. The words relationships increase access to the system's vocabulary and ease the entry of patient data while disease independent relations between findings allows the system to make medical logic inferences (e.g, biopsy findings of Crohn's disease and ulcerative colitis are mutually exclusive) and demonstrate a measure of common sense (e.g., pregnancy in males).

3.3 The user Interface

Through the use of pull-down menus and windows, the user may control the operation of the program to meet his/her needs. To add information in Iliad, user has to type one or more words describing the new symptoms. Up to five findings may be entered in the same window. Iliad uses a stripping algorithm to try to identify a suffix in each word and then from the stem terms looks in its dictionary for a concept matching the terms in each entered string. If the corresponding term is not recognized, Iliad displays a lexicon of terms that start with the entered letters. Another way to enter patient data is via the list hierarchy pathway so any relevant patients findings within a category may be selected. On user's request Iliad is able to determine what the next optimal information to gather in the patient workup. This can be done globally or by category : history (Hx), physical exam (PE) or lab exam (LE). This is achieved by ranking each item in each frame under consideration according to an algorithm which takes into account the probability of the frame provided by the item, and the cost of that information. In a window, findings entered by the user are displayed at all times and their review is enhanced by a medically relevant organization: each category of data is underlined (e.g., Hx, PE, LE), attributes of the same concept are intented and pertinent positive findings are highlighted. If the user selects one findings in this list, an explanation of this findings is presented in the form of an ordered set of intermediate decisions and diseases which most likely account for this abnormality. In the same way, explanation of the logic of the decision frame is obtained from a menu option or in selecting any disease in the differential diagnostic list present in the left lower window.

4. French version development

In early 1990, two of the authors (OB and EL) produced a French version of the Iliad system by translating all the dictionary terms and recompiling the knowledge base. Since all processing involves only the hierarchical codes, this was all the efforts required to obtain a first version in French. The translation of the user interface (i.e. menu and command names, prompt, and help messages) was accomplished by translating the resource files of the Iliad application using the ResEdit Macintosh utility. However, the development and validation of Iliad knowledge base follows an evolutive process with many modifications taking place during the bi-weekly knowledge engineering sessions in each of the 9 internal medicine subspecialities. These refinements often require dictionary changes. To maintain the English and the French version synchronized, a set of tools was developed around the concept of a master dictionary file where aliases representing the different translations are represented [1]. With each new release, the translation table is required for the terms that have seen their textual information altered (e.g., text, keywords, hierarchical address) since last update of the French version. This has reduced the translation efforts to a minimum. Afterwards, the French dictionary is rebuilt with the new modifications and the knowledge base is recompiled into a updtodate French version.

5. Implementation

Iliad is implemented on the Macintosh personal computer. The program is menu driven and easy to use. A tutorial and documentation are provided with the program which is presently being commercialized by Applied Informatics Inc (Salt Lake City, Utah). Iliad is an integral part of Utah school of medicine curiculum. It has also been integrated in various ways in 30 medical schools programs in the US. A French version has been developped and is presently tested in Lariboisière Saint-Louis Faculty. A joint experimentation between Lariboisière Saint-Louis Faculty and Utah University is concurrently conducted to evaluate the transferability of the medical content as well as compare French and American students behavior. The collaboration between the French and American Universities would provide a measure of the amount of modifications needed before an expert system's knowledge base is accepted by non-developers as a reliable reflection of how they practice or teach clinical problem-solving skills.

6. Conclusion

Computer based problem solving is becoming a useful tool for accessing to a medical knowledge in continuous evolution and for testing acquired knowledge by students or physicians in training. Iliad program objective is to provide students and practicing physicians quick and easy access to the medical knowledge. Iliad serves as a diagnostic consultant for solving actual cases and as a case simulator for learning. Its structure permits easily development in other foreign langage. Evaluation of french and american behavior should permit to confirm the possible implementation of such system in locations outside the American country.

REFERENCES

1. Bouhaddou O, Lepage E, Warner H Jr, Warner H. (1991): An approach to producing and maintaining translations of a Diagnostic Medical Expert System. (submitted for publication)
2. Warner HR. (1978): Computer-assisted medical decision making. Academic Press, New York.
3. Miller RA, Masarie F., Myers J. (1986): Quick Medical Reference (QMR) for diagnostic assistance. MD Computing, 3:34-48.
4. Barnett GO, Cimino JJ, Hupp JA and Hoffer EP (1987): DXplain: Experience with knowledge acquisition and program evaluation. Proceedings of the 11th Annual Symposium on Computer Applications in Medical Care (SCAMC), 110-115.
5. Bouhaddou O, Lepage E, Warner H Jr, Warner H. (1989): An approach to evaluating the completeness of a medical knowledge base. Proceedings of the 13th Annual Symposium on Computer Applications in Medical Care (SCAMC), 110-115.

The authors thank Apple Computers Inc France for their help in french Iliad evaluation.

VISUALIZING MEDICAL KNOWLEDGE -

an "intelligent" textbook based on graphical browsing

K. Kuhn[1], P. Kottmann[2], U. Holderer-Kottmann[1], T. Zemmler[1], W. Swobodnik[3],
H. Ditschuneit[1]

[1]Medizinische Klinik und Poliklinik der Universität Ulm, FRG
[2]Systemhaus GEI, Ulm, FRG
[3]Medizinische Klinik und Poliklinik der Technischen Universität München, FRG

ABSTRACT

In the process of exploring a method of presenting medical knowledge in a mainly graphical way for an "intelligent" textbook, a system has been implemented on a graphics workstation. The intention was not to build a consultation system, but rather to improve access to knowledge by visualizing complex relationships: the main feature is graphical browsing through a semantic net displayed on the screen. Nodes represent diseases, pathophysiological states, and findings; detailed information about the nodes may be displayed via pull-down menues. The main links represent "is-a", "causes" (with variants like "causes with delay" or "predisposes-to"), "is-associated-with", and "excludes" relationships. The first application domain of the system is gastroenterology. To date, 100 diseases, 100 pathophysiological states, and 400 findings have been entered.

1. OBJECTIVES

The idea of providing access to medical knowledge through computers has to take into account several problems inherent to this knowledge. Medical knowledge itself is extremely complex and it is rapidly growing; for many diseases, on the other hand, it is only shallow and there are inconsistencies and competing hypotheses.

Consequently, an adequate structuring of knowledge is one of the major challenges. Several systems have been developed to make medical knowledge easily available for the user (usually a physician or a medical student) and easy to maintain for the medical author. Important approaches use hypertext methods [1,8] and artificial intelligence [4,7] or try to combine different paradigms [2].

During our work in constructing intelligent frontend workstations including a teaching component for a clinical database system [3], we tried to add functions of an "intelligent" textbook for physicians and medical students. The intention was not to build a consultation system, but to improve access to knowledge by visualizing complex relationships. The system should be easy to maintain and update. Instead of displaying single entities of knowledge (usually "cards" in a hypertext system), we explored the idea of primarily displaying the semantic links between these entities of knowledge.

2. LOGICAL DESIGN

The main feature is graphical browsing through a semantic net displayed on the screen. Nodes and edges are labelled. Nodes can be activated by clicking a mouse button and selecting features of interest via pull-down and pop-up menues in a structured way. For diseases and pathophysiological states, these features can be symptoms, complications or therapy, while findings are described in terms of characteristics and causes. Frisse [1] points out, that the efficiency of finding information in a graph-traversal approach depends on the similarity of the vocabularies used to label links and nodes by the author and the user. The semantics of our nodes are the dimensions disease, pathophysiological state, and findings, which are familiar to physicians and medical students. The main links represent "is-a", "causes" (with variants like "causes with delay" and "predisposes-to"), "is-associated-with", and "excludes" relationships. Different types of nodes and links are displayed by different symbols and/or colours. For a better overview, two levels of information are used. "Cardinal" diseases, pathophysiological states, and findings are shown permanently, while additional nodes and edges can be displayed by clicking the mouse on a node and requesting "more details". By browsing, the medical student or the physician in training can look up the typical symptoms of diseases and pathophysiological states and see the main consequences of diseases. In the opposite direction, it is possible to find the causes of certain findings and pathophysiological states. The main emphasis of the system therefore is not on finding information in an emergency situation. Instead, it is used to assist in studying medical knowledge in an environment showing causal and nosological relationships with the option of changing the focus of interest quickly. A dictionary is used to support the finding of a starting point. As a 19" monitor is not large enough to show all relevant links in a subdomain of internal medicine, the net can be "zoomed" and (via mouse) moved over the screen. A schematic illustration of the approach is given in the figure below.

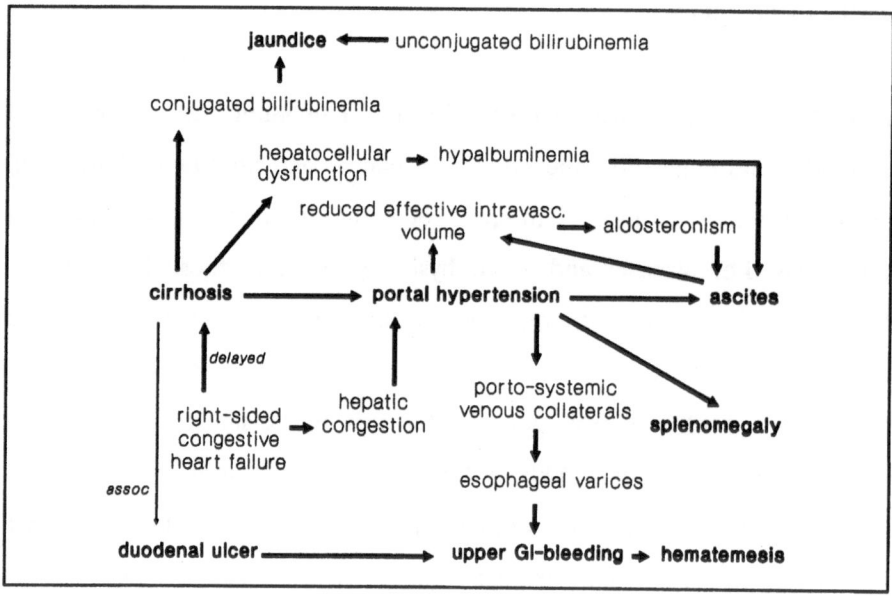

Figure: Schematic illustration of the network structure, demonstrated for the disease node cirrhosis (1 out of 100). The disease node cirrhosis is shown here together with two related disease nodes (duodenal ulcer and congestive heart failure) and related pathophysiological states (portal hypertension, hepatocellular dysfunction...). Findings derived are jaundice, ascites, splenomegaly, and hematemesis caused by upper GI-bleeding which is caused by esophageal varices. The shown links are causal except for the association between cirrhosis and duodenal ulcer. For illustrational purposes, most links to and from the displayed nodes have been omitted (e.g. most causes of cirrhosis, types of cirrhosis connected via "is-a" links, other causes of splenomegaly, complications of duodenal ulcer). The implementation uses different colours, fonts, and graphical symbols to discriminate between types of nodes and links and to highlight important nodes (here: bold print).

3. IMPLEMENTATION

The system has been implemented on a graphics workstation. Based on the X11 system, two object-oriented tools, a window-manager and a tool for handling vector graphics, have been employed. Nodes and edges of the net are mouse-sensitive. After selection of a node, several pop-up and pull-down-menues allow the description of diseases according to the categories etiology, associated diseases, clinical symptoms, findings in physical examination, laboratory findings, x-ray and ultrasound findings, results of other examinations, complications, therapy, together with literature references. Images are displayed under the X11 environment. Subnets showing more details can be loaded from each node.

Knowledge can be added to the system using the same interface as used for browsing. The mouse is used to select between types of nodes and edges and between categories describing the nodes. Nodes and edges may be added, altered, moved, or removed. The first application domain of the system is gastroenterology. To date, 100 diseases, 100 pathophysiological states, and 400 findings have been entered. Knowledge is acquired by medical students or by physicians and revised by senior members of the faculty.

4. RESULTS

A method of presenting medical knowledge in a mainly graphical way for an "intelligent" textbook has been explored, and a system has been implemented. It runs on a graphics workstation and uses the same interface for knowledge acquisition as for the intended visualization. The display of diseases, pathophysiological states, and findings together with their semantic links improves the overview and facilitates memorization. The structure of the knowledge is based on a causal/nosological network as discussed by Pople [6]. The intention of our system is different, however: it has not been built to optimize inference processes but to support fast and structured access to medical knowledge. Detailed knowledge is stored "behind" the nodes. Like QMR [5], our system can be used as a low- or intermediate-level information retrieval or management tool; unlike QMR, however, it displays relationships graphically which may be more time-consuming but offers a new kind of global overview. The integration of the actual stand-alone system in our medical workstation [3] will add an important feature to the spectrum of electronical support facilities for the physician or medical student.

REFERENCES

[1] Frisse M.E.: Searching for Information in a Hypertext Medical Handbook. Comm ACM 31, 1988, 880-886.
[2] Greenes R.A.: "Desktop Knowledge": A New Focus for Medical Education and Decision Support. Meth Inform Med 28, 1989, 332-339.
[3] Kuhn K., Doster W., Roesner D., Kottmann P., Swobodnik W., Ditschuneit H.: An Integrated Medical Workstation with a Multimodal User Interface, Knowledge-Based User Support and Multimedia Documents. Proc 3rd IEEE Symp CBMS, 1990, 469-476.
[4] Miller R.A., Masarie F.E., Myers J.D.: "Quick Medical Reference" for diagnostic assistance. MD Computing 3, 1986, 34-48.
[5] Miller R.A., McNeil M.A., Challinor S.M., Masarie F.E., Myers J.D.: The INTERNIST-1/QUICK MEDICAL REFERENCE Project-Status Report. West J Med 145, 1986, 816-22.
[6] Pople H.E.: Heuristic Methods for Imposing Structure on Ill-Structured Problems: The Structure of Medical Diagnosis. In Szolovits P. (ed): Artificial Intelligence in Medicine. Westview Press, Boulder, Col., 1982.
[7] Reggia J.A., Pula T.P., Price T.R., Perricone B.T.: Towards an Intelligent Textbook of Neurology. Proc 4th SCAMC, 1980, 190-199.
[8] Shultz E.K., Brown R.W., Beck J.R.: Hypermedia in Pathology - The Dartmouth Interactive Medical Record Project. A J C P 91, 1989, Suppl 1, 34-38.

RESEARCH AND EPIDEMIOLOGY

C.Beguin[1], R.Van den Heuvel[2], B.Winkeler[2], M.C.Closon[1], F.H.Roger[1]

Abstract

HOSCOM project organised a EuroHealth-database with hospital data from
seven countries. Comparisons were possible on 199516 inpatients records.
The most frequent pathologies were cardiovascular and respiratory
diseases. Admittance rates in emergency varied between countries. Death
rate was higher for neonatal pathologies in one country, for respiratory
diseases in another one.
DRGs, refined DRGs and Disease Staging have been tested with a specific
database on diabetic patients (4297 records). Diabetes without
complication was the most frequent main diagnosis in the three case-mix
systems. Variance in length of stay was better explained by the refined
DRGs than by the two others.

Introduction

A major objective of the HOSCOM (Hospital comparisons in Europe) project
of AIM ("Advanced Informatics in Medicine") was to obtain a
EuroHealthDataBase for hospital comparisons. Three main steps were
followed : "designing a uniform model for medical data, designing a
uniform model for resources and costs data and testing these uniform
models of reference for medical data as well as for resources and
costs". In order to validate reference models, two groups of studies
were performed. The first one, called "macrostudy" was devoted to test
its feasibility and to obtain international comparisons of hospital data
in the limits of the project. The second one called "microstudies" was
devoted too more medical aspects with a larger data set on fewer
patients in three pathologies : diabetes mellitus, cardiac valve
replacement and hip fracture. In the present report, we will describe
the microstudy on diabetes mellitus and its link with the Eurohealth
database.

Method

A questionnaire was designed and sent to representatives of all EEC
countries in order to define formats and to clarify definitions,
classifications and record lay-outs of the MBDS (Minimum Basic Data Set)
items available in their country. Based on results from this
questionnaire, the European MBDS (1) recommended in 1982 for hospital
acute inpatients was revised in order to obtain a more up to date MBDS
to be tested in a EuroHealthDataBase, located in Utrecht. Marital status
was made optional, and few items were added (medical specialty, type of
admission and discharge, identification of the country...). Each item
was defined and a specific format has been required. Each HOSCOM
partner was asked to send data samples.

1.Centre for Medical Informatics, University of Louvain, 10 av.Hippocrate, B1200
Brussel
2.SIG Services, Maliebaan 50, 3508 Utrecht, Nederlands
This project has been supported by the Commission of the European Communities,
DGXIII F

This database was made of 57057 records from Belgium, 35687 from Denmark, 34289 from Germany, 53489 from Great Britain, 53283 from Italy, 50974 from Netherlands, 23674 from Spain, with a total of 308453 records.

The selection of patients for the microstudy on diabetes was also based on a questionnaire in order to define what data (physiological, administrative and resource data) could be made available in supplement to the items contained in the revised MBDS. In the limits imposed by the exploratory phase of AIM (6 months for a validation phase), three countries agreed to participate, Belgium with 6924 records, Denmark with 3427 records and United Kingdom with 1230 records. It was also decided to test and analyse the data available in the revised medical MBDS, as defined by the HOSCOM project.

Results

A first part of results concerns the data collection for the Eurohealth database and the microstudy on diabetes. The second one describes inpatients comparisons.

1 Need for harmonisation revealed by the EuroHealth Database :

"Some countries did not provide DRGs and DRGs could not be added because other classification systems than ICD-9-CM were used, and could not be mapped to standard groupers". Comparisons had therefore to be restricted during the exploratory phase to sets of data that were comparable. Further diffusion of EuroHealth data requirements is needed.
In the microstudy on diabetes the same difficulty in data dissimilarities has been observed. One country sent incomplete data for some items like sex, type of admission, and discharge status. Another sent erroneous values that had to be corrected for one item. An analysis of diagnostic accuracy showed that 14% to 24% of the diagnoses were not precise enough.

2 Results from inpatients comparisons in the macro and the microstudy

Table I shows the comparisons made in the macrostudy into four countries, where DRGs could be obtained and compared. This table gives the proportion of records in the five most frequent MDCs, with their rate of admittance in emergency and their death rate. The greatest proportion of records is found for cardiovascular and respiratory diseases in the four countries. The proportion of records with admittance in emergency was most often lower in country A. Such difference makes the comparisons difficult between countries and needs further explanations. Death rate was only available in two countries, A and D. In country A, the most frequent cause of death was myeloproliferative diseases and poorly diffentiated neoplasms (MDC 17), neonates pathologies (MDC 15), as well as respiratory diseases (MDC 4). In country D, death rate was highest for respiratory diseases (MDC 4), neurological diseases (MDC 1), myeloproliferative diseases and poorly differentiated neoplasms (MDC 17).

Table I : Distribution, emergency and death rate for the five most
frequent MDC in four countries

	Distribution				Emergency			Death rate	
MDC	A	B	C	D	A	B	C	A	D
1	6,9%	6,3%	7,7%	3%	15,6%	76%	64,1%	7%	6,3%
3	4,7%	4,3%	4,1%	10,3%	1,9%	41%	32,1%	0,5%	0,4%
5	15,3%	9%	10,9%	10,3%	2,4%	75,9%	73,6%	5%	4,4%
6	9,2%	11,6%	8,9%	11,9%	3,3%	59,2%	57,7%	2,7%	1,5%
8	12%	11,3%	6,7%	5,7%	13,4%	51,3%	37,5%	3,5%	0,7%

MDC 1 = Neurological Diseases
MDC 3 = Ear, nose, mouth and throat diseases
MDC 5 = Cardiovascular Diseases
MDC 6 = Digestive Diseases
MDC 8 = Muskulo-squelettal Diseases

Table II shows a comparison of length of stay for the ten most frequent
DRGs in these countries. DRGs are classified by decreasing frequency.
In country D, length of stay is systematically lower than in the other
countries.

Table II Length of stay in the ten most frequent DRGs in four European
countries

DRGs	Country A		Country B		Country C		Country D	
	F	LOS	F	LOS	F	LOS	F	LOS
470	411	14,8	1806	5,7	5089	9,5	9179	5,4
373	2214	6,7	853	4,6	1215	6,6	829	4,6
183	725	6	617	3,9	762	7,6	1915	3,2
467	582	4,5	1909	5	496	5,3	273	4,7
125	2995	4	-	-	32	8,6	824	3,8
390	165	12,7	161	4,8	75	8,5	2717	4
381	188	2,6	956	1,8	607	2	797	1,6
243	793	6,9	585	10,6	623	11,6	348	10
468	810	18,4	453	13,6	575	15,6	385	9,3
82	713	11,6	300	8,3	682	13,9	428	9,2
Total	9596		7640		10156		17695	

F = frequency, LOS = length of stay

```
470 = Ungroupable
373 = Vaginal delivery
183 = Esophagitis, gastroent.digest. diseases
467 = Other factors influencing health care
125 = Circulatory disorders,except acute myocardial
      infarct, with cardiac catheterism
390 = Neonates, with other significant problems
381 = Abortion, curettage, hysterotomy
243 = Medical back problems
468 = Unrelated operating room procedures
82  = Respiratory neoplasms
```

In the microstudy on diabetes mellitus, three case-mix systems have been
tested : DRGs (2), refined DRGs (RGN) (3) and Disease Staging. Table III
gives the distribution of patients in the major categories of these
three case-mix.

Table III Frequency of patients (in percent) belonging to major
categories in three case-mix

Case-mix	Country A	Country D
MDC		
1	7,6%	2,6%
2	6,9%	0,8%
5	6,8%	9,8%
9	1,7%	1,1%
10	74,1%	80,4%
11	2,9%	3,7%
RGN		
0	67,5%	–
1	25%	–
2	5,8%	–
3	0,8%	–
Disease Staging		
1	51,9%	53,23%
2	36%	26,51%
3	10%	18,97%
4	2,1%	1,29%

MDC = major category of diagnosis
RGN = refined DRG

RGN could not be applied in country D because mapping to DRG was
performed to grouper III and was not possible to grouper VI.
Table III demonstrates the feasibility to apply different case-mix
methods on diabetic inpatients in Europe, and the difficulty to obtain
adequate and comparable data in the different countries, if not planned
in advance. The same trends are observed mainly for the most frequent
conditions (MDC 10, RGN 0 and 1, DS 1 and 2).

The percentage of variance in length of stay explained by the three
case-mix in the two countries is 18,8% for DRGs, 23,3% for RGN, 11% for
Disease Staging in country A and 16,7% for DRGs, 12,3% for Disease
Staging in country D.
Length of stay is the most commonly available indirect resource
indicator in Europe, in absence of sufficient availability on procedures
costs by patient in most countries. This result shows that DRGs and
mainly RGNs were better explaining resources use in hospitals for
diabetic patients than Disease Staging that could be better used for
patients outcome appraisal.

Discussion

Three important problems have restricted results in the present study : the data availability, some variations in definition for each item and the retrospective character of data analysis.

Data availability included exhaustivity as well as delay to furnish the data. These difficulties could be overcome by procedures established in order to assure availability and timeliness in future. Data availability interfered with patients selection. It introduced therefore a bias in the epidemiological analysis of the data. In our sample the majority of records in countries A and C dealt with cardiovascular diseases, while digestive diseases were more frequent in countries B and D.

The definition of each item is also important in order to interprete results. There was a lower rate of records with admittance in emergency in country A. What was the exact meaning of emergency?

The most frequent cause of death was neonates problems in country A and respiratory diseases in country B. Death rate must be carefully interpreted because there is no mention of the type of care and of the severity of cases.

In the ten most frequent DRGs appear the DRG 470 "ungroupable" and the DRG 468 "operating room not related to the principal diagnosis". This highlights the problem of the quality of coding and its consequences on the grouping system.

The microstudy on diabetes mellitus allowed us to compare different case-mix systems. The majority of patients had no complication. The most frequent complications were neurological in country A and vascular in country D. Refined DRGs and Disease Staging appear to be promising method in order to measure severity of cases. When using the different case-mix systems to explain variance in length of stay, the refined DRGs explained a greater proportion than the two other methods. However, these comparisons were limited to length of stay and do not taken into account other types of charges.

Lessons from these preliminary studies should help us for future hospital comparisons in order to measure efficiency of care, quality of care and to perform epidemiological studies. We would recommend to work prospectively, to improve the quality of the data by implying physicians in these analyses and by developping tools for the measure of severity, costs and resource of health care.

References

1 Lambert P.M and Roger F.H
  "The Minimum Basic Data Set for Hospital Statistics in the CEE"
  Hospital Statistics in Europe, North Holland, 1982, p 83-112

2 Fetter R.B. et al.
  "Case-mix definition by DRG"
  Med Care Rev 18 (suppl) 1980, p 1-53

3 Fetter et al.
  "DRG Refinement with Diagnostic specific comorbidities and complications: a Synthesis of current approaches to patient classification"; Final report, Yale University, 1989

The Eurohealth Database -
Handling Personal Data Without Access to Personal Identification

Barry Barber[1], Francis Roger-France[2], Bart Winkeler[3] and Peter Olsen[4]

AIM HOSCOM Consortium

[1]NHS Information Management Centre, BIRMINGHAM, UK

[2] Cliniques Universitaires St-Luc, UCL, Bruxelles, Belgique

[3] SIG Services BV, Utrecht, The Netherlands

[4] Kommunedata, Hospital Computer Centre, Copenhagen, Denmark

This paper discusses the Data Protection issues of developing a European Health Database from information supplied by hospitals across Europe as a basis for making comparisons about hospital activities. The review is, which is based on the Council of Europe recommendations and UK legislation, develops the approach used by the AIM HOSCOM project for the Eurohealth Database.

1   Introduction

There is a well established general public interest, as well as a clear professional health care interest, in ensuring that Health Information provided to Health Care Professionals within the confidence of their professional activities should remain confidential to those concerned with their care and the administration of their care. However, because the provision of health care within the present day context of very complex technical activities requires some disclosure of information, a number of specific disclosures beyond the clinical team are accepted as being necessary in order to make these complex arrangements work.

The AIM HOSCOM project investigated the possibilities for comparing hospital activities. It did not require or seek any disclosure of Personal Information in order to make these comparisons. The Data were supplied without the identifying information but with a local code known only to those supplying the information in order that any queries relating to the data could be confirmed by those supplying the data. The absence of any local identifier would have made it impossible to check on the correctness of the data. The work of IMIA WG4 (Griesser et al 1980, 1983, Barber 1988) provide a background to this work. However, it should be noted that the draft EC Directive on Data Protection is likely to herald a major development of the European Data Protection and Information Systems Security environment.

2   General Data Protection and Computer Security

There are many issues relating to Data Protection and Computer Security which govern the degree to which information can be kept confidential. This paper discusses one set of issues relating to Personal Data entered into a central database from which there are no authorised uses of the identified information about individuals. The proposals made below relate to one set of issues but it is assumed that the data will be kept secure at the originating centres [this is likely because they have greater security issues to address because they hold the identified Personal Information], during transit to the central database and at the central data centre. Careless and inadequate computer security in these areas can, of course, negate the value of the steps discussed below.

3   Identified Personal Health Information Held Centrally

There are many valuable reasons for assembling a central data bank of Personal Health Information. It enables studies to be made in respect of specific diseases and to explore variations in Health Care delivery with geographical areas. In addition, by linking all episodes of care resulting in a record in the central data base, it is possible to establish a complete pattern of individual care. Such data bases are valuable for Medical Research and Epidemiology and for Health Care Planning purposes. In many cases such data bases are viewed with some concern by the general public as a possible source of a breach of confidentiality. Where these data bases have been established considerable efforts have been expended to ensure that patient confidentiality is not breached, that the data are kept secure and that the data bank is not misused. This overhead to the data bank can be quite considerable and, hence, it is worth considering the situation where no such identification is required - as is the case with the AIM HOSCOM project.

4   UK Data Protection Legislation

The UK Data Protection Act 1984 (HMSO 1984) was drafted in the context of the UK ratification of the Council of Europe's Convention "For the Protection of Individuals with Regard to Automatic Processing of Personal Data". This act defines "**disclosing**" in part I section 1(9) as including information extracted from the data held and it goes on to note that:-

> "where the identification of the individual who is the subject of the Personal Data depends partly on the information constitution the data and partly on other information in the possession of the Data User, the data shall not be regarded as disclosed or transferred unless the other information is disclosed or transferred."

The definition of "Personal Data" is somewhat wider than this as

> "Personal Data means data consisting of information which relates to a living individual who can be identified from that information (or from that and other information in the possession of the data user), including any expression of opinion about the individual but not any indication of the intentions of the data user in respect of that individual."

The Data Protection Registrar's Guideline 2 The Definitions (1989) amplifies this legal definition as follows in sections 3.1, 3.2 and 3.5:-

> "The Act is only concerned with information which relates to a living individual. If the subject of the information is dead then the information cannot be personal data. If the subject is not an individual, for example, if the information relates only to a limited company or other artificial legal person then it is unlikely to be Personal Data.
>
> The individual must be identifiable. If the data include the individual's name, that will usually be sufficient to make the information Personal Data. Sometimes, even though the data do not contain a name, they will be Personal Data because they relate to an individual whom the data user can identify from other information in its possession. This will be the case where, for example, the data contain an account number or employee number and the data user keeps a separate list, whether on the computer or on paper, from which the individual can be identified."

Within the UK legislation there is no problem about holding information about individuals that cannot be identified - it is just not Personal Data and hence is not governed by the Data Protection Act 1984 - nor is there any problem in transferring Personal Data without the identifying details as it is not a "disclosure". However, in keeping with the aims of the Data Protection legislation in the UK perspective we would wish to ensure that the chance of any recipient of such data having, or acquiring, the additional information required to convert the non-Personal Data into Personal Data was reduced to a very low level.

5   UK Registration of Personal Data Held Without Identification Information

Within the UK such information is frequently stored by Regional Health Authorities or centrally by the Department of Health or the Office of Populations, Censuses and Surveys [OPCS]. The identification information is not supplied with the data so that individuals cannot be identified, except possibly by sophisticated methods. Considerable care is taken with the security of the information but it does not need registration with the Office of the Data Protection Registrar as it is not Personal Data within the meaning of the UK legislation. The only reason for registering such data is precautionary to emphasise the security issues and to cover the possibility that someone in the organisation might inadvertently acquire the information to decode the patient number thus converting a record into Personal Data.

If such an organisation acquires, deliberately or otherwise, information that would enable it to identify any of the individuals, it would need to register the data holding whether or not it had actually done so. There are no "Chinese Walls" within the context of the UK legislation; if anyone legally responsible to the Data User within any part of his organisation has the information to identify individuals within the data, then the organisation is deemed to be holding Personal Data. The restriction of identification information to a particular part of the organisation that requires access is a desirable security procedure not a barrier to registration.

6   Handling Local Identification Numbers

The only functions of the identification codes is to allow for error correction, quality control of the information and record linkage. This can be achieved as follows:-

1   sending the information with the local identification number such as the patient record number but without the name and address

2   the allocation of new code numbers to each individual which are kept secure in the originating institution, eg available only to a single person, but which can be used to translate back into the local identification number when this proves necessary. This would involve extensive look-up tables and would be cumbersome for large volumes of data.

3   The local record number can be encrypted in some convenient fashion and the encrypted number used to identify the information between the two organisations. The appropriate selection of encryption techniques should reduce the chance of obtaining two local record numbers with the same encrypted numbers. This should prove very convenient as there is no need for the receiving organisation to decrypt these number so that there is no need for the transmission of keys. It is merely necessary to keep a record of the keys used and the material for which they were used. The encryption keys can be changed as frequently as desired without inconvenience if record linkage is not required.

4   All identifying numbers can be removed and then the record can only be identified between the two organisations as a result of an exhaustive search to find matching records. This is likely to prove inconvenient and time consuming. It would be particularly important that adequate quality control procedures should be implemented in order to reduce the chance of the occurrence of duplicate or inaccurate records.

Within the European context it would appear that the best choice would be the third one in which the data is supplied together with an encrypted local identification number as no-one elsewhere would have access to it so that the person could be identified. This approach goes beyond the strict requirements of the UK Data Protection Act 1984 but this extension would seem to offer additional security without unreasonable difficulty that is consistent with the aims of the act.

7   Intrinsic Identification

Within any collection of data about an individual there is always the possibility that some particular set of characteristics allow an individual to be identified. This involves a match between a variety of features in such a fashion that the individual in question is the only one satisfying all these criteria. This is most easily achieved where the individual in question has some very special and well known characteristic that effectively identifies him or her. In this case, this characteristic effectively identifies the individual. However, it is difficult to see how such a convenient identification can be achieved with the HOSCOM minimum basic data set unless one were dealing with a hospital that was so small that the date of admission virtually identified the individual.

For those with ready access to the hospital, it might be possible to assemble a selection of information to identify an individual by linking the date of admission,sex, specialty, date of birth and area of residence code. However, it would usually be easier to access the hospital's own records directly rather than attempting to access a remote database held in another country. On the other hand, for those with access to the statistical database, it would be unlikely that they could establish the necessary data for a specified individual to carry out an effective unauthorised search.

8   Detailed Area of Residence Codes or Post Codes

The real problem would be likely to occur with detailed area or post codes as they allow an individual residence to be pin-pointed to within 50-100 individuals. This together with the knowledge of an attendance at a specific hospital effectively identifies an individual. Intrinsic identification or identification using post codes cannot be ruled out as impossible but merely rather unlikely in the circumstances. Accordingly, it is important that the database for HOSCOM should be treated with all security measures that would normally used for the MBDS when it has the full identification information attached. This will then certainly ensure that the information is protected adequately.

9   Council of Europe Convention

Without a detailed investigation of the national Data Protection legislation of each country in conjunction with other relevant legislation governing confidentiality, health care professional ethics and the "duty of care", it is impossible to establish the precise situation. However, an examination of the Council of Europe Convention "For the Protection of Individuals with Regard to Automatic Processing of Personal Data" (1981) shows the following approach that is likely to be acceptable in many European countries as the council's convention has become a world standard in this area.

The following examination cannot, of course, be exhaustive but it attempts to explore the most important issues that emerge from an examination of the text of the Council of Europe Convention and the relevant Recommendations. The view has been taken that although HOSCOM is not technically dealing with Personal Data within the meaning of the convention currently, the data bank holds data that is quite close to being Personal Data and that many of the measures required for handling Personal Data might be appropriate.

The definition of Personal Data is given in Article 2 and it "means any information relating to an identified or identifiable individual" ("Data Subject") and the explanatory notes [28] indicate that "identifiable persons" means a person who can be easily identified; it does not cover identification of persons by means of very sophisticated methods".

Article 6 indicates that "Personal Data concerning Health....may not be processed automatically unless domestic law provides appropriate safeguards". Article 8 states that:-

"Any person shall be enabled:

a   to establish the existence of an automated personal data file, its main purposes, as well as the identity and habitual residence or principal place of business of the controller of the file;

b   to obtain at reasonable intervals and without excessive delay or expense confirmation of whether Personal Data relating to him are stored in the automated data file as well as communication to him of such data in an intelligible form;

c   to obtain, as the case may be, rectification or erasure of such data if these have been processed contrary to the provisions of domestic law giving effect to the basic principles set out in Articles 5 and 6 of this convention;

d   to have a remedy if a request for confirmation or, as the case may be, communication, rectification or erasure as referred to in paragraphs b and c of this Article are not complied with."

Article 12, dealing with trans-border flows of Personal data and Domestic Law, indicates that a party to the convention

"shall not, for the sole purpose of the protection of privacy, prohibit or subject to special authorisation trans-border flows of Personal data going to the territory of another party"

except where:-

a   ".....its legislation includes specific regulations for certain categories of Personal Data or of automated Personal Data files, because of the nature of those data or those files except where the regulations of the other party provide an equivalent protection."

b   "when the transfer is made from its territory to the territory of another non-contracting state through the intermediary of the territory of another party in order to avoid such transfers resulting in circumvention of the legislation of the party referred to at the beginning of this paragraph."

This article allows parties to derogate from paragraph 2 but it would be valuable to examine whether any of the European countries had, in fact, done so.

This examination of the convention, thus, establishes that, like the UK legislation, the data required for HOSCOM is explicitly not Personal Data under the Council of Europe Convention as Article 2 specifically excludes the data requiring sophisticated methods for identification purposes. The problem of Intrinsic Identification is thus a security issue rather than a legal issue. The approach of encrypting the local identification number is, thus, more than adequate for the purpose. Furthermore, even if the data were Personal Data, it could not be prevented from being transmitted across EC country boundaries unless the particular countries had entered a derogation from paragraph 2 in Article 12. There are no problems relating to Subject Access provided that the identifying information is withheld from those responsible for the central data bank.

10   Recommendations Regarding Medical Data Banks [R(81)1]

The Council's recommendations regarding Medical Data Banks carries more detailed requirements for handling Personal Health Data. Generally, these regulations require that:-

Specific regulations governing the scope and purpose of a Medical Data Bank should be drawn up (Rec 1);

These regulations (Rec 3) should include, inter alia, details of how the Data Bank is to be run, who has access to it, what disclosures are made and the security of the data and the installation;

Public notice should be given of the existence of a Medical Data Bank (Rec 2);

Identification information should be separated from the administrative, medical and social data held (Rec 4.2).

Since the data held is not Personal data there is no specific need to observe these requirements but an acceptable set of specific regulations seems desirable governing the handling of the Data Bank with particular emphasis on security issues. There is no reason to leave out public notice of its existence. The matter of separating identifiers does not arise because the Data Bank does not hold identifying information.

11 Recommendations Regarding Scientific Research and Statistics [R(83)10]

The specification in this recommendation of "identifiable" is developed from the previous definition as not covering identification of persons by "means of very sophisticated methods" to not covering identification that requires "an unreasonable amount of time, cost and manpower".

This later definition will have the effect that as some very sophisticated search procedures can be implemented easily and cheaply with improved software and much more powerful hardware some types of "non-Personal Data" will become "Personal Data". Therefore it will be necessary to review current computing facilities from time to time to ensure that a data bank that originally was deemed to hold unidentifiable Personal Information has not, as a result of technological improvements, become an identifiable data bank.

Recommendation 4.3 requires that:-

"Both public and private bodies should have the right to use for their own research purpose the Personal data which they hold for administrative purposes. If in the course of such research Personal Data are added to files already held by the administrative body, or its files are altered, these new files should not be made available to administrative personnel dealing with individual cases, except with the consent of the person concerned."

Recommendation 7.1 requires that:-

"Research projects should make express provision for technical and organisational measures to ensure the security and confidentiality of data."

12 Conclusion

From the foregoing, it is quite clear that there should be no Data Protection impediment to developing the HOSCOM database unless it is embodied in specific requirements of a particular nation's domestic legislation. The following approach should be adopted:-

1 **The local identification number should be encrypted** locally and the keys should not be made available elsewhere. This gives the originating site control of their own security. The central site will only use the encrypted local identification number and this will only be de-crypted at the local site when there are specific queries regarding the accuracy of the data.

2 **Specific Regulations Governing the HOSCOM Data Bank** should be drawn up and publicised as appropriate.

3   **Effective HOSCOM Computer Security Arrangements** are needed
        for the Data Bank governing access, disclosure and responsibility.

4   **No arrangements are required to handle Subject Access.**

5   **Care must be exercised regarding developments** which might turn
        non-Personal Data in the HOSCOM Data Bank into Personal Data.

These recommendations were adopted by the HOSCOM project for its prototyping work and it
appears that the guarantees given to participating hospitals were considered effective and
satisfactory. Work is currently going on in Working Party 12 of the Council of Europe in
respect of updating Recommendation 81(1) on Automated Medical Databanks which will need to
be examined and the draft Directive of the European Commission concerning the Protection of
Individuals in relation to the processing of Personal Data could have significant implications in
terms of the environmental protection for Personal Health Data. However, it is believed that the
regime utilised by the HOSCOM consortium would provide adequate safeguards for the Personal
Health Data.

References

Barber, B NHS Data Protection Handbook, ed Information Management Centre, Birmingham,
        England 1988

Barber, B Current Issues in Data Protection, MIE-88, Oslo, 1988 Medical Informatics, vol 3,
        207-209, 1989

Council of Europe Convention "For the Protection of Individuals with Regard to Automatic
        Processing of Personal Data" No 108, Strasbourg, 28/1/81 ISBN 92 871
        0022 5
        Explanatory Report on the Convention for the Protection of Individuals with Regard to
        Automatic Processing of Personal Data Strasbourg 1981
        Regulations for Automated Medical Data Banks Recommendation No R [81] 1
        Strasbourg 1981
        Protection of Personal Data used for Scientific Research and Statistics,
        Recommendation No R [83] 10 Strasbourg 1984 ISBN 92 871 0317 8

Data Protection Act 1984, HMSO, London 1984, ISBN 0 10 543584 8

European Commission, draft Directive Concerning the Protection of Individuals in Relation to
        the Processing of Personal Data, COM(90), SYN 287, 13 September 1990

Griesser, G, Bakker, A, Danielsson, J, Hirel, J-C, Kenny, D J, Schneider, W and
        Wassermann, A I (ed), Data Protection in Health Information Systems: Considerations
        and Guidelines, ed for IMIA Working Group 4, North Holland Publishing Co, 1980,
        ISBN 0 444 86052 5

Griesser, G, Jardel, J P, Kenny, D. J. and Sauter, K (ed), Data Protection in Health Information
        Systems: Where do we Stand?, ed for IMIA Working Group 4, North Holland
        Publishing Co, 1983, ISBN 0 444 86713 9

HMSO, The Data Protection Act 1984, London, 1984

Office of the Data Protection Registrar Guideline 2 The Definitions, February 1989, Springfield
        House, Water Lane, Wilmslow, Cheshire, England SK9 5AX

ADAMS: Data-base management as a decision support system for epidemiologists

Fernando FERRI^, Patrizia GRIFONI*,Leonardo MEO-EVOLI*, Fabrizio L. RICCI*

*Istituto di Studi sulla Ricerca e Documentazione Scientifica del CNR
Via Cesare De Lollis 12, 00185 Rome
^Dipartimento di Informatica e Sistemistica, Università di Roma "La Sapienza"
Via Salaria 113, 00198 Rome

ABSTRACT

The aim of this paper is to describe a system for the creation, management and manipulation of a statistical database. The ADAMS system is designed as a decisions support system that supports the user work in leading up to statistical analysis. The paper includes descriptions of the various models used to represent statistical data and the manipulation thereof.

key words: statistical databases, man-machine interfaces, decision support systems.

1 INTRODUCTION

The work of epidemiologists consists of acquiring, assessing and interpreting data, and thus of making decisions. Decision support systems therefore perform a vital function in helping the epidemiologist to identify significant data describing trends in a given disease. This function extends to data-interpretation and to decisions affecting the socio-economic factors associated with the trends displayed by certain pathologies.

The ADAMS system presented here is a system for Statistical Database (SDB) management providing the possibility to manipulate statistical tables according to two approaches; the first is based on a visual interaction and the second on a key-word language. The ADAMS system is intended to offer help in defining the context of statistical analysis and in identifying data of significance in working hypotheses. In fact, when such data are scattered over various Statistical Tables (ST), the system offers the possibility of drawing up one single table containing the relevant data only. The table thus obtained may then be subjected to statistical analysis with the appropriate statistics packages. The data appearing in each ST do not concern single events but rather trace out trends associated with phenomena (macrodata) such as mortality due to viral hepatitis according to age and sex, or the distribution of viral hepatitis according to countries and years. In each ST we may distinguish between the statistical data themselves and the data used to describe them (metadata). We may then identify within the metadata a set of variables, a set of variable domains and a data type. The variables provide unique identification of the ST; each variable is in turn associated with a set of values (modalities) constituting the variable domain. Finally, the data type identifies the aggregative function generating the values contained in the ST. An example of an ST on the distribution of cases of viral hepatitis by countries and years is shown in fig. 1:

"Disease distribution" is the name identifying the ST while "countries" and "years" represent the variables. The year modalities are "1980, 1981", the modalities of the country variables "USA, Canada, Austria, France". Finally, "Abs" identifies the ST data type, indicating that the values contained are absolute values obtained with counting functions.

Abs   Disease Distribution

	years	
countries	1980	1981
USA	2148	2542
Canada	1523	1982
Austria	1263	1525
France	1695	2032

fig. 1: Disease distribution by years and countries

2 THE GRASS MODEL

The GRASS model describes the SDB with a direct, acyclic and orientated graph (Ra83); the graph nodes are: S nodes: identifying statistical phenomena associated with the ST's; T nodes: identifying the ST in the SDB and relevant data type; A nodes: nodes indicating the cartesian product of all variables present; C nodes: each of these nodes indicates a variable; M nodes: each of these nodes indicates one of the values (modalities) to be associated with a variable. Precise rules must be respected when linking GRASS nodes. Below is an example of an SDB represented by means of a GRASS graph (fig. 2).

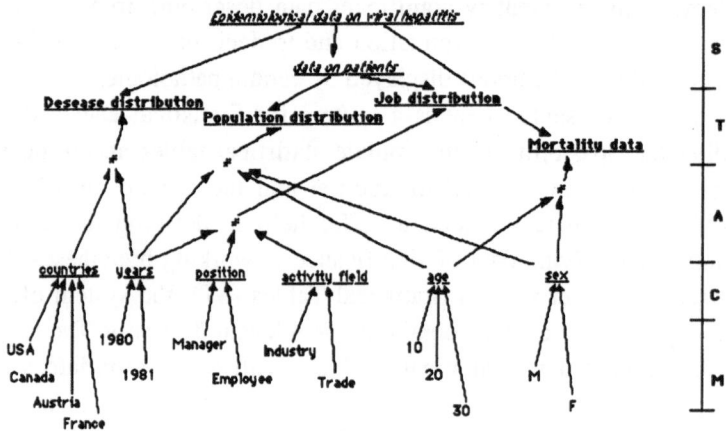

fig. 2: representation of the database using the GRASS graph

The structure of the ST is described in the sub-graph associated with the descending T node, which represents the table. In terms of interface, an alternative form of display was preferred to GRASS for the modes corresponding to each variable.

3 MANIPULATION

Before beginning data analysis the user must generate the ST starting from the ST's stored in the SDB; the fundamental manipulations on STs are "Summarization" and "Reclassification" (Ra90).

Summarization: produces the data aggregation of a ST eliminating a variable. For example the summarization produces the ST "Disease Distribution by years" starting from the ST "Disease Distribution by countries-years" showed in fig.3 and in fig.1

Abs Disease Distribution

years	
1980	1981
6629	8081

fig.3: Disease distribution by years

Reclassification. Substitutes a variable in a ST. Let us again take the example of the table in fig. 1 and assume we wish to know the "Disease Distribution by years-continents". Reclassification can be performed classifying the "countries" in "continents" throught the relation "r1" in fig. 4. The resulting table is shown in fig. 5.

r1

countries	continents
USA	North America
Canada	North America
Austria	Europe
France	Europe

fig.4:Relation countries/continent

Disease Distribution

	years	
continents	1980	1981
North America	3671	4524
Europe	2958	3557

fig.5:Disease Distribution by years and continent

3.1 MANIPULATION OF TABLES

It is possible to interact with the System in various ways according to the user-profile (Br88) and his/her level of experience. For non-experts we adopt a visual interaction that guide the user in the query editing task. For the expert user we adopt the key-word language, STAQUEL (Me90).

The windows available to the user for SDB manipulation are: the GRASS window, the STAQUEL window and the QUERY-GRAPH window. The GRASS window displays the logical structure schema of the SDB (GRASS graph). In the STAQUEL window all queries are expressed with STAQUEL syntax. At last, in the QUERY-GRAPH window queries are expressed with a graph whose nodes represent manipulations and leafs represent arguments. Note, too, that the interface provides a window called GUIDE window, which displays help messages. Queries are edited interactively under the control of the system that automatically checks the syntax and the semantic of queries. The system prevents the user error activating or disabling on the screen the icons that represents data and manipulations. Edited questions are displayed in the STAQUEL and in the QUERY-GRAPH windows regardless of the type of interaction. For example, suppose we wish to use the epidemiological data on viral hepatitis memorized in the SDB in fig. 2 to obtain the numbers of viral hepatitis sufferers according to years and age groups. Fig. 6 shows the query expressed as a QUERY-GRAPH and a STAQUEL expression.

3.2 PRINTING TABLE COMPOSITION

The system allows the database tables to be exported using the formats of the commercially available spreadsheets most frequently used by PC users, so that all the functions

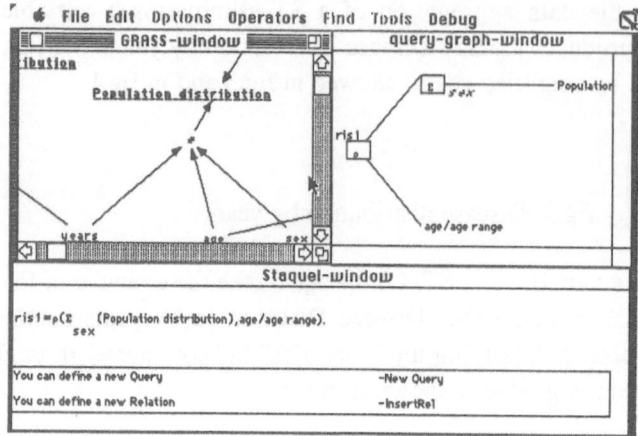

fig. 6: staquel interface

of the latter (histograms, pie charts,...) are available. Furthermore, all the most important statistics packages can be used on these formats. The printing format of STs may be specified by means of an editor which defines the position of each ST and variable. Let us examine the SDB shown in fig.2. Having specified in the GRASS window the ST required to be displayed, the user defines the printing format using the editor showed in fig. 7.

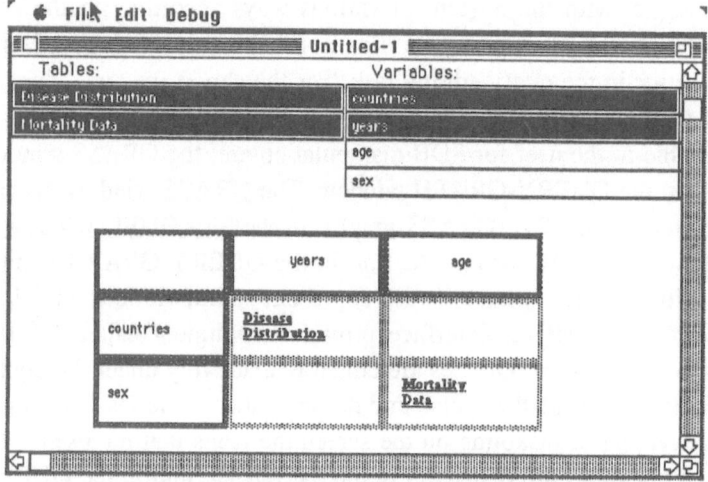

fig. 7: interface for the definition of a printing table

Then the system places the modalities and values in spreadsheet interface (fig. 8) on which the required analyses may be performed.

HEALTH ADDED VALUE OF THE SYSTEM

In order to evaluate epidemiological data accurately it is important to have the data in formats more suitable for statistical analysis. In this sense the Adams system allows the

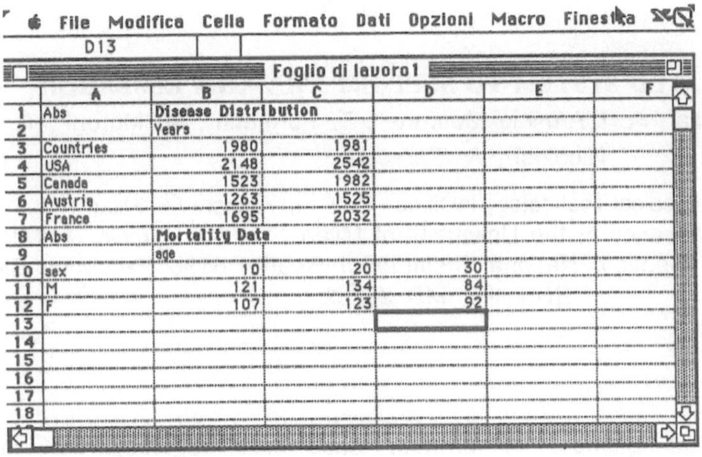

	A	B	C	D	E	F
1	Abs	Disease Distribution				
2		Years				
3	Countries	1980	1981			
4	USA	2148	2542			
5	Canada	1523	1982			
6	Austria	1263	1525			
7	France	1695	2032			
8	Abs	Mortality Data				
9		age				
10	sex	10	20	30		
11	M	121	134	84		
12	F	107	123	92		
13						
14						
15						
16						
17						
18						

fig. 8: printing table

information contained in the statistical tables to be represented in the format with which the user is most familiar and one which is more useful for analysis purposes. In fact, it:
provides useful help during the phase of preparing the statistical data for analysis
allows the data contained in each table to be displayed for examination in different ways (pie charts, histograms, etc.) in order to make it easier to extract the information on which to base the decisions relating to an appropriate policy of prevention and resources management.

CONCLUSIONS

ADAMS is added to the environment of systems which allow significant links to be inferred between the pathology being investigated and the parameters affecting it. In particular ADAMS must be viewed as a system which allows a preliminary analysis to be performed on which the decisions required for effective preventive action may be based. The system runs on Macintosh II and has been developed in an MPW environment in Pascal object oriented language using the Mac App program library.

REFERENCES

[Br88] G. Bracaglia, Currò, A. D'Atri, P. Di Felice, F. L. Ricci, "Man-Machine interfaces to medical information system", VI IASTED International Symposium on Applied Informatics, 1988.

[Da89] A. D'Atri, L. Tarantino,"From Browsing to querying", Data Engeneering Bulletin, IEEE Computer society, vol.12, n°2, June 1989.

[Me90] L. Meo-Evoli,"An aggregate database management system", Proc. VIII IASTED International Symposium on Applied Informatics, 1990.

[Ra83] M. Rafanelli, F. L. Ricci: "Proposal of a logical model for statistical data base", Proc. of the II International Workshop on Statistical Database Management, 1983.

[Ra90] M. Rafanelli, F. L. Ricci: "A functional model for statistical entities", Proc. Database and Expert Systems Applications, 1990.

AN INTEGRATED SYSTEM TO SUPPORT THE AIDS RESEARCH

F. Sicurello*, M. Villa*, A. D'Arminio Monforte°, T. Formenti°, M. Moroni°, A. Nicolosi*, A. Saracco^

* Advanced Biomedical Technology Institute - CNR via Ampere 56, Milan
° Clinic of Infectious Diseases of the University of Milan , via G.B. Grassi 74, Milan
^ Viral Epidemiology Section, National Institute of Health, 6130 Executive Blvd. Rockville, MD 20852

INTRODUCTION

The intelligent management of clinical data base together with an appropriate use of the knowledge on pathologies and their evolution can give the physicians a valid support in defining tempestively both early diagnosis and correlations between objective parameters (clinical symptoms, diagnostic tests, etc.) and clinical course. This is true expecially for those topics whose knowledge is poor, and where information and knowledge can be generated from data properly recorded and analyzed. This may be the case of the Acquired Immunodeficiency Syndrome (AIDS), for which an effective therapy does not yet exist [1].

The problem is to provide physicians and reserchers a tool which can help them on two important points:

1) having an accurate classification of the pathology's development stages, related with clinical and lab parameters, in order to obtain a more effective therapy;

2) charaterizing new markers, in particular at the pre-AIDS stage, which specify the passage to the symptomatic AIDS and inferring from observable data possible hidden parameters.

To this purpose an automatic system which could be able to integrate different functions (data and knowledge management, statistics and A.I. applications) will be surely useful to the clinician and the researcher.

The system is built up by three integrated models: a Data Base Management System, a Knowledge Base and a Statistical Software.

MATERIALS AND METHODS
First Module: the DBMS

The core of the system is the data base, which consists of the clinical information taken during hospitalization or from the seropositive, symptomatic or not, outpatients' clinic examinations.

The patients are those under treatment at the Clinic of Infectious Diseases of the University of Milan [2].

The data, collected through a clinical sheet, are organized in cards (clinical staging, lab tests, anamnestic, instrumental examination, etc.); the clinical staging is set up on the basis of CDC (Center for Diseases Control) criteria:
- stage 1: acute infection
- stage 2: asymptomatic infection
- stage 3: lymphoadenopathy
- stage 4: symptomatic infection (furtherly classificated according to diseases diagnostic of AIDS and other diseases).

The lab tests can be classified into the following groups:
- ematology and biochemestry
- immunology
- viral infection serology
- other infection serology
- HIV serology
- bacterial cultures.

Information relative to the single patient is stored into a MUMPS file (global) which includes private data, anamnesis, case history with related data, and patient classification in respect to his clinical stage.

Afterwards the data management system has been integrated with a query language in order to implement queries and reports, which are important because they allow the physician to find easily and fast the previously stored information, to manage and print selected data, in such a way to generate lists and graphics.

A lack of this tool compromises the usefulness of the system, because the physician can hardly retrieve information about remote visits and tests, and this involves a great waste of time: the capability of the system to generate reports and queries for a particular pathology or for every information about the specific patient spares the physician to waste time in skimming through the clinical sheets.

The system realizes different kind of queries. The easiest ones includes information about a single visit. Another useful information retrieval concerns the summary card, which summarizes the most significant data of the patient's clinical history. The system allows an immediate retrieval of the stored information through queries and a wide flexibility in generating clinical tests. In fact it is very easy for the physician to generate customized reports to summarize collected data.

That is basic in medical field, where it is impossible to forecast the queries which will be useful on the stored data. Only few reports are predefined and included into the application.

Furthermore we have queries carried out on the whole data base (not on the single patient), useful to have a complete outline of the ward's situation or to stress the course of some lab data.

The report "private card", the report "correlation between risk factor (homosexual, drug addict, etc.) and sex (F or M)", the query "CD4 versus opportunistic infections" belong to this class of reports.

The tool adopted to implement the data base is M/SQL ([3]) which is a IV generation language. M/SQL is an integrated environment set up by two ANSI standard languages: MUMPS programming language and SQL (Structured Query Language).

The integration between MUMPS and SQL allows to develope hardware indipendent applications and to unify the MUMPS features to the relational structure and the query capabilities of SQL ([4]).

Second Module: the Knowledge base

The second module of our workstation is built up by the Knowledge Base on AIDS. The Knowledge Base is composed by the information collected from medical papers, written by American researchers or by Italian ones (different epidemiological data based on different rates of patients at risk and on different prevalences of specific HIV-related infection) and by the interaction with the physicians.

This knowledge concerns the predictive factors of the development of symptomatic AIDS by non-symptomatic patients: therefore it includes the causal connections which occur among the parameters collected in the data base as well as between parameters and pre-clinical stages.

On the base of the occurrence of particular diseases (i.e. herpes zoster, pneumonia, etc. CD4 < 400 * 10 3/1 and antigen P24 +) it is possible to classify the patient (in this case CDC IV C2) and to deduce a predictive factor of development of open AIDS (<3 years: 80%, >3 years: 20%).

Since the complex structure of the knowledge Base needs an A.I. language, a system has been built which integrates M/SQL and PROLOG ([5]) and transfers data from the Data Base to the Knowledge Base.

This integrated system allows to overcome the limits of MUMPS (hierarchical information structure, lack of query language, poor logical knowledge management) as well as the poor extension of the PROLOG data base and its sequential retrieval system.

Third Module: the Statistical Software

The third Module of the system is built up by the Statistical Package SPSS ([6]). The records are time oriented, as the relevant information concerns oupatient's and hospitalization data: for each patient the sequential values of more than 200 parameters are stored, where all the variables are dependent on time and patient.

Therefore on such a structure it is possible to both perform descriptive statistics on data. In future the Data Analysis should have to find regularities in the scatterplots through clustering indexes and the search for correlations within particular patients' subsets (e.g. patients with out-of-range parameters).

SPSS provides a wide choice of statistical tests, from the descriptive analysis to the inferential analysis to advanced multivariate techniques (discriminant analysis, cluster analysis, etc.).

CONCLUSION AND FUTURE DEVELOPMENTS

The Clinic of Infectious Diseases of the University of Milan, where the workstation has been installed, gives the availability of studying the widest number of seropositive patients in Italy, but it was not endowed with informatic support to process the data collected.

A correct and intelligent data management can instead simplify and improve data collection, storing and retrieval, and offers a knowledge source for peculiar problems, which can be used to support of A.I. techniques ([7]).

Currently the system has been installed and we are developing methods for the integrated use of data and knowledge bases through A.I. and statistical techniques.

In fact it is possible to amplify the Knowledge Base through new causal associations, by drawing new correlations among variables by statistical data analysis.

For example it is possible to explore the knowledge base (enriched with the new causal relationships) through logical programming methods ([8]).

Our aim is to develop techniques of logical exploration together with a set of discovery heuristic rules. We are studying cognitive methods which lead toward the formulation of new scientific hypoteses in terms of clinical events and causal relationships between disease's agents and organic functions.

Finally from the point of view of information technology the problems is to integrate the modules (M/SQL-PROLOG-SPSS) in one workstation (under MS-DOS, XENIX or UNIX environment) with a friendly interface man/machine.

REFERENCES

[1] Gallo R.C., Montagnier L., AIDS IN 1988, Sci. Am. 59,4,1988:41-48

[2] Moroni M;, Lazzarin A., Galli M., et al. ASPETTI CLINICI ED EPIDEMIOLOGICI DELL'AIDS E DELLE SINDROMI CORRELATE IN MILANO, Microb. Med., 1, 1986:31-34.

[3] Intersystem, M/SQL REFERENCE MANUAL, Intersystems 1988

[4] Baker, SQL: A NEW STANDARD, Computerworld O, 7/A, Feb. 1986: 55-58

[5] Dahl V., PROLOG MUMPS AND FIFTH GENERATION COMPUTING, MUG Quarterly, Vol.15, N.3,1986

[6] Norusis Marija, SPSS/PC+ for the IBM PC/XT/AT, SPSS Inc. 1986

[7] Gale W.A., KNOWLEDGE REPRESENTATION IN DATA ANALYSIS, Proc. IV Int. Symp. on Data Analysis and Informatics, INRIA ed. 2, 1985:721-738.

[8] Glymour C., Scheines R., et al. DISCOVERY CAUSAL STRUCTURES:A.I., PHILOSOPHY OF SCIENCE AND STATISTICAL MODELLING, Academic Press 1987

AN INTERNATIONAL NEUROLOGY DATABASE LINK, ALLOWING GLOBAL RESEARCH QUERIES ACROSS LANGUAGES.

Manfred W. LÜDTKE, Satish C. DUTT [1], Richard C. BURGESS [1],
The Anh VUONG

Epilepsie-Zentrum Bethel, Präoperative Diagnostik,
Maraweg 21, D-4800 Bielefeld 13, Germany
and
[1] The Cleveland Clinic Foundation, 9500 Euclid Avenue,
One Clinic Center, Cleveland, Ohio 44195-5221, USA

An epilepsy database has been ported from a US clinic to a german one.
The use of consistent terminology and a common view of the database in
both institutions allow medical research to be based on the common data
pool. Key problems of the database portation are described and automated
mechanisms for the sharing of data are presented.

1. LINKING DATABASES OF DIFFERENT CLINICS

This project aims at enhancing the significance of statistical research
based on a combined pool of patient records from different hospitals,
using digital database and networking technology. Standardized classification schemes and use of consistent terminology are prerequisites
as well as transparency to native languages.

Our institutions, the Epilepsy Center Bethel and the Cleveland Clinic
Foundation (CCF), have established a partnership which includes mutual
training of medical and technical staff as well as ongoing efforts to
exchange computer programs and data, namely the EBASE neurology database. This database has been ported from the CCF (USA) to Bethel
(Germany). Procedures and tools have been developped allowing database
queries to be run at both the local and the remote institution, with
the systems automatically taking care of the differences between the
two databases.

In this paper we discuss experiences and features of our joint database
project that might be of general interest:

- Effect of the database system and application design on the portability;
- Level of compatibility that can be reasonably achieved among institutions and databases using different native languages;
- A scheme for running queries across institutions and languages.

2. THE "EBASE" DATABASE

The EBASE database, originally developped by the CCF, supports on-line access to patient records which include:

- demographic data,
- history information,
- parameters and results of neurological tests[1] (EEG/Video-Monitoring, Evoked Potentials, O_2 Saturation etc),
- results of other relevant tests (radiology, laboratory, etc).

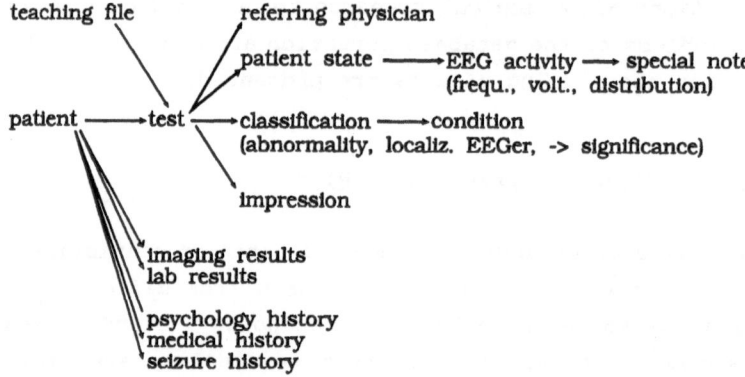

Fig. 1 EBASE database structure (purely administrative entities ommitted)

Main objects of classification are morphological features of the recorded EEGs, rather than seizures[2] or epilepsies[3] in general.

In addition, EBASE supports the scheduling of patients, rooms and staff and generates printouts of reports to be sent to the referring physicians and to the paper-based hospital patient file.

EBASE is a multiuser system. Users are secretaries, technicians, physicians and administrators of the hospital unit (Fig. 2). In order to enforce a standard terminology in the database, all critical entries are to be choosen from selection lists according to the predefined classification scheme and terminology in the units.

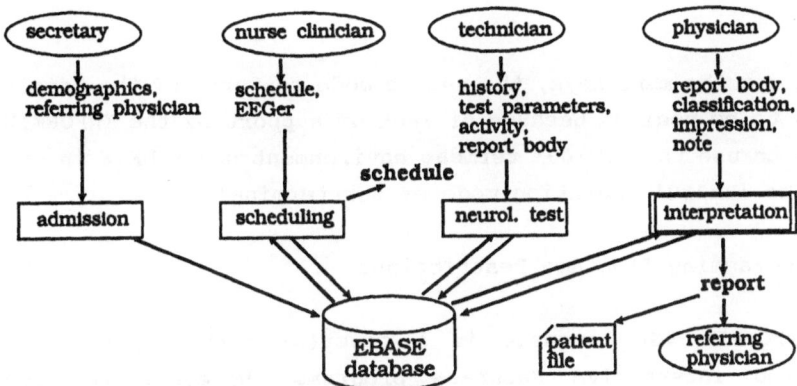

Fig. 2 Organizational scheme supported by EBASE

The EBASE database application runs under INFORMIX and UNIX on an HP9000/800 minicomputer. It is mainly written in INFORMIX-4GL and consists of 30.000 lines of code - more than 4 man-years worth.

3. SYSTEM DESIGN AND PORTABILITY

3.1 Native Language Character Sets

While the default character set for our computer configuration is Roman-8, which is the best supported by our german Hewlett Packard 700/92 keyboards, the USASCII 8-bit character set is required by the german version of the INFORMIX product underlying the EBASE application. The selection of USASCII is also in line with the character set used in the database of the CCF partner institution, and with the demands of another international product being used here (WordPerfect textprocessor).

We discourage the use of the Roman-8 set in the context of international data exchange. If USASCII is not well supported on national keyboards, users with sophisticated demands - like computer staff - do better with english keyboards.

3.2 Hardware Dependency

The EBASE application utilizes user menu keys on the terminal. Although this introduces some hardware dependency, it is an excellent tool for keeping the application program independent from native language menu texts.

Except for the menu keys, the native mode features of the terminals (HP) proved to be useless because of lack of support by the INFORMIX system. We had to use the 'VT100' termcap environment under UNIX in conjunction with the 'EM220' emulation mode of our terminals.

3.3 Programming Language Restrictions

The INFORMIX 4GL language is a powerful "4th generation" tool in designing interactive database programs. However, its syntax has several constructs that require strings to be specified as constants rather than variables, thus prohibiting an elegant native language support. Consequently, adaptation to german language had to be done on source code level.

3.4 Database Scheme

National conventions and customs led to modifications and extensions of the database schema during the portation of EBASE. Examples are: adress format, the "race" attribute, etc.

INFORMIX 4GL is a state-of-the-art relational database product which facilitates modifications of the schema. However, it does not completely isolate database table structures from program code and screen form definitions, thus leading to program modifications in consequence of schema modifications.

4. COMPATIBILITY BETWEEN REMOTE DATABASES

Since there are slight differences between the database schema of each institution, the EBASE application can not directly access a remote database (see 3.4). At the source code level however, modules can be exchanged without or with only minor changes (see 3.3).

A compatible view of the database schemas is achieved by agreeing on a common set of tables and attributes for each table. Local extensions are possible.

SQL queries that conform to the common view of the databases can run locally and remotely without any formal changes.

5. RESEARCH QUERIES ACROSS INSTITUTIONS AND LANGUAGES

Initially, queries are expressed in SQL in a joint effort of physicians and computer staff. Some queries might become preprogrammed and parameterized later on.

A query source file is sent to the other other institution via electronic mail or by file transfer during a remote login. For transfer between the systems the english version of all medical terms is used. The non-english system provides the necessary translation through an utility program. Translation is based on bi-lingual tables which reflect the selection tables used during the data input. For the result tables the same procedure applies. Another utility accomplishes the merger of the result tables.

If the communication is accomplished via electronic mail (BitNet in our case), low transmission cost is counterbalanced by the need of support at the remote site for running the query and returning the result.

CONCLUSION

Although we do not have a true distributed database, we feel our approach to international sharing of data for research and patient care is a reasonable compromise. It preserves the autonomy of each organisationally independant site as well as the full responsibility of the respective database administrators.

With a modest effort for adaptation (approx. 4 man-months) it is possible to adopt an efficient and flexible neurology database, and gain mutual access to a remote data base. This approach might be attractive for other groups to follow.

REFERENCES

(1)   Burgess, R.C., Jacobs, E.C.: Computer Analysis of Epileptiform EEG Abnormalities. Cleve Clin J Med, vol. 56 (1989), p. 240-247.

(2)   Internation League against Epilepsy: Proposal for Revised Clinical and Electroencephalographic Classification of Epileptic Seizures. Epilepsia, vol. 22 (1981), p. 489-501

(3)   Internation League against Epilepsy: Proposal for Revised Classification of Epilepsies and Epileptic Syndromes. Epilepsia, vol. 30 (1989), p. 389-399

AN EPIDEMIOLOGICAL APPROACH TO COMPUTERIZED MEDICAL DIAGNOSIS: THE AEDMI PROJECT, A MULTICENTER DESIGN TO WHICH DIFFERENT ARTIFICIAL INTELLIGENCE SYSTEMS MAY BE GATHERED.

L. Alonso-Vallès *, P. Ferrer-Salvans *, R. Rubio-García **,
O. Juan-Babot *, E. Vidal-Casas *
* Unitat de Farmacologia Clínica. Ciutat Sanitària de Bellvitge.
Hospital Duran i Reynals, Autovia Castelldefels Km 2.7,
08907 Hospitalet de Llobregat, Barcelona, Spain.
** Andersen Consulting, Madrid, Spain.

Abstract:

A project to develop a clinical decision aid system is proposed, based on a multicentric design and on the application of epidemiological methods to the analysis of clinical data bases and clinical judgment. The knowledge of the prevalences of the most common diseases in the treated virtual population allows the assessment of diagnostic predictivities, and the provision of objective probabilities as a reference for the expert system. The characteristics of the system proposed are be described.

Introduction

The AEDMI program -Epidemiological Approach to Computerized Medical Diagnosis- (1), is being developed in the Bellvitge Hospital and other associated hospitals in Barcelona. The Bellvitge Hospital is a public health care centre with more than 1,000 beds that depends on the autonomous government of the Generalitat de Catalunya.

The objective of the project is to develop a 'general-purpose' expert system, following an epidemiological approach and using clinical trial methodologies. Standard items obtained on a multicenter basis form a large-scale data base. Simultaneously, the reasoning of clinical experts in each real case is analyzed to obtain a knowledge-rules data base. The methodology of the program combines Bayesian systems, expert systems, and other new lines of research such as neural networks or case-based reasoning.

The multicentric design gives the opportunity to establish an international collaboration which we are kindly requested. The first 1-year experience of the program and the general framework of the project are discussed in another presentation at this Congress (2).

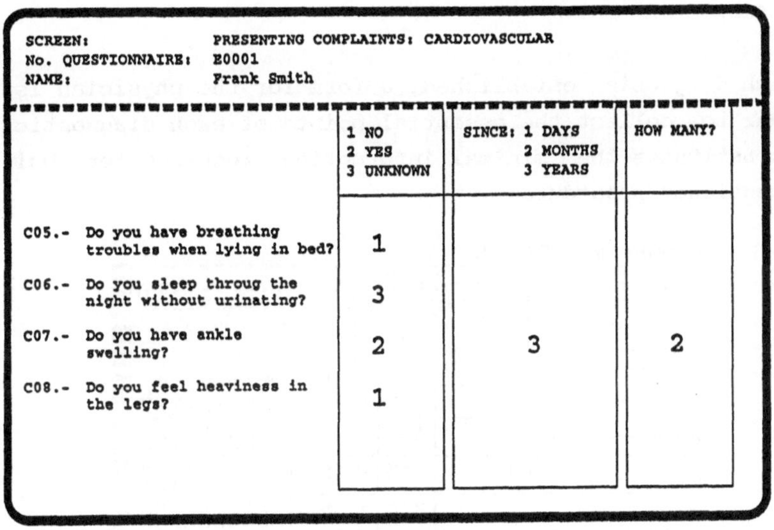

Figure 1.- Hard copy of a screen of the computer program.

Clinical data

To collect clinical data two procedures have been developed, a structured medical interview which can be run on IBM compatible personal computers (Figure 1) and a printed questionnaire of this interview adapted to computerized optical reading (Figure 2) with the same questions answered in the first kind of anamnesis. This permits the accumulation of data on a large scale. Data from both types of anamnesis are stored in the same data base, and are retrieved and interpreted using a program capable of producing a written summary of the pathological findings of each patient. Time evolution of current symptoms (see 3-5) is analyzed. In order to speed up the entry of data, functions have been developed for the automatic codification of hospital services, geographic sites, occupations, IDC-9-CM diagnoses, drugs registered, and hospital services.

Medical knowledge

Provision is made for different forms of eliciting medical knowledge (6). Procedures have been developed on a case-to-case basis, i.e. interviews with the doctor who was attending the patient, analysis of the information of the free answers contained in the program (7,8), and review of conventional clinical records, or in groups of cases, i.e. analysis of statistical patterns, discussions with doctors on clinical sessions, and information collected from the medical literature.

For each diagnosis established, a form for the physician is provided
in order to collect the essential points of each diagnostic process.
This constitutes the minimal information required for building the
afore-mentioned procedures.

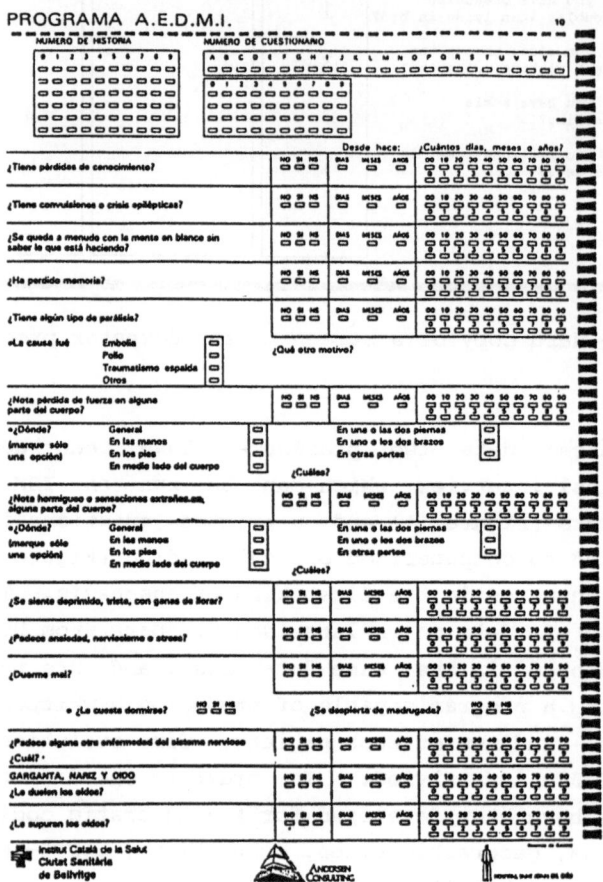

Figure 2.- Reduced copy of the a page of the optical reading form.

Epidemiological methods

An epidemiological approach is used to analyze the two data bases
obtained (clinical variables, medical knowledge) to produce a system
which can either apply numerical methods, such as statistical
analyses or neural network models, or qualitative methods, such as
inductive or knowledge-based systems.

By studying the clinical data base, the sensitivity, specificity and predictivity of signs and symptoms can be calculated either individually or in terms of more or less complex patterns (9). A sufficiently large clinical data base permits the determination of the prevalence of disease in populations attended by the hospital and the calculation of objective probabilities with which to counterbalance findings. The multicenter design (10) of the project facilitates the creation of a large scale data base as well as to analyze and compensate the bias introduced by each institution.

By studying the medical knowledge data base, the necessary rules to construct the expert system are obtained. The original feature of the proposed method lies in the fact that the experience of not only one expert is taken into consideration, but that of all the experts who contribute to the construction of the system. The analysis of the knowledge of groups of experts will be carried out by epidemiological methods in order to study the clinical judgment (11) and the consensus on diagnostic patterns.

The phase of collection of clinical information and the generation of a summary of pathological data constitutes a pre-expert system. The management of the over 1,000 rules of medical knowledge resembles a data base more than a symbolic programming system. At present, this knowledge is being put into a shell, so as to be able to use artificial intelligence techniques to enter data. Other systems have also been chosen to implement knowledge step-by-step while offering a practical framework to physicians (12).

The questions in the present program distinguish between normal and abnormal conditions. According to their location in the general sequence of the program, it is possible to determine which apparatus or system they belong to. Once the system or apparatus to which the possible pathological data has been identified, continuing the diagnostic process with such an extensive approach is not advisable. For this reason, the diagnostic process is limited and interrelated with artificial intelligence-based procedures. An example of a possible model of this kind is offered in another presentation at this meeting (2). Once the context of the illness has been defined, the proposed methodology may integrate different types of expert systems even of different research groups.

Overall integration of the AEDMI system

The diagnostic aid system under consideration is based on the communication between physicians and the expert system, and on the analysis of the coincidences and divergences between the opinions of both. It is designed for use in clinical research and requires, above all, an interface which includes interactive programs, with or without artificial intelligence, and the entry of data using instrumental or optical reading techniques. The analysis of discrepancies permits the continuous updating of the system.

References

[1] Ferrer Salvans P, Alonso Vallès L. An epidemiological approach to computerized medical diagnosis: the AEDMI program. Comput Biol Med 1990; 20: 433-43.

[2] Alonso-Vallès L, Ferrer-Salvans P, Juan-Babot O, Rubio-García R, Vidal-Casas E. Experiences in the application of a computerized medical interview as the basis of an expert system: the AEDMI project. Proceedings of Medical Informatics Europe '91. Lecture Notes in Medical Informatics. Springer-Verlag. Berlin 1991.

[3] Fagan LM, Shortliffe EH, Buchanan BG. Computer-based medical decision making: From MYCIN to VM. In Clancey WJ, Shortliffe EH. Readings in Medical Artificial Intelligence. The first decade. Addison-Wesley 1984.

[4] Adlassning KP, Kolarz G, Scheithauer W, et al. CADIAG: Approaches to computer-assisted medical diagnosis. Comput Biol Med 1985; 15: 315-35.

[5] Miller RA, Pople HA, Myers JD. INTERNIST-I, an experimental computer-based diagnostic consultant for general internal medicine. N Engl J Med 1987; 307: 468-76.

[6] Olson JR, Reuter HH. Extracting expertise from experts: methods of knowledge acquisition. Expert systems 1987; 4: 152-68.

[7] Glowinski A, O'Neil M, Fox J. Design of a generic information system and its application to Primary Care. In Hunter J, Cookson J, Wyatt J (eds.). Proceedings AIME '89. Lecture Notes in Medical Informatics, n 38. Springer-Verlag, Berlin 1989, pp 221-33.

[8] Fox J, Ginzler M, Glowinski A et al. Technicalities and practicalities of logic engineering in medicine: the LEMMA project. Proceedings of the AIM EUROFORUM, Sevilla 1990, 79-86.

[9] Bernardo JM. Bayesian linear probabilistic classification. In Gupta SS, Berger JO, eds. Statistical decision theory and related topics. Springer-Verlag, New York 1988, n 4, pp 151-62.

[10] Sedano-Monasterio E. Cooperación multicéntrica en el diagnóstico médico informatizado. Novática 1990; 87: 58-61.

[11] Chaput de Saintonge DM, Cookson MJ. The role of clinical judgment analysis in the development of medical expert systems. In Hunter J, Cookson J, Wyatt J, eds. Proceedings AIME'89. Lecture Notes in Medical Informatics, n 38. Springer-Verlag, Berlin 1989, pp 3-13.

[12] Howkins TJ, Kay S, Rector AL et al. An overview of the PEN & PAD project. In O'Moore R, Bengtsson S, Bryant JR, Bryden JS (eds.). Proceedings of Medical Informatics Europe '90. Lecture Notes in Medical Informatics n 40. Springer-Verlag, Berlin 1990, pp 73-8.

BIOCELL:
AN INTEGRATED AND INTERACTIVE TOOL
FOR THE MANAGEMENT OF LINGUISTIC AND EIDETIC BIOLOGICAL DATA

F. Beltrame, G. Marcenaro and M. Sassoli*

Department of Communication, Computer and System Sciences,

University of Genoa, Genoa, ITALY.

* Author to whom all the correspondence should be addressed (first author).

Abstract

An exhaustive description of most biological data requires, beside a set of analytic information, an eidetic representation of the data itself. BIOCELL is a sort of biological atlas containing the linguistic and eidetic description of cell lines, plus a set of tools to correlate, insert, update, manipulate, display and delete such data.

Linguistic data are stored in the tables of a relational data base (ORACLE) and include items such as karyotype, culture medium, taxonomic classification and bibliographic references. Eidetic data are stored as an unstructured data base of images (files) of cells cultured "in vitro" and acquired by a standard TV camera via optical microscopy in absorption, fluorescence and phase contrast.

A furnished set of software tools manages the access to the two data bases, both for enquires and updates, takes care of the consistency and completeness of stored data and realizes an image processing shell. With such tools, the user may correlate linguistic and eidetic data, search the relational data base tables for entries that meet various criteria, compare a laboratory image with cell images stored in the eidetic data base and even perform cell image processing in order to extract additional information such as morphometric and densitometric measurements.

1. Introduction

BIOCELL is a sort of biological atlas composed of two major parts.

The first part includes information related to cell lines identification and cataloguing, realizing a sort of electronic cell lines catalogue. Cell lines distributors, parameters furnished by official distributors as well as by private laboratories and related bibliography are stored in the tables of the relational data base allowing for a quick, flexible and friendly data retrieval and update.

The second part has been conceived as an electronic note book where biologists may record every step of their experiments, starting from cells thawing up to cell images acquisition. The target is to offer the biologist a flexible instrument to memorize, formalize and compare his experimental materials, methods and results. Each experiment is described reporting the starting environment, the fixation, staining and cleaning procedures, and the microscope and TV camera set-up. A built in software application computes morphometric and densitometric parameters of acquired images, extracts statistical parameters (such as average value, variance and histogram) and automatically stores them inside the relational data base together with a few typical images per slide.

ORACLE was chosen as RDBMS both because it is becoming a standard for biological applications and because of its reliability.

User interface is based on a WIMP (Windows, Icons, Mouse and Pointers) environment (X-Window) to allow for a simultaneous display of images, free text and data base forms. Particular care has been taken to satisfy biologists and clinicians requirements and to realize a friendly and self-explanatory environment.

BIOCELL is now running on a HP 9000/360 SRX under UNIX, but can be easily ported on other hardware and operating systems, since portability through both hardware and software has been one major design constraint.

The present report is organized as follows: section 2 introduces multimedia data bases, section 3 and section 4 describe, respectively, the cell line catalogue and the note book, section 5 gives some insights on the data base design and section 6 discusses user interface.

2.   Multimedia data bases

While conventional data bases are largely diffuse and at present many of them are industrial products and important working tools, multimedia data bases have been long neglected. Only recently, new attention has been turned to multimedia data bases, mostly thanks to remarkable technological advances, such as, for example, large capacity optical disks. A common approach is to expand and to rebuild current commercial data bases. This approach uses a relational data base to store textual data and a special purpose image system to store and manage images; the relations describing the image files and their pathnames constitute the bridge between the two systems. This solution presents several practical advantages:

a)   relational data bases allow for the formulation of complex queries and for an easy updating of the data base structure by modification or addition of new attributes;

b)   textual data may be stored in high speed access magnetic disks, while images may be stored in high capacity optical disks;

c)   relational data bases may rely on industrial products, such as ORACLE, which represents an important guarantee for the handling of a large amount of data and for system reliability.

The main drawback of such technique is the non homogeneous handling of texts and images. This is unacceptable for pictorial data bases used by researchers in computer vision and image processing, where textual aspects are minimal and consist mostly of linguistic encoding of pictorial features. Still, it is appropriate for textual data bases where pictures occur only as attributes of a logical record.

Many other approaches are under development to overcome this problem, but most of them are still at research stage.

3. The cell lines catalogue

As anticipated, the first part of BIOCELL is mostly concerned with cell lines identification and cataloguing. Its main topics are cell lines distributors, distribution parameters and annotations, and bibliography. Distribution parameters, in particular, include: source organism, strain, organ and tissue; taxonomic classification and karyotype; viability, plating efficiency and growth characteristics of thawed cells; passages number and maximum number of serial subcultures; freezing and culture media; functional, histochemical, tumorigenic and species confirmation markers; sterility tests and virus susceptibility; qualitative morphology; source tumour or transforming agent. Moreover, each cell line may be associated to one or more keywords and applications for quick cell lines selection.

Images involved at this stage are cell colony images acquired via optical microscopy in phase contrast, usually at low magnification. These images should be delivered by cell distributors as an eidetic description of living cells appearance in the suggested culture medium, for a quick and rough cell line recognition and check. Much textual information can be deduced from these images, such as qualitative morphology parameters.

4. The note book

The second part of BIOCELL is mainly concerned with the description and formalization of the various steps of an experiment, starting from cell thawing up to cell images acquisition. These steps include: the starting environment (culture medium, temperature, pH, etc.); the fixation, staining and cleaning procedure; any used mechanical support; the microscope set-up (optical and geometrical resolution, magnification, light source, illumination type, field diaphragm, lens and filters); the TV camera set-up (gain, offset and linearity); plus a free text description of the experiment (materials, methods and results). Such data are important for repeatability but still incomplete. In fact, quantitative morphological parameters are not included. The main difficulty in extracting meaningful quantitative parameters is that the analysis of a few cell images, particularly for high magnification images, is poorly representative of the cell colony features. In fact, morphometric parameters, such as area and perimeter, and densitometric parameters, such as integrated or average optical density, are meaningful only if computed on a population of at least a few hundreds events. The adopted solution is to acquire hundreds of images per slide and to compute, for each image, the morphometric and densitometric parameters. Only the statistical description of the acquired parameters (average value, variance and histogram), plus a few significant images per slide, are stored in the data base.

Summing up, this part of BIOCELL includes a module to acquire morphometric and densitometric parameters, evaluate their statistical description and automatically store the computed values in the tables of the relational data base, together with the name of a few representative images. Images managed at this level include slide images acquired by a standard TV camera via optical microscopy in absorption, fluorescence and phase contrast at high magnification.

5. Data base design

In a relational data base, both data and relationships between data are represented as tables. Each column of a table represents an attribute of the related entity or relationship and each row a different specimen. The tables of BIOCELL, 49 altogether, are in third normal form, which makes possible both saving of memory occupancy and check of data base consistency and completeness. Tables have been provided also for educational topics and for help messages and menu choices, so that all of them may be updated on line.

The representation of each entity includes, beside its name and other formatted attributes, a free text comment. Such comments may be short (up to 240 characters) or long (up to 65536 characters), depending on the relevance of the entity in the context of cellular biology.

For an easier identification of columns contents from columns name, a standard suffix is added to the name of each column, such as _NAME for names, _DESCR for comments and _ID for unique identifiers.

Tables have been provided of three distinct access levels for a differentiated access to the data base and of indexes for faster data retrieval. The typical query takes about 3 seconds for a data base with about 1000 cell lines.

A detailed description of BIOCELL tables is outside the scope of this paper but may be provided upon request.

6. User interface

User interface is based on a window environment (X-Window). The main window manages the access to the data base through a form-oriented application while other windows display related images and texts (see figure 1).

Forms are tools for data retrieval and update, which may be used without any preliminary knowledge of data structure and even of data base query language. The user simply fills-in or reads the form exactly as if it was a sheet of paper. It is up to the form manager to translate each user operation into the correspondent data base query statements. The form manager displays related images and texts, helps the user to correctly fill-in the forms, checks errors and even automatically fills-in predetermined fields.

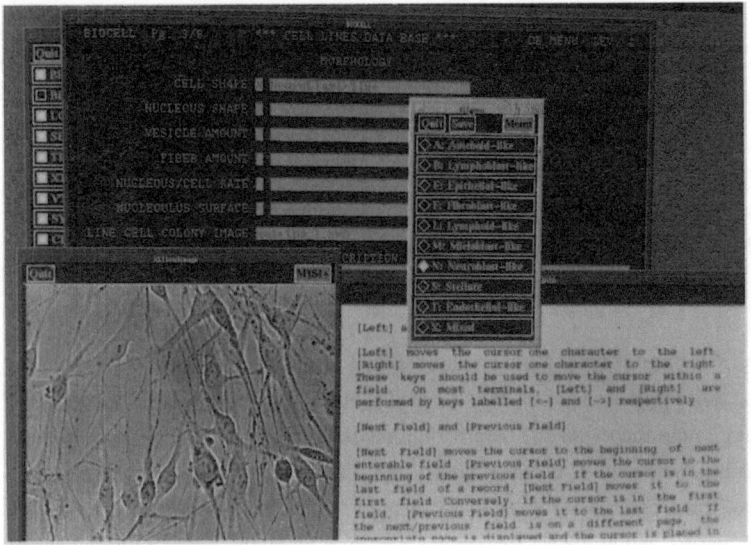

Figure 1

References

G. Burger, J.S. Ploem and K. Goerttler editors, "Clinical Cytometry and Histometry". Academic Press, 1987.

A.M. von Ginneken, J.P.A. Baak, W. Jansen and A.W.M. Smeulders, "Evaluation of a Diagnostic Encyclopaedia Workstation for Ovarian Pathology". Human Pathology, vol. 21, n. 10, pp. 989-997, 1990.

J.P.A. Baak and P.H.J. Kurver, "Development and Use of a RULE-BASED Pathology Expert Consultation System". Analytical and Quantitative Cytology and Histology, vol. 10, n. 3, pp. 214-218,1988.

S.B. Yao editor, "Principles of Database Design". Prentice-Hall, 1985.

A. Della Ventura, "Electronic Image Banks: State of the Art and Market Requirements in Europe". Official Publication of the Commission of the European Communities, EUR 11736, Contract DOCMIX, Final Report ,1988.

The practical design and implementation of Thesauri for primary care information retrieval applications

A.W.Eliasz

Department of Computer Science
University College London

Ann Mason and L.Malcolm

Information Resources Centre
Royal College of General Practitioners

Abstract

The importance of well designed Thesauri for information retrieval purposes is discussed. The design of a practical Thesaurus for use with the GP Literature bibliographic database ,(GP-LIT), developed at the Royal College of General Practitioners is described and an outline of the implementation given.

Retrieving information from online bibliographic databases is known to be a difficult and inefficient process for the inexperienced user [WALKER 87], [WALKER 85]. This is because the searches are often performed by untrained users, rather than with the help of intermediaries, the subject coverage is often wide and the subject description in the records is often inadequate, and may even be absent. The Information Resources Centre of the Royal College of General Practitioners is developing a large online bibliographic database of research papers and articles, monographs and grey literature, dealing with General Practice and related Primary Health Care issues, [MALCOLM 89], [MASON 89]. As well as storing information about authors, journal, title, abstract and the like, each entry is also indexed by subject area and various specialisations of that area. Thus for example a given paper might be dealing with "audit" - of some particular practice in general practice. In this case the major subject area would be the particular activity being audited, with audit as a secondary descriptor denoting the methodology being applied. On the other hand, a paper dealing primarily with audit would be indexed with audit as the major subject area. This approach can form the basis of a powerful indexing system for information retrieval. In order to be useful, however, it is important that a consistent indexing scheme is developed. A consequence of this is that a given preferred subject term such as "audit" may have a number of synonyms in the literature (and in user's minds) such as, for example, quality control. Furthermore the meanings of given key words may be context dependent. The need for a Thesaurus linking various words and phrases together is therefore obvious. Such a Thesaurus is being developed by the Information Resources Centre. The existing system is based on a commercial package and has rather limited facilities and a poor user interface. The Thesaurus itself contains a large amount of data, and cannot be readily interfaced with the online information retrieval system.

The logical structure of the existing Thesaurus is that of an ordered list of records, each record corresponding to a particular word or term. As such it follows the standard approaches to constructing Thesauri [AITCHISON 87], [BSI 87]. Each record contains a brief definition or explanation (called a scope note) and a number of associated words or terms. The type of association between the given word or term and the associated word or term is also specified for each word. Currently used associations (which are described below as a general description given in quotes, followed by the technical word or words in angle brackets) include " is a synonym " <use for / use> , " is a specialisation of " <narrower>, " is a generalisation of " <broader>, " is a contextual modifier of " <narrower>, " occurs in connection with " <related>. In the record these associations are represented as two letter codes (see glossary). Thus, starting with a given word or term it is possible to explore the network of words or terms associated with it. At present this has to be done manually, and it would be very useful to be able to generate such networks and subnetworks automatically. Another useful facility would be to be able to generate, given a list of words or terms, a subset of the main Thesaurus containing only those words or terms and preserving only those relationships involving the words or terms in the given list. Such "micro" Thesauri have many useful applications in handling medical information. Thus, for example, a Thesaurus for use by a general unit manager would differ considerably from that needed, for example, by a district nurse, or by a general practitioner. The existing Thesaurus lacks a substantial collection of acronyms and abbreviations. To date, not much need for this sort of data in the context of the literature being indexed has been found. However, the methodology described can readily be extended to include such things. All that is required is to decide whether the acronym should be the preferred term and the full expression the non-preferred term or vice versa.

An important problem in connection with Thesauri is the number and variety of phrases they support. An important aspect of designing Thesauri is knowing when to split phrases into simpler terms. The British Standards Institute and Aitchison and Gilchrist [AITCHISON 87]recommends "post co-ordinate indexing" - which is a scheme whereby non phrase single word terms are brought together at the time of search, wherever possible. The other approach [ORNA 83] is to pre-co-ordinate terms to produce phrases (compound terms). In our experience, the more specialist the Thesaurus the greater will be the need for compound terms. However, for a very large database such as MedLine, the number of phrases that would have to be included would be astronomical. It is no surprise, therefore, that MedLine does not support many compound terms. A consequence of this is that many database searches would be "poor" in the sense that they would turn up large numbers of unwanted references. It would then be up to the skill of the searcher to put relevant terms together to produce useful phrases on which the database could be searched. The RCGP database is more specialised and provides quite a lot of support for compound terms such as "referral rate" and "consultation reason".

In the ideal, theoretical, world information is unambiguous and easily accessible. In the real world, searching for information generally involves the help of a subject specialist who has the necessary indexing and Thesaurus skills. Such specialists are not always available, and it would be useful to develop computer systems that go some way to making the skills possessed by such specialists more readily available. Various reports have shown that most in-house searches have a high probability of failure. Either they do not find anything at all, or they do not find anything useful, or they produce huge, and thus not very useful, lists of bibliographic references. [MARKEY 84], [MARKEY 83], [BATES 77], [BATES 86]. Attempts to improve on this state of affairs have included spelling correction facilities. Spelling problems are due not only to keyboard errors, but also to such things as differences in spelling between American and English terminology (e.g. gynecology and gynaecology) and to differences in the use of abbreviations (e.g. US, USA, United States of America). They have also included features such as automatic truncation and stemming facilities as well as cross referencing and various other lookup facilities. Automatic truncation is a function of how the database is indexed. It is therefore helpful to provide a pop-up window containing a list of all associated terms and allowing the user to select one or more of these terms as needed. One of the situations our Thesaurus tries to cope with is that where certain concepts are simply "too broad" to be useful. Concepts such as "attitude" are organised around terms such as "doctor attitude" or "patient attitude". The choice of terms has been purely empirical. A refinement of the Thesaurus would be to provide a "tree structure" facility such as that provided by MeSH [MESH 91] which would allow the user to perform broad searches and subsequently to narrow them down.

The purpose of the Thesaurus described here was to help searches by generating "go/see" lists [MITEV 85] , facilities for narrowing or broadening the concept being searched on, facilities for choosing the most appropriate modifiers/adjectives and facilities for handling acronyms and abbreviations.

The literature relating to Thesaurus construction and use is rich and varied. The classical references are, of course, [AITCHISON 87] BSI 5723 [BSI 87], [ORNA 83]. Supporting literature concerned with indexing techniques includes the report by the International Organisation for Standardisation [IOS 85], and the more recent work of the Cleavelands [CLEAVELAND 90]. A more informal guide is provided by [BATTY 89]. Good reviews of problems arising with the construction of medically oriented Thesauri are given by [RADA 88] and [HUMPHREYS 89]. Recent developments in information retrieval include approaches based on data dictionaries [LINNARSON 89], hierarchical concept graphs [KIM 90] and techniques for speeding up searches based on parallel computing techniques [STEWART 87].

The design of the Thesaurus involves three main areas - namely the design of the user interface, the design of the data structures and algorithms underlying the Thesaurus, and finally the design of a collection of tools to support the retrieval and organisation of different kinds of information from the Thesaurus, as well as tools for automatically constructing a micro Thesaurus from a large "master" thesaurus, tools for merging two Thesauri together, and tools for constructing a Thesaurus from Thesauri given as "flat" ASCII text files. The design of the user interface depends on observations of user behaviour with existing indexing schemes [HANCOCK-BEAULIEU 90] as well as theories of the mental processes underlying information retrieval [GREER 65], [FROHMAN 90], and an appreciation of the limitations of relationships in Thesauri [MANIEZ 88] .

A rapid prototyping approach is being used. Prototypes running under both UNIX and MSDOS are being developed. The programming languages chosen are C and C++. In addition various UNIX tools (also available as programs running under MSDOS) such as grep and awk are being used, C libraries for building up extendibly hashed databases of key/content pairs and RDBMS (Relational Database Management System) - ORACLE in this case, using both a UNIX and an MSDOS version of ORACLE. The user interface is being prototyped using appropriate C++ libraries supporting either X Windows or Windows 3.

References:

[AITCHISON 87] Aitchison J. and Gilchrist A. Thesaurus Construction: a Practical Manual (2nd Ed.) pub. Aslib (1987)

[BATES 77] Bates M.J. Factors affecting subject catalog search success Journal of the American Society for Information Science Vol. 28 No. 3 May 1977 pp 161 - 169

[BATES 86] Bates M.J. Subject access in online catalogs : a design model Journal of the American Society for Information Science Vol. 37 (1977) pp 357 - 376

[BATTY 89] Batty D. Thesaurus Construction and Maintenance: A Survival Kit Database February 1989 pp 13 - 20

[BSI 87] BRITISH STANDARDS INSTITUTION British Standard Guide to Establishment and Development of Monolingual Thesauri (BSI 5723 : 1987, ISO 2788-1986) pub. British Standards Institution (1987)

[CLEAVELAND 90] Cleaveland D.B. and Cleaveland A.D. Introduction to Indexing and Abstracting (2nd Ed.) pub. Libraries Unlimited (1990)

[FROHMAN 90] Frohman B. Rules of Indexing: A Critique of Mentalism in Information Retrieval Theory Journal of Documentation Vol. 46 No. 2 June 1990 pp 81 - 101

[GREER] Greer F.L. User Vocabulary in Thesaurus Development Perceptual and Motor Skills Vol. 21 No. 3 December 1965 pp 827 - 837

[HANCOCK-BEAULIEU 90] Hancock-Beaulieu M. Evaluating the Impact of an Online Library Catalogue on Subject Searching Behaviour Journal of Documentation Vol. 46 No. 4 December 1990 pp 318 - 338

[HUMPHREYS 89] Humphreys B.I. and Lindberg D.A.B. Building the Unified Medical Language System Symp. Comput. Applications Med. Care Procedures 1989 pp 475 - 480

[IOS 85] INTERNATIONAL ORGANISATION FOR STANDARDISATION Documentation - Methods for Examining Documents, Determining their Subjects and Selecting Indexing Terms International Organisations for Standardisation (1985)

[KIM 90] Kim Y.W. and Kim J.H. A model of Knowledge Based Information Retrieval with Hierarchical Concept Graph Journal of Documentation Vol. 46 No. 2 June 1990 pp 113 - 136

[MANIEZ 88] Maniez J. Relationships in Thesauri: Some Critical Remarks International Classification Vol. 15 No. 3 1988 pp 133 - 138

[MARKEY 83] Markey K. Online catalogue use : results of surveys and focus group interviews in several libraries Final report to the Council on Library Resources Vol II OCLC Online Computer Library Center (1983)

[MARKEY 84] Markey K. Subject searching in library catalogs : before and after introduction of online catalogs OCLC Online Computer Library Center (1984)

[MALCOLM 89] Malcolm L. The Essential Reverence Tool GPLIT RCGP News No. 1 January 1989 pp 10

[MASON 89] Mason A. RCGP Thesaurus - ' An Extremely Important Retrieval Aid' RCGP News No. 2 February 1989 pp 10 - 11

[MITEV 85] Mitev N.N., Venner G.M. and walker S. Designing an online public access catalogue : Okapi, a catalogue on a local area network (Library and Information Research Report 39) London: British Library (1985)

[ORNA 83] Orna E. Build Yourself a Thesaurus: A Step by Step Guide pub. Running Angel (Norwich England) (1983)

[RADA 88] Rada R., Hafedh M. Letourneau G. and Johnston D. Creating and Evaluating Entry Terms Journal of Documentation Vol. 44 No. 1 March 1988 pp 19 - 41

[WALKER 85] Walker S. The free language approach to online catalogues In: Keyword Catalogues and the Free Language Approach Bryant P. (Ed) University of Bath Library (1985)

[WALKER 87] Walker S. and Jones R.M. Improving Subject Retrieval in Online Catalogues British Library Research Paper 24 pub. British Library (Boston Spa UK)

Glossary:

The following is a brief glossary of some of the terms used in the RCGP Thesaurus for the GP Literature bibliographic database (GP-LIT).

bt Broader term

This indicates that there are terms that cover a wider range than the one being currently looked at. This is useful to broaden a specific search or to allow indexing to include a broader, more general concept.

nt Narrower term

This indicates that there are terms that can be considered as subsections of the term that is currently being looked at. They allow the search to be narrowed and make indexing more specific.

rt Related term

This indicates that there are other terms that, whilst not directly of the same class or species as the term currently being looked at, may be found useful for consideration for either search or indexing purposes.

SN Scope note

This indicates the usage of a particular term within the context of the Thesaurus.

uf Use for

This indicates that these terms are non-preferred terms and are considered (for the purposes of the given thesaurus) to be similes of the preferred term

us Use/See

This indicates that the term in lower case is a 'non-preferred' term, that is it has not been selected as an indexing term, and the term to be used is the term indicated after 'us'.

Non-preferred term

This is a word that is a simile of a term that has been chosen as the indexing term. For example, the RCGP GP-LIT Thesaurus indexes under the term 'elderly' with 'aged','pensioners' and 'old people' entered as non-preferred terms, with a 'us' note directing the user to see

Preferred term

This is the term selected fo indexing purposes and the term to be used to either search the Thesaurus of index material for it. Preferred terms are entered in upper case.

INVESTIGATIONS OF DEPENDENCIES IN THE USSR STATE COMPUTER INFORMATION SYSTEM "POPULATION HEALTH - ENVIRONMENT"

Alexander B. Jornitsky[1], Vladimir I. Tsurkov[2]

[1]USSR Scientific Research Institute for Automation of Management
in the Non-industrial Sphere, 4-2 Sivashkaya Str., 113149 Moscow, USSR

[2]Computer Center of the USSR Academy of Science
40 Vavilova Str., 117963 Moscow, USSR

ABSTRACT

The State Computer Information System "Population Health - Environment" (SCIS - "Health") has been functioning in the USSR since 1983. Every month the data on environment pollution factors and the population health indexes from 153 industrial centers enters the database of the system. The system ist based on the complexy of models for a process of influence "environment - health". The application of the suggested method of modelling allows to exclude the essential influence of non-controlled factors and to ensure obtaining stable results.

1. INITIAL DATA FOR MODELLING

Every month the real information from 153 large industrial centers of the USSR enters the database of the system SCIS-"Health". From one to four districts of observation with populations of about 30000 persons in a district have been selected in each town. Environment data represents average monthly concentrations of air pollution, standard indexes of drinking water quality, noise levels and values of meteofactors. The health of the twenty population groups (according to sex and age) is characterized by the diseases indexes "according to addressing" (cardiovascular, oncological, endocrinological diseases, diseases of lungs and sensory organs, diseases of the skin and others D 13 groups of disease), indexes of pregnancy pathology and others [1].

Hygienic settlement of the project is carried out by the specialists in medicine, in particular by the specialists of the All-Union Center of Prophylactic Medicine.

2. PARADOX DESCRIPTION

One of the main variants of the dependencies investigation in the SCIS-"Health" system is realized by the following: 1. The population group (according to sex and age) is fixed by the user. 2. The single diseases index (output variable) and the set of environment factors (input variables) are fixed. 3. The set of territories (subset of observation districts of the SCIS-"Health") and the time intervals (arbitrary set of months) are fixed. 4. The data on the months mentioned by the user, territories, factors, health indexes and the group (sex and age) is read from the database. 5. The equation of linear regression, expressing the correlation of the given output variable with input ones within the read data set is built.

The coefficient of this regression equation at the environment factor indicates an "average" increase of disease when the level of influence of the factor increases by one unit of measurement.

At the initial stage of functioning of the system during a short time interval of observation, the regression equations were formed for the fixed month. The following paradox occurred: for some months and sex/age groups, the majority of coefficients at the factors of air pollution (according to a number of diseases indexes) appeared to be negative [2].

3. PARADOX INVESTIGATION

The reason for obtaining the negative coefficients at the factors in the situation described above may be the following: 1. The low reliability level of the initial data on health showing and environment factors, occurrence of casual and systematical errors. 2. The violation of an a priori assumption of the correlation and regression analysis on the character of distribution for the investigated values. 3. A non-linear and even non-monotonous character of a real relation between the level of pollution and diseases. 4. The casual occurrence of negative coefficients as a result of insufficient sample volumes. 5. The used diseases indexes according to addressing does not sufficiently connect with the level of population health and does not reflect the influence of pollution. 6. The entire structure of investigation—health indexes, environment factors, the observed contingents and observation periods—was incorrectly selected (for example, the annual data of mortality would be used). 7. The levels of factor influence are so low that they cannot exert any essential influence on public health and the level of addressing. 8. The different factors of air pollution have negative correlation with each other, in this case the small number of the most dangerous factors "overshadows" the influence of less dangerous ones. 9. The different diseases indexes have negative correlation with each other, and the "sensitive" indexes are in the minority. 10. The negative coefficients in the regression equation can be explained by the influence of non-controlled factors, such as the availability of medical service or the migration factor.

4. THE STRUCTURE OF THE SET OF NON-CONTROLLED FACTORS

The detailed analysis of the situation, particularly with the use of dispersal diagrams [2], showed that the paradox can only be explained by an influence of non-controlled factors.

The total set of factors influencing population health of the town's territories includes three groups: 1. Factors that depend essentially on territory, and only slowly (or episodically) change in time as well: medicosocial service, the cast and characteristics of the contingent, etc.. 2. Factors that depend essentially on time, but simultaneously and almost act at nearby territories: weather and other and climatic or seasonal factors, simultaneous beginning of vacations, holidays, etc. The third group consists of all factors which depend essentially on both territory and time. This group includes the factors of environment pollution and the factors of local catastrophes.

5. EXCLUDING THE INFLUENCE OF NON-CONTROLLED FACTORS

Now let us suppose that the diseases represent the sum of three functions, each of which expresses the influence of the corresponding group of factors. Let us take the first function to depend exclusively on territory, and the second exclusively on time; the third one has a zero sum, according each territory and each moment in time. Then the algorithm for investigating the influence of pollution can include two stages: 1. Substract the average level of diseases for a given territory from the level of diseases, and then substract the average level of diseases for a given month. Thus we can obtain the function expressing the third group of factors. 2. Investigate the correlation dependencies between the obtained remainder (the third function) and the pollution factors.

Another two-stage algorithm is also possible: 1. Pass from diseases (as a function of territory and time) to the increase of diseases in comparison with the previous month. Use the same operator for each factor in the space of two variable functions—the transition to the function "increase in comparison with the previous month". 2. Investigate the correlation dependencies between the new input variable and the new output variables.

In the two previous paragraphs we mean two different models of the process of influencing the environment pollution factors on the diseases.

6. OPERATOR METHOD

As distinct from the classic approach to the investigation of dependencies, our SCIS-"Health" system allows to study the correlations not only between the functions from input and output variables. The correlations between the images of different input and output variables under the action of different transformations—operators in the space of functions of two variables: territory and time. The used set of operators includes the time shear operators, operators of transitions to the increase for a unit of time, to the deviation from the average level for that territory, or to the deviation from the average for a given moment in time; operator of the transition to the devisation from time smooth level; superpositions of the mentioned operators, etc.

The selection of models of the process for different groups of diseases and the identification of these model parameters is realized with the use of real data from the system. This method, based on the use of operators, is described in more detail in [1–4].

7. EXAMPLE

The influence of the level of atmospheric air pollution by soot (variable x) on the special index of sickness: diseases of the respiratory tract among grown-up population (variable y) was studied from the data of the 1985–87 period in 19 observation areas of SCIS-"Health". The models

$$ln\ y(s,t) = a_1 + b_1 ln\ x(s,t), \qquad (1)$$

$$ln\ y(s,t) - ln\ y(s,t-1) = a_2 + b_2(lnx(s,t) - lnx(s,t-1)), \qquad (2)$$

(s - territory, t - time) were compared for two groups of cities and for three groups from 12 months of every year. In model (1) the estimated value of the coefficient of pair correlation (r) varied from $+0.17$ to -0.24 (the number of observations varied from 52 to 49). In model (2) value (r) varied from $+0.26$ to $+0.61$ (the number of observations varied from 44 to 30).

Of course, a lot of multidimensional models were also investigated.

8. MAIN RESULTS AND CONCLUSIONS

The application of the operator method allows to obtain the stable results appropriate to the a priori assumptions. The constructive description of the whole set of factors influencing the resulting indexes allows to build a wide spectrum of the investigated process models. The further process of modelling "environment - health" may be connected not so much with investigations of the correlations "factors - health indexes" as with investigations of the correlations between different factors and social ones in the first place.

REFERENCES (IN RUSSIAN)

[1] J.E.Kornejev, A.B.Jornitzky, V.M.Volovich. Hygiene and Sanitation, 1986, N 11, pp. 8–11

[2] A.B.Jornitzky. Designing the Automated System of Investigating the Correlations of the Complex Process Characteristics. Autoabstract of Dissertation. Computer Center of the USSR Academy of Science (CC SU AS), Moscow, 18 p.

[3] A.B.Jornitzky, V.I.Tsurkov. Mathematical Model of Making Decisions on Medical-Ecological Arrangements / Packages of Applied Programs: Mathematical Modelling (series "Algorithms and Algorithmical Languages"). Moscow "Science", CC SU AS, 1989, pp. 63–72

[4] A.B.Jornitzky, V.I.Tsurkov. A Formalised Approach to the Problem of Disengagement in the Study of Relationships / Mathematical Modelling, 1990, N

HEALTH CARE SYSTEMS AND SERVICES

HARMONISATION OF HEALTH DATA ON THE INSTITUTIONAL LEVEL
THE CASE BASED MODEL AS AN EUROPEAN APPROACH TO HEALTH CARE SERVICES PLANNING AND MANAGEMENT

J.M. RODRIGUES*, J. CATTERALL**, J. HOFDIJCK***, J. MEADOWS**,
F. MENNERAT* and I. VERIN*.
* Département de Santé Publique, Université de Saint Etienne Jean
Monnet, Faculté de Médecine, 15 rue Ambroise Paré 42100 SAINT ETIENNE
FRANCE.
** C International Limited, LONDON, UNITED KINGDOM.
*** BAZIS, LEIDEN, THE NETHERLANDS.

ABSTRACT
Following AIM Exploratory action CAMAC consortium is proposing as
main outcome a COMMON NUCLEUS OF STANDARD ARCHITECTURES AND MODELS
(for data and processes) ABLE TO ENSURE THE CONSISTENCY AND
TRANSFERABILITY OF HOSPITAL INFORMATION using advanced information
technology and telematic for clinical data and for cost data ; we
stress the benefits which can be expected from this harmonisation.

1') INTRODUCTION

Health care services are becoming more and more complex in term
of institutional organisations, information systems within and
outside the organisation, existing health care technologies, health
policy making bodies, social and economic acceptability to users and
to community.

Management, Planning , Quality Assessment require increasing
exchanges of data between different users, different organisations
and for different goals : these data must be harmonised.

2') HARMONISATION OF CLINICAL DATA

    2.1 MEDICAL TERMINOLOGY

    There are three critical points to a broader use of medical data:

1 - The different kinds of complementary tools required by different users to respond to a precise purpose : classifications, nomenclatures, thesaurus and glossaries.
The situation being far more confused by the non specific utilisation of these tools and their multipurposes unvalidated transformation using tables of cross-references.

2 - The lack of ability to handle the richness and ambiguity of information used in clinical medicine and to map it into coded data which are the only informations computers and computer-computer communications can cope with.

3 - The dependence of the natural medical language from different national languages within Europe.
As stated by the IMIA working Group on coding in the conference of Ottawa in 1984 the long term goal must be to obtain a unique conceptual schema:In the short term nevertheless it is necessary to make progress from available classifications, nomenclatures, glossari and thesauri to a unique conceptual schema for specific and different priorities in health care.

    2.2 DATA SETS

It appears that 4 extensions (including a redefinition) of hospital mbds are required to reach different goals.

1 - Extension of the field :

    There is a consensus to extend the hospital mbds to all hospital activities and namely to rehabilitation, long term, psychiatric, ambulatory and day care.

2 - Redefinition of the concept.

    The initial definition of mbds provided by Roger et al was not the data set required for goals like quality and outcome of care assessment, process of care management, etc. Henceforth there is a need for refined definition of mbds with two different data sets :

    1 - Minimum data set MDS

    The smallest data set necessary to enable a particular activity to take place.

2 - Common data set CDS

The set of data required to enable all desired activities to take place (or at least for more than one activity).

3 - Extension of the content

Following point 1 and 2 the following updating of hospital mbds content is proposed :

Severity variables for all the areas (functional health status, nursing work load, Admission data,Process of care) and specific variables for Obstetric and newborn, Rehabilitation, Psychiatric care, Long term care and Intensive care unit.

The workload related to this extension can be fairly evaluated by the total number of items required compared to the initial mbds :

FROM 13 TO 20 ITEMS FOR ALL THE AREAS

FROM 13 TO 25 ITEMS FOR SOME SPECIFIC AREAS

4 - Extension of the concept

There is a need for data set linkage between encounter data sets either at a level of a Plan of care (all the encounters managed by a leading health care practitioner)
either at a level of Episode of illness (all the encounters managed by one or several leading health care practitioners during an illness). This implies to use Information Technology data transfer and security and protection methods to relate safely data between different encounters and in some cases different health care practitioners.

2.3 PATIENT CLASSIFICATION SYSTEMS (P.C.Ss.)

Patient classification system following Hornbrook is a categorisation of patients specific to one or more precise objectives : The different classifications needed are specific for the objective of the exercice :

This implies :

1 - Several PCSs are needed due to the area of patient care concerned, the level of decision the main intention of the assessment, the orientation.

2 - A common european PCS framework must be based not only on a standard data set but too on flexible data sets which can be either unidimensional indicators either detailed data.

A minimum PCS framework requires 7 (6+1) PCS.

A common European PCS framework (for a precise set of goals or benefits) can require 14 (11+3).

3') HARMONISATION OF COST DATA

   3.1 METHODOLOGY

   Five steps must be followed to satisfy the different needs.
1 - To examine the required outputs and goals of a cost model rather
than the existing data sets which are so different between countries.
2 - To define a set of MINIMUM STANDARD DATA REQUIREMENTS in relation
with the goals which would ensure that any country can produce its
own costs comparable only within countries.
3 - To specify a subset of this data requirements to produce a LOWEST
COMMON DENOMINATOR from the national data sets which would serve as
the first STANDARD REFERENCE VERSION of an INTERNATIONAL COMPARATIVE
DATA SET mapped to the national data sets on the basis of on an
agreed set of definitions.
4 - To develop a comprehensive FINANCIAL SUPPORT SYSTEM able to
perform the different functions on the institutional level.
5 - To follow a case-mix costing development path planned in time and
space. This approach can be applied to the most advanced pilot
hospitals information systems using patient based costing as well as
to the crude information systems developed in other hospitals.

   3.2 DATA SETS
   3.2.1 MINIMUM STANDARDISED COST DATA SET (MSCDS)
   The following headings are required :
1 - CHART OF ACCOUNT
   - medical staff, (senior staff, junior staff); nursing staff,
(permanent staff, agency nursing staff; other staff; consumables;
prostheses; drugs.
2 - COST CENTRES
   - diagnostic and therapeutic departments; operating theatres
services; support services; general institution overheads.
   3.2.2 COMMON COMPARATIVE EUROPEAN CASE-MIX COST MODEL
Four models do exit : RVU CASE-MIX COST MODEL, STANDARD COST
APPORTIONMENT MODEL, EVENTS APPORTIONMENT MODEL, PATIENT BASED MODEL
(events standard costs and care profiles).
The first model only is available to day for comparison, the fourth
requires HIS development and the second and the third can be
developped as a mid term goal.

4') BENEFITS

The advocated harmonisation of health data on the institutional level is a CRUCIAL move from a supply side and technology driven health services model to a demand side and PATIENT BASED APPROACH model with a comprehensive information system related on one side to institutions and on the other side to EPISODE AND PATIENTS by data set linkage.

SUCH A DEVELOPMENT CAN BE A MAJOR CONTRIBUTION FROM EUROPEAN STATES AND EUROPEAN INSTITUTIONS FOR APPLICATION OF WHO POLICY FOR HEALTH FOR ALL 2000.

5') REFERENCES

1) Bergner M; Quality of life,health status and clinical research. Med Care 1989 27 S148.

2) Brook RH; Studies of process-outcome in medical care evaluations; Ann Arbor, MI : Health Administration Press 1985.

3) CAMAC .Final report .AIM EEC BRUSSELS 1991.

4) CHIC .Final report .AIM EEC BRUSSELS 1990.

5) Cote RA ; International Classification For Health and Disease : the expandable common care concept : Med Inf. 1983 8(1) 5-16.

6) Hornbrook MC. Hospital case mix: its definition, measurement and use.Part I.The conceptual framework. Part II. Review of alternative measures. Med Care Review 1982 39 1-43 73-123.

7) Lambert PM ; The minimum basic data set for hospital statistics in the EEC ; Commission of the European Communities Brussels 1981.

8) Mc ACE. Final report.AIM EEC BRUSSELS 1990.

INFORMATION MODELLING IN THE DUTCH HEALTH CARE

A.J. ten Hoopen, J. Nutma & P.F. de Vries Robbé
Dept. of Social Medicine & Epidemiology/
Dept. of Medical Information and Decision Science
State University/ University Hospital Groningen
P.O. Box 72, 9700 AB Groningen, The Netherlands

Abstract

An introduction is given on the underlying concepts and motivation for information modelling in the past decade in Dutch Health Care. An overview of achieved results on the development of reference models is presented, some critical questions are raised, and a few remarks on future developments are made.

Introduction.

In Medical Informatics as elsewhere the determination and analysis of user needs takes a more and more important place in the first phases of the development of information systems. Extensive knowledge of user needs might be the most important success factor in building systems, or as Van Bemmel stated it recently: 'for the development of programmes not only knowledge is required from computer science, but in the first place from medicine itself: about the functioning of the hospital, about diagnostic and therapeutic processes and on how people provide medical care' (Van Bemmel, 1990).

There are at least two very good reasons to concentrate on the analysis of information requirements (IRs) of users. Firstly to develop information systems which not only improve organizational efficiency, a complete inventory of IRs has to be made and analysed in the context of the userprocess (which is contributing in a certain manner to the goals of the business). Doing for example a thorough classical data analysis is certainly not enough, because as Galliers stated so nicely: 'Data analysis is a very useful tool for efficient database design. It is much less useful as a means of identifying IRs (especially where these are "fuzzy" and unstructured), or in allowing different viewpoints to be taken into consideration. Too often based on an analysis of current situations, data analysis - in the extreme case - is a great way of encapsulating organizational ineffectiveness in the resultant database!' (Galliers, 1987).

Secondly the successful development of (large) information systems depends heavily on the complexity of such a system. One of the most difficult (and often ignored) problems in system development is the handling of a large collection of requirements (see e.g. Neumann, 1990). So analysis of user needs should at least result in stating non-redundant IRs, to avoid unnecessary complexity.

In this contribution the development in the Dutch Health Care of models and techniques to achieve a complete description of non-redundant IRs (in the context of the process to which they belong) is described.

Methods.

The initial reason for developing what has been called the Hospital Information Model (HIM, ZIM in dutch, Geurts-de Haas et al., 1984) was the need for some basic description of <u>all</u> hospital IRs and for a (conceptual) datastructure from which these IRs could be fulfilled. This description was initially needed as a reference framework for comparing Hospital Information Systems (and their functional specifications and databases), and in the end for system development.

Such a reference framework (also called Reference Information Model) should contain a precise description of the 'core' information, e.g. the maximum set of IRs which is common to all hospitals. Because differences in organizational structure tend to confuse discussions, distract from the main points to concentrate upon (and should be dealt with at the level of specific organizations), it was decided that the description would <u>not</u> contain anything in detail about the organizational structure. Naturally the framework contains some common elements on which the structure of organizations can be based: the business model. This consists of three levels:

on the 'lowest' level the <u>primary</u> and <u>ancillary</u> activities (processes) are described, on an intermediate level the activities of (managerial) <u>control</u>, and on the highest level a description is given of '<u>goal setting</u>' activities.

The primary and supporting activities are in an ad hoc way clustered into what has been called 'functional areas'.

For every activity (on the lowest level) IRs are described. Each IR is linked to the datastructure by summing up the entities which are needed to fulfil the IR. The control process is basically a feed back loop and consists of the following steps: 1. observation of (process

relevant) signals, 2. explanation of deviations, 3. taking appropriate
measures/steps/actions to correct, then back to 1. (see upward and
downward arrows between 'control' and 'primary & ancillary activities'
in figure below). The IRs of the control activities are described for
each functional area. The goal setting process is not extensively
described. Instead a division in subject (or focal) areas and (the
main part of) the IRs for goal setting activities are listed per
subject area.

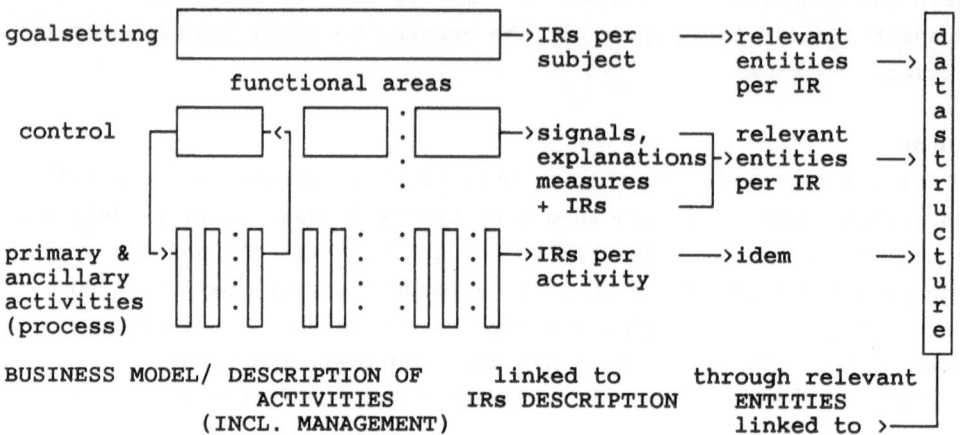

BUSINESS MODEL/ DESCRIPTION OF   linked to   through relevant
              ACTIVITIES   IRs DESCRIPTION   ENTITIES
          (INCL. MANAGEMENT)   linked to >

The development of a reference framework like the HIM is basically
done by interviewing a great number of experts on all kinds of
subjects throughout the country. It consists of three main steps.
The development starts with creating a description of activities on
which there has to be some agreement among the experts (which is
tested in interviews).
After that per activity or small set of activities all (non-redundant)
IRs are determined using the business model described in the last
paragraph, the description of activities obtained in the first phase,
and some quality assurance techniques to structure the interview. The
synthesis of these results of two rounds of interviews is aiming at a
comprehensive, consistent and (in the way Neumann, 1990, used the
word) elegant description of the complete conceptual level of the
information service needed in the hospital area.
The third step creates the datastructure. This datastructure is the
result of a 'classical' data analysis and consists of the usual
definition of entities, listing of attributes per entity, graphical
presentation of (key) relations between entities and some overviews
like the create/use matrix between activities and entities.

So in the end all relations between activities (processes) and data that are important for decisionmaking on planning and developing information systems can be derived from the resulting framework.

To summarise:
> an Information Model like HIM is a description of a business model with an explicit managerial concept, linked through the description of IRs to a datastructure (containing all relevant entities, attributes and key relations), independent of the organizational structure, intended for use with informationplanning (like Business Systems Planning) and Information System Development.

Results.
After first standards being set by the development of the HIM, a lot of work on information modelling for Health Care has been done in the Netherlands. The HIM-project was continued to include the specific topics of Academic Hospitals (education and research) as well. In the mean time similar, though a bit less extensive, models had been made for Nursing Homes, and Institutions for the Mentally Handicapped. This range of models was then extended to cover non-residential areas of health care like Public Health Organizations, Institutions for Ambulatory Mental Health Care, Physiotherapy Practice, and an other type of residential organization: the Mental Hospital.
Recently a model to cover all of the Regional Health Care activities was completed (Ten Hoopen et al., 1990a & 1990b), in which all the foregoing work was incorporated and in which the field of Primary Health Care and some of the Social Services is included (for an overview of available models and references see Ten Hoopen et al., 1990a). This last model is itself available as a database with the following underlying structure:

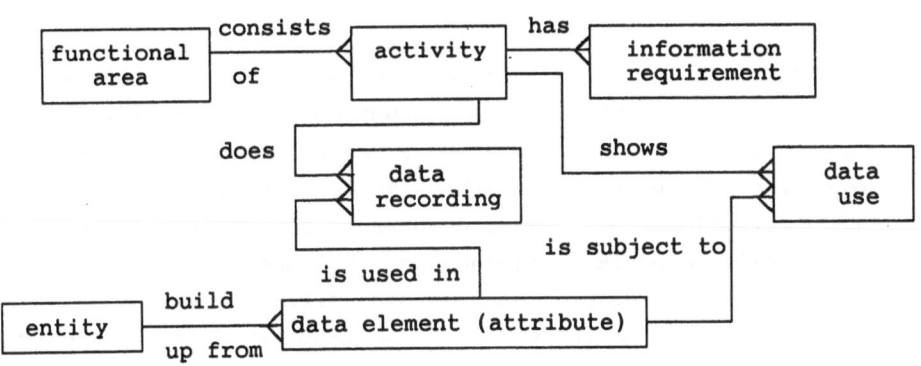

During the development of the HIM ideas on possible use of the model
were extended. Explicitly some way of evaluating (part of) an existent
information service was added to the final report on HIM. Also
included was a method to use HIM as an aid in developing an
information policy and a development plan for information services
(various example forms to use with such applications can be found in
Geurts-De Haas et al., 1984). The HIM has been included in workbench
like software to support the information managers planning activities.
Although it is not known that the HIM has explicitly been used for
integral system development, it started (recently) to influence
Hospital Information Systems development in the Netherlands.
Furthermore there are complete systems developed in the Public Health
sector which are exclusively build on a HIM type of model.

Discussion.
Although the HIM has been the explicit (methodical) reference for all
developed models in the Dutch Health Care (and though the Ministry of
Welfare, Health and Cultural Affairs has always connected conditions
aiming at uniformity to the financing of projects), there are some
points on which the models differ.

Firstly of course due to the different parts of Health Care they
cover, which causes differences in terminology, but also differences
in the way 'functional areas' have been distinguished within the
models.

And secondly due to the sometimes smaller or larger area a model deals
with, the level of detail in descriptions differs.

Thirdly sometimes different data analysis approaches have been used
(so that for example cardinality of relations is added, and some
object model exists).

Fourthly the development process has not always been structured the
same way: trained layman interviewers conducting structured interviews
on a relatively large scale aiming at a large number of interviews per
kind of expertise, delphi methods with a limited number of experts
(with unknown selection/bias), small numbers of carefully selected key
informants interviewed by IR-Determination (IRD) specialists, all has
been used in some of the developments causing differences in the
description/ content of the IRs of which the importance is not clear.

And last there are several minor differences, for example sometimes
the goalsetting activity (process) is not dealt with at all, and some
projects did use a supporting computerised development tool (CASE)
which probably improves consistency, while other projects didn't.

Some important extensions to the way of developing the HIM have been
established during the development of the overall (regional) Health
Care Information Model. Basically four questions were raised in that
project:
1) how do you get a **valid and sufficient detailed** description of
   processes in (regional) Health Care?
2) how do you get a **good** IRD?
3) how do you **integrate** all kinds of descriptions from already
   existing Reference Information Models?
4) what's "valid and sufficient detailed" and "good" in respectively
   questions one and two if you consider the **use** of a Reference
   Information Model in applications like the informationplanning
   process (which develops among other things an information
   architecture), or to put the central question in an other way: how
   do you ensure the quality of the model developed regarding the
   needed quality in applications?

Future developments.
The extension to still other areas of Health Care and Social Services
continues. Some modelling will be done or has already started on the
activities of rehabilitation centres; care, nursing and family aid,
delivered at the (family) home by various organizations; centres for
primary health care; social service institutions; care for the
addicts; regional 'protected living' residences; and medical
specialist practice.

It is considered to do some work on the existing models. They should
all be made available and in some form on disc. And in a number of
them the datastructure could be extended with use/ recording and
coding characteristics of entities and attributes, and with
constraints on various levels to facilitate database definition.
Furthermore IR descriptions could be analysed to deliver (main parts
of) the functional specifications of information Systems.
An update of the contents of the existing models (even the oldest one,
the HIM) does not seem to be necessary at this moment (an opinion
based on recent application experiences).

For some well defined areas in Health Care the model development will
be embedded into a complete system development cycle (for example
areas 'home care' and 'centres for primary care' mentioned above).

Finally the Dutch experience on development and application of these
models could, because for example the way confusing discussions on
differences in organizational structures are avoided, be very useful
in some unifying or standardization activities on an European level.
Discussions with the National Health Services' Information Management
Centre have recently been started about the properties on the 'meta
level' of this kind of models, confronting their Common Basic
Specification method for development of information services in Health
Care with the developments described in this contribution.

Literature

Bemmel, J.H. van (1990). Communication in Health Care - New
developments. In: Preprints of the Proceedings of the IMIA Working
Conference on Telematics in Medicine 18-21 november 1990 EUR Rotterdam
The Netherlands (Proceedings will appear with North Holland, in the
IMIA series).

Galliers, R.D. editor (1987). Information analysis: selected readings.
Addison-Wesley Publishing Company.

Geurts-De Haas, G.E., Oorschot, H.P.F. van & Vondel, H. van (1984).
Ziekenhuis Informatie Model. Nationaal Ziekenhuis Instituut, 84.382,
Utrecht.

Hoopen, A.J. ten & Nutma, J. (1990a). Gezondheidszorg InformatieModel.
Een gebruikshandleiding. Rijksuniversiteit Groningen/ Projekt
Gezondheidszorg Almere. (a translation into the english language is in
preparation)

Hoopen, A.J. ten, Nutma, J., Smit, C.A.C., Loop, L.A.M. & Vries Robbé,
P.F. de, (1990b). Gezondheidszorg InformatieModel. De ontwikkeling.
Rijksuniversiteit Groningen/ Projekt Gezondheidszorg Almere.

Neumann, P.G. (1990). Beauty and the Beast of Software Complexity -
Elegance versus Elephants. In: Beauty is our business: a birthday
salute to Edsger W. Dijkstra. W.H.J. Feijen et al. Springer-Verlag New
York Berlin Heidelberg.

EXECUTIVE INFORMATION SYSTEMS FOR NHS SENIOR MANAGEMENT

Yitzhak Peterburg, MD, DrPH, MSc (London School of Economics);
Steve Smithson, PhD (London School of Economics);
Victor Peel, PhD (University of Manchester)

ABSTRACT

Executive Information Systems (EIS) have grown very popular in the last
few years, serving as a tool for senior management to cope with the
increasingly complex business of the 1990s. The health care industry
has been one of the latest to follow suit. Our project, focusing on the
seventeen members of the Management Support System General Managers
Panels, aims to identify what is expected of the EIS, what are their
most important capabilities and especially, what are the training
needs. Practical implications for the introduction and implementation
of such systems, based on the results of the survey, are discussed.

———

The proposed changes of the White Paper 'Working for Patients' have
highlighted the value of information in addressing key management
issues of general managers within the British National Health System
(NHS). The Management Focus Group (MFG), a multi-disciplinary task
group, composed of general managers at all levels of the NHS, declared
the establishment of Management Support Systems (MSS). Those systems
are almost identical to Executive Information Systems (EIS) or
Executive Support Systems (ESS), which have drawn remarkable attention
and interest in many industries and across borders in Europe and USA
(Friend, 1986; Garelick, 1987). They are "based on the premise that
more reliable and timely information makes for better decisions, and
that better decisions make for better, healthier businesses (Friend,
1986; Jones, 1989). The EIS provide consistent, immediate information
regardless of location or time, give management a chance to dig deeper
into corporate databases, facilitate communication among a fast-moving
management team and link executives to other employees and online
services (O'Shea, 1989; Raths, 1989). The retrieved information is
defined by the style in which the executive is used to work, rather
than attempting to redefine his job. It helps the senior manager to
track key changes, using time-series data to illustrate trends, in his

organization and sometimes in the outside competitive world as well
(Jordan, 1988; Miller, 1989). Moreover, it is argued that ESS provides
better mental models for executive decision making by allowing
'what-if' and 'what-best' questions, discussing various decision
alternatives and the resulting business scenarios (Jones, 1989).

THE STUDY - MATERIALS AND METHODS

The study was originally undertaken to address only the issue of the
training requirements for the implementation of the Management Support
Systems, discussed above. The objectives were enlarged to also
encompass the desirable capabilities and users' expectations of these
systems. Executive Information Systems are pretty new in the British
healthcare field. Meaningful discussion of the above objectives
require some prior knowledge of these systems, and it was therefore
decided to focus on the highly selective General Managers Panels of the
Management Focus Group. those are composed of seventeen (17) members,
all General Managers, distributed among an Acute Unit Panel (5), a
Community Unit Panel (5), and a District Panel (7).

A questionnaire was prepared and piloted with some of the Panels'
members. After minor changes, 16 questions were chosen for the final
version of the questionnaire. After all questionnaires were answered
and analyzed, six members, two from each Panel, were interviewed to
validate their answers and elaborate on the issues under consideration.
Because of the small number of participants, no statistical
significance analysis was done.

FINDINGS

Out of the seventeen participants, eight had either a computer terminal
or a personal computer at their desk. It was used mainly for
word-processing and database management, for less than 30 minutes
daily, on average. As explained above, the participants were a highly
selective group, and therefore all of them were at least aware of the
existence of EIS or ESS applications. Twelve (71%) had either seen EIS
used, or had used it themselves.

The most important expectations of these sophisticated EIS applications
were better analysis of the resources used by the organization, better
future planning, and the ability of instant overview of the whole

organization. Some participants emphasized the use of EIS systems, especially their forecasting capabilities, for dealing with the required contracting processes. Competitive advantage, and the most feared control of mid-management were the least desired capabilities. No significant differences were noted among the various Panels, although for the District Panel, instant overview of the organization seemed more important and future planning was regarded as less important in comparison to the other two Panels. When user expectations were analyzed according to the ownership of a personal computer or terminal, the results again were very similar in the two groups, with better analysis of resources and better future planning heading the list of preferences.

Half of the participants expressed their belief that only senior managers should have access to the EIS systems. Another five were willing to extend EIS use to mid management as well. The most interesting suggestion, in some ways opposite to the definition of EIS/ESS, was to make those systems open to everybody in the organization, on a network. When asked to rank the capabilities of such an EIS/ESS system in order of their influence on the manager's decision to use them, the analytical capability of the system was perceived as the most important capability, with user friendly interface following. In the case of the Acute Unit Panel this ranking was reversed. Better graphic presentation, usually the most prominent feature of EIS was ranked only third in importance, which was similar to the ranking of the capability of producing better reports and presentations in prior questions. All Panels agreed that security capability, i.e. restricting access of unauthorized personnel to the sensitive information, was least important. Preferences of EIS capabilities were almost identical in the group that had their own terminal and the group that did not. No significant differences were noted when those groups were analyzed among each Panel, separately.

The majority of participants (12) preferred at-work training, arguing that it was more convenient and fruitful, if the training was post implementation of the EIS in their organization. Moreover, if training of all the management team was preferred, it seemed to be feasible only at work. Only one manager preferred a 'private' lesson, and on the other extreme, four (24%) had no preference with whom their training was going to be. The latter group was almost exclusively composed of the Acute Unit Panel. Nevertheless, most senior managers (59%) preferred their training to be with managers from a similar level, either from their own organization (35%), other organizations (6%), or from both (18%). Only two participants were willing to share their training with mid-management as well. Ownership of own terminal had no obvious influence on the participants' training preferences.

Most participants (59%) preferred a training programme, up to three days long. Four (24%), wanted a more concise version of one day long intense' workshop. The majority of the latter group came from those who did not have a computer terminal of their own. The remaining three (17%) were willing to study slower, on a three hours weekly basis. It should be emphasized that in the interviews, when this issue was further elaborated on, almost all interviewees said that their answers referred only to the introductory phase in the EIS implementation, and that refresher courses, 'consolidation events', and on-going training should continue to explore all potential uses and realize all the benefits of these highly sophisticated applications.

DISCUSSION

The importance of information systems for general managers within the NHS, especially in the post Review era, seem to be unquestionable and self-evident. The respondents, representing the different aspects of healthcare delivery systems, were not only unified in the realization of the need for timely and accurate information, but also in their commitment to the development of such systems. Three major issues are identified by this survey, which are most probably even more applicable to the general population of senior management within the NHS. Those include what the user expects of Executive Information Systems, regarding his perceived needs and the system capabilities, who should use and have access to such a system, and what training is needed to maximize the promised benefits.

The answer to whom the EIS is targeted at, senior management exclusively or lower levels as well, have direct bearing on the final product. Some argue that while you start implementing an EIS system usually at the top management, there is even more benefit to the whole organization by applying the technology further down, to the mid-management level (Kelly, 1988; Nelson, 1990). The survey does not supply the answer to this issue, but it clearly shows that the participants, all senior managers in the NHS, are confused and hold different opinions, ranging from open systems on a network to systems for only the very top management. This question should be addressed before any systems are actually developed. While some argue that you need no training with EIS ("after about 15 minutes of training, turn

him loose"), most of our survey respondents were rightly less
enthusiastic about it and preferred either a training of 1-3 days long
or a one day long 'intense' workshop. Although at-work training was the
most favoured place (71%), further discussions in the interviews lead
me to suggest that two types of training should be offered. The first
one, prior to installment of the particular EIS at a specific site,
should be done outside work-place premises. This should focus on the
general characteristics of EIS applications, what they have to offer,
and will try to help the managers define their needs and expectations.
The forum should be that of fellow senior managers. It was argued that
in order not to jeopardize their credibility, the teams should be
brought along only after their senior managers have some prior
knowledge about the systems. On the other hand, after the EIS system
is installed, training should be aimed at the management team as a unit
by itself, so that most options and benefits are realized. This is
at-work training, including on going refreshers, workshops, etc. One
unresolved question is whether a more homogenous forum, e.g. acute
units managers or DGMs, would prove to be more beneficial.

REFERENCES

1.   Frenkel K.A.: Executive Information Systems: war for the executive
     desktop. Personal Computing 14(4): 56-64; 1990.
2.   Friend D.: Executive Information Systems: successes and failures,
     *nsights and misconceptions. Journal of Information Systems
     Management 3(4):31-36; 1986.
3.   Garelick H.: Executive Information Systems: marketing hype or
     invaluable management aid? Industrial Management & Data Systems,
     March-April 1987. pp. 20-22.
4.   Jones K.: Executive Support Systems come of age. Modern Office
     Technology 34(10): 78-82; 1989.
5.   Jordan M.L.: Executive Information Systems make life easy for the
     lucky few. Computerworld 22:51,55-57; 1988.
6.   Management Focus Group: Key management Issues for Healthcare. A
     Monograph. October 1989.
7.   Miller R.: Executive Information Systems help you conduct your
     business. Today's Office 23(11): 16-24; 1989.
8.   Nelson R.: Executive Information Systems: culture clash at the top.
     Personal Computing 14(4): 76-77; 1990.
9.   O'Shea T.J.: Low-cost approaches to Executive Information Systems.
     Journal of Information Systems Management 6:34-41; 1989.
10. Raths D.: The politics of Executive Information Systems. InfoWorld
     11(20): 47-52; 1989.

A Generic Model of Clinical Practice - the COSMOS Project

T Cairns[1], H Timimi[2], M Thick[1], and G Gold[2].

1 Transplant Unit, St Mary's Hospital, London, UK;
2 NHS Information Management Centre, Birmingham, UK.

ABSTRACT

One of the aims of the COSMOS project is to develop a generic model of clinical practice intended to provide a logical design which will form the basis for the development of a comprehensive computer record of any chosen clinical activity. The model, intended to become the clinical view of the UK NHS' Common Basic Specification, forms part of a functional specification enabling systems to be developed as integral parts of much larger, complex systems of health care.

INTRODUCTION

The COSMOS project is jointly funded by the UK NHS Information Management Centre (IMC) and Parkside Health Authority, London, and is part of the IMC programme to develop the Common Basic Specification (CBS)[1], which aims to cover all aspects of running a Health Service. The CBS will specify a solid foundation for the development or procurement of information systems supporting and integrating clinical practice and general management. The practice of medicine as a whole involves the collective knowledge and action of countless individuals in both formal and informal organisations. The application of information technology to enhance this activity demands the development of information systems as integral parts of the practice of organised medicine[2]. The early work of the CBS project has been to establish the use of disciplined methods to produce both the basic specifications and the computer systems derived from them, that satisfy the need for integration in clinical practice.

The COSMOS Clinical Process Model (CCPM) is one of the early results of the clinical projects attached to the CBS. Although the CCPM does not provide designs for diagnostic expert systems, as such, it is intended, however, to specify how such specialised systems should fit into the general framework of the CBS.

METHODS

The CCPM has been produced using Ptech[3], a technique developed by Associative Design Technology. The model aims to provide part of the functional specification for an implemented system, namely a description of the data file structure, and a description of the data analysis required for alterations to and use of the knowledge base. The model does not specify screen design, maintenance and back-up procedures, security requirements, or other related issues. It does not specify the activities for correcting erroneous data or adding data files.

The model is described using three types of Diagram:

Activity Diagram

The Activity Diagram is a comprehensive process view of the chosen clinical activity. Each Activity represents a discrete collection of operations that reflects the way in which the work considered is organised. The result of an Activity is known as its Product. The Activity Diagram illustrates the Products that are exchanged between each Activity and forms a framework for the functional specification.

Event Diagrams

The Event Diagrams illustrate the causal sequence of events both within each Activity, and in the exchange of Products between Activities. Events represent changes to the knowledge base, but they may occur on the basis of a series of Queries. Queries represent the handling, and Events the recording, of information within the system. Together they represent the detail of the functional specification outlined in the Activity Diagram.

Concept Diagrams

Concept Diagrams contain all the elements which are both necessary and sufficient for a record of Events to be complete. In this way they represent both the Product of an Activity, and the elements necessary for its production. The Concept Diagram contributes to the functional specification by specifying the information that can be recorded and manipulated, and how it is to be stored.

THE MODEL AS A FUNCTIONAL SPECIFICATION

As stated, the conceptual model and its description constitute the functional specification. The Activity Diagram provides a structure for the functional specification; the Concept Diagram specifies the data files. The knowledge of human health and disease necessary for all of the Activities considered is specifically represented in the Concept Diagram.

The Event Diagrams describe the points at which the knowledge base is altered by Events, or used in Queries. Events and Queries are represented in a well-defined context that will determine both the software modules and the options available to the user in the implemented system. The detailed description of Events and Queries is used by those who will build the data management functions, and those who will use the system. It should provide a common starting point for discussion of final screen design, since the Concepts described for each Event or Query represent the data items that will need to be entered or displayed on the screen.

THE COSMOS CLINICAL PROCESS MODEL: CONCEPT DIAGRAM

In the CCPM Concept Diagram, clinical activity is represented by Concepts grouped either at a knowledge level or at an operational level.

The Concepts expressed at the knowledge level represent what is known about human health and disease, what can be measured, how measurements and other observations can be made, and what protocols can be used to intervene.

The Concepts at the operational level are used to record occurrences of these measurements, observations and interventions in relation to specific cases, whether populations or individuals, known within the model as Objects Of Care.

It will be shown how, in the model, the state of health of any Object Of Care (OOC) is described through Observations made about it. Observations are Actions that recognise or note that instances of knowledge level Observation Concepts apply to the OOC. In this way the observer can relate what is known about an OOC to the rest of his knowledge, which includes other Observation Concepts. Observations are not instances of Observation Concepts; they are the Procedures of recording that specific Observation Concepts apply to an OOC.

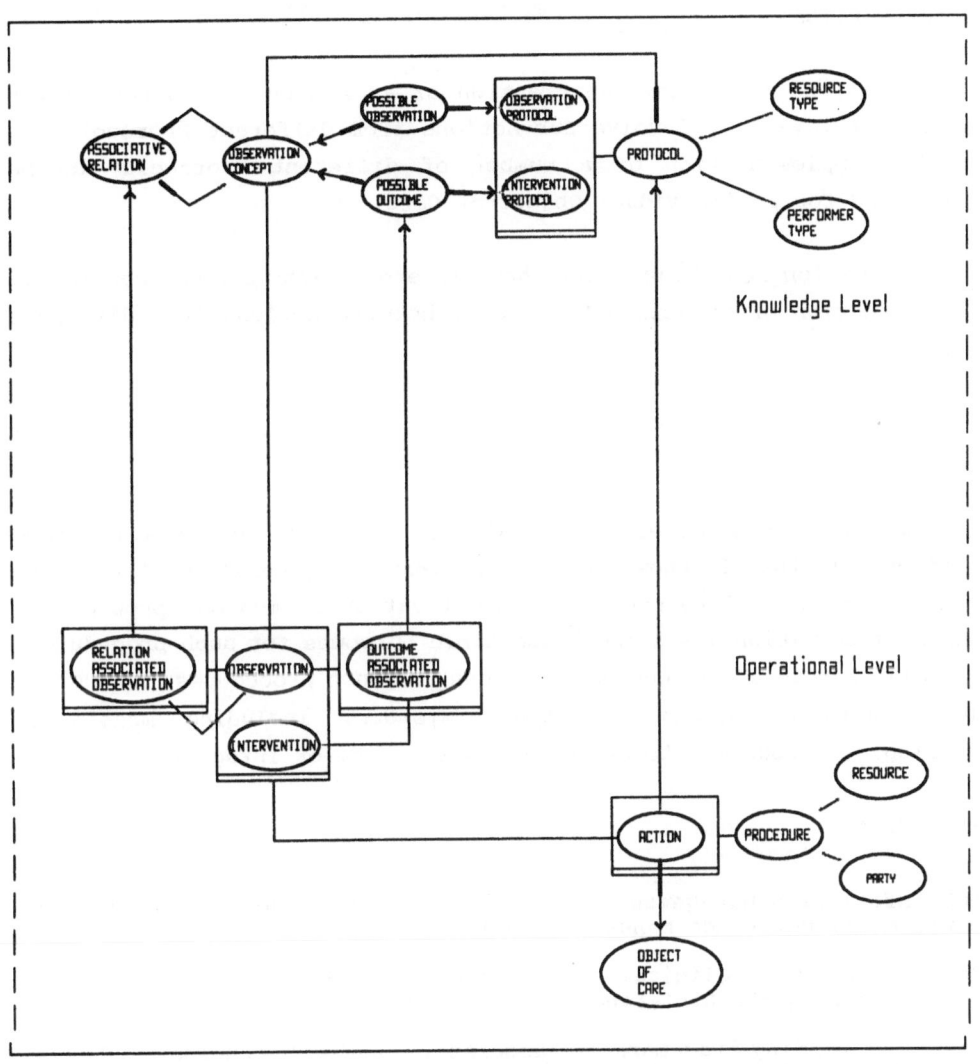

THE COSMOS CLINICAL PROCESS MODEL CONCEPT DIAGRAM (Figure 1)

Actions are recorded at the operational level and represent the implementation of Protocols. Protocols are part of a performer's knowledge and skills. Protocols describe, at a general level, the characteristics that an implemented Action will have. They can also be thought of as the means that can be used to achieve certain ends from given starting points.

Protocols can be characterised by the Performer Types, Resource Types and Technique required and their given starting points. A Protocol therefore unites Resource Type, how a Resource Type is to be used (Technique), and who is qualified to use it (Performer Type). A classification of Protocols can be developed from consideration of these characteristics.

It will be shown how the creation of an Action Dependency at the operational level may involve Sub-Actions from different Protocols, so that the implementation of a number of different Protocols can be coordinated for an individual Object of Care.

In addition it will be shown that different Plans can be coordinated by the creation of an Action Dependency between Actions from different Plans.

CONCLUSION

A model has been developed in which clinical events can be recorded to reflect all that is known about such events in general; whether it be a reflection of an international classification of medical procedures, a contrast to nationally agreed acceptable outcomes for such procedures, or locally agreed use of costed resources for such procedures. The model allows decision support or expert systems, including models of physiological processes to be developed from it, or integrated with it.

REFERENCES:

1.NHS Information Management Centre. Common Basic Specification. The Generic Model Reference Manual, CBS001_1.0. 1990

2.Gold, Gerry. The Clinical View of the Common Basic Specification. Health Computing '91 Conference Proceedings. ISBN 0 948198 11 7

3.Ptech - a pending trademark of Associative Design Technology (US) Ltd. Two Westborough Business Park, Westborough, MA 01581-3199, USA

BUILDING A NATIONAL HEALTH INFORMATION SYSTEM

Carmel White and Tony Carroll

Rotunda Hospital ,

Dublin, Ireland

Abstract

The provision of Health Services is an enormous undertaking for all countries. Services are usually distributed through a maze of statutory and other bodies established by government. The information cycle between these agencies is vital, particularly at management level. Often there is no comprehensive Health Information System available to health care managers and staff. As a result, the decision-making process for them can be precarious because the necessary information available is often disjointed, inaccurate or out of date. In addition such information can be time-consuming to obtain. All of this is extremely wasteful and very costly both in terms of managerial time and constructive results. There is a great need therefore for a Health Information System on Computer. This paper explores the possibility of developing such a system called HISk.

INTRODUCTION

The organisation and management of any enterprise is a complex task requiring specialised skills. Not least of these skills is the ability to be able to communicate with people. However, excellent communication skills are of little use if good information channels are not in place. For example, the managing director of a large company employing thousands of people will not be able to communicate with each employee on a personal level every day but through effective communication channels such as internal memoranda, notice boards and news letters, his workforce can receive his messages clearly at any time. This same kind of clarity is perhaps far more crucial to his departmental heads who have to interpret his instructions and implement his policies. But private enterprise is unique from a standards point of view and not just in terms of the information cycle. There are a host of infra-structures which are automatically in place., almost as acceptable as the expectation of profit at the end of the day. Such is not always the case in the public sector. A dramatic expansion in the scope of information systems in the public sector is a crucial precondition for developing information for goal/objectives and strategy formulation and the management control involved in the implementation of strategies (Hally, Page 234). The development of an National Health Information System could be a significant step for propelling one of the major public sector spenders into cost effective management

Overview

Information may be defined as a quantum which precipitates a change in the current structure of knowledge; it is necessary for decisions and generates change (Wainwright,Page 398).The kind of information which would be included in an national health information system will have to be diverse in order to meet general requirements. An integral part of the system should be to promote cost-benefit awareness. Therefore HISk would have to include modules on the following: General Information, Financial Information, Purchasing Management, Personnel Management, Patient Services Management, and Epidemiological Information. This selection of modules is by no means comprehensive but they are offered here as key modules which are essential in order to build the system. For example, the General Information Module would contain the following information: 1.A guide to Health Legislation including Statutory Instruments. This would take the form of a collection of abstracts. The menu would display the titles of the legislation, any of which could be accessed   by reference number displayed. European Community legislation on   health matters would also be included. 2.The contents of The Civil Service Directory. 3. The contents of the Registers from Professional Registration Bodies. 4. Directives from the Minister for Health. A complete data bank of all Directives and circulars issued to date would be put into the   system.   5.A Summary of Entitlements to Health Services. 6.A complete guide to Private Health Insurance Regulation 7. A directory of Medical Practitioners providing free services.   8.A guide to Private Hospitals, Nursing Homes and Voluntary Group associated with health care, including the names of contact persons. 9. Relevant Statistical Publications from The Central Statistics Office. 10."Who is saying what about the Health Services"! A list of Publications about health services' management with abstracts and references.

This Module will be of general use and would be frequently updated as new information comes on stream.

Building HISk

The concepts of the GUIDE system and HYPERTEXT in general are well established. GUIDE has had major success with large corporations wishing to create electronic reference works. A lot of U.S. colleges are insisting that their students run GUIDE on their Macintosh computers. Lecturers give out course notes in GUIDE format and the students enhance, append and, delete the contents to suit their own requirements. Although not purpose-built as a text outliner, in many ways GUIDE is more useful because of the range of connections that can be made (Tebbut, Page 148). The University of Kent has also produced a number of on-line textbooks using the concept. This kind of software could be adopted for a national health information system like HISk.

It would have many advantages for the users and would simplify the whole process of updating information in the   modules.

Implementation

In developing a HISk one has to assume that all health care agencies throughout the country have computers and systems which would be capable of linking in to such a grande system. However, it could also be possible to store these modules on CD-ROM or possibly even floppy disk, so that cheap stand-alone micros could be installed in smaller health agencies throughout the country. Periodic updates could be circulated when necessary. Alternatively, the system could be launched through AERTEL, the R.T.E. data network, or VIDEOTEL, the teleshopping system which is being piloted in Ireland at present. This system requires only a telephone with a telemonitor and keypad. A similar type of system called STATUM is being marketed by Irish Medical Systems of Blackrock Clinic, Dublin. This is used by general practitioners to access data bases on a range of subjects such as drug interactions..

Cost Benefits

The introduction of HISk could realise significant savings for the Health Services. These include the following:

1. The absence of published material relating to the amount of time health care managers spend on extracting important information makes it difficult for the writer to quantify in monetary terms ,the cost benefits of the system. In a Swedish study, Andersson et al states that information handling in health care is estimated to take roughly 30% of the working hours of all staff (Andersson, Page 234). If we were to translate this figure into Irish terms, the savings arising from HISk for the health services would be enormous.

2. The Purchasing Information Module would contain a wealth of information which is vital for health agencies to combat escalating prices.

Quite often, an agency is paying the top prices for products which are discounted to other agencies, but the agency concerned may have no proper means of getting up to date information on prices being paid in general, throughout the health services. This situation can result in huge losses to the Health Services as a whole. HISk would help redress the problem and lead to more aggressive bargaining on the part of health agencies.

3. The third major saving would be in "consumables", such as photocopying, publishing, postage ,labour and general distribution costs incurred centrally. These would be abolished with HISk. .

4. Directives could be implemented more quickly. If these were of a monetary nature or involved the immediate rationalisation of services, all the relevant bodies would be notified simultaneously, and could therefore take the action required. This could result in immediate savings being realised .

5. The HISk concept would promote and maintain high standards of professionalism right across the board. Everyone would be at the same level in terms of information requirements. Errors of misinterpretation, which are often costly to correct, would be eliminated.

6. An Expert System in the Personnel Information Module could lead to better decision-making on the part of Personnel Officers, thus reducing the industrial relations workload and the likelihood of work stoppages.

7. A Computer-Aided Learning Package in the Patient Services Module would lead to more accurate data being collected, and give a much-needed boast to the Hospital Inpatient Enquiry Scheme. This type of information is vital for health care planners and if its accuracy could be increased, the savings to the Exchequer would be significant.

Managers cannot manage if they do not have comprehensive management information available to them. They can merely "keep things going" rather than "make things go".

References

Andersson, L. et al (1986) A Computer-Aided Medical Information System in a local health district in the county of Uppsala, Sweden. In: Economy in Health Care- the proceedings of the 6th European Conference On Health Records, Malta, May 5-7, 1986. C.O. Kohler, R. Zwick, U. Hoffman (eds). Economed, Lech, 234-237.

Hally, D. L. (1980) Accountability and the Public Sector. In: Journal of Institute of Public Administration, vol. 28, no.2, 224-234

Huffman, E. K. (1985) Medical Records Management. Physicians Record Company, USA, 393.

Tebbut, D.   (1988) Guide. In: PCW, June, 1988. 144-148

Wainwright, L. et al (1984) Training for Information in Health Care. In: Lecture Notes in Medical Informatics- the proceedings of Medical Informatics Europe, Brussels, September 10-13, 1984. F. H. Roger, J. L. Willems, R. O'Moore and B. Barber (eds), Springer-Verlag, Berlin, Heidelberg, New York, Tokyo. 396-404.

HealthPROMPT - A new Initiative in

Providing Information for Health Promotion

A M Woodward, BSc FIInfSc
Health Promotion Authority for Wales, 8th Floor
Brunel House, 2 Fitzalan Road, Cardiff CF2 1EB, Wales, UK.

J B Hepworth, MA FLA MIInfSc
G A Vidgen, BLib
Department of Library and Information Studies,
University of Wales Aberystwyth, Llanbadarn Fawr,
Aberystwyth, Dyfed SY23 3AS, Wales, UK.

ABSTRACT

The paper describes a pilot project for the delivery of an integrated set of information services on-line to health promotion workers in Wales. The services include information on resources, organisations and lifestyle data which can all be searched and retrieved using the same software and techniques.

INTRODUCTION

Changes in our perceptions of health and the ways in which the general health of the population can be improved are leading to changes in the way that health care is being managed. In particular, there is an increasing emphasis on health promotion as a means of obtaining value for money in health care. In the United Kingdom, specific requirements to undertake health promotion are prominent in the recent changes in the way that contracts for general practice are operated. The Health Promotion Authority for Wales (HPAW) has had significant successes with its own health education campaigns such as HeartBeat Wales in recent years.

The HPAW, and its predecessor, Heartbeat Wales, has, over the past six years, been collecting data on life styles and some measures of underlying health in Wales in the general community, in young people and in the workplace, in order to guide its own activities and those of others in creating healthier lifestyles in the population of Wales. This information has also been used to evaluate the success of its own policies, activities and campaigns. As a result the HPAW has a large store of information which would be valuable for the work of health promotion and health education workers. The major results and conclusions of these surveys have been presented in reports on a district by district basis in Wales in for example a series of reports entitled "The

Pulse of .....", but the limitations of the printed report means that only a fraction of the total data collected can be presented in this way.

It has been recognised by the HPAW for some time that health promotion workers and other associated workers such as voluntary organisations, public health consultants etc would have need to gain easy access to the professional literature on health promotion. Other health workers need to be able to locate information on voluntary bodies and other organisations active in health promotion. This has resulted in the development of a library at HPAW and the provision of an enquiry answering service.

However, these services are expensive to operate and it was felt that electronic services could be developed to provide an integrated information service on a self-service basis to provide the basic information to potential enquirers and to free up staff time to answer more complex enquiries. In particular it was our contention that there are many professional people such as service planners who have a wide need for simply presented statistics which are up to date and who do not have the resources to commit for the sophisticated analysis of the data that are currently available.

It was therefore decided to see whether an integrated set of information services could be provided including bibliographic references, information on organisations and retrievable statistics on lifestyles and underlying health which would be simple to use and provide useful information to potential clients. Developments in computing and telecommunications meant that electronic access was becoming easier and cheaper for many different kinds of organisation within the health service and associated sectors. A major factor in Wales has been the development of the NHS All-Wales X.25 network which will provide a universal telecommunications facility for all NHS sites in Wales and therefore gives access to good telecommunications to a wide range health locations in the Principality.

THE HealthPROMPT PILOT EVALUATION PROJECT

The HPAW requested the Department of Library and Information Studies (DILS) at the University of Wales, Aberystwyth to assist in the development of information services for health promotion workers. The two bodies consequently established a joint project under the banner title HealthPROMPT to assess the information needs of health promotion workers in Wales and to evaluate the mechanism of providing information over electronic links (1). This received support from the British Library in funding the research component at Aberystwyth and from the Welsh Office in providing the technical infrastructure at the HPAW.

Two District Health Promotion Units in Wales were invited to become pilot sites. During the first phase of the project, the DILS research team carried out assessments of the information needs of these two sites using Soft Systems Methodology (SSM) (2,3). The second phase saw the development of pilot databases by HPAW for subsequent evaluation by the pilot sites and the DILS team.

Three pilot databases were established:

HPAWMAIN, a database of resources based around the library catalogue of the HPAW with additional information on materials produced by HPAW and some on-going projects;

HPAWVOL, a database of voluntary organisations and self help groups in health care, based in large measure on the "Help for Health" database developed by Wessex RHA with the addition of some information on Wales based organisations.

HPAWSTAT, a database based on HPAW's own statistical information.

The HPAWMAIN and HPAWVOL databases are conventional bibliographic databases constructed using one record per item and with a number of searchable fields. The HPAWSTAT database was designed in the same way but the core of each record is a pre-processed table of statistics prefixed by a searchable title field and suffixed with other useful searchable fields.

Archive datasets of the main surveys conducted by the HPAW, and previously by HeartBeat Wales, were used to create standard tables. The surveys used were the 1985 Heartbeat Wales Community Survey, the 1988 Interim Community Survey and the Youth Surveys carried out in 1986, 1988 and 1990. Topics were selected as those most central to health promotion issues and giving consistent results. Each topic is presented by standard breakdowns and for districts or counties within Wales. Each table is presented as a set of simple percentages (see fig. 1) together with certain other information which is indexed and used for retrieval i.e. a unique reference number, descriptive title, age range covered, source of the data and whether weighting had been used. A further field shows how to retrieve descriptive records outlining the design and sample size of the survey in question so that actual numbers can be reconstructed from the percentage tables. The techniques used have been described elsewhere (4).

All three databases are made available using the STRIX text retrieval package. STRIX offers high functionality as a text retrieval system and is flexible in its input requirements. STRIX can also be tuned in a number of ways to optimize searching for different needs and to facilitate searching by inexperienced users.

```
HPAW Search Listing      HPAWSTAT

Set     1    Record No. 1545                      1 of 1

TTL YOUTH 1988 - TASTED ALCOHOL BY FORM IN POWYS
TAB

    ┌─────────────┬────────────────────────────────┐
    │ POWYS       │         Tasted Alcohol         │
    │ YPY0008     ├──────────┬──────────┬──────────┤
    │             │   Yes    │   No     │ Not Sure │
    ├─────────────┼──────────┼──────────┼──────────┤
    │ 1st         │  86.9%   │   9.2%   │   3.8%   │
    │ 3rd         │  89.8%   │   7.9%   │   2.4%   │
    │ 5th         │  99.1%   │    .9%   │          │
    └─────────────┴──────────┴──────────┴──────────┘

SAM Search "SAMPLE" or "DESIGN"
        and "SOU=YUTH88" for details
        of conduct of the survey
AGE 11-16
SOU YUTH88 - HPAW YOUTH SURVEY
DAT 1988 SPRING
WEI NO
SUB ALCOHOL
BKD FORM
GEO POWYS
REF YPO0008
```

EVALUATION AND CONCLUSIONS

At the time of writing, the evaluation studies have only just been completed and therefore the detailed examination of the way in which these information services have been used and the further development of the services has only just started. However, the range of data in the statistics database coupled with the ease with which it may be identified, displayed, downloaded and/or printed out locally has raised a lot of interest in the pilot. As a result, in the new year the pilot system will be extended to two further sites in Wales and to all nine District Health Promotion Units in Wales during 1991 as well as other potential users.

The novel way in which the statistical information is processed, retrieved and presented has led to the examination of other sources of data and other ways in which the system can be used for statistical information. Other ways of presenting the data will also be tested for feasibility, including simple bar charts and graphs using the extended ASCII character set so that the displays can be sent over public networks without noticeable time delays.

The advantages of this system are that up-to-date information is always available to users, especially data from current surveys as the information is released. A range of tables, charts and graphs in different presentations can also be made available on demand and individual presentations can be quickly and easily located and the resultant data downloaded for incorporation into documents or other local systems etc.

The advantages over paper based systems are clear; for the user, permanent availability, up-to-date data, low cost; and to the HPAW, savings in staff time, postage, and long print runs etc. In time it is anticipated that the service would be a candidate for a CD-ROM product though there would be delays in providing such a compendium of current statistics. The potential market for such a product may not be sufficient to justify the investment in CD-ROM, either at the producer end or the user end, but with a constantly changing market, this is an option that needs to be borne in mind.

REFERENCES

1. Vidgen, G.A. et al "How IT is improving access to health promotion information" Paper submitted to HealthCare Computing, Harrogate 1991

2. Vidgen, G.A.; Hepworth, J.B. "Yesterday's philosophy" British Journal of Healthcare Computing v 5 (Sep) pp. 19-30, 1990

3. Hepworth, J.B.; Woodward, A.M.; Vidgen, G.A. "Improving access to health promotion information" In: Moore, R.O et al, eds Proceedings Medical Informatics Europe 1990, Glasgow. Berlin: Springer-Verlag pp. 535-8, 1990

4. Woodward, A.M.; Nugent, Z.; Hepworth, J.B. "Statistics for Health Promotion - Making more data more available" Paper submitted to Journal of Information Science.

The authors would also like to acknowledge the assistance of Ms E M Griffin, Research Assistant, Department of Library and Information Studies, University of Wales Aberystwyth for her work in the evaluation and to Dr Z Nugent, formerly Statistician, HPAW for her work in devising the routines to process the statistical information to present in the retrieval database.

AN ELECTRONIC PATIENT INFORMATION SYSTEM IN MENTAL HEALTH -
An Integrated Solution for Better Care and Management

Michael J. Rigby

Lecturer in Health Planning and Management, University of Keele,

Keele, Staffordshire, ST5 5SP, United Kingdom

Abstract

This paper describes a project undertaken by Plymouth Health Authority with support from the author. The special needs and requirements of mental health services have been studied, and a networked integrated patient-based information system has been designed and is now being implemented. It is intended to ensure quality of service, optimum use of resources, and management control of a dispersed service.

Background

Mental health services form special problems in their organisation and delivery. Though they have been a priority in the United Kingdom for many years (1), they have nevertheless failed to attract the degree of management attention offered to acute hospital services, and to a lesser degree to community services. Yet mental health services have many complexities not common in other forms of health care - in particular they should have a number of access points to accommodate preferences or sensitivities of clients; they must have a variety of professions and agencies involved; they must be localised as far as possible; and they must span hospital and community services. Many of the service components may operate on a semi-autonomous basis, or be contractually linked independent facilities. Above all, they must provide personalised care plans for the clients involved. Particular emphasis has been placed in the United Kingdom, as elsewhere in Europe, on modernising services by moving away from centralised institutions, in favour of supporting individuals wherever appropriate in their own homes or elsewhere in the community (2) (3). At the same time, this Care in the Community initiative has been recognised as having its own special problems, not least in matching clients with appropriate services and ensuring continued service delivery (4). Above all, it is recognised that mental health service clients are particularly vulnerable to failures of service and to their own failure to comply with agreed service plans. By the nature of mental health problems they may lack drive or motivation, yet at the same time resist an over-dominant form of professional supervision.

Opportunities for Innovation

General pressures for service development, and the specific Care in the Community initiative, have encouraged services to become more progressive. However, these pressures have not themselves stimulated information initiatives. More recently, though, the Department of Health has launched the Resource Management Initiative (5). The purpose of this has been to make better use of health service resources, in terms of efficiency and effectiveness, but also in terms of quality of outcome. The Resource Management Initiative has laid emphasis on specific critical success factors, the most important of which are a devolved management structure, devolved budgets matched by devolved service objectives, and the necessary information resources to enable effective management against objectives to be accomplished successfully.

The latest emphasis has been on Medical Audit and Clinical Audit (which latter is multi-disciplinary). In the latest NHS reforms following the White Paper "Working for Patients" (6), there is a specific requirement that all service providers shall operate a form of audit.

The Plymouth Health Authority Initiative

Having already implemented the main components of a progressive mental health service, Plymouth Health Authority realised that its principal weakness lay in the lack of any monitoring arrangements or effective information system. Within Plymouth there are a range of important service components in different locations within the city - these including day hospitals, a walk-in Psychiatric Advisory Service, consultant psychiatrist out-patient sessions in a variety of locations, and in-patient wards in small hospitals. The main acute in-patient psychiatric beds, together with the principal component of the rehabilitation service and a range of long stay beds, are currently located in a rapidly reducing base psychiatric hospital in a rural setting 15 miles from the city centre.

The Authority was concerned that patients might fall between gaps within services, or for other reasons fail to have their care plans delivered or complied with; that different components of the service might treat the same person in different ways, particularly with regard to emergency or respite care; that there was insufficient evaluation of medium-term and long-term outcomes of alternative patterns of care; that there was insufficient study of referral patterns and thresholds; and that management information was extremely scarce. It decided that the appropriate way forward was a real-time patient-based information system which would assist all health professionals in managing treatment.

Instigating the Initiative

The Authority studied its requirements carefully. It also obtained designation as a community services pilot site under the Resource Management Initiative, thereby attracting a small sum of Government money. It was the first authority to indicate that it would use this initiative to address mental health services (7). In 1988 it issued an invitation to tender for the supply of a computerised patient information system, with outline user requirements. It recognised that the Authority itself did not have the full competence to design such a system, though the experience of its health professionals meant that it could play a positive lead in such design. The author became involved at this stage, initially to assist in appraisal of the tenders, and then to advise in the ongoing development. The tender was awarded to Protechnic Computers Limited of Cambridge, who had previous experience of developing a psychiatric inpatient system.

Design Approach

It was a fundamental objective from the beginning that the system should be patient-based, networked, and real time. It was also intended that the data recorded, as processed and presented by the information system, would support and improve the care delivery processes. Data are recorded and displayed in user-friendly screens, with pop-down option lists being available for every coded item. Patient identity is displayed at the top of each screen, and relevant history at the foot of each screen, so that decisions and recording are in an informed setting. However, the data can also be accessed and analysed on a staff basis, to show the workload, responsibilities, and activity of any staff member.

Design Objectives and Process

It was recognised that introduction of a shared information system, with a necessary degree of standardisation of terminology, would itself be challenging for the organisation and for operational staff. A structure was therefore established with three components - a managerial Steering Group to give overall direction to the design process; a Core Group representative of clinical areas and professions; and access to Care Teams to discuss new issues.

Core System Components

This section gives a brief summary of the key components of the Information System for Psychiatric Services, as currently being implemented in Plymouth:

Registration: The patient's name and address, aliases, date of birth, next of kin, most interested relative or friend, informal carer, and general medical practitioner are recorded. As appropriate a Case Manager is appointed and logged.

Referral: The source and location of the referral or self referral are logged, together with the staff member initially dealing with the referral and the action taken.

Presenting Problem: Traditionally, health information systems record clinical conditions, normally diagnosis according to ICD 9 and operations according to a classification such as OPCS 4. These are inappropriate for mental health. The system therefore collects information as it becomes available to three levels:-

> Presenting Problem - as seen by the client or referrer (eg Depression) together with any essential Underlying Factors (eg Bereavement)

> Need - as perceived following professional assessment

> Diagnosis - by ICD if this is relevant, or required for national statistics

Care Plans: The core of the system, and the part involving most original thinking in systems terms. They comprise the following levels:-
> Aim
> Needs
> Goals
> Interventions

Aim is the long term target for the patient, but may not be established until part way into the therapeutic programme. It might indicate, for instance, that a patient ought to be rehabilitated to a sheltered apartment. **Needs** are recorded following multi-disciplinary assessment, and record the purposes of treatment, such as Improved Self Care Skills, or Establish Self Confidence. Each of these is referred to a specific service or profession, such as Rehabilitation or Psychology. When each service accesses the patient's record it will see displayed the reason for the referral, and it will be able to set **Goals**. These are steps along a care plan which will normally be achieved in approximately 4-6 weeks. Review dates are set for each goal, and the system will signal if these reviews are not undertaken. At the review the success in completely, partially, or not at all achieving the goal is recorded. Therapy towards goals is achieved by **Interventions**. Initially at least these will not normally be recorded within the system, through a recording facility has been designed to enable some key interventions to be recorded and monitored, such as Day Hospital attendance or Depot Injection.

Scheduling, Monitoring and Coordinating

With the recording of this key information, the system can undertake some important tasks. For activities such as outpatient appointments, Day Hospital attendances, or Community Psychiatric Nurse visiting, it can arrange schedules and issue appointments. It can prompt when these are not achieved. Thus for instance failure to review a case, or to administer a depot injection, can be sent as an alert to the case manager. Finally, and of great importance, whenever a person presents to any branch of the service on a planned or unplanned basis, it will be possible immediately to see not only if that person has had previous contact with the mental health services, but also any current treatment plan.

Hardware Environment

The information system has been designed to operate on the Health Authority's existing DEC VAX cluster, and DEC Ethernet district network. Remote sites are assessed by a case communications network; there are thus no site restrictions. (The supplier anticipates providing the system to other localities in Unix and other environments to suit any common hardware platform). The initial installation has 40 VDU terminals on seven sites, with a printer close to each terminal. Even in the first six months, the configuration has been adjusted to match changes in service provision.

The next technical development being sought is a hand-held version for community-based staff. A small user group is currently defining the exact requirements, but it is envisaged that a portable PC will hold a user defined subset of the patient database and a subset of the full functionality, with regular dial-up cross-updating.

Ethics and Security

In such a sensitive service as mental health, great attention has to be paid to ethics and security. The system is tightly controlled by passwords, and each authorised operator has personalised read or write access to individual categories of patients, and fields within patient records. The system has been designed to comply with the British Data Protection Act 1984.

Implementation Process

Implementation of such a comprehensive system in a new business area has not been without its tensions, even though a training strategy was drawn up well in advance, and key trainers identified for each principal service component. Four issues arose. First, the number of staff who needed training, to cover all professions and service activities. Second, the need to produce training materials, and handouts related to training and operational processes. Third, and arising from this, the need to ensure clear and standardised operational policies across the service to support the much more integrated (yet devolved) service pattern. Fourth, and by far the most significant, the common recording and appropriate sharing of information has challenged pre-existing departmental practices. Assessments, processes, and terminology are exposed to scrutiny and stress when shared across the service. Discussion, development, and corporate ownership have been shown to be vital to success, but also have intrinsic benefits of professional education and team building. Without a sensitive implementation process the information system would be threatening, and liable to misinterpretation.

Audit and Outcome

The health professionals of Plymouth Health Authority Mental Health Service have had an enlightened attitude to Resource Management throughout this project. They believe service effectiveness should be monitored in the interests of patients, community, and staff. However, unlike some aspects of acute services such as surgery, it is impossible at present to define anticipated standard outcomes. Similarly, in terms of evaluating resource consumption, standardisation of case mix fails to fit into Diagnostic Related Group categories. It is believed that this system will give a unique comprehensive research base to enable long term psychiatric epidemiological studies to be undertaken. However, it has been designed round two initial concepts. First, that the best measure of outcome is success against the objectives which therapeutic staff share with patients, namely care plan Aims and Goals. Second, by recording patient-based data together with presenting problem and underlying factors, it will be possible to evaluate alternative therapeutic approaches. At the same time, the operational database will form an ideal and rare platform for meaningful Clinical Audit, in that it will not only record patient condition and all significant components within the patient's history, but it will also relate these to both short-term and long-term outcome.

Conclusion

The information system now being implemented in to Plymouth forms a major step forward in delivery and management of mental health services. It brings to these services the principles have already been applied in the United Kingdom to acute and community services, yet the need in mental health services is much greater. It also integrates hospital and community services. Implementation will have its own immediate benefits, but at the same time will form a starting point for evaluation of resource utilisation and service outcomes, thereby generating a second phase of service improvement.

References

(1)   Secretary of State for Health: Better Services for the Mentally Ill; Cmnd 6233, HMSO London 1975
(2)   Department of Health and Social Security: Health Circular (83)6: Care in the Community and Joint Finance; Department of Health, London, 1983
(3)   Mangan SP (ed): Mental Health Care in the European Community; Croom Helm 1985
(4)   House of Commons Social Service Committee: Community Care with Special Reference to Adult Mentally Ill and Mentally Handicapped People; HMSO London 1985
(5)   Department of Health and Social Security: Health Notice (86) 34; Department of Health, London 1986
(6)   Secretary of State for Health: Working for Patients; Cmnd 555, HMSO London 1989
(7)   Resource Management Unit: Resource Management in the Community Health Services Department of Health, London 1991

COMPUTERS IN PRIMARY HEALTH CARE
The Bhorugram Experience - INDIA.

A.K.Singh[1,2,3], Khalid Moidu[1,2], B.S.Rathore[3], Erik Trell[2], Ove Wigertz[1].

[1] Dept.of Medical Informatics, Faculty of Health Sciences, Linköping University, S - 581 83, SWEDEN.
[2] Dept. of General Practice, Faculty of Health Sciences, Linköping University, S - 581 83, SWEDEN.
[3] Bhorugram Rural Dispensary, P.O. Bhorugram, District Churu, Rajasthan, INDIA

ABSTRACT

The primary health care concept holds the key to make "Health for All by the year 2000 AD" a reality and not remain just a slogan. If an effective health care service is to be provided to the larger population mass living in the rural areas of the developing countries. Then the primary health care delivery must be strengthened. The information infrastructure strengthened through computer implementation would support the care providers, as for example in monitoring the target population to follow-up the drop-outs from the immunisation programme. The administrators would receive accurate reports and have a factual base to study the outcomes of the interventions. In the preparatory phase to implement a computer-based system to support the Mother and Child Health Programme, a base line study was started, and a cohort group for immunisation followed. A dropout rate of 72% was seen in the immunisation programme and not a single pregnant lady had till then received any antenatal care. A computer-based system will make the programme delivery effective through follow-up and monitoring, thus introduce quality assurance in the care.

1. INTRODUCTION.

To attain the global goal of "HEALTH FOR ALL BY THE YEAR 2000 AD" the delivery of health care by the Primary Health Care (PHC) concept has been accepted (1). The World Health Organisation (WHO) global review report of 1987 emphasizes that "a major constraint reported by practically all countries is inadequate information support for the managerial process" (2). Research to strengthen the information infrastructure in primary health care delivery with computer technology is needed, including for developing countries (3). The objective of such research must be closely linked to the health care delivery process, as Bertrand states "the solutions to the basic public health problems are known, it is the socially acceptable and economically viable delivering capability that requires research" (4).

A recent study was conducted by the Indian Council of Medical Research to assess the quality of family welfare services [that includes Family Planning and the Mother and Child Health (MCH) programmes]. The report states the services are in most instances poor. It recommends a continuous monitoring and evaluation system that provides feedback to the health care professionals involved in primary health care (5). Computers enhance the value of information systems and their support at the primary health centre level is advocated (6)

In India, like other Developing countries, 70-80% of the population lives in rural areas. The MCH project is being conducted at a number of sites, some in rural India. The aim is to increase the potential for the care providers to follow-up and monitor the target population of the MCH programme with the use of a computer-based information system. The information system will assist the PHC centre staff in their day to day work. Generate on demand administrative reports or the epidemiological profile of the population registered. It has been reported that approximately 20 to 40 % of the working time of the PHC staff is used in collating and compiling to prepare the reports and returns (7).

In this paper the experiences gained during the early preparations for computer implementation are described.

2. MATERIALS AND METHODS

A software has been developed at the Department of Medical Informatics, Linköping University to support the Mother and Child Health System (MCHS). It was developed under a contractual service agreement from the Programme of Quality in Care and Technology, World Health Organisation (European Region) based at Copenhagen. The software is based on a preliminary *essential data set*, which was derived from existing Peri-natal forms, fulfilling the following criteria: easy to collect, that provides information related to health status, assists in assessment of risk and prediction of outcomes.

The data input format was based on an analysis of forms filled in by care providers, to make the data entry design acceptable to the care providers. To ensure quality in data collected, measures to validate the data have been incorporated in the software. A trivalent logic is used to distinguish between *No & Not Known*, a requirement for statistical analysis. In preparation to implement the software, a base line study was undertaken at this rural site.

SITE

The dispensary is in Bhorugram, a village with a population of 1200, lies in the Thar Desert of Rajasthan, India. It is the health care delivery facility of Bhorugram Charitable Trust (BCT), an organisation working at the grass roots (village) level to improve the quality in life of the people in the community. The activities of the trust are varied and cover approximately 101 villages in the area. The Bhorugram Charitable Trust runs Non-formal education centres in each of the 101 villages in the area..

A primary health centre of the State health services operates in the area, but due to the poor transportation facilities, their services are restricted. The Rajasthan state health services regularly conduct immunization camps, eye camps, and family planning camps in collaboration with the BCT dispensary, in the BCT dispensary catchment area

MANPOWER RESOURCES AND TARGET POPULATION

At the BCT dispensary there are two physicians who provide medical cover. The physicians and the pharmacist (compounder) were identified as the potential system end-users. The Non-formal education teachers are another manpower resource. Typically a teacher is a female, most often from the village where she works. They are all educated till the formal high school level. The dispensary serves the people from the village and surrounding villages, a population of approximately 150,000.

METHOD

The approach plan, was to start with a baseline survey of the community with the assistance of the non-formal education teachers. The data collection forms designed at Linköping have been translated, adopted and printed in the local language by BCT. On completion of the baseline survey the target population will be identified and the baseline data of the community to available. To assist monitoring and measure the programme outcome. Then the MCHS software will be used to enter data collected on visits for perinatal care, family planning and Immunisation, at the Bhorugram rural dispensary by the physicians, or at the community level through the peripheral health worker and the non-formal education teachers. The data entry is to be performed by the physicians or the compounder (pharmacist). The outputs for follow-up of antenatal cases who missed appointments and dropouts from the immunization programme, will be given to the peripheral health workers (Multi-purpose Workers and the Auxiliary Nurse Midwifes). The non-formal education teacher will also be used as a channel to contact these persons and to advise them to attend the antenatal or the immunization clinic. The project will be carried out in a phased manner and may be summarized as:

Phase I - Baseline survey with the assistance of the non-formal education
programme teachers based at the dispersed villages.
Phase II - Implementation of computer for monitoring of the antenatal cases among
the target population and track dropouts from the Immunization programme.
Phase III- Evaluation of the impact of the system after the it has been in use for at
least 24 months.

3. PRELIMINARY RESULTS

Some early observations from the project are reported here, as the project was only initiated in September, 1990. The attitude of potential end-users was first assessed. Despite no prior experience or even having seen a computer, their enthusiasm to use the computer as a "tool" was high. The physicians were more positive than the compounder (pharmacist).

The baseline survey provided interesting insights about the health status of the community, and it will be the record of the initial state of problems in the community. An essential element to study the impact and outcome of an intervention. Some findings are summarised in Table 1.

Table 1. Findings of social factors and utilization of family welfare services

The Number of Villages covered		20
Literacy rate	Total	24%
	Males	37%
	Females	11%
Number of women Interviewed		320
Mean age of women at marriage		16 years
Number of women pregnant at the time of survey		92
Number of women who are pregnant and attend an antenatal clinic		0
The last delivery of the respondent was at	Home	110
	PHC centre	0
	Hospital	5
The last delivery was conducted by	Traditional Birth Attendant	110
	Nurse (with Midwifery training)	5
Number of women who currently use any Family Planning method		0

During the period of baseline survey we were able to monitor the immunization programme, which was conducted by the State Health Services in collaboration with the BCT Dispensary. The preliminary data exemplifies the problem of drop-outs from the immunization programmes (see Table 2). A single cohort group of infants who received the 1st three doses of Oral Polio vaccine (OPV) and the Diphtheria, Pertusis and Tetanus (DPT) vaccine were followed during the period from September 1990 to November 1990 in 6 villages of the same area.

Table 2 Immunization Drop Outs

	IMMUNISED	DROPOUTS
1st Dose DPT and OPV	108	†
2nd Dose - a month after the 1st Dose DPT and OPV	57	51 (47% of those who took 1st dose)
3rd Dose- 2 months after the 1st dose DPT and OPV	30	27 (further 47% of those who took) (2nd Dose)
TOTAL	30 (28%)	78 (72%)

†Total number of the target children population in the villages at the time was not known

4. DISCUSSION

The MCH programme is a global programme implemented in almost all the countries in the world with a high priority. Despite the importance given and the expenditures being incurred, the continuing high incidence of maternal mortality makes it a major public health programme. A statistical estimate of the magnitude of the problem puts a figure of 350 deaths per 100,000 live births are due to complications related to the pregnancy status (8). The World Health Organisation estimates that approximately 500,000 women die each year from pregnancy-related causes, more than 98 % of these deaths occur in the developing countries (9). In developing countries hospitals, maternal mortality is among the ten most common causes of death, the decline if any is not perceptible as the figures are still very high. Conversely the infant mortality rate in these very same countries has shown a marked decline (10). Perhaps the success relates directly to the impact of the immunisation programme.

Many of these maternal deaths are preventable even in the developing countries, through antenatal screening, safe obstetrical practices and post-natal care (11). We have thus selected this programme for developing a software tool to assist the care providers. In the MCH project we provide a software system to support the information management related to the activities to protect the vulnerable group of the mother and the child. Improved information management will help reduce the drop-outs from the immunisation programme. In antenatal care through follow-up and close monitoring of the high risk reduce unfavourable outcomes.

The baseline survey has revealed that the extension of the health services in the area are restricted to the villages around the PHC centre. It has provided us insights into the existing state and will help to monitor the change over time. Bamisaiye has reported the use of similar baseline survey to collect data (12). We found that the majority of this population is illiterate, they lack access to the health education programs and the awareness to utilize the available facilities for preventive action is just not there. Participation by this major portion of the community in the health care is negligible. Thus, the entire responsibility of providing health care falls on the primary care providers. They must monitor the norms of care and follow-up the high risk among the target population in the community. The baseline survey therefore also serves the purpose of health education, since at the time of the interviews the women are informed about the availability of health care services for the pregnant women at the BCT dispensary and it its potential value.

5. CONCLUSION

The role of timely and accurate information is well recognised and documented, however, at present in PHC centres and especially in developing countries it is not available. Provision of effective quality in care for the population under a PHC centre cannot be achieved without an effective information system to support the activities at these centres. A significant reduction of mortality and morbidity can be achieved, only if timely information is made available for action to the PHC centre staff or even directly to the community.

6. ACKNOWLEDGEMENTS

The authors wish to express their gratitude for the collaboration, support and assistance provided by Dr Ashok Agarwal, Chairman and other members of the Bhoruka Charitable Trust. The support and the constructive discussions in the development of the MCHS software from the staff of the Programme for Quality in Care and Technology, World Health Organisation, European Regional Office, Copenhagen, is also acknowledged.

7. REFERENCES
1. World Health Organization, Geneva. ALMA - ATA (1978). Primary Health Care. Health For All Series No 1. WHO, Geneva.
2. World Health Organization. (1987) Assessment of Achievement In: Evaluation of the strategy for health for all by the year 2000. Seventh report on the World Health situation. Global Review. WHO, Geneva. 1, 109-116.
3. Moidu K, Trell, E, Wigertz O. (1990). Primary Health Care: Medical Informatics to Strengthen the Delivery. Submitted to the *Scandinavian Journal of Primary Health Care*.
4. Bertrand, W.E. (1987). Use of microcomputers in health and social service applications in developing nations. *CRC Critical Reviews in Medical Informatics*. 1; 3: 229-240
5. Indian Council of Medical Research. (1989) Evaluation of quality of maternal and Child health and Family planning services at primary health centres. New Delhi, Indian Council of Medical Research.
6. Moidu K, Wigertz O. (1989). Computer-based informations systems in Primary Health Care — Why ?. *Journal of Medical Systems*. 13; 2: 59-65.
7. Helfenbein, S. Sawyer, H.Sayer,P.Wijesinghe.(1987). Improving management effectiveness and efficiency. In Eds. Favin, M.Dunn, C.Rajasingham,D.- Technologies for Management Information Systems in Primary Health Care. World Federation of Public Health Association, Washington D.C. - 52-57.
8. Högberg, U. (1985) Maternal Mortality in Sweden, Doctoral Dissertation 156, University of Umeå.
9. World Health Organization. (1987). Maternal mortality: the dimension of the problem. Presented at the Safe Motherhood Conference; February 11,1987; Nairobi, Kenya.
10. Högberg, U, Frostesson, L, Sterky G, Talle A. (1987). Maternal Health Care and Developing Countries. Karolinska Institutet, Stockholm.
11. Petros-Barzavian A. (1984) World Priorities and Targets in Maternal and child health for the year 2000. *Int. J. Gynaecol. Obstet.* 22: 439 - 448.
12. Bamisaiye A, .Johnson T.O. (1988) Planning PHC for a community: a baseline survey provides essential data. *Tropical Doctor*, 18,36-37

COMPUTERS AND WORKING CONDITIONS IN NURSING: EXPERIENCES FROM GERMAN HOSPITALS

J. John

GSF-Institut für Medizinische Informatik und Systemforschung (MEDIS)

Ingolstädter Landstraße 1, D-8042 Neuherberg, F.R.G.

Abstract

The results of a recent survey on hospital data processing in Germany reveal a rapid increase of computer applications in hospital care. The use of computers in medicine is expected to produce not only considerable effects on quality of health care, but likewise drastic changes in the working conditions of the health care professions. Additional evidence for this guess is presented coming from a recent study dealing with real and virtual impacts of computer applications in nursing. To get some detailed insight into these effects, about 100 hospital staff members confronted or experienced with the new technologies have been interviewed in six hospitals. The results demonstrate that introduction and use of computers require appropriate implementation and project management strategies, effective further education and training, and a mutual adaption of the computer system and its organizational environment in order to improve the "quality of working life". Substantial research and development is necessary to meet these requirements.

1.   State and future development of hospital data processing in Germany

The use of computers is being more and more generally adopted in all fields of economy and society. The hospital sector has been seized by this diffusion process as well, but until very recently with a clear focus on single particular tasks of the hospitals. But now there is a development towards a much broader spectrum of computer applications in hospitals which is documented by the results of a new hospital survey carried out in 1989 [1] and gathering, among other subjects, information on data processing in 369 German hospitals. Hospital administrators were asked about the current and the future use of computers by supported hospital functions and occupational groups. The data on future use reflect concrete plans and projects in the field of data processing, referring, as a rule, to a time horizon of 1 to 3 years and thus looking ahead till about 1992.

Looking at the activities of nurses in the hospital wards the survey results show that at present, computer support of nurses' activities is the exception. Only in 7% of the hospitals computers are used by this occupational group, especially for administrative tasks; as a tool of clinical nursing practice, the computer plays no role so far. According to the hospitals' plannings, this situation will change soon: All things considered, in the near future nurses will use computers already in every fifth hospital (see Table 1).

Table 1. Current and future use of computers at the hospital ward by supported activities of nurses (in % of hospitals; n = 369)

Activities	Current use (1989)	Future use (1992)
Nurses' activities among them:	7.0	19.0
- nursing care administration	3.5	11.4
- nursing care planning	0.3	6.2
- nursing care documentation	1.1	9.0
- communication with ancillary units	1.4	10.1
- staff scheduling	1.6	12.5

2. Computers and working conditions in nursing

2.1 Study purpose and design

As use of computers in nursing is not widespread until now in Germany, impact research on computers and working conditions in nursing is still in its infancy, too. As a first step in this area, actual and possible impacts of new information and communication techniques on the working conditions of hospital nursing staff were explored by a series of oral interviews with hospital staff: In six selected hospitals, differing by size, level of care provided, by hardware systems and computer applications, and being in different phases of implementation and use of the systems, about 100 persons from different units and in different positions were interviewed individually or in groups. The computer applications used by nurses in these hospitals included patient administration systems, order entry systems with and without results reporting, order entry and patient scheduling systems, and staff scheduling systems, all being in routine use, furthermore nursing care planning and patient classification systems in pilot testings. Additionally, there was a workshop held with floor nurses about their experiences with computers. All interviews and the workshop were conducted between October 1989 and February 1990.

2.2 Study results

The interviewed persons' experiences made with computer systems are summarized among three labels: (1) system implementation and project management; (2) education and training; (3) work and working conditions. A more detailed presentation can be found in [2]. The short summaries of experiences are complemented by a number of questions and problems for which satisfactory and suitable solutions could not be found till now.

2.2.1 System implementation and project management

Experience

Even now, computer systems are sometimes seen by health care professionals as `general problem solvers' and even now they are sometimes presented by the vendors as a panacea for all the financial, organizational and management problems of the hospitals. Until now only a minority of hospital administrators, physicians, and nurses are able to identify the ways in which computer technology can be used. This lack of competence results in giving computer specialists full authority in decisions about computer systems, and in poor communication between users and those persons who assume responsibility for the design and the initial implementation of the computer system.

Generally, hospitals are lacking know-how in the process of innovation management: Nowhere timely efforts were made to approach the widespread resistance to the use of computers by common managerial measures of information, communication, and education; planning techniques were only applied to the technical aspects of system installation, not to the use of the systems; no hospital had carried out a structured ex ante evaluation, which is a very useful activity for intra-institutional evaluation [3]; efforts towards ex post evaluation were made only if serious problems of acceptance occurred and compelled management action.

User participation in the selection and design of systems, and in the appropriate reshaping of work organization was, with one exception, not practised. Of course, there was involvement of the users if the time of crisis management had come.

Introduction of information systems affects many different units and groups of individuals in various ways. Thus project management has to handle with conflicting interests of professional groups and departments. The profession-oriented and multiple-tracked hospital organization and the high degree of departmental autonomy makes it difficult to identify and to implement stable solutions for those conflicts.

Open questions

This last point leads directly to the first of the following two questions to which until now satisfactory answers cannot be given:

- How to bring nurses, physicians, and hospital administrators in a more balanced position and how, at same time, to make the hospital more capable of planning and managing technical and organizational innovation?
- How to introduce and insure staff participation in those innovational processes? This includes the questions for appropriate organizational models as well as for the necessary qualification measures to make all parties participating in this process competent and able for fruitful cooperation.

2.2.2 Education and training

Experience

In all hospitals training was limited to transmit the skills required to operate the system. As a rule, this training was assessed by the users as insufficient. Poor training programs and measures have caused serious conflicts and substantial loss of system acceptance in some hospitals. The organizational concept of training which is usually applied, is the concept of multiplicators. Some nurses are trained by the vendors during courses of one or several hours duration and they are charged to train their colleagues at the wards. Apparently this concept does not work very well; frequently the knowledge required for system use is transferred only in part; thus, operating the system makes often problems for long time and is very time-consuming. To some extent this is also the effect of lacking teaching skills of vendor's training staff as well as of the multiplicators. From the viewpoint of the nurses these problems can be solved by creating a new job for all the data inputting, storing, and retrieval activities, and this has actually been done in two hospitals. One problem of this solution is that these new jobs are of rather doubtful "quality of working life".

Open questions

There are a lot of open questions in this area requiring further analysis the most important perhaps being the following four:

- What are exactly the additional skills required for participation in systems development and in shaping of technological change?
- What are the appropriate educational strategies and techniques taking into account the specific working conditions in the hospitals, as for example shift work, unpredictable periods of extreme work load, and a high rate of staff fluctuation?
- How can the trainers in the enterprises and especially in the hospitals be made more competent for teaching activities?
- Is computerizing nursing administration and practice not the case for specialization within the nursing profession instead of knowledge and job expansion for all?

2.2.3 Work and working conditions

Experience

In the six hospitals visited, routine use of computer systems in nursing so far was restricted to the processing of supportive and administrative data; professional information in the narrower sense was not processed by the computers. Therefore, the most relevant benefit to be expected from these systems is time-saving through reduction of clerical work, telephone calls, and handwritten documentation or information transfer. Patient administration systems are generally assessed by the nurses as actually time-saving. This did not hold in all hospitals for order entry systems. But if both systems were running well, nurses reported substantial time savings. Surprisingly, there was no clear picture of how the time saved is used. There are very different observations, the most frequent perhaps being that all things are running more calmly. The feeling that this type of rationalization has led primarily to devote more time to the direct contact with the patient was not widespread.

Experiences with order entry system are mixed. One problem is that the redesign of the work process may reallocate portions of tasks to the disadvantage of the nurses. There was, e.g., the tendency to shift reporting functions for administrative and management purposes from the ancillary units to the wards. In general, order entry systems require more discipline, and create transparency and possibilities of comparison and control, and if individuals or staff groups feel that this is to their disadvantage they fall out of the system. For the nurses this means the parallel use of traditional ways of communication and of the computer system, causing additional workload and trouble, and, in consequence, increasing loss of system acceptance.

Open questions

In order to identify the impacts of computers in nursing on work and working conditions more precisely and completely the following questions should be made topical issues of further analysis:

- Time budget studies are necessary on how the patterns of work activities are really changed by the introduction of computer systems.
- Careful analysis in various contexts of action is necessary to determine whether the use of computer systems results in increasing or decreasing flexibility, and in smaller or greater scope for individual planning and initiative.

- It has to be analyzed why computers are an additional source of stress, as many nurses have assured, and what would be the appropriate measures of computer system design and working place design to avoid this.

3.   Conclusions

There is increasing consensus in society that the steering of selection, design, and introduction of new technologies should be based on the weighing of alternative technological options with regard not only to their effects in terms of costs and quality of the products or services provided by the use of these technologies, but as well to their impact on the "quality of working life". "Quality of working life" is a multidimensional concept comprising a set of general principles of what might be regarded as an improvement of work contents and working conditions including, e.g., reduction or elimination of adverse health effects, job expansion and enrichment, maintenance and growth of communication and cooperation, greater scope for individual planning and initiative, safeguarding of existing skills and acquisition of additional skills, and participation of employees in operational planning.

In this perspective computer system implementation and project management, education and training, and the mutual adaption of the computer system and of the work organization have proven to be critical issues in the use of computers in nursing. There is substantial additional need of research and development which should focus primarily on the following areas:
- Methods and tools in support of technological and organizational processes of innovation allowing for participation of nurses in these processes;
- concepts of staff development and of education and training including not only the transmission of operating skills, but the knowledge required for competent participation in systems development and in the shaping of technological change, as well. Training concepts have to take into account the specific working conditions in hospitals as shift work, unpredictable periods of extreme workload, and a high rate of staff fluctuation;
- development and testing of computer systems integrating the new informations techniques into the work of nurses in a task oriented manner, making possible a user oriented interface design, avoiding a restrictive division of labour and a reduction of human skills required for nursing care, and enabling a sufficient psychosocial, non-technical care of and communication with the patients.

4.   References

[1]   M. Baumann, J. John, W. Riedel, U. Zell: Neue Wege in der stationären Krankenpflege: Umstrukturierung der Arbeitsorganisation und Entwicklungstendenzen des EDV-Einsatzes. In: Das Krankenhaus 86 (2) 1990, 79-84.

[2]   H. von Benda, V. Wohlmannstetter: Auswirkungen des EDV-Einsatzes im Pflegebereich des Krankenhauses. Neuherberg (Gesellschaft für Strahlen- und Umweltforschung mbH München) June 1988, unpublished report.

[3]   H. Peterson, U. Gerding Jelger: Evaluation: A mean to better results. In: M.J. Ball, K.J. Hannah, U. Gerdin Jelger, H. Peterson (eds.): Nursing informatics. Where caring and technology meet. New York Berlin Heidelberg (Springer-Verlag) 1988.

CLASSIFICATION AND CODING

ACCURACY OF HOSPITAL DIAGNOSTIC AND OPERATIVE PROCEDURE CODING

E. J. Wilkinson, BSc.,MBBS.,MRCGP., Registrar in Public Health Medicine, South Glamorgan Health Authority.

I. Harvey, MB.,MRCP.,MFPHM., Senior Lecturer in Public Health Medicine, University of Wales College of Medicine.

ABSTRACT

The quality of Hospital Activity Analysis [HAA] data needs to be assured if it is to be relied upon as a basis for planning services and setting contracts in the new National Health Service. Accuracy and completeness are important measures of the quality and our study assessed the accuracy of inpatient clinical coding in the three main teaching hospitals in South Glamorgan.

A professional medical record specialist overcoded 120 randomly selected admissions at each of the three hospitals. The results were encouraging and showed that at least 80% of the codes chosen were in complete agreement with codes chosen by local coders [A=82.9%; B=80.3%; C=84.1%]. ICD - 9 + OPCS - 4 were used throughout. Differences were mainly accounted for by codes put down by the coding specialist alone.

The nature of these omissions and ways to improve accuracy further have been considered. Quality control measures are already integral to the system of coding in the U.S.A.; future monitoring of accuracy will be needed locally in South Glamorgan.

INTRODUCTION

In 1969 a Hospital Activity Analysis [HAA] system was introduced in England and Wales that brought together administrative, personal and clinical details of acute hospital inpatients. The quality of clinical activity information must be assured if it is going to be of any real value in assessing health needs, planning services, medical audit, resource management, research and contracting.

Several published studies [1 - 11] have been carried out over the years looking at the accuracy of the HAA diagnostic and operative procedure coding.

As a prelude to the introduction of formal contracting within the N.H.S., we have undertaken an assessment of the accuracy of inpatient clinical coding at three Teaching Hospitals in South Glamorgan Health District [population about 400,000].

METHOD

A professional medical record specialist working on an All Wales record project [S.F.] was employed to overcode 120 randomly selected admissions in each of the three largest acute Hospitals in South Glamorgan.

The overcoding was performed without prior knowledge of the codes already chosen by the coding clerks .   ICD - 9 and OPCS - 4 [12 and 13] were used throughout.

The professional coding by S.F. was used as a "gold standard" against which other codes were compared.

RESULTS

The results are shown in Tables 1 - 3.

TABLE 1

HOSPITAL [no.of notes overcoded]	TOTAL NO. HOSPITAL CODES	TOTAL NO. S.F. CODES (a)	TOTAL NO. OF CODES AGREEING (b)	TOTAL NO. (%) OF CASES AGREEING
A (120)	227	251	208	86 (71.7)
B (115)	225	244	196	82 (71.3)
C (120)	270	289	243	87 (72.5)

The differences were analysed to see whether they existed at the 1st, 2nd, 3rd or 4th digit/position level of ICD - 9/OPCS - 4 or whether they were totally different.

TABLE 2

HOSPITAL (No.of notes overcoded)	Differences (no) at positions				Codes (no) noted by hospital only	Codes (no) noted by S.F. only
	1	2	3	4		
A (120)	3	1	4	8	3	27
B (115)	0	1	3	15	10	29
C (120)	4	5	3	4	11	30

These differences are expressed as percentages in Table 3.

TABLE 3

ANALYSIS	HOSPITAL		
	A	B	C
% agree at 4th digit level *	82.9	80.3	84.1
% differ at 1st digit level #	7.0	0	8.7
% differ at 2nd digit level #	2.3	2.1	10.9
% differ at 3rd digit level #	9.3	6.2	6.5
% differ at 4th digit level #	18.6	31.3	8.7
% noted by S.F. only #	62.8	60.4	65.2

Key * - b divided by a in Table 1
     # - denominator is a - b in Table 1

Five overcoded results were lost from the hospital B data leaving 115 overcoded notes for analysis.

DISCUSSION

At least 80% of codes showed complete agreement at the 4th digit level [A=82.9%; B=80.3%; C=84.1%]. Differences were mainly accounted for by codes that S.F. had put down that the hospital coders had not [A=62.8%; B=60.4%; C=65.2%]. This will have underfunding implications in an internal market. Other differences were mostly at the 4th digit level [A=18.6%; B=31.3%, C=8.7%] but the numbers were small.

Lockwood[2] carried out one of the first studies to assess accuracy of coded data in 1971. He found few errors with primary codes but greater inaccuracies with secondary codes; primary diagnostic coding was about 94% correct and primary operative coding about 90% correct. It was not possible to assess differences at primary and secondary code level in our study as this had not been separately noted. S.F. did note sequencing errors when they were thought to be significant i.e. when a secondary code should have been put as a primary code [A=5; B=4; C=12].

Recurrent errors included:-
(a) Omissions by hospital coders of:-
  - endoscopy, sigmoidoscopy, lumpectomy of breast, skin biopsy.
  - complications eg. patient having to go back to theatre, urinary tract infection, post-operative wound infection, adult respiratory distress syndrome.

- old conditions relevant to the present episode eg. old myocardial infarction.
- positive results eg. E.Coli from urine sample.

(b) Codes noted by hospital only:-

- symptoms coded as primary diagnostic code.
- local codes not in I.C.D. - 9/OPCS - 4 used.
- aberrant local rules eg. previously corrected congenital abnormalities.
- old conditions not applicable to present admission.

CONCLUSIONS

Much of the miscoding occurs due to difficulties extracting the relevant data from the case notes. The records themselves are often poorly structured. This can make it difficult to differentiate between episodes and important diagnoses and procedures can be missed as the coders have to work through poor handwritten entries and disordered records.

The coding clerks usually work in isolation from the medical staff. Better communication between coders and clinicians should improve the accuracy of coding. This may involve the coding function being carried out closer to the clinician either by the medical secretary or by coders who are allocated to particular wards or specialities. Diagnosis and operative procedures should be clearly noted by the clinical staff on the summary sheet.

The results of this study have indicated a reasonably good standard of coding along with areas of potential improvement; over 80% of codes showed complete agreement. Over 60% of the differences occurring can be accounted for by codes noted by the medical record specialist alone.

As the U.K. moves towards a developed internal market in health care accuracy of data will remain of key importance and if such data is to be used to assess needs, plan services and set contracts, quality control measures need to be applied which should include regular local monitoring of accuracy.

REFERENCES

1. Alderson M. Mortality, morbidity and health statistics. Basingstoke : Macmillan, 1988 : 254.

2. Lockwood E. Accuracy of Scottish hospital morbidity data. Brit. J. Prev. Soc. Med. 1971; 25 : 76-83.

3. Patel A R, Gray G, Lang G D, Baillie F G H, Fleming L, Wilson G M. Scottish Hospital Morbidity Data 1. Errors in diagnostic returns. Health Bull. (Edinb.) 1976: 34 : 215-220.

4. Martini C J M, Hughes A O, Patton V A. A study of the validity of the Hospital Activity Analysis information. Brit. J. Prev. Soc. Med. 1976; 30 : 180-186.

5. Lennox B, Clarke J A, Drake F, Ewen S W B. Incidence of salivary gland tumours in Scotland : accuracy of national records. Br. Med. J. 1978; 1 : 687-689.

6. George A M, Maddocks G B. Accuracy of diagnostic content of Hospital Activity Analysis in infectious disease. Br. Med. J. 1979; 1 : 1332 - 1334.

7. Rees J L. Accuracy of Hospital Activity Analysis data in estimating the incidence of proximal femoral fracture. Br. Med. J. 1982; 284 : 1856 - 1857.

8. Whates P D, Birzgalis A R, Irving M. Accuracy of Hospital Activity Analysis operation codes. Br. Med. J. 1982; 284 : 1857 - 1858.

9. Hole R. Accuracy of Hospital Activity Analysis operation codes. Br. Med. J. 1982; 285 : 210.

10. Crawshaw C, Moss J G. Accuracy of Hospital Activity Analysis operation codes. Br. Med. J. 1982 : 285 : 210.

11. Butts M S, Williams D R R. Accuracy of hospital Activity Analysis data. Br. Med. J. 1982; 285 : 506 - 507.

12. World Health Organisation (1979). International classification of Diseases. Manual of the International Statistical Classification of Diseases, Injuries and Causes of Death, Ninth revision. Geneva WHO.

13. Office of Population Censuses and Surveys (1990). Classification of Surgical Operations and Procedures. Fourth revision. London. OPCS.

ACKNOWLEDGEMENT

I would like to acknowledge the help of Stephanie Freyaldenhoven, Medical Records Specialist for CASPE Healthcare Knowledge Systems Ltd., in overcoding the records at the three hospitals mentioned.

GIANO: a decision aid
to represent the semantics of medical terms

Domenico M. Pisanelli, Angelo Rossi Mori, Valentina Coacci

Reference Centre for Terminology and Coding for Healthcare Informatics
Istituto Tecnologie Biomediche, CNR
V.le Marx 15, 00156 Roma, Italy

Abstract

In this paper we are concerned with the issue of representing medical terms by means of a synthetic code belonging to a classification system. In particular we focus on the International Classification of Diseases (ICD) and present GIANO, a decision aid for choosing the ICD code that best expresses the semantic of a term appearing in a medical document.

The decentralization of health-care management and planning and the proliferation of clinical information systems are making evident the need of decentralizing coding activities as well. GIANO is a system designed to support non-medical staff in the activity of coding, especially at a local level, where they might not be experienced enough to carry out the coding task effectively.

GIANO was designed for a specific class of non medical users, and induces them to use all the information present in a document in order to reach the code that expresses the maximum of details considered statistically relevant by ICD. The delivery version is implemented on personal computer for processing Italian terms, but search engine, thesaurus management, user interface and utility routines are language independent. The approach does not require medical manpower to revise the ICD database, and thus it is easily re-customed for different languages and other classification systems or nomenclatures having an extended index of terms available, as in the case of ICD.

Keywords: Classification, Coding Assistance, Decision Aid, Health-care data management

1. Introduction

The diffusion of clinical information systems and computerized medical records requires an adequate formalization of the medical concepts expressed in the original documents. We envisage that in future it will be possible to process medical language routinely, but at the moment clinical information management needs tools to make this information portable and easily processable.

Portability of medical information is needed to allow comparisons and transfer of data. On the other hand, the need for an *easy processing* comes from the large amount of data and information involved in the health-care field. In Italy, for example, 10 million hospital discharge summaries are compiled each year, while death certificates are more than 500 000.

Classifications and coding are used to organize and process medical data. Applying and extending ISO 1087 [2,6], we define a MEDICAL CONCEPT as a conventionalized unit of thought, independent from any particular language (e.g., the concept of "cirrhosis of the liver" in Western medicine). A medical concept may be expressed by several MEDICAL TERMS (each term is represented by one or more words, or word parts, e.g., "kidney", "nephro-"): one of these terms may be declared as the PREFERRED TERM for this concept, the others being synonyms. In a CLASSIFICATION, elementary concepts are grouped together in CLASSES (e.g., "maxillary hyperplasia" may be considered as one term of the class "major anomalies of jaw size"), and CODES are labels assigned to classes to simplify (statistical) data processing. Terms may be joined together in a DESCRIPTION (like in the case of "hepatitis in malaria"). Usually this join will not be registered as a new term but sometimes – when relevant for statistical purposes - a special class is produced in a classification starting from a composite description.

Therefore *classification* (as the process of classifying) and *codification* (the assignment of a label) are actually two different conceptual processes consisting respectively in:
   • aggregation of elementary concepts in classes;
   • expression of the aggregates by means of a unique identifier: the code.

To avoid confusion, the term "coding" will be used below to designate the whole process, whereas "classification" will be reserved to the organization of concepts purposively designed by an institution such as the World Health Organization (WHO).

2. The need of a decision support for ICD coding

In this paper we are concerned with the issue of representing single- or multi-word medical terms by means of a synthetic code belonging to a classification system. In particular we focus on the International Classification of Diseases (ICD [7]) – issued by WHO and officially adopted by a large number of countries – and present GIANO, a decision support system for choosing the ICD code that expresses at best the semantic of a term reported on a medical document.

The task of a coder is to recognize a term, written by a certifying physician in a specific field of a document. Sometimes (s)he has to decide if information in other fields (*co-text*) may affect the coding, e.g.: "thyroid dysfunctions" (240-246) are coded under 648.1 if complicating pregnancy.

ICD is essentially organized on three levels: the top one is that of *sectors* (general topics) consisting in *categories* (3 digit codes) divided in *sub-categories* (4 digit codes). Codes are provided to account for incomplete information, allowing to express always a code, the most generic being 799.9: "Other unknown and unspecified cause". In Italy the WHO's Manual is translated and published by the National Institute for Statistics (Istituto Centrale di Statistica: ISTAT) [3]. According to the law, ISTAT is in charge of coding all certificates of death (physicians are obliged to fill them in), and a sample of hospital discharge summaries. This process is carried out at central level. In the meantime, however, the decentralization of health-care management and planning and the proliferation of clinical information systems are making evident the need of decentralizing coding activities too. Coding assistance may be provided by a set of tools to input and formalize medical terms, each tool tuned to the requirements of a different class of users.

GIANO is a system designed to support non-medical staff in the activity of coding, especially at local level, where they might not be experienced enough to carry out the coding task effectively.

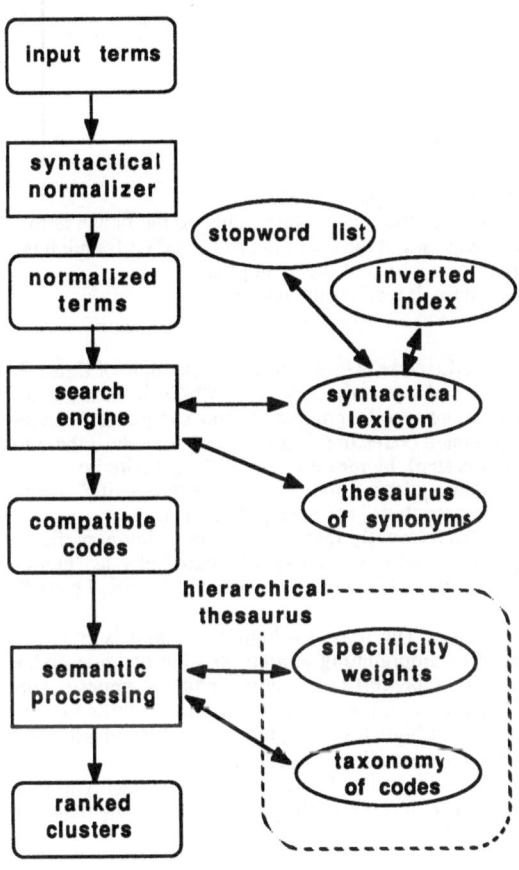

Fig. 1 Selection of compatible codes and ranking through semantic processing (steps 1 and 2, §3).
Rectangles denote processes, ovals refer to databases, rectangles with smoothed corners are data

3. The system GIANO

The aim of GIANO is to find the ICD code to represent a medical term given in input. This is achieved in 4 steps:
1) selection of compatible codes, i.e.: those pointed by the words belonging to the term;
2) grouping and ranking of selected codes, according to pre-defined criteria;
3) disambiguation and validation of residual alternatives;
4) assistance in considering co-text information in the original document.

Step 1 and 2 are totally automatic (they are represented in figure 1), steps 3 and 4 require user-interaction: the whole interactive process can be regarded as a decision aid to the task of coding.

Step 1. The system looks for the codes pertaining to the significant words of the phrase, and retrieves the one pointed by every word, as in the printout reported in figure 2. It disregards words less relevant to the semantic of the input phrase, like articles or prepositions.

This kind of process is comparable to a search by keywords in information retrieval systems (IRS). However, a relevant difference is due to nature and structure of the elementary information item to be retrieved. Whereas the user looks for documents in a typical IRS, in GIANO the atomic units to be found are codes. Each code corresponds to a *cluster* of terms: those pointing to it in the ICD index (figure 3).

The output of step 1 involves two reasons of redundancy:
- ambiguity and errors of interpretation (e.g. produced by homography);
- co-presence of codes related to the same topic, but involving different aumount of details.

The latter may be dealed automatically and is tackled first.

```
> tumore maligno della coda del pancreas

tumore       tumor        636
maligno      malign       424
coda         coda         12
pancreas     pancreas     26

             1 codice(i)  soddisfa(no) la richiesta

157.2        Tumori maligni del pancreas: Coda del Pancreas
```

Fig. 2. Step 1: the retrieval of compatible codes
In this printout, reproducing the actual computer output, the code corresponding to the Italian term "tumore maligno della coda del pancreas" ("malignant neoplasm of the tail of the pancreas") is found: it is the only one common to the four significant words of the input phrase.
Being the input a very specific term, it recalls only one code.

Step 2. If a query is sufficiently specific, only a specific code is found, as in the example of figure 2. If the input term is not specific, ICD assures the existence of a generic code (e.g., 490.0 "bronchitis, not specified if acute or chronic") and step 1 locates also the more specific compatible codes (e.g., all the other 22 codes involving "bronchitis"). Therefore, we group related codes in a "family" and we reduce them to the most generic one (the only one shown to the user in this step), by means of two different criteria:

a) a specificity weight is associated to each code, ranking from 1 to 5, e.g.: 490.0 "bronchitis", being very generic has a weight of 5, 491.2 "obstructive chronic bronchitis" has a weight of 1 [1];

b) a hierarchical thesaurus, i.e.: a taxonomy of codes (currently implemented for pulmonary diseases), where each node is linked to a more generic "parent" node (e.g., an explicit chain links, as "grandchild", 491.2 to 490.0); at the top of the taxonomy there is 799.9, "Other unknown and unspecified cause".

```
bonnier, sindrome di
neuronite _ vestibolare
nistagmo _ benigno parossistico
sindrome _ otoliti
vertigine _ auricolare
vertigine _ labirintica
vertigine _ otogena
vertigine _ parossistica benigna
vertigine _ periferica
vertigine _ uditiva
vertigine _ epidemica
```

Fig.3 A cluster of Italian terms from the ICD-9 index.
They are all the items that refer to the class "Vertiginous syndromes and other disorders of vestibular system; other and unspecified peripheral vertigo" identified by the code 386.1

Step 3. The role of a human operator is essential that of disambiguating among possible residual codes that might be retrieved, being equally generic and compatible with the sentence in input. A skilled coder easily disambiguates through the title of the classes. An optional routine allows him/her to browse in the clusters of terms, to examine their content and eventually to find and validate the code of the parent of the family that best matches the input.

Step 4. In absence of other information, the code is correct. If co-textual information is available in the original document, it may be considered to focus on specific codes. Interaction is therefore required to go deep in the "family tree" (defined in step 2) and the system presents to the user more specific codes that might apply.

The development of GIANO required a pre-processing of data on a mainframe (IBM 3090 at the computing centre of the University "La Sapienza" in Rome). GIANO was implemented in a personal-computer environment using the programmable relational data-base management system DBase-IV under MS-DOS. The delivery version (4.5 Megabyte, or 8 Megabyte with the optional routine to browse in the clusters of original terms) is currently implemented for processing Italian terms, but search engine, thesaurus management, user interface and utility routines are obviously language independent.

4. Discussion

Concept formalization is not only a complex task, but requires different tools for different actors who perform it in different contexts. Four types of contexts can be identified:

1) <u>Care provision units</u>. They are formed by people carrying on a well defined task, using a subset of concepts on a narrow domain; typical contexts are: clinical laboratory, patient assistance, general-practitioners' ambulatory. Classifications, such as ICD, are too broad in their scope and not detailed enough to satisfy the needs of routine data processing; specific extensions are often adopted. Given the dimension of the teams, nobody can be employed full-time only for data coding. Computerized data entry should be based mainly on mnemonic keywords and pre-defined menus, since the work concentrates on a limited number of medical concepts.

2) <u>Divisions</u>. They group units operating in the same structure and having different tasks or performing the same task on separate groups of patient. The numerical consistency of personnel justifies the presence of data processing operators, but not their formal training as professional coders (an extremely time-consuming training).

3) <u>Hospitals / Local Health Authorities</u>. This is the first level of aggregation in which some operators can be full-time employed for data processing, either depending directly from the structure, in specialized departments, or as external contributors (there are actually firms specialized in providing these services). However the clerical staff - being full-time EDP operators, but only part-time coders - might not be experienced enough to carry out the coding task effectively.

4) <u>Regions / State</u>. This aggregation level deals essentially with health-care programming and management. The presence of full-time coders is justified and the amount of data they manage can give them an adequate experience.

GIANO was designed to be employed at the second or third level of this scale, where it can be effective and close to the needs of those classes of users. It was conceived to be interactive: the aim is not to replace the human expert, but to give a support in the decision phase.

Portability was considered an essential feature in its design, therefore a delivery version in a personal-computer environment was realized. User-friendliness was also stressed in the building of the system: it is one of the most crucial factors for its acceptance and certainly its improvement is a near goal. GIANO is part of a general-purpose framework of systems conceived for formal representation of concepts in medical documents [5]. It prepares the formal input for a knowledge-based system which applies WHO's rules on death certificates and is based on stereotypical medical knowledge [4].

The present version of GIANO is able to manage only simple descriptions (combinations of terms registered by ICD in one code), but not description leading to more ICD codes (e.g.: "asthma in cardiopathic"). But more often the problem is the reverse: the combinations of terms considered by ICD as statistically relevant - and thus requiring one code - are actually present as two separate terms on different parts of the form (e.g.: if the primary diagnosis is "cirrhosis of the liver", and the secondary is "chronic alcoholism", the proper code will be 571.2 "alcoholic cirrhosis of the liver"). In GIANO, the step 3 routine, suggesting possible specifications to the selected diagnosis, allows for careful coding of further details.

The order of words is disregarded by GIANO; the meaning and the restriction of possible combinations of significant words in multi-word terms are so powerful, that efficiency of the system is not affected. Homographs (e.g. "tumor" can mean "swelling" or "neoplasm") and the rare cases of ambiguity that we generate with our algorithm (e.g. of the type: "kidney pelvis" and "pelvic kidney") are normally disambiguated by the other words in the term; very few are to be solved by the user.

A pre-processing routine is envisaged to cover most of these problems, when more experience with them and with the system will be gained.

5. Conclusions

Coding activity covers a fundamental role in the management of health-care information. The task is far from being trivial and error-free and adequate supports should be given to those who have to perform it. Inaccuracy of codes hampers full exploitation of clinical data for epidemiological, audit and planning purposes.

The usefulness of a tool to assist the coder in the decision process is evident. Compared to the manual's use, not only it offers more rapidity and can be readily and constantly updated and customized, but allows a better retrieval of all pertinent codes and permits the browsing of a conceptual cluster of terms.

GIANO is conceived for a specific class of non medical users, and induces them to use all the information present in a document, to reach the code that express the maximum of details considered statistically relevant by ICD.

The approach does not require medical manpower to revise the ICD database, and thus it is easily re-customed for different languages and other classification systems or nomenclatures having an extended index of terms available as in the case of ICD.

References

[1] Cislaghi C, personal communication, 1990.

[2] International Standard Organization, *Terminology - Vocabulary (ISO-1087)*, Geneva, ISO.

[3] Istituto Centrale di Statistica, *Classificazioni delle Malattie Traumatismi e Cause di Morte*, IX Revision, Rome, ISTAT, 1984.

[4] Pisanelli D.M., Rossi-Mori A., "Converting the Representation of Medical Data: Criteria to Code the Underlying Cause of Death", *Methods of Information in Medicine*, **29** (3), pp. 220-235, 1990.

[5] Rossi-Mori A., Chiappetta P., Pisanelli D.M., Riccardi M., "MeDEA: Modular Knowledge-Based Systems to Support Coding of Medical Documents", to appear in: Dal Monte P.R., D'Imperio N., Giuliani-Piccari G. (eds.) *Imaging and Computing in Gastroenterology*, Berlin, Springer Verlag, 1991.

[6] Rossi-Mori A., Thornton A.M., Gangemi A., "An Entity-Relationship Model for a European Machine-Dictionary of Medicine", in: Miller R.A. (ed.), *Proceedings 14th Annual Sysmposium on Computer Applications in Medical Care*, Los Alamitos, California, IEEE Computer Society Press, pp. 185-189, 1990.

[7] World Health Organization, *International Classification of Diseases. Manual of the International Statistical Classification of Diseases, Injuries, and Causes of Death*, 9th Revision, Geneva, WHO, 1977.

CLASSIFICATION WITHIN HIOS+

Francois M.H.M. Dupuits, Arie Hasman and Patrick C.M.H.F. Jansen
University of Limburg, Dept. of Medical Informatics
P.O. Box 616, 6200 MD Maastricht, The Netherlands
Telephone: +3143888412

Abstract

This paper deals with a research conducted by the University of Limburg in order to investigate and evaluate search & disclosure processes concerning ICPC criteria. Research aims are: (1) the development of a new consistent criteria list belonging to the Dutch ICPC and the implementation of this list in a medical information and research system, and (2) a more active disclosure of Dutch ICPC criteria. The new criteria list will be implemented in HIOS, a system already equipped with ICPC search algorithms and capable of presenting criteria. Part 2 of our research involves the development of tools which enable interpretation of free text into a query and usage of this query to give decision support during coding. For these purposes, two tools have been designed as separate modules within decision support system HIOS+: the Free text Formaliser (FF) and the Formal Interpreter (FI).

Keywords are: ICPC, Free text Formalisation, Formal Interpretation, Decision Support, Queries.

Introduction

In 1986 we initiated the development of HIOS, a GP Information and Research System. The aim was to come up with a system which supports GPs in their daily practice activities and in research. For some years now, HIOS has been operational within several general practices. It is being used as a registration system for basic and medical data of patients and enables research concerning these data. HIOS consists of modules which have been extended with several facilities throughout the years.

At the end of 1989, the development of HIOS+, a Decision Support System (DSS) for use in general practices and hospitals, was started within the project 'Decision Support System in Health care' (DSSH). In this development, use is made of a Phased Development Method (see [4]). General information on DSS is given in [8]. HIOS+ consists of the modules Information Facility (IF), Model Maker (MM), Advice & Warning (AW), Free text Formaliser (FF), Formal Interpreter (FI) and makes use of the HIOS data bases. IF, MM and AW are described in [2] and [3]. FF and FI enable the use of free text in a coding environment and are the main subjects of this paper.

HIOS+: the classification process

One of the prerequisites for successfully applying information systems in research is the use of codes. With these codes a user is enabled to classify and register data efficiently. Within HIOS and HIOS+, codes are used to classify and register diseases. A code used (national policy) is the International Classification of Primary Care (ICPC). General information about the ICPC is given in [7] and [10]. Use of codes is preferred to free text entry because information and research systems, like HIOS and HIOS+, presently are not yet capable of successfully interpreting free text. Misinterpretations are e.g. caused by semantic problems, negation difficulties and the absence of proper criteria which describe diagnosing of diseases.

In the Netherlands, a national study is conducted to create an algorithm for searching codes within the ICPC and to investigate the use of criteria by GPs during coding within medical information and research systems. In this study, several universities have joined forces: the University of Leiden (RUL), the Erasmus University of Rotterdam (EUR) and the University of Limburg (RL). RUL is engaged in translating the ICPC into Dutch. Creation of the ICPC search algorithm is the task of EUR. RL is investigating and evaluating search & disclosure processes about criteria belonging to ICPC codes. The presently available Dutch ICPC translation and the search algorithm have been tested at several general practices during the first months of 1991. First results in the matter of the RL research task within the national ICPC study will be gathered from May 1991 onwards; detailed results will be made known after a second test (September - October 1991). It has already been stated that it is the task of the RL to investigate and to evaluate search & disclosure processes concerning criteria in use within the ICPC. It is our aim to achieve a universe of discourse for all diseases in the Dutch

ICPC by disclosing criteria. Our task first of all involves the development of a new consistent criteria list belonging to the Dutch ICPC and the implementation of this list within a medical information and research system. Since HIOS is already capable of presenting criteria and is equipped with ICPC search algorithms, we intend to implement the Dutch criteria list into this system. After having entered an ICPC code and having activated search algorithms, a user is presented a subset of hits in a window. Every code on which criteria are present in HIOS+, is marked by a '*'. Criteria of such a code are presented in a second window after the user has activated criteria presentation by pressing function key F1. Criteria representation is shown in figure 1. This concludes the first phase of our task. The second phase involves a more active

```
VERSION 010291    PATIENT ENCOUNTER MODULE    05-04-91 15:32:59   (MI&S)
 MIS 010885 Mr.    ERT    Med  * R70 002 PLEURA EXUDATE TUBERCULOSIS TB
                                * R70 003 PLEURA FLUID TUBERCULOSIS TB
 Annalaan 60              641   * A70 014 MENINGITIS TUBERCULOSIS
                                * R70 001 HYDROTHORAX TUBERCULOSIS
 S   COD SEQ             DES    | A27 009 FEAR FOR TUBERCULOSIS
                                * A70 001 TUBERCULOSIS BONE
 S1  R02 001 PAIN IN THE BA     * A70 002 TUBERCULOSIS IN GENERAL
 S1  No further information
 A1          tube

 IC2  TUBERCULOSIS, ALL LOCATIONS
      INCL. LATE EFFECTS, RECENT POSITIVE TURNING OF
      TB SKIN TEST
      THIS DIAGNOSIS NEEDS ONE OF FOLLOWING CRITERIA
      A) EVIDENCE OF MYCOBACTERIA TUBERCULOSIS
      B) CHARACTERISTIC X-RAY
      C) CHARACTERISTIC HISTOLOGICAL PICTURE
      D) RECENT TURNING TO POSITIVE TUBERCULIN SKIN

 1:HELP    2:SEARCH    4:PRBLST    6:MEDIC.    7:F_TXT    10:OTHER      MUT
```

Figure 1. Representation of criteria

disclosure of Dutch ICPC criteria. In this context, we first had to decide whether to achieve such an active disclosure manually or automatically. On the basis of aspects like consistency and security of data, ability to make use of a standard for sharing information, validation of data entry and creation of suitable data structures, we chose for the automated option. Another decision which had to be taken concerned the make-or-buy aspect of software. We decided to make our own application, because of the versatility of the required software, the availability of HIOS+ sources, the fact that HIOS+ had been operational and the need for an integrated HIOS+. After having taken these decisions, we investigated the development boundaries and the basic features of the tools which are needed to reach our active disclosure objective. It became apparent that tools would have to be developed which enable interpretation of free text into a query (logical expression) and usage of this formalised representation to support users in their decision making during coding. One of the tools which has since been developed is HIOS+ FF. The purpose of HIOS+ FF is to enable interpretation of criteria into a query. In this, FF needs the help of a user to identify and logically combine topics within criteria. When a user is presented criteria of an ICPC code within FF, he/she first has to identify topics within the presented text. Next, the selected topics are checked against ICPC codes stored in HIOS+.

Valid topics are then presented to the user in a window along with certain formal commands by means of which these topics can be logically combined. Within FF, use is made of formal commands which are provided by the Arden Syntax, a standard for sharing medical information. This syntax focusses on knowledge which is represented as a set of independent modules, the Medical Logic Modules (MLMs), which provide therapeutic suggestions, alerts, diagnosis scores, etc. A typical MLM consists of three categories: maintenance, library and knowledge. In FF, every free text of criteria is constructed into an MLM. Created queries constitute the knowledge category in an MLM. The decision to use the Arden Syntax was taken on the grounds that this Syntax is a for our purposes suitable, medical-oriented, international standard and ICPC criteria are admirably suited for the purpose of being converted into MLM structures. The process of constructing queries in a formal (natural language) representation is also described in [1], [5], [6] and [9]. The interpretation of criteria is shown in figure 2.

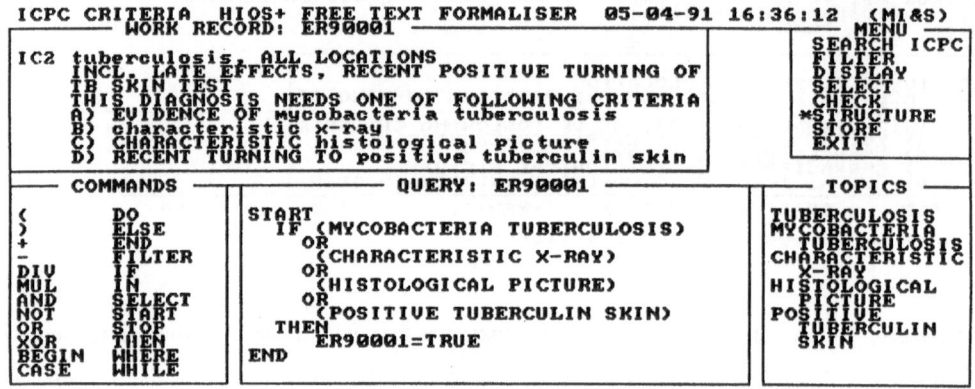

Figure 2. Construction of query within FF

The development of HIOS+ FF is on its way; the first version became operational in February 1991. Some positive and negative preliminary remarks about FF can be made. Negative aspects are e.g.: a user has to learn how to operate FF, automatical creation of an MLM takes longer than manual creation, and an application built with a third-party standard product can be developed faster than own software. Positive aspects are e.g.: readability, consistency and security of data are assured, an MLM is built according to agreements, an international standard for sharing information is used, the data structure ensures usage by FF and FI, the software is tailored to the specific needs of the users, data entry is validated, knowledge can be exchanged using several media, and queries can be linked with ICPC codes. A query created by FF is used by a tool called HIOS+ FI. The purpose of FI is to interpret queries with regard to actual facts stored in the HIOS data bases. A warning will be presented in case a user wants to use a certain ICPC code of which the logical expression has not yet been ascertained by FI as being true. The user is confronted with the violation. The development of HIOS+ FI has not yet been initiated. It is our intention, however, to be able to use FI during the second test of the Dutch ICPC and the search algorithm.

Conclusions about HIOS+

Although the development of HIOS+ is still in progress, we are certain of the fact that this DSS will be of enormous value to GPs and medical specialists. Success and usefulness of HIOS+ depends on two aspects: the reliability of data stored in the HIOS data bases and the correctness of queries. These aspects are ensured by providing users with classification codes, like the ICPC and criteria belonging to ICPC codes. An active disclosure of criteria is provided by FF and FI.

References

[1] Donini FM, Lenzerini M, Nardi D. Using Terminological Reasoning in Hybrid Systems. The European Journal on Artificial Intelligence September 1990; Vol. 3 No. 3: 128-138.
[2] Dupuits FMHM. A General Practitioners' Information and Research System with Decision Support Facilities (HIOS+). International Conference 'Doctors at work' Utrecht The Netherlands May 1990.
[3] Dupuits FMHM, Hasman A, Schoonbrood GGM. Decision Support in a General Practice. In: O'Moore R, Bengtsson S, Bryant JR, Bryden JS, eds. Lecture Notes in Medical Informatics - Medical Informatics Europe '90 Proceedings - MIE 90, Glasgow, UK, August 1990. Berlin Heidelberg: Springer-Verlag, 1990: 40, 231-235.
[4] Dupuits FMHM, Hasman A, Ulrichts EMJJ. The Designing of HIOS+. Software Engineering in Medical Informatics (SEMI), Amsterdam The Netherlands October 1990.
[5] Heidorn GE. Automatic Programming Through Natural Language Dialogue: A Survey. In: Rich Ch, Waters RC, eds. Readings in AI and Software Engineering 1986. Los Altos California, U.S.A.: Morgan Kaufmann Publishers Inc., 1986: 203-214.
[6] Hripcsak G, Clayton PD, Pryor A, Haug P, Wigertz OB, Lei van der J. The Arden Syntax for Medical Logic Modules. SCAMC proceedings, 1990, 200-204.
[7] Lamberts H, Wood M. International Classification of Primary Care. In: Oxford Medical Publications, World Organisation of National Colleges, Academies, and Academic Associations of GPs/Family Physicians, Oxford University Press, 1987.
[8] Turban E. Decision Support and Expert Systems - Managerial Perspectives. New York USA: Macmillan Publ. Co., 1988.
[9] Wald JA, Sorenson PG. Explaining Ambiguity in a Formal Query Language. ACM Transactions on Database Systems June 1990; 15 (2): 125-161.
[10] Wood M. The New International Classification of Primary Care: Genesis and Implications for Patient Care and Research. The Journal of Family Practice 1987; 24 (6): 569-571.

The design and implementation, using an object oriented methodology, of a user friendly primary health care patient management system based on the ICPC classification.

A.W.Eliasz

Department of Computer Science
University College London

Abstract

The widespread acceptance of medical nomenclature coding schemes depends on their relevance and ease of use. This paper considers one such scheme, the ICPC scheme and discusses some of the user interface issues involved in implementing a patient management system based on this scheme. The design of the system uses an object oriented design methodology which is strongly oriented to tackling user interface problems.

In a previous paper [ELIASZ 90] the applicability of the object oriented paradigm to the data modelling and retrieval of medical information was discussed. This paper is a report on a particular case study attempting to apply some of these ideas. The system to be described here has as its goal the facilitation of the the entry, storage and retrieval of medical data according to the ICPC (International Classification of Primary Care) Model. [LAMBERTS 87] We chose to study this application for the following reasons:

1. Much of the preliminary data analysis and classification has already been done

2. Trials with a manual version of the system have already been carried out successfully

3. The application and the underlying data model lends itself to an object oriented approach

4. In order for the ICPC approach to become more widely used it will be necessary to make data entry, data coding ,and data retrieval much more efficient by providing a good human computer interface (HCI) and by incorporating facilities for coping with synonyms and ambiguities.

5. The ICPC classification scheme is of a manageable size for a pilot project of the sort described.

This paper is divided into several sections. In the first section "objects" and their properties will be reviewed. In the second section the ICPC scheme will be briefly described. In the third section the methodology followed will be described. Finally we will describe some of the design problems which had to be overcome and why the particular solutions described were chosen.

1. Objects and the Modelling of Medical Information

The process of object-oriented software construction has been well described by Bertrand Meyer [MEYER 88] and only a brief outline will be given here.

Objects, in the object oriented programming sense are software objects which couple data structures and algorithms in a tightly knit fashion. These objects can be thought of as engines which store data and can performed predetermined actions when "sent a message" to do so. The predetermined actions, or operations, define the visible interface to the object, the underlying data structures and implementation of the operations are hidden.

Developing software according to the object oriented paradigm involves the following steps:

1. Identify the objects (or entities) of interest and the data (attributes) to be associated with them

2. Specify the operations that are going to be performed on each object

3. Examine the objects of interest to see if they can be grouped into hierarchies of classes and subclasses.

The mechanisms of encapsulation provided by object oriented programming languages provide means for creating multiple object instances, behavioural sharing via inheritance mechanisms, strong typing to provide verification of correct object usage and the ability to structure resources when developing concurrent applications.

When using object classes it is important to be aware that an object class specifies a set of visible operations, a set of hidden instance variables, a set of hidden operations that perform the operations, and that every new instance of an object class has its own instance variables and shares the operations methods with the other instances of that class. Object classes should not be confused with prototypical objects. These differ from Object Classes in that they serve as templates from which new instances are developed. They are useful, however, in situations where objects evolve rapidly and have more differences than similarities.

When choosing an object oriented programming language it is important, amongst other things , to understand the inheritance mechanisms provided by that language. In particular it is necessary to know whether inheritance occurs statically (fixed in advance) or dynamically (at runtime). Who inherits the properties - classes or instances of classes? as well as What can be inherited e.g. instance variables methods values? Which inherited properties are visible? Whether inherited properties be overidden or suppressed? In systems where multiple inheritance is allowed it is also important to know how are conflicts resolved?

In modelling medical information the major difficulties arise because this information is multidimensional, has many viewpoints, large amounts of data need to be processed and also the relations between the various data items may be very complex.

2. The ICPC scheme

The ICPC scheme [LAMBERTS 87] is concerned with primary care problems. It provides a fairly comprehensive classification of these problems. The various modes in which it can be used are

- the reason for encounter mode where the aim is to record and classify reasons for a particular medical consultation

- the diagnostic mode where the aim is to record and classify the various diagnoses made , and , finally

- the process mode in which the various treatments are recorded and classified.

The ICPC scheme is centred around patient "episodes of illness", and aims to provide summarised information of the patient's movement through the health care system during his or her various episodes of illness. Movement through the health care system involves places such as the home or workplace, the physician office, the hospital, the outpatient clinic and so on. Data elements are associated with events occurring at each of these places. These elements may include things such as symptoms or cause of injury, reason for encounter at the physician's office, reason for admission to hospital and so forth. These data elements, in turn may be stored on various files such as the physician's record files, the hospital record files etc.

ICPC has a biaxial structure consisting of 17 "chapters" covering major organ systems as well as psychological and social problems and each chapter has 7 components covering such matters as e.g. "symptoms and complaints", "treatment procedures, medication" and "Administrative". For each component of a given chapter there are tables describing the possible entries and their respective ICPC codes. ICPC aims to provide a means whereby the various encounters and treatments a patient undergoes during the various episodes of illness occurring during his or her life can be recorded.

3. System design issues:

The methodology followed in developing the application is based on work carried out by Winnie Pun for her PhD [PUN 90] thesis together with Russel Winder. I will therefore refer to it as the Pun - Winder methodology. The methodology works at three levels. First is the conceptual level, which produces a Conceptual Model. The conceptual level is made up of two layers, the User Interface Level and the User Transparent Level. Next is the system level which produces the Implementation Model and finally there is the specification level which produces a specification in the form of Class Structure Charts and Message Structure Charts. Of the two layers of the Conceptual Level the User Interface Layer contains application objects which communicate and interact directly with the user, and it provides a visual presentation of what the system is to the end-users. The User Transparent Layer contains application objects which are transparent to end-users, the users do NOT directly interact with these objects.

The interactions between objects are captured by means of Object Interaction Diagrams. These contain "circles" - which denote objects involved in the system and "arcs" - which denote interactions between the objects. These diagrams make use of levelling, so that an object at one level of abstraction can be expanded into a more detailed object interaction diagram at a lower level. The relationships between objects may be of several types. Important types of relationship are the "Contain" relationship, the "Use" relationship and the "Inherit" relationship. The "Contain" relationship is a one to many relationship between objects. Identifying such a relationship may help highlight other implementation objects and may reveal the underlying structure of an object. The "Use" relationship is a one to one relationship between objects. It denotes the fact that an object A communicates with an object B (distinguishes between sender and receiver). Identifying such a relationship may help identify other implementation objects and may highlight which operations are required for a particular object. The "Inherit" relationship is one to one if only single inheritance allowed but is one to many for multiple inheritance. Identifying such relationships is very important in production of reusable code. Further discussion of these types of relationship may be found in [GORLEN 90] and in [WINDER 91]. On the basis of the various relationships that are identified between objects and the Conceptual Level analysis an implementation model can be described. This model is formalised at the specification level. One of the outputs at the specification level is a collection of Class Structure Charts which is a series of documents containing detailed information about a given class, namely, its description, its attributes [data and operations], its class hierarchy and its inherited attributes. The other output is a collection of Message Structure Charts. A Message Structure Chart is a graphical description describing the method of a message/operation for a given class. It contains rectangular boxes - representing an individual object or class, dashed rectangular boxes - denoting the fact that the message sender and message receiver belong to the same class, curved rectangular boxes - to denote the superclass of the class which is of current interest, diamonds - to denote an alternative paths and elliptical loops to denote iteration constructs.

4. Design and Implementation Issues

The system is implemented in C++. The shortlisted languages were Smalltalk/V, Objective C and C++. C++ was chosen because of the availability of compilers running on a large range of machines from PC's through to Workstations and the perception that it is becoming the language of choice for developing object oriented systems. The availability of class libraries of graphical interface objects and data abstraction objects is proving to be of considerable help in developing the system. Versions of the system are being developed to run under Windows 3.0 on PC's and under X-Windows on Sun Workstations. The starting point for system development was the availability of a computerised version of ICPC [OXFORD]. The availability of a case study of a much simpler GP Patient Record Management System carried out as part of Winnie Pun's PhD was also very helpful. The biggest design problem was how to make the process of entering data into the encounter forms described for ICPC in [LAMBERTS 87] as straightforward as possible. The initial system allowed entry of data and text into a standard form directly. The codes had to be entered explicitly by the user. The initial system for finding the correct codes for a given situation was also simple. By selecting a given component and chapter the contents of that section of ICPC were displayed in a window and could be examined in sequence by the user. The user can also search for codes via the ICPC alphabetical index. Thus , for example, if the user types in abuse in the prompt window he will obtain a list of the various types of abuse such as alcohol abuse, drug abuse, child abuse and either the correct code or an indication that he has to search another level down.

The full details of the design of the first prototype will be available as a technical report [ELIASZ 91]

References:

[ELIASZ 90] Eliasz A.W. and Kostrewski B.J. Data Modelling: Medical Informatics and the Object Oriented Environment Medical Informatics Europe '90 pp 638 - 644 Eds. O.Reinhoff and D.Lindberg pub. Springer Verlag (1990)

[ELIASZ 91] Implementation of a Patient Record Management System Conforming to the ICPC system technical report in preparation UCL

[GORLEN 90] Gorlen K.E., Orlow S.M. and Plexico P.S. Data Abstraction and Object Oriented Programming in C++ pub. Wiley (1990)

[LAMBERTS 87] Lamberts H. and Wood M. (Eds) ICPC - International Classification of Primary Care pub. Oxford University Press (1987) Reprinted with corrections (1989)

[LAUREL 90] Laurel B. (Ed) The Art of Human-Computer Interface Design pub. Addison-Wesley (1990)

[MEYER 88] Meyer B. Object-oriented Software Construction pub. Prentice Hall (1988)

[OXFORD] Oxford Electronic Publishing Oxford University Press Walton Street Oxford OX2 6DP UK

[PUN 90] Pun W.W.Y A Design Method for Object Oriented Programming PhD Thesis Department of Computer Science University College London (1990)

[WINDER 91] Winder R. Developing C++ Software pub. Wiley (1991)

CHIC: Community Health Information Classification and Coding[1]

Results of A Project of the Commission of the European Communities

Reli Mechtler
AG Gesundheitspolitik an der Universität Linz
Altenbergerstr 69, A-4040 Linz

Abstract

This project had the objectives of developing an European Minimum Basic Data Set (MBDS) for Ambulatory Care identifying and defining all the data items which are relevant of health services outside the acute hospital environment, producing an extensible structure for the MBDS, conducting a survey of the acceptability of the MBDS, and developing specifications for supporting software.During the course of the project there was recognised the need to investigate the legal requirements and ethical constraints of different countries on the MBDS specifications. This statement is focused on describing the MBDS for Ambulatory Care. [2]

1. Project Objectives

The specific objectives are as follows: [3]
To identify the MBDS which will support the effective and efficient delivery of individual clinical treatment and health services within the primary and community health sectors of a number of countries, using methods which can be replicated in all countries in the Community.
To produce an extensible structure for the MBDS identified above, compatible with the tools in use in hospital settings and having acceptance at the international level.
To carry out a survey of the acceptability of the MBDS within the countries of the Community.
To develop specifications for software to support the use of the MBDS.
In the longer term, the objective of the participants is to produce and validate a common European basic set which defines all the data items which are relevant to the management of health services outside the acute hospital environment and which is capable of supporting:
- linkage between related hospital and community service episodes to create an individual health career;
- the validation of alternative treatment regimes based upon common diagnostic criteria;
- the construction of cost models of alternative community health service processes;
- the development of international standards for the analysis of the epidemiological characteristics of morbidity and the implications of these for health services.

2. The Minimum Basic Data Set for Ambulatory Care

As conventional definitions of a MBDS (i.e. Roger's definition 4)for hospital use) are inadequate for use in ambulatory care the MBDS- AC was defined as follows:

"The smalles set of data items which is required to describe the interaction between a health care practitioner and a patient at a single encounter, sufficient to differentiate between one patient and another, and to define the practitioner, date and location, the results of the previous encounter, the reasons for this encounter, and the services provided and planned with their objectives."

The ambulatory encounter is frequently no more than a part of a bigger process. In the health care systems of many European countries, the patient is free to seek medical treatment and advice on an ambulatory basis from the practitioner of his/her choice, and thus a succession of health care practitioners (HCPs) may become involved in the treatment of what is essentially a series of related conditions or one condition. So the data required to summarize following kinds of event:

- **Encounter(s)**
- **Health Plan(s)**
- **Episode(s)**

An episode may consist of a number of encounters (at the surgery, a home visit, or even advice during a telephone conversation) during which examination, clinical assessment, referral decisions, prescriptions or other diagnostic and therapeutic procedures are undertaken.These could be with different HCPs, each one of whom will have developed a health plan.

Other encounters might similarly complete in themselves, but lead the HCP to initiate some further course of action.

It has to be recognised that an encounter may occur at any stage during an episode and that the presented problem may or may not be already known to the practitioner.

However, the encounter is the only opportunity for data collection. Thus the MBDS-AC can only be derived from information available during the encounter, but must place that information in the context of the episode. Like that the MBDS-AC must contain information that will identify the following:

- Patient	- Health care practitioner,
- Payer(s)	- Episode reference,
- Health plan reference	- Encounter date,
- Location	- Results achieved,
- Problems and diagnoses	- Services provided,
- Goals to be achieved	

The Minimum Basic Data Set for Ambulatory Care (MBDS-AC) which meets the above criteria has been identified and is described in the following table 1:

Entity No.	Entity	Attribute No.	Attribute
1	PATIENT	1.1	Patient's identity number
		1.2	Health insurance number
		1.3	Sex
		1.4	Age or date of birth
		1.5	Post code
		1.6	Household structure
		1.7	Social and medical characteristics verified? (y/n)
2	HEALTH CARE PRACTITIONER	2.1	HCP identity (including profession)
		2.2	Provider's address
		2.3	Contact location
3	PAYER	3.1	Payer's identity number
4	HEALTH PLAN	4.1	Episode reference number
		4.2	Health plan category / number
		4.3	Problems (<5)
		4.4	Principal / secondary diagnoses (<5) (provisional if goal is assessment)
		4.5	Goals to be achieved
		4.6	Initial contact
			4.6.1 Date of contact
			4.6.2 ADL score
		4.7	Services provided - For each:
			4.7.1 Service code
			4.7.2 HCP identity (if third party)
			4.7.3 Date provided
			4.7.4 Results of tests
		4.8	Medicine prescribed - For each:
			4.8.1 Product code
			4.8.2 Unit dose prescribed
			4.8.3 Route of administration
			4.8.4 Date prescribed
			4.8.5 Duration of course
			4.8.6 Results (including reactions)
		4.9	Results achieved
			4.9.1 ADL index at final contact
			4.9.2 Goals attained (% score)
			4.9.3 Date of final contact
		4.10	Resources
			4.10.1 Duration of contact
			4.10.2 Charges payable
		4.11	New health plan? (y/n) If yes:
			4.11.1 New plan category and number

Table 1: Minimum Basic Data Set for Ambulatory Care

3. The Extensible Structure - Ambulatory Care Data Sets

Some encounters would have a close causal relationship with other health events, while other encounters might not, one approach is to collect a sufficiently large volumne of encounter based data using an MBDS to describe encounters of all kinds, and subsequently develop clinically and statistically sound methods of characterising indentifying and grouping together encounters which were causally related and separating them from encounters which were not. The scrutiny to which the CHIC Project has subjected this argument has led to the identification of a hierarchical framework stretching from the individual encounter to the health career, (summary health record or PRDS) which will enable encounters of different kinds to be characterised a priori rather than post hoc. This will be expanded in this chapter.

3.1. The Encounter

This has already been covered in chapter 2 and presented in table 1.

It was recognised that for the specific purpose of reimbursement and as a legally acceptable minimum record of the encounter, a summary of the MBDS-AC could be produced. The CHIC Projects recommendation for the Encounter (or Contact) data set: it has to include information of the Patient, HCP, Payer, data which describe the Care Plan and the Contact.

Having identified that the encounter is the only level for data collection and that the provision of ambulatory care is potentially a complex process.

Following diagrams show the handling of the MBDS. As well as the contents of an encounter are summed up by the MBDS-AC, the contents of one or a series of contents are summed up by the Health Plan and the contents of a completed health care process, comprising one or many Health Plans, are summed up by an Episod.

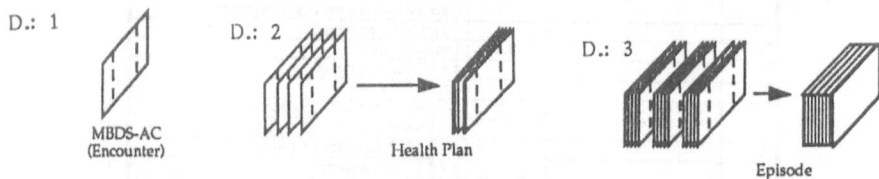

Diagram 1 has been used to graphically indicate the MBDS-AC, how it can be extended, and its relationship with the other data sets describing the components of ambulatory care.

3.2. The Health Plan

A Health Plan is defined as a planned care process, comprising one, or a series of, encounters or contacts between a HCP and a patient, initiated by the formulation by the HCP of a health plan in response to the patients perceived or actual problems which defines the process through which the goals of the health plan will be achieved and the date by which results will be assessed. Like That the Health Plan Data Set must include additional items, that will indentify the Health Plan:

- Episode reference   - Health plan category / number
- Problems (<5)   - Principal / secondary diegnoses (<5)
- Goals to be achieved   - Initial contact
- Services provided   - Medicine prescribed
- Results achieved   - New health plan? (y / n)
- Death

The Health Plan is something which is initiated on the first encounter by a HCP, and updated on subsequent encounters with that practitioner. It is HCP related. In terms of the data that is collected, it consists of data from each encounter (MBDS-AC) as indicated in diagram 2.

3.3. The Episode

But health plans themselves may need to be grouped into further cluster, this time characterised by the problem, its date of onset, and the date on which it is finally considered to be resolved. It is from such clusters that episodes are formed.

An episode is thus a completed health care process, designed to cure or alleviate a health care problem or suite of related problems, comprising one or many health plans, initiated by the detection of the principal of those problems and terminated by cessation of treatment or at the patient's or HCP's initiative, or death. The episode data set is then a summary of all care plans (see diagram 3) sufficient:

for comparisons and for future reference by HCPs.

The Episode Data Set includes following additional items:

- Episode reference number
- Data of first encounter
- Number and category of care plans in this episode
- Episode strategic goals
- Diagnostic of problems following assessment
- Secondary diagnoses
- Treatments and interventions

- Episode category
- ADL index (first encounter)
- ADL index at final encounter
- Diagnostic results (with dates)
- Results of the episode
- Referrals (with dates)

3.4. The Personal Health Career

Data sets which summarise health episodes, require additional data to produce a summary of person's health career. Thus the Patient Related Data Set (PRDS) is a summary of a patient's medical record, consisting of:

basic patient demographics, background medical data, current medical history (incomplete episodes).

The definition of the PRDS is the **minimum set of data about a patient which is necessary for the global assessment of the patient's health by an HCP who has had no prior contact with the patient.** As such the PRDS record is intended to be portable and interpretable by a wide range of practitioners.

The structure of the PRDSD is shown in diagram 4 and shows the relationship to the episode, health plan and encounter (MBDS-AC) data sets.

The PRDS must contain information that will identify the following:

- **Personal characteristics**
  general characteristics
  allergies and intolerances
  lifestyles
  environmental/social risk
- **Permanent health characteristics**
  permanent health deficits
  vaccination / immunisation record
  health screening
  summary of completed episodes
- **Current medical history**
  incomplete episodes
  completed health plan(s)
  uncompleted health plan(s)

As each health plan is completed, it is summarised and forms part of an incomplete episode. As each episode is completed, it becomes a completed episode (and produces an episode data set).

The PRDS must be seen in the context of a computerised clinical information system. It is a standardised sub-set of the records which responsible HCPs would keep about their patients.(See diagram 5).

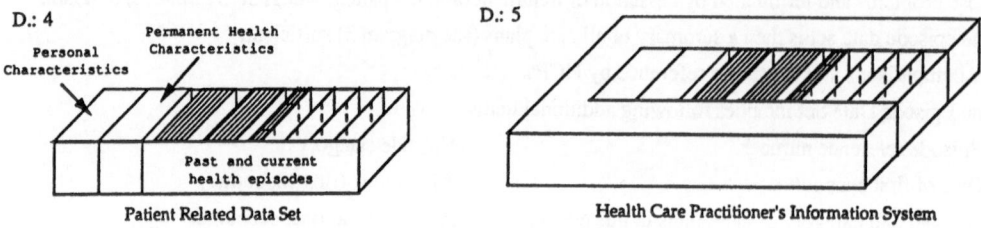

D.: 4

Personal
Characteristics

Permanent Health
Characteristics

Past and current
health episodes

Patient Related Data Set

D.: 5

Health Care Practitioner's Information System

3.5. Record Linkage

An individual data set record (for example an MBDS-AC from an ambulatory encounter, or an episode summary data set) can only be linked to other records if the event which generated the data set is set in the overall context of the healthcare the patient is receiving. The only reliable way to do this within the complexities of ambulatory care, is to recognise the hierarchical relationship of encounters, health plans and episodes, and to accept that the common element is the patient - hence the patient related data set (PRDS). Record linkage can only work in the context of the PRDS.

4. Acknowledgements

I wish to acknowledge the involvement of the other members of the CHIC project without whom this work could not have been achieved. They are STC Technology Ltd, Zentralinstitut für die kassenärztliche Versorgung in der Bundesrepublik Deutschland, University College of Wales, Universite Catholique de Louvain, Universite de Saint Etienne, and East Dyfed Health Authority.
I would also like to acknowledge the Advanced Informatics in Medicine (AIM) programme of the CEC DGXIII for part funding this work.

References

1) COOPER, P., (editor); CHIC: Community Health Information Classification and Coding (A 1026). FINAL REPORT, 1990, Advanced Informatics in Medicine, DG XIII. With contributions of: Bott, F.; James, S.; Deliege, D.; Mercier, M; Taylor,J.; Griew, A.; Savill, A.; Brenner, G; Rodrigues, J.M.; Mennerat, F.; Mechtler, R.
2) Cooper, P.; (editor); The CHIC Project - Abstract, 1990
3) European Community goal T221
4) Roger, F.H.; The minimum basic data set for hospital statistics in the EEC, 1981

AIM(ING) FOR THE RECORD

A.W. Savill, S.D. James and J.E. Taylor
Institute for Health Informatics
UCW Aberystwyth, Llanbadarn Fawr
Aberystwyth, Dyfed SY23 3AS

Abstract

The paper describes how the results of the CHIC (Community Health
Information Classification and Coding) Project of the AIM
(Advanced Informatics in Medicine) Programme have been used to
produce the Prototype Personal Health Summary. This summaries a
patients general and clinical details into two logical databases.
The first - the Resident Population Index (RPI) records
administrative data for a patient and the second - the Personal
Health Summary (PHS) records clinical data in the format suggested
by the CHIC Project. The two databases can be used in conjunction
by a clinician to provide an individual clinical summary, or in an
aggregated annonymised format for use by epidemiologists and
managers.

Introduction

AIM in the title refers to the AIM Programme which ran from June
1989 till May 1990. Record refers to one of the chief desires of
those engaged in Health Informatics, namely the creation of a
comprehensive summary of the health care given to a patient from
whatever source, ie a computerised clinical record.

Amongst the problems bedevilling the creation of a summary
clinical record (which is to encompass both Ambulatory and
Hospital Care) has been the lack of a structure which could
incorporate all the diferent health care events, - however these
are to be defined.

Other problems such as the need for a comprehensive classification
and coding system appear, in the U.K. at least, to be addressed by
the increasing adoption of the Read Clinical Classification.

Extending the aiming metaphor to a practical dimension, the
creation of the clinical summary could be represented as a game of
darts, Figure 1 shows:

FIGURE 1   AIMING FOR THE RECORD

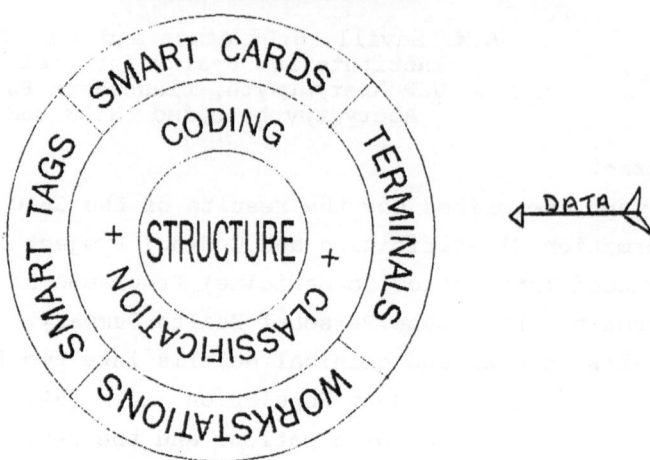

Within the AIM Programme, the Community Health Information
Classification and Coding (CHIC) project, postulated a structure
for a clinical summary based on a Minimum Basic Data Set (MBDS)
for Ambulatory Care. The CHIC project had as two of its
objectives:-

> To identify the Minimum Basic Data Set (MBDS) which will
> support the effective and efficient delivery of individual
> Clinical treatment and health services within the primary and
> Community health sectors of a number of countries within the
> European Community, using methods which can be replicated in
> all countries in the Community.

> To produce an extensible structure for the MBDS identified
> above, compatible with the tools in use in hospital settings
> and having acceptance at the international level.

> The project defined four data sets in an extensible structure
> of Ambulatory Care Data Sets, having identified that the
> encounter is the only level for data collection.

1. THE ENCOUNTER - MBDS-AC

Defined as the smallest set of data items which is required to
describe the interaction between a health care practitioner and a
patient at a single encounter, sufficient to differentiate between
one patient and another, and to define the practioner, date and

location, the results of the previous encounter, the reasons for
this encounter, and the services provided and planned with their
objectives.

This extended definition is required because of the difference
between a hospital spell and an ambulatory encounter.

2. THE HEALTH PLAN

Defined as a planned care process, comprising one, or a series of,
encounters or contacts between a Health Care Practitioner (HCP),
and a patient, initiated by the formulation by the HCP of a health
plan in response to the patient's perceived or actual problems
which defines the process through which the goals of the health
care plan will be achieved and the date by which results will be
assessed.

3. THE EPISODE

Defined as a completed health process, designed to cure or
alleviate a health care problem or suite of related problems and
terminated by cessation of treatment or at the patient's of HCP's
intiative, or death.

4. THE PATIENT RELATED DATA SET (PRDS)

Having identified data sets that summarise health episodes, it
requires little additional data to produce a summary of a person's
health career. Thus the PRDS is a summary of a patient's medical
record consisting of:

> basic patient demographics
> background medical data
> current medical history (incomplete episodes)

It is defined as the minimum set of data about a patient which is
necessary for the global assessment of a patient's health by an
HCP who has had no prior contact with the patient.

PROJECT METHODOLOGY

The PRDS and its associated data sets form the basis of a project
being carried out on East Dyfed Health Authority, subcontracted to
the Institute of Health Informatics, Aberystwyth; on behalf of the
Welsh Office. The Prototype Personal Health Summary (PHS) project,

due to Complete in mid 1991, has as one of its objectives, the task of demonstrating the validity of the CHIC Ambulatory Data Sets.

The structure for the Prototype PHS is essentially that defined by the PRDS. Additionally the project will use a patient index which will have a similar structure to the District Health Index which is in operational use in East Dyfed Health Authority.
The Prototype PHS has three categories of possible user - clinical, epidemiological and managerial. Clinicians will be able to link patient identifiers (from the patient index) to an individuals PHS record to obtain a clinical summary for an individual patient. Epidemiologists and managers will have access to aggregated anonymised data from the PHS and demographic type data from the patient index.

Clinical Data for the project will be supplied in three ways, which are described later. The data will be coded within the database using READ 5 with additional codes where necessary eg Strategic and Technical Goals.
The technical environment for the PHS is based on a client/server configuration using SUN Sparc Station 2s and an Open Systems UNIX platform, an ICL DRS6000, running the INGRES Relational Database.

Ancillary objectives of the Prototype project will include examination of the security and confidentiality issues which can have a critical impact on systems dealing with patient related data.

It is also hoped to demonstrate the value of a Geographical Information System(GIS) using the health data available in the Prototype PHS. ARC/INFO has been selected in view of its general use.

RESULTS

A total of 26,000 patient (some 10% of the Disctrict Population) taken from the DHI have been loaded with the RPI, thus providing the necessary patient registration data, all of the records have been scrambled so as to avoid identification.

There have been three sets of clinical summary records created for the project:

a) 14 Patients Records created from all records available on existing computer systems.

b) 6,000 Patient Records obtained from a download of a GP Practice Management System.

c) 20,000 Patient Records which have been created from data provided in the Royal College of General Practitioners, survey "Morbidity Statistics from General Practice, 1981-2.

Rules have been constructed for converting the records of type a) and b) into the structure proposed by the CHIC Project.

DISCUSSION

The only other project the authors are aware of in the UK which seeks to provide a summary of clinical "events" is that proposed within DISS - District Information Support System Project.
However this only sought to provide a list of "events" and did not seek to incorporate them into an overall structure.

SUMMARY

A successful Prototype PHS Project using the CHIC datasets should thus alter the debate from AIMING FOR THE RECORD ie the creation of a clinical summary, to AIMS OF THE RECORD ie how best to use it to improve the delivery and quality of the Health Care needed.

REFERENCES

1. Advanced Informatics in Medicine Programme - Commission of the European Communities - CHIC:Community Health Information Classification and Coding (A1026) Project Final Report 30th June 1990.

THE READ CODES AND NATIONAL AND INTERNATIONAL MEDICAL DATA INTERCHANGE

Dr James D Read FRCGP, Director
NHS Centre for Coding and Classification
Woodgate, Loughborough, Leicestershire, LE11 2TG, UK

1. Origins and Aims of the Read Codes and the General Practice Experience

The Read Codes started back in 1982 when James Read, as a General Practitioner decided to write a simple coding system for recording his practice's clinical data. Initially there were 25 codes! There are now some 100,000 codes with 150,000 synonyms covering all areas of medicine.

A key step in the development of the Read Codes was the endorsement, in 1988, by the Joint Computer Group of the British Medical Association's General Medicine Services Committee and the Royal College of General Practitioners. They recommended that the Read Codes be adopted as the standard for general practice, and that the implications be considered throughout the National Health Service (NHS).

Following this, the Read Codes were acquired by the Secretary of State for Health, and became Crown Copyright in April 1990(1). The Department of Health also established the National Health Service Centre for Coding and Classification (CCC), with James Read as its Director, to maintain and develop the codes for the NHS. The Centre has a Supervisory Board, comprising mainly of representatives of the medical profession to oversee the further development of the Codes.

Whereas the aim behind the original 25 Read Codes was to produce a brief problem listing for the general practice, the current aim is to support a totally computerised medical record, appropriate to, and communicable between, all healthcare sectors and all medical specialities.

Today some 10,000 GP's in the UK are routinely using the Read Codes in their consultations, and the Codes are available on most GP systems. It has been concluded by Pringle(2) that by 1992 over 90% of practices will have a computer system and that "the Read clinical classification is the only coding system to offer full cover for the symptoms, procedures, and events of primary care".

2. Read Codes in National Health Service Hospitals

In the secondary sector, the Read Codes were first implemented at Huddersfield Royal Infirmary where they have now been in use for more than two years. They have enabled the clinical teams, with the support of Resource Service Managers, to produce a wide range of audit and management reports based on clinically-valid data.

More recently the Read Codes have been implemented in several major hospitals in the UK, including St James's, Arrowe Park, Belfast Royal Infirmary, Pontefract, Airedale, York and Inverclyde. The next six months will see some 20 more implementations with another 20 planned, with all major resource management systems now offering Read. Scotland have adopted the Read Codes as the standard medical coding system across all sectors of the Health Service in that country, and all the major medical audit systems either have adopted or are about to adopt the Codes.

2.1 Changing the culture and the National Health Service Reforms

The advantage of the Read Codes is that they are designed BY clinicians, and FOR clinicians. Thus clinical information recording can be primary, with use for management purposes being a secondary application 'piggy backed' onto the clinical information system. This is part of the 'cultural' change that is taking place in the NHS at the moment, primed by the Resource Management Initiative, and carried along by the NHS Reforms. But if it is to succeed it must involve clinicians being responsible at both ends of the information line - as COLLECTORS of data, and as USERS of that data. In this sense, hospital clinicians are following the same path that GPs have been travelling along for some time now.

2.2 Data interchange

Read Codes are also vital for data exchange between primary and secondary care. In the not too distant future, GPs will be sending Read-coded data to hospitals as part of the referral process, and Fund Holding practices will be expecting to be able to cost and assess care based on Read Codes recorded by the hospital. For this reason, all sectors of the NHS will need to standardise their clinical language for the electronic communication of data.

The Read Codes look set to become the standard nomenclature for communicating within the NHS, a view shared by Radford and Wallace(3) in a recent review of coding systems.

> "It seems likely that the Read system will become the standard medical classification system for national use, and as such will become the mainstay of clinical information services both for clinicians and hospital management. The benefits of this should then be seen in terms of better hospital records, better patient care, and better statistics for research, planning, audit and resource management. It is vital that hospital information systems currently under development around the country take account of it."

3. New Developments

3.1 Coding Developments and Clinical Specialties

The new NHS Centre for Coding and Classification (CCC) has major ongoing work to maintain the Read Codes. Each month the drug and appliance codes are updated as are the other chapters to take into account user feedback.

Some chapters are undergoing major redevelopment, particularly where the take-up in the hospital sector is resulting in new requirements from clinical specialties. The CCC is now working with national groups of most of the specialties. The aim is for each group to make sure that the terms and synonyms they require are defined and included in the Read Codes. For many of these specialties a 'specialty flag' is being linked to their terms in the Read Code database for use by them as a dictionary, for example for audit.

Work is also underway with paramedical groups such as the Chartered Society of Physiotherapists, Dieticians and the Disablement Services Agency.

3.2 Technical Developments

A key feature of the Read Codes is that they are a dynamic system, being updated at frequent intervals. To this end, users can submit requests for new codes or synonyms for processing by the NHS CCC. If accepted they are distributed with the next set of Release disks. From early in 1991 the new releases will be available as a file of additions and changes (Read Codes are never deleted, they can only become inactive, if for example a drug is withdrawn). In addition each user licence will have a unique serial number and each Read Code update will have a unique code to denote the version.

Early in 1991 a new file structure is also being introduced. This contains some important new fields. The medical terms will be offered in three different length fields, 30, 60 and 198 characters. A 'specialty flag', to denote a code as a member of specialty subset, will be included, and a 'language field', to support the automatic translation into other languages, will be introduced.

The 'key' (usually part of a term or an abbreviation for the term) which is to search for a term and its Read Code will be extended form 4 to 10 character in length.

A 'term code' field will also be introduced. This will enable the system to store a unique reference to the language with which the user chose to select a term (eg a common synonym such as **heart attack**), so that when the code is output, for example in a discharge letter, the original language of the clinician can be preserved.

4. The Future

The Read Codes are more and more evolving essentially into a coded nomenclature of medicine, each term having a unique code identifier for transmission purposes, that provides a 'gateway' to enable each user to reconstruct the data received or stored into the format of every other system to which the nomenclature is cross-referenced - including other languages. The Read Codes are, or will be by 1992, cross-referenced to every other commonly-accepted classification system used in the NHS.

The incorporation of ICD-10 and the appropriate mappings will be in place in time for the 1993 release and every system using the Read Codes will have no work to do to incorporate the change - they will merely receive and load the new mapping field.

Moreover, by 1993, the Read Codes will be in a position to support all medical implementations within the NHS, including all feeder systems.

We could have a truly common vehicle not only for communicating clinical information throughout the National Health Service in the United Kingdom, but also throughout the world.

Projects are planned or underway for collaboration in many standards initiatives in the EEC, the Nordic countries, Canada, Australia and New Zealand. The introduction of the Read Codes into all of these countries is also being discussed with the relevant professional and governmental bodies.

REFERENCES

1. Chisholm R. The Read Clinical Classification. British Medical Journal 1990; 300: 1092

2. Pringle M. The new agenda for general practice computing. British Medical Journal 1990; 301: 827

3. Radford P, Wallace A. The code war. British Journal of Healthcare Computing 1990; 7 (Nov): 22-4

Towards a European Classification of Procedures in Medicine (ECPM) - AIM-SESAME and the Dutch and German Approach -

Rudolf Thurmayr[1] and Bernd Graubner[2]

[1]Institut für Medizinische Statistik und Epidemiologie (kommissar. Direktor: Prof. Dr. R. Thurmayr), Technische Universität München, Ismaninger Str. 22, D-8000 München 80
[2]Abteilung Medizinische Informatik (Vorsteher: Prof. Dr. C.-Th. Ehlers), Georg-August-Universität, Robert-Koch-Str. 40, D-3400 Göttingen

Summary

The SESAME project, a part of the AIM programme, surveyed existing procedures and results of standardization on semantical aspects in the fields of primary health care, medical procedures and drugs. In Germany the ICD-9 is obligatory e. g. for the coding of causes of death, or in hospitals, for the coding of diagnoses. On the other hand in Germany and in the German speaking countries no single classification is used for the coding of medical procedures. On the basis of the preliminary work of SESAME, the Working Group on Surgery of the German Society of Medical Documentation, Informatics and Statistics (GMDS) proposed the translation and adaptation of the 1990 Dutch Extension (ICPM-DE) of the International Classification of Procedures in Medicine (ICPM), originally published by WHO in 1978, and using this for the German general classification of medical procedures. The Dutch authors consented to the German translation, the first version of which is now available. The Working Group expects this to be the first step in Germany towards a European Classification of Procedures in Medicine (ECPM). Its structure is one of the tasks in the draft workplan of the Technical Committee 251 on Medical Informatics (TC 251) of the European Committee for Standardization (CEN) and also a suggested proposal for an AIM main phase project (European Classification of Medical Procedures [Euclamep]). The paper discusses some of the international and German classifications of medical procedures and concentrates on the actual German development. In our opinion, the Dutch ICPM-DE is actually the best choice for Middle European purposes. To avoid further self-made developments in this field in Germany it would be useful, if the government or at least scientific bodies, would strongly recommend using in general for medical documentation a single classification of medical procedures.

1. Approaches towards a standardized classification of medical procedures within the European Communities

The Commission of the European Communities planned the programme "Advanced Informatics in Medicine" (AIM) for strengthening Medical Informatics. The preliminary phase was during 1989/90, and the decision to establish the main phase is expected in 1991. One of the basic projects of this programme was the project A 1031 "Standardization in Europe on Semantical Aspects of Medicine (SESAME)" managed by Pieter F. DE VRIES ROBBÉ, NRV/WCC Zoetermeer and University of Groningen/The Netherlands (now: University of Nijmegen). Co-workers came from Germany, Italy, the Netherlands and the United Kingdom [1].

The special aim of the SESAME project is to develop a standardization framework. A first step was to collect, analyze and compare some existing classifications in the fields of primary health care, medical procedures and drugs. The following issues were prepared for each topic: a list of existing classifications, criteria for selection of the most important classifications, criteria for their evaluation, proposals of universal structures for classifications in these fields and mapping of selected classifications with this structure.

This paper focuses on classifications of procedures in medicine because an international accepted classification of procedures (especially of surgical operations), beside the International Classification of Diseases (ICD) as the world classification of diagnoses, is of prime importance for medical documentation. The result of SESAME in this area was a list of 13 classifications of medical procedures. Seven of them were selected for extensive evaluation. These are ([1]: Deliverables 3 and 6):

1. Catalogue des Actes Medicaux (CDAM). (France, Le Ministere des Affaires Sociale et de l'Emploi. French, 1987),
2. Classification of Surgical Operations and Procedures. 4th Revision (OPCS-4). (United Kingdom, Office of Population Censuses and Surveys. English, 1990),
3. International Classification of Diseases. 9th Revision. Clinical Modification. Volume 3: Procedures (ICD-9-CM Procedure Classification). (USA, Department of Health and Human Services, Health Care Financing Administration. English, 1990),
4. Nordic Operation List. (Scandinavian countries, Nordic Medico-Statistical Committee [NOMESCO], Copenhagen. English, 1989),
5. READ Clinical Classification (RCC). (United Kingdom, J. READ / National Health Service Centre for Coding and Classification. English, 1990),
6. VESKA-Operationsschlüssel 1986. (Switzerland, Vereinigung Schweizerischer Krankenhäuser (VESKA). German and French, 1986),
7. WCC-standaardclassificatie van medisch specialistische verrichtingen. (The Netherlands, Nationale Raad voor de Volksgezondheid, Werkgroep Classificatie en Coderingen [NRV, WCC]. Dutch, 1990). Its English name is ICPM-DE (= Dutch Extension), because this classification is mainly based upon the International Classification of Procedures in Medicine (ICPM), published by WHO in 1978. (The ICPM-DE was selected in SESAME instead of the original ICPM, as today the latter does not represent the state of art.)

Because of its restrictive or extensive contents and also because of a lack of labour and time, only short evaluations were given for the following two classifications:

8. Manual for Laboratory Workload Recording Method. (USA, College of American Pathologists. English, 1989),
9. Systematized Nomenclature of Medicine (SNOMED). (USA, R. CÔTÉ / College of American Pathologists. English, 1986. German translation [F. WINGERT], 1984).

The "International Classification of Clinical Services (ICCS)", published 1990 in the USA by the Commission on Personal and Hospital Activities, could not be taken into consideration in SESAME because it was available only when most of the other work was finished. This classification is designed for most of the hospital procedures outside the operation room and will form a substantial contribution to the further development in this field. Classifications which are not in use outside its country of origin or developed only for financial purposes were excluded (see some German examples in paragraphs 2.2 and 2.3).

ICD-9-CM Procedure Classification [10] is a modification of chapter "5. Surgical procedures" of ICPM [11] and was also used for the preparation of the ICPM-DE ([1]: Del. 3 and 6]). The Dutch ICPM-DE [18] is derived from ICPM too, from which in the actual version the chapters "1. Procedures for medical diagnosis", "8. Other therapeutic procedures" and especially the already mentioned "5." were translated, adjusted and updated. In addition, some classes were also selected from "4. Preventive procedures" (contraceptive measures only) and "9. Ancillary procedures". The figures of 3, 4, 5 and 6 digit code numbers in the several chapters can give an information about the scope of the ICPM-DE: chapter 1: 1 106 codes, chapter 4: 6 codes, chapter 5: 5 568 codes, chapter 8: 838 codes and chapter 9: 75 codes; the total is 7 593 codes (not counting codes for variable use, e. g. in addition to codes from 5-760 to 5-859 for topography).

Some examples of "appendectomy" will attempt to give an impression of the most important classifications discussed here (the more extended examples see in [9]):

ICPM (1978):
 5-47 Operations on appendix
 5-470 Appendectomy (includes: Appendectomy with drainage)
 5-471 Drainage of appendix abscess

ICD-9-CM Procedure Classification (1989):
 47 Operations on appendix
 47.0 Appendectomy
 47.1 Incidental appendectomy
 47.2 Drainage on appendiceal abscess (excludes: that with appendectomy [47.0])

ICPM-DE: WCC-standaardclassificatie van medisch specialistische verrichtingen (1990):
 5-47 Operatieve verrichtingen aan appendix
 5-470 Appendectomie
 5-470.0 appendectomie via wisselsnede
 5-470.1 appendectomie via mediane laparotomie
 5-470.2 appendectomie incidenteel, tijdens laparotomie om andere redenen
 5-470.9 niet gespecificeerde appendectomie
 5-471 Incisie en drainage van appendiculair abces

First draft of the German translation of the ICPM-DE (1991):
 5-47 Operationen an der Appendix
 5-470 Appendektomie
 5-470.0 Appendektomie mit Wechselschnitt
 5-470.1 Appendektomie durch mediane Laparotomie
 5-470.2 Gelegenheitsappendektomie während einer Laparotomie aus anderen Gründen
 5-470.3 Appendektomie mit Pararektalschnitt
 5-470.9 nicht näher bezeichnete Appendektomie
 5-471 Inzision und Drainage eines Appendixabszesses

VESKA-Operationsschlüssel 1986:
 380 Appendektomie
 380.0 Abszess-Drainage
 380.1 Gelegenheitsappendektomie

Operativer Therapieschlüssel (SCHEIBE / THURMAYR, 1990):
 In the "special part" combination of the extended code of topography 4868 (= appendix) with
     one of the following procedures (example: 48689 Appendektomie o.n.A.):
 ....0 Darmoperation o.n.A. [= ohne nähere Angabe]
 ....1 Enterotomie
 ...
 ....9 Radikaloperation, Exstirpation, Ektomie eines Darmabschnittes

2. The situation in the field of German classifications of procedures in medicine

The use of the International Classification of Diseases (ICD) is obligatory in Germany for mortality statistics and some morbidity statistics. It is mandatory for the annual hospital statistics on
diagnoses since 1968 in the former German Democratic Republic and since 1986 in the old
Federal Republic of Germany [12]. In contrast to this no single classification of medical procedures is in use. The following two classifications are used only in some hospitals in Germany,
Austria and Switzerland.

2.1 VESKA-Operationsschlüssel 1986 (Code of operations)

The Swiss VESKA-Operationsschlüssel was introduced in 1972 and is available since 1986 in its
third revision in German and French ([13], [1]: Del. 6). All Swiss hospital departments participating in the VESKA operations documentation and statistics and some hospitals in the Federal
Republic of Germany, in Austria and in France use this classification. During the last years a co-

operation of VESKA with the I&D Company in Berlin started, among others with the intention of implementing the VESKA-Operationsschlüssel in the ID DIACOS programmes for semiautomatic encoding of textstrings (available in 1991). The VESKA-Operationsschlüssel contains nearly 3000 code numbers and covers nearly all relevant surgical and anaesthetic procedures for indexing of medical records. The code which is numeric only has the same structure as the ICD-8 or ICD-9 code: three digits and one decimal digit. A second decimal digit is used only for the more detailed localization of bone operations. The first 10 chapters are classified by topography, only chapter 11 (Anaesthesia, resuscitation) is classified by the type of procedure performed. Quite often, the four digit subcategories are not specified sufficiently, so that the users themselves have to classify a certain operation. Only few nonsurgical procedures are present. - The VESKA-Operationsschlüssel is intended for medical documentation, in Switzerland other lists are in use for billing purposes.

2.2 Operativer Therapieschlüssel (Code of surgical therapies) of O. SCHEIBE

The classification of surgical procedures of Otto SCHEIBE ("SCHEIBE classification") was published first in 1961. The second edition [14] was published in 1982 by the Working Group on Surgery of the German Society of Medical Documentation, Informatics and Statistics (GMDS) under the responsibility of R. THURMAYR. The numerical code consists of 6 digits. The first 3 digits are strictly formed according to the topography of the human body (e. g. vessels, nerves, bones, soft tissue; = "general part" of the classification), whereas the second three digits (4-6) indicate the type of procedure performed. The user has to combine the codes of topography and of the type of procedure like facets. In this general part 420 topography and 260 procedure codes can be combined theoretically. In contrast to this, in the field of organ systems (e. g. digestive, urinary or genital system) each organ has its own classification of procedures, formed with the digits 4 - 6. In this "special part" the 5 or 6 digit codes are fixed. The special part contains 2 374 codes (not counting the distinction of right and left). Because of its high differentiation this classification is used only in some more scientifically interested hospitals.

2.3 Other German classifications of medical procedures

Two classifications are derived from the SCHEIBE classification. The "Bad Godesberger Schlüsselsystem" [2] stopped using the possibility of combining codes in the common part of the SCHEIBE classification, thus avoiding errors caused by combining. The "Nürnberger Schlüsselsystem" [16] eliminated the distinction of the right and the left side. This and the removal of procedures seldom performed shortened it to a more handy classification. Several hospitals and a few scientific medical societies use other self-made classifications, and in most cases there are no connections between these solutions (references e. g. in [3] and [12]).

Beside this, some other lists are available for financial purposes, but they are not so well suited for medical aspects due to their other principles of classification and their often very detailed description of single activities. Nevertheless, some hospitals use these "classifications" for documentation as they cause no additional workload because these codes are collected for accounting first. These lists are namely: "Gebührenordnung für Ärzte" (GOÄ, 1988 [7]), "Tarif der Deutschen Krankenhausgesellschaft für die Abrechnung erbrachter Leistungen ..." (DKG-NT, 1990 [17]), "Bewertungsmaßstab für kassenärztliche Leistungen" (BMÄ, 1990 [4]) and "Ersatzkassen-Gebührenordnung" (E-GO, 1990 [6]). (GOÄ and DKG-NT on the one hand and BMÄ and E-GO on the other hand are more or less compatible but have different functions.)

The situation in Austria is similar to that in Germany. Beside lists for financial purposes, the already mentioned classifications and separately developed classifications are in use (e. g. [5]).

In summary no single classification of medical procedures is used in Germany nor in the German speaking countries. The internationally recommended ICPM was only introduced in parts in the former German Democratic Republic, where a German translation, revision and enlargement of most parts of its chapter 5 (= surgical operations) and some other chapters is used in nearly 50 hospitals.

The situation in this field in the old Federal Republic of Germany is shown in an inquiry within the GMDS Working Group on Surgery in 1989: 4 hospitals used the VESKA-Operationsschlüssel, 4 the SCHEIBE classification and 8 had developed their own classification. It can be summarized, that the VESKA-Operationsschlüssel is more suitable for practicioners and the SCHEIBE classification more for scientists. Actually, there is no German classification of medical procedures which can be used for both purposes, that means especially with more rough short codes on the one side and with detailed extended codes on the other side.

3. Actual standardization activities in Germany

The situation already described in the field of classifications of medical procedures in the German speaking countries forces activities towards standardization. We are convinced that there is no need for a new classification, but rather for the adoption of an international standard. The preliminary work of SESAME has given detailed references to the appropriate classification.

The ICPM-DE, since 1990 obligatory for all Dutch hospitals, combines the advantages of ICPM and ICD-9-CM Procedure Classification and reflects the present Middle European standard in medical science and practice in the best way. This classification offers the possibility of coding on different levels, is very specified and includes also non-surgical procedures.

The GMDS Working Group on Surgery, which is mainly formed by interested physicians, decided therefore in 1990 to translate and adopt the ICPM-DE and to publish a German draft. The first version of this draft was distributed in December 1990 and discussed first in April 1991. The Dutch colleagues are very interested in a co-operation. The VESKA demonstrated its interest too. The I&D Company in Berlin also intends to use this classification in its semi-automatic encoding system ID DIACOS, and the first demonstration in April 1991 looked hopeful.

The Working Group is convinced that the chance will grow to introduce a single classification of medical procedures in Germany. This is the precondition that medical statistics will become more comparable at the national and international level. Finally, this German effort may contribute to the target of a European Classification of Procedures in Medicine (ECPM). The structure of such a classification is one point in the draft workplan of the newly established Technical Committee 251 on Medical Informatics (TC 251) of the European Committee for Standardization (CEN) and is also a suggested proposal for an AIM main phase project (European Classification of Medical Procedures [Euclamep]) ([1]: Del. 22 and Executive Summary].

4. Discussion

Most comments on the first German draft of February 1991 welcome the translation and stress the good opportunity to come to a standard classification of medical procedures in Germany. There is some criticism of the structure which has mainly to be discussed with the Dutch originators and is indeed to some extend already under discussion among them. This refers to the original structure of ICPM, but also to the enlarged structure of the ICPM-DE. Some areas are very specified, e. g. vessels, other fields are rather small or insufficient, e. g. procedures in Orthopedics or the differentiation of forearm and hand. The differentiation between uni- and bilateral is not carried out consequently and should be better coded, separately if necessary. The topography in the field of fractures should be more homogeneous. The differentiation between biopsy with and without incision is rather irrelevant and causes confusion. Some codes of the original ICPM are missing, e. g. 5-05 and 5-190, but this may be only an editorial problem or is caused by an other structure of the ICPM-DE in details.

It is always necessary to find a good compromise between the diverging meanings of the different experts. It would be better to prepare enlarged and differentiated compatible extracts of the classification for or within the several medical specialities, than to swell up the whole classification to an unwieldy book for all users.

It is very useful that the ICPM-DE is limited to procedures and does not also contain indications and diagnoses. Procedures which usually are named as eponyms are explained or the proper name is set in parentheses, thus they are also understandable at international level (e. g. "5-437.0 partiële gastroduodenectomie volgens BILLROTH II" or "5-433 Pyloromyotomie [RAMSTEDT-WEBER operatie])". The alphabetic index is only available in the form of the more commercial SIG edition of both the Tabular List and the Alphabetic Index [18]. It could be advantageous to have one body responsible for both.

A classification of medical procedures needs to be updated in short intervals of one or two years. Because the World Health Organization was not able to do this for the ICPM, WHO has still not decided to publish a second version. A very short classification with 100 - 200 classes is planned in future [15] and for this a conversion table into and from the ICPM should be prepared. Since the Dutch ICPM-DE has no fixed revision cycle and the last update was in 1989, it is not surprising that German experts found some obsolete procedures and made proposals for some recently created procedures. Further updates could become a joint task of Dutch and German scientists.

To avoid further self-made developments in this field in Germany it would be useful, if the government or at least scientific bodies [8], would strongly recommend using in general for medical documentation a single classification of medical procedures (similar to the introduction of the ICD-9 in clinical documentation by the "Bundespflegesatzverordnung" of 1985 [12]).

5. Conclusions

In our opinion, from all discussed and available classifications of medical and especially surgical procedures the Dutch ICPM-DE is actually the best choice for Middle European purposes. The lively discussion about the German draft elucidates a strong interest in an international accepted classification of medical procedures in Germany. The GMDS Working Group on Surgery forces their efforts towards the German translation and adaptation of the ICPM-DE and finally its introduction in medical documentation. Further comments and co-operation are welcome by the Working Group and specially by the authors of this paper.

References

[1] AIM project No. A 1031: Standardization in Europe on Semantical Aspects of Medicine (SESAME). 1989/90. All documents ("Deliverables") are available by the projectmanager Prof. Dr. Pieter de Vries Robbé, Dept. of Medical Informatics and Epidemiology, University of Nijmegen, P.O.Box 9101, NL-6500 HB Nijmegen (formerly: Groningen). The following deliverables are of special importance: 13 (Standardization framework in Europe, code of practice for standardization, vocabulary), 17 (Proposal for national standardization organizations on medical terminology and classifications [with an overlook about concerning institutions and persons within the 12 EC-countries]), 22 (Outline for an AIM main phase program on semantical aspects of medicine), Executive summary. The deliverables 3, 6, 10 and 15 relate to classifications of medical procedures: 3 (evaluation criteria and a list of classifications), 6 (evaluation), 10 (structure) and 15 (mapping).
[2] Bad Godesberger Schlüsselsystem: R. Haunhorst: Entwicklung von Schlüsselsystemen für Diagnosen, Komplikationen und Therapien. Medizinische Dissertation, Universität Bonn. 1990. 3 Volumes. - Dr. R. Schunck, Ev. Krankenhaus Siloah, Wilferdinger Str., D-7530 Pforzheim.
[3] Basiswissen ICD-9 für Morbiditätsstatistiken: mit Übungen. Ed. by DIMDI. Prep. by Elisabeth Berg-Schorn. Köln etc.: Kohlhammer. 1989. 69 pp. (pages 54-66: survey about editions of ICD-9 and other classifications).
[4] Bewertungsmaßstab für kassenärztliche Leistungen (BMÄ). Stand 1.7.1990. Ed. by Kassenärztliche Bundesvereinigung. Köln: Deutscher Ärzte-Verlag. 1990. 284 pp. (loose-leaf ring binder).

[5] CHIDOS Chirurgisches Dokumentationssystem. Maria Anna Puchner EDV-Organisation, Ehrenfelsgasse 14, A-1120 Wien (more than 30 installations are reported; the classification of medical procedures in the "Schlüsselbuch" is an enlarged VESKA-Operationsschlüssel).

[6] Ersatzkassen-Gebührenordnung (E-GO). Stand 1.7.1990. Ed. by Kassenärztliche Bundesvereinigung. Köln: Deutscher Ärzte-Verlag. 1990. 286 pp. (loose-leaf ring binder).

[7] Gebührenordnung für Ärzte (GOA 88) mit Gebührenverzeichnis für ärztliche Leistungen. Stand: 1.7.1988. Köln: Deutscher Ärzte-Verlag. 1988. 301 pp.

[8] GMDS-Memorandum zum Aufbau und Betrieb eines medizinischen Klassifikationszentrums. Ed. by R. Klar. In co-operation with B. Graubner, J. Michaelis, R. Repges and H. E. Wichmann. Stuttgart, New York: Schattauer. 1991. (Schriftenreihe der Deutschen Gesellschaft für Medizinische Dokumentation, Informatik und Statistik e. V.) In press.

[9] Graubner, B. and R. Klar: Standardisierung medizinischer Klassifikationen in Europa und Deutschland. In: Quantitative Methoden in der Epidemiologie. Proceedings of the 35th Annual Meeting of GMDS. Berlin, September 1990. Ed. by Irene Guggenmoos-Holzmann et al. Berlin, Heidelberg, New York etc.: Springer. 1991. (Medizinische Informatik und Statistik.) In press.

[10] International Classification of Diseases. 9th Revision. Clinical Modification (ICD-9-CM). Vol. 3: Procedures. Tabular List and Alphabetic Index. Ed. by Health Care Financing Administration, Department of Health and Human Services. 3rd ed. 1988, annual addenda. Washington, D.C. 20402-9371: Superintendent of Documents, U.S. Government Printing Office. XXIX, 519 pp. (loose-leaf ring binder). - Parallel edition by the American Medical Record Association (AMRA), P.O.Box 97349, Chicago, IL 60690-7349.

[11] International Classification of Procedures in Medicine (ICPM). Published for trial purposes in accordance with resolution WHA29.35 of the Twenty-ninth World Health Assembly, May 1976. Geneva: World Health Organization. 1978. Vol 1: 1. Procedures for medical diagnosis. 2. Laboratory procedures. 4. Preventive procedures. 5. Surgical procedures. 8. Other therapeutic procedures. 9. Ancillary procedures. IX, 310 pp. Vol. 2: 3. Radiology and certain other applications of physics in medicine. 6. & 7. Drugs, medicaments, and biological agents. V, 147 pp.

[12] Klar, R., B. Graubner and C.-Th. Ehlers: Leitfaden zur Erstellung der Diagnosenstatistik nach § 16 Bundespflegesatzverordnung (BPflV). In co-operation with R. Hartwig, Barbara Schmidt-Rettig, H.-J. Seelos and S. Eichhorn. Ed. by Der Bundesminister für Arbeit und Sozialordnung (BMA). 2nd, rev. ed. Bonn: BMA. 1988. 105 pp. (Forschungsbericht Gesundheitsforschung. 135.). - Reprint in: Internationale Klassifikation der Krankheiten, Verletzungen und Todesursachen (ICD), 9. Revision. 2nd, rev. ed. Köln etc.: Kohlhammer. 1988. Vol. I part A, pages 651-762. - Actualized reprint in: Medizinische Dokumentation und Information. Handbuch für Klinik und Praxis. Ed. by C. O. Köhler. Landsberg/Lech: ecomed. 1983 ff. 9th suppl.: 1989. Chapter X-3.3.3, pages 1-104.

[13] Operationsschlüssel 1986. Ed. by Vereinigung Schweizerischer Krankenhäuser (VESKA), Kommission für medizinische Statistik und Dokumentation. Prep. by Jana Stutz, M. Steck, H. Ehrengruber and I. Balmer. Aarau: VESKA. 1986. 72, 34 pp. (loose-leaf ring binder).

[14] Operativer Therapieschlüssel. Zusammengestellt von O. Scheibe. 2nd ed., rev. 1990. Ed. by Arbeitskreis Chirurgie der Deutschen Gesellschaft für Medizinische Dokumentation, Informatik und Statistik. Chairman: R. Thurmayr, München. 83 pp. (Available from Prof. Dr. Rudolf Thurmayr, Institut für Medizinische Statistik und Epidemiologie der Technischen Universität München, Ismaninger Str. 22, D-8000 München 80, tel. +49.89/41404320.)

[15] Proposal of Procedures. Presented by DES Unit of the World Health Organization at the Meeting of Heads of WHO Collaborating Centres for the classification of diseases, Paris, 28.2.-7.3.1989. 26 pp. (DES/ICD/C/89.23).

[16] Remmel, E.: Ein topographisch-hierarchisches Schlüsselsystem zur Verschlüsselung chirurgischer Diagnosen, Therapien und Komplikationen. Special issue "EDV in der Orthopädie" of the journal "Orthopäde" (Berlin) 1991 [(n press). - This "Nürnberger Schlüsselsystem" is implemented in the system "ratiodoc" of Grün-Data Gesellschaft für Datentechnik mbH, Gustavstr. 16, D-8510 Fürth.

[17] Tarif der Deutschen Krankenhausgesellschaft für die Abrechnung erbrachter Leistungen und für die Kostenerstattung vom Arzt an das Krankenhaus (DKG-NT), zugleich vereinbarter Tarif für die Abrechnung mit den gesetzlichen Unfallversicherungsträgern (BG-T). Stand: 1.7.1990. Stuttgart: Kohlhammer. 1990. 318 pp. (loose-leaf ring binder).

[18] WCC-standaardclassificatie van medisch specialistische verrichtingen (ICPM-DE [see text above, paragraph 1]). Ed. by Nationale Raad voor de Volksgezondheid (NRV), Werkgroep Classificatie en Coderingen (WCC) [Postbus 7100, NL-2701 AC Zoetermeer, tel. +31.79/517644]. Version 2.0. 1990. 241 pp. (Tabular List only. An edition with Tabular List and Alphabetic Index was edited by Stichting Informatiecentrum voor de Gezondheidszorg [SIG], Postbus 14066, NL-3508 SC Utrecht, tel. +31.30/345611.) - English translation of the introduction to this classification in: Annual Report 1989 of WCC, Dutch classification and terminology committee for health. Zoetermeer, 1990, pages 28-32. Report on the further work in: Annual Report 1990 etc. (edited 1991), pages 12-14. - German translation of the classification: First draft, prepared by R. Thurmayr. 1990/91. 173 pp. (address see [12]).

Acknowledgement

Parts of this work were supported by the Commission of the European Communities: AIM Project Number A 1031 (SESAME). The authors also wish to thank the Werkgroep Classificatie en Coderingen (WCC) of the Dutch Nationale Raad voor de Volksgezondheid (NRV) and especially Prof. Dr. Pieter F. de Vries Robbé and Dr. Willem Hirs.

A MULTIAXIAL MODEL FOR THE DESCRIPTION OF MEDICO-SURGICAL PROCEDURES

Burgun A., Le Beux P., Lenoir P.
Département d'information Médicale
CHRU Pontchaillou
35033 RENNES CEDEX

SUMMARY

Nomenclature management is essential for the analysis of medical data. A multiaxial model gives a flexible tool to represent medical terms and we applied this method to the medical procedure classification used in France for the standardized medical summaries

INTRODUCTION

The University Hospital of Rennes has developped for the last ten years an integrated data base system for medical record summaries called RMS (1). This system is able to produce automatically standardized medical summaries used for the DRG classification (2).
It is connected with a RSS/DRG system based on a UNIX sub system using a relational data base . Specific tables in this data base describe the nomenclatures used by the archivists staff. Diagnosis are coded using the ICD 9 (3) . A French specific procedure classification. : the CDAM (4) has been built under the management of the Ministry of Health in order to:
- compensate for the lack of precision and exhaustiveness of the ICD-9 and the NGAP (5) which was designed in France and used to reimburse treatments by the insurance and thus is not well-adapted to the description of medical activity.
- evaluate the cost of each procedure in terms of human and material resources.

The Department of Medical Information needs a flexible and easy to use tool for nomenclature management and it is obvious that decisions about nomenclature building and data representation are crucial determiners of the capabilities and performance of the system (6).

Two main types of nomenclature structures can be considered :

- <u>classifications</u> which are tree-structured nomenclatures . An element of a classification represents a complex object : a disease (ICD9) or a medical procedure (CDAM) and objects are linked together by arbitrarily defined hierarchical relations . The relation between a node of the tree and its children may represent for example precisions about the anatomic site, or precisions about the physiological mecanism, or precisions about the etiology . Despite the fact that all these relations are "isa" links, they are quite different when they are regarded as semantic links.

- <u>multidimensional nomenclatures</u> based on a decomposition into fields that must reflect as well as possible the dimensions of medical concepts according to a semantic structure . SNOMED (7) is an example of such a lexicon and studies of automated indexing based on SNOMED have been performed (8,9).

It should also be noted that the National Library of Medicine has initiated the Unified Medical Language System (UMLS) project to develop methods to facilitate automatic translation of medical terms from one vocabulary into another (10) . Thus it will facilitate integration of information from a variety of information sources (biomedical litterature, clinical records databases, medical knowledge bases) using disparate vocabularies .

A standard way of representing medical terms using semantic description has been proposed (11) and international standardization efforts are currently undertaken in the US and Europe.(12)

Other works such as the Linguistic String Project (13) are applied for converting narrative portions of patients records into structured form for code enhancement.

In this context, our aim is to study and improve nomenclature management using a multiaxial representation of medical procedures. We may emphasize that we incorporate specific French nomenclature and classification using a French dictionary interface designed for the consultation of the large medical knowledge base called ADM (14) that has been developed in the laboratory .

THE STRUCTURE OF THE CDAM

The general structure

This classification has been designed by the French Ministry of Health in 1985, in order to have a more precise classification of medical or surgical procedures to be used by all the hospital medical information departments in the country.

This nomenclature contains seven fields:
- ALPHA = diagnostic and therapeutic procedures (surgery, endoscopy...)
- BETA : Anesthesia
- GAMMA : Imaging
- MU : Radiotherapy
- RHO : Pathology
- TO : Laboratory
- OMEGA : Intensive care.

The current study only concerns the first field which is the most important for DRG grouping. A hierarchical model is used to describe each field.

The ALPHA field is made up of seventeen chapters which represent either physiological systems (e.g. nervous system) or specialities (e.g. obstetrics). Inside each chapter, elements are usually arranged first by topography (organ) and then by method or technique applied for the procedure.
But these rules are not always enforced : for example under "Urinary system" we can find "Endoscopy" or under "Obstetrics" we can find "Pregnancy".

The representation of the objects in the CDAM

An element of the CDAM is referenced by a unique alphanumeric code which has no significance related with its place in the tree-structured nomenclature.
An object is supposed to have a unique place in a classification. In fact, we have to adopt a poly-hierarchical organization : a concept, which is represented by a node of the tree structure may be related to more than one parent term. For example some procedures concerning the spinal column may be members of the chapter "musculoskeletal system" or members of the chapter "nervous system".

Two types of procedures can be identified : elementary procedures and complex procedures.

As we choose to describe procedures using a multiaxial approach based on four classes : TOPOGRAPHY, METHOD, DISEASE and TECHNIQUE, we define an elementary treatment as made up of at most one component belonging to each axis, the METHOD class attribute being mandatory.

A complex procedure is composed of several elementary procedures : for example "peritoneoscopy with guided transhepatic cholangiography with biopsy" .

The computerized management of complex objects can be implemented :
- inside axis management but it would imply that the contents of each axis had been defined so that any nomenclature could refer to it.
- by specific tables in each nomenclature management subsystem.

As we used a relational data base model to manage the nomenclatures, this last solution was easier to implement, and consequently we chose it.

A MULTIAXIAL MODEL FOR PROCEDURES

The nomenclature is partitionned into lists which represent a semantic categorization of the terms and each list is structured according to semantic links between its components.

An element of a class represents a single information unit, an elementary concept: for example "ectomy" or "oesophagus".

A procedure is defined by its attribute values and ought not to inherit keywords from his father in the nomenclature tree if the structure of the axis contains this property.

With such a model, it is possible to execute either a query which appears to be simple and/or global (e.g. all the endoscopies) or a very specific one which is supposed to bring an accurate answer.

By using such a structure, it becomes very easy to add a new term.

But these advantages are balanced by a tedious indexing process for a human user ; so we will try to extract the attribute values of medical procedures using an automatic and computer aided method from keywords which are kept out from the utterances by the existing ADM dictionary and thesaurus programs.

Choosing the axis

A review of the procedures in CDAM showed that they can be described by two main features : the method applied (insertion, destruction...) and the topography. We added two axes : "diseases" and "technique" (electrocoagulation...)

We found a lot of problems to represent the temporal dimension : for example the treatment of recurrent diseases, a sequence of treatments.....

Instead of creating an axis " temporal description", we shall try to reconsider this problem at an upper "aggregation level" by adding a column "link attribute" in the table which describes complex procedures.

Some other semantic components of a procedure might be identified such as patient characteristics for example . As probably each of such classes may be made of few elements, we decided to manage these information categories by a comprehensive method which considers keywords related with the ADM dictionary.

Another problem is that, at the first sight, one concept could belong to one semantic category or another. The variety of points of view suggests that natural semantic categories, even in such a small area, are not juxtaposed but partly surimposed one on another.

For example if we consider the procedure "treatment X by endoscopy"
- if endoscopy belongs to the field METHOD this procedure will be defined as the association of two basic procedures : "treatment X" and "endoscopy".
- if it belongs to the field "TECHNIQUE" this procedure is an elementary one.

In a multiaxial model, one term must appear in only one class but its definition may include a notion from another category. For example, we could describe cross references between DISEASE and TOPOGRAPHY such as relations between "hiatus hernia" and "stomach".

The description of the links between semantic types should require the definition of a semantic network.

Representation of the axis.

We have to define the best representation for each class according to the links between its related terms and the computerized tasks we want to implement.

We considered first the topography field and defined a polyhierarchical model describing the two usual representations for anatomy : classification by systems and classification by anatomic areas.

Thus, one element of the topography field is related with two elements of the upper level : one link represents the fact that it is a member of a system and the other one the fact that it is a part of an anatomic area or is related with an organ (vascular elements).

With the aim of a partially automatic extraction of the attributes of a medical procedure, the problem of synonymy should be treated by integrating a morpholexical analysis module into the ADM dictionary program. The problem consists in studying the minimal meaningful units which can be words or morphemes together with the synonymy relations between them and the arrangement of morphemes in formation of terms, that produces French utterances such as "oesogastroduodenoscopie".

Polysemia is another difficulty (for example "cyst" in cystographie and cholecystectomie) which may be reduced by either defining rules of choice based on morphemes or considering context that is the place of the medical procedure in the nomenclature for topography.

Furthermore procedure utterances may be not significant such as for example "putting a sus-pubic catheter".

Another problem remains : two attribute values of a field may be necessary for describing procedures such as anastomosis or plasty and the two values have different meanings.

CONCLUSION

Despite several obstacles, it is obvious that a multiaxial approach used for constructing formal representations of medical terms brings a powerful method for nomenclature management.
It must be applied only for describing elementary medical procedures. Complex procedures have to be represented by relations in the specific nomenclature management module. These relations describe which are the basic procedures and which kind of links between them make up the complex procedure.

Only four semantic fields were defined in our multidimensional model . Other semantic categories such as patients characteristics should be required for giving this model exhaustiveness . We did not define other descriptors but considered other terms as keywords so that we can use the existing ADM dictionary interface.

A prototype based on the rules described above has been developed on MacIntosh using Oracle relational database system and HyperCard. Further efforts are needed to improve it ; however such a method is expected to be powerful.

References

1. Cornillet D., Lenoir P.
RMS documentation, CRIH Rennes, 1988

2. Fetter R.B., Shin Y., Freeman J.l., Averill R.F., Thompson J.D.
Case Mix Definition by Diagnosis Related Groups. Medical Care ,Feb.80, Vol18

3. International Classification of Diseases, ninth revision, OMS,1975

4. CDAM . Catalogue des Actes Médicaux . Direction des Hôpitaux, Ministère de la Santé , Bulletin Officiel No 87-21bis,Paris,1987

5. NGAP. Nomenclature Generale des Actes Professionnels . Union des Caisses Nationales de Sécurité Sociale, 3-1989

6. Packak M.G.,Dunham G.S.
Computers and medical language, Med. Inform.,4,1,13-27,1979

7. Systematized Nomenclature of Medicine . Second edition. Skokie , College of American Pathologists, 1979

8 . Wintgert F.,
Automated Indexing based on SNOMED, Meth. Inform. Med,24, 27-34, 1985

9 . Wingert F.,Rothwell D.,Coté R.
Automated indexing into Snomed and ICD
in Computerized natural medical language processing for knowledge representation.pp 201-239
IFIP- IMIA WG6 Sherrer J. R., Coté R.A., Mandil S. H editors North Holland 1989

10. Lindberg D. A. Humphreys B. L.
Computer systems that understand medical meaning
in Computerized natural medical language processing for knowledge representation. pp 5-17
IFIP- IMIA WG6 Sherrer J. R., Coté R.A., Mandil S. H editors North Holland 1989

11 . Cimino J.J., Barnett G.
Automated translation between medical terminologies using semantic definitions , M.D. Computing,7, 2, 104-109, 1990

12. Benson T.
The challenge of standardized terminology
in Computerized natural medical language processing for knowledge representation. pp 41-45
IFIP- IMIA WG6 Sherrer J. R., Coté R.A., Mandil S. H editors North Holland 1989

13. Lyman M.,Sager N.
The New York University Experience in the computer processing of medical language
in Computerized natural medical language processing for knowledge representation.pp 195-200
IFIP- IMIA WG6 Sherrer J. R., Coté R.A., Mandil S. H editors North Holland 1989

14. Le Beux P.,Rammal M., Burgun A., Riou C,Frangeul C.,Cador F.,Lenoir P.
"ADM:a diagnostic aid knowledge base for general practitioners"
IMIA Working Conference Medical Informatics and Medical Education.
Prague Czechoslovakia Sept 90

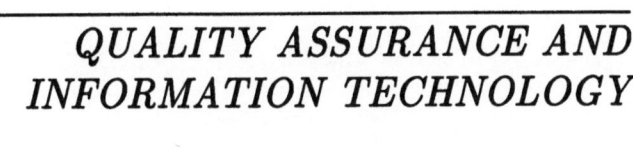

QUALITY ASSURANCE AND
INFORMATION TECHNOLOGY

HOW TO INDUCE PHYSICIANS TO ENGAGE IN QA ACTIVITIES IN A UNIVERSITY HOSPITAL ENVIRONMENT:**

Alexandra Giraud MD, MPH

Direction de la Stratégie
Assistance Publique-Hôpitaux de Paris
3, avenue Victoria, 75100 Paris RP France

Assistance Publique (AP) is a large University Hospital system that serves as a teaching hospital for Paris and the Greater Paris area. It comprises 52 hospitals, 32,000 beds and 76,630 staff among which about 11,000 physicians and 6,832 medical students. There were 71,586 admissions in 1989, 72% of which in acute care. AP's physicians are among the better known in the country. In 1987, the Director of Planning in the central management of this institution created a small Quality Assurance unit to which he entrusted the mission of developing quality assurance among AP physicians.

The Context

Contrary to other European countries like Germany, Italy and Belgium and to the United States, there is no legal or customary obligation in France for physicians to engage in quality assurance (QA). Much emphasis has nonetheless been put of late by the goverment on the importance of developing what is

---

* This paper is adapted from an article forthcoming in Quality Assurance in Health Care, 1991.

currently called *évaluation médicale,* and a new Agency was created in 1989 for the diffusion of quality assurance methodology .

Faced with the increasing costs of health care, government and management hope that QA activities will entail economic savings. The medical profession is aware of this, and being less familiar, at least in France, with the nature and scope of QA, as opposed to the constant theme of cost containment, is instinctively distrustful of any efforts to promote it, rightly suspecting governments and hospital administrations to have financial goals.

Further, developing QA in a teaching hospital context presents a number of specific difficulties. Medical university careers are built, in France as they are elsewhere, on research publications more than they are on the actual quality of the care delivered. The latter in any case is not measured, therefore not known, and not rewarded but by virtue of the dogma of medical infallibility (1) assumed by those who deliver it to be excellent. As a consequence, the intellectual interest and stimulus of physicians leans essentially towards clinical research. Further, as previously stated, the medical staff of Assistance Publique is among the most illustrious in the country. For them, quality assurance, or, stated otherwise, quality control of the care delivered seems at best superfluous.

In AP, this situation was aggravated by the fact that, as previously stated , the initiative towards developing QA came, in this instance, from the Direction of Planning of AP's central management headquarters, and not from the physicians themselves.

The elements of the context we have described shaped the policy we adopted.

The Policy

The team consisted of four members: a public health physician, acting as head; one methodologist: a practising physician experienced in clinical research; a head nurse trained in management and hygiene and one secretary.

The doctrine of the QA unit was very much inspired by that of the Netherlands' CBO (2). It consisted essentially in stressing the medical importance of QA as opposed to its possible financial benefits. Indeed we believe that stressing the possible financial benefits of QA can be misleading, since if some aspects of QA such as the review of diagnostic testing can entail savings, many other QA studies may not. We therefore tried to stress that QA had to be undertaken for medical reasons, i.e. the complexity of modern medicine, its potential dangers for patients, and the difficulty of individual medical decision-making in the face of the inflation of medical knowledge. QA, or medical evaluation as we have called it, mus be conducted for qualitative and not for quantitative reasons.

We insisted that medical evaluation be conducted by the physicians themselves, based on the model of **peer review**, and performed on a **voluntary basis**. Assistance Publique, like many other large medical administrations, has already experienced that it is difficult if not impossible to impose QA on physicians as is any form of behaviour modification that does not originate from inside the profession, and we realized that if medical evaluation was to be developed, it would be by the contagion of example. We believed that in time, publication of QA studies of scientific standing in respected medical journals would be an incentive for university physicians to engage in the activity.

Therefore, the assignment of the Unit was to act as active consultants, to **inform** physicians about the existence and methods of medical evaluation, **promote** QA studies within AP, and **assist** the clinical departments that would engage in such studies. The assignment was not to evaluate, it was to help physicians develop quality assurance themselves.

INFORM. We created an internal **newsletter** after the model of CBO's international newsletter. It contained abstracts of the main publications on QA translated into french and information about QA activities in the world, in France when there were any, and in AP when there began to be some. We inserted a technical addendum (*fiche technique*) that contained the abstracts of consensus conference recommendations. This newsletter was issued 3 times a year, and distributed free to all physicians in AP, students included. We organized a **clearinghouse** on all kinds of QA documentation: books, journals, by specialty and in general. After little more than a year, we wrote an **Introductory Guide** to QA approaches in hospitals, that was distributed free to all fulltime physicians in AP.

We also presented QA principles and methods in teaching **seminars** that AP regularly organized for all its categories of physicians, students included.

PROMOTE. We chose to promote medical evaluation in AP through a **horizontal strategy** that aimed to spread knowledge about QA through different hospitals, as opposed to acting on a hospitalwide basis. We assumed that when a sufficient amount of individuals would be concerned by different studies in one hospital, they would then organize their own hospitalwide QA. A key point in this strategy is that due to the large number of its hospitals, there are several departments of all medical subspecialties in AP. We thus proceeded by calls for participation in our newsletter asking for the participation of voluntary physicians in **multicentric QA studies** by **topic**: diagnostic test ordering (4 hospitals, 14 departments (2)) or **specialty**: emergency departments (19 departments), AIDS clinics (12 clinics in 9 hospitals), smoke cessation clinics (12 clinics). These studies were initiated either at the suggestion of the unit, or at the demand of physicians. When this was the case, we systematically asked them to engage as many of their colleague specialists as they could in the study.

We organized a **Consensus conference program** at the AP level. The program was introduced with a conference that presented the concept and methods of consensus conferences to AP physicians (3) . Three conference were organised on topics that were suggested by physicians: Diagnosis of pulmonary embolism, Use of imaging in non-surgical common vertebral sciatica, and Prevention of thromboembolism in surgery.

The main objective of this horizontal strategy was to bring AP to work more closely as an organization rather than as separate and often conflicting departments and thus enhance homogeneity and quality of care.

ASSIST. Essential limiting factors for physician activities are time and manpower. We realized that it would have been irrealistic to ask physicians to engage in medical evaluation, an extra activity they were not asking for, without providing assistance and support.

The assistance we offered was in **methodology** for the study design; we constructed **software programs** for the different studies with the help of the Informatics Division of AP. **Hardware** equipment was also lent to unequipped departments. Most importantly, the general management provided the Unit with a yearly pool of 92 monthly fees that could be attributed to clinical departments to allow them to get help for data collection and entry. In this way, we only asked physicians for a few hours of their time to agree on objectives and protocols. All material assistance was limited to the duration of the study, and conditional to the presentation of a project entailing effective improvement of patient care.

INCENTIVES. This is an important aspect of QA promotion among groups that are not primariliy interested in its development. Though **financial incentives** come to mind first and are of course very popular in times of financial constraints, the problem is that all QA studies are not productive of financial savings, and that financial incentives to perform quality assurance deters physicians from the true spirit of QA which is medical, and must ultimately be performed on a routine basis, just as any other clinical activity, independently of any consideration of personal or collective financial profit. We therefore beleive other types of incentives have to be found, for instance in our context, the provision of integrated medical information systems.

AP has considerably delayed in developing integrated information systems. Up to now information policy focused essentially on the collection of administrative data such as number of admissions, length of stay, occuppation coefficient etc. The reason for this is that traditionnally, evaluation of hospital activity and financing relied on such data. As a result, the construction of medical information systems was entirely left to the initiative of individual physicians, and developed, where it did, independently, without coordination or compatibility between departments and hospitals.

We therefore thought that the **provision of integrated information systems** in priority to departments and/or specialties that engaged in quality assurance would be an incentive that would meet more than one objective. Medical information is needed by both physicians and management. By physicians for their own research; by management because they need information on medical activities. Furthermore, information is a prerequisite for quality assurance, but the data needed for quality assurance are not always the ones physicians wish to collect. In the absence of any medical information, all our quality assurance studies began by the definition of a set of data to collect and the construction of a program to collect it.

We beleive that, on the occasion of a QA study, such data definition can be expanded to include data wanted by physicians for clinical research, the necessary hardware and software provided when it does not exist, and in that way, begin to contribute to the design of the larger information system that will inevitably some day be in use, wherever it comes from. Up to now in France, the most significant effort towards the construction of a medical information system has come from the government with the implementation in French hospitals of diagnosis related groups (*groupes homogènes de malades, GHM*) in view of "medicalising" hospital information systems (*Projet de médicalisation du système d'information, PMSI*). We beleive the medicalisation of hospital information must come from physicians and that, in a context such as the one we have described, quality assurance can be the occasion for them to do so, if the corresponding systems are provided as an incentive. But this is a political decision.

Conclusion

In the space of three years, by informing our university hospitals about quality assurance, promoting multicentric studies and assisting the clinical departments involved with methodologic and material support, the unit engaged 60 departments in 25 hospitals in medical evaluation. One hospital constituted an evaluation committee and has engaged in ongoing hospitalwide quality assurance.

References

(1) EDDY D. The challenge, JAMA 1990; 263:287-290

(2) REERINK E. Improving the Quality of Hospital Services in the Netherlands. The role of CBO - The National Organization for Quality Assurance in the Netherlands. Quality Assurance in Health Care Vol.2 No.1, pp 31-36, 1990.

(3) GIRAUD A, FOURNIER V, GERBAUD L, JOLLY D. Rationaliser la prescription diagnostique de routine.Une expérience. La Presse Médicale, 30 mars 1991, 20, no. 12, pp. 535-538.

(4) GIRAUD A, JOLLY D, Eds. Le Consensus en Médecine. Méthodes et Bilan des Conférences de Consensus dans le monde. Paris, Doin , 1991.

CHILD HEALTH QUALITY ASSURANCE - A PRACTICAL APPROACH
Using the Child Health System and Focusing on Pre-School Screening

Diana Osborne   Business Training Consultant
6 Penleonard Close, Exeter, Devon EX2 4NY, U.K.
Pat Lambert Principal Medical Officer (Child Health), Basingstoke & North Hampshire H.A.

ABSTRACT
A UK Quality Assurance Project Group has been developing a QA programme both for all aspects of the British National Child Health System, and for all aspects of the community-based immunisation, screening and surveillance child health services which are administered via the computer system [1].   This paper describes the Project Group's initial theoretical work and focuses on the application of this theory to pre-school screening and surveillance programmes.

1. BACKGROUND

The National Child Health System is a National Health Service (NHS) computer system which provides most of the Health Authorities and Boards in England, Wales and Northern Ireland with a powerful and flexible tool for the management and administration of community-based child health services. The foundation of the System is the Child Register, with three service-delivery Modules - Immunisation, Pre-School Health and School Health - and statistics and information derived directly from the service data [2]. In the new NHS arrangements, child health services are the joint responsibility of District Health Authorities or Boards, family doctors, and the Family Health Services Authorities. The QA Project aims to help all these System users assure the quality of their child health services, and to ensure that we comply with WHO European Regional Target 31, ' all Member States should have built effective mechanisms for ensuring quality of patient care within their health care systems' [3].

2. THE QA PROJECT METHODOLOGY

The QA programme has been about formulating QA principles and devising QA measures - measures of what is *best* and what is *right* - and the work has been a series of steps:-
- dividing the whole subject matter into manageable areas or topics; the topics are quality assurance *per se;* the computer system; confidentiality, security and data protection; performance indicators; services management, planning and epidemiology; running the System; client facets; immunisation; screening & surveillance programmes; vision & hearing testing; height & weight, growth measurement; and the child register:
- agreeing an approach for the programme; the agreed approach is based on the four groups of people involved - the clients, the health professionals, the managers, and the computer staff:

- considering each topic in relation to the four groups of people:
- establishing principles for any QA measures; these principles are - accuracy and completeness, timeliness, effectiveness, efficiency and economy, acceptability and value:
- devising a suitable QA model, a model which is relevant and practical:
- devising measures and means of applying the model to each topic:
- and testing the proposed solutions in a number of differing pilot sites.

Most of these steps have been completed during the work of the last couple of years. The Project Group includes all professions, mostly System users, so individual members with relevant experience were selected as topic leaders; Dr. Lambert leads on screening and surveillance programmes, and Mrs. Osborne on confidentiality, security and data protection.

3. THE QA MODEL

The Project Group sees the QA process as continuous and evolutionary, so there is obvious relevance in the circular conceptual QA model proposed by Dr. Norma Lang, adapted by the American Nurses' Association, and widely used in nursing QA [4]. Our QA model (in the Figure below) must be flexible and adaptable to the needs of a variety of users; based on a computer system, it has the System data as its hub, surrounded by a number of steps to be carried out within an agreed limited time-scale, after which the process recommences. The model accords with Dr. Lang's definition of *values* as 'the level of quality health care we are willing to support in terms of personal behaviour, professional behaviour, and public policy'.

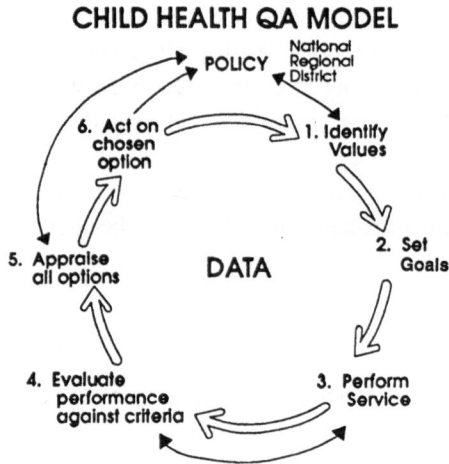

CHILD HEALTH QA MODEL

4. PRE-SCHOOL SCREENING AND SURVEILLANCE PROGRAMMES

4.1. Background. The agreed QA methodolgy was applied to each topic, using the Model to define values, standards and criteria, and to devise practicable QA measures. While matters such as health policy, clinical activities, administrative procedures and inter-professional communication are outwith the actual computer System, their importance is noted and appropriate references made, because of their relevance to desired outcomes and the quality of child health services. For example, Dr. Hall's Report "Health for All Children, a Programme of Child Health Surveillance" [5] is the basis for our topic of Screening and Surveillance programmes; and System users are always referred to the body of excellent work on professional standards.

4.2. QA for Pre-School Programmes in general. The QA methods and model were considered first for the Pre-School Programmes as a whole, to provide a useful framework for individual tests or programmes.

Preliminary Policy; policy on child health services may be set at national, regional and district levels. The policy operating locally must be defined and agreed by all the practitioners concerned, including precise definition of target population, timing ands type of contacts and tests, by whom tests will be done and the acceptable qualification and training levels. The established policy must be recorded, regularly reviewed, and updated as appropriate. An expert committee should be set up to examine outcomes.

1. Values will be the specific level of resources set and committed for the agreed period (the timescale should never exceed twelve months) of each specific QA cycle; these values must be realistic, so that goals are attainable in the given period.

2. Goals should then be set to effect improvement in the quality of uptake, information, equipment and conditions, and test performance, using the QA principles already listed.

3. Perform programmes and tests, including clear and accurate recording of outcomes.

4. Evaluate performance against the goals set - uptake achieved against target population, results (including false positives and negatives, and late positives), noting any problem areas. There is the opportunity for personal evaluation by the practitioner against previous contacts, for managerial evaluation of the efficacy of the general pre-school programmes, and for evaluation of the efficiency and effectiveness of the System.

5. Appraise options for the next QA cycle, including the resource implications, and specifying possible outcomes and benefits. Option appraisal should reflect the goals set and should include items such as training needs.

6. Act on chosen option(s) which may need a change in policy, and which always indicate the start of the next QA cycle.

4.3. QA for Individual Tests or Programmes There are parameters - usually incorporating QA principles such as timeliness, efficiency and effectiveness - which are generally professionally agreed for diagnosis of specific conditions to ensure the optimum opportunity for successful treatment. For example, timeliness is a crucial factor in the diagnosis of sensori-neural deafness by the age of eleven months. At the Preliminary Policy stage, the essential parameters for each specific screening or surveillance programme should be clearly agreed by the involved health professionals with the appropriate Health Authorities or Boards. Performance can then be monitored in relation to these parameters and outcomes can be audited through the System. Key outcomes should be selected for each contact, for example the hip test at six weeks and the hearing test at eight months. Timings of notifications to Local Education Authorities of children with special needs should always be monitored. Where performance falls outwith the agreed parameters, the expert committee should examine the particular circumstances and give appropriate advice, and the related action should then be included in the options chosen for the following QA cycle.

5. THE QA PROCESS - THEORY AND PRACTICE

The development of our QA programme thus far has concentrated on theory and methodology, but there has been constant dialogue with System users, and some aspects of the work have been tested informally. Three initial conclusions can be drawn. First, there has been no need to convince people of the need for a QA programme, as there is general agreement that quality assurance of health care information technology is essential. As Francis Roger succinctly expresses it, 'when [data sets] are used for financial purposes and quality control, their accuracy, reliability and comprehensiveness become imperative. This phenomenon appears to be due to the scarcity of resources and the availability of new technologies. Both lead to the definition of new indicators of productivity and of quality of care.' [6]. Second, our essentially practical approach has been welcomed, as users are certain that the quality assurance process must be simple and feasible, because health workers do not want additional unnecessary pressures and because they recognise that "superlative results invariably come from focusing your energy and resources on those few crucial details that allow you successfully to implement change .. without letting yourself get swamped by trivia" [7]. Third, the 'people-based approach of our programme is welcome for, as Donabedian has recognised, the judgement of quality is not simply a technical, professional matter, the interpersonal aspects are extremely important. [8]

The next phase of the project is a thorough, controlled and evaluated pilot of our proposals in a representative selection of U.K. System user authorities, and hopefully in a number of European sites which do not yet use the System. The pilot will first cover four topics in depth - the child register, running the System, immunisation, and data protection, confidentiality and security - with initial surveys establishing the current practices in the pilot sites, then the QA model being operated for each topic in a limited timescale. When the findings for the four topics have been analysed, conclusions will be applied to the other topics, which will then be piloted on a more limited scale. The outcomes will be incorporated in a series of Notes of Guidance for System users, and in Recommendations for any appropriate System enhancements.

CONCLUSIONS

The main conclusion of the Project Group is that implementing such a comprehensive QA programme is both feasible and desirable. It may bring to light differences in understanding, both of what the objectives of the service and the System and of how these are carried out in practice. Desired changes in relationships between client and health professional, health professional and manager, may need to be reflected in the ways that the System is run and the services provided. Perhaps the ultimate goal of the QA Project Group is not to promise unachievable perfect quality, but rather to help those involved in child health services to appreciate that quality assurance enables them 'to err and err and err again, but less and less and less'. [9]

ACKNOWLEDGEMENTS

For encouragement and information the authors thank Bud Abbott and the staff of the King's Fund Centre, London. We particularly acknowledge the contribution and support of the other members of our QA Project Group.

REFERENCES

[1] Osborne, Diana, Badminton, M., Churchill, S., Quality Assurance and Child Health; in: O'Moore, R., Bengtsson, S., Bryant, J.R., Bryden, J.S. (Eds), Medical Informatics Europe 90, Proceedings (Springer-Verlag, Berlin 1990).

[2] Walker, C.H.M., Rigby, M.J., The British Child Health Computer System, in: Roger, F.H., Gronroos, P., Tervo-Pelikka, R., O'Moore, R. (Eds), Medical Informatics Europe 85, Proceedings (Springer-Verlag, Berlin 1985).

[3] European Regional Targets, Health for All by the Year 2000, WHO.

[4] Lang, Norma M., Quality Assurance - How Technology can help, in: Fokkens, O., et al (Eds), Medinfo 83 Seminars, Proceedings of the Medinfo 1983 Amsterdam Seminars, (Elsevier Science Publishers B.V., Amsterdam 1983).

[5] Hall, D.M.B., Health for All Children - A Programme of Child Health Surveillance, (Oxford University Press 1989).

[6] Roger, F.H., New Trends in Medical Informatics in Europe, Opening Address, in: Medical Informatics Europe 85 (Springer-Verlag, Berlin 1985).

[7] Hickman, C.R., Silva, M.A., Creating Excellence (Unwin, London 1985).

[8] Donabedian, A., The definition of quality and approaches to its assessment: (Health Administration Press, Ann Arbor, Michigan, 1980).

[9] Hein, Piet, Gruks, (Hodder), also, More Gruks, and, Still More Gruks.

NURSING

C.N.I.S. - Innovation into practice.

Ruth Roberts

Nursing Department, East Dyfed Health Authority, c/o C.H.I.P. Office, St. Davids Hospital, Carmarthen, Dyfed, Wales. SA31 3HB

ABSTRACT

Kimberly defines an innovation as a departure from existing practices or technologies which represent a significant departure from the art at the time it appears. The development and implementation of a Clinical Nursing Information System (C.N.I.S.) is an innovation for Wales. The thought of trying something new is often viewed with caution or fear, and the use of the computer by ward nurses represents a significant departure from their previous practice of record keeping. A literature review identified several papers which considered the introduction of innovations, Hage and Aiken examined the innovation process and sequence of events in relation to organisational change. This work appeared to provide an appropriate theoretical framework to apply when developing and implementing C.N.I.S.

This paper describes the development of C.N.I.S. and discusses how the evaluation, initiation and implementation stages of the innovation process have been applied.

1. INTRODUCTION

1.1 Background

During 1984 the Chief Administrative Nursing Officers in Wales identified their priorities for computer developments; care planning was their top priority. The clinical nurse views care planning as a way of using and documenting a systematic approach to care; the nurse manager sees the care plan as the most complete record of care given to individual patients and, therefore, of great value in resource management. A care planning system will only be acceptable in the nursing environment if it improves the quality of patient care, eases communication, does not increase the amount of time that nurses are away from the bedside and assists in the management of resources. Specific objectives for a Clinical Nursing Information System (C.N.I.S.) were identified [1] and used as the basis for an option appraisal of nursing systems available; none were deemed to meet the requirements. It was, therefore, decided to develop a Clinical Nursing Information System for Wales.

1.2 Innovation

Kimberly [2] defines an innovation as a departure from existing practices or technologies which represents a significant departure from the art at the time it appears. Innovations can take a variety of forms; they can be developed within an organisation or can be imported from outside. Innovations can be things that are totally new and never tried before or things that are new only to a particular organisation. Hage and Aiken in 1970 [3] and Hage in 1980 [4] examined the innovation process and sequence of events in relation to organisational change, they divided the innovation process into four periods or stages: evaluation, initiation, implementation, routinization. The development and implementation of a Clinical Nursing Information System is an innovation for Wales.

2. METHOD

2.1 Development

The Welsh Computer Strategy Committee approved funding for a project to be developed by the Welsh Health Common Services Authority Computer Services Department in collaboration with East Dyfed Health Authority. A Steering Group was established to oversee the project and to ensure that the objectives set were achieved within the timescales and a project leader (the author) was appointed.

The development of C.N.I.S. has been in three phases. Phase One - a pilot study and development of a ward based system; Phase Two - expansion of the system to other wards, specialties, enhancements to the software and the use of bedside terminals; Phase Three - validation on other, new, sites. The input of the project leader in the implementation is also being reduced in order to establish whether the system is successful in its own right and not just as a result of the project leader's influence and direct involvement.

Gibson [5] identified that user acceptance of computerisation is crucial to success. Encouraging the users to participate in the design, implementation and evaluation can help feelings of ownership and commitment to the system.

Although the pilot project made use of data modelling, the ward nurses could not visualise what the system would be like. It was agreed that a prototype, based on one topic, would be produced for the nurses to obtain a feel about the system. Following viewing of the prototype comments would be incorporated into the system design and this system tested for a small group of patients, further comments would be taken on board for the final system. This prototyping approach was seen as essential, as by using in-house systems development the users had a clear understanding that revisions could be readily incorporated so that the system would accurately reflect their nursing practice.

2.2 Evaluation

There is a need to assess whether any system developed meets the objectives set. Although the project leader undertook baseline studies and six monthly personal appraisals of the pilot system, it was deemed essential to have a more formal, independent evaluation. For Phase One, a professional and technical study was undertaken in August, 1988.

Involvement of the users in Phase Two was not as intensive as the pilot. The users perspective was considered important - might fresh users, lacking the pioneering spirit reject it? An independent professional evaluation was completed in May, 1989.

For Phase Three a benefits study is being undertaken on the transfer sites. There are three sections to the study: A staff based questionnaire - to establish the saving in time on administrative and clerical recording and staff perception of care planning and computers. A sampling study of patient based nursing activity - to establish the changes in the use of time used for nursing duties. An evaluation of the documentation for Care Planning - to establish the accuracy, completeness and consistency of the documentation. The before studies have been undertaken and the post studies will be completed by June, 1991.

3. RESULTS

One of the requirements of C.N.I.S. was for it to be an "expert" system. When viewing the initial prototype the nurses stated that if this approach was used for all aspects of nursing it would be very frustrating as it was slow to work down the pathways. Work on nursing expert systems in the USA has also identified this [6]. A modified "expert" approach was used in the construction of the knowledge base files. The knowledge files follow a hierarchial structure, the starting point is the nursing model. The system allows the nurse to select the most appropriate nursing model for the care of the individual patient. Each problem is related to relevant outcomes, and each outcome is related to relevant interventions.

Phase One evaluation concluded that C.N.I.S. is a prototype Nursing Process system which appears to meet its objectives. It was deemed well designed and presented and seemed popular with the users at the pilot site.

Phase Two external evaluation report stated "The heart of a nursing information system is the careplanning facility. And at the heart of careplanning is the Knowledge Base. Given this dual importance, it is gratifying to state with little equivocation that careplanning in C.N.I.S. is a major strength and achievement." In acute general hospitals patients are cared for at the bedside; this is where the health professional, especially nurses, need to have access to the computer system. Nurses and patients readily accepted the use of bedside terminals. Nurses stated that the size of the portable computer did not inhibit the nurse-patient relationship, something they had been concerned about.

4. DISCUSSION

Involvement of the users has been the key to the success of the development of C.N.I.S. Experience with the Resource Management Initiative in England has raised some questions over the way information is obtained; by whom, for whom and for what purposes? The Department of Health [7] reported nurses as expressing dissatisfaction at entering data into a computer which seems to have no direct relevance to their clinical practice. They felt they were providing information without getting anything in return. In our experience, initially the mature, experienced ward nurses can not see any value in having a computerised care planning system, but after a couple of months use they are the strongest supporters of the system.

The evaluation, initiation and implementation stages of the innovation process have been applied to each phase of C.N.I.S. Normally evaluation is seen as the last stage of any process, however the initial evaluation (option appraisal) had to be undertaken before a decision to develop the system could be made. Following the evaluation of each phase the initiation stage of the next phase had to be undertaken. The initiation stage has two aspects, the search for financial support and the appointment of people with the requisite skills and training "to fill the occupational slots" created by the innovation. Hage and Aiken comment that health, welfare and education may be able to obtain limited central funds but as this source is frequently temporary, alternative sources for support may not be available once the central funds cease.

The decision whether to recruit from outside the organisation or to select individuals from inside the organisation has to be made. Bringing in a stranger increases the likelihood of resistance to the innovation by organisational members. The danger of recruiting internally for a radical innovation is that the individual selected may be unaware of the full potentialities of the innovation. The Steering Group had decided that the project leader was to be an experienced clinical nurse rather than a systems analyst. The person appointed had not previously worked in Wales.

The implementation stage starts with the first attempt to manufacture the new product/service. The more radical the change the longer the stage lasts because, frequently, the first trials fail. At the project level, the three Phases of C.N.I.S. are clearly three iterations of the innovation process loop. Alternatively, at the macro level the three Phases can be seen as a single implementation stage, with the iteration being the implementation by other authorities, and other nursing specialties within user sites. It has been easier to obtain funding for the smaller phases, but the simultaneous macro view has been important in ensuring strategic consistency.

At some point the elite of an organisation must decide whether the innovation is meeting the organisational need for which it was designed. If the organisation decides to keep the innovation a period of consolidation is begun. Hage and Aiken comment that perhaps the best sign of the routinization of the "new program" occur when the people who were originally involved in the implementation are replaced. "If the program remains essentially the same, that is, it does not trigger another process of change, we can then say that it has been stabilized." The reduced input of the project leader in Phase Three has not, yet, triggered any additional requests for change other than those identified by the project leader.

At the end of Phase Three it may be confirmed that the system meets nurses needs in different health authorities and that C.N.I.S. will be available for other health authorities. Using Kimberly's definition of an innovation, each time the system is introduced to other health care settings it will be viewed, by that organisation, as an innovation. Ward staff will probably perceive it as a radical innovation as it represents a significant departure from their previous practice of record keeping. The evaluation, initiation, implementation and routinization stages of the innovation process ought to be applied by each health authority in order to accommodate the organisational issues associated with the introduction of an innovation into practice.

References:

1. Roberts R, Taylor JA. Computerized clinical nursing information system. In: Bryant JR, Roberts J, Windsor PG, editors. Conference Proceedings - Current perspectives in healthcare computing. 1987. 196-202
2. Kimberly JR. Managerial Innovation. In: Nystrom PC, Starbuck WH editors. Handbook of Organizational Design. Vol. 1 1981 Oxford University Press.
3. Hage J and Aiken M. Social Change In Complex Organizations. 1970 Random House.
4. Hage J. Theories of Organizations. 1980 John Wiley and Sons.
5. Gibson SE. Managing Computer Resistance. Computers in Nursing. 1986 Vol. 4/No. 5 (September/October) 201-4
6. Ozbolt JG. Knowledge-Based Systems for Supporting Clinical Nursing Decisions. In: Ball MJ, Gerdin Jelger U, and Peterson H editors. Nursing Informatics - Where Caring and Technology Meet. 1988 Springer-Verlag.
7. Department of Health, Nursing Division and Operational Research. The resource management initiative and ward nursing management information systems: a review of issues and progress to date. 1988 Department of Health, London. (unpublished)

NOMENCLATURE, CODING, CLASSIFICATION and STANDARDS for NURSING INFORMATION SYSTEMS.

Joyce Wiseman
Nursing Consultant
United Kingdom

Abstract

The paper presents the case for a structured nursing language within an electronic data base. It will promote the Knowledge of Nursing through a systematic and scientific language framework.

1. Introduction

"Nursing has been defined as an art, a science and a profession" (1). An ongoing debate continues in Nursing; is Nursing an art? A science? A profession? The questions arise because of gaps in nursing knowledge, and a lack of evidence to answer these questions. Greenwood (2) defines "Systematic Theory" as one of the five key components which has to exist in a Professional Body. This factor is lacking within Nursing as identified by Wilson (3) who states that "No evidence has been found which provides a basis for the establishment of criteria regarding the standard of knowledge of the biological sciences required by the practising nurse."
Research through its "formal, systematic and intensive process of carrying on a scientific method of analysis (with its) purpose of discovery and development of a body of knowledge" (4) is the activity which will promote nursing knowledge so that the boundaries of "art", "science" and "professionalism" can be identified and further defined.

3. The Nursing Record and its Facility to Contribute to Knowledge.

The constant words in the various definitions are: Systematic and Scientific. Scientific Measurement can only be performed within a Systematic Framework, and which, crucially, includes language. Grobe (5) states that "The absence of a research based nursing language and a taxonomy of nursing interventions seriously compromises research on nursing practice; such compromise affects collaborative research activities dependent upon unambiguous and comparable standardised terminology and codification schema".

Records are "......one of the four methods of collecting (research) data, providing a readily available and valuable source of data....(6)"...Good records are of vital importance: to patients and clients, to nurses, midwives and health visitors.......Such records are a visible evidence of care given. They provide basic information for the development of nursing, midwifery and health visiting practice and research..."(7).

Ambiguous words do not provide reliable interpretations of the patient/client care, and free text writings are not conducive to means of scientific measurement. Little motivation has existed to alter nurse recording practices, but now, with the computer becoming an every day tool in the workplace the nursing profession has a purpose in determining its own terminologies of Nomenclature, Coding and Classifications.

3. Nomenclature, Coding, Classification and Standards.

According to The Oxford English Dictionary (8) Nomenclature is "a catalogue of systematic naming - a termninology of science", Coding "a systematic collection such as to avoid inconsistency" whilst Classification is to "assign to a class".

Standards are seen as "to obtain by analysis specific values for the purpose of comparisons".

Thus, it is shown that standards can be measured through the rigid rules set in the shema of Nomenclature, Coding and Classification.

The first systematic collaborative effort to systemise medical terminologies was initiated in Vienna in 1891 at The International Statistical Congress (9). Since that time medical codings have received a central focus and ongoing work has continued to refine and develop their depth and their contribution to interpreting in a structured format medical diagnoses, so assisting with a scientific presentation of comparative medical data.

There are the international ICD-9-CM codes and, more recently, The Read Codes (10) initiated from a Family Doctor source.

4. The Rationale for Interfacing Medical and Nursing Nomenclatures Codings and Classifications.

Medical systematic terminologies need to be interfaced with Nurse codings which reflect underlying Patient Problem(s) through a Nursing Diagnosis.

Using the specimen Medical Read Codes from the reference (10) above, chapter heading "A Hierarchical Classification" para 3, p.3.

Selection: "Level 3. Rubella   Read code   A56   ICD Code 056"

"Rubella" is the Medical Diagnosis.

The Nursing Interface: A Community Nurse, requested to visit the patient by the Family Doctor, will have to carry out a Nursing Diagnosis into the Patient Problem(s).

What could be the Patient Problem in the case of Rubella? Is it ITCHING SKIN? STREAMING EYES? PHOTOPHOBIA? a FEBRILE DISTRESSED INFANT? an AGITATED MOTHER? IGNORANCE on INFECTION CONTROL?

The words in block capitals can be identified as Key Words, describing the Patient Problems, and which are a Nursing Diagnosis.

From such assessments the nurse will have to determine the interventory measures for her plan of care, and which will depend on various factors, such as age, understanding of illness, environment, physical/intellectual and emotional states and family /neighbour support networks.

All these facets of care have implications to quality of care and the cost effectiveness of care. A discipline of language will facilitate research, and enable hitherto hidden patient care needs to be measurable.

Grobe (11) in her paper "Nursing intervention lexicon and taxonomy study: Language and classification methods" reveals the dichotomy of a language discipline so that it is sufficiently fexible to allow the nurse freedom to fully express the ever present variables in patient care, and at the same time Nursing takes full advavantage of electronic data bases to amass meaningful words which enable the Nursing Diagnosis and the resulting Interventions to be quantified in statistical patient population terms.

Grobe considers "A good example of the use of controlled vocabulary and standardized terms exists in Medline's automated bibliography retrieval system", and she indicates that this type of system could be used by the practising nurse "who typically expresses ideas using the fullest range of terminologies."

5. Information Technology and The Nursing Record.

The author since 1984 has been leading a comprehensive computerised community nursing information system (12). The System adapting to take advantages of the latest technological developments as they arise. During the total trials some 900 patients have had their record maintained on their own respective computerised patient data card. The experience has highlighted the inadequacies of literal usage within an electronic data base; differing means of literal inputs producing an unproductive, unscientific jumble of words and terminologies as shown below:

Literals	Numbers
Poor Mobility	25
Poor Mobility.	02
Poor Mobty	02
Immobility	06
Immobility.	03
Very Immobilised	01
TOTAL	**39**

The community nurses in the sample have identified patients with a total of 39 mobility problems which are written in six different ways and so there is a variety of six statistical outputs. It can be seen that the placing of a full stop after "Poor mobility" produces another statistical output, whilst other varieties of collation occur through mis-spelling or different wording.

6.Discussion.

Decisions have to be taken in Nursing on terminologies for Nursing; what words should be used; how they are to be displayed; how they are to be structured; how they are to be coded. Comparative data will be collated and nursing will be moving forwards in the discipline of a scientific framework.
There is much to do, and by working collaboratively, we, in Nursing, will promote the International understanding of the Profession of Nursing.

REFERENCES:

1.& 6. Treece E W, Treece J W 1973 "Elements of Research in Nursing"
   C V   Mosby & co, USA.
2. Greenwood E 1957 "Attributes of a Profession" Social Work 2 (3)
   July 1957.
3. Wilson K J W 1976 "A study of the Biological Sciences in Relation
   to Nursing" Churchill Livingstone, Longman Group Ltd.
4. Best J W "Research in Education" 1970 Prentice Hill Inc pp 8-9.
5. Grobe S J 1989 "Nursing Intervention Lexicon & Taxomony Study:
   Description of a Conceptual Framework" University of Texas School
   of Nursing, Austin Texas 78712 USA.
6. Treece & Treece (see 1)
7. CNO Letter 1988 Nursing Records Parliamentary Commissioner for
   Administration: Health Service Commissioner Report 1986 - 87 PL/CNO
   17 DHSS.
8. The Concise Oxford English Dictionary 1966. Edited by Fowler HW &
   FG, Oxford Clarendon Press.
9. Gabrieli E R 1989 "A New Electronic Medical Nomenclature" Journal
   of Medical Systems vol 13, No 6 1989 pp 355-373.
10.Read J D "The Read Clinical Classification" (undated) Computer
   Aided Medical Systems Ltd, 26-28 Leicester Road, Loughborough,
   Leicestershire. LE11 2 AG.
11.Grobe S J 1990 "Nursing Intervention and Taxonomy Study:
   Language and Classification Methods" Advances in Nursing Science,
   Dec.1990, pp 22-33.
12.Wiseman J 1989 Memory Cards Portable Micro-computers and
   Community Nurse Recording" Medinfo '89. Edited by Barber et al,
   North Holland, pp 647-649.

A NURSING MINIMUM DATA SET IN PRODUCTION
Facilities and Training

Delesie L., L.Croes, W.Sermeus, A.Tanghe, G.Vanden Boer, J.Vanlanduyt

Department of Hospital Administration and Medical Care Organization

Catholic University of Leuven, Belgium

Abstract

Patient data and patient care data is catching up with cost data in the national and local management of hospitals. This development demands for adequate tools to make the information accessible to all management levels, for an organizational structure in which to discuss this information and for lear ning and training facilities. Belgium is doing this for its 311 general hospitals, its 1232 medical departments and its 2700 nursing units. This paper reports on the state of affairs.

1. Introduction

Modern hospital management demands for the utilization of patient- and patient care information alongside cost data and traditional structural data such as number and type of beds. The hospital law of august 7,1987 in Belgium anticipates this in its article 86 (1) and a royal decree of august 14,1987 identified a first minimum data set: 23 minimum nursing activities, major diagnosis (I.C.D.-9-C.M.,3 digits), some data on age, sex and hospital stay, an activities-of-daily-living or ADL index on a voluntary basis and some data on the nursing unit and its personnel. This data set is called the "nursing minimum dataset". The authors have been involved with the implementation of this decree since its origin.

Most patient classification systems such as the Diagnostic Related Groups or DRG's in the US or the Groupes de Diagnostic Homogänes or GDH's in France reduce the great variety of hospital patients to a fixed set of some 400 types of patients. Moreover for each type of patient, the wide range of actual hospital practice patterns is summarized to one figure, usually a national average. Examples are: one amount of dollars, one length of stay deemed acceptable or one amount of nursing time minutes deemed refundable by type of patient. This approach allows for easy understanding and simple application but foregoes the rich reality of hospital life and hospital practice.

Our approach has been to highlight the contribution of each additional angle of incidence to our gradual understanding of the hospital product and to look at nursing units, medical specialties, departments, hospitals and hospital regions in a holistic way rather than the weighted sum of some idealized types of patients. Belgium has three regions -- Flanders, Brussels and Wallony -- and three cultural communities -- Flemish, Walloon and German community -- which moreover do not coincide. Belgians by tradition beware of magic formulas and simple solutions.
This paper reports on our experience with the "nursing minimum data" collected as of january 1, 1988 and for the first time available on a national level after much concerted effort by many as of january 1991. An additional "minimum clinical data set" has been launched on october 1,1990 but these data are not yet available.

2. Development of the "Nursing Minimum Dataset" (NMDS) (2)

The NMDS has been developed in cooperation with the government and the national nursing association starting from a list of 111 activities which they had defined (3). Two research projects were involved. By 1987 agreement was reached on the sample of 23 activities and the periodic sampling procedure. The items are divided into fundamental care (e.g.hyginic care), technical nursing care (e.g. drawing blood specimens) and typical activities (e.g. decubitus preventive care). From the start equal attention went to the development of relevant feedback to all levels of management: the utilization of information is as important as the collection of reliable data. Proper statistical techniques and standardized reports were developed. Field trials were run to test every aspect of the operation with the active participation of the national government and the professional nursing associations.

Some opposition arose from the hospital administrators as well as from the hospital physicians: the administrators were reluctant to start justifying their costs on the basis of their patient mix, while the physicians were cautious to start sharing their monopoly on patient care decisions with other categories of professionals. This reluctance was founded as the financing of the hospital budget as of 1991 explicitly takes into account medical procedures and nursing activities.

3.Tools of the "Nursing Minimum Data Set"

The NMDS is collected on every nursing unit in each Belgian general hospital daily during a 15-day sampling period four times a year. The basis of the collection is the nursing care plan which, just as the medical record, is part of the patient record obligatory for each hospital admission. Five days per registration period are selected by the ministry of health for further data processing. These data are collected in many different ways by each hospital dependent on its computer facilities and organization but results in a diskette or tape which is sent to the ministry on a quarterly basis.

A **first tool** is data entry and cleaning software made available to all hospitals on a voluntary basis.

A **second tool** is the Feedback Programme. This programme is written in interpreter Basic. This takes into account very heterogeneous computer facilities and allows each hospital to integrate the programme into its own information system. Minimum facilities (XT type computer) are needed which again put the programme within reach of every nursing unit. Again this programme was developed with the active participation of the professional nursing associations (4) and is distributed by the ministry of health. For the reasons indicated above, the unit of observation of this programme is the nursing unit. This is the smallest management entity in the hospital and this allows to respect the privacy of individual patients and care providers. The target group for the information is the head nurse who manages the unit. The programme extracts indicators and trends based on administrative, nursing and medical data relevant for the management of the unit in a standardized way. No comment nor conclusions are drawn, all attention is focused on the information provided. The programme presents three parts: the patients, the personnel and the nursing activities. The dynamic character of the nursing unit is presented by comparing two different periods of registration. The comparison of two different nursing units altogether is also possible. The Feedback Programme is demonstrated in this M.I.E. 91 congress.

A **third tool** is a Ministry Feedback by the ministry of health which validates the data by indicating unacceptable data and signaling data which diverges significantly from expected patterns on a nationwide basis.

A **fourth tool** are the National Statistics. These are developed after pooling all the data nationally and by use of especially developed statistical procedures. The statistics are twofold. The first part concentrates on the variables. National "fingerprints" of the 23 nursing items, the diagnostic profile and the ADL index are published by type of hospital department and by region. An example is given in Figure I. The second part concentrates on the national group of nursing units and hospital departments. Using multidimensional scaling techniques and graphical representation techniques, the location of all unit and departments is displayed in two national maps. One map uses the fingerprints of all units with respect to the 23 nursing items; one map uses the diagnostic profile of all hospital departments. Each map is zoned into 'city blocks' and for each block some relevant data is presented: length of stay and age of the patients, number and qualification of nursing personnel. Figure II shows the map of all intensive care nursing units in Belgium on the basis of their 23 nursing items

These maps emphasize the different ways in which hospital care is provided. They show for instance to what extent two departments with the same patient mix as measured by their diagnostic profile may differ with respect to their nursing activities. These maps have to be presented in such detail as indeed, by amalgamating units or departments into hospitals one does obtain the profile of a hospital but by the same token one loses all interesting management information: two hospitals may have similar internal medicine nursing units but be quite different with respect to maybe some surgical units. Any patient classification such as DRG's can easily substitute the I.C.D.-9-C.M. classification used sofar in our approach.

A fifth tool is again a programme. It allows each hospital to calculate the fingerprints of every nursing units or group of units of its choice with respect to the 23 nursing items, the diagnostic profile and the ADL-index and compare these fingerprints to national figures by use of box plots. The same programme also allows to calculate the position on the "minimum nursing data" map and the "diagnostic profile" map and to compare length of stay, age and personnel indicators with national figures.

4. Training with respect to the "Nursing Minimum Data Set"

The implementation of hospital management information in new areas such as patient classification and patient care including nursing care not only demands tools and organizational forums but also learning and training programmes. Hence, in march 1990 a national training programme was started to reach the 60000 nurses in the Belgian hospital sector. The target group are directors of nursing, middle managers and head nurses. They learn the purpose and meaning of the operation and the different tools of NMDS. To safeguard the uniformity of the training a strategy was developed: The government instructed us to train 7 coordinators appointed by the 7 medical faculties of Belgium. These coordinators on their turn train 3 persons designated by each Belgian hospital. Overal, 340 hospitals and about 900 persons participate in the training programme. These hospital trainees will bear responsibility to start teaching NMDS and developing applications in their own hospital within a national and regional context. Several applications have already been started.

Also in cooperation with the ministry and the 7 coordinators, we are developing a uniform teaching packet. Some lessons are being learnt the hard way. Within the group of participants the disparity in factual knowledge, in experience with information and in interest in management information is enormous and demands for gradual but continuous effort. The training in two languages -- dutch and french - demonstrates the difficulties towards the development of a common patient and patient care language. It also highlights time upon time the cultural differences in handling patient information for management purposes and the actual hospital practice differences prevalent between each region and within each region. The cooperation of the ministry helped to solve all problems along the way. Also, workshops and meetings are organized to allow as many as possible to get familiar with all aspects and tools. During the training a motivation to use the NMDS as a management instrument in nursing is slowly replacing the feelings of uncertitude and purposeless registration which were characteristic in the first months.

5. Conclusions

The introduction of medical informatics is no easy task. When the aim is a national operation many difficulties arise. These are as well of an organizational and educational nature as of a technical and instrumental nature. Though simple solutions exist which are highly popular, our efforts show it to be worthwhile to look not only at the patient mix but also at the practice patterns of nurses and hospitals in a coherent way. Our experience in bi-cultural Belgium gives an interesting preview of what lies ahead for a multi-cultural Europe.

1. Hospital Law of August 7, 1987, Belgian official Journal of october 7, 1987.
2. Delesie (L.), P. De Becker, W. Sermeus, Hospital care financing, Hospital Management International, International Hospital Federation, 1989, 219-226.
3. U.G.I.B.-A.U.V.B., Profiel van de verpleegkundige zorgvezrlening en de minimale verpleegkundige gegevens, Cahiers nr.1 en nr.2 1986, pp. 72
4. Delesie (L.), C. Fontaine, B. Dierckx, P. De Becker, A. Tanghe, Statistische gegevens over medische en verpleegkundige activiteiten, systematische beleidsinformatie, K.U.Leuven, Centrum voor Ziekenhuiswetenschap, 1990, pp. 33, Dutch and French versions.

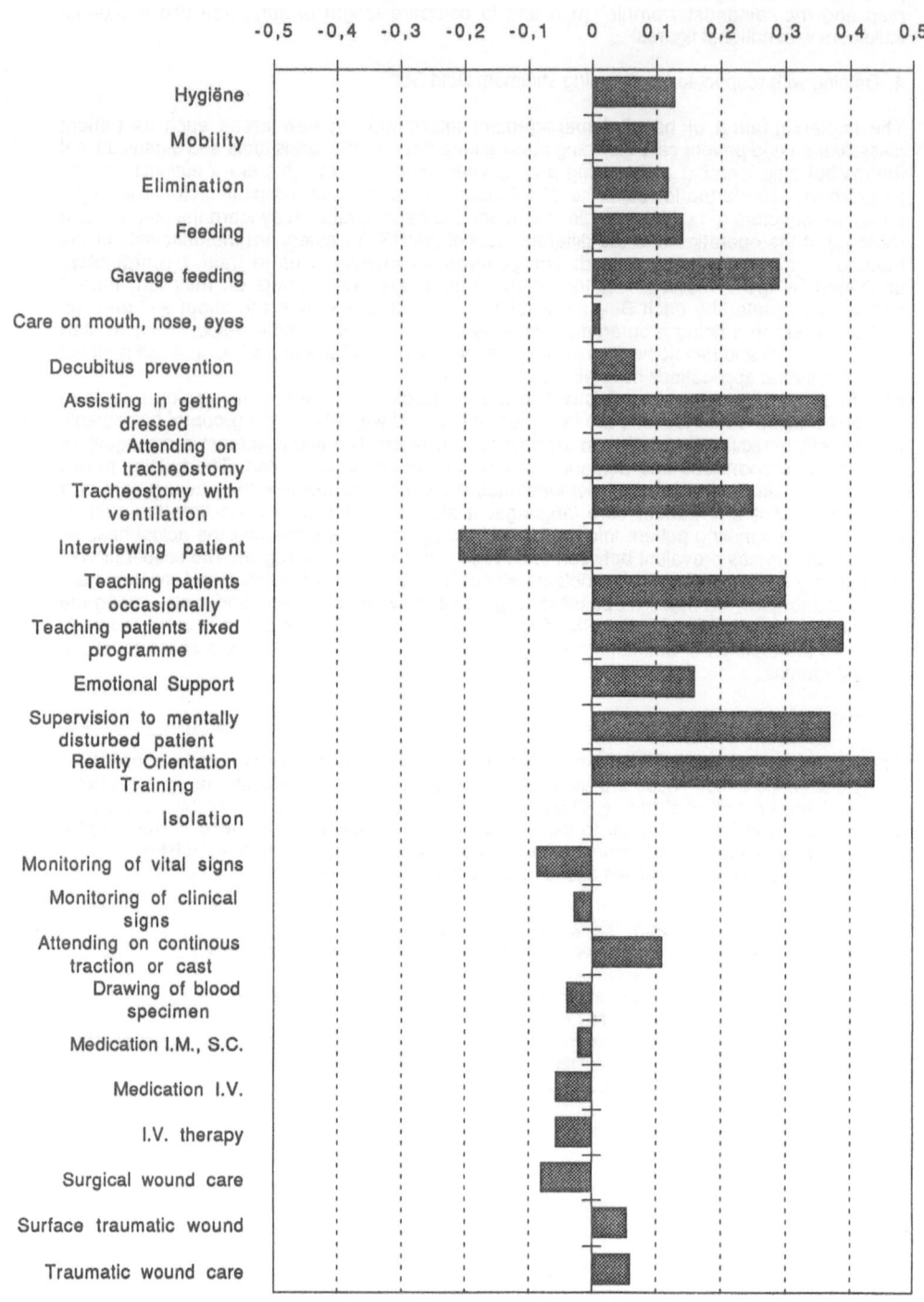

Figure 1. AN EXAMPLE OF A FINGERPRINT FOR A GERIATRIC NURSING UNIT

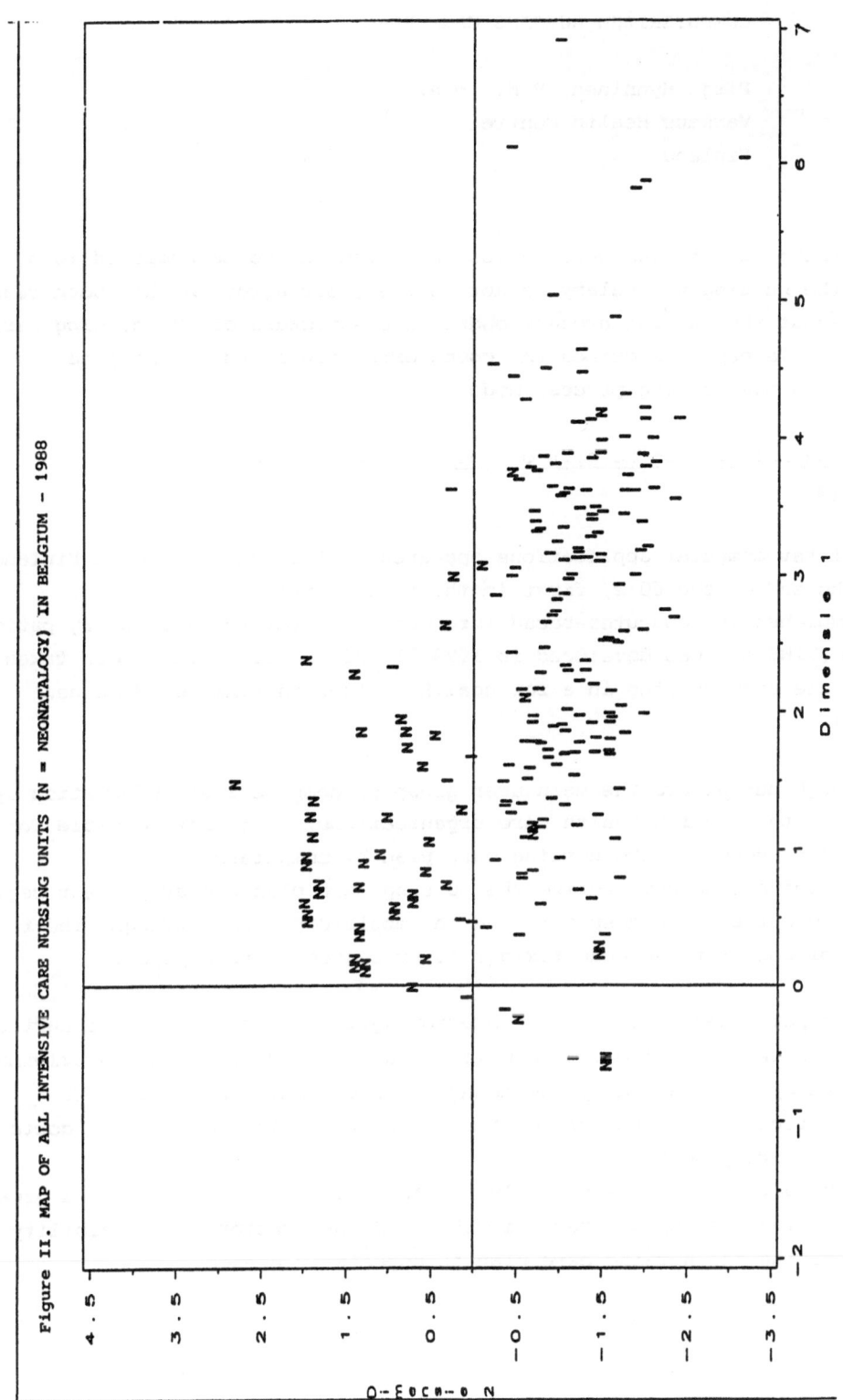

Figure II. MAP OF ALL INTENSIVE CARE NURSING UNITS (N = NEONATALOGY) IN BELGIUM – 1988

COMPUTERIZED NURSING CARE PLAN

Pirjo Hynninen, R.N., M.A.
Varkaus Health Centre
Finland

Abstract: In Finland nursing documentation has no established forms,
and the nursing vocabulary is not unified, but agreement has been reached about the nursing process model as a structure of the nursing care
plan. This paper describes the computerization of the nursing care plan
based on the nursing process model.

Nursing information as part of the computerized patient record

The first computer applications appeared in the health care in Finland
at the end of the 60's, first in the major university hospitals.
A comprehensive computer-based information system for ambulatory patient
care (FINSTAR) was developed in 1979-81 and has since then been taken
into use step by step in a few health centres in Finland (Hynninen
1981).

Although nurses are the main user group of computerized information systems in the Finnish health care organisations, it is not possible for
nurses to document the nursing care plan by computers.
Some projects to computerize the nursing care plan are at present beging
carried out both in hospitals and in ambulatory care settings. The result of one of these undertakings is presented in this paper.

The computerized nursing documentation system described here is part of
the computerized patient information system FINSTAR, which was originally developed to make easy the managing of medical record data. The
terms, topics and structure of the information flow follow the doctors´
patient care process.
Though doctors and nurses partly use the same concepts there is a great
need to include nursing terms in the FINSTAR-directory. A possibility to
computerize the nursing care plan is especially needed.

In spite of the shortcomings of the FINSTAR-system, nurses have been obliged to use it for documentation of the nursing process. Nurses have entered the assessment of patients' needs as well as planning of a care under medical headings such as anamnesis and status.

The basic registration data of every inhabitant in the area of the health centre are despatched to the FINSTAR-system four times a year on computer tape by the Population Register Office. Additional information needed in the care of a patient (primary nurse, next of kin, address of next of kin etc.) is entered to the personal details table, which is the starting point in the documentation, because the patient records are stored under the patient identification number.

To document the implementation of care, nurses have used various terms for procedure (injection, dressing change) or non-medical treatment concepts (diet-counselling). There is no medical heading for the evaluation of the care. That is why one cannot usually find any evaluation data in patients' records.
Even if all nursing data have been entered to the patient record it has been buried under medical headings so thoroughly that it is quite impossible to get a clear idea of the actual nursing care plan.

The limitations of FINSTAR were most pronounced in the work of the district nurses, where the focus is on nursing instead of medical care. The district nurses were the first to get fed up with documentation difficulties and began to demand the development of a computerized nursing care plan.

Description of the computerized nursing care plan

The nursing care plan option, added to the topics of FINSTAR-program, was developed by district nurses in conjunction with a computer programmer.
The computerized nursing care plan gives structure in documenting the nursing process. It it not based on any nursing theory or theoretical model, but on a common decision making process (Simon), which can be observed in the background of the nursing process model by Yura and Walsh (1988) and in the Medium-term Programme in Nursing/Midwifery by WHO (1976). Some nursing theorists prefer to speak of a professional decision making process in nursing rather than a nursing process model (Lauri).

Yura & Walsh regard patient as holistically integrated being with 35 human needs. The goal of nursing is to fulfill the patient's unmet needs. Gordon (1982) designs an assessment format according to 11 functional health patterns, which derive from various nursing theorists (Orem, Roy, Rogers, Johnson). In human sciences, such as nursing a way of viewing man is holistic, with three aspects: physical, psychological and social. Since holism consists of three parts some theorists call this way of analysing human beings monopluralism (Rauhala).

The computer program for the nursing care plan only gives a structural framework for documenting nursing, it does not presuppose any nursing theory. However, nurses have been used to observing patient's needs for defining the problem. The development of nursing vocabulary is not within the limits of this project.
Whatever name has been given to the process it consists of the same basic phases: assessing the problem, planning the nursing interventions, implementating the planned care and evaluating the care given (Yura & Walsh).

In the assessment phase the nurse consentrates in finding nursing problems rather than of checking through long lists of needs. Experience has brought out the most common problems in the care of long-term patients. The most common problem areas are shown in the assessment table. If some problems are not included it is possible to add, as needed.

After defining the nursing problems, the next step in the process is the planning of care, i.e. setting goals and stating a date by which the goals should be reached.
To document nursing interventions nurses can either use concepts from a list of non-medical treatments and procedures or use text, or a combination of both.

The data of an intervention with the observations are entered after every visit to the patient.
When the date set for a goal is approaching the system reminds the user, and it is not possible to proceed without completing the evaluation.

The nursing care plan is one of the basic options in the FINSTAR index. Under this heading any doctor or nurse can access nursing care plan when required (the FINSTAR-system functions 24 hours a day seven days a week, and there is a video terminal in every doctor's and nurse's office) (Figure 1).

SMITH, JOHN 150226-099X M 64 YEARS
Medical diagnosis: Ca ventr.

DATE	PROBLEM	GOAL	DATE OF GOAL	INTERVENTIONS
23.10.90	RISK OF NOT GETTING ENOUGH FOOD RELA- TED TO THE NUTRI- TIONAL PROBLEM	NOT TO LOOSE WEIGHT	23.11.90	MASHED FOOD, NUTRITIVE FLUIDS, SMALL MEALS OFTEN
	EVALUATION: WEIGHT LOSS 2 KG			
23.10.90	CONSTIPATION	EMPTIES BOWEL TWICE A WEEK	9.12.90	ENEMA 2 TIMES A WEEK IF NEED- ED, FIBROUS SUBSTANCES IN FOOD
	EVALUATION:	BOWEL DOES NOT EMPTY WITHOUT AN ENEMA		
23.10.90	RISK OF LONELINESS RELATED TO A PHYSICAL WEAKNESS TO MOVE	NOT TO FEEL LONELY	9.12.90	MAKE SURE THAT RE- LATIVES VISIT AS BEFORE
	EVALUATION: NOT LONELY			

Figure 1: Nursing care plan

Though the computerization of the nursing care plan was designed by
district nurses, it can be used in any nursing field. The content may be
modified to fit the client`s situation. The program has been tested du-
ring 1990 and has been taken in everyday use in the beginning of 1991.

References

Gordon,M., (1982) Nursing diagnosis, McGraw-Hill Book Company, New York

Hynninen, P.,(1983) A comprehensive computer-based system for patient information in primary health care in: Scholes, M., Bryant, Y., Barber, B., The impact of computers on nursing, North-Holland Publishing Company, Amsterdam

Lauri,S., (1986) Hoitotyön ammatillinen päätöksenteko, Sairaanhoitajien koulutussäätiö, Helsinki

Rauhala,L., (1986) Ihmiskäsitys ihmistyössä, Gaudeamus, Helsinki

Simon,H., (1979) Päätöksenteko ja hallinto, Weilin & Göös, Espoo

WHO, (1976) The nursing process, Report on the first meeting of the Technical Advisory Group, Nottingham

Yura, H., Walsh, M.,(1988) The nursing process, Appleton & Lange, California

Nursing Workload Measurement - Computer Support

Christine Greenhalgh, Jean Roberts

Greenhalgh & Company Ltd.

Chatham House, Church Street West, MACCLESFIELD, UK, SK11 6EJ

Abstract

There is a requirement to periodically capture the workload profile of areas of the healthcare delivery process, analysing the efficacy of the resources used and monitoring any effects of changes made since the last review. A service is described which uses hand-held data capture devices and extensive computer support to evaluate the nursing activity in a busy acute hospital and to compare this activity profile with national normal values.

Audit for Healthcare Delivery

In this instance, an activity-based audit of the nursing function is the focus for the audit service. This is only one of a number of audit processes applicable to nursing. The methodology, equipment and processes used can readily be transferred to other healthcare delivery agents. The work study of hospital based nurses, a skilled and costly resource, is increasingly in demand in the UK due to the changes being made as a result of the 1989 NHS White Paper 'Working for Patients'[1] and subsequent moves towards healthcare delivery within a business context.

Objectives and Goals

The objective of the Activity Audit in Nursing study is to answer the following questions :

* how is nursing time spent
* are nurses appropriately deployed
* are the skills that are available used appropriately

The evaluation of the data captured is in two parts. Firstly an interpretation of the raw data to give standardised utilisation rates, workload profiles by staff grades, specialities and locations. Secondly, a preliminary interpretation of the reasons for the profiles observed - in discussion with the nursing, clinical and management staff of the area under study.

As a result of the discussion on the outputs from the study, changes in working practice are identified and implemented with an expected direct or indirect benefit to patient care through effective healthcare management.

A post-study repeat of the datacapture and analysis exercise assists in the quantification of the benefits of the changes made. It must be recognised that there are also intangible benefits to the process which are more difficult to identify and evaluate.

A number of UK studies to date have addressed the area of nursing audit in an operational context with very positive local outcomes [2]. GCL are in collaboration with a UK health authority to derive a transferable process that is of general applicability in order to effect the consistent comparability of processes across the NHS [3]. The generic core processes can then be made available in a wider domain.

Requirements

The process requires :

* Skilled data capture staff who do not impact detrimentally on the operation of the ward(s)

* Facilities to aggregate data from a number of operational locations within the Unit

* Functionality to analyse the data, mapping current situations onto previous positions, and indicating trends

* Report presentation of the audit information suitable for different levels of the organisation

* Confidential handling of clinically / operationally sensitive data pertinent to a particular delivery area

Comments

Whilst workstudy is a commonly used service, its use in routine activity analysis of nursing is not extensive in the UK. The principles have been adapted for a specific purpose and have been extended to include resampling and interpretation by highly skilled personnel. As further studies like the one outlined in this paper are carried out, the cumulative database will provide increasingly valid normal / standardised values for activity comparative purposes.

Future Developments

As the 'Internal Market' extends, hospitals in the UK will be compared and will have patients referred to them on the basis of their performance, efficiency and effectiveness. The criteria of value for money, positive outcomes and service availability will need to be marketed in order to secure further business. Those who commission these organisations to deliver care to their patients will require audit processes to monitor quality before referring patients to a particular establishment. Thus the Nursing Workload Monitoring package and Audit Service has wider market applicability in subsequent development phases.

Subsequent phases of the project will be developed to provide :

* Electronic data transfer to authorities from ourselves for statistical purposes

* Skills transfer / training of authority staff in the audit process

Conclusions

The audit process is still evolving. The core analyses and reports are emerging from such studies as described and the ad-hoc analyses being added to the formal studies as a result of the continuing nursing, clinical and management debate.

It is felt that such studies are of benefit to Healthcare Provider Organisations whether self governing Hospital Trusts, Private Hospitals and Directly Managed Units within the NHS or internationally.

References

1. NHS White Paper 'Working For Patients', HMSO 1989

2. Hulland, S.M., Smith, P.M., Clwyd H.A: Nursing Activity Audit Report (1987)

3. Greenhalgh, C.A., Clinical Audit Guidelines, GCL, 1990

CRITICAL CARE NURSING INFORMATICS:
PROMOTING THE QUALITY OF LIFE DURING CRISIS

Nancy J. Gantz
Good Samaritan Hospital & Medical Center
1015 N.W. 22nd Avenue, T230
Portland, Oregon 97210

ABSTRACT

The need to meet the technical challenges for the future of Critical Care Medicine and Nursing Practice is upon us. Never before has the complexity of clinical problems presenting in patients been greater, as well as the crucial need for high levels of nursing productivity, intervention and resource allocation. When acutely ill patients' clinical management become the driving force of the expert clinician, a strong support system must be available. This system must produce speed and accuracy, be convenient, show a reduction of repetitious tasks and produce a superior quality product. This system must be an electronic chart thus computerization of the medical record. The future must be a totally automated environment in critical care areas.

I. INTRODUCTION

The superior level of nursing practice that has evolved is directly proportional to the complexity of the multi-system failure patients that are presented in our hospitals. There must be a "High-Touch" in practice and a "High-Tech" in management if the acutely ill are to survive and promote the quality of life. As the level of nursing practice advances, it becomes more difficult to provide that sensitive aspect of touch and concern through the decreased man-hours or amount of time, resources available, governmental factors and fiscal constraints. It is at this point where directing technology toward an automated environment will help to address the dichotomy.

All areas of the United States of America as well as selected world countries are seeing a shortage of clinically competent and committed nursing practitioners. This is especially relevant in the area of Intensive Care and Critical Care Nursing. Nursing leaders, managers and educators must concentrate on various ways to retain the competent nurses already in practice. By creating an automated environment, nurses can practice with decreased paperwork, less frustration and inadequate documentation, thus creating more time for patient care. This, in turn, results in the highest quality of patient care and practice during the patients' episode of life-threatening illnesses.

II. RESULTS AND BENEFITS

This presentation will specifically illustrate the benefits for bedside informatics to the practicing clinical care clinician, manager, physician, ancillary personnel and, most importantly, the critically-ill patient. Through the formation, refinement and now sophistication of the Computer Implementation Committee (CIC) in our critical care units at our hospital, most of the problems or concerns that have arisen during the past five years have been addressed. The nursing staff praises and depends upon its:

- speed and accuracy of treatment, medication documentation
- quality assurance tracking
- concise bedside reporting
- lack of "hand-written" records
- ability to "scroll" through the patient's record (i.e., electronic chart) rather than having "screens" to paste together
- integration of all data that is collected on the complex patient.

The managers glean numerous advantages from this computerization, the most critical being that of increased utilization of nursing care time, effective conservation of health care dollars and resources, advancement as well as an enhancement toward a unified patient care delivery system, retrieval of vital information for risk management benefits--these have been a few of the components that the managers have seen with returning to a personalized, humanizing touch in patient care at the bedside.

The physicians in the hospital have seen many advantages that have assisted them in their day-to-day treatment and care using computerization. They were first very skeptical about the system, but now use it daily for medical grand rounds, data retrieval such as for hemodynamics, lab, drugs, IV's, as well as summarizing that into a 24-hour/48-hour picture. Additionally, due to the teaching status of the hospital, it is accessed for teaching rounds in a well-organized form in order that no vital information is neglected that could aid in the patient progress.

Ancillary personnel such as respiratory therapy, dietary and pharmacy all access the system and use the electronic chart to record their specific department statistics that, in turn, integrate with other patient information.

During the orchestration of the patient electronic information chart, concerns and glitches arose which were addressed individually and all resolved. Currently, the major project is the integration with the other hospital computer systems.

The benefits for the patient have shown to be numerous. It puts the nurse at the bedside with "high touch" and time to adequately care for their critical needs. This computerization system focuses on preserving and enhancing the quality of life for the critically ill. Quality of life is the gap between what the patient would like or needs and what he is able to achieve or retrieve. And the goal of nursing intervention and informatics is to narrow that gap.

III. CONCLUSION

The nursing profession has begun to look closer at their essential applications in the health care arena. Critical Care has had computerized clinical physiological data for over twenty years, but must now look at moving that technology even further into a vast network within the individual system. Critical Care Units must be able to have laboratory data, admission information, x-ray interpretations, quality assurance retrieval, audit capabilities, achieving, data selection, billing information--all within a single system. This system must be in the physicians office, transfer to the patient's admission to the hospital and follow them all the way to discharge and rehabilitation at home. The bedside clinician must never again see a piece of paper for each discipline, study, procedure or test result. Instead, the Critical Care practitioner will not only utilize a stethoscope but a computer for every aspect of that multi-system failure, critically ill patient intervention, treatment and life quality.

IV. REFERENCES

Ball, M.J. and Hannah, K.J.   Using Computers in Nursing (Prentice-Hall, Virginia, 1984).

Ball, M.J.; Hannah, K.J.; Gerdin Jelger, J. and Peterson, H. Nursing Informatic: Where Caring and Technology Meet (Springer-Verlag, New York, 1988).

Christensen, W.W. and Rupp, P.R.   Guide To Computers (Aspen, Maryland, 1986).

Cox, H.C.; Harsanyi, B. and Dean, L.C. <u>Computers and Nursing:</u> <u>Application to Practice, Education and Research</u> (Appleton & Lange, Connecticut, 1987).

Blum, B.I. <u>Information Systems for Patient Care</u>. (Springer-Verlag, Inc., New York, 1984).

Saba, V.K. and McCormick, K.A. <u>Essentials of Computers for Nurses</u> (Lippincott, Philadelphia, 1986).

Saba, V.K.; Rieder, K.A. and Pocklington, D.B. <u>Nursing and Computers: An Anthology</u> (Springer-Verlag, Inc., New York, 1989).

WOUND CARE MANAGEMENT

Elizabeth A. Butler, RGN, ONC, MChS, MBCS
Senior Nurse (Computing), St. Thomas' Hospital, London

Angela E. Jeune, RGN, RMN, CMS
1988-9, Specialist Nurse - Computer Liaison, St. Thomas' Hospital.
Analyst, Computer Centre,
South West Thames Regional Health Authority, London

ABSTRACT

This paper describes a computer system to aid nurses in the decision making process of selection of treatment and dressings for particular types of wound.

INTRODUCTION

The initiator of this system was a senior staff nurse on an acute surgical ward at St. Thomas' Hospital, London. Her interest in wound care arose from what she saw as the apparent confusion and at times disagreement amongst nurses and doctors in making decisions on the treatment and dressing of wounds. She realised that there was a lack of awareness of the wide range of products available and a lack of knowledge of what the products were and when and how they should be used. Many of these products were not being used despite the increase in research being published supporting their advantageous use. Her first priority was to increase her knowledge through reading the literature available. As Chairman of the Wound Care Review Group, she decided to attempt to increase the knowledge and awareness on this subject amongst her colleagues.

The Group decided that an information source was needed to which nurses could refer, which would enable them to be more aware of the products that could be used for a particular wound. The decision was also made not to advocate a particular product for use. This would allow room for preference and the individual patient's needs. It was also felt that there was a need to include research references which would encourage nurses to carry out research-based care.

A protocol was drawn up (ref. Bibliography 3) so that research references could be included. Initially the protocol was devised in order to have an information folder available on each ward. However, the Group were encouraged when their approach to the hospital Computer Services Department to develop a new wound care system received an enthusiatic response.

DEVELOPMENT OF THE COMPUTER SYSTEM

A collaborative group of nurses and computer professionals was formed to analyse, develop, pilot trial, and implement the required system.

The Wound Care Management system was planned to be included in the General Ward menu of the Patient Administration System, and to be one of several systems available on terminals placed in forty-one wards and outpatient departments in St. Thomas' Hospital.

OUTLINE DESCRIPTION OF THE COMPUTER SYSTEM

Upon entering the system a list of six questions is displayed, each with a reply box at the end of the line (see Fig. 1).

```
        Wound Care Management Checklist
        -------------------------------

                                          Y or N (E to End)

    1. Is there any black necrotic tissue present?        [ ]

    2. Is there any yellow/creamy coloured slough present? [ ]

    3. Are there any signs of an acute wound infection?
       eg inflamation, copious yellow pus, offensive
       odour, green slough, increase in body temperature. [ ]

    4. Is the wound producing copious amounts of exudate? [ ]

    5. Has the wound been surgically closed and is healing
       by primary intention?                              [ ]

    6. Is the wound filled with healthy red granulating
       tissue and healing by secondary intention?         [ ]
```

Figure 1

The permitted answers are Y if the question describes the particular wound, N if not, and E for end and exit the system. For example, Question 2 extracted from the list of questions is:

```
2. Is there any yellow/creamy coloured slough present? [ ]
```

A Y answer categorises the type of wound to be investigated. If an N answer is given, the cursor moves to the next question on the list whilst a Y answer brings a screen of recommended preparations, where they can be obtained and the references in which their use has been described (see Fig. 2). It was hoped that all details of the preparations and references could be fitted onto a single screen (or page). However, one question required two screens, and in this case the user can move forward or backward between the two pages. Both pages must be viewed as it is considered important that all items should be shown for a particular question.

```
Black necrotic tissue is present.
----------------------------------

Need for Debridement:-

  i) Surgical Debridement

 ii) Enzymatic Debridement

        Varidase - (European Journal of Clinical
        ========   Pharmacology, 1983,24:623 628
                   *Order from Pharmacy

iii) Chemical treatment

        Use of Hydrogen - (Nursing Times Community Out-
        Peroxide           look, April 1987, 30-34
        ===============   *Order from Pharmacy

              Next Action.[ ] E = End, C = Checklist
```

Figure 2

Once all the details have been viewed, the user can choose to either exit or continue with the next question on the checklist. After the sixth question, the user will be returned to the first question if the transaction is not ended.

The screens and questions may be edited by the programmer to keep the information up to date and the second revision is being prepared at this time.

The program is written in COBOL and runs on a mainframe T85 (Telefile Dual Configuration) using the AMPS operating system and distributed via the Ethernet Net 1 to ward terminals at St. Thomas' Hospital. A version is available on a PC written in BASIC using the same information with a minor modification that the questions are presented one at a time for reply.

IMPLEMENTATION AND EVALUATION OF THE SYSTEM

It was recommended that a pilot trial of the system should be carried out on the ward where the Chairman of the Wound Care Review Group was available for advice and guidance. The pilot trial commenced in the week of the 7th March 1988 for a four-week period.

After a favourable evaluation, it was agreed that the system should be released to the thirty-five wards in the Acute Unit on the 24th May 1988.

Implementing a 'user friendly' system to nurses who were already competent in the use of computers was achieved rapidly.

The Specialist Nurse - Computer Liaison took responsibility for the implementation across the Acute Unit. Most wards required only one visit, to advise them on the availability of the system and how to access it. Some wards had already investigated the new transaction on the menu before the arrival of the Computer Liaison Nurse, and had found it most helpful.

Whilst ongoing support was available, very few requests were made. The quick acceptance and smooth implementation of this system was very rewarding for all staff who were involved in the development.

EVALUATION BY MEANS OF A BEFORE-AND-AFTER QUESTIONAIRE

Before the system was released to the wards, it was decided that by the use of questionaires it would be possible to obtain unbiased and valuable feedback for research purposes.

The questionaires revealed that at the time of the introduction of the wound care management system the ward staff felt confident of their knowledge on this subject. But having used the system they discovered that their knowledge was incomplete and that they had therefore benefited from this new source of information.

The complete analysis is contained in a separate report (ref. Bibliography 5).

CONCLUSIONS

Two years have elapsed since this system was introduced. In that time it has been free from problems and extensively used. It is currently running throughout St. Thomas' Hospital as six wards in the Maternity Unit have recently been included in the system.

This is an example of a successful system devised by nurses for the use of nurses which was guided and supported by nursing and computing staff with the Computer Services Department.

BIBLIOGRAPHY

1. Adhami, Z., 'Surgical dressings', Journal of Hospital Infection, (1983) 6 123-7.
2. Draper, J., 'Make the dressing fit the wound', Nursing Times, Oct. 9, 1985, 32-5.
3. Monson, M., 'Priorities in wound management, Part I', The Professional Nurse, Aug. 1987, 352-5.
4. Monson, M., 'Priorities in wound management, Part II', The Professional Nurse, Sept. 1987, 402-7.
5. Rawlings, S., Analysis of the Wound Care Management Questionaire. Report issued by the St. Thomas' Hospital Computer Services Department, Aug. 1988, revised Oct. 1988.

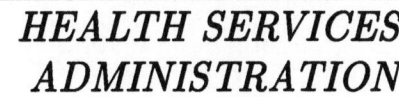

HEALTH SERVICES
ADMINISTRATION

IDENTIFICATION OF GROUPS OF PATIENTS CONSUMING EQUAL RESOURCES FOR A HOSPITAL FINANCING SYSTEM BY REGRESSION TREES

K.P.Pfeiffer[1], A.Maier[1], K.Malli[1], C.Buchegger[1], H.Spann[2],
D.Klingler[3], G.Embacher[4], M.Pregartbauer[4], E.Peer[4]
[1] Physiologisches Inst., Universität Graz, Austria
[2] IFU-Mangment, Wien
[3] Neurologische Abteilung, AKH Linz
[4] Österr. Bundeskanzleramt, Wien

SUMMARY

Regression trees have been used to identify groups of patients which
consume a similar amount of resources. As classification criteria the
main diagnosis, additional diagnosis, expensive medical intervention
and some other factors have been used. To find statistically robust
solutions different parametric and nonparametric methods have been
examined. A comparison of the old subsidies with the ones based on the
new system has been performed.

INTRODUCTION

Similar to the methods used for the construction of diagnosis related
groups (DRG's) [Fett80], we tried to classify patients into groups
which consume the same amount of resources, where resources are
expressed in monetary terms. A classification system which is based on
patterns of diagnostic, therapeutic and demographic variables was
developed. The aim of this system is the development of a diagnostic
and performance related hospital financing system.
Because of the complexity of the classification process a special
computer program has to be developed. The basic strategy of this
program and some statistical aspects of classification problems using
regression trees are discussed.

DOCUMENTATION, DATA, DATA QUALITY
Since 1989 it is obligatory in Austrian hospitals to document a
minimal basic data set for each patient. This data set consists of:
- main diagnosis (ICD-9-VESKA)
- up to nine additional diagnosis
- expensive medical interventions, operating room procedures
- age
- sex
- length of stay
- type of reception
- type of discharge.

For a sample of 20 hospital, which is the learning sample, also the costs for each patient are available. This sample includes about 340000 stationary patients from 1989.

To get more homogenous results from a medical viewpoint the whole ICD-9-VESKA-code was partitioned into 23 major diagnostic categories (MDC). Each MDC has been analyzed separately.

A fundamental problem of this study is the data quality. Different types of data errors, like insufficient documentation (only main diagnosis, no additional diagnosis), misspecification of diagnosis (only three positions of the ICD-9-VESKA code are used instead of the more precise four positions), mixing up main and additional diagnosis, expensive medical interventions are reduced to yes/no and some other may occur. Only few of these errors can be identified by a posterior reliability check.

REGRESSION TREES

Because the variables can be splitted into independent (minimal basic data set) and dependent (cost) ones, regression trees [Brei84] have been constucted to identify groups which are consuming equal amounts of resources, that means groups of patients with approximately equal costs. The classification process consists of two elementary procedures, namely split and merge.

Split: During the split process a group is diveded into two subgroups, called leaf, according to a certain variable from the minimal basic data set.

Before a "split" is performed, the means of the two resulting subgroups have to be compared and only if a significant difference for a given type I error (P_{split}) has been found, this split is considered purposeful. Furthermore in each subgroup the number of observations has to be greater equal N_{min}.

Merge: During the merge process two groups, which have been formed by a preceding split processes are merged together. An essential condition for merge is that the means of the two groups are not statistically significant different.

As a global criterion, similar to the DRG-methods, a sum of squares criterion has to be minimized:

$$SSQ = \sum_{i=1}^{p} \sum_{j=1}^{N(i)} (y(i,j) - y(i))^2$$

y(i,j).......dependent variable, cost of leaf i, patient j
y(i)..........mean of leaf i
p............number of leafs
N(i).........number of observations in leaf i

This criterion is used for the stepwise selection of the best variable for split respectively to select the two best groups for merge.

To identify groups, which consume a homogenous amount of resources, a sequence of split and merge procedures are applied (fig.1).

An analysis of the distribution of the dependent variable shows, that most leaves constructed by this procedure are contaminated by outliers, mainly patients with very high costs. It is well known, that a criterion, like SSQ, is very sensitive to outliers. The same problem arises for the statistical tests during split and merge. Therefore as a first step for the reduction of the influence of outliers, the values of the upper δ-tail of the distribution function of a possible leaf are reduced to the $(1-\delta)$-quantile of this leaf. Usually δ is choosen 0.05 or 0.10.

This limitation of the influence of outliers resulted in more homogenous groups from a medical viewpoint. Furthermore it is considered as a first step to handle insufficient documentated patients.

To circumvent these problems and to find a statistically more robust solution a nonparametric approach is considered. The main point is, that the absolute distance from the median (MAD) is used as model evaluation criterion:

$$MAD = \sum_{i=1}^{p} \sum_{j=1}^{N(i)} |y(i,j) - y(i)|$$

y(i)...median of leaf i.

Furthermore for the comparison of two leaves nonparametric rank tests, which compare the distribution and not the mean are applied during split and merge.

MODEL EVALUATION

Statistical evaluation: Not only one of the two model evaluation criteria, SSQ or MAD, has to be optimized; for a "good" model the distances between terminal leaves should be large, whereas the variance within leaves should be small.

Medical evaluation: Each statistical classification result was evaluated by a group of medical doctors. Medical plausibility criteria are mainly:

- the comparability of the resources used by patients with different diagnosis in one leaf
- the usefulness of a split of a main diagnosis according to additional criteria like age, sex, length of stay.

This medical evaluation leads to interactive modifications and furthermore to a critical inspection of the data base.

External validity: But the most important point of all evaluation criteria is the external validity, that means the correctness and in consequence the acceptance of a system for hospital financing. It is well known that for example the acceptance of the DRG-system [Pacc90] is not very high, because it is a very crude system and does not consider the complexity of dignostic and therapeutic procedures.

A comparison of the old subsidies for each Austrian hospital with the subsidies based on the new system shows winners and losers, where for some hospitals the amounts are rather high. Therefore the acceptance of this model was not very high too. Winners and losers have to be analysed with respect to external factors like hospital type, number of beds, structur quality, performance quality and outcome quality Furthermore it seems necessary to include additional variables or more detailed information into the model.

DISCUSSION

The aim was to construct a small number of homogenous diagnostic and performance related groups for a hospital financing system with a small but representative number of variables. Regression trees have been used to identify groups of patients which use the same amount of resources. First experiences with a learning data set from 1989 with 340000 patients and the application of the classification results to 158 Austrian hospitals shows some weak points which should be removed in a next study:

1) Data quality: Many medical doctors are not aware of the importance of documentation. This results in insufficient or incorrect documentations. Training in documentation and informations about the value of documentation for internal communication, external information and hospital planing are the first steps for an improvement of documentation. Further steps are expansions of the documentation programs, especially the inclusion of redundant information for a posterior reliability check [Grau90].

2) Data volume: The catalogue of expensive medical interventions and operating room procedures has to be expanded and it is necessary that all hospitals document these informations. It may be necessary that additional variables have to be included into the documentation, to consider the complexity of diagnostic and therapeutic processes.

3) Statistical methods: Robust model evaluation criteria and characteristic parameters of distributions, which are not so sensitive to outliers have to be used.

In the next few years we hope to identify a minimal data set and to develop classification procedures for a diagnostic and performance related hospital financing system, which is sensitive enough to reflect the necessary resources. To achieve this aim the first step is an improvement of the data quality and than it should be easy to construct appropriate classification trees.

Fig.1:

LDF Classification algorithm

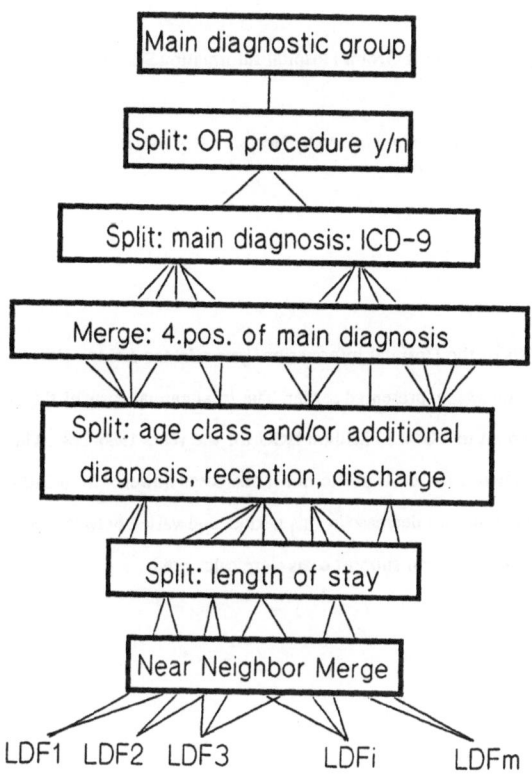

REFERENCES

[Brei84] Breiman L. et al.: Classification and Regression Trees. Wadsworth Int. Group, Belmont, Ca., 1984

[Fett80] Fetter R.B., Shin Y., Freeman J.L., Averill R.F., Thompson J.D.: Casemix definition by Diagnosis Related Groups. Med.Care, 18, 1-53, 1980

[Grau90] Graubner B.: Klinische Basisdokumentation und ICD-9. In: Medizinische Dokumentation in Forschung und Praxis. Augsburg 1990 (Tagungsband: Deutscher Verband d. med. Dokumentare).

[Pacc90] Paccaud F., Schenker L. (eds.): Diagnosis Related Groups. Verlag Hans Huber, Bern, 1990

UNIFORM HIS-COST MODELING:

EXPERIENCES AND FIRST RESULTS FOR THE LEIDEN UNIVERSITY HOSPITAL

W. Willemsen[1], E.M.S.J. van Gennip[1], A.R. Bakker[1], C.P.Louwerse[2]

1: BAZIS Central Development and Support Group Hospital Information System, Schipholweg 97, 2316 XA Leiden, The Netherlands.

2: Central Data Processing Department, Leiden University Hospital, Rijnsburgerweg 10, 2333 AA Leiden, The Netherlands

For the years 1986-1989 the costs of the Hospital Information System in the Leiden University Hospital were calculated using the cost allocation system presented earlier. The total annual costs of the HIS, including software, support and operating costs, amount to 2.08-2.33 Million ECU for the years 1986-1989. These costs represent 1.6 to 1.8 of the hospital budget respectively. The costs per terminal decreased however from 3100 ECU to 2300 ECU. The percentage of equipment costs did not decrease in this period, and varied between 33 and 36%. For various groups of applications, the software costs and support costs were calculated.

1. INTRODUCTION

Hospital Information Systems may require substantial investments. Cost and benefit analyses of these systems are scarce (see Collen for a review of the studies carried out for the USA (1)), and their conclusions diverge. For instance the estimates of the costs of the systems vary between 1.5 and 4.5% of the hospital budget (2,3). However a good comparison of these data is difficult, as often neither the way the results have been derived, nor the definitions are explicitly mentioned. A need for evaluation studies has been observed during a recent IMIA-ISTAHC workshop (October 1990, Montpellier (4)). (Inter)national cooperation and exchange of data among institutes is recommended.

The development of uniform models will facilitate (inter)national cooperation. In an earlier paper, presented at the MIE conference in 1990, we have suggested an uniform model for HIS cost modeling (5). This model is now being applied in a number of Dutch Hospitals. The present paper reports on the experiences and the first results for the Leiden University Hospital. In this hospital an extensive, integrated Hospital Information System is being used in the daily routine already since 1974 and it is gradually expanding. At present, more than 1000 terminals are in use for a large range of applications. For this hospital the costs of the HIS have been analyzed for 8 successive years (earlier results have been published (3)). This paper presents the results of the analyses for the period 1986-1989.

2. MATERIALS AND METHODS

The cost model

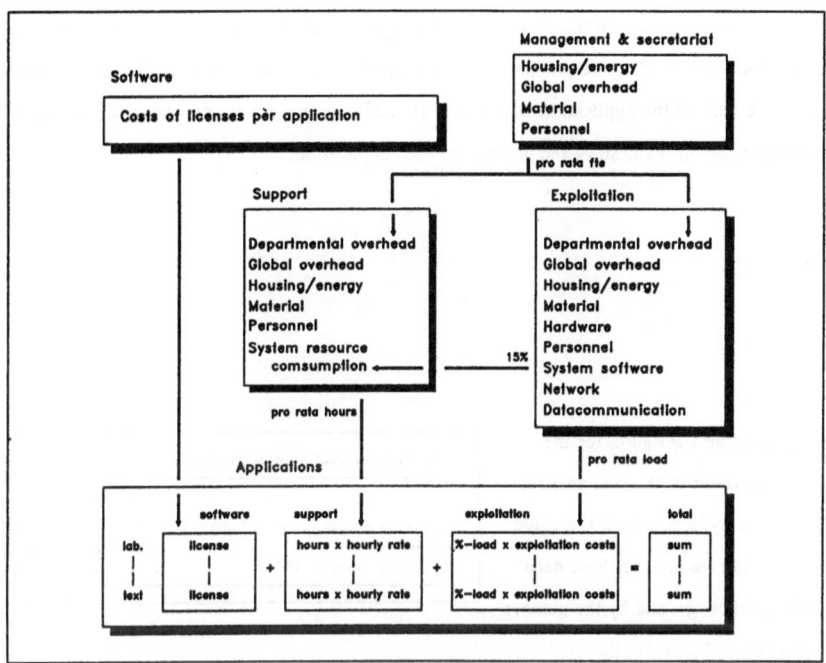

Figure 1: Cost allocation scheme

The cost model which is applied follows the model suggested earlier (5). This cost model allocates all the costs which have been made in a given year to the applications. First, all the costs are grouped into *cost centers*. Four cost centers are distinguished (Fig. 1): management and secretariat, support (including implementation and small scale local development), exploitation (of computer facilities) and software. Each of these cost centers takes into account a number of *expense elements*. The costs of system software (i.e. of the operating system) are included in the cost center exploitation. With regard to small scale local development, both the costs of software and of support are included in the costs center support. The costs are allocated to groups of allocations as indicated in Figure 1. As a consequence of the allocation scheme (Fig. 1), three cost categories can be distinguished for each group of applications: software costs, support costs and exploitation costs. For the allocation of the costs of *exploitation*, a detailed registration of the consumption of the various applications is required, i.e. an accounting system. As this accounting was not adequate, such an allocation could not be carried out.

The sources of information

The general ledger is the main source for the cost-figures for the various elements of expense. As not all the costs could be found in the ledger in sufficient detail, we were obliged to make estimations of the costs of housing and energy, costs of overhead for personnel, and costs of the network and data communication. All costs are expressed here in ECU (1 ECU = Dfl. 2.32 = US$ 1.23, dd April 9, 1991). The costs of *software* were estimated by projecting the current license system to the years 1986-1989. (Since 1990 the hospital pays an annual license fee for each software product it uses and a tariff for other services of BAZIS (like consultancy, implementation support and training). To scale the results, they are related to production figures from the hospital. These figures were derived either from the annual reports of the hospital, or from departmental administrations. To allocate the costs of the cost center *support* to each of the applications the records of manhours spent per product/project are used. The costs of *software* were allocated on the basis of the licenses for each application.

3. RESULTS

Table 1 gives some key figures for the hospital. The overall results of the cost analyses for the Leiden University Hospital are presented in Table 2. To scale the results, they have been divided by the hospital budget and by the number of terminals. The Figure 2 specifies the total costs for the three different cost categories (i.e. software, support and exploitation). The Figures 3 and 4 present the distribution of the costs of software and support among the groups of applications (5) (local development is not taken into account). These groups are Laboratories (Lab), Administrative (Adm), Logistic Applications (Log), Medical Records (MR), Personnel & Payroll (Pers), Other General

Table 1: General production figures

	1986	1987	1988	1989
Hospital budget (millions ECU)	130	129	124	128
# terminals	675	825	900	1030
# patient days (x 1000)	237	231	218	212

Table 2: Overall results cost analysis

	1986	1987	1988	1989
Total costs (millions ECU)	2.08	2.21	2.23	2.33
Costs as a % of hospital budget	1.6	1.7	1.8	1.8
Costs per terminal (x1000 ECU)	3.1	2.7	2.5	2.3
Costs per patient day (x1000 ECU)	8.8	9.5	10.2	11.0
Equipment costs % total costs	38	34	33	36
# hours spent support (x1000)	13.8	18.5	13.6	15.3

Applications (Gen), Radiology (Rad), Pharmacy
(Pharm), Appointment Scheduling (App), Nursing
(Nurs), and Text Editing (Text). One should
however bear in mind that this grouping does not
indicate whether the dataprocessing offers a
superficial support or a support in depth. Further
refinement in this respect should be considered.

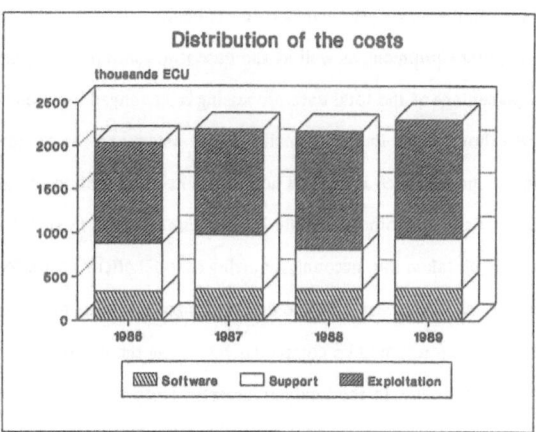

Fig. 2: Distribution of costs dataprocessing.

4. DISCUSSION

During the period 1986-1989, the costs of
data processing as a percentage of the total hospital
budget have increased from 1.6% to 1.8%. The
increase in the costs may be attributed to an
increase in the intensity of use of the system.
Between 1986 and 1989 the functionality of the
Hospital Information System increased.

For instance in 1989 a new generation of a large
laboratory information system has been installed.
Moreover the number of terminals increased by
more than 50% during this period. It has been
stated that HIS costs in the USA may amount to
4.5% (2). Hence, the outcome for the Leiden
University Hospital, 1.6-1.8%, can be considered
low. However, in order to make a full comparison
of the results, also the performance and
functionality of the system should be taken into
account. In our opinion, the system at Leiden sets a
high standard in both of these respects. The
exploitation costs (i.e. the costs of operating and
hardware together), amount to more than 50% in
the Leiden University Hospital. Instead of declining,

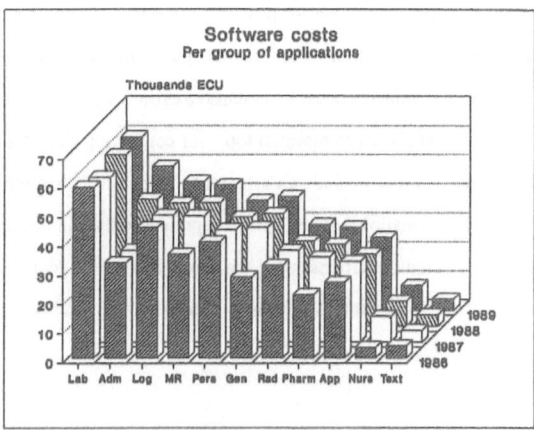

Fig. 3: Software license costs (excluding local development)

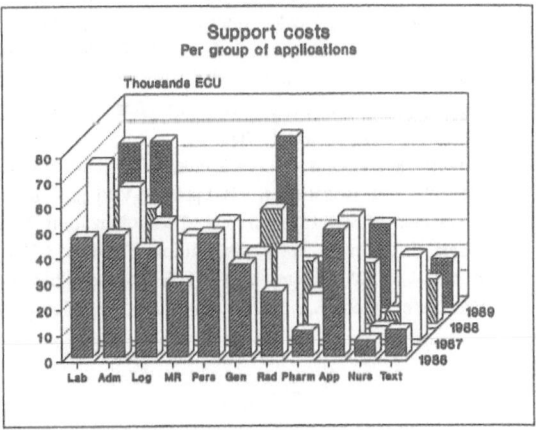

Fig. 4: Support costs (excluding local development).

as is often assumed, the hardware costs tend to stabilize. This hardware-componentincludes the costs of the central computer equipment, as well as the decentral computer equipment. In the period 1986-1989, the costs of hardware, as a percentage of the total data processing costs ranged between 33 and 38%. The costs of support remain stable too, even though both the functionality of the system and the number of terminals have increased.

In the model which is applied here, costs have been allocated to groups of applications, as a first step to facilitate the comparison with other Hospital Information Systems. In such a comparison also the functionality of the applications should be taken into account, requiring cost-benefit or cost-effectiveness analyses. The current allocation of the costs to applications reveals that the distribution of the costs of software and support vary widely among applications. The cost allocation should be completed, by adding the exploitation cost-component. For that we must find a suitable distribution code. In the Leiden University Hospital an accounting system records the consumption of resources for each application (indicated by the starting modules), during the day-shift (i.e. from 7.30 a.m. until 17.15 p.m.). Several items are measured, e.g. swap outs, disk accesses, and cpu(time). These data, however are not sufficient to distribute the load as firstly the load for processing during the night is not included in the present numbers, secondly in an integrated Hospital Information System applications interrelate, thirdly the item "disk accesses" refers to "logic disk accesses", and fourthly there is no consensus on how to balance the different measured items.

Cost analyses are essential tools for comparing Hospital Information Systems and to guide future developments. In this paper we have made an attempt to carry out an analysis, following a model which may be applicable for any Hospital Information System (5). We experienced that an accurate ledger, a registration of manhours spent and accounting modules are essential. We would like to challenge other groups to apply this model to their Hospital Information System and to inform us about their experiences.

5. REFERENCES

1. M.F. Collen, 1991: Assessing Medical Information Systems: a historical review of the United States experience. In: "Assessment of Medical Informatics Technology Joint Working Conference Montpellier, October 22-26, 1990", C. Flagle, F. Gremy, S. Perry, eds. Editions ENSP: 179-209.
2. R.M. Coffey, 1980: How a medical information system affects hospital costs: The El Camino Hospital experience. NCHSR Research Summary Series, DHEW Pub. No (PHS) 80-3265, Washington D.C.: Department of Health, Education and Welfare.
3. A.R. Bakker, H.G.M. van der Zanden: Five years of total HIS accounting, analysis and prognosis. In: MIE 85 Helsinki, F.H. Roger et al. eds, Springer-Verlag, Berling, Heidelberg, New York, Tokyo: 59-64.
4. Assessment of Medical Informatics Technology Joint Working Conference Montpellier, October 22-26, 1990, C. Flagle, F. Gremy, S. Perry, eds. Editions ENSP: 553-558.
5. A.R. Bakker, W. Willemsen 1990: HIS cost modelling; a suggestion for uniformity. In: MIE 90 Glasgow, R. O'Moor et al. eds, Springer-Verlag, Berlin, Heidelberg, New York, Tokyo: 143-148.

One Approach to Assessing Experience/Price
Levels at Hospitals

Jana Dale
BUPA, Provident House, Essex Street, London, WC2R 3AX

Abstract

Comparing the levels of hospital charges made between different hospitals is by no means a straight forward excercise. This is because hospitals may carry out vastly different mixes of procedures and treat patients who may require longer/shorter stays in hospitals. So it is necessary to take account of procedure mix and patient mix when assessing charges in order to ensure that 'like with like' comparisons are made.

A number of approaches were considered by BUPA and comparisons of episode and daily charges studied into some depth. Both episode and daily charge comparisons have a number of advantages and disadvantages. A decision was made that for practical applications comparison of the daily charges adjusted for length of stay and procedural complexity mix would be used.

1. Introduction

In the U.K. private healthcare provision developed alongside the National Health Service as a complementary service providing care for some 10 percent of the population. The early eighties noticed a large increase in people purchasing private healthcare cover. With some two years delay the costs of providing this care rocketed.

During the eighties the level of medical inflation has been running substantially above the retail inflation. As every increase in healthcare costs inevitably finds its way into health insurance premiums, BUPA saw the need to foster a role of its 'members champion' rather than just a simple payor of claims. As a part of this new role BUPA started to scrutinize where the majority of costs were being incurred with a view of excercising some control over them.

Over half of all the claims paid consist of hospital bills for inpatient admissions. Hospital costs were therefore the first area BUPA decided to analyze in some depth.

2. Hospital Charges

Hospital charges incurred during a hospital stay (so called episode of treatment) can be broken down into four basic elements: accommodation and nursing; theatre fees; drugs and dressing; diagnostic and ancilliary charges (pathology, radiology, physiotherapy etc.). The consumption of these services however does not follow a uniform pattern.

During a surgical episode of treatment there would be one visit to the theatre, one set of radiological and pathological tests, and also the majority of drugs, dressings, and other consumables would be used at the beginning of the hospital stay. Accomodation and nursing and relatively small amounts of drugs would then be consumed on a daily basis.

3. Comparison of charges

There are a number of factors that affect the level of hospital charges. Hospitals carry out vastly different mixes of procedures and treat patients that may require longer stays in hospital, perhaps due to their age, chronic conditions or poor general state of health.

From the insurers point of view, we want to compare 'like with like'. The aim is to compare the cost of the same treatment between different hospitals without penalizing those hospitals that concentrate on more complicated surgery, or have a patient population with a higher age profile.

3.1 Episode approach

One method would be to look at how total episode charges, perhaps by procedural surgical complexity category, vary between hospitals. However this approach yields several problems:

(i) Episode charges for different procedures, even within one procedure category, can vary considerably due to longer/shorter lengths of stay required.

(ii) Hospitals treating large numbers of elderly patients would be penalized due to the longer lengths of stay required.

(iii) One very long length of stay could severely affect average episode charges at smaller hospitals with few BUPA patients.

3.2 Per Diem approach

Another possible approach would be to compare hospital average average daily charges.

This approach would remove the length of stay problem. However this would be unfair to hospitals with generally shorter lengths of stay as their fixed costs i.e. theatre fees, drugs and dressings, and other ancilliary charges would be spread over a smaller number of days, thus making them appear expensive.

Consequently an approach was required which allowed for longer lengths of stay when necessary but allowed for fixed charges on an episode basis.

This is the basis of our "adjusted daily all-up charge".

3.3 Length of stay adjustment

Total theatre fees, drugs and dressings and ancilliary charges made by the hospital are divided by what would have been the total expected (standard) length of stay during the period in question. This gives a daily figure which is then added to the standard bed charge to give an "adjusted daily all-up charge".

Example:

Suppose a patient had a major procedure and was charged as follows:

Accomodation & nursing	(A)	10 nights at 120	= 1200
Theatre fees	(G)		= 135
Drugs and dressings	(H)		= 200
Pathology	(F)		= 100
Radiology	(F)		= 50
Physiology	(F)		= 50
Total			= 1735

A daily charge for this 10 days hospital stay would be:
1735 / 10 = 173.5.

Suppose BUPA's expected length of stay for a major procedure is 7 days.

Then the adjusted daily all-up charge would be

    (A) + ((G+H+F) / Expected Length Of Stay)

    120 +   (535 / 7)   = 196.4

This example covers one procedure only but in practice costs for all episodes performed are combined together. This removes any possible unfairness envisaged due to one patient requiring large amounts of drugs for instance.

Thus hospitals with generally short lengths of stay or hospitals carrying out relatively major procedures as daycare are not penalized. Expected lengths of stay rather than actual lengths of stay are used in the calculation.

Similarly hospitals requiring long lengths of stay due to their patient mix are not penalized as the accomodation charge is still allowed and only the fixed charges are adjusted.

No judgements are made at this stage with regards to the appropriateness of a particular length of stay as this would be a subject of utilization review not considered here.

3.2 Complexity adjustment

BUPA classifies procedures into 5 main categories (and a further 25 sub categories) according to surgical complexity: Minor, Intermediate, Major, Major Plus and Complex Major.

One argument used against this method is that some procedure types could be expected to cost more per day than others.

Whilst it may be true of individual procedures, on analysis of the data it has been established that daily charges by procedure category are very similar. Minor procedures for instance cost much the same per day (on average) as major ones.

Thus those hospitals performing more or less complex procedures than others are treated fairly given the reasonable assumption that a fairly standard mix of procedures within each category is undertaken.

However there is one exception to this finding. Complex Major procedures e.g. open heart surgery do cost significantly more per day than other procedure types. In fact they cost about 50% extra per day.

This is taken into account in a hospital assessment. If the hospital performs more or less Complex Major procedures than average the extra costs or the reduced costs are taken into account and the daily charge adjusted accordingly.

4. Discussion

At the end of the day, "adjusted daily all-up charges" at different hospitals should be comparable regardless of procedural and patient mix, and it is felt that this method provides the fairest possible assessment of prices at hospitals, as experienced by BUPA.

If it is felt that experience differs significantly from expectation (given base price lists etc.), special investigations are carried out to establish whether there may be specific reasons for adopting some special adjustment. In practice special adjustments are rarely justified.

This approach could be extended to make it more sensitive to specific procedures and this has been on accassions undertaken e.g. in cases of specialist centres. Other factors can also be taken into account e.g. the age of the patients, geographical location etc. These areas are currently being studied at BUPA.

5. Sources

BUPA data 1983 - 1990.

NOSOCOMIAL INFECTIONS AND LENGTH OF HOSPITALIZATION ACCORDING TO DRG

An evaluation based on the bacteriological laboratory and the PMSI data at the University hospital of Nancy in 1989.

B. Legras, A. Patris, J-C. Burdin, D. Mayeux, L. Feldmann

Service d'informatique médicale, Hôpital Marin, Nancy, 54000, France

Abstract : We took the informations of the discharge summaries (GHM : French equivalent of DRGs) with those of the bacteriology (evaluation of nosocomial infections) in order to estimate the increase of the average length of stay when there are acquired infections. For the 18 GHMs with a sufficient size, the length is multipliedd by a factor which varies between 1.3 to 3.1. We propose a correction because natural "longer" stays have more risk of acquired infections. Then the variation factor is smaller, from 1.1 to 2.8, and the increase the length of stay reaches 7.1 days in average.

Introduction :

The present situation in the French hospitals leads to the fact that the practitioners do not often declare acquired infections. Thus, their cost is difficult to appreciate. At the University Hospital (UH) of Nancy, two complementary computerized data bases allow us to study this problem:

- the records of bacterial sensitivity to antibiotics allows a satisfactory estimation of the nosocomial infections (1, 2).
- the discharge summaries (DS) inform on the pathology of the patients and their GHMs (French equivalent of DRGs).

Bringing together these two data bases makes it possible to evaluate the influence of a probable nosocomial infection, on the average length of hospitalization (ALH) of the GHMs, .

Methods :

The first step consists first in selecting the bacteriological analyses corresponding to nosocomial infections. The Central Laboratory of Bacteriology of the UH receives every sample taken in the hospital. The software, elaborated by the authors (3), allows the entry, recording and reporting of these explorations. In order to obtain a data base on the "suspected" germs supposed to be a reasonable image of the acquired infections of the UHN, we carry out different selections:

- the first-one checks only the germs with record of bacterial sensitivity to antibiotics. This selection takes into account the type of the sample, the results of the direct examination (existing leukocytes), and eventually the numeration of the involved germ (as for the cultures of urine and of the respiratory tract).
- the data base must not include "doubles". Thus, for a specific patient, it counts a defined germ only once, even if it has been isolated in different samples (for

example in blood and urine cultures) during a fixed period (now set at two months). In addition the bacterial sensitivity profile is taken into account for each germ : when several strains are isolated, we admit to different germs when there is an important difference for an antibiotic (for example the strain going for sensitive to resistant or inversely; on the contrary, changing from sensitive to medium, or from medium to resistant, is not considered significant).
- we only take into account the samples taken after two days (classical definition of the nosocomial infection).
- some particular samples are not selected, for example the examinations done in order to control the effectiveness of a digestive decontamination.

The second step consists in bringing these informations together with the data of the discharge summaries' base. From 1985 on, the UHN experiments the French Program for Medicalisation of the Information System (PMSI). The Department of Medical Information collects the DS filled up by the clinical units, enters them and uses them with an original software locally developed. For each DS, the system calculates the length of hospitalization (LH) and the GHM. As the key is the same, it has proved quite easy to update the DS with the bacteriological informations : suspected germ, sampling date, sample type. We can then compare, globally and by GHM, the ALH of the patients supposed to suffer from a nosocomial infection (I category) and those supposed not to have (S category).

Material :

The initial bacteriology data base concerns 12,169 records of bacterial sensitivity to antibiotics, managed in 1989. Every missing incoming date has been completed later on. After removing the "doubles" and the before-two-days samples, we obtain 5,655 suspected germs. The more frequent one are: staphylococcus aureus (19 %), escherichia coli (19%), pyocyanic (11%), the other staphyloccocci (9%), proteus (6%), klebsiellae (5%). That same year, we collected 51,905 DS in 44 units (over 50) of "short-stay type" hospitalization units. We consider only the stays lasting more than two days, in order to compare judiciously between I and S categories, because the less-than-two-days stays are not taken into account in the I category. We exclude the multiple-unit stays, because the rate of exhaustivity is not satisfactory and they are more difficult to analyze. Thus, we are lead to studying 34,367 mono-stays.

The junction of the two data bases leads to 1774 stays of the I category, which corresponds to 2932 of the 5655 suspected germs (52%). The difference arises from the non-PMSI units, the exclusion of the multiple-unit stays, and the moderate exhaustivity of some PMSI-units. We will compare this group to the stays of type S, including 32,580 stays. In the joined data base, we keep the information on the first germ detected, and especially the date of the first sample. By comparing the lengths of stays without infection and those before the first sample, we tried to find out if "natural" longer stays could explain in part the increase of the length of the stay. We compare the lengths of stays using the t Student's test, with a 5 % risk. We indicate, in addition to the averages and standard errors, the relative length, which is the rate between the ALH of the I category and that of the S category.

Results :

There is an important difference between groups I and S : the ALH I is 2.50 longer than the others (table 2). The difference is a little higher for the surgical GHMs (2.57) than for the medical GHMs (2,35).

However the ratio of stays of the I type is not the same considering the GHM. We study separately the 18 GHMs with more than 20 stays of group I, in order to have a more acurate idea about the influence of the infection on the ALH. These GHMs concern 618 stays (35% of the total). The average of their relative length of stay is 2.1, which is shorter than the average of the whole. The majority of relative lengths (10 out of 18) is in between the interval [1.6 - 2.4]. They are all over 1.3. Every difference is highly significant with p <0.01.

In these 18 GHMs, we study the average of the length of stay before the first sample. It is around 0.4 times the total length. For most of the GHMs (9 out of 18), it is between 0.75 and 1 of the length of stay of the S group (fig. 1).

Considering the small size of the GHMs in the I category, we have grouped the surgical GHMs and the medical GHMs in order to compare the length of stay before sample and that of the group S. To study this, we divided the lengths into periods of five days, except for the last class including from 40 to 300 days. In each of these classes, we calculate the number of days of hospitalization (NDH) concerning the group S stays. For the group I, we determined then the number of stays (NS), for which the first sample was taken during the period concerned. We then calculate the ratio R = 1000 * NS/NDH.

We show the results in table 1. For the medical GHMs, R is the higher from 20 to 34 days. Considering that the ALS is equal to 10.3 days, we can suppose that the I group includes patients who would have stayed longer than the average time, even without infections. The result is less evident for the surgical GHMs, where R is higher from 10 to 24 days. We can obtain a more concise indicator in calculating the "estimated average length of hospitalization" (EALH) :

$$EALH = \frac{1}{n} \sum_{i=1}^{k} n_i * ALH_i \qquad \text{where :}$$

    n is the size of the GHM (or the group of GHMs) studied in I group,

    n_i patients have had their sample at i day,

    ALH_i is the ALH of the patients of the same GHM (or of the same group of GHMs) without infection, and having a length of at least i days.

EALH is the average length of hospitalization of patients chosen by groups which size is n_1, n_2, ..., the n_i of the "i"th group being chosen randomly over the stays of the S group having a length of at least i days. We obtain an adjusted relative length in calculating the ratio between the ALS of I group and the corresponding EALH. The results figure in the column "Adjusted Relative Length" of table 2.

Discussion and conclusion :

We cannot specify the diagnosis of nosocomial infection without medical informations. By themselves, the laboratory data lead to false positives and false negatives. The analysis, proposed here, reduces these errors without suppressing them. Its evaluation is going on. In spite of these reserves, the obtained results are very clear: the rough increase of the ALS is globally at a level of 2.1. For an economic point of view, the study using the GHMs allows the estimation in each category. Among the 18 studied GHMs, the rough increase rate varies between 3.4 and 1.3, 2.8 and 1.1 after adjustment. The relative length of stay with infection decreases when we use the more comparable stays as a reference. After adjustment, the increase of the length of hospitalization is divided by 2 to reach 7.1 days, in average on the 18 studied GHMs , value comparable with the results of others studies (4).

References :

1-LEGRAS B, PATRIS A, LEGRAS J et al. : Une aide automatisée à la détection des infections nosocomiales à partir d'un fichier central de bactériologie. Méd. et Mal. Infect. 1989, 19, 728-733.

2-LEGRAS B, BURDIN J-C, FELDMANN L et al. : Evaluation des infections nosocomiales à partir des examens de bactériologie. Revue de Santé Publique, 1990, 6, 6-12.

3- LEGRAS B, LEGRAS J , BURDIN J-C Bactério : un logiciel sur microordinateur pour la bactériologie avec une validation des antibiogrammes et une aide à la détection des infections nosocomiales. Revue française des Laboratoires, 1991, 217, 47-51.

4-WENTZEL R : Nosocomial infections, DRG and study on the efficacy of nosocomial infection control. JAMA, 1985, 78, 3-7.

Days	R. Med	R. Surg
3-5	4.71	6.77
6-9	4.07	8.72
10-14	3.96	9.82
15-19	4.06	9.23
20-24	6.11	9.41
25-29	6.60	8.71
30-34	6.22	7.04
35-40	1.54	5.42
40-300	4.45	2.67

Table 1 : Rate of first sample over 1000 days and by length
R. Surg = 1000*NS/NDH for the surgical GHM   R. Med. = 1000*NS/NDH for the medical GHM

	group I			group S			relative lengths	
	(n)	m	±s	(n)	m	±s	real	adjusted
All GHM	(1774)	26,8	±0,53	(32593)	10,7	±0,06	2,50	1,81
Surg. GHM	(990)	28,8	±0,81	(13400)	11,2	±0,10	2,57	1,89
Med. GHM	(767)	24,2	±0,62	(18891)	10,3	±0,06	2,35	1,66
GHM 1	(71)	28,2	±2,14	(243)	14,1	±0,47	2,00	1,25
GHM 2	(37)	31,9	±2,60	(69)	12,9	±0,72	2,47	1,24
GHM 18	(65)	30,7	±2,24	(386)	16,0	±0,49	1,92	1,41
GHM 113	(36)	36,6	±4,89	(116)	19,4	±1,44	1,89	1,40
GHM 128	(33)	29,5	±3,85	(356)	12,2	±0,60	2,42	1,70
GHM 129	(31)	25,1	±3,16	(150)	17,2	±0,84	1,46	1,29
GHM 136	(26)	23,5	±2,40	(221)	14,1	±0,67	1,67	1,32
GHM 139	(51)	28,0	±2,67	(247)	13,5	±0,58	2,07	1,50
GHM 159	(22)	34,7	±5,46	(107)	21,4	±1,16	1,62	1,24
GHM 160	(24)	30,2	±5,00	(515)	9,0	±0,38	3,36	2,30
GHM 184	(29)	25,5	±2,75	(319)	13,6	±0,51	1,87	1,50
GHM 302	(23)	18,1	±2,37	(1099)	8,2	±0,12	2,20	1,35
GHM 429	(27)	25,6	±1,45	(11)	19,1	±3,82	1,34	1,20
GHM 432	(35)	19,3	±2,40	(148)	12,6	±0,40	1,53	1,10
GHM 589	(32)	34,3	±2,80	(107)	16,7	±1,34	2,05	1,77
GHM 593	(24)	30,9	±3,76	(486)	9,1	±0,44	3,40	2,79
GHM 622	(30)	34,7	±3,08	(177)	17,3	±0,91	2,00	1,55
GHM 675	(22)	26,0	±3,30	(316)	9,7	±0,39	2,68	1,75

Table 2 : Comparison of the length of hospitalization (days) of the I and S groups
(n=size, m=average, s=standard error)

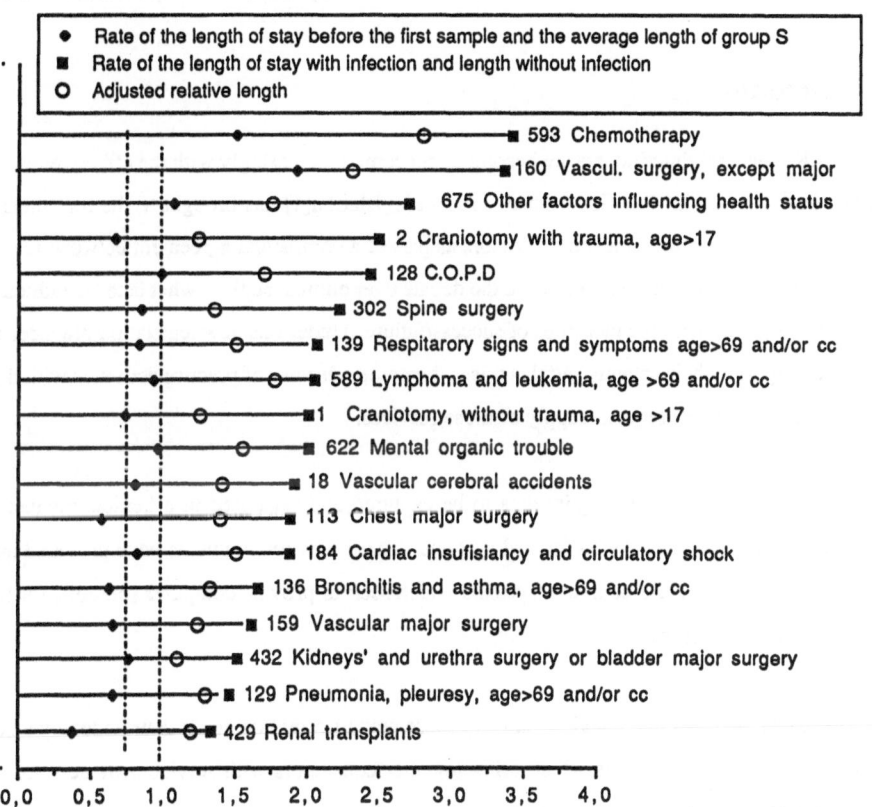

Fig 1: Standardized length on stays without infection for the 18 studied GHMs.

Appointment Systems — an Information Resource for General Practice

T.J.Howkins

Medical Informatics Group, Department of Computer Science, University

of Manchester, Manchester M13 9PL, U.K.
Tel +44-61-275-6159, Fax +44-61-275-6280

Abstract

The majority of British General Practitioners organize their patient contacts through appointment systems. This paper examines the central position of appointments systems in a practice's information system and examines the information resource which such system control. It is suggested here that the information resource can be classified as practice-centred, clinician-centred or patient-centered and that in each of these domains, the appointment system can be a powerful tool for providing information.

1 Introduction

In the U.K., General Practitioners are becoming concerned increasingly with the effectiveness of what they do and how they do it. The Government's recent legislation[1] has brought to the fore measures of performance which must be achieved by doctors as part of a contractual agreement between the state and the doctor. These measures have accentuated the debate over clinical audit — what is to be audited, how it is to be audited together with the measures of success/failure. Under this new legislation practices must supply an annual report to their patients and this raises the *consumer view* of practice activities with their demands for services and the consequent supply of those services.

These information needs require data to be captured and organised in a flexible manner which have cost implications, particularly on manual systems. These new requirements have provided an impetus in the sale of commercial GP computer systems which seek to provide computer solutions for the emerging needs of general practice.

This paper suggests that a major source of these new information needs is provided by a computerised appointments system. Systems which bring together consumers with service providers are an everyday occurrence, for instance, airline reservations, mail order companies, theatre bookings to name but a few. In the U.K., appointment systems provide the main contact mechanism between doctor and patient. In

1981, the Royal College of General Practitioners produced a report[2] which stressed the importance of an appointments system in uniting all aspects of a practice's information system.

A prototype system was designed and has been in use since 1986 in a practice in Manchester with the financial support of the U.K. Department of Health. The features and facilities of this system have been described more fully elsewhere[3, 4]. The following diagram illustrates the overall architecture of the system:-

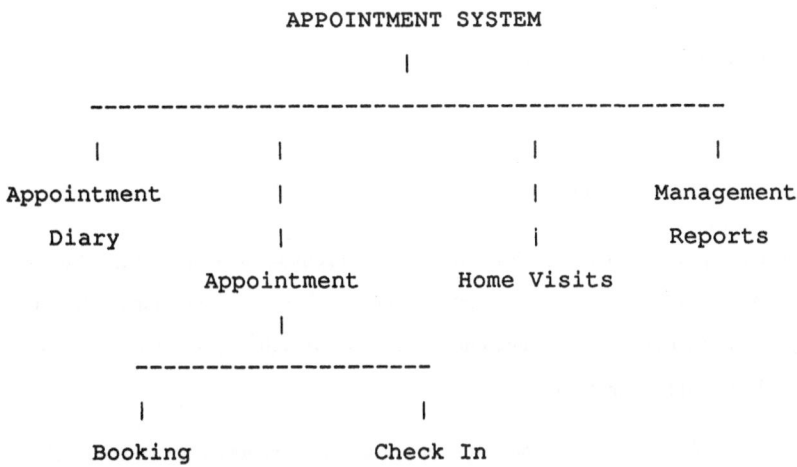

One important feature of this system is the ability of the computer system to capture data *at no cost to the practice*. This data has considerable potential for information provision. This paper examines this potential for meeting the emerging information needs of general practitioners in this new decade by discussing three major perspectives of such systems, namely *Practice-centred, Clinician-centred and Patient-centred*.

2 Practice-centred information

The Appointment System is the fulcrum of the practice's activity. It is the system which brings together demand for services together with their provision. In a business sense, there is much data available which describes the take up of services on offer, the nature of the 'customer' and the quality of the services provided. This can yield valuable management information and can provide flexibility in coping with the information needs of the practice.

It is important to have an overall control of *appointment capacity* — i.e. the number of appointments which are available for booking in a specified time period. This is an important measure of capacity and should help identify times where there is under-provision of appointments. This allows the Practice Manager to take action to plan additional capacity and thereby avoid turning patients away. In the practice in which the prototype system was installed, 85% of patients' demand for appointments is for the next four working days. Whilst this will vary from practice to practice and indeed from country to country, it raises an important issue. The patient expects to be given an appointment in his/her own timescale and is disappointed if this is not possible. In countries where mobility between practices is possible — i.e. where practices *compete* for patients then this is of crucial importance. Differential booking periods for appointments may be desirable to regulate the supply of appointments. For instance, the appointment system allows the practice to specify booking periods as:-

- Normal — available throughout a forward period.

- Standby — available up to 14 days before the appointment date.

- Urgent — available on the day of appointment only.

An Appointment System can provide *workload* information which can enable both the Practice Manager and Clinicians to keep an activity profile of the practice. The Appointment System can provide this because the data captured to describe such a transaction can yield much useful information. For instance, a booked appointment may be described by the following data:-

- Patient's identification and thereby access to patient data — e.g. name, address, age and other characteristics.

- Date and Time of the appointment.

- Clinician's identification.

- Reason for the appointment (if known)

Furthermore, when the patient arrives for the appointment, a *check-in* procedure ensures that additional important data can be captured automatically — time of arrival, time of departure etc. This gives the opportunity to examine the behavioural aspects of patients attending surgeries, — e.g what percentage of patients do not turn up for an appointment or are late?

Workload information can be provided in the form of appointments and home visits serviced by each clinician in the practice over a given period. With access to patient data, it is possible to build age-sex profiles of each session and thereby analyse the patient population which presents.

3 Clinican-centred information

An Appointments System provides the opportunity for clinicians to monitor the timekeeping aspects of their sessions by showing details of all waiting patients with their appointment time and their time of arrival. It also enables them to examine their punctuality in keeping appointment times. Unpunctuality is unpopular with patients but may have many legitimate causes. It is possible to analyse sessions by an age-sex profile but it should be possible to link the appointment to an encounter/diagnosis/treatment record which shed light on cases of persistent overrunning. It would also enable the clinician to examine presentation patterns with particular regard to patterns of disease. This opens an important door to *research uses* of this data which would be helpful to a practice which has research objectives.

4 Patient-centred information

Patients often regard appointments systems as a *barrier* to obtaining the service they need. A computerised appointment system must anticipate this and provide patient-friendly methods of responding to the patient's needs. In such a way, patients may come to regard appointment systems as cooperative rather than obstructive.

Patients should have a *reasonable* probability of gaining an appointment which suits their need. The provision of suitable appointments, together with warnings of under capacity are therefore crucial in maintaining an *adequate* supply to meet patient demand.

A major source of patients' complaint is excessive waiting time for their appointment. It follows that waiting times should be kept under review. The Appointments System checks in patients on their arrival for an appointment and records automatically the time of arrival. This allows the practice to analyse waiting times and examine the following problems:-

- Late arrival for appointments.

- No show patients.

- Average waiting times.

- Clinicians whose sessions regularly run behind schedule.

This would allow more 'fine-tuning' of session/appointment lengths to minimize the problem. If a patient has a persistent history of 'no show', it may guide the receptionists in giving future appointments.

5   Conclusions

The need is evident for more pertinent information flows to help in the delivery of healthcare. This paper has drawn attention to the role of a computerised appointment system as a powerful information provider enabling practices to monitor their activity more closely and tune it to patients' needs. With the emergence of more sophisticated methods of making enquiries and retrieving information from practice-held data, the real prospect opens up of providing a system which responds to ad hoc requests for information. This will be crucial to practices in the 1990s.

References

[1] *Working for Patients* HMSO Cm555, London 1989.

[2] *Computers in Primary Care*, Occasional Paper 13, Royal College of General Practitioners, London 1982.

[3] Howkins TJ & Kay CR *A Computerized Appointment System for General Practice*, Proceedings of MEDINFO89 Singapore, December 1989 pp 991-4.

[4] Howkins TJ *Computerized Appointments System in General Practice: Responding to the Challenge* Proceedings of the Royal Australian College of General Practitioners 6th Computer Conference, Sydney 1990.

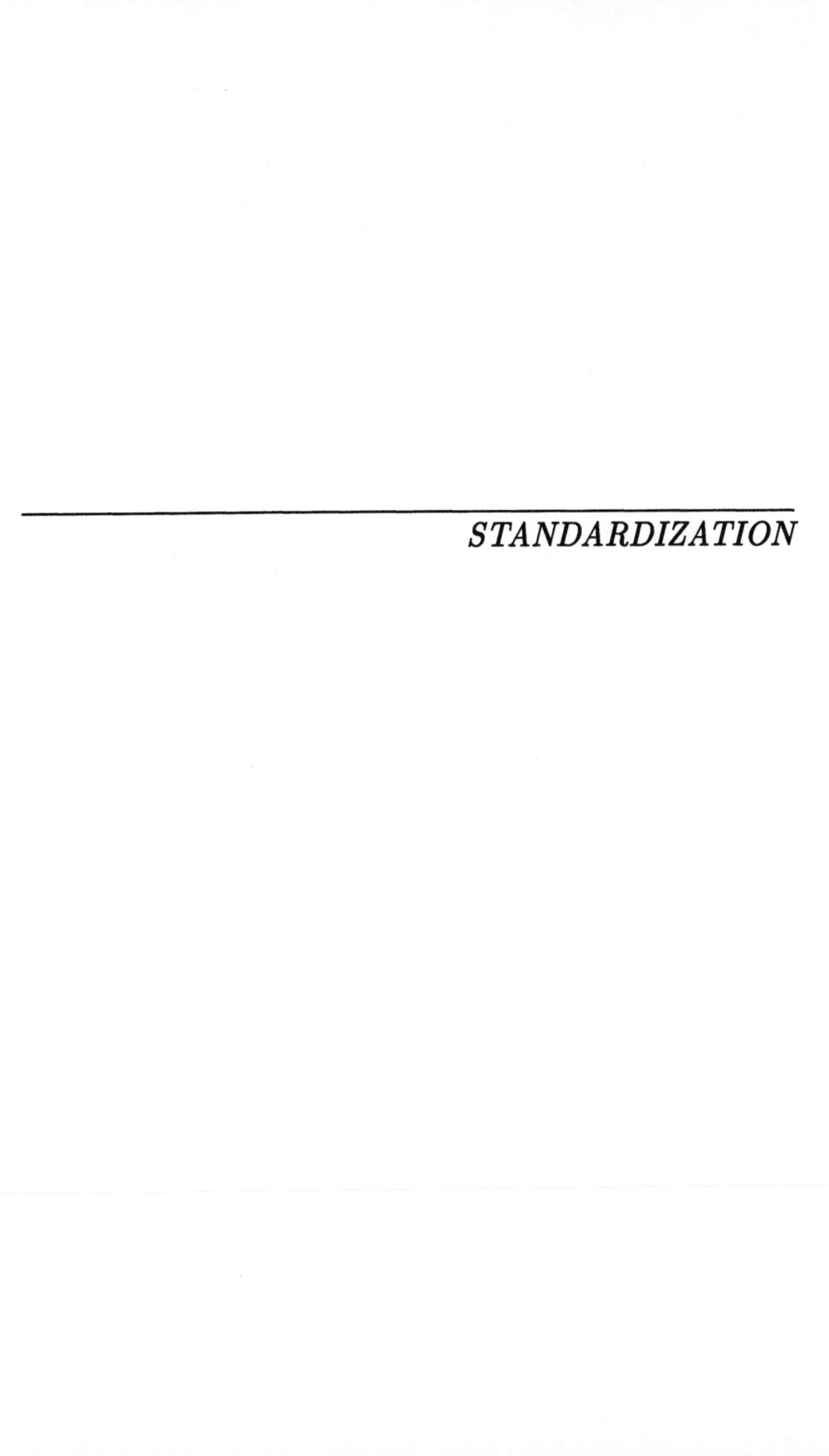

STANDARDIZATION

INTER-INSTITUTIONAL INFORMATION EXCHANGE IN HEALTHCARE

A. Hasman, A. Ament, P.G. Arnou, A.C.A. van Kesteren

Foundation 3I, c/o Dpt. of Medical Informatics and Statistics,

University of Limburg, Maastricht, The Netherlands.

Abstract.

In this paper the results of the standardization efforts of the 3I-project are described. Electronic data interchange needs standardization of exchanged messages. In the 3I-project ten different types of messages were defined. The use of these messages for exchanging information between hospitals, GP's and pharmacies is described. It is concluded that the electronic data interchange between hospitals and GP's can be cost-effective. The electronic communication of recipees between GP's and pharmacies is not cost-effective at the moment.

INTRODUCTION.

Communication forms an essential part of the healthcare process. This is especially true in countries where different types of care providers are working on different aspects of healthcare. In the Netherlands patients e.g. always first have to visit a general practitioner (GP). This GP can then, when necessary, refer the patient to a hospital. Usually the GP cares for the patient and will use the services of the hospital for ordering lab tests, X-rays, etc. The referral of patients or the ordering of tests or X-rays is accompanied by the exchange of information. The information is usually available in digital form although it is exchanged in print. The relevant data therefore have to be re-entered in the information system of the receiver. Therefore research is being performed to assess the possibilities of electronic data interchange (EDI). When evaluating a new technology in an early phase one has to consider the fact that such an ex ante assessment carries a risk: it is evident that through the use of a new technology one may become aware of new applications which can make the technology much more worthwile. But since several hospitals and GP's are now already willing to spend money to enhance the quality of information exchange it was felt that an early assessment of EDI would be worthwile. In the Netherlands the 3I-project was initiated to investigate the potential of integrated information exchange between the autonomous systems of different types of care providers. The goals of the 3I-project were to develop standard messages and to test their adequacy in a large enough environment. In this way one also could obtain an insight in the costs and benefits of this new technology.

In Europe EDIFACT (Electronic Data Interchange For Administration, Commerce and Transport) is an accepted standard for defining messages. This standard was adopted by the 3I-project. In the project only messages that are care orientated are developed.

Parts of this project were described earlier [1,2,3]. In may of 1991 the standardization and evaluation part of the 3I-project will be completed. In this contribution the results of the project are presented and discussed.

THE 3I-PROJECT.

After a preliminary study [3] it was decided to develop standard messages to replace existing high frequency data flows between hospitals, GP's and pharmacies. Because of the frequency of exchange the senders and receivers have already a lot of experience with the current way of information exchange so that they are in a good position to state which data are needed to be exchanged.

Several organizations were involved in the project: the Dutch PTT, Unisys, developers of GP, pharmacy and hospital information systems, the DIV (an EDP organization in Tilburg serving a number of hospitals), the SIG (Dutch Centre for Health Care Information) in Utrecht, the Province of Limburg, the University of Limburg and the Academic Hospital Maastricht. The project was carried out in two regions: one around Tilburg (under the auspices of the DIV) and one around Maastricht. In both regions a number of hospitals and GP's were involved. In the region around Maastricht also pharmacists were participating. The DIV was involved in the MIRAGE project (aimed at the development of communication software), a project of the BAZIS organization, supplier of the BAZIS hospital information system. In the 3I-project the implementation of standards was performed via four pilots:

o communication between hospitals and GP's   o the evaluation pilot
o communication between GP's and pharmacies   o the standardization pilot

Within the 3I-project three working groups were concentrating on the technical, standardization and evaluation aspects respectively.

Because of privacy reasons the PTT MEMOCOM electronic mail system was chosen to transport the data. The electronic mail system provides a mail box facility. Because of this the GP information system does not have to be connected to the telephone network continuously.

Those GP practices that did not have a computer system were offered a Unisys system during the period of the project. The GP's selected and bought the software themselves. The suppliers of the software committed themselves to developing the communication software.

The total project management was performed by van de Bunt, a firm of consultants that was also involved in the preliminary study.

EVALUATION.

The costs and benefits of EDI were evaluated. First a baseline study was performed concerning the cost of the traditional system (communication via telephone and mail) and concerning the time delays occurring between the request for and the receipt of the information. The physicians were asked which benefits they expected from the use of electronic communication. Then a similar study was performed involving electronic data interchange.

It could be established that for the hospital electronic data interchange of care orientated messages was at most as costly as the traditional way. A large spread in the cost of the traditional system was observed in the four hospitals that were investigated. This had to do with the size of the hospital, whether the mail handling was done centrally or by a department itself, whether the mail was sorted by physician and collected until the end of the day so that the post tariff could be relatively low and even with the fact that in one hospital GP's collected the letters when visiting that hospital.

The cost of electronic communication depends on the size of the messages. By combining several messages an optimal use of the network is made. The developed messages are rather large (in the order of 0.5 to 1.5 kbytes). This is due to the fact that quite a number of data elements have free text values.

A model was developed that can be used by hospitals to calculate the net costs of electronic communication. The model takes into account the costs of the traditional mailing system (on the average between f. 1000,- and f. 1500,- per year per GP), the expected number of messages of different types (determined from national statistics), the costs of exchanging these messages, etc.

The electronic messages were received earlier than the corresponding letters. The gain in time depended on the type of message. A time gain of three days was observed for ADT messages. These time gains are mainly due to organizational aspects of handling the mail in the hospital.

In the traditional system specialists pay the hospital a certain amount of money for mail handling. The electronic message sent by the specialist to the GP is still rather long and therefore electronic data interchange is still more costly.

Also the GP's do not gain financial benefits from the use of EDI. In the traditional system the patients take the letter to the hospital or specialist and letters coming from the hospital are paid by the hospital or the specialist. However with EDI they receive the messages in a form that can be directly stored in their information system. The quality of the data is higher, the time devoted to reading letters, to indicate which parts should be entered into the information system by the doctor's aide and the time needed for archiving the letters is reduced. On the average 12 letters were received per physician per day. In the old system about half an hour is needed for handling these letters. In the new system the GP can directly read the message and store it in the information system with one key stroke.

The GP's indicated that in 10% of the messages the earlier arrival was important. Especially the much earlier arrival of ADT messages was well appreciated.

GP's also send recipees to the pharmacy electronically. For the patients electronic communication can have the advantage that the drugs are ready when they visit the pharmacy (they also do not have to visit the GP first in case of repeat prescriptions). The pharmacist can better spread the workload when good arrangements are made with the GP's. For GP's that have a practice at some distance from the pharmacy electronic communication has advantages. Since the GP's are the senders of the messages they are charged. The electronic communication of these messages appeared to be very costly. At the moment faxing the recipees is less expensive. Another problem appeared to be that the pharmacy information systems could receive the messages but not automatically store them. In this area further research should be performed.

Changes in the organization of healthcare that will allow maximum utilization of the advantages of EDI in our opinion mainly concern tuning the work of the different healthcare providers.

CONCLUSIONS.

In the study reported here standard EDI messages were developed to replace existing high frequency data flows between three types of institutions (hospitals (including specialists), GP offices and pharmacies). Use was made of an electronic mail system. Although such a system is designed for interpersonal communication it can also support EDI. The advantage of a message handling system is that it provides a mail box. GP's can empty the mail box at the time it suits them. Because their information system does not have to be connected to the telephone network continuously the chance that hackers break into their systems is minimized. The standard messages at the moment contain still a lot of free text. Therefore the messages are relatively large. This has consequences for the current costs of electronic communication. The electronic communication of care orientated data must not be considered from the point of costs alone, however. The quality of the data in the GP information systems will increase because the data do not have to be re-entered. Also when electronic communication will be more widely used this facility will certainly be used for other applications as well. It was not possible to evaluate the impact of EDI on the quality of health care. EDI certainly will improve the services of the GP to the patient.

REFERENCES.

[1] Arnou, P.G., Bouman, P.C., Hasman, A. and Ferwerda, P.H. A computer communication network for hospitals and general practice. In: Proceedings Medinfo '89, (Barber, B., Cao, D., Qin, D. and Wagner, G., Eds.), North Holland, 1989, p. 1121-1124.
[2] Hasman, A., Arnou, P.G. and van Kesteren, A.C.A. In: Proceedings Medical Informatics Europe '90, (O'Moore, R., Bengtsson, S., Bryant, J.R. and Bryden, J.S., Eds.), Springer Verlag, 1990, p. 135-140.
[3] Hasman, A. Telecommunication in medicine - the 3I project. Int. J. Biomed. Comput, 26 (1990) p. 229-236.

EUCLIDES : A European clinical laboratory
data exchange standard (AIM-project : A 1033)

Georges J.E. DE MOOR
Department of Medical Informatics
State University Hospital Gent, BELGIUM

1. **Abstract**

EUCLIDES has been supported by the Commission of the
European Communities (CEC DG XIII - F) in the framework of the AIM (Advanced Informatics in Medicine)
programme.

The goal of the EUCLIDES project has been to provide
a much-needed European standard for clinical laboratory data exchange between independent and heterogeneous Medical Information Systems.

EUCLIDES will be an open standard i.e. freely available to all, and unbiased towards any manufacturer's
hardware or software. By convergence with other emerging standards, it could develop into a world standard. It could also be extended to encompass other
specialties in medicine.

EUCLIDES addresses the data exchange problem in a
three-pronged approach :
1. the transfer-mechanism, 2. the message syntax, and
3. the medical coding systems used within the message. Moreover, the EUCLIDES system offers through its
'bridge' a user-friendly software solution for interfacing with existing local systems at both the sender's and receiver's ends.

2. **Keywords**

EDI - Clinical Pathology - X.400 - Syntax - Coding-
system - Bridge software.

3. **Introduction**

Extensive study of the questionnaires sent to a large
community of general practitioners and medical specialists in Europe indicates that connections and exchanges of information are mostly required between
clinical laboratories and them.
This requirement is evident through the fact that
many laboratories, at least in Europe, already make
extensive use of electronic data interchange but

unfortunately in a basic and heterogeneous way, simply by using proprietary message formats and less efficient communication facilities. All the various experiments conducted on local scales inevitably and unfortunately resulted in the proliferation of incompatible solutions.

Careful study of the best known solutions proposed by other teams worldwide, have shown that the essence of the matter – the approach – is usually incomplete and hence less adequate. This may be due to the fact that this inter-disciplinary field is vast and presents difficulties in matching both medical knowledge and informatics with obvious results such as good analysis of the medical problem but wrong choice in informatics solutions or vice versa.

Euclides also adopted the principle that defining systems which look good in the form of specifications but are difficult or even impossible to implement are of little use. This is why <u>great emphasis was placed on prototyping at a very early stage of the programme</u>.The main area of application is two-way routine transmission of laboratory messages (orders, requests, results) between remote computers of medical offices, hospitals and laboratories (hospital, university and private laboratories).

4.   <u>The EUCLIDES Syntax</u>

The EUCLIDES syntax unambiguously defines and identifies the message structure, all message components and their behavior.
In EUCLIDES, an <u>Information Exchange Unit</u> (I.E.U.) is a structured set of messages communicated between the dialogue partners.
A <u>message</u> should be understood as an aggregate that serves a specific information exchange purpose (e.g. a test request).

EUCLIDES uses two distinct classes of messages (aggregates) :

<u>a</u>.   <u>System messages</u>, e.g. for the transfer of metadata (e.g. syntax-specifications).
<u>b</u>.   <u>Data messages</u> containing the Laboratory Related Information (L.R.I.), e.g. a test report.

The rather unique concept of a dedicated information carrier for metadata exchanges (the "<u>system</u>" <u>messages,a</u>), enables the transmission of all the syntax specifications and/or modifications, and this, on a request basis only (only when needed and where needed).

The majority of Euclides I.E.U.'s are transmitting subjectmatter data. These data messages (b) correspond with the following EUCLIDES-aggregates :

- Information Exchange Unit Header (I.E.U. Header)
- Test request message
- Test result message
- Test query message
- Test query response message
- Pick-up message
- Technical message
- Billing message
- Comment message
- Information Exchange Unit Trailer (I.E.U. Trailer)

One of the other characteristics of the EUCLIDES syntax is its object oriented approach and the principle that the data (and not the functions) were the chosen foundation to build the syntax.

The chosen EUCLIDES objects are well identified and described. Each EUCLIDES object represents only one real world concept (no overlapping). Seen from a general medical viewpoint (cf. Health Care Information Model) the objects could easily be reapplied in other contexts, i.e. usable for other health applications (e.g. radiology, anatomopathology...) without modification.
The dominant characteristics of laboratory messages are the extreme variabilities of information structures and contents. The EUCLIDES syntax allows to eliminate all unpredictable syntax-overhead caused by these extreme variabilities.

Another main characteristic of the EUCLIDES is the direct tagging of each data-element (aggregates, objects, attributes) in the messages (down to the bottom-level). The identification of the elements is not position-bound nor based on the use of special delimiters or separators, as is the case in ASTM 1238 records with their fields, subfields and sub/sub-fields or in UN/EDIfact, where below a certain level, i.e. in the segments, data elements -, and component data elements - separators (e.g. + and:) are used.

EUCLIDES unique combination of direct tagging for identifying data-elements on the one hand, and the availability of syntax-messages for exchanging meta-data on the other, results in the obvious advantages of easy upgradability when new elements have to be added or easy maintainability (no reprogramming efforts).

5. The EUCLIDES Transfer Mechanism

Euclides adopted MHS, which is a set of specifications known as the CCITT X.400 series of recommendations, dedicated to guide the system implementor towards archieving a complete, secure and open messaging system.

6. The EUCLIDES Coding System

There was a critical need for the immediate development of lists of codes to support electronic information exchange in clinical pathology. It is not sufficient to have a message transport system available
and also an agreed message syntax specification when
several different coding systems and/or terminologies
are still being handled within the messages. Good
codes (standards) are more than ever needed now we
have entered the era of telematics in medicine.
Existing schemes for clinical pathology are not message oriented. Most of these lists are classifications intended for other purposes (billing, statistics,
management etc) and inappropriate for exchange of
routine data in clinical pathology since they are
either not specific enough, or contain inconsistencies or overlaps, or have other deficiencies.

The vectors of the EUCLIDES coding system are :

1. Tests :   - analytes
                 - procedures
                 - function tests
                 - ratios
                 NB Not batteries/panels/profiles/re-
                 port headings etc.

2. Specimens : - specimen types
               - specimen origins
               - specimen collection procedures

3. Lab. Procedures :   - (basic) analytical proce-
                       dures
                       - reagents
                       - temperatures
                       - equipments

4. Units :   - denominators
                 - numerators

5. Kinds of quantities

6. Coded comments

The EUCLIDES Conversion Utility (E.C.U.) (coding software) allows access to the EUCLIDES Semantics Database in a user-friendly way. It enables the user to map his locally defined codes with the EUCLIDES standard codes. The E.C.U. database includes all elected terms, synonyms and abbreviations currently supported.

7.   **The EUCLIDES Bridge and its subsystems.**

The software package, called the EUCLIDES bridge, facilitates the communication from, or to, any local information system (ambulatory care information system, laboratory information system, hospital information system) installed on what so ever platform.

The subsystems of the EUCLIDES bridge are : the I.E.U.-compose, the I.E.U. decompose, the database-manager, the encrypt/decrypt, the compress/decompress, the deliver, the directory manager, the error handling, the syntax maintenance, the system maintenance subsystems

The result of the concepts behind the EUCLIDES BRIDGE is easy maintenance since each subsystem (corresponding with a group of coherent functions) can be replaced by a new version without touching any other subsystems' functionality.
The bridge is written in C for easy portability to UNIX and MSDOS.

8.   **FUTURE**

The EUCLIDES foundation (international) will be responsible for the maintenance of the coding system, the syntax-specifications and the bridge. It will also act as a conformance testing center and give legal and commercial support to interested parties in CEC and EFTA countries.

Linking Medical Data Standards, Knowledge-Based Systems
and the technique of Partial Evaluation

Hammond, P.*, Aye, L.K.S.A.* and Kay, J.D.S.+

*School of Computer Science, University of Birmingham, PO Box 363, Birmingham B15 2TT.
+Dept. of Clinical Biochemistry, John Radcliffe Hospital, Oxford, OX3A 9DU.

Abstract The ASTM specification is a standard for transferring clinical observations between independent computer systems. It is employed in a knowledge-based front-end to a biochemistry laboratory information system using the technique of partial evaluation.

Introduction

As the scope of medical knowledge-based systems widens and underlying computer power increases steadily, the prospect of a desktop medical workstation is rapidly approaching. To be broadly applicable such a system will need to be integrated with other in-house hospital information systems. In addition to the obvious hardware compatibility and communication capability, there is the problem of the representation and transfer of data from laboratories, image processing sources, computerised pharmacies and patient record database management systems. Standards for the specification of medical data are slowly being introduced after many years of uncoordinated and independent development of biomedical systems [6, 7]. The ASTM specification [5] is a standard for transferring clinical observations between independent computer systems. This paper describes how the ASTM specification is used in a knowledge-based front-end (KBFE) to a biochemistry laboratory information management system (LIMS) by exploiting the technique of partial evaluation. The approach is applicable to other medical information systems and specification standards.

Under funding from the UK Department of Health (IT Branch), the authors are currently developing a KBFE [2] on Apple Macintosh computers using MacPROLOG [4]. The KBFE retrieves patient data from a laboratory computer and provides controlled annotation using rule-based application of population reference intervals and tabulated effects of drugs on laboratory tests. The highly graphical interface provides more rapidly assimilated output which is used like an "intelligent" notepad from which the user selects and highlight points on graphs, data in tables and text in display windows to request their further analysis. The system uses its dual representation of data, as graphical objects and instances of answers to earlier queries to the knowledge base, to interpret the user's actions and undertake further analysis. This KBFE can be thought of as a component of the medical workstation we hope to build in the future.

In parallel with the development of the KBFE, there have been significant developments in the electronic transfer of laboratory test results. At a set time, on a daily basis, the biochemistry laboratory "force feeds" test results to computers used by doctors who have submitted specimens for biochemical analysis. The data is transferred in ASTM format, although only a subset of the full specification needs to be used for the data generated by the laboratory. The main advantages offered by a structured and formally defined data representation are reliability of interpretation and flexibility for further manipulation.

In order to be compatible with this new arrangement, the KBFE must be able to receive and transmit ASTM representations of patient data as well as manipulate its own internal logic-based representation in PROLOG. Since only part of the complete ASTM specification is used a simple approach would be to represent this subset as a translator program directly in PROLOG itself. However, this solution would restrict the use of the implemented translator to this particular LIMS. We advocate a more general approach by representing the entire ASTM specification as a set of grammar rules in PROLOG and use a technique called 'Partial Evaluation' to "specialise" the representation to the LIMS specific data. The general ASTM representation can then be used by other laboratory information systems needing only the identification of those parts of ASTM required for the task at hand.

The ASTM standard specification

ASTM E1238 is a standard specification for bi-directional, electronic transfer of clinical observations and requests between independent computer systems, typically between laboratories and specialised units producing observations and hospital wards or medical practices. The specification provides a format for sending requests for analysis to, and receiving results from, diagnostic services. It covers general information about diagnostic testing as well as specific data useful for clinical practice, administration, and research. Currently, ASTM is the only standard to offer this functionality.

```
H`(I)\```PATH LABS`OXFORDSHIRE HAIJOHN RADCLIFFE HOSPITAL\OXFORD\OX3A`9DU``(0865)817380``
AAH1238`LAB(4816)`D`AAM02`199001191732
C`1`L`MESSAGE SENT ON EVENING OF FRIDAY 19TH JANUARY
P`1``R000003``RABBIT\ROGER```M`````MCVITTIE```````````LAB(4816)```````
OBR`1``10002Y````199001190000````````199001190000`BLOOD`MCVITTIE``````A`1990901191732```F``````````
OBS`1`1III45F7.IUREAIL}READ5`5.9`MMOL/L`(2.5-6.7)``AIS`F
C`1`L`COMPATIBLE WITH PREVIOUS SPECIMEN'S RESULTS
OBR`2``10001V````199001190000````````199001190000`BLOOD`MCVITTIE``````A`199001191732```F``````````
OBS`1`1III45N1.ISODIUM(L)READ5`140`MMOL/L`(135-145)``AIS`F
OBS`2`1III45N2.IPOTASSIUM(L)READ5`3.9`MMOL/L`(3.5-5.0)``AIS`F   L`1
```

Figure 1: An Example of an ASTM message for a single patient with two specimens

An ASTM message consists of 9 record types arranged in a hierarchical form (see figure 2) and always comprises a header and a trailer record, and may contain one or more record types in level 1. The records in level 2 appear as part of the patient record, and those in level 3 appear as part of the test order record. Comments and error records may appear at any point. The ASTM message format is designed to cater for a wide variety of uses and contains a total of 125 fields in the 9 record types above. It is very unlikely that all 125 fields will be applicable to a particular laboratory information system in which case some fields are omitted. For example, the biochemistry laboratory computer at the John Radcliffe Hospital uses only 40 fields. This also explains the multiple sequences of the ` separator symbol in the example in figure 1 indicating missing or blank fields.

0	Message header and Message trailer records
1	Patient, Request result and Scientific records
2	Test order (specimens) record
3	Results (test results) record
unspecified	Comment and Error records

Figure 2: Field Types in ASTM

ASTM representation in a grammar formalism

PROLOG is commonly used for Natural Language Processing applications and many implementations provide a built-in grammar formalism, the Definite Clause Grammar (DCG). Typically, programmers enter grammar rules for the language they are interested in defining and the PROLOG system automatically converts them to PROLOG parsing or translation programs. Obviously, ASTM defines a very restricted subset of Natural Language augmented with various separator symbols and so a grammar based representation can be produced relatively routinely. Two grammar rules in the ASTM representation are

```
astm(records(Head,Body,Last)) --> header(Head), body(Body), trailer(Last).
header(head(Head_Id,Sender,Misc)) --> head_id(Head_id), head_sender(Sender), head_misc(Misc).
```

Given that the LIMS employs only 40 of the 125 fields in ASTM, a complete representation contains considerable redundancy and hence results in computational inefficiency and unnecessary complexity. We would like to specialise the full representation without explicitly writing the specific sub-grammar that corresponds to the fields we are interested in. The technique we employ is to allow the user to specify which fields are to be omitted from messages and to partially evaluate (compile) this description into the ASTM grammar to generate automatically one specific to the ASTM subset used.

Partial Evaluation

Partial evaluation is a program transformation technique originated in Functional Programming. It was introduced to Logic Programming by Komorowski [3] and has been further developed for specialised meta-interpreters for logic-based inference engines and knowledge-based systems [9]. For pedagogical reasons, we illustrate the technique with an example less esoteric than the ASTM specification. Consider the knowledge base K with two rules expressed as PROLOG clauses [1] and where strings beginning with upper case letters denote variables:

```
K = {should_take(Person,Drug)  if  complains_of(Person,Symptom)
                                and  suppresses(Drug,Symptom)
                                and  not unsuitable(Drug,Person)  ,
         unsuitable(Drug,Person) if  aggravates(Drug,Condition)
                                and  suffers_from(Person,Condition) }
```

The knowledge base K can be transformed in two ways. Firstly, if we can assume that there are no other rules defining the relation *unsuitable*, then we can partially evaluate the reference to it. Such "hand compiling" results in a single rule version, K', of K

$$K' = \{ \text{should\_take(Person,Drug) if complains\_of(Person,Symptom)} $$
$$\text{and suppresses(Drug,Symptom)} $$
$$\text{and not(aggravates(Drug,Condition)} $$
$$\text{and suffers\_from(Person,Condition)) } \}$$

Furthermore, if our interest is confined to only two drugs described by, say, four facts in D

$$D = \{ \text{suppresses(aspirin,pain), suppresses(lomotil,diarrhoea),} $$
$$\text{aggravates(aspirin,peptic\_ulcer), aggravates(lomotil,impaired\_liver\_function) } \}$$

we can partially evaluate K' with respect to D to obtain two specialised drug prescribing rules:

$$K'_D = \{ \text{should\_take(Person,aspirin) if complains\_of(Person,pain)} $$
$$\text{and not suffers\_from(Person,peptic\_ulcer) ,} $$
$$\text{should\_take(Person,lomotil) if complains\_of(Person,diarrhoea)} $$
$$\text{and not suffers\_from(Person,impaired\_liver\_function) } \}$$

In general, the partial evaluation will be performed by a suitably constructed meta-program (also expressed in PROLOG) which compiles away some of the generality and complexity of the original knowledge base. Typically, the transformed program or knowledge base will execute more efficiently. In this exagerratedly small example, we might not perceive such benefit. However, for a much larger program, for instance one comprising a large knowledge base and a complicated inference engine, such partial evaluation can have considerable benefit [8].

One obvious drawback that can be seen even in this small example is the loss of explicit and separate descriptions of different facets of drug behaviour. However, with a suitable programming environment both versions of the knowledge base could be made available, one used for efficient computation and the other for explanation or for amending drug data without changing the generalised procedure for drug prescription. Of course, for the sake of consistency, the program or knowledge base used for efficient computation is always derived by partial evaluation from any new version of the original.

A LIMS specific ASTM subset

We can apply the same partial evaluation technique used in the example above to the ASTM specification. To do this we need the DCG representation (as PROLOG clauses) of the complete ASTM specification and a description of those fields which are to be omitted from messages sent and received by our particular LIMS. In parsing terminology, the latter set is the collection of terminal symbols which will be represented simply as null strings. The result of the partial evaluation will be a translator program specific to the LIMS and set of message types we are interested in. With a different LIMS or different standard or message requirement we can reapply the partial evaluation technique to produce a revised translator specific to the new LIMS and/or standard (see figure 3 below). The benefits of this approach are improved efficiency of computation, reduction in programming effort and the concomitant improvement in program correctness.

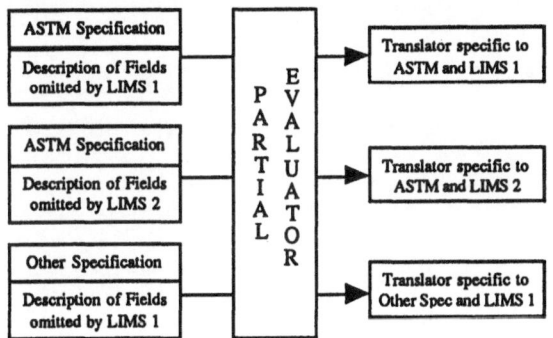

Figure 3: Generation of Translators for specific Standards and LIMS

References

1. Hammond, P. 'micro-PROLOG for Expert Systems' in micro-PROLOG : Programming in Logic (eds K.L.Clark and F.G. McCabe) (1984) Prentice-Hall.
2. Hammond, P., Kay, J.D.S. 'Knowledge-Based Assistance for Interpreting Biochemical Data'. (1989) The Fourth International Symposium on Computer and Information Sciences, Çesme, Turkey; 909-919.
3. Komorowski, H.J. 'A Specification of an Abstract Prolog Machine and its Application to Partial Evaluation'. Linkoping Studies in Science and Technology Dissertations (1981), No 69, Software Systems Research Centre, Linkoping Univ., Sweden.
4. MacPROLOG, Logic Programming Associates Ltd,Studio 4, RVPB,Trinity Road, London, SW18 3SX.
5. 'ASTM 1238-88 Draft Specification, Revision 2' (1990). (C.J. McDonald (Chairman), Regenstrief Institute for Health Care, Indiana University Medical Center, Indianapolis, Indiana)
6. McDonald, C.J. 'The Search for National Standards for Medical Data Exchange'. M.D. Computing (1984), 2(1); 3-4.
7. McDonald, C.J., Hammond, W.E. (1989) 'Standard Formats for Electronic Transfer of Clinical Data'. Annals of Internal Medicine, 110(5); 333-335.
8. Sterling, L., Beer, R.D. (1989) 'Meta-interpreters for Expert System Construction'. Journal of Logic Programming, 6 (1-2); 163-178.
9. Takeuchi, A., Furukawa, K. (1985) 'Partial Evaluation of PROLOG Programs and its Application to MetaProgramming'. ICOT Tech. Report, Tokyo, Japan.

POSTER PRESENTATIONS

POSTER PRESENTATIONS

INFORMATION SYSTEMS
AND HEALTH CARE

A DATA BASE MANAGEMENT SYSTEM FOR
AN OBSTETRICS DEPARTMENT

J. F. Luís, M. Filomena Cardoso, J. Bernardes,
J. P. Marques de Sá, L. Pereira Leite

Departamento de Engenharia Electrotécnica e de Computadores
Faculdade Engenharia, Universidade do Porto
Rua dos Bragas, 4099 Porto Codex

ABSTRACT

In this paper a Data Base Management System (DBMS) suitable for handling the clinical data of an Obstetrics Departement is presented. This system was developed and is being used at the Obstetrics Service of the Oporto S. João Hospital (main Oporto Hospital). The DBMS structure as well as the method used to introduce and search the data, are described. This system has already brought important benefits to the departmental organization.

INTRODUCTION

As it is well known the application of a DBMS in a medical department can drastically improve the efficiency of the administrative tasks as well as the data storage, retrieval and analysis both for clinical practice and research. This is particularly true for an hospital like ours where all the patient records are stored in a large central manual archive, not linked to the Obstetrics Service. Retrieval and search tasks become therefore very difficult and time consuming when using only that central archive.

The main objectives that we had in view with the development ot this DBMS were both the improvement concerning clinical data management especially in the assistance to diagnosis and therapy and also the possibility of its use for research purposes.

DESCRIPTION OF THE DBMS

The system was developed in Dbase III Plus and is composed of six data bases (person.dbf, clinical.dbf, surgery.dbf, bebe-lif.dbf, bebe.dbf, dequitad.dbf), wich are related by the hospital identification number. It allows the storage, retrieval and analysis of clinical data concerning the pregnancy, the delivery, the newborn and the puerperium.

The system relies on information collected manually by professional staff. Data are entered by them after discharge of the patient. The access to the system is made by a password in order to maintain the confidentiality.

The system is menu driven to make it as easy as possible, and the screen views are similar to the patient record used in the department.

Next Table I summarizes the contents of the data bases:

TABLE I

Data Base	Description
Person	Identification Data
Clinical	Medical History Menstrual History Gynaecological History Previous Obst. History Present Pregnancy History
Surgery	Surgery Description
Dequitad	Delivery Data
Bebe Bebe_lif	Neonatal and Newborn Data

The total number of variables used by the system are approximately 240, and they consist in all the fields present in the clinical record.

The surgical activities are transfered to the computer using coding forms (International Classification of Diseases Codes).

The accuracy of the recorded information is enhanced by some logical fields (yes/no answer) that must be filled in for stepping to the next screen. Once per week there is also an off-line error detection made by the system manager to control the accuracy of the information.

Information retrieval was made easy through a specially developed menu driven program for the construction of the search command. The program checks for the correct syntax of the command and also identifies each variable with its data base. For example if the user wants to know the number of single and housekkeping mothers that gave birth to male children, he will have to proceed as follows:

i) Choose the HOSPITALIZATION option, in order to get the
mother's civil status;
ii)   Chose the NEWBORN option, to select MALE;
iii) Finally, chose the DELIVERY option, in order to select the
delivery type;

the LOGIC menu is used to relate the options as it is shown for the above example in Figure 1.

As it is also shown in Figure 1 this information retrieval section of the DBMS was built in such a way that the pertinent fields are displayed in structured pull down menus.

There is also a free text field to allow the expert user to construct a search command. With this alternative the expert user can enter directly, and probably in a quick way, the search specification, using the appropriate syntax (logical operators, variable identifiers, etc), circumventing the step by step selection process of the pull down menus.

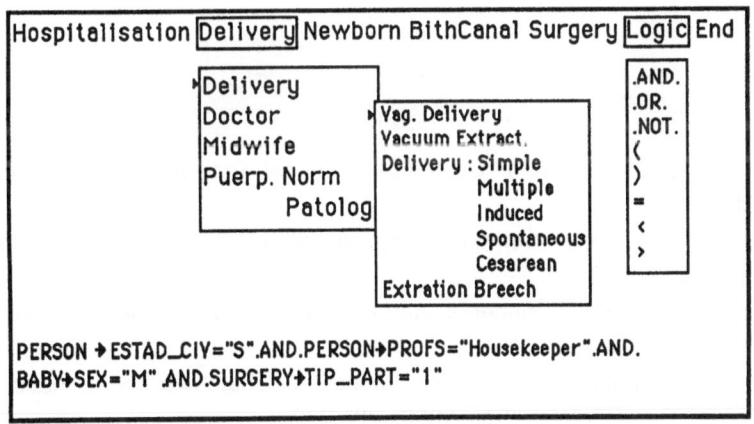

Figure 1 - Example of DBMS search screen

CONCLUSIONS

The described DBMS allows data storage and analysis in an easy, quick, precise and orderly way. Its use in the Obstetrics Service of S. João Hospital, still in a preliminary phase, has already largely demonstrated its benefit to the Service organization and its contribution to the analysis and scrutiny of the clinical activities.

After having analysed all the data entered until now, and gained more experience with the type of tasks that the DBMS is supposed to perform, we became aware that a great number of variables were not relevant for the main aim of this DBMS, which is mostly intended in a retrospective analysis. For example, the arterial pressure and the weight of the preganant women are very important in an on-line system, but in an obstetrics retrospective analysis their importance is much lower.

We now realize that there are too many variables on the DBMS, a great portion of them unused, wasting space and time resources. We are therefore in the process of selecting a minimal set of variables.

In the near future we also pretend to use the DBMS in a Local Area Network (LAN) configured system allowing therefore the remote access to the data bases. This distributed configuration will justify and stimulate the on-line use of the DBMS. We shall also connect the DBMS to the Ecographic Data Base and to an Automatic Cardiotocographic Analysis program that we have developed and is being used in the Obstetrics Service.

REFERENCES

1 - Chard, T. "Computerization of Obstetrics Records" Progress in Obstetrics and Gynaecologic., 1986: 3-22.

2 - Catanzarite & Jelovsek. "Computer Applications in Obstetrics" Am J Obstet. Gynaecologic., May 1987, 1049.

3 - Carapuça et al. "First Concepts About Systems of Information and Data Bases", INESC 1985.

4 - Lilford et al. "Computing and Decision Support in Obstetrics and Gynaecology", Clinical Obstetrics and Gynaecology, Dec 1990: 723-742.

A HEURISTIC APPROACH TO A COMPUTERIZED DATABASE IN A GYNECO-ONCOLOGIC OUTPATIENT CLINIC

E. Hanzal, G. Hoffmann, G. Gitsch, A. Reinthaller, H. Kölbl
2nd Department of Obstetrics and Gynecology University of Vienna, Austria
Head: Prof. Dr. H. Janisch

Abstract:

In our recently installed gyneco-oncologic outpatient clinic an EDP-documentation system has been established to facilitate data management. Instead of a PC-system a mainframe (IBM 3090) based solution has been chosen for the following reasons: (1) almost unlimited capacity of mass storage, (2) efficient data protection, (3) centralized backup facitlities, (4) on-line access to data in other departments connected to this system, (5) data processing using implemented statistical software. The basical WAMIS (Vienna General Medical Information System) software is in use in our department since 1975, thus allowing a heuristic approach developing the new database. Components and development of the system are presented in this paper.

Introduction:

Gynecologic oncology is a widespread medical field. Especially during follow-up numerous different parameters are required to diagnose remission, progression or relapse of gynecologic malignancies. Moreover the therapeutic approach includes a large variety of procedures, such as surgery, different types of chemotherapy or radiation therapy. Thus, documentation using simple record charts is time consuming and complicated, since many investigations are performed by other departments (e.g. radiologic assessment, several laboratory findings etc.).

For the recently installed general gyneco-oncologic outpatient clinic at the 2nd Department of Obstetrics and Gynecology a computerized database system was established. The existence of previous computer based documentation systems and a long term experience in this field was essential for the heuristic approach.

Material and methods:

Since 1975 a mainframe based (IBM 4381, currently replaced by an IBM 3090 supercomputer) so called Vienna General Medical Information System (WAMIS) provided by the University hospital of Vienna represents a helpful tool to develop databases suitable for the specific demands of various University departments connected to this system.

The CICS/VS (1) based WAMIS software has been developed by the Institute of Medical Computer Sciences (IMC) mainly for scientific purposes (2).

Initially, WAMIS was used at the 2nd Department of Obstetrics and Gynecology for obstetric documentation only, but soon medical databases for several other subdivisions (e.g. histology, surgery, laboratory, etc.) were established (Tab. 1).

Table 1 Subdivisions of the 2nd Department of Obstetrics and Gynecology with mainframe-based documentation systems

Subdivision	Computerized documentation (WAMIS) since:
Obstetrics	
Pregnancy follow-up	1975
Labor record chart	1976
Obstetrical history	1977
Delivery documentation	1975
Patient's history	1977
Medical report	1978
Gynecology	
Patient's history	1977
Surgical report	1979
Outpatient breast investigation	1980
Breast cancer follow-up	1983
Cervical dysplasia	1989
Urogynecology	1989
Cytology	1979
Histology	1982
Radiologic assessment	1986
Ultrasound investigation	1980

However, these applications were restricted to the specific needs of these subdivisions. Thus, data retrieval and computation for statistics were very time consuming and required substantial support of an EDP-specialist. Therefore the aim of the database created was to facilitate data input and management for the clinic staff and to integrate existing software applications rather than to develop a completely new system.

Creation of a relevant database was carried out as follows: The existing applications for patient's history and indoor radiologic assessment were entirely integrated. Computerized surgical report, histologic database and indoor laboratory findings had to be adapted to the new system. Input tools for general examination, gynecologic examination, therapy-protocol and side-effect-report had to be newly developed. Moreover a package of program routines was created for projected integration of data assessed by other University departments (e.g. Computed Tomography and Magnetic Resonance Imaging findings, laboratory parameters, etc.) (Tab. 2).

Table 2   Components of the Gyneco-oncologic Database

Patient's history	integrated
Radiologic assessment	integrated
Surgical report	adapted
Histologic database	adapted
Laboratory findings	adapted
General examination	developed
Gynecologic examination	developed
Therapy protocol	developed
Side-effect report	developed
Laboratory findings (other Dept.)	on-line (projected)
Computed tomography	on-line (projected)
Magnetic resonance imaging	on-line (projected)

In order to improve data handling and to reduce input errors, we tried to integrate on-line data whenever possible. Data input is performed on a multiple choice screen by selecting listed data items with a light pen.

Results:
Individual patient's data are retrievable at any time. For every follow-up-patient a conclusive hardcopy containing complete diagnosis, including stage of disease, histologic findings and hormonal receptor status, previous therapy and current state of disease is available. In addition every single assessed variable is presented on a report. In order to visualize the course of laboratory parameters or tumormarkers, values may be displayed as graphs (Fig. 1.).

Fig. 1   Tumormarker course (CA 125) of a patient with ovarian cancer displayed by the mainframe

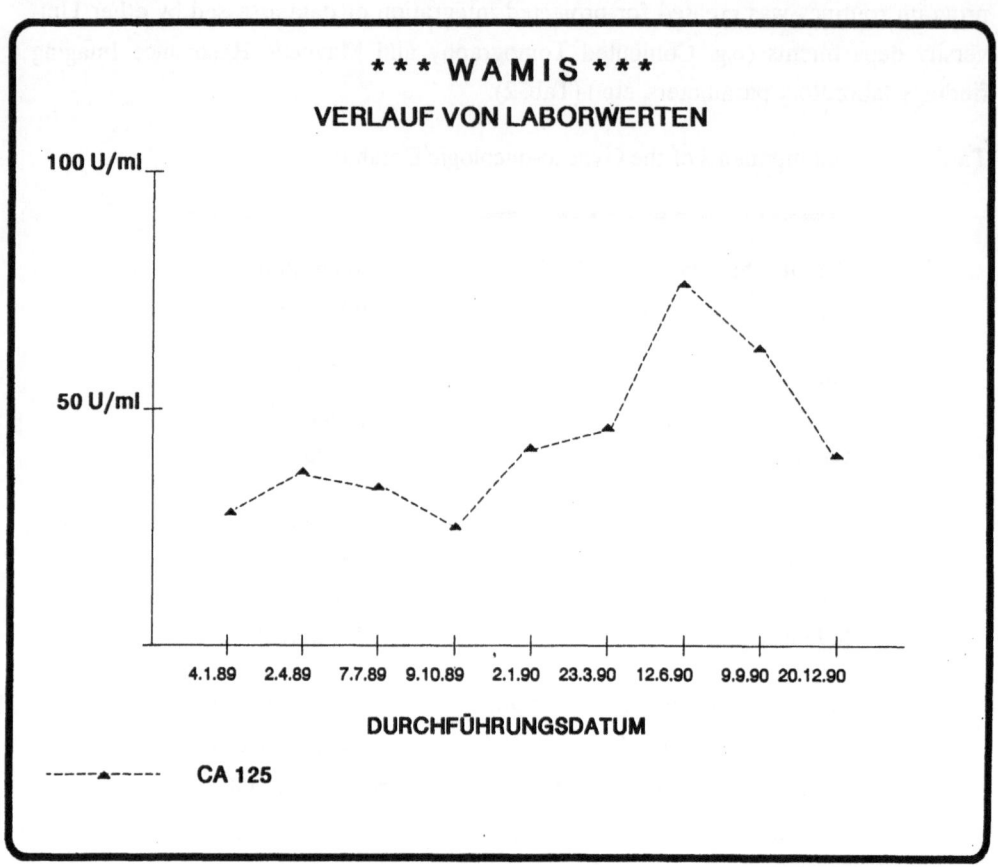

Above the advantage of easy data input, the multiple choice design offers the possibility of improved computerized statistics because nearly all relevant parameters are present as numeric or ordinary variables. Thus, statistical analysis as well as quality control is available at any time. Even evaluation of time depending data (e.g. survival times) can be easily computed on the mainframe with the help of implemented statistical software e.g. SAS (Statistical Analyzing System) (3).

Discussion:

In recent years a rising amount of data had to be managed in gynecologic oncology, due to increasing numbers of patients, shorter follow-up intervals and longer survival times as well as additional diagnostic and therapeutic procedures. In order to deal with these large data accumulations computer based documentation systems have been established in this medical field.

We decided to choose a mainframe based solution instead of a PC-system for the following reasons: 1) existing hard and software provided by the University of Vienna resulting in minimal costs for development; 2) almost unlimited capacity of mass storage; 3) on-line access to data in other departments; 4) centralized data protection and backup facilities; 5) data processing using implemented statistical software on the mainframe.

The main problem of multiple choice EDP-documentation is, that in order to avoid input of textfields, characteristics of variables have to be predefined as ordinary scaled values. Therefore questionnaires and input screens are either too extensive, or documentation may be incomplete. This prompted us to partly continue written documentation on record charts. Findings or conditions which are inadequate for appropriate computation are entered into these charts, which are supposed to serve as a pool for further modifications of the system.

The heuristic approach was essential as shortcomings in previous mainframe based systems could be avoided by the long experience with this computer and software. It could be demonstrated, that the system is quite flexible and capable of modifications whenever needed. However support of an EDP-specialist is necessary in any case, in order to continue optimized step-by-step development.

In conclusion, our computerized gyneco-oncologic data storage and retrieval system offers complete documentation, easy retrieval of individual data, improved patient's administration and standardized statistics including quality control and evaluation of survival times for research purposes. It is time saving and economic and thus allows the clinician to spend more time on patient's care.

Literature:

(1)   Customer Information Control System (CICS/VS) Version 1.6: Application Programmer's Reference Manual, Command Level (1983)

(2)   Grabner, H., et al.: WAMIS: A medical information system. Conception and clinical usage. J. Clin. Comp. 10,154-169,1981.

(3)   SAS-User's Guide, SAS Institute Inc., North Carolina 1985.

ARZTBRIEF: generating medical reports in a multimedia environment

Dirk Kraus
RG Expert Systems,
CT Biomed,
Center for Technology Transfer
Biomedicine
Brahmsstr. 2,
W-4970 Bad Oeynhausen

Eckart Miche
Heart Centre Northrhine-
Westphalia
Department of Cardiology
Georgstr. 11
W-4970 Bad Oeynhausen

Abstract

The ARZTBRIEF system supports the generation of medical reports to the referring practioner by the physician in the cardiological ambulance of the Heart Centre.

A main characteristic of the system is that it consequently exploits the possibilities of multimedia techniques both for user input and output. For example, the user may click on icons or graphical schemes, select from menus, draw / colorize simple forms, talk into a sound digitizer or use a keyboard. The system is now in routine use and has shown that it decreases the time until the referring physician receives the report considerably.

Goals of the project

The system was implemented in order to accomplish the following goals:

a) economize the work of both physicians and secretaries by
- avoiding multiple recording of identical text fragments,
- enabling fast input of frequent and common formulations,
- making it possible to work on the records of different patients alternately

b) yield a good compromise between a necessary standardization and individuality of style
- by providing a large amount of predefined fragments, which can nevertheless
- easily be modified or extended by every user according to his preferences

c) provide a basis for further integration of various clinical data which are multimedial by nature, and thus

d) set an anchorpoint (in the form of hardware, software, user interface and expectations of users) for a projected clinical information system.

It is easy to see that all these goals serve the long term goal of improving medical care.

User interaction

The greatest challenge in building such a system lies in the design of the user interface. Existing glossary based systems (see, for instance, [1]) suffer from major drawbacks which lower the acceptance and usability drastically. These include:

- limited number of glossary terms which are not/not easily modifiable,
- tedious and clumsy access to these terms via number codes which have to be memorized or retrieved from a manual,
- the user has still to use a keyboard to a large extent,
- frequent large patterns of findings have to be "assembled" every time,
- impossiblity to enter graphical information.

In order to overcome these problems, it is unavoidable to resort to a environment based on a graphical user interface (GUI). The workers in the PEN/PAD project [2, 3] have come to a similar conclusion. As our goals was not as ambitious as those of the PEN/PAD project we had very short development times, allowing for various prototyping phases. These revealed that an integration of the dictaphone was imperative, as it seems to be impossible to provide a still time saving means of entering very complex findings.
It may be interesting to have a closer look at the following (slightly clipped) screen shot

of the "main card" used in the cardiological physical examination:

It contains several "interaction elements".

For instance, the **o.B.** button is used to state that the head-throat region is o.B.=NAD.

A short click on the "button" (Atmung=breathing) indicates that breathing is normal. Holding down the mouse for a short period of time brings up a menu, from which common breathing abnormalities can be chosen. Selecting

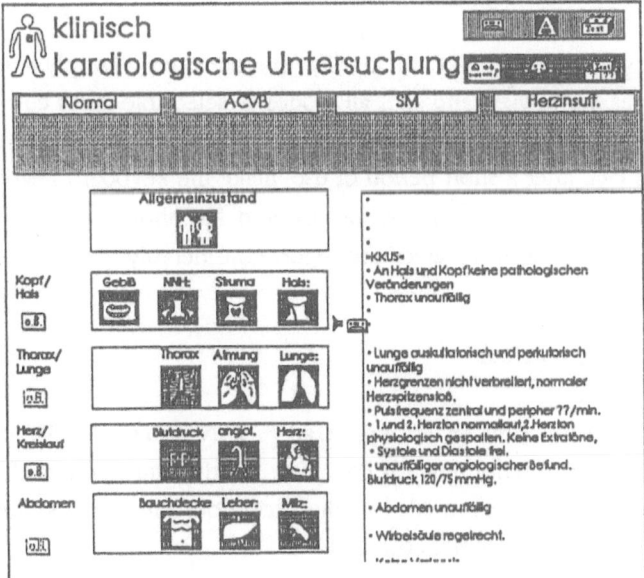

"Other..." from this menu or by simply "double-clicking" the icon pops up yet another card (fig. 2) in which still more detailed information can be entered in the same manner, i. e. merely by clicking on graphical schemes and icons.

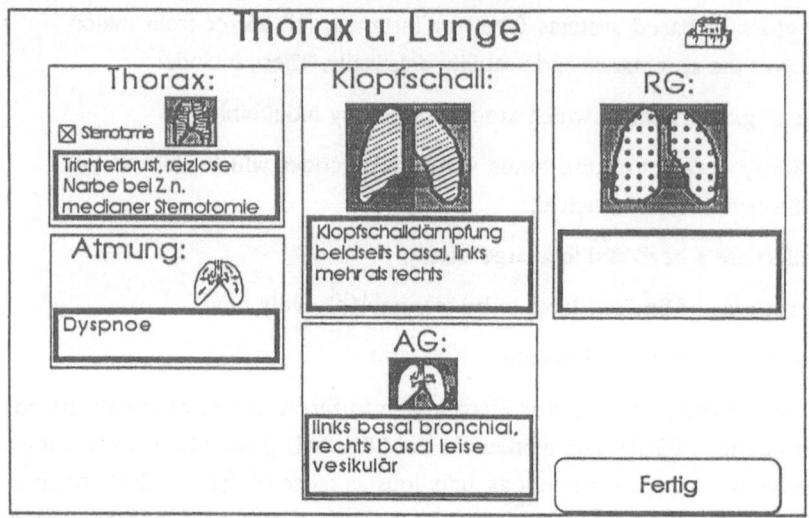

This information instantaneously shows up in the window ("field") on the right hand side of the card. It is possible to select fragments of text in this window that occur frequently and to bring up a button such as `ACVB` which, when pushed, puts this very fragment of text into this window whenever desired. Common patterns of findings can thus easily be remembered and reproduced.

"Play/record"-buttons can be generated wherever the user likes to talk into the sound digitizer, typically when a finding is present which occurs very seldom and /or is very complex.

Should the user like to modify the selections, simply clicking on the -button enables her to view and alter all groups of selectable items currently in the system.

It is important to note that all facilities which allow for the customization of the system do in fact, after a short period of use, make the keyboard nearly obsolete.

The system is now in routine use and has shown that it decreases the time until the referring physician receives the report considerably.

Configuration

ARZTBRIEF runs in an AppleTalk™ LAN under TOPS™, connecting several Apple® Macintosh™ computers (SE/30, IIx), partly equipped with full page screens, and a LaserWriter™. The modules in the reception, the doctors´ rooms and the typists´ office are implemented in HyperCard II™ .

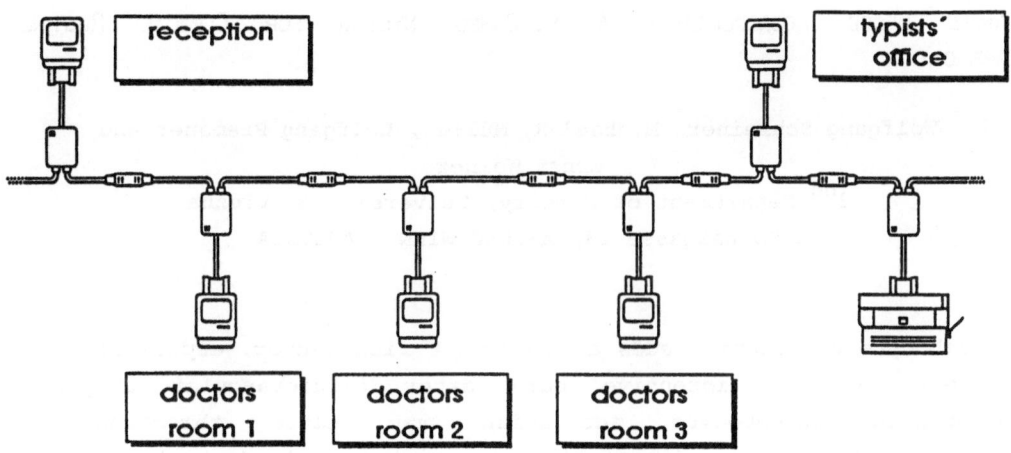

reception

typists' office

doctors room 1

doctors room 2

doctors room 3

Flow of data

In the reception office the secretary enter the patients' basic data. These are visible to all doctors who then decide to take over a patient for examination. All findings may then be entered in the way described above. Once a record is finished it may be "sent" (on the push of a button) to the typists office. Since switching between the patients' records is possible, it is not necessary to finish the first before proceeding with the second record, as is the case when working with a dictaphone.

The secretary in the typists office after accepting the record of a patient simply types in all the passages which where dictated into the sound digitizer, without bothering where they have to been placed in the document. Once this is completed the whole report may be sent to the laser printer.

Bibliography:

[1] **Cordes C, Rötz M, Frey N, Müller A:** Texthandbuch zum programmierten Arztbrief in der kardiologischen Diagnostik und Therapie, perimed Fachbuch Verlagsgesellschaft, Erlangen, 1984

[2] **Horan B:** Intelligent Clinical Data Entry for General Practice: The PEN Project, in: Perspectives in Health Computing, Cambridge University Press, 1990

[3] **Howkins TJ, Kay S, Rector AL, Goble CA:** Improving the Doctor Computer Interface, in: Current Perspectives in Health Computing, Cambridge University Press, 1988

[4] **Kay S, Horan B, Goble CA, Howkins TJ, Nowlan A, Rector AL, Wilson A:** User-Centred Design and Strategic Medical Informatics for Health Care, in: proc IMIA 1990

[5] **Rector AL:** The knowledge based medical record IMMEDIATE-!, in: proc. AIME 85

WHOLE BLOOD AGGREGOMETRY: A PC-BASED SYSTEM FOR CLINICAL ROUTINE APPLICATION

Wolfgang Schreiner, Michael R. Müller, Wolfgang Premauer and
Ernst Wolner
2nd Department of Surgery, University of Vienna
Spitalgasse 23, A-1090 WIEN / AUSTRIA

Thrombocyte disfunction adds an important risk factor, especially for patients in the intensive care after cardiovascular surgery. Unintended thrombocyte activation may cause thromboembolic complications, whereas insufficient aggregability leads to bleedings, regardless of normal coagulation parameters. Whole blood electrical aggregometry (1), designed to assess thrombocyte function, is therefore a valuable diagnostic tool, capable of rapidly screening thrombocyte ("platelet") function (3).

In the present work we describe a personal computer setup, which closely cooperates with the aggregometer and finally yields standardized "numerical diagnostics".

2. PHASES OF DATA-ACQUISITION

After program start, an interactive menue is displayed for entering the parameters of each measurement such as patient-identification, age of blood sample, type and dose of the aggregating substance used, the patients' hematocrit and the dilution factor for the probe.

Following the preparation and insertion of the blood sample, the aggregometer yields a voltage proportional to the impedance between two electrodes immersed in the blood sample. Throughout the time of measurement, this analog signal is converted to digital at 10 samples per second and displayed on the screen in real time. However, depending on the phase of measurement, values are treated differently. First, the initial decline of impedance is monitored and checked against a lower limit. A/D-converted values are displayed and then discarded. As soon as the trend has come to a standstill, the user is informed to calibrate the probe via a pushbutton on the aggregometer.

The calibration step-function, issued by the aggregometer superimposed on the impedance signal, is automatically detected and analyzed in height. Following successful calibration, the program reports to wait for the start of the aggregation proper. The user then adds the aggregans to the sample and initiates the measurement via the keyboard. Beside being displayed, 10 successive a/d-converted values are then subaveraged, calibrated and stored in memory. Thus, 10 minutes of aggregation result in 600 data values to be submitted to further analysis.

The software is in fact capable of performing the above procedure simultaneously on up to four different channels of the aggregometer, even if measurements are started in arbitrary succession and, e.g. the search for a stable baseline on one channel should overlap with the calibration procedure on another channel.

3. Calculation of Diagnostic Quantities

The subaveraged values, representing an aggregation curve, are numerically analyzed as follows, see figure 1.

Starting from several intuitive criteria, formulated by physicians experienced in the visual interpretation of aggregation curves, mathematical quantities have been selected and defined, which can readily be computed from the acquired data.

A most simple quantity is the overall amplitude of the curve, $y_{ampl} = y_{max} - y_{min}$. Alternatively, the total area,

$$A_{0-end} = \int_0^{t_{end}} \left(y(t) - y_{min} \right) dt \qquad (1)$$

between the minimum value and the aggregation curve may be considered. However, results to be compared have either to be based on equal periods of acquisition (t_{end}), or, more favourably, A_{0-end} has to be normalized by duration: $A^*_{0-end} = A_{0-end} / t_{end}$.

Aggregation dynamics can be characterized by the maximum slope (S_{max}) or by the time t_{smax} when S_{max} was found. A more stable criterion is, however, an area ratio such as $A_{0-end} / \left((y_{max} - y_{min}) \cdot t_{end} \right)$. It represents the portion of area under the curve against the area corresponding to amplitude. The earlier and faster impedance rises, the larger this portion will be. In contrast to slopes, being calculated via derivatives, integrals are less sensitive to data irregularities.

Another feature frequently addressed in the phenomenological discussion of aggregometry is the fact whether or not impedance declines after the initial rise. A decline is usually interpreted as a "tiring effect". A corresponding quantity

$$A_{tired} = \int_{t_{max}}^{t_{end}} \left[y_{max} - y(t) \right] dt \qquad (2)$$

can be defined to quantify if and how much of tiring occured.

4. HARDWARE SETUP, SOFTWARE IMPLEMENTATION AND DATA EXPORT

The package was developed on an IBM-compatible 4.7 MHz XT-Computer, equipped with a DASH-8 analog/digital conversion card (METRABYTE). Turbo Pascal 5.0 and the Turbo-Tools (2) (for accessing the DASH-8 card) were used to display menues, perform the analog/digital conversion (including real-time graphic display of curves) and to characterize curve shape via diagnostic quantities. A file management module has been included to output experimental parameters and calculated quantities to appropriate "study result-files", to which one record is appended after each measurement of four probes. Similarly, original data my be output, automatically routed into the data file belonging to the study in question.

All data output on disk conform the a format readable by MICROSOFT EXCEL. Both, original and calculated data may be imported and reproduced in high quality graphics; or else, a basic statistical analysis can be performed. Of note that the data format also allows for a transfer of study result-files to the IBM-3090 mainframe of the Institute for Medical Informatics, University of Vienna, for statistical analysis within the package SAS (4).

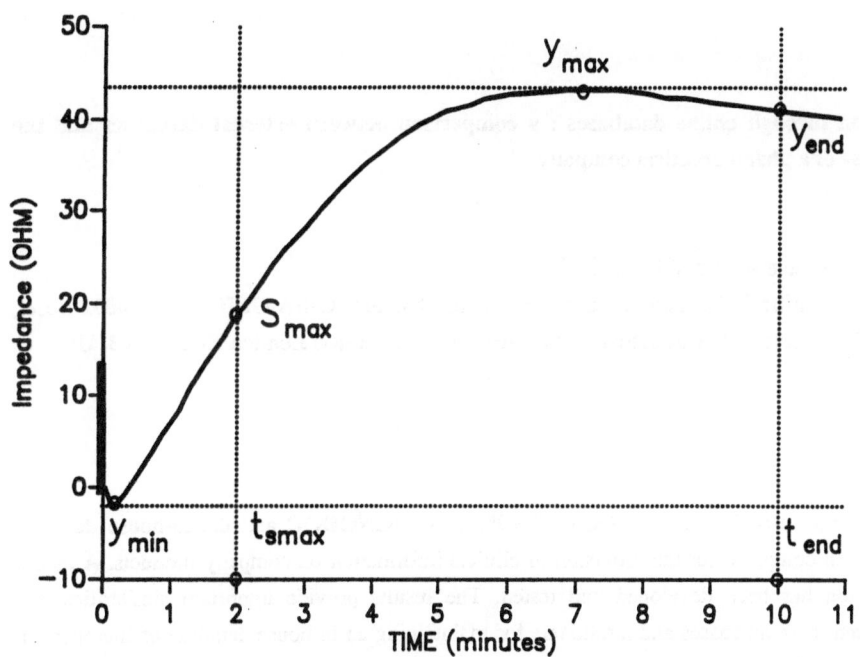

Figure 1: A typical aggregation curve with calculated diagnostics.
The heavy bar on the left represents the calibration signal.

REFERENCES

(1) BORN, G.V.R., M. HUME: Effects of the numbers and sizes of platelet aggregates on the optical density of plasma. Nature 215 (1967)
1027-1029.
(2) MACKIE, I.J., R. JONES, S.J. MACHIN: Platelet impedance aggregation in whole blood and its inhibition by antiplatelet drugs. J.
Clin. Pathol 37 (1984) 874-878.
(3) QUINN-CURTIS: Turbo pascal data acquisition and control tools for
metrabyte das-8 and das-16. Quinn-Curtis Newton MA USA, 1989.
(4) SAS INST.INC.: SAS User's Guide Version 6. SAS Inst. Inc. Cary,NC
USA, 1989.

Drug information through online databases : a comparison between external databases and the in-house database of a pharmaceutical company.

R. J. Sodha[1], B. J. Kostrewski[2] and O. Schier[1]

[1]Department of Scientific Information, Pharmaceuticals Division, CIBA-GEIGY AG, 4002-Basel, Switzerland and [2]Department of Information Science, City University, London EC1V 0HB, UK.

Abstract

The external databases **BIOSIS, EMBASE, MEDLINE,** and **RINGDOC** and the in-house database **CG-DOC** have been compared for the provision of clinical information on company products. A model of drug information has been developed and tested. The results provide important similarities and differences between these databases and a rationale for maintaining an in-house database of literature on company products.

Introduction

The pharmaceutical industry must maintain rigorous monitoring of drug information for several reasons- to keep-up with current drug development of the company's own products as well as products of their competitors, and to meet drug safety regulations [Bawden 1986; van Putte and Peperkamp, 1987; Kruse, 1983]. Company's own research staff need information on literature references, patents, chemical structures, etc.

In the CIBA-GEIGY in-house database of drug literature, detailed information on drugs is available, e.g. minimal/maximal dosage, the number of cases reported in the publication. The records are searched with controlled vocabulary consisting of four thesauri, general terms, indication terms, side effect terms, and substance terms, which are loaded as a VAX file and can be consulted on screen. In the present communication, the external databases **EMBASE, MEDLINE, BIOSIS** (searched via DATA-STAR) and **RINGDOC** (searched via DIALOG) have been compared with the company database **CG-DOC** (searched via DATA-STAR) for the provision of clinical information on one of the company products, diclofenac (VOLTAREN).

Methods

Retrievals were limited to years 1983-1987 inclusive and to English language citations. A set of diclofenac papers that could be retrieved in all five databases (overlap) was identified and the indexing in each paper thoroughly analysed. From this, a model of drug information was developed (Table 1). The performance of the databases was determined by searching a set of questions on diclofenac in each database (Table 2). The model was tested on a second set of questions on company products other than diclofenac (Table 3). Relevance judgement assessment was made by a colleague from the clinical development department. The drug model was independently tested on 20 clinical publications by two physicians.

Results and discussion

A comparison of all five databases for retrieval of diclofenac clinical papers is shown in Table 4. The number of papers exclusively retrieved from a database was also determined (Table 5). CG-DOC not only contributes more papers than the other databases but a high number of papers are exclusively retrieved from this database. Almost 25% of the retrieval from EMBASE was considered irrelevant. MEDLINE's output was remarkable in that there was not a single irrelevant citation. All records exclusively found in BIOSIS were from proceedings of meetings/symposia etc and none had an abstract. RINGDOC, although a smaller database in size, had quite a few citations exclusive to it.

In order to test the model, a series of diclofenac queries were selected relating to each facet of the model and the queries were searched in the databases (Table 6). The model was tested further with a set of questions on a number of CIBA-GEIGY drugs excluding diclofenac (Table 7). The exclusive contributions for diclofenac and the other drugs are described together in the figure. A third of the output from CG-DOC was not present in the other databases.

The present results show important similarities and differences between the biomedical databases widely used in the pharmaceutical industry. No biomedical online database provides complete retrieval of clinical information. The in-house database CG-DOC proved to be best in terms of quantity and provided references not present in the external databases.

References

Bawden, D. (1986). Ten years of Online Information for Pharmaceutical Research. In: *10th London Online Meeting*, Oxford. and New Jersey: Learned Information, pp. 249-254.

Kruse, K. W. (1983). Online Searching of the Pharmaceutical Literature. *American Journal of Hospital Pharmacy* 40 (2) 240-253.

van Putte, N. W.; Peperkamp, H. A. (1987). Online or In-house? The Advantages of an Internal Retrieval System for the Literature on the Products of a Pharmaceutical Company. In: *11th London Online Meeting*. Oxford and New Jersey: Learned Information, pp. 207-211.

Table 1
A schematic model of drug information

Route of Administration.	Dosage Schedule.
Indication.	Side Effect.
Pharmacokinetics.	Drug-Drug Interaction.
Drug Combination.	Contraindication.
Drug-Drug Comparison.	Drug Toxicity.
Patient Information.	Type of Study.

Table 2
Diclofenac questions searched online

1. **Topical administration of** diclofenac in **sports injury.**
2. **Intravenous administration** of diclofenac for **post-operative pain.**
3. Diclofenac in the treatment of **painful shoulder syndrome.**
4. Diclofenac for the treatment of **pain in cancer patients.**
5. Incidence of **intoxication** with diclofenac.
6. **Oral bioavailability** of diclofenac in **children** and **adults over 65.**
7. **Interaction** between diclofenac and **histamine H$_2$ blockers.**
8. **Interaction** between diclofenac and methotrexate.
9. Incidence of **hypotension** with diclofenac.
10. Diclofenac and **allergic reactions.**
11. Diclofenac *versus* naproxen in **ankylosing spondylitis.**
12. Diclofenac *versus* indomethacin in **gout.**
13. Use of diclofenac **suppositories** in **children.**
14. Diclofenac and the incidence of **agranulocytosis.**
15. Is diclofenac **contraindicated** in **pregnancy?**

Table 3
Search queries on drugs besides diclofenac.

1. **Oral administration** of deferoxamine in thalassemia (1983-1989).
2. **Maximum tolerated intravenous infusion dose** of deferoxamine? (1987).
3. Use of metoprolol in **migraine.** (1987).
4. Incidence of **pancreatitis** with carbamazepine treatment. (1983-1989).
5. **Pharmacokinetics** of cefsulodin during pregnancy. (1983-1989).
6. The **interaction** between maprotiline and clonidine. (1983-1989).
7. The **combination** of hydrochlorothiazide and a β-blocker. (1988-1989).
8. Is carbamazepine **contraindicated** in pregnancy? (1986).
9. Efficacy of maprotiline *versus* amitriptyline: Double-blind clinical trials (1983-1989).
10. **Dependence liability (abuse potential)** of methylphenidate. (1988).
11. Double blind clinical trials of carbamazepine in **school children.** (1988).
12. **Double blind clinical trials** of carbamazepine in school children. (1988).

Table 4

A comparison of retrieval of all English language clinical papers on diclofenac for the years 1983-1987.

	Number of papers retrieved from this database (% of the total number of different clinical papers)*				
	83	84	85	86	87
EMBASE	48	23	38	64	49
	51.1%	29.1%	32.5%	59.8%	38.6%
CG-DOC	88	64	94	75	113
	93.6%	81%	80.3%	70.1%	89%
MEDLINE	17	18	27	38	30
	18.1%	22.8%	23.1%	35.5%	23.7%
BIOSIS	12	11	22	31	31
	12.8%	13.9%	18.8%	29.0%	24.4%
RINGDOC	38	25	23	55	59
	40.2%	31.6%	19.7%	51.4%	46.5%

*The sum of all different clinical papers from each year was set as equal to 100% and the distribution in each database determined. The numbers were: 1983 = 94; 1984 = 79; 1985 = 117; 1986 = 107; 1987 = 127.

Table 5

A comparison of retrieval of diclofenac clinical papers exclusively found in each database.

	Number of papers exclusively retrieved (% of the total number of different clinical papers)*				
	83	84	85	86	87
EMBASE	9	2	1	17	11
	9.6%	2.5%	0.85%	8.7%	8.7%
CG-DOC	29	22	24	34	32
	30.8%	27.8%	20.5%	31.8%	25.2%
MEDLINE	0	1	1	1	0
	0	1.3%	0.9%	0.9%	0/0
BIOSIS	1	0/0	1/0	5/3	2/0
	1.1%	0	0.9%	4.7%	1.6%
RINGDOC	2	1	4	10	12
	2.1%	1.3%	3.4%	9.3%	9.5%

* See legend in Table 4

Table 6

Testing the model on diclofenac.

	EMBASE	CG-DOC	MEDLINE	BIOSIS	RINGDOC
	\multicolumn{5}{c}{Number of Papers}				
	Total Contribution / Exclusive Contribution				
Administration*	37/9	52/28	14/0	16/5	12/1
Indication	43/17	72/24	17/0	20/3	29/9
Side Effect	35/12	42/21	11/1	4/0	37/13
Pharmacokinetics	15/4	34/11	8/0	7/0	5/0
Drug Interactions	11/4	17/5	2/0	7/3	16/6
Drug Toxicity	3/0	9/5	2/0	1/0	2/1
Contraindication	3/1	3/2	2/0	1/0	5/3
Drug Comparison	4/1	21/15	1/0	5/1	10/2

*The questions are combined to give the following drug-related information (see **Table 2** for questions): Administration: questions 1, 2, 6, 13; Indication: questions 1, 2, 3, 4; Side effect: questions 9, 10, 14; Pharmacokinetics: questions 6, 13; Drug interaction: questions 7, 8; Drug toxicity: question 5; Contraindication: question 15; Drug comparison: questions 11, 12;

Table 7

Testing the model on other drugs.

	EMBASE	CG-DOC	MEDLINE	BIOSIS	RINGDOC
	\multicolumn{5}{c}{Number of Papers}				
	Total Contribution / Exclusive Contribution				
Administration**	9/3	9/6	5/2	7/3	3/1
Dosage Schedule	--	3/3	--	--	--
Indication	10/3	7/2	1/0	2/0	4/1
Side Effect	6/3	3/2	1/0	3/1	2/0
Pharmacokinetics	1/0	2/1	1/0	1/0	1/0
Drug Interaction	3/2	3/2	2/1	0/0	1/1
Drug Combination	5/1	4/2	6/3	4/3	6/1
Contraindication	20/7	15/4	7/2	0/0	10/4
Drug Comparison	2/1	13/6	5/2	1/0	5/2
Toxicity	5/1	8/4	6/0	0/0	4/1
Patient Data	2/0	4/3	2/0	0/0	4/2
Type of Study	2/0	4/3	2/0	1/0	4/2

** The actual questions are described in **Table 3**.

Figure
Exclusive contributions of the databases

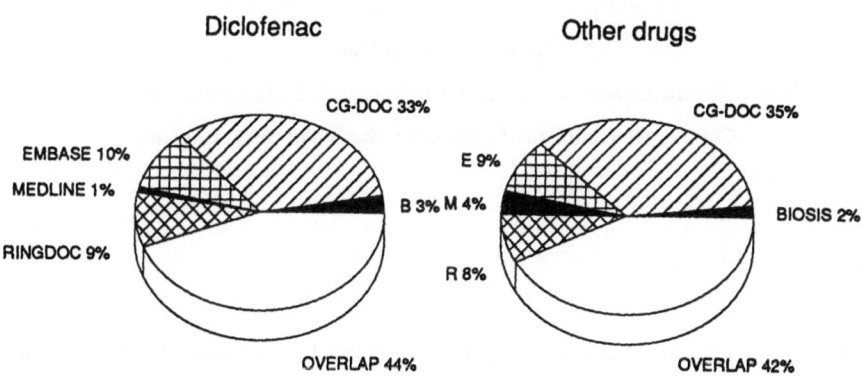

Diclofenac

Other drugs

CG-DOC 33%
EMBASE 10%
MEDLINE 1%
RINGDOC 9%
B 3% M 4%
OVERLAP 44%

CG-DOC 35%
E 9%
BIOSIS 2%
R 8%
OVERLAP 42%

E = EMBASE; R = RINGDOC; M = MEDLINE; B = BIOSIS.
The overlap is between any two databases.

ELECTRONIC TRANSFER OF DATA FOR SURVEILLANCE OF COMMUNICABLE DISEASE

Dr Michael Catchpole

Public Health Laboratory Service Communicable Disease Surveillance

Centre, 61 Colindale Avenue, London NW9 5EQ, England

ABSTRACT

Over the last three years the Communicable Disease Surveillance Centre (CDSC) has developed, in collaboration with other sections of the Public Health Laboratory Service, electronic information systems for communicable disease surveillance. The systems include an application that permits the extraction of data from a wide variety of different laboratory systems and the recoding, manipulation, and electronic transfer of data to CDSC, and a communication and information system based on a wide area network of micro-computers. The systems have strengthened CDSC's surveillance function through improvements in the speed with which the surveillance cycle of collection, collation, analysis and interpretation of data, and dissemination of information can be completed.

INTRODUCTION

This paper outlines the electronic communications systems that have been developed by the Public Health Laboratory Service (PHLS) Communicable Disease Surveillance Centre (CDSC) as part of a national system for communicable disease surveillance in England and Wales.

The underlying principals of communicable disease surveillance are that it provides timely information that will permit the early detection of changes in trend or distribution of disease and that this information is distributed promptly to those responsible for the control of such disease (1). Many of the characteristics of electronic communications systems, in particular speed and accuracy of data transfer, make them ideally suited to meeting the specific requirements of surveillance information systems, which should be distinguished by their accuracy, practicability, uniformity, and rapidity (2).

Over the last three years CDSC, which has the national responsibility for the surveillance of communicable diseases in England and Wales, has developed, with other sections of the PHLS, a number of electronic information systems for the purposes of collection, storage, and analysis of data, and dissemination of information. The systems that have been developed represent a deliberate attempt to strengthen communicable disease surveillance in England and Wales through the application of electronic communication systems to key stages, identified through critical path analysis, in the surveillance process.

METHODS

Collection of Data

CDSC receives routine surveillance data every week from 52 Public Health Laboratories (PHLs) and approximately 300 National Health Service laboratories. Urgent reports, either of outbreaks or of the identification of important organisms, are also received from laboratories and public health physicians on an *ad hoc* basis.

1991 saw the introduction of electronic transfer to CDSC of laboratory data from PHLs, following either automated extraction of data from laboratory computer systems or keyboard entry of data into a dedicated microcomputer database and communications application. The use of a dedicated application (figure 1) permits the extraction of data from a wide variety of different laboratory systems and the recoding, manipulation, and addition of further epidemiologically useful data prior to file transfer to CDSC. Standardisation of data items and associated coding structures is achieved through data validation checks which have been built into the system for organism names and other key fields. Duplicate reporting, arising from multiple specimen reports for individual patients, is avoided by the incorporation into the system of an algorithm for aggregating laboratory data into organism-illness episodes for each patient prior to transmission to CDSC. Following file transfer to CDSC, laboratory data is subjected to further checks for duplicate reports arising from different laboratories and then loaded into the main surveillance database for analysis.

Urgent reports of outbreaks and of identifications of important pathogens are transmitted to CDSC by microbiologists and public health physicians using a communication and information system, known as Epinet, which is based on a wide area network of micro-computers.

Figure 1

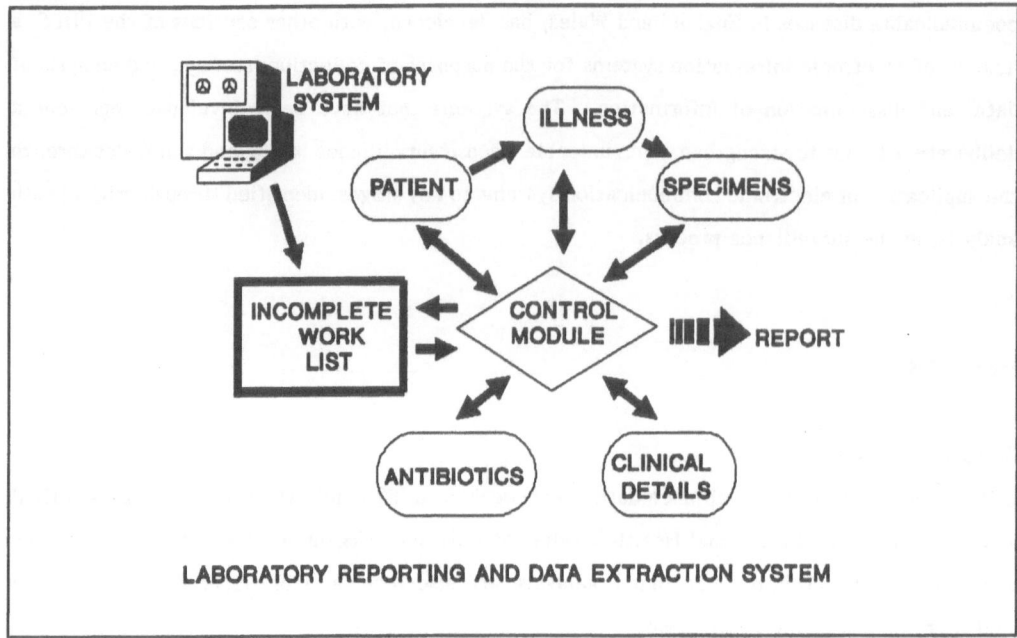

LABORATORY REPORTING AND DATA EXTRACTION SYSTEM

All Epinet communications are controlled by dedicated microprocessor and storage units (Arcoms) and data is transmitted via the Public Switched Telephone Network (PSTN). Arcoms manage view-data pages for non-urgent messages, an urgent messaging service, and file transfer. At the centre of the network is a Host Arcom, which controls the editing and transmission of viewdata pages to Satellite Arcoms based in laboratories and Departments of Public Health. Password-protected text and tabular data may be transferred direct to CDSC or to other users connected to the network using Epinet.

Dissemination of Information

Electronic dissemination of information by CDSC is effected through two separate electronic information systems: an electronic library accessed through a telephone dial-up facility, and messages delivered to users connected to the Epinet system. The electronic library at CDSC is a menu-driven application containing viewdata pages of text and tables providing up-to-date surveillance information based on laboratory reports and notifications of clinically diagnosed communicable disease. The library also contains mortality data, population estimates, reports of current outbreaks of communicable disease, medical advice for travellers, and information on vaccines. Many of the surveillance tables held in the library are automatically written and updated as routine reports generated from the database of laboratory reports.

The Epinet system provides a means for sending urgent messages, such as environmental hazard warnings or reports of possible outbreaks of local or national significance. Such messages may be broadcast to all Epinet users or to specified groups of users connected to the network. Messages are stored in RAM in the satellite Arcoms, and recipients of urgent messages are alerted to the arrival of the message by a warning light on the Epinet satellite unit. Future developments are to include the activation of bleeps in addition to the warning light mechanism for alerting users to the arrival of important information. Messages, which are password protected, are accessed through a PC link to the Epinet satellite unit. Less urgent messages, such as update reports on outbreaks and key surveillance tables, are transmitted as viewdata pages to all Epinet satellite units, where they are stored for access at any time, via a PC link.

RESULTS

Over 200,000 patient-illness episodes were recorded on the routine laboratory reporting system operated by CDSC in 1990. Approximately 50% of these reports were made by Public Health Laboratories, all of which will report data to CDSC through electronic file transfer by the end of 1991. The use of electronic extraction of records from laboratory computer systems and automated file transfer of laboratory reports has enabled CDSC to produce weekly analyses that are based on laboratory identifications made during the preceding week in those Public Health Laboratories already running the dedicated application (figure 1).

A wide variety of surveillance information, including national surveillance tables based on laboratory reports made during the preceding week, are made available to public health physicians, microbiologists, and others responsible for the control and prevention of communicable disease through the electronic library maintained by CDSC.

The Epinet system has already proved to be a valuable tool in the investigation and control of acute outbreaks of communicable disease, having been used successfully by CDSC in requesting early information on cases in a number of outbreaks (CDSC, unpublished data).

DISCUSSION

The use of electronic communications systems for data transfer, both from laboratories to CDSC and from CDSC to those responsible for the prevention and control of communicable disease, has improved the speed with which CDSC can complete the surveillance cycle of collection, collation, analysis and interpretation of data, and dissemination of information. Automated extraction of data from laboratory systems has also reduced administrative workloads and should improve the completeness and accuracy of laboratory reporting. The Epinet system developed within the PHLS also provides a rapid and reliable means of alerting authorities to public health hazards.

The applications described have significantly strengthened the surveillance of communicable disease in England and Wales. Standards for electronic transfer of data on clinically notified infectious disease are being developed by the Office of Population Censuses and Surveys in England, and electronic reporting systems for clinically notified infectious disease have been developed in Wales by the CDSC Welsh Unit. Future developments in electronic reporting systems for communicable disease are likely to include the automatic identification and reporting of notifiable diseases by computerised general practitioner record systems.

REFERENCES

(1)   Galbraith NS. Communicable disease surveillance. In: Smith A, (ed.) Recent advances in community medicine No.2, pp 127-142. Churchill Livingstone, London. 1982.

(2)   Last JM. A Dictionary of Epidemiology, 2nd edition. New York: Oxford University Press 1988.

COMPUTER-AIDED CLUSTER ANALYSIS OF CITATION NETWORKS AS A TOOL OF RESEARCH POLICY IN BIOMEDICINE

Sergei G. Burchinsky, Yuri K. Duplenko
Institute of Gerontology AMS USSR
Vyshgorodskaya St. 67, 252655 Kiev-114, USSR

ABSTRACT

The method of mapping a research trend involving citation analysis allows to quantify the development of a particular research area and, more importantly, to establish its interrelations with other areas and thus to create the map proper. In our investigation we have tried to create the map of current trends in the neurobiology of aging by using computer-aided cluster citation analysis. It was found that this map of interrelations, both between separate research trends and within each of the trends in neurobiology of aging and Alzheimer's disease, in particular, has provided us with the quantitative "portrait" of this area. In addition, we managed to assess the most cited and most significant investigations and hence to evaluate the contributions made by each research center to the development of this field.

INTRODUCTION

Among the methods to be used for studying information processes and particularly document classification is that of citation analysis. It allows to track the development of a given field of research over time and its penetration into related fields (Porter et al., 1988; McRoberts and McRoberts, 1989). Price (1965) noted that citation of scientific papers produces a network connecting all papers in a single system. Each paper appears as the basis of other papers and in turn becomes itself the basis for other papers. According to Price (1965), the system of scientific references ensures an insight into the nature of science research as a whole. Concerning the objectives of classification of a particular area of knowledge, it is essential that a study should involve all publications related to this particular research field. The obtained results of the quantitative evaluation of citations are to be subjected to a qualitative analysis as well. The purpose of the present investigation was to visualize the structure of a concrete research area—neurobiology of aging—and to assess the interrelations among separate publications pertinent to this area.

METHODS AND MATERIALS

We have used the Science Citation Index developed at the Institute for Scientific Information (USA) to carry out formal analysis on the development of a particular field of science, i.e. to track its separate research trends and to study the classification and reclassification. The essence of classification with the help of the above-mentioned index lies in finding a conceptual relationship between the paper cited in the reference list and the present paper. In other words, the paper is classified by means of its bibliographic references.

The classification study enabled us to establish the relationships between documents based on common citations in other papers. The documents A and B are considered to be interrelated provided that there is a sufficient number of papers that cite simultaneously document A and document B. According to Small et al. (1985) and Marshakova (1988), such a relationship can be called prospective or co-citation. The prospective relationship between cited documents depends to a great degree on the development of the science and represents a great interest for scientometry. The intensity of relationships between two publications, as defined by the co-citation method, is proportional to the number of papers citing simultaneously both of these publications. The process of setting the relationships between publications on the basis of co-citation leads to the formation of a citation network. After establishing the co-citation threshold, which is dependent on the value of mathematical expectation about the number of common references to a given paper, the citation networks break into separate clusters. Such thorough, comprehensive analysis of the results obtained in cluster formation allowed us to visualize the structure of the study research trend, the thematic profile of each cluster, the contribution made by different authors to this area, the determination of a succession of ideas, and establishing interrelations among periodical publications, etc.

RESULTS

In our investigation we have employed the computer-aided cluster analysis of citation networks in order to track modern trends in the development of gerontology, which is a relatively new and intensively developing branch of biomedical sciences, and one of its perspective fields, the neurobiology of aging. Computer-aided cluster analysis of the database was performed using an IBM PC/XT and the DataEase system program (USA), the latter having been adapted for solving the task of citation network construction. The information input procedure consisted in loading the basic publications (cited papers) and the corresponding prospective publications (citing papers) into the computer. Thus we selected the document pairs from basic publications, which were characterized by a definite strength of links between them, as determined by the number of citing papers. We broke an overall amount of basic publications into clusters and formed the citation networks, this being performed as the man-machine classification procedure. Thus we created the cluster map of the research field under study. The scheme for a part of the cluster map for the neurobiology of aging, representing internal and external interrelations between publications dealing with Alzheimer's disease, is shown in Fig. 1. These interrelations characterize, from a quantitative point of view, the links between different aspects of this problem (A,B,C,D) and ascertain the main research centers and "invisible colleges" of specialists working in this field.

DISCUSSION

Having assessed the most prospective research trends with the help of this map, it may well be possible to resolve many questions pertaining to scientific policy such as funding, the development of national and international research projects, evaluation of the contribution made by leading scientific schools, etc. In summary, cluster analysis was found to be an operational tool in the organization and management of research in biomedicine.

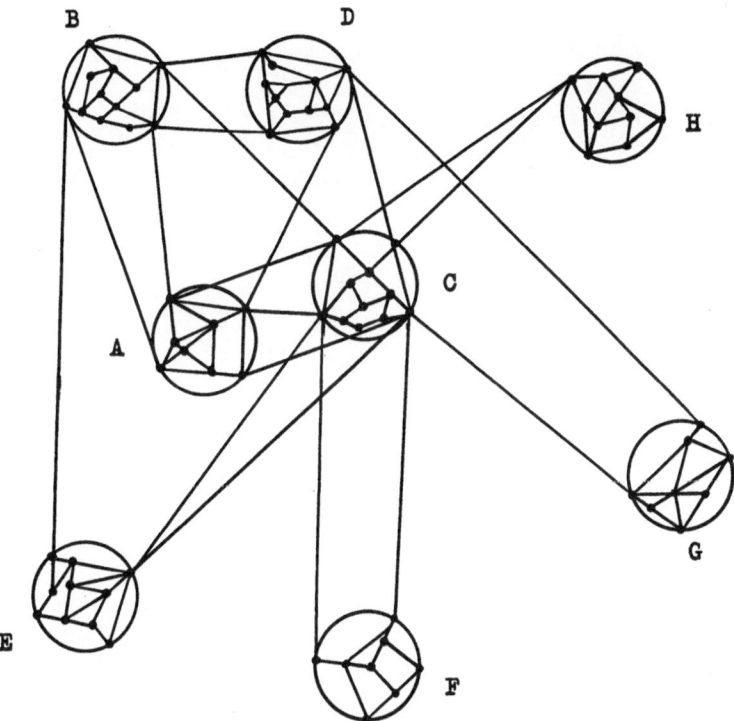

Figure 1: Scheme for a part of the citation network of the cluster map for the neurobiology of aging, reflecting research on Alzheimer's disease.

Points inside clusters reflect concrete publications, lines between clusters reflect links between these publications resulting from co- citation.

Names of the clusters: A - molecular biology and genetics of Alzheimer's disease; B - cytology and histochemistry of Alzheimer's disease; C - morphology of Alzheimer's disease; D - neuropeptides and neurotransmitters of Alzheimer's disease; E - morphology of the aging brain; F - clinical psychology of the aging brain; G - metabolism of the aging brain; H - neuroimmunology of the aging brain.

REFERENCES

I.V.Marshakova. Citation System of Science Literature as a Tool for the Control of Science Development in: Nauka, Moscow 1988

M.H.McRoberts, B.R.McRoberts. Problems of Citation Analysis: A Crit- ical Review in: J. Amer. Soc. Inform. Sci., 1989, vol.40, n5, pp. 342-349

A.L.Porter, D.E.Chubin, Xiao-Jin Jin. Citations and Scientific Progress: Comparing Biblio- graphic Measures with Scientist Judgements in: Scientometrics, 1988, vol.13, N 3-4, pp. 103-124

D.J.Price. Science of Science in: Bull. Atom. Sci., 1965, vol.21, N 10, pp. 3-7

H.Small, E.Sweeney, E.Greenlee. Clustering the Science Citation Index Using Co-Citations. II. Mapping science in: Scientometrics, 1985, vol.8 N 5-6, pp. 321-340.

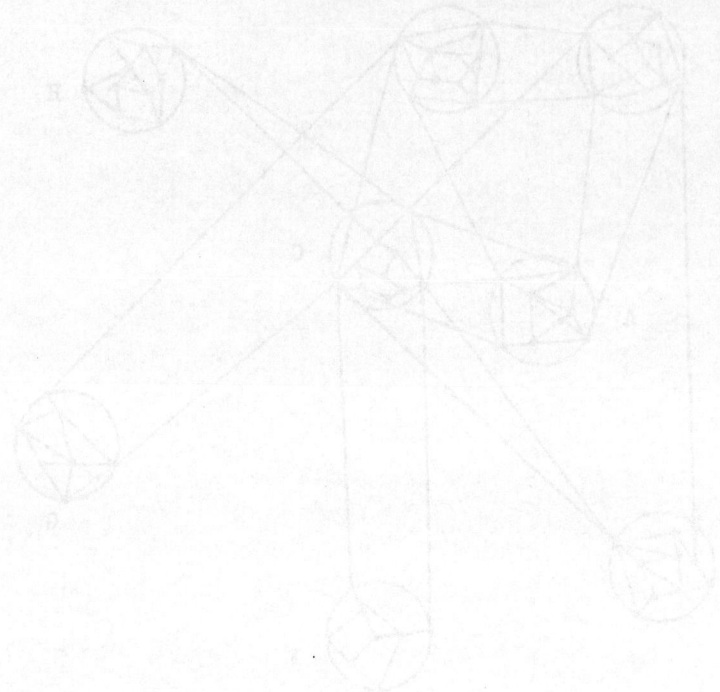

EXPERT SYSTEMS AND DECISION MAKING

SOME ASPECTS OF THE IMPLEMENTATION OF DECISION MONITORING LOGIC WITHIN A HETEROGENEOUS HOSPITAL INFORMATION SYSTEM

Michel, A., Sebald, P., Dudeck, J.
Department of Medical Informatics, University of Gießen
Heinrich-Buff-Ring 44, D-6300 Gießen

Abstract

The following article describes strategies for the implementation of a decision monitoring system within the heterogeneous computer environment of a german university hospital. After a short discussion about different types of computerized decision support in medicine, it presents selection criteria for the integrated commercial software and design goals for the main components of the decision support software. At last, the current state of the system implementation is described.

Introduction

At the University Hospital of Gießen, Germany, there is currently a hospital information system (HIS) under development, which consists of a mixture of commercially available and self developed software. The software resides on a network of departmental Unix machines and MS-DOS local area networks (LAN's), connected to a central Tandem host computer for ADT and communication management /6/. One goal in the development of this HIS is the integration of decision monitoring as a type of medical decision support. Many aspects of decision monitoring have been recognized during a three year test installation of the HELP-System's kernel at our site from 1984 to 1987.

Decision support in medicine

Decision support systems can be grouped into two categories, according to their interaction with the user:

- Consultation Systems

  This type of decision support systems is representated by a number of standalone medical expert systems, mainly for the support of differential diagnoses in a variety of medical fields. Most of these systems have failed to reach a state of practical acceptance by the physicians /8/.

- Decision Monitoring Systems

  This type of decision support has been successfully implemented in the well known HIS HELP /7/ and CARE /3/. These systems communicate with their users typically by sending alert messages to predefined destinations. Only this type of decision support has been accepted for routine use by the clinicians. This is well documented in some studies in the field of drug ordering /2/ and lab test ordering /4/. The knowledge base of these systems is organized in highly independent modules and therefore simply expandable and potentially shareable between different systems. A standard format for the sharing of such medical logic modules is currently under development /1/. As a major benefit, the language for such shareable medical logic modules allows a simple interface to common relational databases.

With regard to the major advantages of the decision monitoring concept and our experience with the HELP system, decision monitoring has been choosen as the preferred concept for decision support.

System development strategies

The decision to build a medical decision support system on top of a set of commercially available software products is based on the following facts:

- Existing HIS that fully include decision support (HELP) are not transferable into the german hospital environment.

- There are rapidly growing needs in all clinical departments for basic support in electronic data processing that could be met by a number of commercially available software products.

- The available clinical software is commonly designed to run on departmental computer systems. To meet the basic requirements of clinical communication, these systems must be interfaced in any case with each other and with the existing host based ADT system.

All these facts lead into the direction, that future activities of the hospital information processing department are mainly concerned with the selection of appropriate departmental software, subsystem interconnection and distributed system and database management. On this base, decision monitoring should be implemented step by step.

To support the later implementation of decision monitoring functions, it is necessary to define selection criteria for departmental hard- and software. The most important of these are:

- Usage of a standard operating system (UNIX) for the departmental computer systems

- Usage of a standard communication protocol (ETHERNET, TCP-IP)

- Usage of relational database management systems (DBMS), which support SQL as a relational language

- Domination of structured data aquisition strategies (e.g. mouse based menu selection) over free text input

The added decision monitoring system consists mainly of two types of software modules:

- Interface software between the different departmental DBMS for efficient distributed data manipulation and compensation of several lacks of the different DBMS software (e.g. domain management and integrity features). This software acts as a bridge between the heterogeneous commercial software products to form a single logical clinical database.

- The management and execution software for the decision monitoring system.

Major design principles for these software modules are:

- Full distribution
  There is no central component which makes a departmental system unable to run in a standalone mode. Instead the software modules are organized as groups of cooperating processes which communicate in a client server mode to perform synchronized system wide tasks.

- Two level architecture
Every software module consists of a system independent part which is very similar on every incorporated system, and a subsystem specific interface module which implements the module specific functions in a highly subsystem specific manner.

Components of the decision monitoring system

The decision monitoring system consists of five basic components:

- The Medical Data Dictionary (MDD) /5/
The main task of this tool is domain management which is a lack of allmost all current DBMS implementations but necessary for decision support. This means, the MDD acts as a thesaurus for all objects that could be stored in the columns of any relation and provides this essential information to the developer of decision support logic. Additionally, the MDD exposes the collected structural information of all subsystem databases (tables, views, domains) in a uniform manner to the designer of the knowledge modules.

- The medical logic module editor (MLME)
The MLME is an interactive editor which allows the editing and testing of the slot structure that comprises the so called medical logic modules. A very important feature is its integrated access to the MDD to define the neccesary database access statements which play a key part in every logic module.

- The medical logic module manager (MLMM)
This module manages compilation, storage, distribution and execution of the medical logic modules /1/, within the heterogeneous clinical computing environment.

- The message router (MR)
This module transfers the generated alerts to all appropriate locations within the HIS including the storage of alerts within the patient database.

- The program control environment (PCE)
Commercial application programs run under control of the PCE which is a window based execution shell and triggered by the logic modules. It allows basic control over the running applications.

Outlook

Today the distributed MDD and decision logic modules written in C have been successfully tested within a prototype system which covers the field of structured data aquisition for clinical examination and drug ordering.

Literature:

1   Clayton, P.D., Pryor, T.A., Wigertz, O.B., Hripcsak, G.: Issues and Structures for Sharing Medical Knowlege among Decion-Making Systems; The 1989 Arden Homestead Retreat, Proceedings of the 13. SCAMC 1989

2   Department of Medical Informatics, University of Utah: Computerized Medication Monitoring System, Salt Lake City, Utah, 1988

3   McDonald, C.J.: Protocol-based computer reminders in the quality of care and the nonperfectability of man, New England Journal of Medicine, 295, 1976, pp. 1351-1355

4   McDonald, C.J.: Use of a computer to Detect and Respond to Clinical Events: Its Effect on Clinician Behavior, Annals of Internal Medicine, Volume 84, No. 2, 1984, pp. 162-166

5   Michel, A., Prokosch, H.U., Dudeck, J.: Concepts for a Medical Data Dictionary, Proceedings MEDINFO 1989

6   Prokosch, H.U., Sebald, P., Michel, A., Dudeck, J., Schroeder, F., Heeg, M.: Integrating the HELP HIS Philosophy into the Tandem Pathway Environment, Proceedings MEDINFO 1989

7   Pryor, T.A., Gardner, Gardr, R.M., Clayton, P.D., Warner, H.R. The HELP System, Journal of Medical Systems 7, 87-102, 1983.

8   Shortliffe, E.H.: Computer programs to support clinical decision making, JAMA, Vol 258, No.1, July 3 1987

TEN YEARS OF COMPUTER SUPPORT
IN A METABOLIC INTENSIVE CARE UNIT

S. Svacina, R. Hovorka, T. Haas, Z. Masek and J. Kabrt

3rd Dept. of Medicine, Charles University, Prague, Czechoslovakia

Abstract. The primary aim of computer support in Metabolic Intensive Care is to improve the quality of care. This paper details 10 years experience with computer support in a Metabolic Intensive Care Unit, during which time numerous programs have been developed and adapted. The main areas where computer support showed to be of particular value and of research interest are described.

INTRODUCTION

The Metabolic Intensive Care Unit was established at 3rd Dept. of Medicine, Charles University, Prague in 1981 and operated in a single room on a standard ward. In January 1985, a separate ward was refurbished and opened as an independent Metabolic Intensive Care Unit. The unit has 8 beds in 5 rooms, a detached laboratory, a diet kitchen and an ambulatory diagnostic room. From the beginning computer support of medical decisions and clinical administration has been performed. Many computer programs were developed in the last ten years to provide this support, some of these programs have already been referred to at MEDINFO 83 [1], and later at IMIA 85 [5] conferences. Currently, a complex set of computer programs is used to support routine metabolic care and special investigation techniques. Other standard clinical programs are also available.

COMPUTER PROGRAMS
Routine programs

1. <u>Drug, infusion and food database</u>. The database of drugs, infusions and food is continuously updated. The database is accessed by several programs as mentioned below.

2. <u>Metabolic balance</u>. The program performs the evaluation of metabolic balance of energy, water, nitrogen, ions, vitamins. A database containing drugs, infusions and food composition is accessed. Daily losses of ions, nitrogen and water are entered and the balance of various items is determined. For some items, e.g. vitamins, only input quantities are processed.

3. Program for enteral and parenteral nutrition planning. A sum of proposed therapy containing energy, ions, water and vitamins is interactively computed. The clinicians may vary the therapy proposal in order to obtain ideal or real metabolic balance. The velocities of fat, protein and carbohydrate infusion are shown as a part of the results.

4. Acid base balance. Evaluation of acid base balance disorders and therapeutic proposal is supported (including programs developed by Kazda et al [4]).

5. Evaluation of indirect calorimetry data. The consumption of oxygen and the production of carbon dioxide is measured by the indirect calorimeter Spirolyt. The non protein respiration quotient is computed. The consumption of energy calculated using this approach is compared with the Harris Benedict formula. The proportion of protein, sugar and fat consumption is calculated.

6. Renal functions. Evaluation of renal functions is adopted from programs developed by Kazda et al [3]. Excretion fractions and clearances of ions, water and other metabolites are calculated. The type of diuresis (osmotic versus water diuresis), and type of renal failure (prerenal versus renal) is determined.

7. Nutritional status assessment. Laboratory and anthropometric data are evaluated and the type of protein or caloric malnutrition is classified and scored.

8. Evaluation of glucose control in diabetic patients. M-value, MAGE and GMW value are computed from daily blood glucose profiles to comment on blood-glucose control.

9. Consultation system for insulin therapy. A system to advise on insulin therapy for diabetic patient has been developed and is currently under clinical evaluation [2].

10. Specific databases. Databases are maintained for in- and out-patients with diabetes and obesity.

Clinical investigation of metabolic disorders using computer programs.

1. Modelling of glycation. Computer modelling of haemoglobin and protein glycation is performed to understand these parameters and to identify kinetic parameters [6].

2. Insulin receptor system identification. Several insulin receptor models are employed to compute binding parameters in radioligand experiments.

3. Computer support of artificial pancreas Biostator Miles. The device is connected to the computer via a serial link and it transmits measured data to the computer for analysis. Biostator-patient interaction was simulated to optimise the initial setting of the device.

4. Quantification of glycoregulation using Bergman minimal model. Different clinical trials were performed to calculate the insulin sensitivity and beta cell secretion in different diseases and after specific therapeutic interventions.

The Metabolic Intensive Care Unit also uses clinical computers programs, e.g. central patient evidence, drug information system, reduction of drug dose in renal failure etc.

EXPERIENCE AND CONCLUSIONS

During 10 years, approximately 1000 patients were treated, 35% with diabetes-related complications, impaired blood-glucose control and acute diabetic coma, 35% with nutritional problems, e.g. long term parenteral nutrition, enteral nutrition, intestinal bowel disease, severe malnutrition. The rest of the patients were admitted due to hepatic coma or decompensation of the liver function, pancreatitis, severe endocrinopathies, morbid obesity, intoxications etc.

The use of computers has become a routine. Metabolic balance determination is performed in about 60% of patients. Several computer programs are used in more than 85% of patients. Three years ago, there was a hardware failure and the Metabolic Care Unit was without the computer support for several weeks . A considerable reduction in the quality of the medical care was observed. Immediately after the computers began to perform again, the quality of the care was restored.

From this experience with computers in Metabolic Intensive Care Unit it may be concluded:

1. The use of computers in metabolic care enables an exact documentation and control of care. For instance, the metabolic balance seems to be necessary. Another important factor is the improvement of the adminstration and medical care organisation (sample collecting and analysis, recording of intake). A similar profit was obtained when the documentation of diabetics records was computerised.

2. There are some situations where exact but simple computations and evaluations are useful, e.g. acid base balance and renal function evaluation. These computations are useful but they are not obligatory.

3. Exact metabolic investigations need dynamic quantification and in this field the use of computers is mandatory - indirect calorimetry, glycoregulation evaluation - minimal modelling, glucose clamp technique.

4. The use of complex programs, e.g. expert consultation systems is not easy and essential in clinics. We have identified insulin therapy of diabetes mellitus as a suitable, well-defined area, where such systems may have practical results. The consultation system for insulin therapy is able to predict blood glucose level and to propose insulin dosage in all therapeutic regimens. The quality of prediction was studied and the similarity of physician and system advice in a retrospective study was observed. However, a prospective study is planned to complete the evaluation of the system performance. In a complex therapeutic and diagnostics field, the physician often prefers his/her own decision as opposed to a complex computation. Such types of program have more advantages in an ambulatory care or in unspecialised wards.

5. Computer support of metabolic care. Our experience show that complex metabolic care cannot be done without calculations and computers. With a user-friendly oriented interface, computers can be used by all medical and paramedical personnel.

REFERENCES

1. BENDA, J. Computer programs in the metabolic intensive care unit. In: *MEDINFO 83*,edited by VAN BEMMEL, J.H., M.J. BALL, and O. WIGERTZ. Amsterdam:North-Holland, 1983, p. 1279.
2. HOVORKA, R., S. SVACINA, E.R. CARSON, C.D. WILLIAMS, and P.H. SöNKSEN. A consultation system for insulin therapy. *Comput. Methods Programs Biomed.* 32:303-310, 1990.
3. KAZDA, A., A. JABOR, and M. ZAMECNIK. Program for renal function evaluation. *Biochem. Clin. Bohemoslov.* 13:221-231, 1984.
4. KAZDA, A., A. JABOR, M. ZAMECNIK, and K. MASEK. Monitoring acid-base and electrolyte disturbances in intensive care. *Adv. Clin. Chem.* 27:201-267, 1989.
5. SVACINA, S., R. HOVORKA, Z. MASEK, and J. KABRT. Computer support of the metabolic intensive care unit. In: *Medical Decision Making: Diagnostic Strategies and Expert Systems*,edited by VAN BEMMEL, J.H., F. GREMY, and J. ZVAROVA. Amsterdam:North-Holland, 1985, p. 133-136.
6. SVACINA, S., R. HOVORKA, and J. SKRHA. Computer models of albumin and haemoglobin glycation. *Comput. Methods Programs Biomed.* 32:259-264, 1990.

APPLICATION OF RULE INDUCTION ALGORITHM IN MEDICAL RESEARCH

Miroslawa Lasek
Department of Cybernetics and Operational Research,
University of Warsaw, Dluga 44/50, 00-241 Warsaw, Poland

Witold Lasek
Department of Transplantology, Institute of Biostructure,
Medical School, Chalubinskiego 5, 02-004 Warsaw, Poland

ABSTRACT

Method aimed at discovering influences of various factors on medical parameters is presented. The method, based on the rule induction algorithm, enables to generate rules representing connections between factors and parameters. Theory of the method is described and illustrated by an example.

1. INTRODUCTION

The aim of medical research is very often to discover and analyse the effect of some factors on tested laboratory parameter in studied population. Usually, the higher number of factors expected to influence the parameter tested the more difficult is the analysis of dependencies. To help in analysis of such dependencies, we propose to use the method with rule induction algorithm, which is based on work by Quinlan [1,2,3] and is suggested as a knowledge acquisition method in expert system software [4,5]. This algorithm enables to find a tree of rules - in the form of IF...THEN clauses - from a given set of data. Such a tree of rules represents relations and connections between factors (attributes) and studied parameter.

In the paper, theory of the method is presented and illustrated by an application. In the example, dependencies between factors as age, sex, cigarette smoking etc. and blood parameter - NK activity (antitumour activity of the subpopulation of white blood cells named NK cells, tested in vitro) are studied in the population of healthy individuals.

2. PROCEDURE OF THE METHOD

Procedure consists of five following steps:
Step 1. Classification of the individuals from the population studied

in regard to analysed parameter criterion,

Step 2. Selection of attributes which can be used to describe particular individuals; categorization of individuals studied in regard to each attribute,

Step 3. Construction of the decision tree, representing relationships between attributes values and classes of individuals.

Step 4. Generation of rules from the decision tree.

Step 5. Analysis of the resulted rules.

On the step 1 and 2 of the method we decided that classification of individuals to subsets or categories, in the case of numeric character of an attribute, would be presented in the form: "low level - normal level - high level" or would be expressed in numeric ranges. Data for analysis were stored in standard dBASE data base in IBM microcomputer.

To construct the decision tree (step 3 of the method), J. R. Quinlan's algorithm was used [1,2,3]. According to this algorithm the decision tree is constructed from the data which specify association between each of the attribute values and the classes to which the individuals from studied population belong. The data, showing the associations between attribute values and classes, are set out in a contingency tables (matrixes) [2], each element of such tables indicates the number of individuals in class j with attribute value i. In the process of decision tree construction, information measure (IM) is employed. The information measure is a statistics for contingency table based on information theory. It is defined as the gain in information resulted from the knowledge about number of individuals with known attribute values and known assignment to classes and can be calculated for each attribute from the data in contingency table, constructed for that attribute [4]. Detailed formulas for the calculations are given elsewhere [4].

The information measures, calculated from a contingency tables, are used to select an attribute which is the best discriminator within the given set of data and for this reason is selected as a succeeding node of the decision tree. Thus, in the procedure, information measure is calculated for each attribute and the attribute with the maximum information measure, as giving maximum gain or increase in information, is chosen as a node of a decision tree. The possible values of an attribute specify branches leaving the decision node. The subnodes (subtrees) are established in the same procedure within the attributes not yet selected in a given path in the tree and within the subset of the data representing values on the branch being examined. The process is continued and terminated for the path when values of attributes on that path indicate explicitly on the class of individual, setting up a leaf of the decision tree or all attributes are examined on that path. For detailed formal discussion of the algorithm see Quinlan [1,2,3].

The main advantages of using Quinlan's information measure for our purposes are (i) usefulness in extracting associations between parameter studied and factors which could influence this parameter, (ii) ensuring the order of the attributes, which will next serve as conditions in the rules, from the most important to the least important (iii) computational simplicity.

Rules were conducted directly from the decision tree and were in the form of IF...THEN clauses (step 4). To evaluate the fitness of the developed rules we used data not applied in the process of generation of the decision tree (step 5). We tested how this data would match the rules. The proposed method is iterative. In the fifth step of the method we can make decision whether it is necessary:
- to change the decision tree (return to step 3),
- to use another attributes to describe particular individuals (return to step 2),
- to apply another classification of the individuals into subset or categories (return to step 1).

3. SOFTWARE

The method of acquiring knowledge from the data describing individuals from the studied population has been coded as a program in Turbo Pascal for the PC DOS operating system. This program can be used in IBM-PC or compatibles. In the program, decision tree was constructed from laboratory data according to Quinlan's algorithm. Thus, in the program, Information Measure - IM for attributes was computed, the attribute with maximum IM was selected as a succeeding node of a decision tree, the tree was constructed and the rules from the tree were generated.

4. APPLICATION

We applied our method to generate the rules representing relationships between some factors characterizing the population studied and the level of NK activity. The population studied consisted of 176 subjects tested for NK activity in a standard ^{51}Cr-release assay [6]. The influence of following factors on NK activity was analysed: sex, age, total volume of blood donated in the past (=blood), white blood cell number per litre (=leuk), cigarette smoking, blood groups of ABO system (=ABO), and Rh antigens. Further details concerning population studied, especially from medical point of view are described elsewhere [6,7].

In the first step of procedure we classified all individuals into subsets (categories) according to the parameter tested, i.e. the level of NK activity. Three groups of individuals were composed. Group the first included those with NK activity in the range 6.05 - 23.91 (values below $\bar{x}$-SD, low level); group the second - with NK activity in the range 23.92 - 59.74 (values $\bar{x}$ ± SD, normal level); and group the third - with NK activity: 59.75 - 83.91 (values higher than $\bar{x}$ + SD, high level).

In the second step of the method, we selected to analysis seven attributes mentioned above (sex, age, blood etc.). Individuals were classified as follows. For sex: males and females, for age: 1) 19 - 25, 2) 26 - 35, 3) 36 - 45, and 4) 46 - 64-year-old, for "blood": 1) 0.00, 2) 0.01 - 4, 3) 4.01 - 10, 4) 10.01 - 20, and 5) 20.01 - 40.50 litres of blood donated in the past, for "leuk": 1. 3.87 and lower, 2. 3.88 - 7.08 and, 3. more than 7.09 G/l, for cigarette smoking: 1) heavy smokers, 2) moderate smokers 3. non smokers, for "ABO": 1) A, 2) B, 3) AB 4) 0 blood group, and for Rh antigens 1) "+" (positive), 2) "-" (negative).

In the third step of the method we set out the data, translated from dBASEIII+, in a contingency tables. In our contingency tables we obtained data which represented an association between the groups of attribute values and classes of individuals.

To construct the decision tree, based on the data in contingency tables, we used Quinlan's algorithm. The results were obtained as a tree, fragment of which is shown in Fig. 1.

```
ABO = A: (75)
|   BLOOD = 0.0: (28)
|   |     SEX = M: (20)
|   |   | NK: low (3)
|   |   | NK: normal (11)
|   |   | NK: high (6)
|   |     SEX = F (8)
|   |   | NK: low (1)
|   |   | NK: normal (5)
|   |   | NK: high (2)
.   .
```

Figure 1. Fragment of a sample decision tree

This fragment of the tree represents relationships between blood groups of ABO system, blood donation, sex and NK activity for individuals studied. Numbers, after each leaf in parentheses, indicate how many of the subjects are covered by that leaf. Rules generation from the tree is automatic. The rule from the sample of the decision tree presented in Figure 1 for men is:

IF "ABO" = A AND "BLOOD" = 0.0 AND "SEX" = M THEN NK = low (3) OR NK = normal (11) OR NK = high (6).

Relatively high number of individuals with high NK activity has been observed. This could suggest that additional statistical analysis should be performed. We found that a number of leaves in the tree confined very few observations, for example only 3, 2 or even 1, while in the beginning we started to consider the large number of individuals. The reason is that during construction of the tree, number of observations - individuals considered in lower and lower levels of the tree - becomes progressively smaller, what was also observed in other applications of Quinlan's algorithm [4]. We found that the optimal number of factors for the analysis of their influence on NK activity, was two or three.

5. CONCLUSIONS

The intention of the described method was to perform an initial analysis of medical/laboratory parameters and to draw attention to possible correlations which may occur between them. The study with real data indicate that the method may be useful for this purpose and making further statistical analysis easier.

REFERENCES

[1] Quinlan J. R., Induction of decision trees, Machine Learning 1 (1986), 81-106.
[2] Quinlan J. R., Simplifying decision trees, Int. J. Man-Machine Studies 27 (1987), 221-234.
[3] Quinlan J. R., Rivest R. L., Inferring Decision Trees Using the Minimum Description Length Principle, Information and Computation 80 (1989), 227-248.
[4] Mingers J., Expert Systems - Rule Induction with Statistical Data, J. Opl Res. Soc. 38 (1987), 39-47.
[5] Vrba J. A., Herrera J. A., Expert System Tools: The Next Generation, IEEE Expert Spring (1989), 75-76.
[6] Lasek W., Plodziszewska M., Jakobisiak M., The effect of blood donation on natural killer activity in man, J. Clin. Lab. Immunol. 22 (1987), 165-168.
[7] Lasek W., Jakobisiak M., Plodziszewska M., Gorecki D., The influence of ABO blood groups, Rh antigens and cigarette smoking on the level of NK activity in normal population, Archivum Immunologiae et Therapiae Experimentalis 37 (1989), 287-294.

A Fuzzy Logical Model of Nutrition Diagnosis

Frank Kretzschmar
Dept. Medical Informatics, St. Georg Hospital Leipzig
Str. d. DSF 141, O-7021 Leipzig, Fed. Rep. Germany

Abstract: A computer model for nutrition diagnosis was developed. The diagnosis is made with the help of a fuzzy logical model on the basis of biochemical, anthropometric and immunological parameters to obtain more differentiated results than before. Variations of the model were suggested and discussed.

Introduction

Malnutrition increases the risk to surgical patients in pre- and post-operative phase. The main causes are malignant growth in the gastroin-testinal tract and chronically inflammatory intestinal diseases. Therefore it is necessary to detect and treat the malnutrition. Different methods have been used to diagnose malnutrition (Chang, 1984; Schmoz, 1986). A fuzzy logical model has been developed to support the detection of malnutrition.

Material and Methods

There were two samples of 170 and 104 patients respectively with car-cinomas of the oesophagus, gastric, colon and rectum. These samples were divided into two nutritional status groups: "normal" and "di-sturbed" (Table 1). Disturbed patients had the diagnoses marasmus, kwashiokor and mixed type (marasmus and kwashiokor).

Table 1: Samples structure

	normal patients	disturbed patients
learning sample	131	39
testing sample	86	18

The mathematical model is based on the first sample (learning sample). It is tested on the second sample (testing sample).
For 6 parameters, namely the biochemical parameter serum albumin,
serum transferrin and haemoglobin, the anthropometric measuring values circumference of the humeral muscle and triceps skinfold thickness, as well as the skin test quotient, the medians and the means of
every group were calculated (Table 2).

Table 2: Medians and means from learning sample groups

parameter median of the normal patients (131 patients):   a
parameter mean of the normal patients (131 patients):   b
parameter median of the disturbed patients (39 patients): c
parameter mean of the disturbed patients (39 patients):   d

----

	a	b	c	d
Serum albumin (g/l)	42.0	41.0	34.0	34.8
Serum transferrin (g/l)	3.0	3.1	2.4	2.4
Haemoglobin (mmol/l)	8.6	8.5	6.7	6.7
Circumference of humeral muscle (%)	100.0	102.0	88.7	86.3
Triceps skinfold thickness				
(Oesophagus/Gastric) (%)	87.0	83.7	47.0	43.3
(Colon/Rectum) (%)	87.0	87.9	74.4	83.7
Skin test quotient	2.5	1.5	0.5	1.2

The procedure of the diagnostic process may be divided into three
steps (Model 1):
- Each of the 6 parameters were described by a membership function
  $m(x) = S(x;a,b,c)$ (see Figure 1) in which the parameter a and c are
  the medians of the parameters of the two groups of nutritinal status
  (by means of the medians a and c: $b = (a+c)/2$):

$$m(x) = \begin{cases} 0 & \text{for } x \geq a \\ 2 * ((a-x)*(a-x))/((a-c)*(a-c)) & \text{for } a > x \geq b \\ 1 - 2 * ((x-c)*(x-c))/((a-c)*(a-c)) & \text{for } b > x \geq c \\ 1 & \text{for } c > x \end{cases}$$

Figure 1:

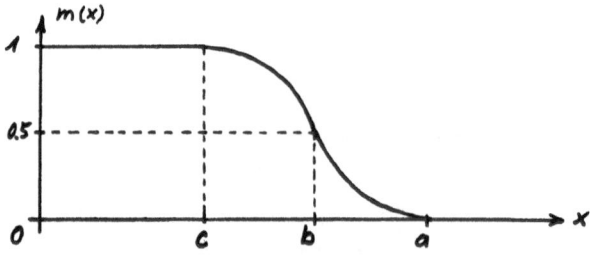

- Based on the frequency of disturbed parameters in the group of disturbed patients, weights were calculated. These weights permit the estimation of the nutritional status on the basis of the following convex combinations:

Biochemistry (serum albumin, serum transferrin, haemoglobin):
$$m_B(x) = 0.36 * m_{ALB}(x) + 0.29 * m_{TRAF}(x) + 0.35 * m_{HB}(x)$$
Anthropometry (circumference of the humeral muscle, triceps skinfold thickness):
$$m_A(x) = 0.52 * m_{UAMC}(x) + 0.48 * m_{TSFT}(x)$$
Nutritional state (serum albumin, serum transferrin, haemoglobin, circumference of the humeral muscle, triceps skinfold thickness, skin test quotient):
$$m_E(x) = 0.19 * m_{ALB}(x) + 0.15 * m_{TRAF}(x) + 0.18 * m_{HB}(x)$$
$$+ 0.16 * m_{UAMC}(x) + 0.15 * m_{TSFT}(x) + 0.17 * m_{STQ}(x)$$

- A diagnostic scheme allows to determine the nutritional status as (without the values includes in paranthesis)

  - no alimentary deficiency:
      1. $m_E(x) < 0.1$ or
      2. $\min(m_A(x), m_B(x)) < \underline{0.5}$ (0.75)
  - diagnostic hint:
      3. marasmus:
         $0.1 \le m_E(x) < \underline{0.9}$ and   (0.95)
         $\max(m_A(x), m_B(x)) = m_A(x) \ge \underline{0.5}$ (0.75)
      4. kwashiokor:
         $0.1 \le m_E(x) < \underline{0.9}$ and   (0.95)
         $\max(m_A(x), m_B(x)) = m_B(x) \ge \underline{0.5}$ (0.75)
      5. mixed type:
         $0.1 \le m_E(x) < \underline{0.9}$ and   (0.95)
         $\min(m_A(x), m_B(x)) \ge \underline{0.5}$ (0.75)
  - proven diagnosis:
      6. marasmus:
         $0.1 \le m_E(x) < \underline{0.9}$ and   (0.95)
         $\max(m_A(x), m_B(x)) = m_A(x) \ge \underline{0.9}$ (0.95)
      7. kwashiokor:
         $0.1 \le m_E(x) < \underline{0.9}$ and   (0.95)
         $\max(m_A(x), m_B(x)) = m_B(x) \ge \underline{0.9}$ (0.95)
      8. mixed type:
         $m_E(x) \ge \underline{0.9}$ (0.95)

The fuzzy logical model was varied by the following three steps:

- Instead of using the medians (a and c from Table 2), the means were used (b and d from Table 2) as membership functions parameters (Model 2).

- Instead of using the weights found by conditional probability in the convex combinations, weights found by standardized canonical discriminant functions coefficients were used (Model 3).
  Biochemistry:
  $$m_B(x) = 0.40 * m_{ALB}(x) + 0.19 * m_{TRAF}(x) + 0.41 * m_{HB}(x)$$
  Anthropometrie:
  $$m_A(x) = 0.55 * m_{UAMC}(x) + 0.45 * m_{TSFT}(x)$$
  Nutritional state:
  $$m_E(x) = 0.25 * m_{ALB}(x) + 0.11 * m_{TRAF}(x) + 0.25 * m_{HB}(x)$$
  $$+ 0.18 * m_{UAMC}(x) + 0.15 * m_{TSFT}(x) + 0.06 * m_{STQ}(x)$$

  and equally distributed weights were also used (Model 4).

- Reduction in tolerance limits in the diagnostic scheme, i.e. the marked values in the scheme, were replaced with the values in brackets (Model 5).

Results

The 5 models were tested by reclassification. These results were compared with the discriminatory analysis results (Kretzschmar, 1991). The estimation of specificity and sensitivity for every model is shown in Table 3.

Table 3: Models specificity and sensitivity.
          Values means: learning sample/testing sample

	Diskr.Model	Model 1	Model 2	Model 3	Model 4	Model 5
Specificity	82/ 80	63/ 63	67/ 64	60/ 66	57/ 56	84/ 85
Sensitivity	95/100	97/100	97/100	97/100	97/100	82/ 78

Reclassification results show that Model 1 is relatively stable in variation by step one or step two.

Conversely the reclassification results are worse in the reduction of tolerance limits in the diagnostic scheme.

Discussion

The discriminatory analysis model specificity is better than the fuzzy logical model specificity.
The fuzzy logical model allows a more differentiated determination of the nutritional status than the discriminatory analysis model. It is relatively stable when varying of the parameter membership functions and the weights of convex combinations.
Contrary to this the reclassification results depend on the tolerance limits in the diagnostic scheme.
In the development of the fuzzy logical diagnostic model, this determination of the tolerance limits should be taken into consideration, i.e. the tolerance intervals should not be set too small.

References:

Chang, R.W.S.: Nutritional assessment using a microcomputer. 1. Programme design. Clin. Nutr. 3 (1984), 67-73.

Chang, R.W.S.; Richardson, R.: Nutritinal assessment using a microcomputer. 2. Programme evaluation. Clin. Nutr. 3 (1984), 75-83.

Kretzschmar, F.; Laue, R.; Hartig, W.; Weiner, R.; Schmoz, G.; Grube, U.: Zur Modellierung von Ernährungsdiagnostik und -therapie. Z. Klin. Med. 43 (1988), 703-706.

Kretzschmar, F.: Zum Begriff der Ungewißheit in der medizinischen Diagnostik und deren Anwendung bei dem Erkennen von Ernährungsstörungen. Diss. A, 1991 (in preparation).

Schmoz, G.: Klinisch experimentelle Untersuchungen zur Erfassung von Ernährungsmängeln bei Patienten mit Karzinomen des Gastrointestinaltracktes. Berlin: Akad. f. ärztl. Fortbild., Diss. B, 1986.

ARTIFICIAL INTELLIGENCE IN CONTACT DERMATITIS: THE CODEX/E SYSTEM

A. Dooms-Goossens, M. Dooms, J. Drieghe, H. Degreef
Department of Dermatology, U.Z. St.-Rafaël
Katholieke Universiteit Leuven
Kapucijnenvoer 33, 3000 Leuven, Belgium

Introduction

In the course of one's life, one is intimately exposed to a vast chemical environment. In exceptional cases, contact of chemicals with the skin gives rise to adverse reactions, such as allergic contact dermatitis (or contact allergy). Clinically, this condition is manifested by eczematous skin lesions that appear several hours to several days after exposure to the allergen or allergens to which the individual has been previously sensitized.

Allergic contact dermatitis can occur in several ways, for example, by directly applied agents, by occasional contact with an allergen or an allergen-contaminated surface, by airborne contact, or by systemic exposure.

In some cases of what are called photosensitivity reactions, the photo-contact allergy is induced by contact with a photo-allergen and simultaneous exposure to sunlight.

Consequently, the identification of the causal allergen or allergens as well as of the sensitization sources (profession, local medication, cosmetics, etc.) may be very complex. Required are not only a thorough clinical examination, a detailed anamnesis, and appropriate skin testing but also a great deal of experience in the field.

Codex/E is an on-line system designed to facilitate the allergological examination. We have been using it in our Contact Allergy Unit since September 1989.

Methods

Codex/E works on three levels, to each of which are coupled rules that refer to potential sources of sensitization, allergenic products and substances, with an accompanying degree of significance.

As the first step in Codex/E, the rules of Level 1 indicating possible sources of sensitization are applied to the sex of the patient and the localization and the nature of the lesions. For example: male + eyelids suggests a professional cause, medication, or airborne agents; a linear lesion configuration on the arms suggests that a plant is the source of the allergy. These rules on Level 1 are derived by means of batch programs from the Codex Patient File, which contains information on some 13,000 patients who have been examined over the last 12 years in various Belgian contact dermatitis units.

In the next step, the dermatologist goes more deeply into the various sources of sensitization. Of the 20 defined sources, we will present three here by way of illustration.

- Professional: For specific professions, such as baking and hair-dressing, the allergens are proposed in function of the products encountered (Level 2), for example, baking fat may contain propyl gallate. For other professions, significant allergens are directly suggested (Level 3) on the basis of positive skin tests recorded in the Patient File.

- Iatrogenic: The establishment of the allergens is based on the Codex Product File, which contains the complete composition of over 7,000 pharmaceutical products that are intended for application on the skin and mucous membranes. This Product File is constantly updated with data obtained from the Belgian Ministry of Health. Each ingredient is automatically assigned an allergenicity score, which is regularly updated (cf. the Patient File).

- Cosmetic: The suggested allergens are retrieved from the Cosmetic Product File, in which the causal cosmetic products have been classified according to certain categories (for example, skin-care products and perfumes). Since the composition of cosmetic products changes very frequently, only information from the previous three years is processed.

On the basis of the patient's sex and the localization, and nature of the lesions and also on the previous exposure to local medication, rules of Level 3 indicating possible allergens are also applied. For example, female + earlobe suggests nickel; leg-ulcer patient suggests wool alcohols.

In order to detect new trends, the data from the last 1,000 patients examined are subject to special processing.

At present, Codex/E contains some 1,200 rules, which are automatically updated in function of ongoing clinical experience. This assures that the system is fully dynamic.

Finally, Codex/E executes "user rules" introduced by the contact allergy expert on the basis of his personal experience and of literature data. Such rules can be applied on the different levels of the system.

Because the total set of possible sensitization sources and allergenic products and substances was and is still increasing in size and complexity, we are continuing to optimize Codex/E.

Materials

The Codex/E system is implemented on an IBM 9370 Computer. The operating system is VM, and the software is written in PL/1. Codex/E, together with its management tools and other facilities, consists of 110 programs, 96 REXX procedures, and 55 files.

Several on-line anamneses and readings can be performed simultaneously, for which four terminals and a printer are available in our Contact Allergy Unit.

Results and Discussion

Over the last two years, we have used Codex/E to assist in the examination of some 925 patients. This experience has demonstrated the following:

- This expert system has attained a high degree of efficiency in the identification of allergens. There is less chance of overlooking factors in the anamnesis and in the determination of suspected allergens because of the on-line guidance. This advantage was expected, since the system is based on previous expertise (internal and external).
- Codex/E, with its broad informational databases, with its specific suggestions of possible sources of sensitization and allergenic products and substances, offers a rapid and efficient way of training dermatology residents. It also provides considerable support for dermatologists with little specific expertise in the field of contact allergy.
- The facilities provided by the system produce standardized and accurate information that is useful for the patient and the referring physician as well as for epidemiological studies.

The positive evaluation is, admittedly, a subjective appreciation of the performance of this expert system. An objective evaluation requires the use of parameters such as ratios of number of positive persons to the number tested and the number of positive tests to the number of positive persons. Unfortunately, the patterns of the particular problems encountered (allergens appear and disappear) and the patient population (particularly in an academic environment) constantly change. Thus, comparisons of the ratios mentioned above are not useful. Parallel examinations with and without the expert system might produce data that would make objective evaluation possible. Due to the large varieties of problems (professional, cosmetic, etc.), more or less reliable results can only be obtained after a large patient series has been accumulated. Our experience in practice indicates that the benefits of the system are so immediately obvious that such tests are unnecessary.

References

Dooms-Goossens A., Drieghe J., Degreef H., et al.: A computer system for contact dermatitis; in Galli C.L., Hensby C.N., and Marinovich H. (Eds.): Skin pharmacology and toxicology: Recent advances, NATO ASI Series, Series A: Life Sciences 1989, Vol. 187, pp. 277-281.

Dooms-Goossens A., Drieghe J., Degreef H., et al.: The "Code-E": an expert system for contact dermatitis. Contact Dermatitis, 1990: 22, 180-181.

ARZNEPH: Computer assisted Drug Dosage in Renal Failure

Michael Giehl, Frieder Keller

Universitätsklinikum Steglitz, Ganzkörperzähler und Abteilung für
Allgemeine Innere Medizin und Nephrologie

Keywords:
pharmacokinetics – renal failure – computer

Summary

ARZNEPH should provide the published pharmacokinetic knowledge
for assisting drug dosage in renal failure. Therefore we set up a relational data base in a **SYMPHONY** spread sheet consisting of (till now)
1,275 drugs from 925 publications documented in **WORD**. There is a
need to develop an apppropriate statistical method for metaanalysis of
the published data. The aim of **ARZNEPH** is to combine a userfriendly
interactive environment and an appropriate data management system
with (preexistent) informatic systems already in use. Algorithms of
dose calculations, individual analyzing and procedures to combine
population derived kinetics with individual data are to be integrated.
ARZNEPH should assist bedside support in drug dosage recommendations and (preliminary) being validated by therapeutic drug monitoring.

Background

An up-to-date compilation proves that elimination of 57 % of 1,027 drugs
depends on renal function (SEYFFART 1990). In renal failure there is a risk
of intoxication due to accumulation of drugs and their metabolites. Therefore
the dosage has to be adjusted to renal function (DETTLI 1977). The appropriate dose can fail in both directions. Especially antibiotics have not only
the danger of toxic overdose but also subtherapeutic lack of effective levels
(MOORE 1987, KUNZENDORF 1988).

In numerous drugs elimination has been investigated in normal and insufficient renal function (BENNETT 1983). All of new drugs - mainly antibiotics
- are examined in view of renal failure. Publications and data are growing in
abundance. There are procedures on the base of BAYES' theorem combining
previous knowledge on population derived kinetics with individual kinetics
(SHEINER 1984).

Pharmacokinetic Concept

The fundamental pharmacokinetic equation in renal failure is the linear dependency of elimination on kidney function (DETTLI 1977). Drug elimination can be quantified by means of clearance (CL). Renal function is to be determined via creatinine-clearance (Cl_{cr}).

$$CL = CL_{anur} + m * Cl_{cr}$$

Such simple a relation is proved for large numbers of drugs by regression of empirical findings. Drug clearance (CL) diminishes in various slopes (m) of the according equation (GIEHL 1990). The clearance (CL = $K_e * V_d$) is the product of volume of distribution (V_d) and elimination rate constant (K_e). The elimination rate constant (K_e) is indirect proportional to the half life time ($T_{1/2} = \ln(2)/K_e$). Appropriate statistics to standardize various data by metaanalysis are still to be developed (CONRAD 1990).

Looking at the pharmacokinetics suggests a single compartment model to reduce the required number of parameters of each drug to only a few. This model facilitates to define peak levels during the distribution phase immediately after dosage and in consequence the loading dose.

Drug dosage in renal failure relies on accumulation kinetics defining the steady state after 4.32 half life times no matter of the application intervals. The oscillation of the blood levels in steady state condition is determined by the peak level (C_{max}), and the though level (C_{min}), dependent on bioavailability (F), dosage (D), distibution volume (V_d), dosage intervall (Tau) and the dominant elimination half life time ($T_{1/2}$).

$$C_{max} = \frac{F*D/V_d}{1 - \exp(-0.693 * Tau/T_{1/2})}$$

$$C_{min} = \frac{F*D/V_d}{\exp(0.693 * Tau/T_{1/2}) - 1}$$

The loading dose (DS) is decisive in adjusting the dosage in renal failure. It is defined as the very multiple of the maintenance dose supplying the steady state in a single shot. The loading dose meets the desired amount of drug in body in terms of therapeutic efficacy. The therapeutically required load is invariant in renal failure. Theoretically, the loading dose (DS) is calculated from distribution volume (V_d), bioavailability (F) and the therapeutic peak level (C_{max}).

$$DS = C_{max}*V_d/F$$

In practice, the loading dose is not a calculated parameter but a clinically determined, empirical quantity. Bioavailability (F) and distribution volume do not use to vary in renal failure and are therefore of no (mathematical) consideration in determining the maintenance dose via loading dose. The desired maintenance dose (D) reduced in renal failure and supporting the therapeutic effect is to calculate from the constant loading dose (DS), an choosen dosage interval (Tau) and a changing dominant half life time $(T_{1/2})$.

$$D = DS \, (1 - \exp \, [\, -0.693 * Tau \, / \, T_{1/2} \,] \,)$$

Extracorporal elimination techiques cause difficulties of dosage adjustment in addition. Drugs are eliminated in hemodialysis, hemofiltration, peritoneal dialysis or plasma exchange (LEE 1984, KELLER 1985, KELLER 1990). The loss of drug has to be replaced in favour of therapeutic effect (KELLER 1982). The subsitution dose (DHD) compensates the expected fraction (fR) of the loading dose (DS) eliminated during extracorporal treatment.

$$DHD = fR*DS$$

Pharmacodynamics (therapeutically desired as well as undesired side effects) require further consideration in dosage adjustment. The clinical parameters essential concerning subtherapeutic, therapeutic or toxic effects are still to be investigated.

Populationkinetic Database

We analyzed medical scientific literature and reveiled 925 citations (figure 1) in an wordprocessor (**MS-WORD**). So we collected and arranged in a **SYM-PHONY** type spreadsheet published data of 1,275 drugs in renal failure (figure 2). The software provides portability in other systems and rapid prototyped evaluation. This should be the first step towards the knowledge base **ARZNEPH** (figure 3).

```
1
  Abernethy DR, Greenblatt DJ, Smith TW: Digoxin disposition in
  obesity: clinical pharmacokinetik investigation. Am Heart J
  1981,102:740-4

  Abshagen U, Koester W, Kaufmann B, Lang PD: Pharmacokinetics of
  bezafibrate after single and multiple doses in the presence of
  renal failure. Klin Wochenschr 1980,58:889-96

  Adir J, Narang PK, Josselson J, Sadler JH: Pharmacokinetics of
  bretylium in renal insufficiency. New Engl J Med 1979,300: 1390-
  1391

  Adler DS: Phenytoin. Clin Toxicol 1979,14:147-150

  Akizawa T, Koshikawa S, Nakazawa R, Yoshida T, Kaneko M, Nitadori
  Y: Elimination of ß2-microglobulin by a new polyacrylonitrile
  membrane dialyser: mechanism and physiokentics. Nephrol Dial
  Transplant 1989, 4:356-365
                                                      LITPHARM.TXT
BEFEHL: Ausschnitt Bibliothek Druck Einfügen Format Gehezu Hilfe Kopie
        Löschen Muster Quitt Rückgängig Suchen Übertragen Wechseln Zusätze
Druckformatvorlage nicht gefunden!
Sel Spl          ()              ?              ZA          Microsoft Word
```

figure 1: collection of medical drug related literature in WORD

```
  ┌───A───────B───────C───────D───────E───────F───────G───────H───┐
  │ 10                 T1/2 (Stunden)              Vd (Liter)       │
  │ 11                                                              │
  │ 12                                                              │
  │ 13                 norm    anur    hd          norm    anur  hd │
  │ 14                                                              │
  │ 15                                                              │
  │ 16  Acebutolol (*)  2.7    7.5     3.2         118.         12. │
  │ 17                  (10.)  (32.)   (7.4)       (141.)      (26.)│
  │ 18                  7.0            HF/HP=0.5                     │
  │ 19    (Roux 1980, Benet 1980, Lenga 1989)                      │
  │ 20                                                              │
  │ 21  Acecainid       6.     40.     22.          91.            │
  │ 22    (Lee 1984) siehe Procainamid                            │
  │ 23                                                              │
  │ 24  Acenocoumarol (*) 10.                                      │
  │ 25                   (24.)                                      │
  │ 26    (Enantiomer)   3.                          21.           │
  │ 27    (Klotz 1984, Dettli 1983)                               │
  │ 28                                                              │
  │ 29  Acephyllin      0.8    1.6                                 │
  └──────────────────────────────────────────────────────────EINS─┘
```

figure 2: SYMPHONY spreadsheet of drug publications

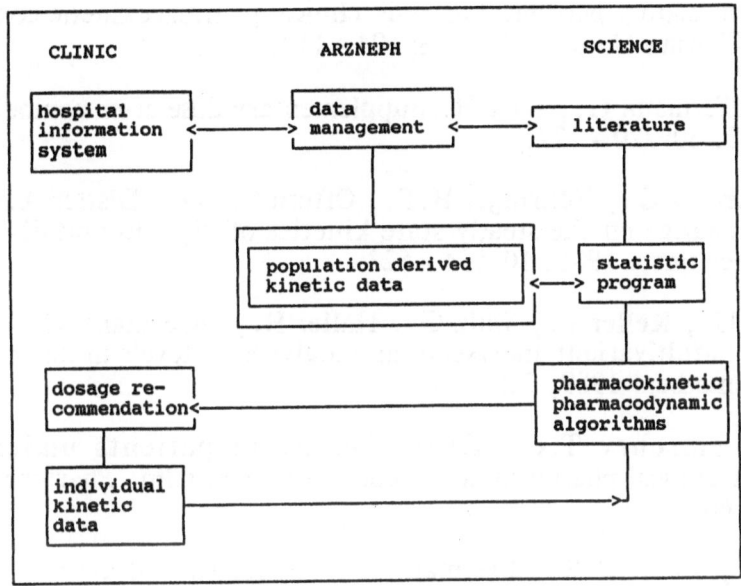

figure 3: diagram of the projected elements of **ARZNEPH**

Address for correspondence:
Priv.Doz.Dr.F.Keller
Klinikum Steglitz
Medizinische Klinik
Hindenburgdamm 30 , W-1000 Berlin 45

Literature

Bennett W.M., Aronoff G.R., Morrison G., Golper T.A., Pulliam J., Wolfsom M., Singer I.: Drug prescribing in renal failure: dosing guidelines for adults. Am. J. Kidney Dis. 1983, 3: 155 - 193.

Conrad P., Büttner P., Keller F.: Metaanalytische Statistik populationskinetischer Daten zur Pharmakokinetik von Netilmicin bei Niereninsuffizienz. Nieren Hochdruckkrh. 1990, 19: 479 - 481.

Dettli L.: Elimination kinetics and dosage adjustment of drugs in patients with kidney disease. Progr. Pharmacol. 1977, 1: 1 - 34

Giehl M., Keller F.: SYMPHONY Makro zur linearen Regressionsanalyse. Software Kurier 1990, 3: 20 - 23.

Keller E., Reetze P., Schollmeyer P.: Drug therapy in patients undergoing continuous ambulatory peritoneal dialysis: clinical pharmacokinetic considerations. Clin. Pharmacokinet. 1990, 18: 104 - 117.

Keller F., Offermann G., Lode H.: Supplementary dose after hemodialysis. Nephron 1982, 30: 220 - 227.

Keller F., Kreutz G., Vöhringer H.F., Offermann G., Distler A.: Effect of plasma exchange on the steady state kinetics of digoxin and digitoxin. Clin. Pharamcokinet. 1985, 10: 514 - 523.

Kunzendorf U., Keller F., Walz G., Haller H., Offermann G., Borner K., Lode H.: Multivariant analysis of aminoglycoside levels in hemodialysis patients. Chemother. 1989, 35: 1 - 6.

Lee C.C., Marbury T.C.: Drug therapy in patients undergoing haemodialysis: clinical pharmacokinetic considerations. Clin. Pharmacokinet. 1984, 9: 42 - 66.

Moore R.D., Smith C.R., Lietman P.S.: Association of aminoglycoside plasma levels with therapeutic outcome in gram-negative pneumonia. Am. J. Med. 1984, 77: 657 - 662.

Moore R.D., Smith C.R., Lietman P.S.: The association of aminoglycoside plasma levels with mortality in patients with gram-negative bacteremia. J. Infect. Dis. 1984, 149: 443 - 448.

Sheiner L.B.: Analysis of pharmacokinetic data using parametric moodels - 1: regression models. J. Pharmacokinet. Biopharm. 1984, 12: 93 - 117.

Seyffart G.: Internationales Projekt: Dosierungsrichtlinien bei Niereninsuffizienz - Aufarbeitung bestehender Erfahrungen und Daten bei 1200 Pharmaka. Nieren Hochdruckkrh. 1990, 19: 473 - 475.

COMPUTER-ASSISTED TRAINING AND EDUCATION

TEACHING ELECTRO AND PHONO CARDIOLOGY
WITH MICROCOMPUTER

W. C. de Lima , R. G. Ojeda,C. I. Zanchin
  Dept.Electrical Engineering
  Univ. Federal de St. Catarina
  Florianópolis, Brazil

J. M. Barreto
Lab. of Neurophysiology & Lab. of Automatics
Université Catholique de Louvain
Belgium

ABSTRACT

A microprocessor controlled system, aimed at the training of cardiologists in the interpretation of phono and electrocardiogram signals, was developed and implemented. The system has two independent modules: the data acquisition module and the generation module. The data acquisition module allows the creation of digital files of ECG and standard cardiac sounds which are processed by a microcomputer and stored in an EPROM. By using these data files, the microprocessor generation module generates the standard signals allowing the user to choose the kind and shape of signal to be generated. These signals can then be visualized in a monitor or plotter and an audio output. The system allows the user to simulate typical heart disease signals at different frequencies and to change the standard signals by software.

INTRODUCTION

A good way of learning how to interpret electrocardiograms and phonocardiograms once the comprehension of the phenomena involved in the production of sounds and the electric activity of the heart is achieved, is a good deal of practice. Records of normal and common pathologies are usually available and the medicine student is confronted with them during his or her training. Since the availability of a particular case is a function of its frequency of occurrence, rare cases are generally not available.

One way of forthcoming this lack of unusual records, for teaching purposes, is to use a computer to generate the electric and audio signals to be presented during a training section. The computer plays the role of a laboratory in this computer assisted learning (CAL), where simulation is used as a paradigm of learning by doing. [2],[4].

To achieve this goal some difficulties exist. If the automatic interpretation of electrocardiograms and phonocardiograms is a challenging problem, here we need the solution of the inverse problem. We need to create with the microcomputer, an electrocardiogram and phonocardiogram corresponding to a precise interpretation. The records must be as real as possible. This means that we must create a model of the cardiovascular system [1], where all the attributes related to the electrocardiogram and phonocardiogram must be retained. In this way, experimenting with this model, i.e., simulating the system, provides the several desired outputs.

Modeling and simulation has been largely used in hemodynamics and several sophisticated models exist [3]. However, to reproduce with sufficient realism an electrocardiogram and the phonocardiogram corresponding to a disease, involves fast transients that must be reproduced during several cardiac cycles. This is a very huge task for a model based on differential equations, that will be stiff.

Considering this difficulty, a pragmatic approach was followed: instead of using a model with internal parameters with physiological interpretation a macro representation based on data base model concepts was used. So, the following approach was followed in building a CAL system to training in interpreting the signals of electrocardiograms and phonocardiograms:

• Construction of a data base corresponding to real electro and phonocardiograms, taken from several different heart conditions.

• Construction of a set of tools to modify individually the attributes of each element of the data base; ex: modification of amplitude and/or frequency of the signals.

• Possibility of build a combination of two or more elements of the data base.

• Possibility of presenting the resulting signals in a usual way; ex: the electrocardiogram seen in a cathode ray tube and the phonocardiogram send to a loudspeaker through an audio amplifier.

SIGNAL CHARACTERISTICS

ECG Signals

ECG signals are a graphical representation of the electric potentials produced in myocardial during the cardiac cycle. They are composed by several parts: P waves, QRS complex and t wave representing the electrical depolarization and repolarization associated with the atrial and ventricular contractions.

This representation called "electrocardiogram" is used in the diagnosis of several cardiac pathologies and indicates the conditions of heart functioning. The diagnosis is performed by careful examination of each characteristic of the ECG, including time intervals between events, polarity and magnitude of each ECG characteristic whose frequency varies between 0 and 100Hz.

Cardiac sounds

The mechanical activity of the myocardium causes the heart to vibrate. These vibrations cover the range from about 1 to 100Hz and occurs in different moments of the cardiac cycle producing heart sounds but it is possible to exist the murmur and in this case the range is over 2KHz.. In the normal person, at least two heart sounds can be detected. The first is closed by the closure of the atrioventricular valves, in synchronism with the

QRD complex of the ECG. The second sound is produced by the closure of the aortic and pulmonary valves, approximately to the end of T-waves. These signals are used in medical diagnosis. These sounds have a correspondence with events of the electrocardiogram.

STRUCTURE OF THE SYSTEM

Considering the desiderata and the main characteristics of the signals, it was chosen to implement the system mainly in hardware, the data base being stored in an EPROM and the manipulation done using a dedicated microprocessor.

The system is composed of two modules, the acquisition module and the generator module.

Acquisition module

The acquisition module (Fig.1) is fed with data from real ECG and cardiac sounds (registered from real patients in a tape recorder coupled to the ECG-meter) as input. The desired output is the data represented in files containing the digitalized data (floppy disk and EPROM in Fig.1). To do so, Butterworth filters for both signals are used. For the ECG it was taken a cut frequency of 100Hz for a 4th order filter and for the cardiac sounds 400Hz for a 2nd order filter. After filtering, an A/D conversion is used.

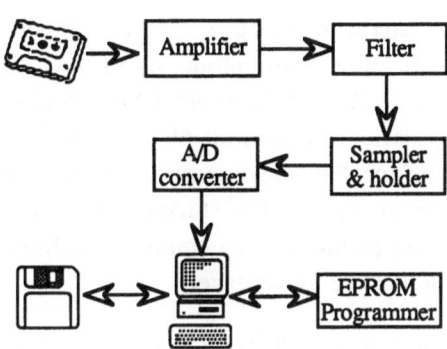

Fig.1 Acquisition module

In the input the system has an amplifier of variable gain to optimize the use of the A/D 8 bits converter. The data resulting from the digitalization is minimized (ex: elimination of the baseline) to obtain the minimal one retaining the main characteristics of the signal, and the data obtained is written in EPROM. These functions are computer controlled.

Generator module

The generator module was designed using a 8085-A microprocessor (a 8 bits precision is sufficient to represent the data with the desired precision). It controls the creation of data files based in codes programmed by the user using digital switches. All the interface is programmable and the real time clock allows to change the frequency between 60 to

130 bmp (beat per minute). As in the acquisition module filters allow to reconstruct the signals after sampling in the 8 bits digital analog converter.

Finally using attenuators it is possible to control the amplitude of the signals and an amplifier to give an audio output of the cardiac sounds. The electrocardiograms can be visualized in the computer's monitor or send to a plotter if a hard copy is desired. The sounds corresponding to the phonocardiogram are produced at the same time as the electrocardiograms and send to a loudspeaker.

The files containing the data recorded during the acquisition phase can be manipulated by the microcomputer to give the result to be presented to the students; Examples of manipulations are:
• multiplication of a signal by a constant,
• a linear combination of two of more signals.

LEARNING BY DOING

The material recorded is used as a laboratory for the students for practical classes on identification of symptoms by electro and phono cardiograms. The instructor can by program combine the several files stored in the ROM in such a way to reproduce rare diseases of combination of diseases. The resulting signals are then presented to the student for diagnostic purposes and the diagnostic compared with the disease simulated by the instructor. The student can also experiment with the system, creating himself complex pathologies by combining different files and observing the resulting outputs in a monitor and loudspeaker.

Examples of signals that can be obtained are:
• in ECG signals: isquemia enfizema, atrial tachycardia, ventricular hypertrophy, etc.
• sounds corresponding to: aortic stenosis, mitral regurgitation, first double sound, atrial sound, second double sound, etc.

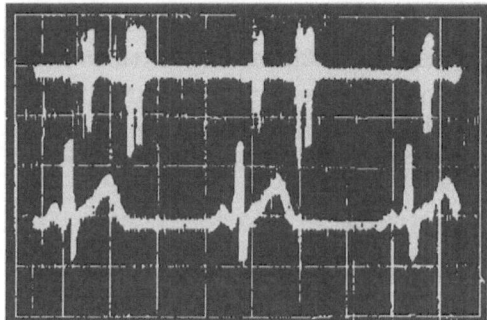

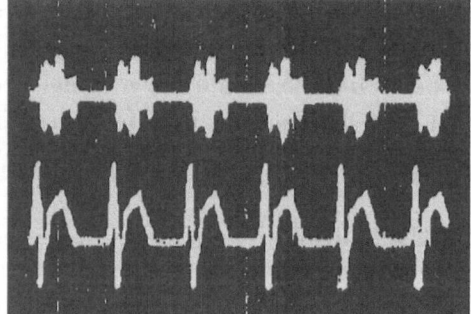

Fig.2 Normal ECG type 0   Fig.3. ECG without P-wave

Fig.2 and 3 shows examples of generated ECG signals taken from the monitor, where noise was introduced to better represent reality. These signals are presented to the student simultaneously with the corresponding cardiac sounds and the student must recognize the possible pathology.

Some additional characteristics of the simulator are, starting from one or several available data files in EPROM to manipulate the data to create new signals, for example:
• elimination or not of P wave;
• inversion of T wave;
• elimination of a cardiac cycle;
• inclusion of a premature contraction;
• full control of cardiac frequency;
• inclusion of a 60Hz noise (distribution frequency of electric energy; it could be changed to 50Hz, as usual, in Europe).
It is possible this way to reproduce easily rare pathologies with great training effect.

CONCLUSIONS

The use of a hardware simulation system based in a general purpose microprocessor allows the creation of a very versatile system. The present implementation uses ECG and phonocardiograms but the methodology can be used to different biological signals. The system is of easy manipulation by the medical surgeon, is very compact (approximately the size of a box of 5"1/4 floppy disks), has high confiability of functioning and, low cost. We hope that the use of hardware simulation starting from real signals could open a new direction in simulating biological phenomena.

ACKNOWLEDGEMENTS: The support of the Belgian National incentive-program for fundamental research in Artificial Intelligence, Prime Minister's Office - Science Policy Programming, is acknowledge. The scientific responsibility rests with its authors.

REFERENCES
[1]–Lefèvre, J. & J. Barreto, "Didactic microcomputer simulation in cardiac dynamics", 5th.Conf. on Frontiers of Eng. in Health Care, (IEEE), Columbus, Ohio, 1983.
[2]–Lefèvre, J., R. Fabri, J. Barreto, "An Authoring System for Computer Aided Instruction and Simulation in Physiology", 7th Annual Conf. of the IEEE Eng. in Medicine and Biology, pp.731-733, Chicago, Illinois, Sept. 27-30, 1985.
[3]–Milnor, W., "Hemodynamics", Williams & Wilkins, Baltimore, 1982.
[4]–Pagano, R. & J. Barreto, "Laboratory Experiment Simulation in Electrical Engineering Education". 3rd European Simul. Cong. Edinburg, Sept. 5-8, 1989

COMPUTER AIDED TEACHING IN NEUROLOGY

Mihaljev-Martinov J[1], Žikić M[1], Matejašev S[1], Nikolić I[2]

1 Institute of Neurology, Psychiatry and Mental Health
  Medical Faculty, University of Novi Sad
2 Institute of Pathophysiology, Medical Faculty,
  University of Novi Sad

ABSTRACT: Our model for computer program support in medical education is based on Suppes project, 1967, recommendations given by WHO Regional Office for Europe in 1974, Computer literacy pool available for assessment, 1984 and a Model clinical neuroscience curriculum suggested by Mancall et al in 1987. Program methodology is based on level principles beginning from a background knowledge up to creating new ideas and values of clinical entities in neurology. Through the application of this program the value of computers in self-instruction and simulation of diagnostic problems can be realized. Students are tought to develop a "diałog" with the computer and have a possibility to create expert systems.

KEY WORDS: medical informatics, clinical neuroscience curriculum,
           computer assisted instruction

INTRODUCTION

The program for support in education of medical students in neurology is based on the principle of basic clinical knowledge and experience. Application of computers as self-instructional devices makes possible for each student to learn how to obtain medical records in neurology, physicial examination, major manifestations and the basis of neurological diseases, laboratory investigations and other diagnostic methods used in neurology. The aim of basic education in neurology is that each student, through acquiring theoretical knowledge and skills, gets a knowledge in this field of medicine as well.

METHODS

Computer supported program (3) is formed on the basis of teaching
plans and programs that are in use at Medical Faculties in Yugoslavia
(1), and the model of Mancall et al (2). In order to create a computer
program applicable in education in neurology the requirements for
computer literacy given by the Advisory Board (4) have been accepted.
These requirements include three types of competence - undrestanding,
knowledge and skills. We have also used recommendations about the role
of computer in the process of self-instruction that were reported on
a Seminar convened by WHO Regional Office for Europe in 1974, (5).

Methodology of computer aided education in neurology is based on
the principle of levels starting from a background knowledge up to
creating new ideas and values of clinical entities. The first level is
supported by a data base consisting of multiple-choice questions. The
second level is formed on data base and knowledge base about topographic localizations and manifestations of neurological diseases and
this level gives a student a possibility to make choice among different diagnostic procedures. The third level will be formed to enable
neurological diseases simulation by using data base and knowledge
base. The basic principle of computer program for all three levels
is a student-teacher relationship.

Technical requirements necessary for implementation of this computer program include personal support for computers PC/IBM and/or AT.
dBase III Plus, Lotus 1,2,3 and Quatro have been used as a software
support.

At the first level students can but do not have to accept initial
solutions and the freedom of program language selection is left to
them. If students' knowledge of software is on a lower level then
teacher's assistance is always required. Students having a higher knowledge in application of medical informatics can create a data base by
using program languages they are familiar with. They are also able to
transfer their knowledge to other students. If students are well educated in medical infromatics the presence of teacher during this part
of education is not necessary. When students ask for continuous help
and advise during their work at the computer terminal then the presence of teacher is essential. A higher knowledge in medical infromatics

enables a student to participate more actively in programe creation and thus the computer becomes a device for assessment, supplementation and enriching of his existing knowledge without a direct influence of his teacher. The student is offered apossibility for individual creating through the levels of practice as it is offered in Suppes project (6).

The part of the program - test questions and answers - is based on knowledge checking system suggested by WHO (7). Data base allows memorizing 8 types of test questions out of an overall number of 4000, as well as their randomized selection for test application. The system can be enlarged if needed in accordance with the concept presented on Fig.1.

Example of multiple choice question:
- Tied questions type:
  Choose the type of epilepsy having no signs characteristic for other four types:
  A) somato-motor (Bravais-Jacksonian epilepsy)
  B) epilepsia continua (Koshevnikoff`s epilepsy)
  C) adversive seizure
  D) absence seizure
  E) aphasic (phonatory) seizure
  Correct choice is: D
  Explanation: D is a type of generalized Petit-mal epilepsy while the rest of four types belong to epilepsia partials (focal e.) of elemental phenomenology.

The second level presents a data base consisting of: a) often occuring diseases in medical practice (i.e. headache, epilepsy, cerebrovascular diseases, multiplex sclerosis, etc.), b) therapeutical principles (i.e. pain, epilepsy, encephalitis, etc.), c) treatment of urgent conditions in neurology. The knowledge base consists of topographic localizations, major symptoms in neruology, indications and contraindiciations for application of diagnostic procedure (i.e. EEG, CT, SPECT, MRI). Data and knowledge base searching can provide a student with all information necessary for diagnostic and therapeutic procedures as well as for short and long term prognoses.

General concept of third level is a problem-oriented or disease-oriented presentation of neurological diesease or specific neurologic disorders. Program system structure of this level in general can be presented as in Fig.2. This system contains following elements:

data base, knowledge base and program support for handling the bases. With the program organized in this way it is possible to fulfill all requirements for both undergraduate and postgraduate students.

CONCLUSION

It is already known that the application of computers in medical education is possible providing that certain conditions are fulfilled. We are of the opinion that the same conditions are also compulsory in computer aided education in neurology. The structure of our model program makes possible its application under following conditions: a possession of a PC with a satisfactory configuration, a possesion of computer programming languages, having an ability for making programs suitable for creation of both data and knowledge bases in the field of neurology, teachers` and students` knowledge bases in medical informatics and skillfullness of program makers in application of existing knowledge and creation of a new one.

REFERENCES

1. Katalog znanja, Med Fak Univ. Zagreb, Studije medicine 1981 37: 157-165

2. Mancall EL, et al: Model clinical neuroscience curriculum, Neurology, 1987, 37:1697-1699

3. Mihaljev Martinov J, Konjović Z, Jovanović M, Jerković M, Vujić M: Računarska podrška u edukaciji iz neurologije, I kongres medicinske infórmatike Jugoslavije, Beograd, Zbornik radova 1990, 329-332

4. Computer literacy pool available for assessment, ETC Developments, New Yersey/Spring, 1984.

5. Modern medical methods, Regional Office for Europe, Copenhagen, 1974, 15-18.

6. Suppes P: On using computers to individualize instruction In: Busnnell DD, Allen DW: The computer in American education New York, Wiley 1967, 11-24

7. Gumbert IJ: Educational handbbok for Helath organizations, Geneva, 1981.

FIG. 1.

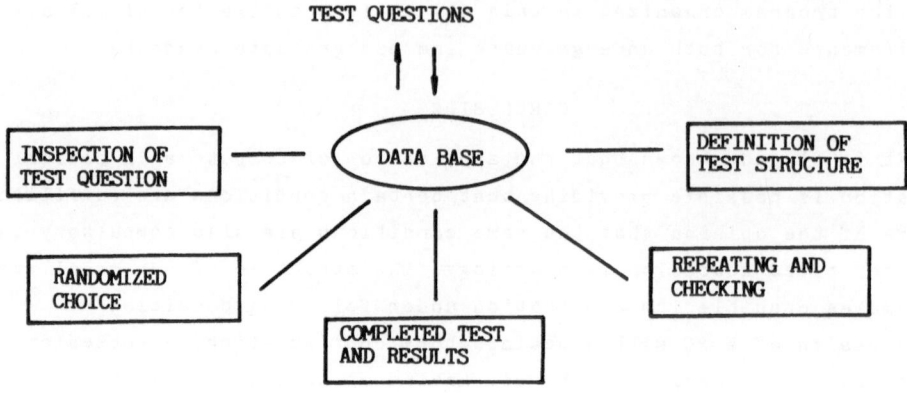

FIG. 2.

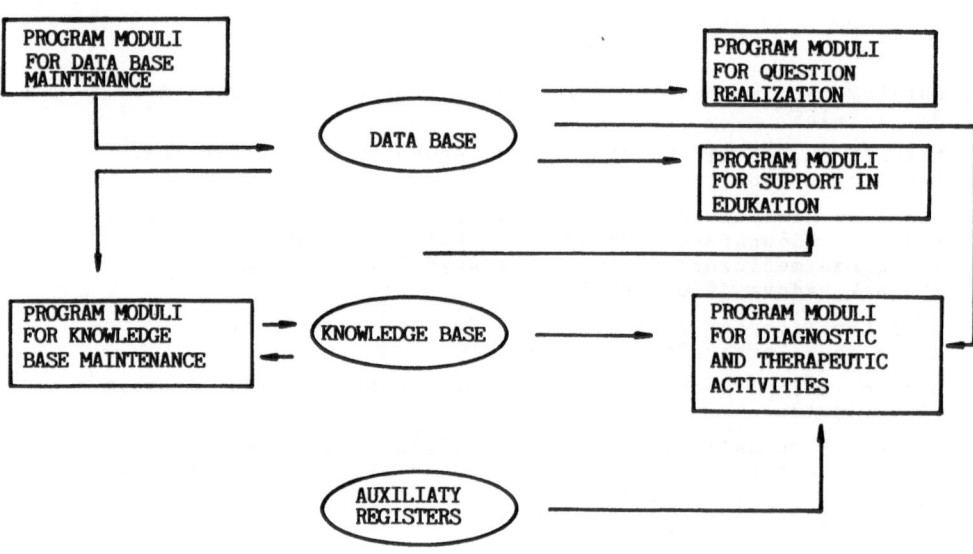

"AN AI - BASED TRAINING FOR NOSOCOMIAL INFECTIONS CONTROL"

Aurora Ramirez Pozo* & Walter Celso de Lima** & Jorge M. Barreto***

     *   F. Universidade Regional de Blumenau -   FURB
           - Blumenau - SC - Brazil

     **   Universidade Federal de Santa Catarina -   UFSC
            - Florianópolis - SC - Brazil

    *** Université Catholique de Louvain - Louvain - La
            Neuve - Belgique)

Address for reprint requests: Prof. Walter Celso de Lima

UFSC - P.O. Box 476 - Florianópolis SC 88049 Brazil

Fax 00.55.482.341524

Abstract - Nosocomial infections are a problem for the entire world. In the United States and Europe about 5 to 10% of the hospital patients get nosocomial infections after a surgical intervention; this rate raises up to 20% within the Brazilian hospitals. Since 1983 the Brazilian Public Health Service has given special attention to nosocomial infection control. All the hospitals in the country must have a committee for this disease control. The committee's main function is to train the hospital personnel on surveillance and prevention of nosocomial infections. To help in this job, a computer training system has been developed using a PC-XT IBM microcomputer and artificial intelligence techniques. Such a system includes a data base to calculate the nosocomial infection rate. The A.I. system is based on four types of knowledge: the knowledge domain, the student's knowledge, pedagogical knowledge and communication. The knowledge domain includes the main theme of nosocomial infections like criteria to identify them, kinds of nosocomial infections, rate computation, prevention of nosocomial infections got through invasion process and others. The system interface is friendly with different ways of theme presentation, like problem-solving, false-true questioning, alternative selection or concept description. The student is led through the different topics which are more or less deepened depending on the student's knowledge. The system has been designed for individual use, aiming at a general view on nosocomial infection, bearing in mind the total lack of knowledge about the subject by most of the personnel working in hospitals (doctors, nurses) who, no doubt, have a direct influence on the nosocomial infections. The system hopes to improve the quality of the assistance given in hospitals. Personnel well informed about the risks and ways of controlling the nosocomial infections, will surely help fighting them.

Introduction - Nosocomial infection control is a preoccupation in all the world. In Brazil all the hospitals must have a committee for nosocomial infection control. The committee's main function is to train the hospital personnel on surveillance and prevention of nosocomial infections.

To help in this job, a computer training system has been developed using a PC-XT IBM microcomputer and a data base to calculate the nosocomial infections rate. In part 2, this methodology is presented.

The instructional part in the knowledge domain includes the main theme of nosocomial infections like criteria to identify nosocomial infections, kind of nosocomial infections, rate computations, prevention of nosocomial infections got through invasive procedures and others.

The system interface is friendly with different ways of theme presentation, like problem-solving, false-true questioning, alternative selection or concept description.

The student is led through the different topics which are more or less deepened depending on the student's knowledge. In part 3, a session teaching example is presented.

Methodology - An Intelligent Computer Aided Instruction or "ICAI" is a personal training, that means, it must be dynamically adapted to the student's knowledge level and need. It should allow an environment that closely resembles what actually occurs when students and teachers face one another and attempt to teach and learn together. To reach its objective, an ICAI system has four components (Figure 1): expertise module, student model, tutorial module and communication module.

The expertise module contains the domain knowledge. This knowledge is used to answer student's questions or to solve problems in order to provide a basis for comparison with the student's responses.

The student model is simply a model maintained and used by the computer tutor of the student's knowledge and capabilities.

The tutorial module has as its job to choose the next strategy for teaching the student, based on the current state of the student model.

966

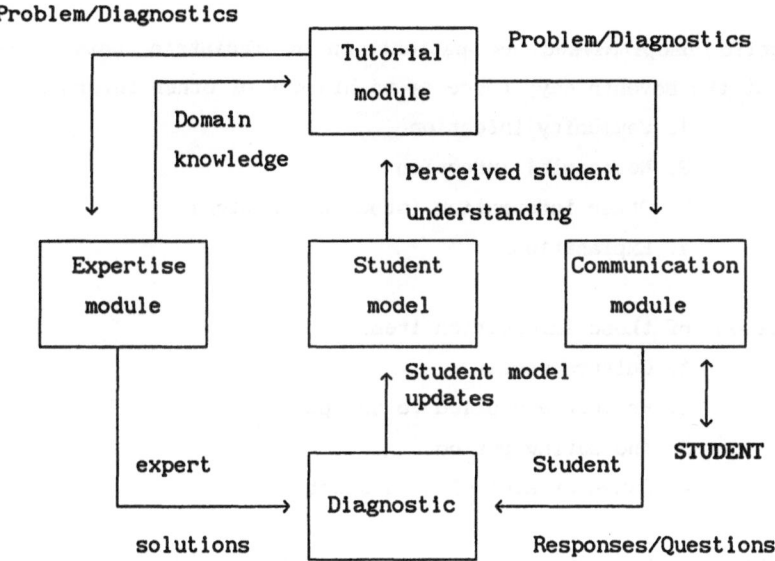

Problem/Diagnostics

Problem/Diagnostics

Figure 1

This includes providing diagnostics, presenting new information, and asking questions or stating problems to the student.

The communication module makes the student-system communication. The system is going to be used by people with no computer knowledge, thus the system must be friendly, in the Portuguese language.

One of the greatest problems faced by the committee for disease control is the maintenance of up-to-date rates. This rate allows a systematic observation and a routine analysis of the infection incidence and its distribution. This information is used for a suitable control action. This is why a data base has been implemented with which we can make an automatic computation of the main rate, and (if it is needed), correlation between data. The data base has been implemented in DBase III Plus, and is part of the expertise module, however it can be used independently. The data for infection rate are obtained from special forms, filled in by the committee of diseases control.

Session Teaching Example - The ICAI development has been made in "INSIGHT", an expert system software based on production rules, with a Pascal language interface for the student and diagnostics.

An important topic to teach is the criteria to identify nosocomial infection. The system defines problems in order to identify the student's knowledge. A session example for this topic is detailed in the following lines.

Example:

System: A child hsopitalised as patient in a pediatric unit, presents
Hepatitis A, at the seventh day, there is no history of other internment.

        1. Community infection

        2. Nosocomial infection

        3. Other information (student's option)

        4. Explanations

System: Choose one of these information items:

        1. Culture result

        2. Procedure applied to the patient

        3. Incubating period

        4. Cause of admission (student's option)

System: In this problem the incubating period is important. The sickness
incubating period is the interval of time between the exposure to an infection
agent and the first sickness sign. For hepatitis A:

        The minimal incubating period: 10 days and

        The maximal incubating period: 30 days.

System: The infection is

        1. Community infection

        2. Nosocomial infection

        3. Other information

        4. Explanation (student's option)

System: The rule to apply is:

IF the inferior incubating period IS GREATER THAN the admission days AND there
is no history of an other hospital internment. THEN IT IS a Community
infection.

Response of the system is dependent of the student's options. If the student's
answer is correct, other questions are asked in order to verify the student's
knowledge.

Conclusion - The proposed system is a useful tool for the committee for
disease control and for the hospitals. Two fundamental points are the focus of
this work:

1. The training of people (ICAI) to prevent hospital infection;

2. Data base to promote a more efficient control action.

The system hopes to improve the quality of the assistance given in hospitals.

Personnel well informed about the risks and ways of controlling the nosocomial infections will surely help fighting them. The data base is a way of getting feedback from the system.

Other problems are going to be themes for future work:

- Graphical interface for the data base;

- Natural language mechanisms for the communication;

- Integral processing of the system, data base and ICAI, in order to integrate semantic and numerical processing.

References

01. Brown, J. & R. Burton & F. Zdybel. "A model-driven question answering system for mixed-initiative computer-assisted construction". IEEE Transaction on Systems Man, and Cybernetics, vol. SMC-3, N. 3, pp: 248-257, May 1973.

02. Burton, R. & J. Brown. "An investigation of computer coaching for informal learning activities". Int. J. Man-Machine Studies, n. 11, pp: 5-24, 1979.

03. Clancey, W. "Tutoring rules for guiding a case method dialogue". Int. J. Man-Machine Studies, v. 11, pp: 25-49, 1979.

04. Dwer, T. A. "Heuristic strategies for using computers to enrich education". Int. J. Man-Machine Systems, v. MMS-11, n. 4, pp: 137-154, Dec. 1970.

05. Kearsley, G. "Artificial intelligence and instruction applications and methods". Addison-Wesley Puplishing Company, June 1987.

06. Koffman, E. & S. Blount. "Artificial intelligence and automatic programming in CAI". Artificial Intelligence, n. 6, pp: 137-154, 1974.

07. Rickel, J. "Intelligence computer aided instruction: a survey organized around system components". IEEE Transactions on Systems, Man, and Cybernetics, v. 19, n. 1, pp: 40-57, Jan-Feb 1989.

08. Stevens, A. & A. Collins & S. Goldin. "Misconceptions in student's understanding". Int. J. Man-Machine Studies, n. 11, pp: 145-156, 1979.

09. Wesler, J. "Information networks in generative computer-assisted instruction". IEEE Transaction on Man-Machine Systems, v. MMS-11, n. 4, pp: 181-190, Dec. 1970.

10. Woolf, B. & D. Donald. "Building a computer tutor: design issues". IEEE Computer, pp: 61-73, sept. 1984.

11. Zanon, U. & J. Neves. "Infecções hospitalares: prevenção, diagnóstico e tratamento". Medsi Editora Médica e Científica Ltda, 1987 (in Portuguese).

BIOMETRY AND
BIOSTATISTICS

CAN AUTOMATIC "SCORING" IMPROVE COMPARABILITY OF CASES AND STATISTICAL RESULTS IN EMERGENCY MEDICINE?

R.Inglis, J.Windolf, A.Pannike

Frankfurt [Main] University Hospital
Dpt. Traumatology
Theodor Stern Kai 7, D-6000 Frankfurt [Main]

Trauma-Scoring today is the main tool to compare severities of injuries and outcome of patients following severe trauma.

As could be shown in additional papers, we presented at the 54th DGU-Congress in Berlin 1990, the results and the precision of trauma scoring depend mainly on the skill of the individual doctor and furthermore are influenced by various factors such as degree of awakeness of the doctor and stress due to work-overload.

That is why results from different hospitals vary a lot and using the same scores do not prevent results from getting full of discontinuities or even unrealized errors. These however "overlay" the results as unknown factors and often kill multicenter-study-results at all.

To keep the individual doctor from scoring differently according to the factors mentioned above we used our modified AO-Classification-Encounter Sheets as checklists to fix bone-injuries in patients after trauma. To fix the soft-tissue and organ injuries we developed a Soft-Tissue-Injury-Classification-Table using a nomenclature similar to the AO-Classification of fractures.

Having put all the items investigated on optical mark reader encounter-sheets doctors now have the complete check-lists at hand to fix the patients' clinical findings only once without any need of 'data-transfer' to the individual personal-computer

Using the optical mark reader (OMR)-encounter sheets 18 anatomic (static) scores are calculated from the same sets of input data and thus results are comparable even statistically.

25 dynamic (physiological) scores are calculated the same way using daily laboratory results at the intensive care unit that are transferred to omr-encounter sheets as described above.

Data analysis is performed after putting the encounter-sheets through an programmable optical mark reader that operates independently from any computer and stores data from up to 1200 encounter-sheets on one 360 kilobyte IBM-compatible floppy disk. Proceeding this way data-input is done without any keyboard entries; data from 1200 sheets are transferred to the personal computer in about three hours without any need for proof-reading.

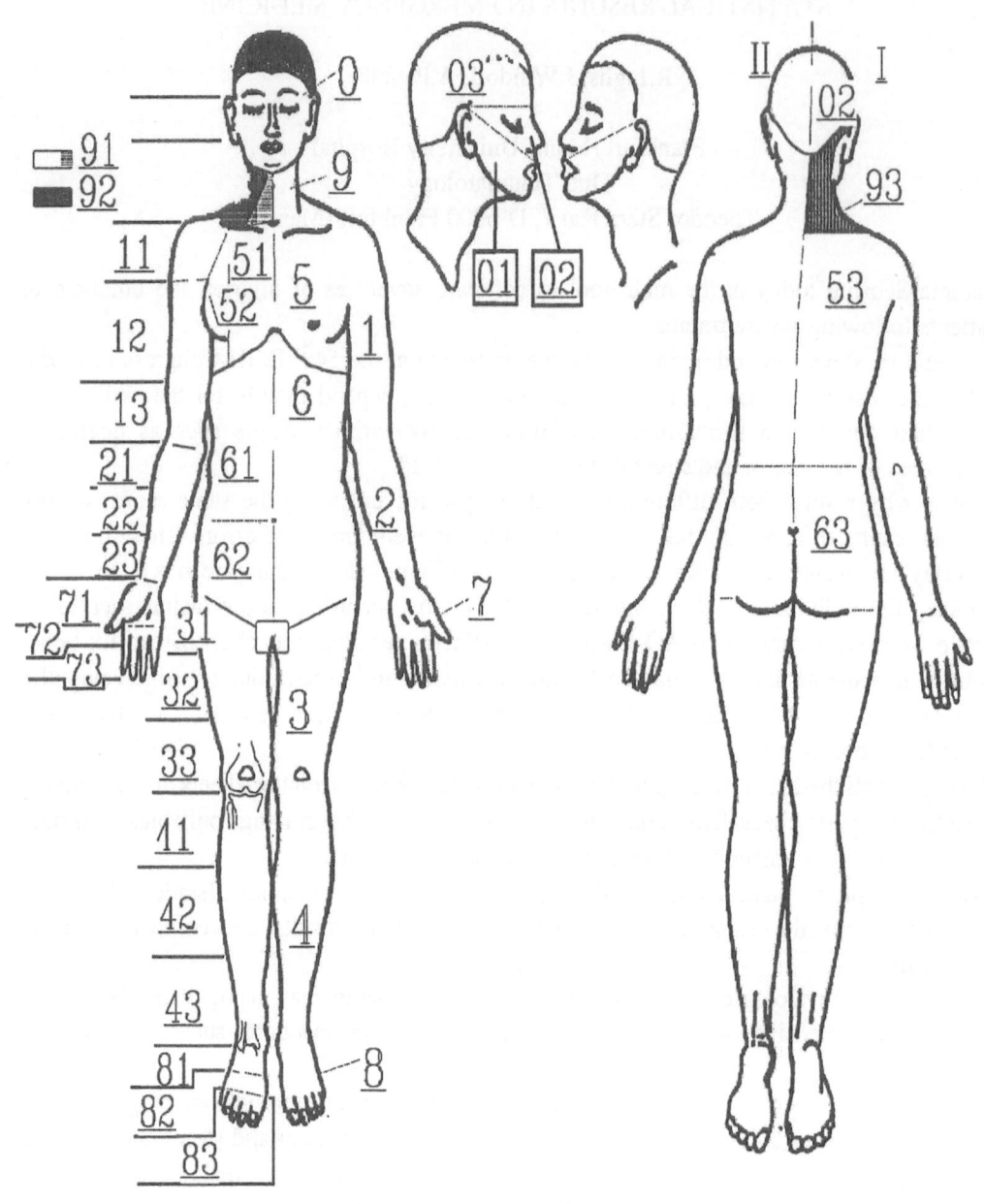

Frankfurt University Soft Tissue Injury Classification Table

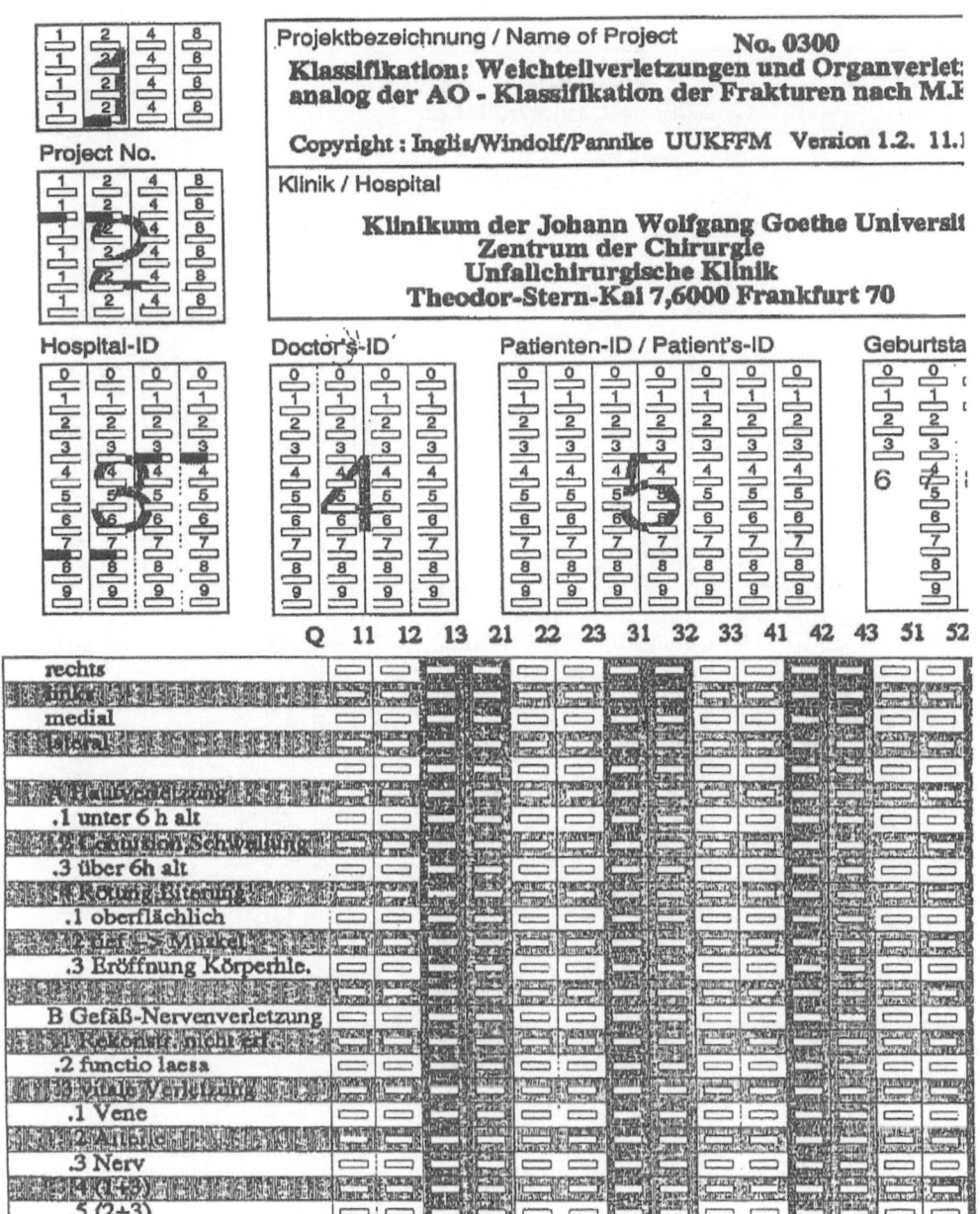

Soft Tissue Injury Checklist

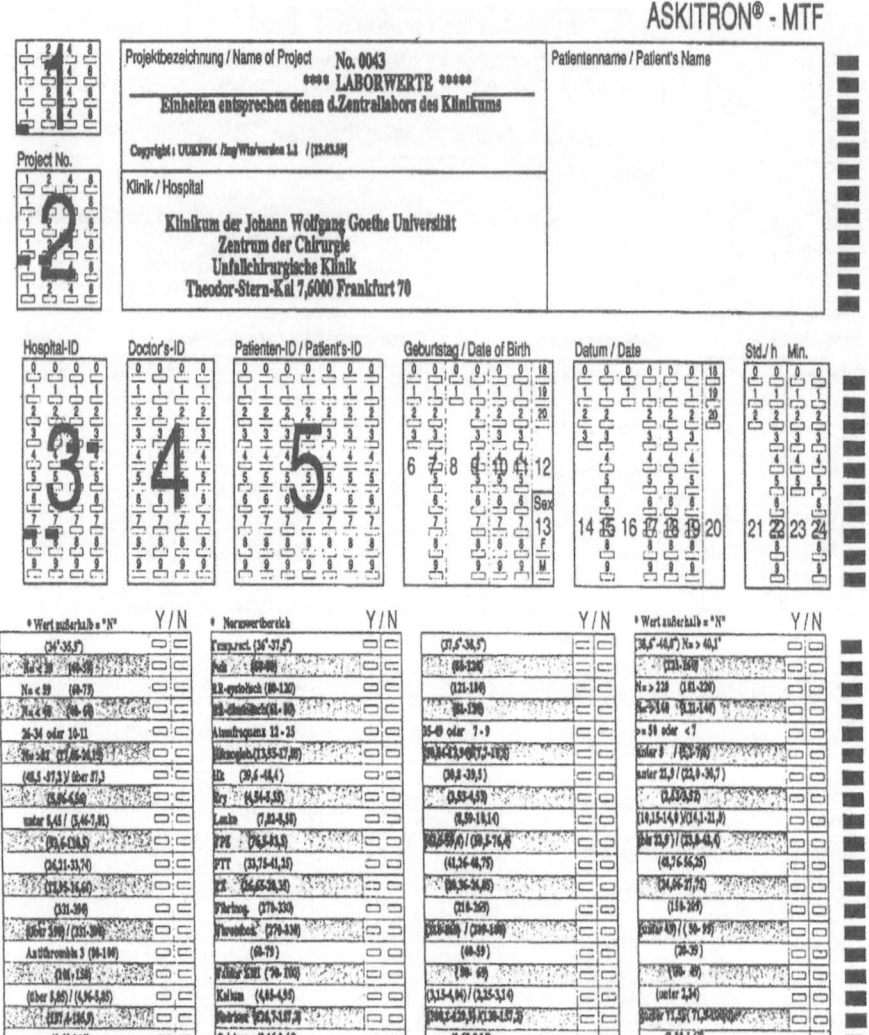

Encounter Sheet for Laboratory Results

The databases used were set up as copies from an empty database structure, thus we called this kind of data handling 'processing with structured empty databases'. This enables us to have only one programm for data analysis { and data transfer to statistic packages } for every stucture of data that can be coded on the type of encounter sheet employed.

As data handling now is free from data input via keyboards we found the doctors' and nurses' acceptance for this procedure higher than for every 'data maneuver' before.

The combination of data input " via pencil " and coded and thus kategorized clinical findings of laboratory data to be gathered is the key to make cases comparable and to calculate scores using the same set of data.

Scoring results until now were depending on the doctors skill, his state of awakeness, interest and stress and depending on interindividual as well as intraindividual bias depending on different investigation times, different timespans from the investigations to the fixation of results, different doctors gathering data for scores to be compared and so on.

Analyzing 1025 sets of data from 98 patients we could prove the applicability and reliability of the new method. However we found that "the best score", that is the score that fits best concerning outcome or survival, still cannot be calculated from our data as data-sets from 50000 patients would be necessary to give statistically reliable result from the more as 50 parameters that were registered for each of the sets of data.

Summary Attributable Risk Estimation
in $2 \times 2 \times K$ – Tables

Olaf Gefeller

Abteilung Medizinische Statistik, Georg-August-Universität Göttingen

Humboldtallee 32, W-3400 Göttingen, F.R.G.

Abstract

Summary attributable risk estimation in the presence of confounding and effect–modification is studied by means of a simulation study in this paper. Seven summary estimators are compared with respect to bias and asymptotic variance. From the results it is concluded that the maximum likelihood estimator resulting from the 'case load weighting' of stratum–specific estimates constitutes the best overall choice.

I. Introduction

Consider a population that is classified into groups according to a dichotomous disease variable D and some dichotomous exposure characteristic E. Let $P(D|E)$, $P(D|\overline{E})$, and $P(D)$ represent the disease probability among the exposed, the unexposed, and the entire population, respectively. The attributable risk according to Levin [1] is defined as

$$AR = \frac{P(D) - P(D|\overline{E})}{P(D)} . \tag{1}$$

From an epidemiological point of view this measure can be interpreted as the proportion of cases of disease due to the exposure among all cases of disease in the population. It constitutes a useful measure in guiding public health administrators to a rational choice of disease prevention strategies. In the statistical literature the estimation of attributable risk has received considerable attention during recent years. In the simple 2×2 – table situation the maximum likelihood estimator and its asymptotic variance can be derived easily under all sampling models [2]. But typically in observational epidemiologic studies the exposure–disease relationship is affected by confounding and/or effect-modification due to other variables. As a consequence the estimator derived from the simple 2×2 – table cannot be interpreted in the way described above. The extension to the multivariable case to allow for potential confounding and effect-modification leads to the situation of a $2 \times 2 \times K$ – table where the third dimension is represented by a stratum variable C with K levels. The distributional assumption in the situation of an unrestricted sampling of subjects is that of one multinomial distribution. This sampling model applies to cross-sectional studies and cohort studies in which the sampling process is independent of the exposure status. Depending on the role of C two different models should be distinguished: (i) homogeneity model (C acts as a confounding variable), (ii) interaction model (C acts as an effect-modifying variable).

Under both models the summary attributable risk to be estimated from the data of the $2 \times 2 \times K$ – table can be expressed analogously to (1) as:

$$ AR_{Summary} = \frac{P(D) - \sum_{i=1}^{K} P(C_i) \cdot P(D|\overline{E}, C_i)}{P(D)} \tag{2} $$

where $P(C_i)$ represents the proportion of the population in the i-th stratum of C, and $P(D|\overline{E}, C_i)$ denotes the stratum-specific disease probability among the unexposed in the i-th stratum of C. Additionally, the following notation is used in the next chapter: N_i refers to the observed number of subjects in the i-th stratum, a_i to the observed number of exposed cases in the i-th stratum, b_i to the observed number of exposed non-cases in the i-th stratum, c_i to the observed number of unexposed cases in the i-th stratum, and d_i to the observed number of unexposed non-cases in the i-th stratum. The quantities N, a, b, c and d denote the sum of the stratum–specific values.

II. Summary Estimators of the Attributable Risk

Different strategies to estimate (2) from the data of $2 \times 2 \times K$ – tables have been proposed. These strategies can be categorized as follows:

Type I: A weighting procedure of the stratum-specific attributable risk estimates is employed.

Estimators of this type have the following form

$$ \widehat{AR}_{Summary} = \sum_{i=1}^{K} w_i \widehat{AR}_i \tag{3} $$

where $\widehat{AR}_i$ denotes the attributable risk estimate from the 2×2 – table of the i-th stratum and $w_i, i = 1, \ldots, K$, is a special set of weights with $\sum_{i=1}^{K} w_i = 1$. The following two weighting schemes have been discussed in the literature:

$$ w_i = \frac{a_i + c_i}{a + c} \qquad , i = 1, \ldots, K . \tag{4} $$

$$ w_i = \frac{\left[\widehat{Var} \, \widehat{AR}_i \right]^{-1}}{\sum_{i=1}^{K} \left[\widehat{Var} \, \widehat{AR}_i \right]^{-1}} \qquad , i = 1, \ldots, K . \tag{5} $$

In (4) the weights are the proportions of cases in the strata among all cases in the sample. The summary estimator resulting from this 'case load weighting' $\widehat{AR}_{CLW}$ can be derived as the maximum likelihood estimator in this situation [3]. In (5) the weights are inverse proportional to the estimated asymptotic variances of the stratum-specific estimates. This 'precision weighting' proposed by Ejigou [4] implies the assumption that the underlying stratum-specific attributable risks are constant across strata to yield an unbiased estimator of a common attributable risk. However, this assumption cannot be fulfilled under the homogeneity model and is only achieved in special situations of the interaction model. As a consequence, the summary attributable risk estimator constructed by employing 'precision weighting' $(\widehat{AR}_{PRW})$ will in general be biased.

Type II: The functional relationship of relative and attributable risk is used to estimate the summary attributable risk via adjustment of the relative risk.

Miettinen [5] discussed first the following fundamental relationships between attributable and relative risk (RR):

$$AR = P(E|D) \cdot \frac{RR-1}{RR} \tag{6}$$

$$AR = \frac{P(E) \cdot [RR-1]}{P(E) \cdot [RR-1]+1} \ . \tag{7}$$

Only (6) can be generalized to the multivariable case, whereas (7) is only applicable in the 2×2 – table situation. Under the homogeneity model we can apply any relative risk estimator of the common relative risk in (6) to get a summary attributable risk estimator. The estimator will be unbiased as long as the applied relative risk estimator is an unbiased estimator of the common relative risk [6]. Under the interaction model this method falls to the ground, because there is no common relative risk which can be estimated from the data. If estimators of this type are used inappropriately in this situation (like e.g. proposed in [7]), the resulting attributable risk estimator $\widehat{AR}_{AHO}$ is biased in general.

Usually, under the multinomial sampling model the following estimators of a common relative risk are employed:

$$\widehat{RR}_{MH} = \frac{\sum\limits_{i=1}^{K} \frac{a_i \cdot (c_i+d_i)}{N_i}}{\sum\limits_{i=1}^{K} \frac{c_i \cdot (a_i+b_i)}{N_i}} \quad \text{or} \quad \widehat{RR}_T = \frac{\sum\limits_{i=1}^{K} \frac{a_i \cdot (c_i+d_i)}{b_i+d_i}}{\sum\limits_{i=1}^{K} \frac{c_i \cdot (a_i+b_i)}{b_i+d_i}} \tag{8}$$

which yield the summary attributable risk estimators $\widehat{AR}_{RRMH}$ and $\widehat{AR}_{RRT}$, respectively. Another popular procedure consists of approximating the relative risk by the Mantel-Haenszel estimator of a common odds ratio. The resulting summary estimator of the attributable risk is referred to as $\widehat{AR}_{ORMH}$.

Type III: Miettinen's factorization idea in the context of relative risk estimation is adapted to the attributable risk setting.

Walter [2] assumed that the attributable risk in the collapsed 2×2 – table, AR_{crude}, can be written as a sum of two components: the component AR_{conf} due to the effect of confounding variables and the summary attributable risk component. By heuristic arguments he suggested to estimate the summary attributable risk as follows:

$$\widehat{AR}_{WAL} = \widehat{AR}_{crude} - \widehat{AR}_{conf} = \frac{c \cdot \sum\limits_{i=1}^{K} \left(\frac{a_i d_i}{c_i} - b_i \right)}{(a+c) \cdot (c+d)} \ . \tag{9}$$

The estimator $\widehat{AR}_{WAL}$ was criticized by Ejigou [4] who pointed out that the heuristic argumentation is incorrect and that the proposed estimator is biased.

III. Simulation Study

In order to investigate the finite properties of the summary estimators discussed in the preceding chapter a simulation study was conducted. Three situations of the homogeneity model (no. 1–3) and two of the interaction model (no. 4–5) were considered. In each situation two sample sizes were analysed. The impact of the confounder and effect–modifier, respectively, was taken into account by stratifying the data into two groups.

The seven estimators were compared with respect to bias and asymptotic variance. 500 simulation trials per situation were carried out. In table 1 mean biases and in table 2 mean asymptotic variances of the estimators are presented in detail.

Table 1: Results of the simulation study: mean biases (in per mille)

Summary Estimator	Situation: 1		2		3		4		5	
	Sample size:									
	1000	5000	1000	5000	1000	5000	1000	5000	1000	5000
$\widehat{AR}_{CLW}$	−5.7	−4.0	−2.2	2.2	2.5	1.7	0.8	0.4	2.6	0.9
$\widehat{AR}_{PRW}$	—	—	−48.0	−44.7	0.6	−0.8	32.7	30.1	59.0	56.6
$\widehat{AR}_{RRMH}$	−6.2	−3.4	−2.3	2.2	2.5	1.7	14.8	13.8	28.5	26.9
$\widehat{AR}_{RRT}$	−6.3	−3.7	−2.3	2.2	2.4	1.7	−2.2	−3.5	19.5	17.9
$\widehat{AR}_{ORMH}$	11.4	17.9	43.1	48.3	98.5	98.3	121.2	120.4	97.2	96.2
$\widehat{AR}_{AHO}$	−5.1	−21.3	−39.8	−36.0	−38.6	−39.6	11.3	10.3	6.3	4.3
$\widehat{AR}_{WAL}$	−16.8	−40.5	−104.3	−111.4	−151.2	−162.0	209.3	200.6	115.6	106.0

Table 2: Results of the simulation study: mean asymptotic variances (in per mille)

Summary Estimator	Situation: 1		2		3		4		5	
	Sample size:									
	1000	5000	1000	5000	1000	5000	1000	5000	1000	5000
$\widehat{AR}_{CLW}$	15.52	3.07	4.91	0.98	1.62	0.33	1.37	0.27	2.21	0.44
$\widehat{AR}_{PRW}$	—	—	5.78	1.12	1.71	0.34	1.89	0.37	2.19	0.43
$\widehat{AR}_{RRMH}$	15.45	3.04	4.66	0.93	1.61	0.32	1.32	0.26	1.97	0.39
$\widehat{AR}_{RRT}$	14.99	2.96	4.71	0.94	1.63	0.33	1.42	0.28	2.10	0.42
$\widehat{AR}_{ORMH}$	22.02	4.22	4.54	0.90	1.09	0.22	2.01	0.40	1.86	0.37
$\widehat{AR}_{AHO}$	10.92	2.16	5.03	1.01	1.83	0.37	1.29	0.26	2.09	0.42
$\widehat{AR}_{WAL}$	10.68	1.87	5.77	0.93	3.11	0.41	10.73	1.82	6.93	1.19

The main results can be briefly summarized as follows:

- In concordance with theoretical considerations $\widehat{AR}_{PRW}$, $\widehat{AR}_{AHO}$ and $\widehat{AR}_{WAL}$ were severely biased in most situations. In general there was no sufficient compensation for the bias in terms of a lower asymptotic variance.

- $\widehat{AR}_{ORMH}$ overestimated the true summary attributable risk in all situations. This is due to the fact that the odds ratio does not approximate the relative risk in situations where the disease probabilities are not low. $\widehat{AR}_{ORMH}$ will perform much better under rare disease models (e.g. in case-control studies).

- Under the homogeneity model no relevant differences between $\widehat{AR}_{CLW}$, $\widehat{AR}_{RRMH}$ and $\widehat{AR}_{RRT}$ could be observed. The bias of all estimators was negligible. The asymptotic variances of the estimators differed only slightly. Under the interaction model only $\widehat{AR}_{CLW}$ remained unbiased, whereas the others revealed remarkable biases.

IV. Conclusions

The multifactorial approaches to allow for confounding and effect-modification in the estimation of attributable risk are often more realistic than the reduction to a simple 2×2 – table of disease and exposure [2,3]. In this paper different estimators were reviewed and compared by means of a simulation study under the unrestricted multinomial sampling model. The summary attributable risk estimator $\widehat{AR}_{CLW}$ resulting from the 'case load weighting' of the stratum-specific attributable risk estimates showed the best overall performance. In addition, a theoretical underpinning of this method with respect to asymptotical properties is given by the fact that this summary estimator can be derived as the maximum likelihood estimator in this situation. In practical applications it should be the first choice, because no assumptions about the structure of the underlying multinomial model have to be made. Under the homogeneity model the type II estimators $\widehat{AR}_{RRMH}$ and $\widehat{AR}_{RRT}$ represent good alternatives. All other estimators revealed remarkable biases in the majority of the situations. Therefore, they should not be used in practice.

At the end, a word of caution is required with regard to the limitations of the comparison. The results of the simulation study apply only to the unrestricted multinomial sampling model. Other simulation studies (e.g. [3]) indicate that the results are different under other sampling models. In addition, the effect of an increasing number of strata on the properties of the estimators has not been addressed in the study.

References

[1] Levin, M. L. 'The occurrence of lung cancer in man', *Acta Unio Int. Canc.*, **9**, 531–541 (1953).

[2] Walter, S. D. 'The estimation and interpretation of attributable risk in health research', *Biometrics*, **32**, 829–849 (1976).

[3] Whittemore, A. S. 'Statistical methods for estimating attributable risk from retrospective data', *Stat. Med.*, **1**, 229–243 (1982).

[4] Ejigou, A. 'Estimation of attributable risk in the presence of confounding', *Biom. J.*, **21**, 155–165 (1979).

[5] Miettinen, O. S. 'Proportion of disease caused or prevented by a given exposure, trait or intervention', *Am. J. Epidemiology*, **99**, 325–332 (1974).

[6] Greenland, S. 'Bias in methods for deriving standardized morbidity ratio and attributable fraction estimates', *Stat. Med.*, **3**, 131–141 (1984).

[7] Cole, P. and MacMahon, B. 'Attributable risk percent in case-control studies', *Br. J. Prev. Soc. Med.*, **25**, 242–244 (1971).

A Comparative Study on Hazard Function Estimators Employing Nearest Neighbour Distances as Bandwidths

Olaf Gefeller, Holger Dette

Abteilung Medizinische Statistik, Georg-August-Universität Göttingen

Humboldtallee 32, W-3400 Göttingen, F.R.G.

Abstract

The behaviour of nearest neighbour (NN) kernel estimators of the hazard function from censored data is studied by means of a simulation study. Particular attention is paid to the problem of defining NN distances in the case of censored data. We propose a new approach to this problem incorporating the full information of censored observations. The results of the simulation study demonstrate the superiority of the new approach.

I. Introduction

In the analysis of survival data from medical studies hazard functions are nowadays in common use. Their nonparametric estimation from censored data via kernel methods has received considerable attention in the statistical literature, particularly under the random censorship model [1]. Usually, the fixed-bandwidth kernel estimator is employed in this situation. Its asymptotic properties have been investigated in great detail by many authors using different techniques [e.g. 2-3]. But one practical problem of this estimator lies in the fact that it is not data-adaptive in the sense that the data play no role in determining the crucial bandwidth. NN estimators represent an alternative approach to the estimation problem revealing the feature of data-adaption. The basic idea of such an estimator has been suggested originally by Fix & Hodges [4] in the context of nonparametric discriminatory analysis. In the context of hazard function estimation from censored data properties of this type of estimators were studied by Tanner [5], Liu & Van Ryzin [6], and Cheng [7]. However, in the case of censored data the problem arises how to transfer the natural definition of NN distances from the uncensored to the censored setting. All articles cited above circumvent this problem by calculating NN distances in the subsample of the uncensored observations, ignoring all information of the censored observations. Schäfer [8] criticized this approach and proposed a method of incorporating the information of the censored observations into the calculation of the NN distances. In our paper we describe another solution to this problem inspired by Schäfer's idea, but not suffering from the drawbacks of his realization. In chapter III results of a simulation study comparing the effects of the different definitions of NN distances on the behaviour of the hazard function estimators in finite samples are presented. In the concluding chapter IV the practical implications of these results are discussed.

II. Methods

Let $T_1, \ldots, T_n$ be i.i.d. nonnegative random variables ("lifetimes") with identical distribution function F and density function f. Let $C_1, \ldots, C_n$ be i.i.d. nonnegative random variables ("censoring times") with identical distribution function G and density function g. Assume further that lifetimes T_i and censoring times C_i are independent for all i. Under this setting of the random censorship model, one observes the bivariate sample $(X_1, \delta_1), \ldots, (X_n, \delta_n)$, where

$$
\begin{aligned}
X_i &:= \min(T_i, C_i) \\
\delta_i &:= \mathrm{I}\{T_i \le C_i\}, i = 1, \ldots, n,
\end{aligned}
$$

with $\mathrm{I}\{\cdot\}$ denoting the indicator function on a set. In this case of randomly right censored data nonparametric estimates of the survivorship function $S(x) := 1 - F(x)$ and the cumulative hazard function $H(x) := -\log S(x)$ are well known. The Kaplan-Meier estimator $\widehat{S}$ of the survivorship function and the Nelson-estimator $\widehat{H}$ of the cumulative hazard function belong to the standard repertoire of survival analysis.

No standard solution exists for the nonparametric estimation problem of the hazard function $h(x) := f(x)/S(x)$. A huge variety of methods has been discussed in the literature. Throughout this paper we restrict our attention to the kernel method using NN distances as bandwidths. Then, the estimator of h can be written as

$$
\widehat{h}(x) = \sum_{i=1}^{n} \frac{\delta_{(i)}}{n-i+1} \cdot \frac{1}{R(k,x)} \cdot K\left(\frac{x - X_{(i)}}{R(k,x)}\right), \tag{1}
$$

where $\delta_{(i)}$ denotes the censoring indicator corresponding to $X_{(i)}$, K is the so-called kernel function satisfying some regularity conditions, and $R(k,x)$ represents the distance of x to its k-th NN among the observations $X_1, \ldots, X_n$.

The problem of transfering the natural definition of $R(k,x)$ from the uncensored to the censored setting has been tackled in different ways:

(i) Most authors [5-7] ignore all censored data and define $R(k,x)$ as the distance of x to its k-th NN among the uncensored observations $X_i, \delta_i = 1, i = 1, \ldots, n$. This definition will be referred to in the sequel by $R_1(\cdot)$. As Schäfer [8] points out these distances have the disadvantage of being "biased" by the censoring distribution G in the sense that they adapt to the conditional density of T_i under the condition $T_i \le C_i$ of being uncensored, rather than to the density function f or the hazard function h to be estimated.

(ii) As a consequence of his criticism Schäfer [8] proposes an alternative definition of $R(k,x)$ in the case of censored data. In the context of variable kernel estimators he suggests to use:

$$
R_2(k,x) := \inf\{r > 0 \mid \widehat{H}(x+r) - \widehat{H}(x-r) \ge \frac{k-1}{n}\}. \tag{2}
$$

This definition of $R(k,x)$ attempts to incorporate the information of the censored observations by using the Nelson estimator $\widehat{H}$. But this proposal suffers from serious conceptual drawbacks, which can be recognized immediately. Even if no censored data were observed in the sample, $R_2(k,x)$ is not identical to $R_1(k,x)$, i.e. $R_2(\cdot)$ does not reveal the natural definition of NN distances in the uncensored setting. In addition, one inherent property of $\hat{H}$ has an awkward effect on the definition of NN distances: the heights of the steps in $\hat{H}$ increase automatically by definition as $x \to X_{(n)}$. Consequently, in the right tail of the lifetime distribution this effect dominates the value $(k-1)/n$ used in the definition of $R_2(\cdot)$. Consider e.g. the situation of an uncensored largest observation $X_{(n)}$, i.e. $\delta_{(n)} = 1$. Then, for all $t \geq (X_{(n-1)} + X_{(n)})/2$ it follows: $R_2(k, t) = |X_{(n)} - t|$ for all $k \in \{1, \ldots, n\}$, where $|y|$ denotes the absolute value of y. In this extreme example $R_2(\cdot)$ is completely independent of k, which cannot be a desirable property of any definition of NN distances. Even in less extreme situations the increasing heights of the steps in $\hat{H}$ influence the actual values of $R_2(\cdot)$.

(iii) To avoid these problems we propose a modification of the following type:

$$R_3(k, x) := \sup\{r > 0 \mid \hat{S}(x - r) - \hat{S}(x + r - 0) \leq \frac{k-1}{n}\}, \tag{3}$$

where $\hat{S}(x + r - 0)$ denotes the limit from the left of the Kaplan-Meier estimate at the point $x + r$. By using $\hat{S}$ instead of $\hat{H}$ the beforementioned drawbacks of $R_2(\cdot)$ are resolved. In the uncensored setting $R_3(\cdot)$ is identical to the natural definition of the NN distances ($\hat{S}$ reduces to 1 minus the usual empirical distribution function.). The heights of the steps in $\hat{S}$ do not show any systematic trend, they adapt to the configuration of the censored observations. Our definition $R_3(\cdot)$ incorporates the information of the censored data in a plausible way. The open interval $I := (x - R_3(k, x), \ x + R_3(k, x))$ constitutes the largest possible interval which covers an empirical mass of at most $(k-1)/n$ given to I by $\hat{S}$. Due to the configuration of censored observations the actual empirical mass of I can be smaller than $(k-1)/n$. This is compensated by a concentration of empirical mass at the boundaries of I. Consequently, the closed version of I covers an empirical mass of at least k/n. This procedure resembles the situation of tied observations in the uncensored setting.

III. Simulation Study

In this chapter we examine how the definition of NN distances affects the properties of the NN kernel estimator of the hazard function in finite situations by means of a simulation study. We have generated independent samples of exponentially distributed lifetimes with varying amount of censoring (0%, 20%, 40%, 60%, 80%) and different sample sizes (200, 500). The true hazard function was given by $h \equiv 1$ in all ten situations. The distribution of censoring times was chosen as special beta distributions. In each design situation 500 simulation trials were carried out. The three NN kernel estimators were constructed on a grid of 50 points using (1) with the different definitions $R_i(\cdot), i = 1, 2, 3$, of the NN distances given in the preceding chapter and a fixed value of k.

Evaluation of the simulation results is based on the mean integrated squared error (MISE),

$$MISE(\hat{h}) := E \int [\hat{h}(x) - h(x)]^2 dx,$$

which can be numerically approximated by the integrated squared error. To avoid problems in this comparison resulting from the well-known boundary effects of the kernel method the attention is restricted to the interval from the 5th up to the 95th percentile of the observed lifetime distribution. Therefore, artificial discrepancies between the estimators in the tails of the distribution cannot influence our comparison.

The computational realisation of the simulation study took place within a special subsystem of the Statistical Analysis System (SAS) called SAS/IML, which provides a flexible matrix language enabling us to employ fast algorithms in computing all estimators. The simulation study was run on a VAX workstation 3100.

Table 1 contains the results of the simulation study with respect to the MISE values. In all design situations the hazard function estimator incorporating our definition of NN distances revealed the smallest MISE (except for the uncensored case, in which $R_1(\cdot)$ and $R_3(\cdot)$ are identical by definition). Therefore, to illustrate the potential gain when using $R_3(\cdot)$ as the definition of NN distances, table 1 shows the relative increase of the MISE when employing $R_1(\cdot)$ and $R_2(\cdot)$, respectively.

Table 1: Simulation results: MISE and relative increase in MISE for NN kernel estimators of the hazard function employing different definitions of NN distances

| Design situation | | Estimators employing the following definition of NN distances: | | |
sample size	amount of censoring (in %)	$R_1(\cdot)$	$R_2(\cdot)$	$R_3(\cdot)$
200	0	$\pm 0\%$	$+219.69\%$	0.04265
200	20	$+11.19\%$	$+93.09\%$	0.04238
200	40	$+23.69\%$	$+53.82\%$	0.04461
200	60	$+35.45\%$	$+30.21\%$	0.05151
200	80	$+40.51\%$	$+4.35\%$	0.07906
500	0	$\pm 0\%$	$+256.42\%$	0.02732
500	20	$+10.15\%$	$+97.67\%$	0.02724
500	40	$+22.50\%$	$+56.34\%$	0.02804
500	60	$+23.16\%$	$+33.64\%$	0.03502
500	80	$+55.31\%$	$+11.54\%$	0.04117

Obviously, ignoring the information of the censored observations in the calculation of NN distances yields hazard function estimators, which are subject to a larger MISE compared to those employing $R_3(\cdot)$. As expected, this effect gets more pronounced as the amount of censoring increases. Comparing Schäfer's realization of incorporating the information of the censored data into the definition of NN distances to ours, we observe an opposite trend. Here, the superiority of our approach becomes weaker but still existing as the amount of censoring increases. These results are nearly stable with respect to sample size.

IV. Discussion

Hazard functions provide useful information for the medical scientist when evaluating the instantaneous risk of some therapy, drug treatment etc. on health–related events (e.g. death, disease occurrence). The usual situation in medical application confronts us with two problems in this context: the lack of any substantiated distributional assumption about the data and the existence of censored observations. Therefore, efficient nonparametric estimation of the hazard function using the full information of censored data should be the ultimate goal. Due to their computational simplicity and other asymptotic properties, kernel-type estimators are popular for this purpose nowadays. The choice of the bandwidth-parameter is crucial for the behaviour of this class of estimators. In this paper we have considered a special subclass of kernel estimators, those in which the bandwidths are determined by NN distances. To our mind the problem of defining NN distances in the case of censored data has not been adequately taken account of in the literature. Intuitively, it is clear that ignoring the information of the censored observations in calculating NN distances, as it is the existing advice in almost all papers on this topic, cannot be the optimal solution to this problem. Therefore, we have developed an approach to comprise the information of all data in the calculation of NN distances inspired by Schäfer's idea, but not suffering from the serious drawbacks of his realization. In the situation of no censoring our method yields by definition identical results as the usual calculation of NN distances. A simulation study comparing the effects of the different approaches on the properties of the resulting hazard function estimators demonstrated that our definition of NN distances leads to an estimator with a MISE smaller than the corresponding MISE of the other estimators in all situations covered in the study. On the basis of these results it seems justified to recommend the usage of our method in practical applications dealing with the estimation of hazard functions from censored data whenever NN distances are involved in the calculations.

References

[1] Padgett, W.J. (1988). Nonparametric estimation of density and hazard rate function when samples are censored. Handbook of statistics, vol. 7., p. 313-331.

[2] Ramlau-Hansen, H. (1983). Smoothing counting process intensities by means of kernel functions. Ann. Statist. 11, 453-466.

[3] Diehl, S. and Stute, W. (1988). Kernel density and hazard function estimation in the presence of censoring. J. Mult. Analysis 25, 299-310.

[4] Fix, E. and Hodges, J.L. (1951). Discriminatory analysis, nonparametric discrimination: consistency property. Report No. 4, USAF School of Aviation Medicine, Texas.

[5] Tanner, M.A. (1983). A note on the variable kernel estimator of the hazard function from randomly censored data. Ann. Statist. 11, 994-998.

[6] Liu, R.Y.C. and Van Ryzin, J. (1985). A histogram estimator of the hazard rate with censored data. Ann. Statist. 13, 592-605.

[7] Cheng, P.E. (1987). A nearest neighbour hazard rate estimator for randomly censored data. Commun. Statist.-Theory Meth. 16, 613-625.

[8] Schäfer, H. (1985). A note on data-adaptive kernel estimation of the hazard and density function in the random censorship situation. Ann. Statist. 13, 818-820.

Asymptotic Variance Estimation of Association Measures: A New Approach to Overcome Computational Problems

Olaf Gefeller[1], Franz Woltering[2]

[1] Abt. Medizinische Statistik, Universiät Göttingen, W-3400 Göttingen

[2] Fachbereich Statistik, Universität Dortmund, W-4600 Dortmund 50

Abstract

The computational problem of calculating measures of association and their asymptotic variances is addressed in this paper. The link between a special modelling approach for categorical data and the estimation of measures of association is delineated. As a consequence, software programs employed for this modelling approach can be easily adapted to the estimation of measures of association. This is explicitly outlined for a procedure of the Statistical Analysis System (SAS). A practical illustration of the method using Cohen's kappa is provided.

I. Motivation

In medical applications a huge number of specific measures of association has been proposed to describe some feature of the relationship between two variables, usually a disease characteristic and some exposure factor. Association measures offer the opportunity to condense the information of the bivariate distribution of the two variables into one value, which provides an application-orientated interpretation. Therefore, these measures enjoy great popularity among medical scientists. Standard procedures in statistical software packages cover only a small portion of these measures. Whereas in general the calculation of the estimator of the measure of association constitutes no problem, the asymptotic variance of the estimator is not easy to procure. The delta method offers a general approach to develop asymptotic variances of the estimators, but the actual derivation of the variance formulas is often computationally cumbersome. In this paper we show for a broad class of estimators under the multinomial sampling model how to use a standard procedure of the wide-spread Statistical Analysis System (SAS PROC CATMOD) to solve the computational problems. PROC CATMOD is originally designed in the context of the Grizzle, Starmer & Koch (subsequently abbreviated GSK) approach [1] to fit linear models to functions of response frequencies and can be used for linear modeling, log–linear modeling, logistic regression, and repeated measurement analysis. In this paper we demonstrate that it can be easily adapted to estimation problems.

II. The GSK–Model

We shall assume the situation that there are s populations of elements from which independent random samples of fixed sizes $n_1, \ldots, n_s$ are drawn. The responses of the n_i elements of the i-th population are classified into r categories with $n_{ij}, j = 1, \ldots, r$, denoting the number of elements classified into the j-th response category for the i-th population. Thus the resulting data can be summarized in a $s \times r$ contingency table. The random vector $\underline{n}_i := (n_{i1}, \ldots, n_{ir})'$ will be assumed to follow a multinomial distribution with parameters n_i and $\pi_i := (\pi_{i1}, \ldots, \pi_{ir})'$, where π_{ij} represents the probability that an element from the i-th population is classified into the j-th response category. The sample sizes n_i are fixed and consequently the relevant product multinomial model is

$$P(\underline{n}_i, i = 1, \ldots, s \mid n_i, i = 1, \ldots, s) = \prod_{i=1}^{s} \left(\frac{n_i!}{\prod\limits_{j=1}^{r} n_{ij}!} \prod_{j=1}^{r} \pi_{ij}^{n_{ij}} \right)$$

$$\text{with } \sum_{j=1}^{r} \pi_{ij} = 1 \quad \text{for} \quad i = 1, \ldots, s.$$

Let p be the compound vector of $p_i := \frac{\underline{n}_i}{n_i}$ for $i = 1, \ldots, s$ defined by $p := (p'_1, \ldots, p'_s)'$. Then a consistent estimate for the covariance matrix of p is given by the block diagonal matrix $V(p)$ with the matrices $V(p_i) := \frac{1}{n_i} \cdot (D_{p_i} - p_i p'_i)$ for $i = 1, \ldots, s$ representing the main diagonal. D_{p_i} is a diagonal matrix with diagonal elements p_i.

The idea of Grizzle, Starmer & Koch [1] consists of fitting a general class of functions of the product multinomial vector $\pi := (\pi'_1, \ldots, \pi'_s)'$ to a linear model which can be expressed as

$$F(\pi) = X\beta$$

where $F(\pi) := (F_1(\pi), \ldots, F_q(\pi))'$ is a set of $q \leq s \cdot (r - 1)$ functions of interest. X is the known $q \times d$ model specification matrix with full rank $d \leq q$, and β is the unknown vector of model parameters. The functions $F_i(\pi), i = 1, \ldots, q$, are required to have continous partial derivatives through order 2 in a open set containing π. The function vector $F := F(p)$ is a consistent estimator of $F(\pi)$. Hence the model can be written as

$$E_A(F) = X\beta$$

where $E_A(\cdot)$ means asymptotic expectation.

The asymptotic covariance matrix of the estimator $F(p)$ can be consistently estimated by $V_F := HV(p)H'$ where $H := \left(\frac{\partial F(x)}{\partial x}\big|_{x=p}\right)$ corresponds to the first derivative matrix of $F(x)$ evaluated at $x = p$. Thus V_F is obtained via the delta–method. It is important to recognize that a necessary condition for V_F to be non–singular is the linear independence of the functions $F(p)$ and the natural restrictions $\sum_{j=1}^{r} p_{ij} = 1$ for $i = 1, \ldots, s$.

Weighted least squares technique is applied to determine a best asymptotic normal (BAN) estimator b of β as obtained from the expression $b := \left(X'V_F^{-1}X\right)^{-1} X'V_F^{-1}F$. A consistent estimate of the covariance matrix of b is given by $V_b := \left(X'V_F^{-1}X\right)^{-1}$. This noniterative procedure is used for testing goodness of fit of the model and for testing hypothesis about the model parameters.

Forthofer & Koch [2] show that a lot of problems in the analysis of categorical data can be formulated in terms of compounded functions involving linear, logarithmic, and exponential transformations. These transformations are of the following types:

(i) $F(p) = Ap$, where A is a matrix with known elements,

(ii) $F(p) = ln(p)$, where $ln(p)$ is the vector of natural logarithmus of p,

(iii) $F(p) = exp(p)$, where $exp(p)$ is the vector of exponential functions of p.

The corresponding first derivative matrices H can be obtained:

$$H_{Ap} = A, \qquad H_{ln(p)} = Dp^{-1}, \qquad H_{exp(p)} = D_{exp(p)}.$$

Thus, the asymptotic covariance matrices of compounded linear–logarithmic– exponential functions can be computed by repeated application of the chain rule for a matrix differentation.

The GSK–approach has been successfully applied in various settings, e.g. in the analysis of repeated mesurement experiments [3].

III. Computational Realisation

Using the GSK–approach complex ratio statistics such as measures of association have to be written as special functions of the probability estimates of the underlying product multinomial model. To generate estimators of this type compounded functions involving linear, logarithmic, and exponential transformations of the form

$$F(p) = \ldots A_5 \left[\exp\left(A_4 \left[\ln\left(A_3 \left[\exp\left(A_2 \left[\ln\left(A_1 p\right)\right]\right)\right]\right)\right]\right)\right]$$

are used. This general framework offers the opportunity to compute complex estimators in which probabilities from different subpopulations are combined.

In the special situation of a single multinomial population ($s = 1$) achieved by unrestricted sampling of elements measures of association can be expressed in the same as illustrated above. The advantage derived in this situation is the chance of using standard software for GSK–models such as SAS PROC CATMOD to calculate the estimators and their asymptotic variances. The device consists of fitting the simple linear model $F(p) = X\beta$, where $F(p)$ is the 1–dimensional response function as specified above, X denotes the degenerated 1×1 matrix consisting of the constant '1', and β represents the 1–dimensional parameter. Then the estimator b of β equals the response function F itself and the variance of b is given by $V_b = V_F$. This analysis is possible in the SAS procedure CATMOD by directly specifying the design matix on the MODEL statement and by using the RESPONSE statement to describe a series of transformations to the probability estimates in order to produce $F(p)$, the function of interest.

At first glance this procedure seems to increase the computational effort by introducing the tedious work of constructing a series of transformations to describe $F(p)$. But in fact the most annoying part of the application of the delta method, the calculation of the asymptotic variance through computation of the first derivative matrix and of additional matrix products, is completly undertaken by the computer program. Thus the computational effort for the user is reduced substantially.

IV. Example

To illustrate the practical application of the method described in the previous chapters the well–known kappa–coefficient [4] is used. Cohen's κ constitutes a popular measure of agreement between two different ratings, e.g. the classification of disease stage by independent physicians. Procedures for the estimation of the kappa–coefficient and its asymptotic variance are not available in standard statistical software packages like SAS or BMDP. To use the SAS procedure CATMOD to do the calculations in the way outlined above, the following steps have to be applied:

(1) transform κ to a compounded function involving only linear, logarithmic and exponential operations (see general form in chapter III, only terms up to A_4 are needed)

(2) set up the 'dummy' MODEL statement consisting of the constant '1' as the design matrix

(3) set up the RESPONSE statement using the transformation constructed in (1)

(4) run PROC CATMOD and look for the 'Analysis of weighted–least–squares estimates'–table in the output, where the estimated value of κ and its asymptotic standard error appears (in addition, the estimated asymptotic variance of

κ can be obtained directly by specifying the 'COVB'–option on the MODEL statement)

This procedure can be easily implemented and results in a convenient way of estimating the kappa–coefficient and its asymptotic variance. No additional programming effort is needed.

V. Concluding Remarks

The analysis of associations between disease characteristics and exposure factors plays an important role in medical applications. The variety of ways to describe the relationship between variables has lead to an immense number of special measures enabling an application–orientated interpretation with regard to some specific feature of the relation. Each year some new measures of association are added to this multitude, and there is no end of this development in sight. Therefore, producers of statistical software packages fight a loosing battle in trying to extend their systems to cover all measures. Our paper points out the link between the GSK–methodology and estimation problems in contingency tables under the multinomial model. As a consequence, software programs designed for GSK modeling of categorical data can be adapted to estimation problems in contingency tables along the lines of our approach. In this paper we have demonstrated how this works for SAS PROC CATMOD, but in principle other software programs like e.g. GENSTAT can be adapted in a similar manner. The advantage of this new approach lies in a substantial reduction of the computational effort for the user. The cumbersome calculation of the asymptotic variance is completely undertaken by the program. For all situations of the multinomial sampling model our method provides a flexible and convenient way of estimating measures of association and their asymptotic variances.

References

[1] Grizzle, J.E., Starmer, C.F. and Koch, G.G. (1969). Analysis of categorical data by linear models. Biometrics 25, 489-504.

[2] Forthofer, R.N. and Koch, G.G. (1973). An analysis for compounded functions of categorical data. Biometrics 29, 143-157.

[3] Koch, G.G., Landis, J.R., Freeman, J.L., Freeman, D.H. and Lehnen, R.G. (1977). A general methodology for the analysis of experiments with repeated measurement of categorical data. Biometrics 33, 133-158.

[4] Cohen, J. (1960). A coefficient of agreement for nominal scales. Educational and Psych. Meas. 20, 37-46.

*BIOSIGNAL PROCESSING AND
BIOMEDICAL ENGINEERING*

INTELLIGENT PERIPHERAL MODULE FOR DATA ACQUISITION AND CONTROL

D. Pavkov, G. Misic-Pavkov, J. Mihaljev-Martinov, M. Pecujlija

Medical Faculty of Novi Sad, Institute for Neurology,
Psychiatry and Mental Health
Hajduk Veljka 1 - 5, 21000 Novi Sad, Yugoslavia

ABSTRACT

Data acquisition and signal generation has proved to be rather difficult. This paper presents a description of IPM (Intelligent Peripheral Module) and its applications in the field of medicine. From technical point of view IPM is single board computer, equiped with analog and digital inputs and outputs, counter and serial communication channel. It is controlled by personal or any other computer over the serial line. Multiple modules can be configured as LAN (local area network).

Keywords: dataacquisition, processcontrol, communication, single board computer

PREFACE

During the past decade the number of computers, especially personal ones, and software packages has increased enormously, but there is a lack of low cost and easy-to-use interfaces to the "real" world. In fact it is still very complicated to connect computer to measure or to generate various analog and digital signals (1). The intelligent peripheral module (in further text

IPM) is developed in order to help solving such kind of problems. The wide area of its applications cut across almost all medical fields, giving the posibility of rather new and flexibile approach in solving different kinds of problems.

TECHNICAL DESCRIPTION

It is designed as SBC (single board computer) comprising 8 digital inputs, 8 digital outputs (relay type), 8 analog inputs (12 bit conversion) (2), 2 analog outputs (voltage 0 - 2.56 V or current 0 - 25.6 mA), one counter (16 bits), serial line drivers, receivers and its own power supply (3,5). It has its own instruction set that was designed having in mind that IPM is to be easy to work with, even when operated in complicated environment. Any action of IPM is initiated and controlled by computer, that sends commands over the serial line. Simple general purpose communication program, as PROCOMM, can be used on main computer for such activity, especially for experimental or laboratory job. In the cases when real-time schedule (4) is known or when process to be controlled is well defined by many if ... then ... else relations, then IPM is much more efficient if it is controlled by dedicated program on main computer. Software is to be written for each process or environment separately, having in mind all specific requirements.

Instruction set comprises following items:

1. READ ANALOG INPUT
2. READ DIGITAL INPUT
3. SET ANALOG OUTPUT
4. SET DIGITAL OUTPUT (BIT FORM)
5. SET DIGITAL OUTPUT (BYTE FORM)
6. START COUNTER
7. STOP COUNTER
8. READ COUNTER
9. READ GLOBAL (ALL) ANALOG INPUTS

The general structure of the command is:

ADDR.COMMAND   N0 N1 N2 N3 CHSM0 CHSM1 EOM

where first byte is module's address, second is command, Nx are numerical parameters, CHSMx are bytes used for checking message validness and EOM is end-of-message character. Some of numerical parameters may be omited, if not needed for a specific command.

COMMUNICATION

The choice of computer is completely up to the end user, because there is no restrictions as far as computer's hardware is concerned. Communication is made according to RS232 standard, but in case of longer distances (up to 1200 meters), current loop or RS422A is used. IPM modules can be connected in LAN (local area network) up to 250 nodes per single serial channel, but optimal number of modules that are connected is to be smaler if faster overall system response is needed.

Exchanging data between computer and peripheral module is performed by strictly observing pre-defined rules. Data are packed in "messages" that comprises both information and control codes, so simple check of its validness can be done. On receipt of the command from computer, IPM first performs checking of it, then if it is recognized as the one from the set of valid commands, it is immediately executed. After that short report is sent back to the computer, so complete status of environment, that is monitored or controlled, is available at any moment. If some interference, due to high level of electromagnetic noise, occur in communication channel and corrupt transmitted data, IPM will detect it, no action will be taken except sending request to main computer to repeat the previous message. Thanks to that there are no unpredictable reactions of IPM module, that is very important for reliable operating of complete system.

APPLICATION

IPM modules can used for:

- remote monitoring of patient's vital functions
- connecting to standard medical equipment (that provides electrical output), in order to collect data and transfer them to computer
- conducting measurement and control in laboratory investigations
- continuous maintaining of ideal environment conditions (temperature, humidity) in hospital
- registration of patient's requests and generating warnings tothe staff

The applications listed above are examples for which purposes IPM might be used, but in fact the only limitating factor is the imagination of the designer or the end user. The next step in this project will be an improvement in software on the main computer. It turned out to be very convenient to store data sent by IPM in the form that is compatible with data base or statistical programs so time-consuming data entering will be avoided. In the view of communication further experiments are to be made with higher speeds up to 1 Mbit/s. This will cut system response time and allow much more modules to be connected in LAN configuration. Special attention will be payed to graphic presentation of the measured values, because it is known that human characteristic is to observe better pictures that reminds them on real instruments than long strings of alphanumerical characters.

REFERENCES:

1. Robert   J.   Bibbero: Microprocessors   in   Instruments   and   Control,
   John   Wiley & Sons, New York, 1977
2. Data acqusition, HARRIS Semiconductor, Melbourne, USA, 1990
3. Microcontroller   Handbook,   INTEL   Corporation,   Santa   Clara,   USA,
   1986
4. Patrick   H.   Garret: Analog   Systems   for   Microprocessors   and
   Minicom   puters,   Reston   Publishing   Company,   A   Prentice-Hall
   Company, Reston,   1978
5. Peripheral   Design   Handbook, INTEL   Corporation, Santa Clara,
   USA, 1981

A SOFTWARE TO ACQUIRE AND TO TREAT HOLTER TEST ANALYSED BY PATHFINDER 3 MK2 MODEL

P. Conti, A. Polzonetti
Centro di Calcolo - Università di Camerino
Via del Bastione 2, 62032 Camerino (Italy)
F. Moretti, B. Coderoni, G. Bocci
Ospedale Civile - Divisione di cardiologia
Via Lili 61, 62032 Camerino (Italy)

Introduction

The informations given back by up-to-now available ecg automatic readers, especially when average price instruments are used, need further treatment by the physicians to eliminate false answers produced by the instruments because of ecg signal noise or because of objective difficulties in analysing data.
It would be better software supported physicians through this delicate phase. The software would be able to carry out some routine work related with the ecg event analysis; moreover these might offer rapid access to the improper data, making inquiring and correction easier. The proposed program helps the physicians in the clinical and therapeutic follow-up permitting comparisons between ecg tests of the same patient as well as comparisons between ecg data of different patients of homogeneous group; it's an useful characteristic to establish standards.
It is important, for a correct diagnostic and therapeutic behaviour, that physicians could access to previous tests in fast and easy way. The dynamic ecg recording is done by the signal acquisition instrument on magnetic tape with a proprietary coding format, difficult to manage with different instruments.
The tape reader we use (Pathfinder 3 MK2 model), allows us to read and to analyse every single test in a detached way, either from the ecg history, or from the anamnesis of the patient.

1000

It was our aim, in first place, to convert the coding format of the data to an easier one suitable for machine-independent software. In second place, we would create a data base, though incomplete, of the ecg patient tests that would be able to improve both quality and clinical use of medical reports, permitting easy and fast editing and comparison of data.

Tools

XT IBM compatible computer with 640 Kb RAM and 20 Mb Hard Disk has been used to develop this work. Our computer is provided with a parallel and a serial RS-232 ports, the letter used to interface the Pathfinder 3 MK2 model Holter tape reader.
All the software, except the acquisition program, has been written using dBase III Plus programming language. The acquisition program has been written using Quick Basic, because the dBase does not permit to manage the RS-232 serial port.

Data treated

Our package allows to acquire and store, on a hard disk, Pathfinder output data. Data acquisition, from the Holter test, may be executed at time interval of 60, 15 or 5 minutes.
Pathfinder ecg output data must be integrated with complementary clinical and personal informations that the single user is going to input whenever he get them. Such data are divided into 3 files jointly controlled by the package.
Univocal codes identify patients and they are used to link those records which refer to the patient, but stored in different files.
Acquiring program stores data on 2 temporary ascii files whose contents are read by dbase procedures and stored in the dbase files.
One of the temporary files is also employed to exchange controlling parameters between Quick Basic program and dbase procedures. A batch program containing Dos operating systems

commands automatically choices either the Quick Basic procedure or the dBase one depending on the problem the user is facing.
Two additional files are used in order to temporarily save the modifications brought about during the data treatment operations. Such two files are deleted when the user decides to make these changes definitive.

Operative scheme

The software always uses the patient name or code as data access key, except when group comparisons are used (Fig. 1). The patient may be selected from a list that the software displays or he may be searched using either his code or his surname and name jointly. When patient is found the computer shows a list of the dates of all tests he undergone, one of which may be selected to obtain related clinical data. Patients clinical data may be treated to correct signal noise or other anomalies; in this operation clinical data are presented and managed as in a work-sheet, i. e. when an entry is changed the correlated ones are automatically updated.
All data, personal anamnestic and clinical ones, can be obtained through printed reports.
It's possible to add a new patient in data bank. It happens firstly through his personal data, then through his subsidiary clinical data that would be useful to understand test data and finally through his test data input (acquired from pathfinder reader).
Whenever you input new Holter test in the data bank, it is possible to compare its data with the ones of a homogeneous group of tests selected by the operator and then attribute a group code to the ecg test under examination. This procedure permits to classify ecg tests, and consequently patients, into groups. It probably allows the cardiologist clinical experience get improved.
Similarity of Holter tests, useful in establishing the therapeutic effectiveness, may be always evaluated comparing the single test both with another test or a homogeneous group of tests.

Comparisons are possible between homogeneous group of tests to establish normality value threshold and value ranges for different types of disease.

A reduced set of the arrhythmias gathered during the Holter test is used to estimate the similarities. These are aberrant QRS complexes summed to premature and aberrant ones, premature normal QRS complexes, minimal and maxima heart rate.

Comparison is based on an hour slice time; in case acquisition of data is made at smaller time period, these values are summed up to the hour.

During comparisons between tests, differences of the values on the hour base are reported with their per cent changes. In case of groups the values considered are the mean values computed from the hour values of each test in the group. Considering the same hour interval all the values of the same arrhythmia are summed and then divided by the number of tests so that we obtain a mean value for the arrhythmia in the considered hour. Standard deviation is also computed on hour base referring to the group.

The main advantage of the data transfer from Holter reader magnetic tape to the hard disk of the P.C. is the flexibility of the personal computer; in particular data are kept in historical form so that the physician may decide to have a larger view of his patient clinical situation analysing all the testing history of him. This could be really important during therapeutic follow-up, improving the patient arrhythmias knowledge.

Conclusions

We do not think, with the system we developed, to solve all the problems of analysis of ecg data. Nevertheless this instrument may help, in their routinely work, all the physicians working in little hospital cardiological services that, because of insufficient money or little staff, do not have at their disposal more expensive and efficient systems.

Data in dbase format are easy transferable into other formats. This makes possible to use Holter data with general purpose software that may be employed to solve specific problems, which is not permitted by Pathfinder data format.

Our proposal, based on low cost machines, does not require great investment nor technical specialists so that physicians or hospital nurses can directly use them.

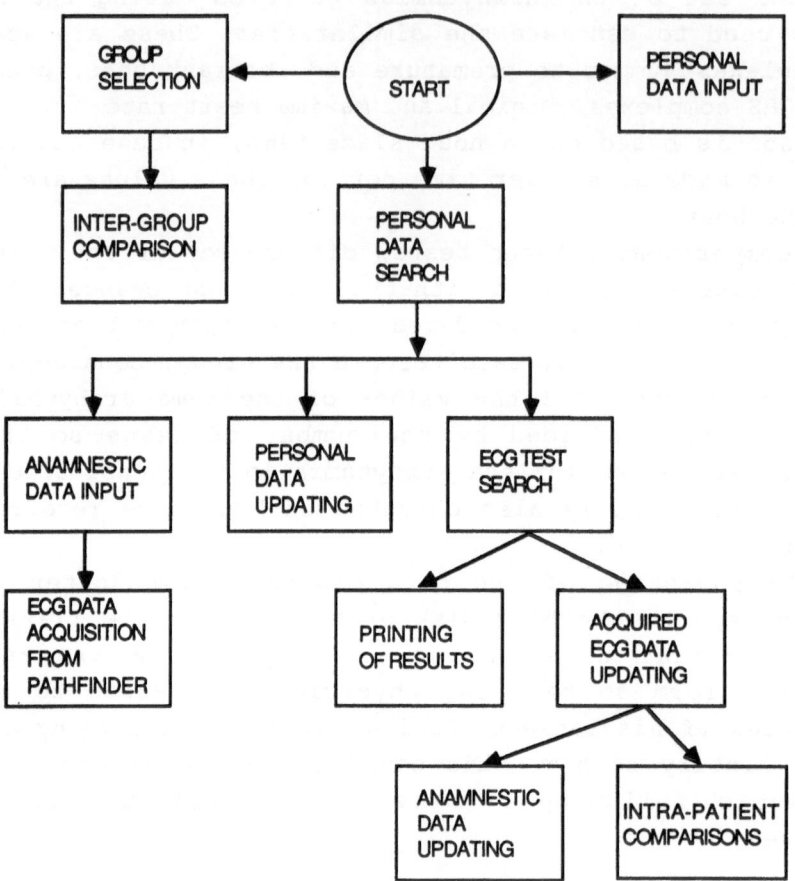

Fig. 1: Software operative scheme.

PC-SUPPORTED 64-CHANNEL DC-EEG AMPLIFIER

G.Lindinger, P.Svasek*, W.Lang, L.Deecke
Neurologische Universitätsklinik Wien, Lazarettgasse 14, A-1090 Wien
*Inst. f. Allgem. Elektrotechnik und Elektronik, TU Wien
Gußhausstr.24-28, A-1040 Wien

ABSTRACT

For investigation of cortical DC-potential shifts a new, computer based multi-channel amplifier system was developed. Because of high input impedance (>50GΩ), low input bias current (<1pA) and low input capacity (<50pF) the amplifier can be used for epicortical, intracranial and intracellular recordings too. There are no analog outputs, the amplified signals were digitalized by a 16-Bit A/D in each channel of the amplifier, then online digitally filtered and after downsampling stored on the hard disk of a PC. All setups, calibration etc. are done by control of the PC. Other important new features are the capability of self testing (preamplifiers, amplifier setup), of testing electrodes (drift, noise etc.) and a computer controlled electrode application system.

INTRODUCTION

Cortical DC-potential shifts reflect excitatory synaptic activity of the cortex. Cognitive and motor brain processes are associated with shifts of the cortical DC-potential [3,4,6]. Investigations of the topographical distribution of DC-shifts offer the possibility to describe task-related spatial and temporal patterns of cortical activity (functional brain topography [6,7]). For calculating current source density (CSD, [5,7,8,10]) on the scalp (a method with the advantage of reference-free datas and of decreased volume conduction effects) and for improved spatial resolution of topographic maps the numbers of amplifier channels had to be increased. Other methods for localizing neuronal sources (e.g. evoked dipol source potential analysis [11], multiple source modeling [2,9]) also needs multi-channel equipments.

Other serious problems, e.g. the difficult measurement of DC-potentials or the time-consuming application of DC-electrodes [1] in a multi-channel equipment also needs improvements. In view of commercial non-availability of all these requirements, a 64-channel computer supported DC-amplifier was developed. The system has a few more new features. So it can also be used for intracraniel, epicortical (e.g. epileptic research) and intracellular measurements.

OVERVIEW OF THE SYSTEM

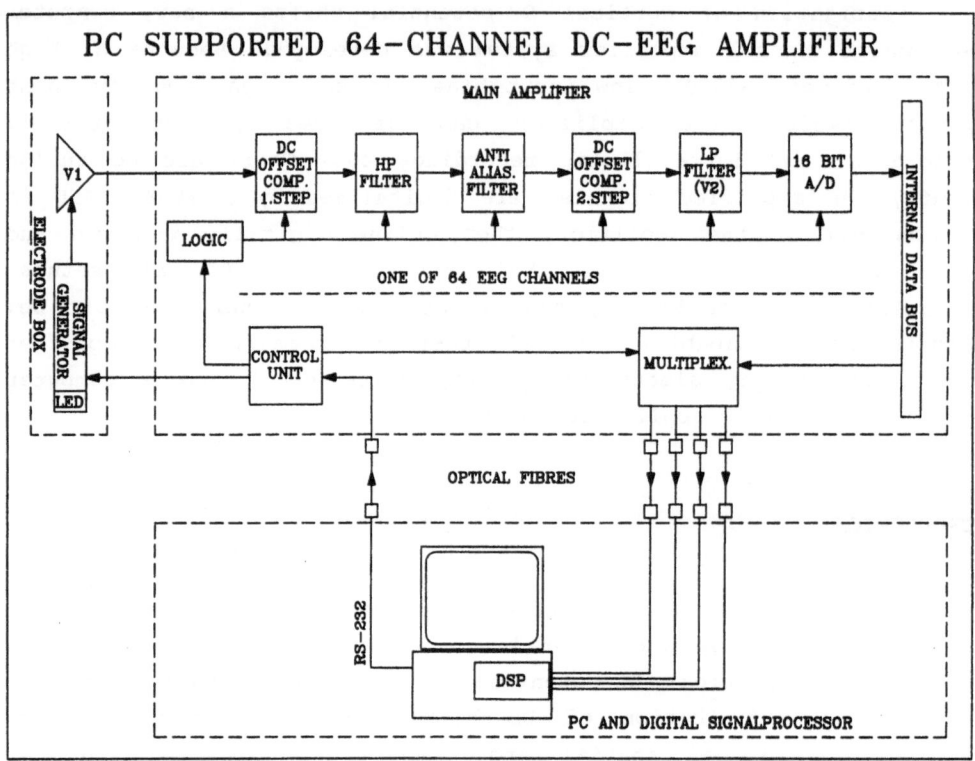

Fig. 1. Principle diagramm of the PC-based amplifier system

Fig. 1 shows the principle of the amplifier: it consists of three parts, the electrode-box, the main amplifier and the PC with a digital signal processor. The electrode box consists of the preamplifiers (amplification V1), a signal generator for testing electrodes and amplifiers and a LED-system for assisting in the application of electrodes.

In the main amplifier the analog-signals were filtered (standard high-pass and low-pass -6dB filters) and amplified (V2), a two step DC-compensation is provided for subtracting DC-offsets. Each channel contains a 16-bit A/D-converter and an anti-aliasing filter. The digital datas of all 64 channels were multiplexed and transfered by optical fibres to digital signal prozessor. There the oversampled datas were digitally filtered and, after downsampling stored on the harddisk of the PC.

The setup of the amplifiers (amplification, filter etc.), the calibration and controlling of sample-parameters are done by the PC, for that purpose, a RS232 optical-fibre connection between the PC and the main amplifier is provided.

Linearity and maximal resolution of the whole system (analog and digital) is about 16 bit.

ELECTRODE BOX AND PREAMPLIFIER

For DC-measurements on the scalp or intracraniel and epicortical recordings, amplifier with high input impedance and low input bias current are necessary. For intracellular measurements with extremly high electrode impedance additional low input capacity is necessary.

The input impedance of preamplifiers and electrode box is about 50 GΩ, the input current is less then 1pA, the overall input capacity is about 500 pF. For intracellular recordings, one part of the electrode-box must be changed, then the overall input capacity is about 50 pF.

DIGITAL FILTER

All datas were digitally filtered online by using a digital signal processor (Burr & Brown signal processor board ZPB34 with the AT&T 50MHz signal processor DSP32C). By using a butterworth filter of 10th order for anti aliasing of oversampled data and linear phase FIR-Filter for digital filtering the overall phase dispersion is less than one sample intervall of downsampling-frequency. Fig. 2 shows the group delay (phase dispersion in sample intervalls) of the Butterworth filter 10th order.

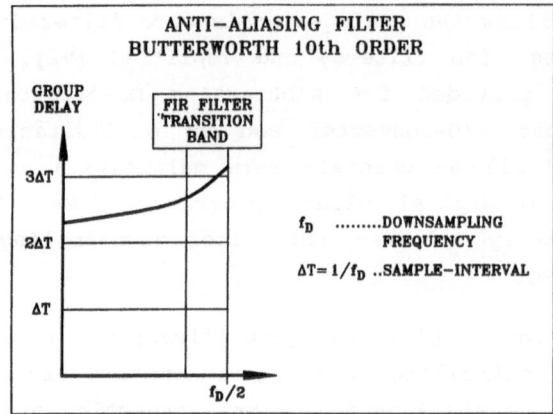

Fig.2. Butterworth filter 10th order: group delay in sample intervalls

Because of filtering in online and down sampling dependend calculation time of FIR Filter there is a limitation of numbers of channels, depending on downsampling frequency:

downsampling frequency [Hz]	numbers of channels	resolution of digital data [Bit]	stopband ripple [dB]
4000	8	12	66
2000	10/16	16/12	90/66
1000	30/40	16/12	90/66
<= 500	64	16	90

ADDITIONAL FEATURES

One feature is an electrode-impedance measurement system combined with a computer controlled electrode application system. Each electrode contains a small LED, which is activated by PC. So the PC can indicate electrodes with to high electrode impedance or bad electrodes. An additional PC-controlled LED system on a symbolic 10-20-system head enables the experimenter to locate the position of each electrode on the subject head.

Other important new features of the system for DC-measurements include: the capabilitys of self-testing (preamplifiers, amplifier-setup) and of testing the electrodes (frequency response, drift, noise and DC-offset and polarisation).

REFERENCES

[1] Bauer H, Korunka C, Leodolter M (1989) Technical requirements for high-quality scalp DC recordings. Electroenceph Clin Neurophysiol 72: 545-547

[2] Baumgartner C, Sutherling WW, Di S, Barth DS (1989) Investigation of multiple simultaneously active brain sources in the electroencephalogram. J Neurosci Meth 30: 175-184

[3] Deecke L (1987) Bereitschaftspotential as an indicator of movement preparation in supplementary motor area and motor cortex. In: Porter R (ed) Motor areas of the cerebral cortex. Wiley, Chicester pp. 231-250 (Ciba Foundation Symposium 132)

[4] Kornhuber HH, Deecke L, Lang W, Lang M, Kornhuber A (1989) Will, volitional action, attention and cerebral potentials in man. Bereitschaftspotential, performance-related potentials, directed attention potentials, EEG spectrum changes. In: Hershberger WA (ed) Volitional action. Advances in Psychology, vol 62, Elsevier, Amsterdam New York, pp. 107-169

[5] Hjorth, B. (1975) An on-line transformation of EEG scalp potentials into into orthogonal source derivations. Electroenceph. clin. Neurophysiol., 39: 526-530

[6] Lang W, Obrig H, Lindinger G, Cheyne D, Deecke L (1990) Supplementary motor area activation while tapping bimanually different rhythms in musicians. Exp Brain Res, vol 76(3)

[7] Lindinger G, Lang W, Obrig H, Deecke L (1990) Topographical analyses of radial current density - Distribution of cortical DC-activation in motor tasks. In: Brunia CHM, Gaillard AWK, Kok A, Mulder G, Verbaten MN (eds) Proceedings of the Ninth International Conference on Event-Related Potentials of the Brain, EPIC IX. Tilburg University, Tilburg

[8] Nunez P (1981) Electric fields of the brain. The neurophysics of EEG. Oxford University, Oxford

[9] Nunez P (1986) Locating sources of the brain's electrical and magnetic fields: some effects of inhomogeneity and multiple sources, with implications for the future. HFOSL technical Note 71-86-12, San Diego

[10] Perrin F, Bertrand O, Pernier J (1987) Scalp current density mapping: value and estimation from potential data. IEEE Trans Biomed Eng BME-34: 238-288

[11] Scherg M, von Cramon D (1986) Evoked dipole source potentials of the human auditory cortex. Electroenceph Clin Neurophysiol 65: 344-360

EEG PROBABILITY MAPPING WHILE LISTENING TO A TEXT: A GROUP AND A SINGLE CASE STUDY[1)]

Rappelsberger P., Lacroix D., Steinberger K., Thau K., Petsche H.
Institute of Neurophysiology and Psychiatry Unit, Währingerstraße 17, A-1090 Vienna

ABSTRACT

An EEG mapping study was conducted in 42 healthy subjects (20 females and 22 males; 25,1a±3,4) while they were listening to a text. EEG changes in the theta and alpha band were observed mainly in the left temporal regions which are responsible for language comprehension.

INTRODUCTION

In the past EEG mapping techniques have proved to be an efficient means in studying cognitive processes. Basically, three different mapping methods may be distinguished. EEG amplitude mapping is mainly applied in evoked potential studies. The second method is based on spectral parameters whereby almost only power or amplitude values of various frequency bands are mapped. In contrast to our method, coherence mapping is hardly found in the literature. Finally, in the third method error probabilities according to statistical tests are mapped.

The conjecture that cognitive processes are reflected in the electrical brain activity goes back till the discovery of the EEG by Hans Berger. However, only in the last decade it was able to proof this conjecture by means of computer aided EEG analysis. Nowadays, the number of papers dealing with EEG related aspects of cognitive performance is considerably increasing, mainly in research concerning hemispheric dominance.

METHODS

19 EEG electrodes were placed on the scalp according to the international 10/20 system. EEG was recorded against averaged signals picked up from both ear lobes (TC 0.3s, Filter 35 Hz). The subjects were sitting comfortably in an arm chair with eyes closed and EEG records were made during listening to a spoken text (VL) presented by ear phones. Additionally, control EEGs were made without presenting a text: the subjects were asked to keep the eyes closed and to relax (AZ). Each record lasted 1 to 2 minutes.

EEG was written out on paper and simultaneously digitised at 128/s and stored on hard disc. Artifacts were eliminated from further computation by visual inspection. All artifact free 2 second epoches of one record were Fourier transformed to compute averaged power- and cross-power spectra with a frequency resolution of 0.5 Hz. 19 power spectra and 38 cross-power spectra were obtained for each record. Averaged cross-power spectra were calculated between adjacent electrodes along the transverse and longitudinal electrode rows and also between electrodes on homologous sites of both hemispheres.

For data reduction averaging of adjacent spectral lines was performed to restrict to the frequency bands: theta (4 - 7.5 Hz), alpha (8 - 12.5 Hz), beta1 (13 - 18 Hz), beta2 (18.5 - 24 Hz)

[1)] Supported by the Jubiläumsfonds der Österreichischen Nationalbank, NB 3580 and beta3 (24.5 - 31.5 Hz). Final computations yielded broad band parameters like amplitude and coherence for the five frequency bands (Rappelsberger and Petsche, 1988).

The results, either absolute values or the changes due to different recordings or task situations, were colour coded and presented as spectral parameter maps.

Statistical evaluations aimed at the detection of significant differences between control (AZ) and task situation (VL) were based on paired Wilcoxon tests in group studies (Fig.1) and on confidence intervals (Rappelsberger et al., 1986) in single person studies (Fig.2). Error probabilities lower than 0.1 were presented as probability maps. The results can be considered as a descriptive approach to yield hints at those of the multiple comparisons for which possible differences between VL and AZ exist.

RESULTS

Fig.1 shows the probability maps obtained for the group of 42 volunteers. The maps demonstrate significant changes of spectral parameters during VL as compared with AZ. As amplitudes are concerned, only decreases can be observed: in the alpha band amplitudes decreased in the frontal parts and in the beta3 band amplitudes decreased in the fronto-central brain area and in the left temporo-occipital region.

Interhemispheric coherence (IC) changes show a different topographic behaviour in the different frequency bands. The most essential finding is the increase between both post-temporal regions in the theta band.

As local coherences (LC) are concerned the most essential findings are the increase in the theta and alpha band in the left temporal regions responsible for language comprehension. However, in theses frequency bands also in the right temporal regions LC increased.

Different topographic distributions of increased and decreased LC can be observed in the three beta bands.

Fig.2 shows an example of the results obtained in a 29 years old female. These probability maps are based on confidence intervals. Amplitudes are mainly decreased during listening to the text. Essential exceptions are observed in the alpha and beta2 bands in the occipital and adjacent regions.

The essential results concerning local coherence were: left temporo-frontal and left temporo-central increase in the theta band, left temporal increase in the alpha band, fronto-central increase in beta1 and beta2 bands and right temporo-parieto-occipital increase in the beta2 band.

The essential findings in the interhemispheric coherences were the frontal increase in the theta band and the occipital and parietal decrease in the alpha band.

DISCUSSION

The methods demonstrated are used to examine EEG changes during cognitive processes. The presented examples show that major changes while listening to a text in a resting state with eyes closed were found in left hemispheric local coherence, mostly in the central, temporal and parietal regions. These changes agree with the traditional role of the left hemisphere in language functions. (Kolb and Whishaw, 1990).

There are several papers dealing with power or amplitude spectral analysis of ongoing EEG records during cognitive processes. However, there are only a few papers in which coherence analyses were employed. In studying functional relationships, coherence analyses yield important new aspects of brain activities which complement the data obtained by power

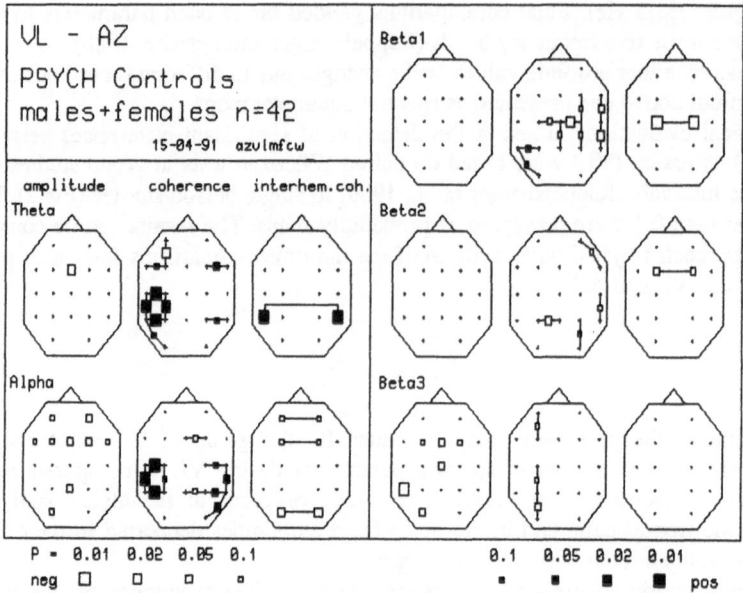

Fig.1: Probability maps. The maps show the error probabilities according to statistical evaluations of the EEG spectral parameter changes during listening to text (VL) and the control situation (AZ). A paired Wilcoxon test was applied.

The five rows relate to the five frequency bands examined. The three columns concern: mean amplitude per frequency band, local coherence, i.e. coherence between adjacent electrodes along the transverse and longitudinal rows, and interhemispheric coherence, i.e. coherence between corresponding sites of both hemispheres.

Significant amplitude differences are indicated by squares at the corresponding electrode positions. A significant transverse or longitudinal coherence change is presented by a square drawn between the two electrodes involved. A significant interhemispheric coherence change is marked by squares at the two electrode locations of homologous sites of both hemispheres connected by a line.

Black squares indicate amplitude or coherence increase and empty squares amplitude or coherence decrease.

spectral analyses, since a change of power does not necessarily mean that the functional relationship or coupling between two signals also changes. It has been argued that coherence between electrophysiological signals from different parts of the brain may depend on structural connectivities or functional couplings between these parts (Busk and Galbraith, 1975).

The value of topographic mapping has been recognised since the 50ies. With the development of computer capabilities in the past decade topographic mapping of cerebral activity, as a means of enhancing the diagnostic capabilities of neurophysiological data, has rapidly advanced in interest and activity. Additionally, as demonstrated in this paper EEG amplitude and coherence mapping have proved to be an efficient tool in studying cognitive processes.

The value of statistical evaluations and probability mapping is demonstrated by considering the increase of interhemispheric central coherence in the beta2 band (Fig.1). Fig.2 shows that this visually significant increase is not significant in the statistical sense and should therefore be interpreted very carefully.

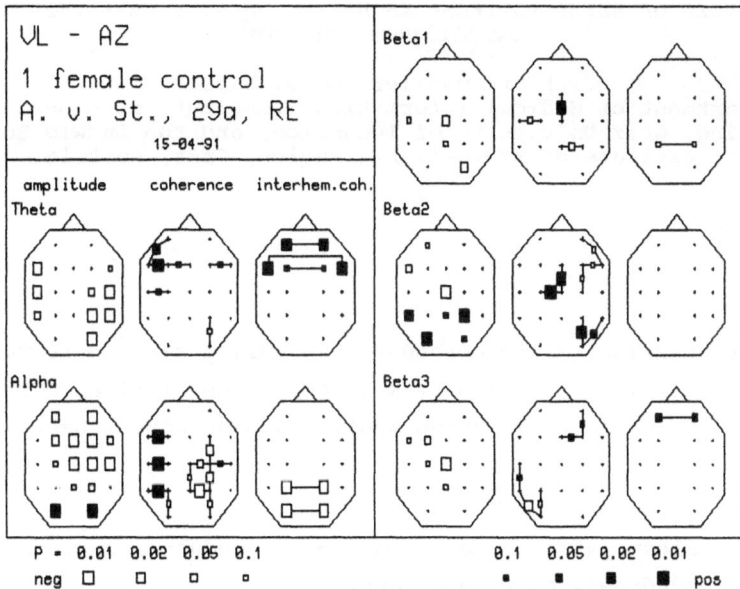

Fig.2: Probability maps of a 29 year old female volunteer. The maps show the error probabilities based on confidence intervals of the EEG spectral parameter changes during listening to text (VL) and the control situation (AZ).

The arrangement of the maps is as in Fig.1.

REFERENCES

Busk, J. and Galbraith, G.C.: EEG correlates of visual motor practice in man. Electroencephal. clin. Neurophysiol., 1975, 38: 415-422.

Kolb B. and Whishaw I.Q., Fundamentals of human neuropsychology, Third edition, Freeman and Co., New York, pp. 568-574, 1990.

Rappelsberger P., Pockberger H., Petsche H.: Computer aided EEG analysis: evaluation of changes during cognitive processes and topographic mapping. EDV in Medizin und Biologie 17(3): 45-53, 1986.

Rappelsberger P., Petsche H.: Probability mapping: power and coherence analyses of cognitive processes. Brain Topography, Vol 1, No 1: 46-54, 1988.

ANALYSIS OF SLEEP PATTERNS IN BABIES USING NEURAL NETWORKS - PRELIMINARY RESULTS[*]

G. Pfurtscheller and G. Litscher
Department of Medical Informatics, Institute of Biomedical
Engineering, Graz University of Technology and the Ludwig Boltzmann-
Institute of Medical Informatics, Graz, Austria.

ABSTRACT

This paper describes a new method for analyzing sleep patterns in
infants. Preliminary results from a comparison of sleep scoring by an
expert and automatic sleep stage analysis using neural networks are
reported.

Key words: Sleep pattern; neural networks; sudden infant death
syndrome; polysomnography

INTRODUCTION

Automatic sleep stage scoring is becoming an increasingly
important tool. It is a more objective and less laborious method than
visual classification. However, in the available studies on adults,
the correspondence between automatic and human classifications is
smaller than that attained with two human observers [1,2]. In
contrast to the large number of systems for automatic sleep detection
in adults, there are only a few systems which are more or less able to
automatically classify sleep stages in infants.

This paper reports preliminary results on a PC-based system for
sleep monitoring in infants and automatic sleep scoring using neural
networks.

[*] This study is supported by the "Fonds zur Förderung der
wissenschaftlichen Forschung (Projekt S49/03) in Austria and is part
of the COMAC-BME project "Methodology for the Analysis of the Sleep-
Wakefulness Continuum".
The babies were selected by the Department of Pediatrics (Head:
Prof. Dr. R. Kurz) and the Department of Physiology (Head: Prof. Dr.
T. Kenner), both of the University of Graz. Visual analyses of sleep
profiles were done by Dr. E. Rebuffat from the Paediatric Sleep Unit,
University Children's Hospital, Free University of Brussels, Belgium.
We would like to acknowledge their support.

METHODS

Infants

In the last 18 months, 57 all-night sleep recordings (8-hour periods) have been performed on infants of ages 6 weeks, 6 months and 1 year in a follow-up study. The babies were separated into a group at risk for SIDS (Sudden Infant Death Syndrome) and a control group.

Data acquisition and processing

To investigate the SIDS phenomenon, different biological signals and their interaction have to be monitored over hours. The following signals have been recorded in the study: electroencephalogram (2 channels EEG), electrocardiogram (ECG), electrooculogram (EOG), electromyogram (EMG), microtremor (2 channels MV, corresponding to actogram - 2 channels M), respiration (3 channels Resp.), temperature (4 channels Temp.), blood pressure (3 channels BP), oxygen saturation (SaO_2), transcutaneuos partial pressure of O_2 and CO_2 and a video signal. After sampling the signals and storing the data on optical disks (8 Mbyte/hour), the processing is done offline, whereby different strategies and methods of analysis can be applied. For the neural network approach, EOG, EMG and microtremor are integrated over 30 seconds and Fast Fourier Transformation (FFT) is applied to 2-second-epochs of the EEG signal and 30-second-epochs of respiration. Furthermore, the heart rate and heart rate variability are calculated from ECG signals. All the data, calculated in intervals of 30 seconds, can be displayed on a video monitor or on a single sheet of paper to obtain a first impression of the data quality over the 8-hour period.

A separate event-marker file is created online by the person performing the recordings, containing the time of occurrence of body movements, artifacts and other observations that are relevant to the recording session.

Sleep classification by a human expert

Visual sleep analysis was performed by an expert in the usual fashion. This was possible offline by scoring the raw data on a video terminal. The scoring was made in 16-second epochs rigidly following the rules of Anders et al. [3] and Guilleminault and Souquet [4] for babies aged 6 weeks and 6 months, and according to the rules of

Rechtschaffen and Kales [5] for infants aged 1 year. The following
parameters were used for the visual classification of sleep stages:
EEG (2 channels), EOG, EMG, ECG, respiration (2 channels) and
actogram.

Sleep pattern analysis by a neural network

For sleep stage classification with a neural network, the multi-
layer PERCEPTRON (back-propagation algorithm) and the self organizing
KOHONEN network in combination with a Learning Vector Quantizer (LVQ)
were taken into consideration. The self-organizing KOHONEN network
[6] needs no supervised learning input and is therefore not able to
classify sleep stages, but allows the study of the organization of
sleep patterns by a sort of cluster process. The data thus obtained
can be classified with the LVQ. Both the multi-layer PERCEPTRON and
the LVQ are supervised learning methods and thus need classified sleep
patterns as learning input.

In this paper, only the KOHONEN net is introduced. Although it
does not directly classify sleep stages, the patterns obtained can be
compared with the expert classifications: a correspondence is
postulated when a specific pattern can be matched frequently to a
specific sleep stage. The network is composed of one layer of
interconnected units, whereby each unit obtains the same n-dimensional
input via adjusting weights. The n-dimensional input is transformed
to a one- or two-dimensional output, whereby input vectors with
continuous values are presented sequentially in time. After enough
input vectors have been presented, the self-organization process
starts with randomized weight vectors and randomly selected input
vectors and consists of 2 steps:

1) Calculation of the inner product between input vector x and
   weight vector m_i and search for the "best-matching" unit.
2) Update of the "best-matching" unit and the topological
   neighbors by the following rule:
$$m(t+1) \ = \ m(t) + \alpha \ \{x(t) - m(t)\}$$
   (where α is the learning factor, decreasing with time)

This self-organizing process has to be repeated several times and as a
result of this, weights will specify clusters or vector centers that
sample the input space in such a manner that the point density
function of the vector centers tends to approximate the point density
function of the input vectors. The KOHONEN net we used is composed of
ten interconnected units and transforms an 11-dimensional input into a
1-dimensional output. Each input vector is represented by 11

variables (EEG band power, EOG, EMG, respiration, etc.) and calculated in intervals of 2 or 8 minutes. In the latter case, the 8 hours of sleep are represented by 60 vectors; in the former case, by 240 vectors.

RESULTS

An example of an offline display from the digitally stored raw data is given in Figure 1, demonstrating EEG_1 (C_z-A_1), EEG_2 (O_z-A_1), electromyogram (EMG), sucking movements, electrocardiogram (ECG), actimeter signals from both forehands (M_1 and M_2), electrooculogram (EOG) and 2 respiratory signals from a nasal thermistor (Resp 1) and an abdominal strain gauge (Resp 2). The data demonstrate a 9-second apnea in an eight-week old infant.

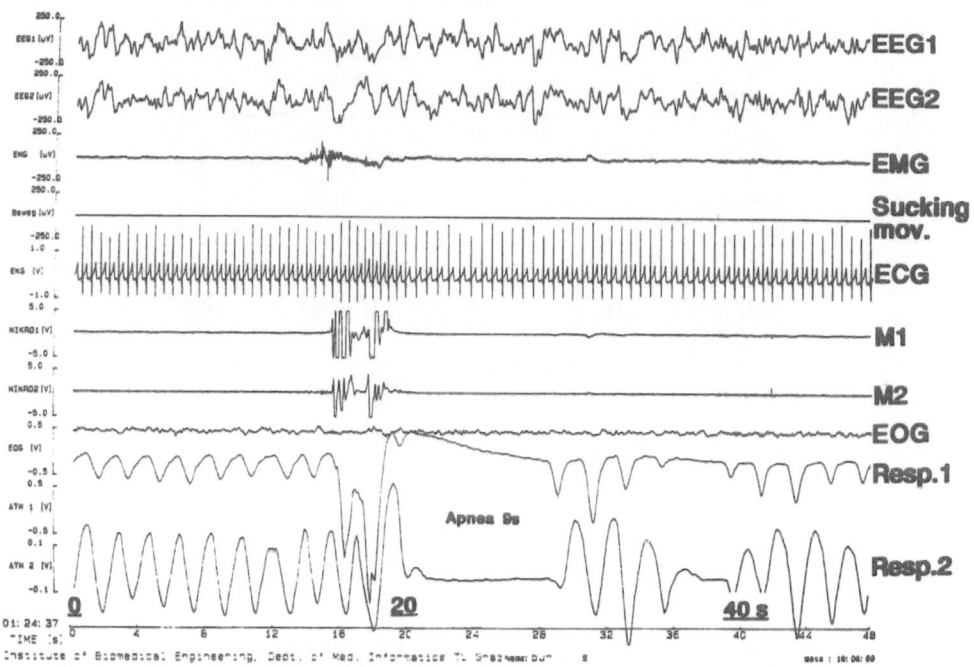

Figure 1: Raw data reconstructed from the digital signals stored on an optical disk.

Examples of 8 hours of preprocessed data (upper panel), sleep scoring results by the expert (middle panel) and the output of the KOHONEN net (lower panel) are displayed in Figures 2 and 3. In Figure

2, the data from a 53-day old baby and in Figure 3, data from the same
baby aged one year are shown.

The signals (parameters) marked by a triangle on the right side
of the upper panel are used for visual sleep scoring and as inputs to
the neural network. The units with the largest output are marked by
horizontal lines. A stable sleep pattern is indicated if the same
unit is active in consecutive 8-minute intervals. As can be seen in
Figures 2 and 3, stable patterns often last 24 minutes (3 intervals of
8 minutes), but can also last up to 32 (4 intervals) or even 40 (5
intervals) minutes.

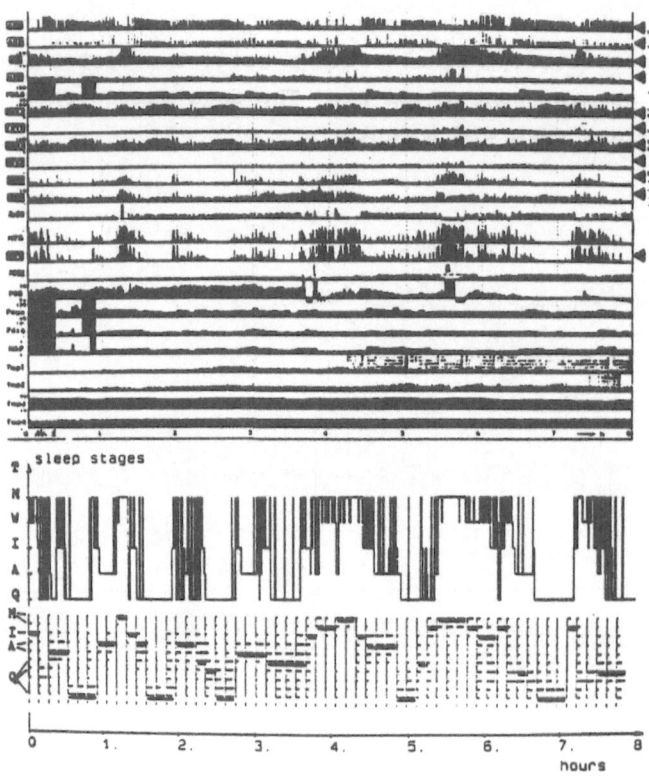

Figure 2: Continuous monitoring in a 53-day-old baby.
    Upper panel: From top to bottom, the following parameters are
    shown: 2 channels of respiration rate, heart rate, heart rate
    variability, pulse rate, EEG_1 (1-4 Hz), EEG_1 (4-10 Hz), EEG_2 (1-4
    Hz), EEG_2 (4-10 Hz), EOG, EMG, sucking movements, 2 channels
    microtremor, pCO_2 and pO_2, oxygen saturation, 3 channels blood
    pressure and 4 channels temperature. Middle panel: visual sleep
    classification. Lower panel: output of a KOHONEN network. Each
    vertical line represents the output pattern from an 8-minute
    interval. The lengths of the horizontal lines represent the
    outputs of each unit.

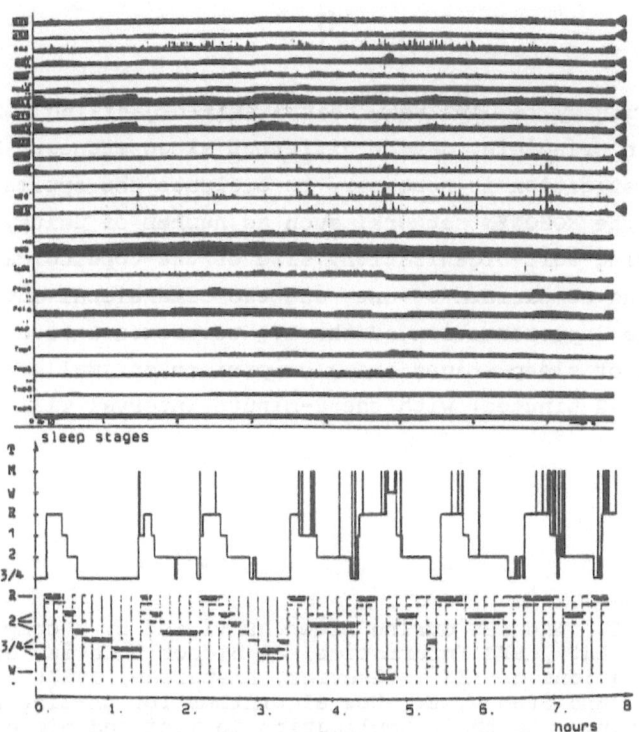

Figure 3: Data from the same baby as in Fig. 2, aged one year.

The visual sleep scoring in Figure 2 reveals 7 intervals with quiet sleep (Q). The neural network also indicates 7 intervals of quiet sleep, of which 5 were undisturbed by movement artefacts (bottom line in the net output in Fig. 2.).

In Figure 3, the first sleep stage 3/4 lasts about 75 minutes (around the first hour), as determined by the expert scoring. The neural network indicates, however, two slightly different 3/4 stages, each lasting 24 minutes (3 intervals of 8 minutes). The EEG delta power (traces No. 7 and 9 from the top of Fig. 3) displays different magnitudes in the first and second half of the sleep stage 3/4, which supports the scoring of the neural network. All eight REM stages scored by the expert (Fig. 3) are also found with the neural network.

DISCUSSION

The preliminary results show that a self-organizing KOHONEN network can, in principle, detect different sleep stages. However, much more investigation is necessary to evaluate the optimal parameters of the KOHONEN network, such as number of units, number of iterations during self-organization, size of the topological neighborhood and comparison of one- and two-dimensional output. In the future, the implementation of the LVQ to obtain a true classification of sleep stages and a comparison of smaller time intervals (e.g. 2 minutes) with the 8-minute interval will be performed.

REFERENCES

[1] Johnson, L.C. The EEG during sleep as viewed by a computer. In: A. Rémond (Ed.), EEG Informatics. A didactic review of methods and applications of EEG. Elsevier, Amsterdam, 1977: 385-406.
[2] Lacroix, B. and Stanus, E. New algorithms for on-line automatic sleep scoring, and their application to mini and microcomputer. Journal A, 1985, 26: 91-97.
[3] Anders, T., Emde, R. and Parmelee, A. (Eds.). A manual of standardized terminology, techniques and criteria for the scoring of states of sleep and wakefulness in newborn infants. Brain Information Service, School of Health Sciences, UCLA, Los Angeles, 1971.
[4] Guilleminault, C. and Souquet, M. Sleep states and related pathology. In: R. Korobkin and C. Guilleminault (Eds.), Advances in Perinatal Neurology. S.P. Medical and Scientific Books, New York, 1979: 225-247.
[5] Rechtschaffen, A. and Kales, A. (Eds.). A manual of standardized terminology, techniques and scoring system for sleep stages of human subjects. Public Health Service, US Government Printing Office, Washington DC, 1968.
[6] Kohonen, T. Self-organized formation of topologically correct feature maps. Biol. Cybernetics, 1982, 43: 59-69.

SPECTRAL ANALYSIS OF BREATHING IN INFANTS IN THE FIRST YEAR OF LIFE DURING QUIET SLEEP - PRELIMINARY RESULTS[*]

G. Litscher and G. Pfurtscheller
Department of Medical Informatics, Institute of Biomedical
Engineering, Graz University of Technology and the Ludwig Boltzmann-
Institute of Medical Informatics, Graz, Austria.

ABSTRACT

In the present study, breathing patterns during quiet sleep were analyzed in 53 follow-up measurements in 25 babies of ages 6 weeks, 6 months and 1 year. Using spectral analysis, respiratory parameters were computed to compare control infants with infants at risk for sudden infant death syndrome (SIDS). SIDS-risk infants show no significant difference in respiratory rate or variability in the state of quiet sleep.

<u>Key words</u>: quiet sleep; respiration; sudden infant death syndrome; infants; spectral analysis

INTRODUCTION

A number of studies in recent years concerning sudden infant death syndrome (SIDS) have investigated aspects of respiratory activity, postulating that abnormal breathing patterns may characterize risk for SIDS [1-5].

In the present paper, we report spectral analysis techniques applied to breathing patterns of babies in the first year of life during periods of 5 X 2-minute epochs of quiet sleep. Data were obtained from 24-channel polysomnographic recodings performed for 8

---

[*] This study is supported by the "Fonds zur Förderung der wissenschaftlichen Forschung (Projekt S49/03) in Austria and is part of the COMAC-BME project "Methodology for the Analysis of the Sleep-Wakefulness Continuum".

The babies were selected by the Department of Pediatrics (Head: Prof. Dr. R. Kurz) and the Department of Physiology (Head: Prof. Dr. T. Kenner), both of the University of Graz. We would like to acknowledge their support.

hours at night, which are stored on optical disks.

METHODS

Infants and data collection

Fifty-three 8-hour multichannel recordings of cerebral and cardiorespiratory data were performed in infants aged 6 weeks, 6 months and 1 year during the period June 1989 to November 1990 [6,7]. Twelve of these infants were recorded three times, one infant in the risk group (P.H.,♂) four times. The fourth measurement with this infant took place at the age of 15 months. When the study is complete at the end of 1991, a total of 90 measurements (30 babies, 3 times each) will have been performed.

The infants at risk for SIDS (near-miss SIDS infants and SAS-infants (sleep apnea syndrome)) as well as the 9 infants in the control group were carefully selected on the basis of clinical investigations and detailed questionnaires. The control babies were infants from volunteers screened by clinical tests, in order to exclude any disturbances. They were also free of a family history of SIDS.

Signal processing and spectral analysis

Sleep monitoring was performed with a multichannel system developed at the Department of Medical Informatics, Graz University of Technology [6-8]. Breathing was controlled by measuring nasal air flow (NAF) with a thermistor (Siemens, Inc.) placed in front of one nostril, and by inductive plesmography (Respitrace, Inc.), which measures thoracic and abdominal diameter variations by the tension on elastic strips placed along the circumferences across the nipple and umbilicus of the baby.

As a first step of data analysis, respiratory wave forms from NAF during quiet sleep were sampled at 4 Hz. The power spectra of the respiratory signals were calculated using Fast Fourier Transformation of 2-minute epochs. In the range of 0.1 to 1.0 Hz of the respiratory spectrum (corresponding to respiratory rates between 6 and 60 breaths/min), a band with a width of 0.06 Hz (P_m) was shifted step by step to search for the greatest power value. We used the relatively broad band width of 0.06 Hz to be sure that a broad respiration peak could be detected. Visual classification of more than 100 respiratory spectra indicated that this band width is practicable. Mean respiratory frequency was defined by the center of gravity in the mean power band P_m.

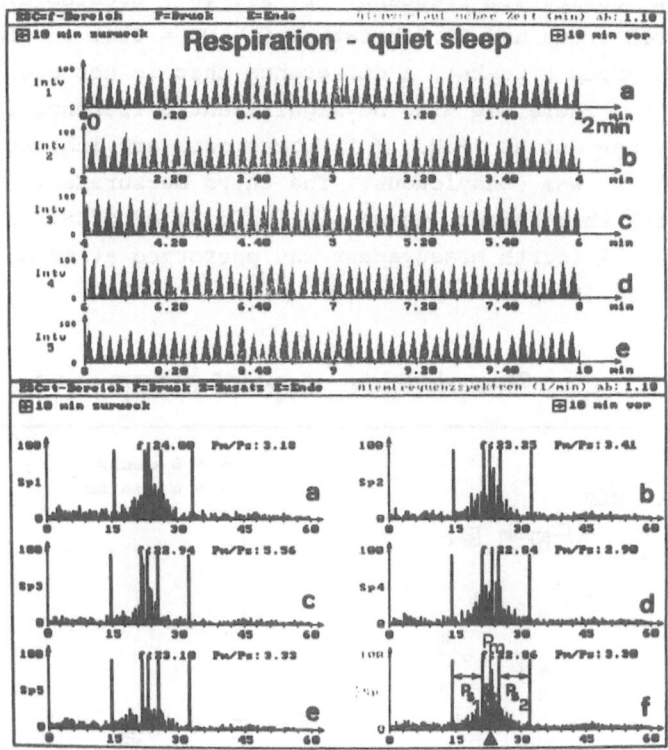

Fig. 1: Upper panel: Respiration signal from the nasal air flow during 5 X 2 minutes (a-e) of quiet sleep.
Lower panel: Respiratory spectra corresponding to the upper panel (a-e); x-axis: frequency in 1/min; y-axis: logarithmic variable. In addition, a mean-spectrum (f) is plotted. The vertical lines in each spectrum mark the band P_m and the lower and upper bands P_{s1} and P_{s2}; additionally, the mean respiratory frequency (f) and the ratio P_m/P_s are indicated.

In addition, two side bands (P_s) were defined, related to the maximum and minimum of the frequency limits of P_m, both with a band width of 0.12 Hz. To obtain a measure for the variability of respiration, the ratio P_m/P_s, where $P_s = (P_{s1} + P_{s2})/4$, was calculated. In order to determine the reproducibility of the analyses, respiratory spectra for five 2-minute epochs of data (a-e) and the normalized average spectrum (f) were calculated.

RESULTS

Figure 2 presents the data of 53 measurements in different age
groups. The respiration frequency f was 40.7 breaths/min (SD = 4.4)
in the control group and 35.7 breaths/min (SD = 6.4) in SIDS risk
infants (age group 6 weeks), a difference that is not significant (p <
0.05; t-Test). There was also no significant difference in the ratio
P_m/P_s. Only one infant (P.H., ♂), whose data are indicated with an
arrow in Fig. 2, was conspicuous. The third measurement (1 year)
performed with this infant, whose sibling died of SIDS, was out of the
normal range. A fourth measurement was performed at 15 months with
the same result (X 15 m).

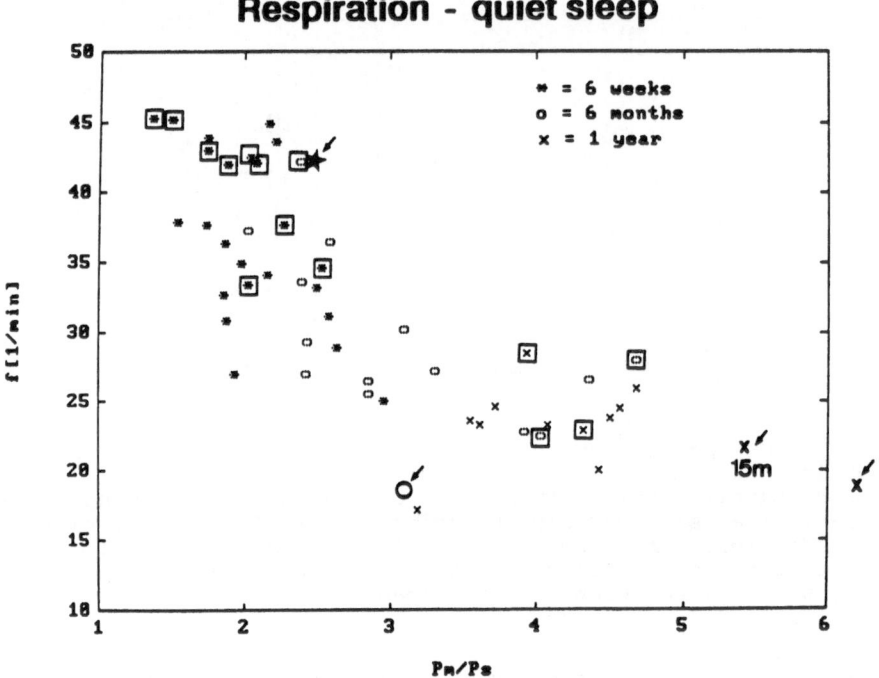

Fig. 2: x-axis: respiratory variability (P_m/P_s); y-axis: mean
respiratory frequency in 1/min. In addition to the different
symbols (* = 6 weeks (n = 25), o = 6 months (n = 15) and x = 1
year (n = 12)), the values of the control group are marked with
squares. Note the values from one infant measured four times,
marked with arrows.

Figure 3 shows a bivariate scatter plot of the ratio P_m/P_s (x-
axis) and the mean respiration frequency (y-axis) for a group of
infants aged 6 weeks (marked by squares) and a group of infants aged 1

year (marked by triangles). The empirical (shaded for the first
group) and theoretical marginal distributions along both axes, the 95%
confidence ellipses and the discrimination line are plotted. The
linear discriminant analysis yields 97.4% correct classifications.

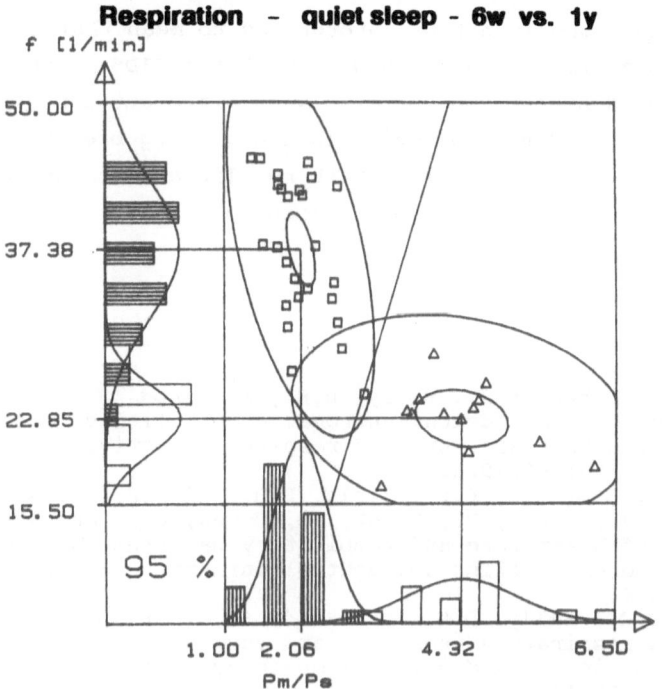

Fig. 3: Bivariate scatter plot of respiratory parameters during
quiet sleep (infants 6 weeks (□) versus 1 year (Δ)).

DISCUSSION

    There are several studies identifying increased respiratory
bandwidth during quiet breathing as a parameter that separates SIDS
babies from controls [1,3]. We applied respiratory spectral analysis
to the data from 16 infants at risk for SIDS and 9 control babies.
There was no infant which subsequently died of SIDS in the data
collection. Most risk infants had a sleep apnea syndrome (SAS). The
diagnosis of SAS was made in general in the presence of clinical
symptoms such as apneas, cyanosis during sleep, poorly coordinated
sucking, swallowing and respiration and gastroesophageal reflux in
combination with an abnormal pneumogram in a one-hour
oxycardiorespirography.

However, it was interesting that one infant, with a history of a near miss event and a sibling who died of SIDS, produced values lying out of the normal range (see Fig. 2). It was also possible to clearly discriminate between infants aged 6 weeks and infants aged 1 year (see Fig. 3).

The findings should not be interpreted to mean that higher values of the P_m/P_s measure indicate a higher risk for SIDS. The results should be used as an impetus for examining different aspects of the SIDS phenomenon. Further investigations analyzing breathing patterns in REM (rapid eye movement) sleep with non-linear methods (chaos theory) are necessary to confirm the results.

REFERENCES

[1] Gordon, D., Cohen, R.J., Kelly, D.H., Akselrod, S. and Shannon, D.C. Sudden infant death syndrome: abnormalities in short term fluctuations in heart rate and respiratory activity. Pediatr. Res., 1984, 18: 921-926.
[2] Gordon, D., Southall, D.P., Kelly, D.H., Wilson, A., Akselrod, S., Richards, J., Kenet, B., Kenet, R., Cohen, R.J. and Shannon, D.C. Analysis of heart rate and respiratory patterns in sudden infant death sysndrome victims and control infants. Pediatr. Res., 1986, 20: 680-684.
[3] Shannon, D.C., Kelly, D.H., Akselrod, S. and Kilborn, K.M. Increased respiratory frequency and variability in high risk babies who die of sudden infant death syndrome. Pediatr. Res., 1987, 22: 158-162.
[4] Kluge, K.A., Harper, R.M., Schechtman, V.L., Wilson, A.J., Hoffman, H.J. and Southall, D.P. Spectral analysis assessment of respiratory sinus arrhythmia in normal infants and infants who subsequently died of sudden infant death syndrome. Pediatr. Res., 1988, 24: 677-682.
[5] Waggener, T.B., Southall, D.P. and Scott, L.A. Analysis of breathing patterns in a prospective population of term infants does not predict susceptibility to sudden infant death syndrome. Pediatr. Res., 1990, 27: 113-117.
[6] Litscher, G., Steller, E., Klug, E.M., Reiterer, F., Schenkeli, R., Einspieler, Ch., Gallasch, E., Maresch, H., Joechtl, G., Haidmayer, R., Loescher, W., Bachler, I., Kurz, R., Kenner, T. and Pfurtscheller, G. Computer-based sleep monitoring in SIDS-risk infants - preliminary results. Biomed. Technik, 1990, 35(Erg.): 92-93.
[7] Pfurtscheller, G., Litscher, G. and Rebuffat, E. Scoring sleep stages in infants using neural networks. Proceedings of the First European Conference on Biomedical Engineering, Nice, February 1991.
[8] Steller, E., Litscher, G., Maresch, H. and Pfurtscheller, G. Multivariables Langzeit-Monitoring von zerebralen und kardiovaskulären Größen mit Hilfe eines Personal-Computers. Biomed. Technik, 1990, 35: 90-97.

ELECTRA 800 DATA MANAGEMENT PROGRAM

CAMBUS J.P.*, DOUSSET B.**, BIERME R*, VALDIGUIE P***

* Laboratoire d'Hématologie, CHU Rangueil, F-31054 Toulouse Cedex
** IRIT Université Paul Sabatier Toulouse
*** Laboratoire Biochimie CHU Rangueil

ABSTRACT

The Electra 800 automatic analyzer performs at high speed and with great precision almost all chronometric coagulation tests. However, the results have to be recopied by hand and if necessary converted using standard graphs if the machine does not have the Data Management option. We therefore developed a data management program for this analyzer, for use with a PC or AT (IBM®) compatible microcomputer.

For standardization of the various tests, the linearity is checked and the points retained are memorized.

All the patients data are grouped on an "electronic worksheet" which allows control, correction of the results and the inclusion of results obtained by another technique.

A printout of each patients file can be produced for the prescribing physician. A daily archive function classifies and prints the whole of the day's work in alphabetical order.

Key words : ELECTRA 800 - COAGULATION TESTER MICRO COMPUTER

INTRODUCTION

The Electra 800, manufactured by MLA, is a semi-automatic coagulation analyzer which carries out almost all chronometric coagulation tests.

As the analyzer only has two peristaltic pumps for the reagents, it can only carry out one type of test at a time. However, it works at a very high speed because of its four photo-optic cells which operate simultaneously. These cells are of excellent quality and their performance is comparable with that of the cells of the Electra 700, considered as being among the best [1,2].

The Electra 800 prints out on a continuous strip of heat-sensitive paper the coagulation times either uncorrected or also converted into percentages, IU/ml or g/l if the machine is equipped with the optional data management module, it is capable of memorizing seven standard curves.

However, this mode has some limitations. Prothrombin time can be given in percentage or INR (after entering a linear curve in a log-log mode) but not both at the same time.

Conversions are carried out between the minimum and maximum points and they cannot be extrapolated above or below these values.

The analyzer is connected to a central computer via an RS-232 communication port. However, it is not possible to enter the patients identification number from the Electra 800. An identification file must therefore be prepared in the central computer before transferring the results, or identification must be made a posteriori from the sequential order of the sample. There is then a risk of error by inversion, or more seriously by shifting of the entire series.

In order to reduce these disadvantages to a minimum, we have written a program to connect the Electra 800 to a microcomputer which will carry out all these tasks.

MATERIAL AND METHODS

1) Microcomputer

The program is written in Turbo C (Borland®) and is suitable for any PC or AT (IBM®) compatible computer with an MS/DOS exploitation system (Microsoft®). It most have 640 Ko random access memory, a hard disk and an RS-232 communication port.

2) Electra 800

The RS-232 communication port of the Electra 800 must be exactly matched with that of the microcomputer (bauds, bits per character, stop bit, parity), using the SW2 block of internal switchs [3].

3) Cable

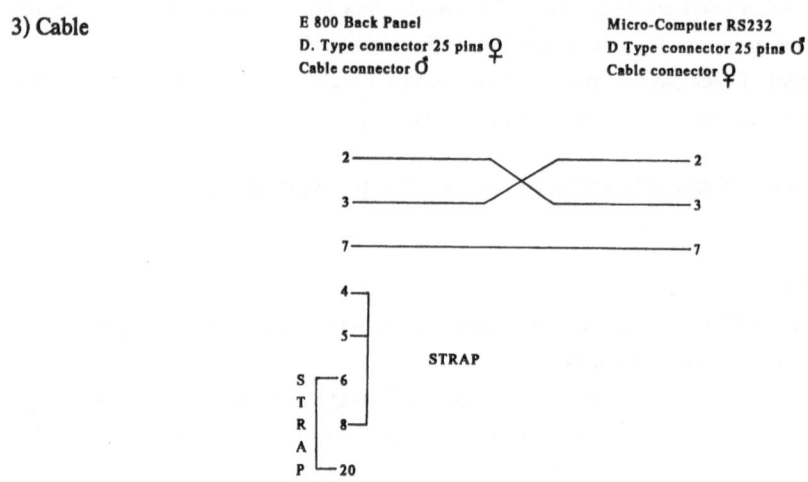

Figure 1 : Electra 800 connecting cable

THE FUNCTIONS OF THE PROGRAM

For ease of use, there is a main menu with only one level of sub-menu according to the option chosen. In order to avoid time-consuming input of codes, the choice is made by moving the cursor on the screen or by typing the code letter which precedes each option.

A help menu, displayed by a function key, permanently indicates the possibilities available to the technician position within the program.

1) Setting of standards

For tests requiring conversion, the introduction of a standard range is followed by a graphic display which allows visual control of the quality of standard curve.

It is possible to select the type of curve (linear, hyperbolic, sigmoid) and the type of scale (linear, log-log or semi-log).

An algorithm deletes the unaligned points, and cancels the standardization, which most be repeated if the number of points falls below three. On the graphic display, the unaligned points are displayed differently.

A particular case is the measurement of fibrinogen using the method of Von Clauss [4]. The limits of linearity of the technique are taken into account. If the coagulation time is below the minimal limit, the result is not converted and a message on the printer indicates that the test must be rerun with a higher dilution. It is repeated with a lower dilution if the time is above the upper limit.

The standards are then memorized on the disc and the graph can be displayed and printed at any time.

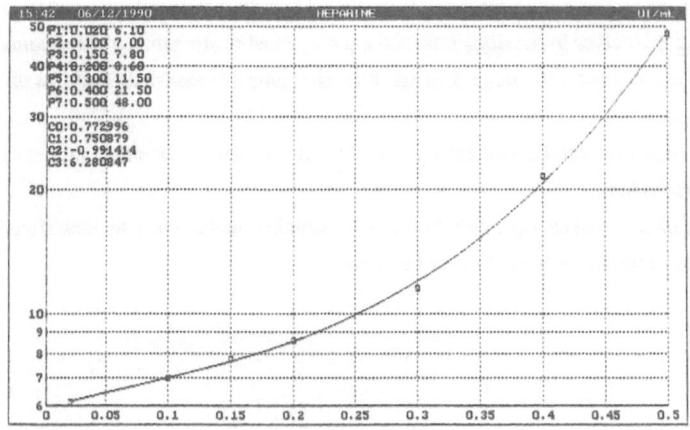

Figure 2 : Example of standard curve

2) Identification of the wells and saving of the results.

After the type of test to be carried out has been selected, the 15 positions of the tray of the Electra 800 are organized in such a way that the technician can enter the identification number of each patient in the space reserved for each reaction well. The double determination mode avoids the possibility of introducing a patient identification number twice by duplicating it.

Different tests can be carried out on a same tray if the same reagent is used in the tests, for example measurement of factors V, VII, X, II.

As soon as the results are obtained, they are recorded on the disc in order to avoid loss. The file is then sorted and the results expressed as percentage or g/l are converted using the memorized standards. Prothrombin time is converted into both PT% and INR.

The technician can use either single or double determination. If double determination is used for a test either simultaneously or later, the mean of the two tests is calculated automatically if the coefficient of variation (CV) between the two tests does not exceed the value introduced when the reference parameters of the test were entered. If the CV is greater, a printed message tells the technician to repeat the test a third. The mean is calculated with the nearest result if the CV is lower than the predefined limit. If the three results differ widely, they are cancelled and the program advises the laboratorian to go through the whole test again, while indicating that the problem may be due to a faulty reagent, thermal instability or a defect of the photo-optic cell.

3) Visualization of the tests

An electronic worksheet presents the results by pages of ten. This enables the technician to assess the coherence of the various results and to carry out checks or complementary tests if necessary.

The results obtained on the Electra 800 by single determination are displayed in normal mode. If double determination is used, the mean is underlined when displayed. If the mean has not been calculated, due to a CV above the security limit, the result is displayed on a flashing mode for operator attention.

By moving the cursor in the divisions of the table, a test result can be deleted, modified or added. Results of tests not carried out using Electra 800 can thus be inserted, such as bleeding time or immunological assays.

Results which are entered manually have absolute priority over other modes of entry and are displayed in reverse video.

A search function makes it possible to find a file quickly, using either its identification number, the name of the patient or the first letters of his or her name.

TEMPS DE THROMBINE: 10 < 19 sec < 99   Temoin=17

			TQ	TP	INR	TCK	FIB	TT	F.V	F.VII	F.X	F.II
DUPONT	P	1	12.0	100	1.22	55	3.22	18				
DURAND	J	2	12.1	100	_D_	42	_D_		_D_	_D_	_D_	_D_
SMITH	L	3	15.0	71	1.42	33						
VALDIGUIE	P	4	12.8	100	1.35			19				
CAMBUS	J	5	_D_	_D_	_D_		_D_	_D_	_D_	_D_		
BIERME	R	6	12.0	100	1.22	35	4.20					
ARAGON	B	7	18.0	46	1.86	55			99	20	19	23
WESSON	P	8	12.5	100	1.30	33		_D_	_D_	_D_	_D_	_D_
MARTIN	R	9	11.9	100	1.21	35						
DUPONT	A	10	16.0	60	1.56	32			100	50	99	99

F1:Aide...   F2:Dossier Complet   F3:Recherche Dossier   F4:Dossier suivant   16:00

Figure 3 : Electronic worksheet

4) Quality control

This function checks for a statistically detectable drift of the automat reagent couple, using a 30 day Levey-Jennings diagram

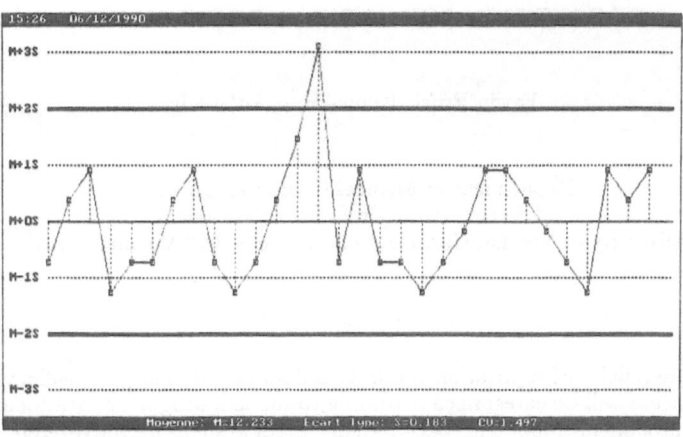

Figure 4 : Quality control curve

5) Patient identification

If there is no central computer, this option makes it possible to add the surname, first name, hospital department or prescribing physician to the identification number. On the electronic flowchart, the tests to be carried out are indicated by the sign --D--.

6) Printout

Using this mode, the results of each patient can be printed out on an individual sheet directly sent for the prescribing physician.

7) Printing of daily archives

This mode prints out in a condensed form all the biological files of the day in alphabetical order.

AVAILABILITY OF THE PROGRAM

This program is available on request from our laboratory. Please send us a floppy disc on which we will copy the program and its documentation (3 1/2" 1.4 Mo or 720 Ko or 5 1/4" 1.2 Mo).

CONCLUSION

The various functions offered by this software increase the usefulness of the Electra 800 automatic analyzer, whose high-quality photo-optic cells and the speed at which it works make it a precious tool.

REFERENCES

1 - Walenga JM, Hoppenstead D, Fareed J, Silberman S, Shevlin P. Automated clot-based methods in coagulation testing : current and future considerations. Seminars thromb. Hemost. 1983 ; 9 : 239-243.

2 - Sher PP. New instrumentation preview Electra 700. J. Clin. Lab. Autom. 1981; 1 : 95-97.

3 - Electra 800 Service Manual. Medical Laboratory Automation, Mount Vernon, N-Y, 1986.

4 - Clauss (Von) A Gerinnungsphysiologische Schnell methode zur Bestimmung des fibrinogens. Acta. Haematol. 1957 ; 17 : 237-246.

ROBOTICS IN MEDICINE: A BRIEF SURVEY

Erwin Ernst, Klaus-Peter Adlassnig

Department of Medical Computer Sciences
(Director: Univ.Prof. Dr. G. Grabner)
University of Vienna, Garnisongasse 13, A – 1090 Vienna, Austria

Abstract

A survey on different fields of application of robots and robot technology in medicine is presented. Robotics applications will be categorized according to the following areas: stationary laboratory robot systems, autonomous robot transport systems, robot systems for the severely handicapped, robot patient simulators, and robot applications in surgery. It is argued that robots and robot technology will be used in medicine at a more rapid pace than anticipated.

1. Introduction

Since the 1950s new technologies have effected major changes in the health field. Beside computerized axial tomography (CAT), scanners, diagnostic sonography, magnetic resonance imaging, thermography, and radioisotopes, we are experiencing today a second wave of development—spearheaded by the computer—in which robots play an ever greater role [25].

However, most industrial robots are designed for a specific purpose and unless subjected to extensive modifications do not lend themselves for use in the medical field. It was only in the last few years that systems with specialized, medically-oriented hard and software have come into more widespread use, sometimes equipped with gripper arms designed especially for various medical applications. Thus the robots can be "reprogrammed" to carry out highly specific tasks, in contrast to systems which cannot be reconfigured ("hard automation") [4,25].

2. Different fields of application of robots and robot technology in medicine

Today approximately 50% of the most common robot applications in hospitals are related to laboratory tasks; another 25% are related to medical care services. According to current estimates, the introduction of robots in hospitals could reduce personnel requirements to 10–15% in the future [1].

Table 1 gives an overview about different fields of application of robots or robot technology in medicine and provides several examples that fall into one of the established categories.

Stationary laboratory robot systems

The use of robots in laboratories is probably the least controversial area of application. The bulk of laboratory work consists of time-consuming steps in the preparation and testing of specimens; procedures that are tedious and often bring the staff into contact with toxic substances.

Procedures such as chromatography, spectral analysis, and infrared spectrography have greatly simplified the analysis of specimens and increased the precision in measuring specimen substances. Additionally improved test procedures such as radio-immunoassays and enzyme-immunoassays, now make it possible to detect a large number of biological substances [6,12,13,14,16, 23,27,34].

Table 1: Application fields of robot systems and robot technology in medicine.

Robot Systems in Medicine

Stationary Laboratory Robot Systems

General descriptions [5,11,34]
Robot system for chromatography tests [12,14,23,27]
Analysis of drugs in biological fluids [13]
Robot system for blood tests [34]
Immunochemical determination of cardiac isoenzymes [6]
Automating extraction methods for food samples [16]

Autonomous Robot Transport Systems

HELPMATE—mobile hospital robot [20]
LABMATE—mobile hospital robot [10]
ROBOTEK—robot assistant for pharmacy [25]

Robot Systems for the Severely Handicapped

Control of prostheses [2,19,24,26,29]
Assistance for quadriplegics in routine functions [7,8,17,33]
SICO—robot for mentally handicapped [25]

Robot Patient Simulators

General descriptions [36]
Mechanical simulation of human body joints [15,28,35,36]
Anaesthesiology and cardiology training [1]

Robot Application in Surgery

Stereotactic neurosurgery [18,21,25,37]
Automated biopsy devices [3]
Surgeon robot prostatectomy [9]
Removal of port wine stains and other angiodysplasias [32]
Robot assistant in microsurgery [25]

To be effective, however, all of these procedures require that the specimens are prepared and handled with the utmost precision. Typical tasks carried out by laboratory robots are: manipulation, liquid handling, separation, conditioning, pulverization, weighing, and measurement [34]. Today the use of robots has highly increased even in such routine clinical tests as determining blood glucose, urea nitrogen, or electrolytes. However, a significant number of other testing procedures have not been automated as yet. Among them are—on the one hand—several routine examinations which are carried out in every large hospital; still, those tests can usually be performed only by specialized laboratories (e.g., serologic tests for hepatitis) and their automation would be rather expensive. On the other hand, these are procedures which are difficult to automate and therefore will be conducted manually for some time until new advances of robotics technology are being made. At present, there are mainly three different robotic systems in practical use: The Minimover-5 (Microbot, Menlo Park, CA, USA), the Puma (Unimation, Inc., Danbury, CT, USA), and the Zymate Laboratory Automation System (Zymark Corp., Hopkins, MA, USA) [34]. The Zymate System is of particular interest because it is a unique system which was developed especially for highly-automated sample handling.

In general, the application of stationary laboratory robot systems makes it possible to increase the number of tests conducted per unit of time, while at the same time the intervals between subsequent tests are reduced [5,11].

Autonomous robot transport systems

Today materials handling systems [22,30,31] are being developed more and more as mobile and autonomous robot systems. For example, HELPMATE [19] is a mobile robot handling meal distribution in hospitals. It is especially suited for tasks where a high quantity (nearly 90% in a certain hospital) of the demanded meals are special orders due to various dietary requirements of patients. HELPMATE is equipped with a vision system, sonar and infrared sensors, enabling it to navigate successfully along the corridors of the hospital. LABMATE [10] is a robot vehicle especially designed for hospital use, consisting of a chassis unit and drive controls as well as extensive sensor equipment. The basic system can be modified by means of interface routines for application programming to suit a wide range of tasks. ROBOTEK [25] is a robot assistant used in pharmacies and hospitals, where it selects automatically (from up to five hundred drugs) and delivers the daily medications for each patient, predesignated by the physician for verification by the personnel. Further applications are, for example, sweeping of hospital corridors, handling and sorting of dirty sheets in the laundry where the staff might be exposed to contamination, or control and inspection of important areas of the hospital, such as the pharmacy [4].

Robot systems for the severely handicapped

There are two basic areas of application:

a) After amputation, arms or legs may be replaced by a prosthesis. These applications are already quite advanced [24]. The aim is to control as many functions of the prosthesis as possible with the few muscles that are still functioning [2]. In this way, some important body functions may be regained [19,26,29].

b) Assistance in necessary routine functions difficult or impossible to perform by the handicapped person. For example, the only way a quadriplegic can eat or drink without help by another person is with the assistance of voice-controlled robot systems [7,8,33]. Some of these systems can also be modified to carry out other tasks [15,17].

SICO [25] is a mobile robot which moves around the room, speaks several languages, and is used to assist in the treatment of the mentally handicapped. Even autistic children are made aware of the world around them by the robot's simple movements and its use of language.

Robot patient simulators

The sequence patterns of human movement must be thoroughly understood [36] to develop the kind of systems for handicapped persons as described above. Systems of this type attempting to simulate certain parts of the human body [28,35] are also often used to train medical students in areas such as anaesthesiology and cardiology. Above all, the cooperation of experts in biomechanics, neurophysiology, biology, and many other fields is necessary to gain more knowledge in this area. For example, the human hand cannot be simulated realistically by a computer unless there is a thorough understanding of its function and its motional sequences, perhaps even an understanding of the human dexterity or skill related to certain kinetic mechanisms [15,35].

Robot application in surgery ·

The main reason for the slowness in introducing robots in the field of surgery is the safety consideration. At present, it is primarily auxiliary functions that robots perform in this area. However, the development of computer tomography makes it possible to establish more precise facts than ever before for example regarding the localization of tumors. In particular for stereotactic operations in neurosurgery, robot systems are being used with increasing frequency [18,21,37]. Here, the stereotactic device is attached to the skull in accordance to its external bone structure. A robot analyzes the CAT data, then drills a hole precisely at the desired spot. Subsequent to this procedure, the system can place a probe inside the skull for a biopsy [3] at exactly the correct angle to the actual targeted point.

Another application which is presently tested is a surgeon robot for prostatectomies [9]. A prostatectomy involves removal of some or all of the prostate gland tissue which has grown to block the urinary tract. This requires the surgeon to continuously view the operation through an endoscope attached to the end of the cutting instrument. This together with the wide angle variations of the instruments can cause the surgeons to develop chronic neck and back pains in their later lives. With the robot system, the surgeon now only inserts the endoscope at the beginning of the operation, the robot makes all necessary movements for surgery. The surgeon has the opportunity to interrupt the operation by pressing a key at any point in the process.

There is also a system currently in use which is able to remove port wine stains and other forms of angiodysplasia [32]. In microsurgery, attempts are now being made to transfer the surgeon's hand movements directly to a robot arm to achieve even finer and more precise movements [25].

3. Discussion

Robotic technology is being used in health care at a more rapid pace than many believed before. Perhaps within the next 10 years, robots and robot technology will be utilized at a greater rate not only in laboratories but also as supplementary systems in clinical medicine and health care. Robotic technology cannot replace human care but it can aid in increasing the quality of care provided by health care professionals to patients [4,25].

Acknowledgement. The authors are indebted to F. Alesch, M.D., for various help.

References

[1] Anderson, J.G. (1987) Hospitals of the Future. In Anderson, J.G. & Jay, S.J. (Eds.) *Use and Impact of Computers in Clinical Medicine.* Springer Verlag, Berlin, 346–347.

[2] Balasubramamian, R. & Scott, R.N. (1981) Pattern Recognition Techniques for Multifunction Prosthesis Control. In *Proc. of the 8th Triennial World Congress*, Japan, 3693–3698.

[3] Bernardino, M.E. (1990) Automated Biopsy Devices: Significance and Safety. *Radiology* **9**, 615–616.

[4] Boissoneau, R. & Anderson, D. (1984) Robotic technology in Health Care Settings. *Hospital Topics* **6**, 8–11.

[5] Boyd, J.C. & Felder, R.A. (1987) Use of a Robotic Arm for Specimen Handling in a Remote, Unmanned Clinical Chemistry Laboratory. *Clinical Chemistry* **33**, 1560–1561.

[6] Castellani, W.J., Van Lente, F. & Chou, D. (1986) Robotic Sample Preparation for the Immunochemical Determination of Cardiac Isoenzymes. *Clinical Chemistry* **32**, 1672–1676.

[7] Cheatham, J.B., Regalbuto, M.A., Krouskop, T.A. & Winningham, D.J. (1987) A Mobile Robotic System as an Aid for the Severely Handicapped. In *IEEE—Ninth Annual Conference of the Engineering in Medicine and Biology Society*, 1100–1101.

[8] Cheatham, J.B., Regalbuto, M.A., Krouskop, T.A. & Winningham, D.J. (1988) A Robotic System for Improved Living by Severely Disabled Persons. In *Proc. of the IEEE Int. Workshop of Intelligent Robots and Systems*, 79–82.

[9] Davies, B.L., Hibberd, R.D., Coptcoat, M.J. & Wickham, J.E. (1989) A Surgeon Robot Prostatectomy—a Laboratory Evolution. Journal of Medical Engineering and Technology **13**, 273–277.

[10] Engelberger, J. (1988) Roboter für Dienstleistungen. *Roboter* **4**, 32–33.

[11] Felder, R., Boyd, J., Margrey, K., Martinez, A. & Vaughn, D. (1988) Robotics in the Clinical Laboratory. *Clinics in Laboratory Medicine* **8**, 699–711.

[12] Fouda, H.G. (1989) Robotics in Biomedical Chromatography and Electrophoresis. *Journal of Chromatography* **492**, 85–108.

[13] Fouda, H.G. & Schneider, R.P. (1987) Robotics for the Bioanalytical Laboratory. A Flexible System for the Analysis of Drugs in Biological Fluids. *Trends in Analytical Chemistry* **6**, 139–147.

[14] Fouda, H.G., Twomey, T.M. & Schneider, R.P. (1988) Liquid Chromatographic Analysis of Doxazosin in Human Serum with Manual and Robotic Sample Preparation. *Journal of Chromatographic Science* **26**, 570–573.

[15] Grupen, R.A., Henderson, T.C. & McCammon, I.D. (1989) A Survey of General Purpose Manipulation. *The International Journal of Robotics Research* **8**, 38–62.

[16] Higgs, D.J. & Vanderslice, J.T. (1987) Application and Flexibility of Robotics in Automating Extraction Methods for Food Samples. *Journal of Chromatographic Science* **25**, 187–191.

[17] Horowitz, D.M. & Hausdorff, J.M. (1990) Rehabilitation Robotics at Tufts New England Medical Center. *Robotics and Automation* **4**, 7–8.

[18] Hou, J., Kwoh, Y., Jonckheere, E.A. & Hayati, S. (1988) A Robot with Improved Absolute Positioning Accuracy for CT Guided Stereotactic Brain Surgery. *IEEE Transactions on Biomedical Engineering* **35**, 153–160.

[19] Khalili, D. & Zemlefer, M. (1988) An Intelligent Robotic System for Rehabilitation of Joints and Estimation of Body Segment Parameters. *IEEE Transactions on Biomedical Engineering* **35**, 138–146.

[20] Krishnamurthy, B., Barrows, B., King, S., Skewis, T., Pong, W. & Weiman, C. (1989) Help Mate—A Mobile Robot for Transport Applications. In *Proc. SPIE—Int. Soc. Opt. Eng.*, 314–320.

[21] Lavallee, S., Cinquin, P., Demongeot, J., Benabid, A.L., Marque, I. & Djaid, M. (1989) Computer Assisted Interventionist Imaging. The Instance of Stereotactic Brain Surgery. *Journal of Medical Engineering and Technology* **13**, 163–169.

[22] Layman, J. (1986) Hospitals Convert Supply Transport. *Robotics World* **12**, 30–32.

[23] Luders, R.C. & Brunner, L.A. (1987) Automated Sample Preparation and Chromatographic Analysis: Determination of CGS 10787B and Related Compounds. *Journal of Chromatographic Science* **25**, 192–197.

[24] Martin, D.A., Zomlefer, M.R. & Onal, A. (1989) Human Upper Limb Dynamics. *Robotics and Autonomous Systems* **5**, 151–163.

[25] Palkon, D.S. (1984) Robotic Technology in Health Care Settings. *Hospital Topics* **6**, 12–17.

[26] Perlin, K., Demmel, J.W. & Wright, P.K. (1989) Simulation Software for the Utah MIT Dextrous Hand. *Robotics and Computer Integrated Manufacturing* **5**, 281–292.

[27] Pivnichny, J.V., Lawrence, A.A. & Stong, J.D. (1987) A Robotic Sample Preparation Scheme for the High Performance Liquid Chromatographic Determination of Ivermectin in Animal Plasma. *Journal of Chromatographic Science* **25**, 181–186.

[28] Raibert, M.H. & Sutherland, I.E. (1983) Maschinen zu Fuß. *Spektrum der Wissenschaften* **3**, 30–40.

[29] Rakic, M. (1989) Multifingered Robot Hand With Selfadaptability. *Robotics and Computer Integrated Manufacturing* **5**, 269–276.

[30] Regalbuto, M.A., Cheatham, J.B. & Krouskop, T.A. (1989) A Model Based Graphics Interface for Controlling a Semi-Autonomous Mobile Robot. In *IEEE EMBS Conf.*, Seattle, WA, USA.

[31] Regalbuto, M.A., Fisher, P.B., Adnan, S., Norwood, J.D. & Weiland, P.L. (1988) A Navigation System Framework for a Semi Autonomous Mobile Robot. In *IEEE Engineering in Medicine & Biology Society, 10th Annual Int. Conf.*, 1511–1512.

[32] Rotteleur, G, Mordon, S., Buys, B., Sozanski, J.P. & Brunetaud, J.M. (1988) Robotized Scanning Laser Handpiece for the Treatment of Port Wine Stains and Other Angiodysplasias. *Lasers in Surgery and Medicine* **8**, 283–287.

[33] Seamone, W (1984) The Application of Robotics to the Patient with High Spinal Cord Injury (Quadriplegia). The Robotic Arm-Work Table. In Brady, M. et al. (Eds.) *Robotics and Artificial Intelligence*. NATO ASI Series, Vol. F11, Springer, Berlin, 645–664.

[34] Severns, M.L. & Hawk, G.L. (1984) Automation of Sample Preparation. In Brady, M. et al. (Eds.) *Robotics and Artificial Intelligence*. NATO ASI Series, Vol. F11, Springer, Berlin, 633–643.

[35] Thompson, D.E. (1981) Biomechanics of the Hand. *Perspectives in Computing* **1**, 12–19.

[36] Tomovic, R. (1989) Transfer of Motor Skills to Machines. *Robotics and Computer Integrated Manufacturing* **5**, 261–267.

[37] Young, R.F. (1987) Application of Robotics to Stereotactic Neurosurgery. *Neurological Research* **9**, 123–128.

DEMONSTRATIONS

EXPERT SYSTEMS AND DECISION MAKING

INTEGRATED MEDICAL DATABASE AND EXPERT SYSTEM HEPAXPERT-II: AUTOMATIC INTERPRETATION OF TESTS FOR HEPATITIS A AND B

Klaus-Peter Adlassnig[1], Wolfgang Horak[1,2], Clemens Chizzali-Bonfadin[1]

[1]Department of Medical Computer Sciences, (Director: Prof. Dr. G. Grabner)
University of Vienna, Garnisongasse 13, A - 1090 Vienna, Austria
and
[2]2nd Department for Gastroenterology and Hepatology, (Director: Prof. Dr. G. Grabner)
University of Vienna, Garnisongasse 13, A - 1090 Vienna, Austria

The HEPAXPERT-II system

HEPAXPERT-II—the successor of HEPAXPERT-I [1]—is an integrated medical database and expert system that stores and interprets the results of routine serologic tests for infection with hepatitis A and B viruses. The following tests are included: hepatitis A virus antibodies (anti-HAV), IgM antibodies to the hepatitis A virus (IgM anti-HAV), hepatitis A virus (HAV) in stool, hepatitis B surface antigen (HBsAg) and antibodies (anti-HBs), antibodies to hepatitis B core antigen (anti-HBc and IgM anti-HBc), and hepatitis B envelope antigen (HBeAg) and antibodies (anti-HBe).

HEPAXPERT-II provides the following database functions: (a) screen input of patient's personal data (patient ID, surname, first name, name at birth, date of birth, sex), administrative data (department requiring the tests, date of specimen sample), and medical data (results of serologic tests where four qualitative results are possible: positive, negative, borderline, and not tested); and/or (b) automatic transfer of patient's personal, administrative, and medical data by connecting HEPAXPERT-II to a laboratory information system, a hospital information system [2], or an automated laboratory analyzer that provides and downloads the respective data.

After screen input or automatic transfer of data, HEPAXPERT-II automatically generates interpretive reports of the obtained serologic findings including an analysis of possible virus exposition, immunity, disease stage, prognosis, and degree of infectiousness. These interpretations are transferred to the department requiring the tests and help physicians explain what are often complex serologic findings.

Since February 15, 1991, HEPAXPERT-II has been routinely used at the Hepatitis Serology Laboratory of the 2nd Department for Gastroenterology and Hepatology of the University of Vienna Medical School (Vienna General Hospital).

Hardware and software

IBM-AT, PS/2 (minimum 80286 processor) or 100% compatible systems, 640 KB RAM, monochrome or color graphics monitor (CGA, EGA, VGA, HERCULES), PC/DOS or MS/DOS version 3.1 or higher or 100% compatible, one diskette drive (720 KB or more) and one hard disk (minimum 1.5 MB disk space for program and initialized database).

Acknowledgements. This research was partly supported by Bender+Co Ges mbH, Vienna, Austria. We would like to thank D. Laner, M.Sc., J. Gamper, M.Sc., and W. Temsch for their excellent programming work and A. Marksteiner, Ph.D., for his manifold assistance.

References

[1] Adlassnig, K.-P. & Horak, W. (1990) Routinely-Used, Automated Interpretive Analysis of Hepatitis A and B Serology Findings by a Medical Expert System. In *Proc. MIE'90*, Springer-Verlag, Berlin, 313–318.

[2] Grabner, G. (Ed.) (1985) *WAMIS — Wiener Allgemeines Medizinisches Informations-System.* Springer-Verlag, Berlin.

VARY – THE FIRST EXPERT SYSTEM FOR ANALYSIS OF GENOME VARIABILITY

Ch. Wojahn, University of Technology, Ahornstr. 55, D-5100 Aachen

R. Hofestädt, University of Koblenz-Landau, Rheinau 3-4, D-5400 Koblenz

H.-P. Müller, University of Bonn, Kirschallee, D-5300 Bonn

Abstract:

In the research field of human genetics one of the important tasks is to consider populations with common with genepools. However, there are many factors that influence the population as a whole and affect the destiny of each individual by passing on genes. Moreover, the coherence between population and environment (including their mutual relationship) is important.

VARY is the first expert system which allows automatic analysis of genetic examinations. The goal of this expert system is to support practical genetic work both by biochemical characterization of the population and by the realization of morphologic and cytologic comparisons.

VARY is based on a well known algorithm which allows the analysis and description of the genepool. This algorithm was developed by Nei /72, 73/. The output from Nei's algorithm are gene diversity and the genetic distance between populations which represent two important goals in gene analysis.

The further development of this algorithm allows the examination of morphological characteristics which describe the phenotype. These morphological features are compared to the genetic diversity and, if a correlation is found, the expert system defines a hypothesis.

The developed software will support and automate the evaluation, analysis and storage of genetic variability considerations. Moreover, VARY is the first system that enables the automation of generation, registration and administration from hypothesis of the genotype-phenotype and genotype-environment correlation.

VARY is implemented in the logical programming language Turbo-Prolog. Execution is possible on any IBM-AT or compatible computer.

Nei, M. (1972):   Genetic distance between populations;
                  The Americ. Naturalist 106, 283-293

Nei, M. (1973):   Analysis of gene diversity in subdivided populations;
                  Proc. Natl. Accad. Sci. USA 70, 3321-3323

PEN&PAD: A Multi-Lingual Patient Care Workstation based on a Unified Representation of the Medical Record and Medical Terminology

WA Nowlan, S Kay, AL Rector, B Horan and A Wilson.
Medical Informatics Group, Department of Computer Science,University of Manchester, Manchester, M13 9PL, United Kingdom.Tel: +44-61-275-6133, Fax: +44-61-275-6236

PEN&PAD is prototype patient care workstation developed using a process of user centred design. Our goal is a radically improved human computer environment for doctors and other clinicians which will be useful and usable in routine patient care. PEN&PAD is a complete clinical record system based on the ideas described elsewhere in this conference [1]. It uses a unified knowledge based representation of the medical record and medical terminology, Structured Meta Knowledge (SMK) [2].

PEN&PAD provides for the recording and display of clinical notes using a graphical user interface. It combines rapid data entry using structured forms with a problem oriented display of the medical record. The aim is to capture all of the clinical information in existing narrative records in a structured representation .

The system has been refined through a process of user centred design which involves cycles of prototype development allied with formative assessment workshops conducted by an external team [3].

The user interface is driven by the underlying representation of medical terminology. This is most easily seen in the data entry forms. The content of the data entry form for any given topic is generated by asking the knowledge base a) what is it medically sensible to say about that topic; b) what are the key associated signs, symptoms and managements,; and c) what is it sensible to say about each associated item.

The information may be appear as graphs, tables, or narrative text. All text items are generated from the underlying representation. Multi-lingual systems are therefore easy to build, since the choice of language in which to generate the text is independent of the information held in the record. Information can be entered on a form generated in one language and displayed in another language. Because the terminology is compact, the effort required to produce and maintain versions in a other languages is minimised.

The user centred design process identified flexibility as the key requirement for clinical information systems. Because the appearance of the PEN&PAD user interface is determined by the information in its knowledge base, the user interface can be easily modified and tailored to the requirements of individual clinicians. SMK provides a uniform way to specify special cases and variations.

References

1.   Kay, S, Rector, AL, Nowlan, WA, Goble, CA, Horan, B, Howkins, TJ and Wilson, A, 1991, "What *Should* we mean by 'An Electronic Medical Record' ?, these proceedings.
2.   Rector, AL, Nowlan, WA, Kay, S, 1990, "Unifying Medical Knowledge using an architecture based on descriptions", in *Proceedings of the Symposium on Computer Applications in Medical Care*, pp.190-194, IEEE Computer Society Press, Los Alamitos, California.
3.   Rector, AL, Fitter, M, Horan, Wilson, A, Kay, S, Newton, PD, Nowlan, WA, Robinson, D, 1991, "User Centred Design and Formative Evaluation in the Design of a Clinical Workstation: The PEN&PAD Experience", submitted to SCAMC'91.

CONSULTATION SYSTEM FOR INSULIN DOSAGE ADJUSTMENT

R. HOVORKA[1,2], S. SVACINA[2] AND E.R. CARSON[1]

[1] Department of Systems Science, City University, London, U.K.
[2] 3rd Medical Department, Charles University, Prague, Czechoslovakia

Insulin treatment belongs to one of the most difficult tasks in the management of diabetic patients. Numerous factors have to be considered before making the therapeutic decision. In order to assist the diabetologist in making the therapeutic decisions and in order to assist an unspecialised clinician or a patient himself to advise and to critique on insulin therapy, a computer system "Consultation System" has been developed. The system comprises three components: model of carbohydrate metabolism, learning module and advisory module.

First a model of carbohydrate metabolism is implemented. It takes into account absorption and kinetics of various insulin preparations, food absorption and physical activity; the model is a discrete time model with a one hour step. Individual parameters are included in the model, e.g. sensitivity parameters and basal insulin profile parameter. Second these parameters are learned from a patient's data on a day-to-day basis. A weighted linear regression analysis is employed. Third using the individual parameters the effect of alternative insulin therapies can be simulated. A risk is assigned to each therapy according to the predicted blood glucose profile. In addition, as the predictions are uncertain due to several simplifications having been made and the nature of the patient's data, an additional risk is added according to the deviation from the previous therapy. The additional risk is weighted according to the precision of model predictions: the more precise the model predictions the less the weight of this additional risk. Finally the therapy with the minimal risk is recommended.

A preliminary retrospective study has been carried out using patients' historic data. Blood glucose was predicted with the mean absolute error of 2.5 mmol/l after 5 days of learning [1].

The system is implemented on PC-based computers, it requires at least 340 kB RAM, a numeric coprocessor is recommended.

REFERENCES

1. HOVORKA, R., S. SVACINA, E.R. CARSON, C.D. WILLIAMS, and P.H. SONKSEN. A consultation system for insulin therapy. *Comput. Methods Programs Biomed.* 32:303-310, 1990.

A METABOLIC PROTOTYPE TO ASSIST IN THE MANAGEMENT OF INSULIN-TREATED DIABETIC PATIENTS

E.D. Lehmann, T. Deutsch, E.R. Carson and P.H. Sönksen

Department of Endocrinology and Chemical Pathology, United Medical and Dental Schools, St. Thomas's Hospital, London SE1 7EH, U.K.

A prototype computer system has been developed to provide advice on the day-to-day adjustment of carbohydrate intake and insulin regimen in the diabetic patient. The prototype is intended to be used as a decision support system by clinical personnel in the context of day-to-day management of insulin-treated diabetic patients. It is designed for use during consultations, as a simulator of patient response following changed insulin and dietary regimen and as a system to provide education on planning insulin therapy. Advice is generated by a qualitative knowledge based system (KBS) which suggests what the next step in improving glycaemic control might be for a given patient, e.g. 'decrease evening medium-acting insulin'. A model of glucose-insulin interaction has been developed to simulate the effects of these adjustments on the patient's blood glucose profile.

An integrated system will be presented which links the KBS and model together with external data collection devices. The system runs under DOS on an IBM PC or compatible. A multitasking version is also available for 80386 based machines running WINDOWS 3.0. This allows the display of multiple windows showing different parts of the system in operation. For example data entry screens can be displayed in one window with advice from the KBS in a second and the results of a simulation in a third; the number of windows displayed at any one time being wholly dependent on the memory capabilities of the machine. All code for the model and connected data processing has been implemented in TURBO PASCAL while the KBS is written in MicroPROLOG using an APES expert system shell.

An overview of the prototype will be provided and its operation illustrated by case studies from insulin-treated diabetic patients. A more detailed description of the system and the results of some preliminary medical validation work are provided by Lehmann et al separately in the Conference Proceedings [1].

Reference:

1. Lehmann et al (1991) Clinical assessment of a computer system for insulin dosage adjustment. in: Lecture Notes in Medical Informatics, MIE'91, (Springer Verlag, Berlin) in press.

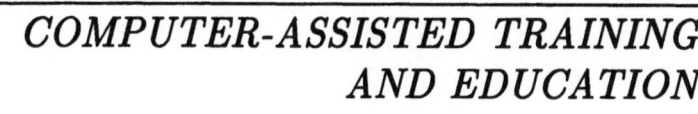

COMPUTER-ASSISTED TRAINING
AND EDUCATION

COMPUTER-BASED CLINICAL TEACHING with MULTIMEDIA TECHNOLOGY

by Mary Anne Sweeney, R.N., Ph.D., Zena Mercer, B.S., Dana C. Randall, M.B.A., The University of Texas Medical Branch at Galveston, TX; Donald McHugh, Ph.D., Northridge Hospital Medical Center, Northridge, CA; Diane Skiba, Ph.D., and Richard Trynda, D.V.M., M.Ed., University of Colorado Health Sciences Center, Denver, CO.

The use of computer-based videodisc technology for delivering instructional information to learners of all ages is gaining widespread acceptance in the United States. The teaching of health-related information is particularly well suited to this technology because of the importance of visual input in clinical instruction. The videodisc has the capability of showing clear views of the patient, equipment, or the setting in which the health care intervention occurs. Still frame pictures and moving images can be combined with computer-generated graphics for the production of interesting and unique learning tools. Since videodiscs store up to 54,000 still frames of visual material with dual audio tracks, developers can freely use their imaginations when creating unique teaching programs. Learners are encouraged to select the order of the instructional sequences by making choices at various menu selection points while moving through the material. The touchscreen capability of the computer monitor and the freedom to make choices throughout the instructional program combine to de-emphasize the technology and place the main focus of the activity on the learning experience itself.

The multimedia programs featured in the demonstration have been used extensively with two groups of learners with vastly differing needs and abilities: 1) health care professionals and 2) patients. The programs include: *Healthcare for Older Adults, Geriatric Nutrition: A Recipe for Good Health, Emergency Surgical Procedures, and Healthy Beginnings: Infant Nutrition and Feeding Techniques.* The programs have been used for instruction and continuing education in medical, nursing, and allied health science schools, in medical centers, and in community health clinics. Key aspects of the development, implementation, and evaluation of this high-tech teaching tool will be covered as it relates to the various target audiences. The technology provides the unique delivery system for teaching the material, but it also permits the instructor to use the computer to implement other functions. For example, a specialized tracking program which resides on the computer can be incorporated in the software to automatically generate a sequential file of all choices made by learners at each menu selection point in the program. The record is used as a key element in the evaluation plan for several of the programs.

The interactive video teaching platform for these applications consists of three elements: a microcomputer, a videodisc player, and a touch sensitive monitor. Alternative hardware platforms for delivering programs can be adapted to the specialized environments as shown in examples from clinics, schools and learning resource centers. The advantages and drawbacks of using a computer network for joining a number of learning stations with one software file server will be covered as well.

All of the videodisc-based programs were grant-supported productions that were developed at The University of Texas Medical Branch in Galveston, Texas and at The University of Colorado Health Science Center in Denver, Colorado. Funding for production-related activities came from sources such as the United States Public Health Service, IBM Corporation, and the W.K. Kellogg Foundation.

MULTIMEDIA AND HYPERTEXT PROGRAMS FOR NURSING EDUCATION

D. Becchio, A. Cavicchioli, M.E. Magnino, I. Berra.,
G.P. Zara, G. Narduzzo, and M. Eandi

Ce.S.P.I. Centro Professioni Infermieristiche
Via XX Settembre 76, 10100 Torino/Italy
MSE Computers s.p.a. Corso Regio Parco 42, 10100 Torino/Italy
Department of Pharmacology, University of Torino/Italy

Professional nursing education depends on the same basic educational principles and processes that apply to any health personnel curriculum; its studying activities should therefore promote "learning how to learn" during and after the basic education.

Hypertext or hypermedia offer a powerful structural model for building such performance support systems.

The use of interactive technology can improve the learning process of the students because they are actively involved in their own education, being able to organize the studying schedule in relation to their personal needs.

We have developed two programs for PC compatible computers. The first is called "The Acute Myocardial Infarction: The First 24 Hours of an Infarcted Patient", written on WISE commercial software (Wicat Interactive System for Education) by Wicat System U.S.A. This author system can handle graphic text, analog images, sound, and interactive simulations. We have also used the Cardiovascular Resources videodisk produced by the Health Sciences Centre for Educational Resources/Washington University. The program is organized in didactic modules: 1) introduction of anatomy and physiology; 2) evaluation of the patient's general conditions; 3) diagnostic tests; 4) nursing plan. The student can select each module from the introduction menu and can move backward and forward through the frames of the module. A vocabulary of specific terms is always available on-line. Storage of the student's answers is also possible for subsequent evaluation of student performance or for correction of mistakes.

The second program was developed using Owl International Guide and is called "Infusion Therapy". This hypertext program utilizes a single screen approach, placing text, graphics and video on the same screen of a PC compatible computer. The nurse can obtain information about the physiology of body fluids, pH and caloric metabolism. Furthermore, she can request clinical pharmacology information about the most common infusion solutions used in the hospital, and she can follow a nursing protocol to assist the patient.

The program can be used in the nursing school; however, it can just as well be used in continuing education projects for practicing nurses.

References

D. Ausubel. Educational Psychology. A Cognitive View. Holt, Rinehart and Winston. New York 1968

J.M. Slatin. Hypertext and Teaching of Writing in: Text, Context, Hypertext. Ed. by E. Barret. The MIT Press. Cambridge 1988

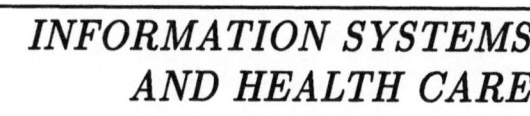

INFORMATION SYSTEMS
AND HEALTH CARE

ARZTBRIEF: generating medical reports in a multimedia environment

Dirk Kraus
RG Expert Systems, *CT Biomed,*
Center for Technology Transfer Biomedicine
Brahmsstr. 2,
W-4970 Bad Oeynhausen

Eckart Miche
Heart Centre Northrhine-Westphalia
Department of Cardiology
Georgstr. 11
W-4970 Bad Oeynhausen

The **ARZTBRIEF** system supports the generation of medical reports to the referring practioner by the physician in the cardiological ambulance of the Heart Centre. A main characteristic of the system is that it consequently exploits the possibilities of multimedia techniques both for user input and output. For example, the user may click on icons or graphical schemes, select from menus, draw / colorize simple forms, talk into a sound digitizer or use a keyboard. The system was implemented in order to accomplish the following goals:

a) economize the work of both physicians and secretaries by avoiding multiple recording of identical text fragments, enabling fast input of frequent and common formulations and making it possible to work on the records of different patients alternately.

b) yield a good compromise between a necessary standardization and individuality of style by providing a large amount of predefined fragments, which can nevertheless easily be modified or extended by every user according to his preferences

c) provide a basis for further integration of various clinical data which are multimedial by nature.

The greatest challenge in building such a system lies in the design of the user interface. Existing glossary based systems suffer from major drawbacks which lower the acceptance and usability drastically. These include:

• limited number of glossary terms which are not/not easily modifiable,

• tedious and clumsy access to these terms via number codes which have to be memorized or retrieved from a manual,

• the user has still to use a keyboard to a large extent,

• frequent large patterns of findings have to be "assembled" every time,

• impossiblity to enter graphical information.

In order to overcome these problems, it is unavoidable to resort to a environment based on a graphical user interface. Prototyping studies revealed that an integration of the dictaphone was imperative, as it seems to be impossible to provide a still time saving means of entering very complex findings.

It is important to note that all facilities which allow for the customization of the system do in fact, after a short period of use, make the keyboard nearly obsolete.

ARZTBRIEF runs in an AppleTalk™ LAN under TOPS™, connecting several Apple® Macintosh™ computers (SE/30, IIx), partly equipped with full page screens, and a LaserWriter™. The modules in the reception, the doctors´ rooms and the typists´ office are implemented in HyperCard II™ .

The secretary in the typists office after accepting the record of a patient simply types in all the passages which where dictated into the sound digitizer, without bothering where they have to been placed in the document. Once this is completed the whole report may be sent to the laser printer.

SPREADSHEETS AS CONVIVIAL TOOLS FOR BIOLOGICAL FOLLOW-UP MANAGEMENT OF HOSPITALIZED PATIENTS

B. Vancraeynest, M.D., Th. Vael, M.D. and P. Baudhuin, M.D.
University of Louvain. Cliniques Universitaires St-Luc
Avenue Hippocrate 10, 1200 Brussels, Belgium.

A generic spreadsheet-based model for medical follow-up applications has been developed. It performs simple processing of raw medical data and it presents synthetic views for selected biological parameters and their evolution, either as tabular or graphical displays. This developement is aimed at facilitating rapid medical decision for treatment adaptation. Moreover, in a LAN environment, communication of informations between users can increase rapidity and security of data entry and transfer: automatic integration of biological results from the hospital's laboratory into the patient spreadsheet files or communication of orders from the doctors' to the nurses' workstations are two examples. Blood glucose follow-up in diabetic patients and hydro-electrolytic balance of intensive care patients are the first two specific applications which were implemented.

Since these applications were implemented for a LAN under a NOVELL 386 operating system on IBM PS/2 microcomputers (MS-DOS® environment), a LAN version of BORLAND's QUATTRO PRO® 2.0 was chosen, on basis of a multi-criteria analysis.

Our model consists of 5 distinct spreadsheet modules, covering the following basic functions: (1) data acquisition, (2) user-defined parameters management, (3) data processing, (4) reports or graphics displays, and (5) storage of patient files on disk. Except for a small specific user interface, most (75%) of each module is common to all applications based on the spreadsheet. Implementation of a new application is thus reduced to instantiation of the generic data structures and definition of parameters of the routines from the 5 standard modules.

Use of advanced features of a widely distributed spreadsheet software saved a large amount of programming time during the prototyping phase, owing to the powerful built-in functions of the spreadsheet. Moreover, maintenance and evolution of applications responding to new user requirements is largely facilitated.

REFERENCES

Burnakis, T.G. 1989. Facilitating drug-use evaluation with spreadsheet software. American Journal of Hospital Pharmacy, 46:84-88.

THE FEEDBACK PROGRAMME FOR
NURSING MINIMAL DATA SET REGISTRATION

Delesie L., Vanlanduyt J., Tanghe A., Sermeus W., Vanden Boer G., Croes L.

Department of Hospital Administration and Medical Care Organization,
Catholic University of Leuven, Belgium

The Feedback Programme reveals to the heads of the nursing units the richness of information in the data collected by the national NMDS registration (1). The programme extracts information for the nursing unit, the smallest entity of the hospital.

The first part presents a description of the nursing unit by giving the length of stay, age, occupancy rate, adl-scores and diagnosis. The registred personnel is discussed in number and qualification. The nursing activities are presented and related to each other: activities attract attention by being present or absent.

The dynamics of the nursing unit can be presented by comparing the information of two different periods. The evolution during the registration period is reflected and compared to the reference period. By comparing two different nursing units the programme gives the dynamical structure of the hospital.

For every item the appropriate selection of presentation has been made. For some items and situations the maximum, minimum and/or mean satisfy. But sometimes only the distribution gives the correct presentation.

The Feedback Programme is accompanied by a second programme which allows every unit to situate itself within a national context.

The introduction of these tools in the nursing units and the training of the different involved persons are of major importance. By using educational examples the users get acquainted with the generated information.

The programme is realized in (interpreter) basic so adoptions to the environment of a specific hospital are simple. The requested computer platform is minimal. The programme works on a two-floppy XT-computer, but in case of lot of data a hard disk may be useful. Knowledge of the basic dos-commands is sufficient to run the programme.

The Feedback Programme is available in Dutch, French and English from the Belgian Ministry of Public Health.

(1) Delesie L., Croes L., Sermeus W., Tanghe A., Vanden Boer G., Vanlanduyt J., A Nursing Minimal Data Set in production: Facilities and Training, M.I.E. 91, Congress Proceedings.

A PC-BASED SYSTEM TO AUDIT RADIOLOGY REFERRAL PRACTICE, COSTS AND EXPOSURE

P.D. Donnelly, W.P. Ennis, C.J. Roberts
University of Wales, College of Medicine
Heath Park, Cardiff CF4 4XN, Wales, U.K.

We will demonstrate a computerised system that we have developed to monitor trends and changes in referral practice for imaging investigations. The objective was to try to help encourage clinicians to comply with guidelines of good radiological practice and thereby achieve the benefits of improved patient care, effective use of resources and reduced radiology dosage. The work has been carried out at the University of Wales College of Medicine under the auspices of the Royal College of Radiologists Working Party on the more effective use of diagnostic radiology and we have been supported by the UK Department of Health and the Kings Fund, London. Six other U.K. Centres have collaborated in the pilot development stage.

The system generates and displays graphically facets and trends in the radiology referral practice of individual consultants, specialties or hospitals, by individual or all imaging investigation categories, over time. Costing and radiological exposure modules have also been developed and these direct implications of clinical referral practice will also be demonstrated.

MEASUREMENT DATA ANALYSIS LANGUAGE "MAL"

Stefan Holzreiter

Forschungszentrum für Orthopädietechnik

Geigergasse 5-9, A-1050 Wien/Austria

The MAL software system is a language interpreter for the scientific analysis of empirical data. MAL is a fully structured fourth-generation language based on a stack concept. It supports fast interactive analysis of measurement data even as the development of complex programs. Like in PASCAL the definition of local procedures and variables is possible. A specific feature of the system is the development environment for new instructions. The implementation can be done in terms of PASCAL of MAL. The present instruction set supports the following topics:

- mathematics
- statistics
- graphics
- database
- handling of menus and masks
- interface drivers
- neural networks

A flexible structure of the internal data representation allows applications in widely different fields, e.g. gait analysis and biomechanics, EMG, EEG, ECG, electrochemistry, vibration tests, etc.

LIMDET: A PROGRAM FOR THE CALCULATION
OF THE DETECTION LIMIT IN CLINICAL CHEMISTRY

Jaime Pérez, Hospital Insular, Las Palmas, Gran Canaria, Spain

Jorge Morancho, EQAS-Spain, AEFA-AEBC, Spain

Introduction

The detection limit is related to the capacity of a given analytical method for the determination of substances pure or present in biological moulds to detect minimal amounts of such substances.

In this draft we present a computer program aimed at calculating the detection limit which is based on the error spread model. It is particularly used in the area of clinical chemistry whenever the condition is a lineal calibration curve.

Methods and System

This program has been written in GW-BASIC on an Amstrad PC 1512 micro-computer, using interpretation of GW-BASIC or BASICA.

The logical system of the program can be divided in four different areas: (a) Files management, (b) Calculation, (c) Results output, and (d) Help system.

Results

The program allows obtaining of primary data as well as of the calculated statistic results, on screen display or as printer hard copy. The meaning of symbols used in statistics and the necessary information to understand the methods used for the calculation is given at any moment on the display.

IMAGE PROCESSING

DIGITAL FILTERS USED TO IMPROVE MEDICAL IMAGE QUALITY

Adrian Radulescu

Institute for Computer and Informatics, Cluj, Romania

Different medical images taken from different medical departments are digitized and stored in an IBM personal computer. The images are taken from medical devices such as angiographs, ecographs, etc., and digitized with an image interface. The image interface contains an analog/digital converter and a 1 MB image memory. The images are stored in different files on the IBM PC, on which image processing is carried out. Different filters are applied on the images. Among these filters are are: smoothing filter, mean filter, shading filter, edge-enhancing filter, etc. The basis for these filters is a 3 × 3 or 5 × 5 pixel matrix. As an example, the smoothing filter is shown in the figure below:

A	B	C
D	E	F
G	H	I

=> E'

$$E' = \frac{1}{16} \times (A + 2B + C + 2D + 4E + 2F + G + 2H + I)$$

Other filters used are:

• the mean filter

$$E' = \frac{1}{8} \times (A + B + C + D + F + G + H + I)$$

• the edge-enhancing filter

$$E' = \frac{1}{2} \times (-2A + B - 2C + D + 6E + F - 2G + H - 2J)$$

After these filters are applied, the image appears on the screen with a program written up at our Institute. A VGA interface with a memory of 256 kB is enough to display the images. Using these techniques, many important medical details may appear. The presentation consists in different primary images taken from radiological devices compared with the images on which various digital filters were used. The difference between them is remarkable.

AUTHOR INDEX

SUBJECT INDEX

Lecture Notes in Medical Informatics

Vol. 24: Medical Informatics Europe 1984. Proceedings, 1984. Edited by E H. Roger, J. L. Willems, R. O'Moore and B. Barber. XXVII, 778 pages. 1984.

Vol. 25: Medical Informatics Europe 1985. Edited by F. H. Roger, P. Gronroos, R. TervoPellikka and R. O'Moore. XVII, 823 pages. 1985.

Vol. 26: Methodical Problems in Early Detection Programmes. Proceedings, 1983. Edited by E. Walter and A. Neiß. VIII, 198 pages. 1985.

Vol. 27: E. Mergenthaler, Textbank Systems. VI, 177 pages. 1985.

Vol. 28: Objective Medical Decision Making. Proceedings, 1985. Edited by D. D. Tsiftsis. VII, 229 pages. 1986.

Vol. 29: System Analysis of Ambulatory Care in Selected Countries. Edited by P. L. Reichertz, R. Engelbrecht and U . Piccolo . VI, 197 pages. 1986.

Vol. 30: Present Status of Computer Support in Ambulatory Care. Edited by P.L. Reichertz, R. Engelbrecht and U. Piccolo. VIII, 241 pages. 1987.

Vol. 31: S. J. Duckett, Operations Research for Health Planning and Administration. 111, 165 pages. 1987 .

Vol. 32: G. D. Rennels, A Computational Model of Reasoning from the Clinical Literature. XV, 230 pages. 1987.

Vol. 33: J. Fox, M. Fieschi, R. Engelbrecht (Eds.), AIME 87. European Conference on Artificial Intelligence in Medicine. Proceedings. X, 255 pages. 1987.

Vol. 34: R. Janßen, G. Opelz (Eds.), Acquisition, Analysis and Use of Clinical Transplant Data. Proceedings. IV, 225 pages. 1987.

Vol. 35: R. Hansen, B. G. Solheim, R. R. O'Moore, F. H. Roger (Eds.), Medical Informatics Europe '88. Proceedings. XV, 764 pages. 1988.

Vol. 36: O. Rienhoff, U. Piccolo, B. Schneider (Eds.), Expert Systems and Decision Support in Medicine. Proceedings, 1988. XII, 591 pages. 1988.

Vol. 37: O. Rienhoff, C. F. C. Greinacher (Eds.), A General PACS-RIS Interface. VI, 97 pages. 1988.

Vol. 38: J. Hunter, J. Cookson, J. Wyatt (Eds.), AIME 89. Second European Conference on Artificial Intelligence in Medicine. Proceedings. X, 330 pages. 1989.

Vol. 39: J. J. Salley, J. L. Zimmerman, M.J. Ball (Eds.), Dental Informatics: Strategic Issuesforthe Dental Profession. X, 105 pages. 1990.

Vol. 40: R. O'Moore, S. Bengtsson, J. R. Bryant, J. S. Bryden (Eds.), Medical Informatics Europe '90. Proceedings, 1990. XXV, 820 pages. 1990.

Vol. 41: J. P. Turley, S. K. Newbold (Eds.), Nursing Informatics '91. Pre-Conference Proceedings. VII, 176 pages. 1991.

Vol. 42: E. J. S. Hovenga, K. J. Hannah, K. A. McCormick, J. Ronald (Eds.), Nursing Informatics '91. Proceedings, 1991. XXV, 820 pages. 1991.

Vol. 43: L. Hothorn (Ed.), Statistical Methods in Toxicology. Proceedings, 1991. IV, 159 pages. 1991.

Vol. 44: M. Stefanelli, A. Hasman, M. Fieschi, J. Talmon (Eds.), AIME 91. Proceedings, 1991. VIII, 329 pages. 1991.

Vol. 45: K.-P. Adlassnig, G. Grabner, S. Bengtsson, R. Hansen (Eds.), Medical Informatics Europe 1991. Proceedings, 1991. XXII, 1089 pages. 1991.